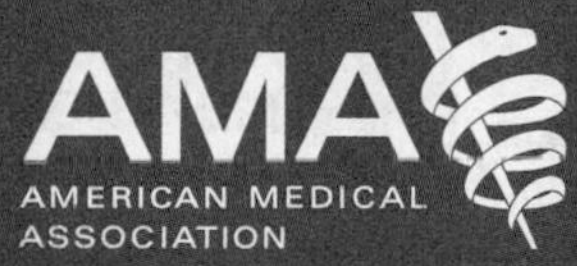

ICD-10-PCS 2021

The Complete Official Codebook

AMA publications fund initiatives that drive improvements in patient health, practice innovation and medical education.

AMAstore.com

Notice

ICD-10-PCS: The Complete Official Codebook is designed to be an accurate and authoritative source regarding coding and every reasonable effort has been made to ensure accuracy and completeness of the content. However, the American Medical Association (AMA) makes no guarantee, warranty, or representation that this publication is accurate, complete, or without errors. It is understood that the AMA is not rendering any legal or other professional services or advice in this publication and that the AMA bears no liability for any results or consequences that may arise from the use of this book.

Our Commitment to Accuracy

The AMA is committed to producing accurate and reliable materials. To report corrections, please call the AMA Unified Service Center at (800) 621-8335. AMA product updates, errata, and addendum can be found at amaproductupdates.org.

To purchase additional copies, contact the AMA at (800) 621-8335 or visit the AMA store at amastore.com. Refer to product number OP201121.

Copyright

OP201121
BQ45: 8/20

Acknowledgments

Marianne Randall, CPC, *Product Manager*
Karen Schmidt, BSN, *Technical Director*
Anita Schmidt, BS, RHIA, AHIMA-approved ICD-10-CM/PCS Trainer, *Subject Matter Expert*
Karen Krawzik, RHIT, CCS, AHIMA-approved ICD-10-CM/PCS Trainer, *Subject Matter Expert*
Leanne Patterson, CPC, *Subject Matter Expert*
LaJuana Green, RHIA, CCS, *Subject Matter Expert*
Stacy Perry, *Manager, Desktop Publishing*
Tracy Betzler, *Senior Desktop Publishing Specialist*
Hope M. Dunn, *Senior Desktop Publishing Specialist*
Katie Russell, *Desktop Publishing Specialist*
Kate Holden, *Editor*

Anita Schmidt, BS, RHIA, AHIMA-approved ICD-10-CM/PCS Trainer

Ms. Schmidt has expertise in ICD-10-CM/PCS, DRG, and CPT with more than 15 years' experience in coding in multiple settings, including inpatient, observation, and same-day surgery. Her experience includes analysis of medical record documentation, assignment of ICD-10-CM and PCS codes, and DRG validation. She has conducted training for ICD-10-CM/PCS and electronic health record. She has also collaborated with clinical documentation specialists to identify documentation needs and potential areas for physician education. Most recently she has been developing content for resource and educational products related to ICD-10-CM, ICD-10-PCS, DRG, and CPT. Ms. Schmidt is an AHIMA-approved ICD-10-CM/PCS trainer and is an active member of the American Health Information Management Association (AHIMA) and the Minnesota Health Information Management Association (MHIMA).

Karen Krawzik, RHIT, CCS, AHIMA-approved ICD-10-CM/PCS Trainer

Ms. Krawzik has expertise in ICD-10-CM, ICD-9-CM, CPT/HCPCS, DRG, and data quality and analytics, with more than 30 years' experience coding in multiple settings, including inpatient, observation, ambulatory surgery, ancillary, and emergency room. She has served as a DRG analyst and auditor of commercial and government payer claims, as a contract administrator, and worked on a team providing enterprise-wide conversion of the ICD-9-CM code set to ICD-10. More recently, she has been developing print and electronic content related to ICD-10-CM and ICD-10-PCS coding systems, MS-DRGs, and HCCs. Ms. Krawzik is credentialed by the American Health Information Management Association (AHIMA) as a Registered Health Information Technician (RHIT) and a Certified Coding Specialist (CCS) and is an AHIMA-approved ICD-10-CM/PCS trainer. She is an active member of AHIMA and the Missouri Health Information Management Association.

Contents

What's New for 2021 iii

Introduction 1
- Number of Codes in ICD-10-PCS 1
- ICD-10-PCS Manual 1
- Medical and Surgical Section (Ø) 4
- Obstetrics Section (1) 7
- Placement Section (2) 8
- Administration Section (3) 9
- Measurement and Monitoring Section (4) 9
- Extracorporeal or Systemic Assistance and Performance Section (5) 10
- Extracorporeal or Systemic Therapies Section (6) 10
- Osteopathic Section (7) 11
- Other Procedures Section (8) 11
- Chiropractic Section (9) 12
- Imaging Section (B) 12
- Nuclear Medicine Section (C) 13
- Radiation Therapy Section (D) 13
- Physical Rehabilitation and Diagnostic Audiology Section (F) 14
- Mental Health Section (G) 15
- Substance Abuse Treatment Section (H) 15
- New Technology Section (X) 16

ICD-10-PCS Index and Tabular Format 19
- Index 19
- Code Tables 19

ICD-10-PCS Additional Features 21
- Use of Official Sources 21
- Table Notations 21
- Appendixes 22

ICD-10-PCS Official Guidelines for Coding and Reporting 2021 25
- Conventions 25
- Medical and Surgical Section Guidelines (section Ø) 26
- Obstetric Section Guidelines (section 1) 30
- Radiation Therapy Section Guidelines (section D) 30
- New Technology Section Guidelines (section X) 31

Index 33

ICD-10-PCS Tables 131
- Central Nervous System and Cranial Nerves 131
- Peripheral Nervous System 151
- Heart and Great Vessels 169
- Upper Arteries 191
- Lower Arteries 215
- Upper Veins 239
- Lower Veins 259
- Lymphatic and Hemic Systems 279
- Eye 297
- Ear, Nose, Sinus 315
- Respiratory System 335
- Mouth and Throat 351
- Gastrointestinal System 369
- Hepatobiliary System and Pancreas 397
- Endocrine System 411
- Skin and Breast 421
- Subcutaneous Tissue and Fascia 439
- Muscles 459
- Tendons 481
- Bursae and Ligaments 495
- Head and Facial Bones 517
- Upper Bones 537
- Lower Bones 557
- Upper Joints 575
- Lower Joints 595
- Urinary System 617
- Female Reproductive System 633
- Male Reproductive System 653
- Anatomical Regions, General 669
- Anatomical Regions, Upper Extremities 681
- Anatomical Regions, Lower Extremities 691
- Obstetrics 701
- Placement 705
- Administration 711
- Measurement and Monitoring 723
- Extracorporeal or Systemic Assistance and Performance 727
- Extracorporeal or Systemic Therapies 729
- Osteopathic 731
- Other Procedures 733
- Chiropractic 735
- Imaging 737
- Nuclear Medicine 767
- Radiation Therapy 777
- Physical Rehabilitation and Diagnostic Audiology 795
- Mental Health 807
- Substance Abuse Treatment 809
- New Technology 811

Appendixes 817
- Appendix A: Components of the Medical and Surgical Approach Definitions 817
- Appendix B: Root Operation Definitions 821
- Appendix C: Comparison of Medical and Surgical Root Operations 827
- Appendix D: Body Part Key 829
- Appendix E: Body Part Definitions 845
- Appendix F: Device Classification 857
- Appendix G: Device Key and Aggregation Table 859
- Appendix H: Device Definitions 869
- Appendix I: Substance Key/Substance Definitions 875
- Appendix J: Sections B–H Character Definitions 879
- Appendix K: Hospital Acquired Conditions 889
- Appendix L: Procedure Combination Tables 909
- Appendix M: Coding Exercises and Answers 931

What's New for 2021

The Centers for Medicare and Medicaid Services is the agency charged with maintaining and updating ICD-10-PCS. CMS released the most current revisions, a summary of which may be found on the CMS website at https://www.cms.gov/medicare/icd-10/2021-icd-10-pcs.

Due to the unique structure of ICD-10-PCS, a change in a character value may affect individual codes and several code tables.

Change Summary Table

2020 Total	New Codes	Revised Titles	Deleted Codes	2021 Total
77,559	544	0	0	78,103

ICD-10-PCS Code FY 2021 Totals, By Section

Medical and Surgical	67,655
Obstetrics	304
Placement	861
Administration	1,336
Measurement and Monitoring	421
Extracorporeal or Systemic Assistance and Performance	51
Extracorporeal or Systemic Therapies	46
Osteopathic	100
Other Procedures	78
Chiropractic	90
Imaging	2,973
Nuclear Medicine	463
Radiation Therapy	2,087
Physical Rehabilitation and Diagnostic Audiology	1,380
Mental Health	30
Substance Abuse Treatment	59
New Technology	169
Total	78,103

ICD-10-PCS Table Changes Highlights

- Device value of Radioactive element added to root operation table of Insertion in several body systems, including:
  - Central Nervous System and Cranial Nerves
  - Peripheral Nervous
  - Lymphatic and Hemic
  - Ear, Nose, Sinus
  - Mouth and Throat
  - Gastrointestinal
  - Hepatobiliary System and Pancreas
  - Endocrine
  - Urinary
  - Female Reproductive
  - Male Reproductive
- New row added to root operation table of Bypass in the Heart and Great Vessels body system for Percutaneous bypass of left atrium to right atrium with synthetic substitute
- New row added to root operation table Fragmentation capturing body part values Pulmonary Trunk, Pulmonary Artery, Right/Left and Pulmonary Vein, Right/Left
- New root operation table of Fragmentation added in the Upper Arteries, Lower Arteries, Upper Veins and Lower Veins body systems
- New rows added to root operation table of Supplement in the Heart and Great Vessels body system
- Qualifier values added to root operation table Bypass in the Hepatobiliary System and Pancreas and Anatomical Regions, General body systems
- Device value of Other device added to root operation table Insertion in the Subcutaneous Tissue and Fascia body system
- Body part values of Lumbar Vertebra, Sacrum, Acetabulum, Right/Left and Coccyx added to root operation table of Removal in the Lower Bones body system
- Device value of Internal Fixation Device, Sustained Compression added to root operation table Fusion in the Upper Joints and Lower Joints body systems
- New root operation table of Transplantation added to Male Reproductive body system
- Approach values of Via Natural and Artificial Opening and Via Natural or Artificial Opening Endoscopic added for body part Pelvic Cavity in the Anatomical Regions, General body system
- Approach values of Open and Percutaneous Endoscopic added to root operation table of Extraction for body part Products of Conception, Ectopic in the Obstetrics body system
- Substance value of Hematopoietic Stem/Progenitor Cells, Genetically Modified and qualifier value of Autologous added to root operation table of Transfusion for Peripheral Vein and Central Vein body system/region in the Administration section
- Qualifier value of High Nasal Flow/Velocity added to root operation Assistance in the Extracorporeal or Systemic Assistance and Performance section
- New root operation table of Other Imaging added to Hepatobiliary System and Pancreas and Anatomical Regions body systems in the Imaging section
- Isotope value of Cesium 131 (Cs-131) added to Brachytherapy tables in the Radiation Therapy section for the following body systems:
  - Central and Peripheral Nervous System
  - Lymphatic and Hematologic
  - Eye
  - Ear, Nose, Mouth, and Throat
  - Respiratory
  - Gastrointestinal
  - Hepatobiliary System and Pancreas
  - Endocrine
  - Breast
  - Urinary
  - Female Reproductive
  - Male Reproductive
  - Anatomical Regions

- Modality qualifier of Intraoperative Radiation Therapy (IORT) added to Other Radiation table in the Central and Peripheral Nervous body system in the Radiation Therapy section
- Many new substances and devices added to the New Technology tables — see New Definitions Addenda — Device and Substance Definitions for more information

New Definitions Addenda

Section Ø — Medical and Surgical
Root Operation

ICD-10-PCS Value	Definition	
Supplement	Delete	Includes/Examples: Herniorrhaphy using mesh, free nerve graft, mitral valve ring annuloplasty, put a new acetabular liner in a previous hip replacement
	Add	Includes/Examples: Herniorrhaphy using mesh, mitral valve ring annuloplasty, put a new acetabular liner in a previous hip replacement

Section Ø — Medical and Surgical
Body Part

ICD-10-PCS Value	Definitions	
Abdominal Sympathetic Nerve	Add	Renal nerve
Hand Bursa and Ligament, Right Hand Bursa and Ligament, Left	Delete	Scapholunate ligament
Wrist Bursa and Ligament, Right Wrist Bursa and Ligament, Left	Add	Scapholunate ligament

Section Ø — Medical and Surgical
Device

ICD-10-PCS Value		Definition	
Add	Internal Fixation Device, Sustained Compression for Fusion in Lower Joints	Add Add	DynaNail Mini® DynaNail®
Add	Internal Fixation Device, Sustained Compression for Fusion in Upper Joints	Add Add	DynaNail Mini® DynaNail®
Intraluminal Device, Branched or Fenestrated, One or Two Arteries for Restriction in Lower Arteries		Delete	Cook Zenith AAA Endovascular Graft
		Delete	Zenith AAA Endovascular Graft
		Add	Cook Zenith® Fenestrated AAA Endovascular Graft
		Add	Zenith® Fenestrated AAA Endovascular Graft
Intraluminal Device, Branched or Fenestrated, Three or More Arteries for Restriction in Lower Arteries		Delete	Cook Zenith AAA Endovascular Graft
		Delete	Zenith AAA Endovascular Graft
		Add	Cook Zenith® Fenestrated AAA Endovascular Graft
		Add	Zenith® Fenestrated AAA Endovascular Graft
Synthetic Substitute		Add	Barricaid® Annular Closure Device (ACD)
		Add	Corvia IASD®
		Add	IASD® (InterAtrial Shunt Device), Corvia
		Add	InterAtrial Shunt Device IASD®, Corvia
		Add	V-Wave Interatrial Shunt System

Section 3 — Administration
Substance

ICD-10-PCS Value		Definition	
Add	Hematopoietic Stem/ Progenitor Cells, Genetically Modified	Add	OTL-101

Section B — Imaging
Type

ICD-10-PCS Value		Definition	
Add	Other Imaging	Add	Definition: Other specified modality for visualizing a body part.

Section X — New Technology
Root Operation

ICD-10-PCS Value		Definition	
Add	Supplement	Add	Definition: Putting in or on biological or synthetic material that physically reinforces and/or augments the function of a portion of a body part.

Section X – New Technology Approach

ICD-10-PCS Value		Definition	
Add	Via Natural or Artificial Opening	Add	Definition: Entry of instrumentation through a natural or artificial external opening to reach the site of the procedure.

Section X — New Technology Device/Substance/Technology

ICD-10-PCS Value		Definition	
Add	Atezolizumab Antineoplastic	Add	TECENTRIQ®
Add	Brexanolone	Add	ZULRESSO™
Add	Brexucabtagene Autoleucel Immunotherapy	Add	Brexucabtagene Autoleucel
Add	Cefiderocol Anti-infective	Add	FETROJA®
Add	Ceftolozane/Tazobactam Anti-infective	Add	ZERBAXA®
Add	Durvalumab Antineoplastic	Add	IMFINZI®
Add	Eculizumab	Add	Soliris®
Add	Esketamine Hydrochloride	Add	SPRAVATO™
Add	Lefamulin Anti-infective	Add	XENLETA™
Add	Lisocabtagene Maraleucel Immunotherapy	Add	Lisocabtagene Maraleucel
Add	Mineral-based Topical Hemostatic Agent	Add	Hemospray® Endoscopic Hemostat
Add	Nerinitide	Add	NA-1 (Nerinitide)
Add	Omadacycline Anti-infective	Add	NUZYRA™
Add	Synthetic Substitute, Mechanically Expandable (Paired) in New Technology	Add	SpineJack® system

List of Updated Files

2021 Official ICD-10-PCS Coding Guidelines

- New guidelines B3.18 and B5.2b added in response to public comment
- Guidelines B3.1b and B3.10c revised in response to public comment and internal review
- Downloadable PDF

2021 ICD-10-PCS Code Tables and Index (Zip file)

- Code tables for use beginning October 1, 2020
- Downloadable PDF: file name is pcs_2021.pdf
- Downloadable xml files for developers: file names are icd10pcs_tables_2021.xml, icd10pcs_index_2021.xml, icd10pcs_definitions_2021.xml
- Accompanying schema for developers: file names are icd10pcs_tables.xsd; icd10pcs_index.xsd; icd10pcs_definitions.xsd

2021 ICD-10-PCS Codes File (Zip file)

- ICD-10-PCS codes file is a simple format for nontechnical uses, containing the valid FY 2021 ICD-10-PCS codes and their long titles.
- File is in text file format: file name is icd10pcs_codes_2021.txt
- Accompanying documentation for codes file: file name is icd10pcsCodesFile.pdf
- Codes file addenda in text format: file name is codes_addenda_2021.txt

2021 ICD-10-PCS Order File (Long and Abbreviated Titles) (Zip file)

- ICD-10-PCS order file is for developers, provides a unique five-digit "order number" for each ICD-10-PCS table and code, as well as a long and abbreviated code title.
- ICD-10-PCS order file name is icd10pcs_order_2021.txt
- Accompanying documentation for tabular order file: file name is icd10pcsOrderFile.pdf
- Tabular order file addenda in text format: file name is order_addenda_2021.txt

2021 ICD-10-PCS Final Addenda (Zip file)

- Addenda files in downloadable PDF: file names are tables_addenda_2021.pdf; index_addenda_2021.pdf; definitions_addenda_2021.pdf
- Addenda files also in machine-readable text format for developers: file names are tables_addenda_2021.txt; index_addenda_2021.txt; definitions_addenda_2021.txt

2021 ICD-10-PCS Conversion Table (Zip file)

- ICD-10-PCS code conversion table is provided to assist users in data retrieval, in downloadable Excel spreadsheet: file name is icd10pcs_conversion_table_2021.xlsx
- Conversion table also in machine-readable text format for developers: file name is icd10pcs_conversion_table_2021.txt
- Accompanying documentation for code conversion table: file name is icd10pcsConversionTable.pdf

Introduction

ICD-10-PCS: The Complete Official Code Set is your definitive coding resource for procedure coding in acute inpatient hospitals. In addition to the official ICD-10-PCS Coding System Files, revised and distributed by the Centers for Medicare and Medicaid Services (CMS), Optum360's coding experts have incorporated Medicare-related coding edits and proprietary features, such as coding tools and appendixes, into a comprehensive and easy-to-use reference.

This manual provides the most current information that was available at the time of publication. For updates to official source documents that may have occurred after this manual was published, please refer to the following:

- **CMS International Classification of Disease, 10th Revision, Procedural Coding System (ICD-10-PCS):**
  https://www.cms.gov/medicare/icd-10/2021-icd-10-pcs
- **CMS Inpatient Prospective Payment System Proposed Rule, FY2021**
  https://www.cms.gov/medicare/acute-inpatient-pps/fy-2021-ipps-proposed-rule-home-page
- **CMS Inpatient Prospective Payment System Proposed Rule, FY 2021 - Proposed, version 38, MS-DRG Grouper software, Definitions Manual files and Medicare Code Editor (MCE) files**
  https://www.cms.gov/Medicare/Medicare-Fee-for-Service-Payment/AcuteInpatientPPS/MS-DRG-Classifications-and-Software
- **American Hospital Association (AHA) Coding Clinics**
  https://www.codingclinicadvisor.com/

ICD-10-PCS Code Structure

ICD-10-PCS has a seven-character alphanumeric code structure. Each character contains up to 34 possible values. Each value represents a specific option for the general character definition. The 10 digits Ø–9 and the 24 letters A–H, J–N, and P–Z may be used in each character. The letters O and I are not used so as to avoid confusion with the digits Ø and 1. An ICD-10-PCS code is the result of a process rather than as a single fixed set of digits or alphabetic characters. The process consists of combining semi-independent values from among a selection of values, according to the rules governing the construction of codes.

	Section	Body System	Root Operation	Body Part	Approach	Device	Qualifier
Characters:	1	2	3	4	5	6	7

A code is derived by choosing a specific value for each of the seven characters. Based on details about the procedure performed, values for each character specifying the section, body system, root operation, body part, approach, device, and qualifier are assigned. Because the definition of each character is also a function of its physical position in the code, the same letter or number placed in a different position in the code has a different meaning.

The seven characters that make up a complete code have specific meanings that vary for each of the 17 sections of the manual.

Procedures are then divided into sections that identify the general type of procedure (e.g., Medical and Surgical, Obstetrics, Imaging). The first character of the procedure code always specifies the section. The second through seventh characters have the same meaning within each section, but may mean different things in other sections. In all sections, the third character specifies the general type of procedure performed (e.g., Resection, Transfusion, Fluoroscopy), while the other characters give additional information such as the body part and approach.

In ICD-10-PCS, the term *procedure* refers to the complete specification of the seven characters.

Number of Codes in ICD-10-PCS

The table structure of ICD-10-PCS permits the specification of a large number of codes on a single page. At the time of this publication, there are 78,103 codes in the 2021 ICD-10-PCS.

ICD-10-PCS Manual

Index

Codes may be found in the index based on the general type of procedure (e.g., resection, transfusion, fluoroscopy), or a more commonly used term (e.g., appendectomy). For example, the code for percutaneous intraluminal dilation of the coronary arteries with an intraluminal device can be found in the Index under *Dilation*, or a synonym of *Dilation* (e.g., angioplasty). The Index then specifies the first three or four values of the code or directs the user to see another term.

Example:

Dilation
  Artery
    Coronary
      One Artery Ø27Ø

Based on the first three values of the code provided in the Index, the corresponding table can be located. In the example above, the first three values indicate table Ø27 is to be referenced for code completion.

The tables and characters are arranged first by number and then by letter for each character (tables for ØØ-, Ø1-, Ø2-, etc., are followed by those for ØB-, ØC-, ØD-, etc., followed by ØB1, ØB2, etc., followed by ØBB, ØBC, ØBD, etc.).

Note: The Tables section must be used to construct a complete and valid code by specifying the last three or four values.

Tables

The tables in ICD-10-PCS provide the valid combination of character values needed to build a unique procedure code. Each table is preceded by the first three characters of the code, along with their descriptions. In the Medical and Surgical section, for example, the first three characters contain the name of the section (character 1), the body system (character 2), and the root operation performed (character 3).

Listed underneath the first three characters is a table comprising four columns and one or more rows. The four columns in the table specify the last four characters needed to complete the ICD-10-PCS code. Depending on the section, the labels for each column may be different. In the Medical and Surgical section, they are labeled body part (character 4), approach (character 5), device (character 6), and qualifier (character 7). Each row in the table specifies the valid combination of values for characters 4 through 7.

Table 1: Row from table Ø27

Ø Medical and Surgical
2 Heart and Great Vessels
7 Dilation Definition: Expanding an orifice or the lumen of a tubular body part
Explanation: The orifice can be a natural orifice or an artificially created orifice. Accomplished by stretching a tubular body part using intraluminal pressure or by cutting part of the orifice or wall of the tubular body part.

Body Part Character 4	Approach Character 5	Device Character 6	Qualifier Character 7
Ø Coronary Artery, One Artery **1 Coronary Artery, Two Arteries** **2 Coronary Artery, Three Arteries** **3 Coronary Artery, Four or More Arteries**	**Ø Open** **3 Percutaneous** **4 Percutaneous Endoscopic**	**4 Intraluminal Device, Drug-eluting** **5 Intraluminal Device, Drug-eluting, Two** **6 Intraluminal Device, Drug-eluting, Three** **7 Intraluminal Device, Drug-eluting, Four or More** **D Intraluminal Device** **E Intraluminal Device, Two** **F Intraluminal Device, Three** **G Intraluminal Device, Four or More** **T Intraluminal Device, Radioactive** **Z No Device**	**6 Bifurcation** **Z No Qualifier**

For instance, table 1 above shows the first row from table Ø27 in ICD-10-PCS. The values *Ø27* specify the section *Medical and Surgical (Ø)*, the body system *Heart and Great Vessels (2)*, and the root operation *Dilation (7)*. As shown, the root operation (Dilation) is also accompanied by its corresponding definition and explanation. Note, a definition of the root operation is provided for every table in ICD-10-PCS; however, an explanation may not always be applicable.

In total, this single row can be used to construct 240 unique procedure codes. The valid codes shown in table 2 (below) are constructed using the body part (character 4) value of Ø, Coronary artery, one artery, combined with all valid approach (character 5) values, device (character 6) values, and a qualifier (character 7) value of Z, No Qualifier.

Table 2: Code titles for dilation of one coronary artery (Ø27Ø)

Ø27ØØ4Z	Dilation of Coronary Artery, One Artery with Drug-eluting Intraluminal Device, Open Approach
Ø27ØØ5Z	Dilation of Coronary Artery, One Artery with Two Drug-eluting Intraluminal Devices, Open Approach
Ø27ØØ6Z	Dilation of Coronary Artery, One Artery with Three Drug-eluting Intraluminal Devices, Open Approach
Ø27ØØ7Z	Dilation of Coronary Artery, One Artery with Four or More Drug-eluting Intraluminal Devices, Open Approach
Ø27ØØDZ	Dilation of Coronary Artery, One Artery with Intraluminal Device, Open Approach
Ø27ØØEZ	Dilation of Coronary Artery, One Artery with Two Intraluminal Devices, Open Approach
Ø27ØØFZ	Dilation of Coronary Artery, One Artery with Three Intraluminal Devices, Open Approach
Ø27ØØGZ	Dilation of Coronary Artery, One Artery with Four or More Intraluminal Devices, Open Approach
Ø27ØØTZ	Dilation of Coronary Artery, One Artery with Radioactive Intraluminal Device, Open Approach
Ø27ØØZZ	Dilation of Coronary Artery, One Artery, Open Approach
Ø27Ø34Z	Dilation of Coronary Artery, One Artery with Drug-eluting Intraluminal Device, Percutaneous Approach
Ø27Ø35Z	Dilation of Coronary Artery, One Artery with Two Drug-eluting Intraluminal Devices, Percutaneous Approach
Ø27Ø36Z	Dilation of Coronary Artery, One Artery with Three Drug-eluting Intraluminal Devices, Percutaneous Approach
Ø27Ø37Z	Dilation of Coronary Artery, One Artery with Four or More Drug-eluting Intraluminal Devices, Percutaneous Approach
Ø27Ø3DZ	Dilation of Coronary Artery, One Artery with Intraluminal Device, Percutaneous Approach
Ø27Ø3EZ	Dilation of Coronary Artery, One Artery with Two Intraluminal Devices, Percutaneous Approach
Ø27Ø3FZ	Dilation of Coronary Artery, One Artery with Three Intraluminal Devices, Percutaneous Approach
Ø27Ø3GZ	Dilation of Coronary Artery, One Artery with Four or More Intraluminal Devices, Percutaneous Approach
Ø27Ø3TZ	Dilation of Coronary Artery, One Artery with Radioactive Intraluminal Device, Percutaneous Approach
Ø27Ø3ZZ	Dilation of Coronary Artery, One Artery, Percutaneous Approach
Ø27Ø44Z	Dilation of Coronary Artery, One Artery with Drug-eluting Intraluminal Device, Percutaneous Endoscopic Approach
Ø27Ø45Z	Dilation of Coronary Artery, One Artery with Two Drug-eluting Intraluminal Devices, Percutaneous Endoscopic Approach
Ø27Ø46Z	Dilation of Coronary Artery, One Artery with Three Drug-eluting Intraluminal Devices, Percutaneous Endoscopic Approach
Ø27Ø47Z	Dilation of Coronary Artery, One Artery with Four or More Drug-eluting Intraluminal Devices, Percutaneous Endoscopic Approach
Ø27Ø4DZ	Dilation of Coronary Artery, One Artery with Intraluminal Device, Percutaneous Endoscopic Approach
Ø27Ø4EZ	Dilation of Coronary Artery, One Artery with Two Intraluminal Devices, Percutaneous Endoscopic Approach
Ø27Ø4FZ	Dilation of Coronary Artery, One Artery with Three Intraluminal Devices, Percutaneous Endoscopic Approach
Ø27Ø4GZ	Dilation of Coronary Artery, One Artery with Four or More Intraluminal Devices, Percutaneous Endoscopic Approach
Ø27Ø4TZ	Dilation of Coronary Artery, One Artery with Radioactive Intraluminal Device, Percutaneous Endoscopic Approach
Ø27Ø4ZZ	Dilation of Coronary Artery, One Artery, Percutaneous Endoscopic Approach

Table 3: Rows from table ØØH

Ø Medical and Surgical
Ø Central Nervous System and Cranial Nerves
H Insertion Definition: Putting in a nonbiological appliance that monitors, assists, performs, or prevents a physiological function but does not physically take the place of a body part
Explanation: None

Body Part Character 4	Approach Character 5	Device Character 6	Qualifier Character 7
Ø Brain Cerebrum Corpus callosum Encephalon	**Ø Open**	**1 Radioactive Element** **2 Monitoring Device** **3 Infusion Device** **4 Radioactive Element, Cesium-131 Collagen Implant** **M Neurostimulator Lead** **Y Other Device**	**Z No Qualifier**
Ø Brain Cerebrum Corpus callosum Encephalon	**3 Percutaneous** **4 Percutaneous Endoscopic**	**1 Radioactive Element** **2 Monitoring Device** **3 Infusion Device** **M Neurostimulator Lead** **Y Other Device**	**Z No Qualifier**
6 Cerebral Ventricle Aqueduct of Sylvius Cerebral aqueduct (Sylvius) Choroid plexus Ependyma Foramen of Monro (intraventricular) Fourth ventricle Interventricular foramen (Monro) Left lateral ventricle Right lateral ventricle Third ventricle **E Cranial Nerve** **U Spinal Canal** Epidural space, spinal Extradural space, spinal Subarachnoid space, spinal Subdural space, spinal Vertebral canal **V Spinal Cord**	**Ø Open** **3 Percutaneous** **4 Percutaneous Endoscopic**	**1 Radioactive Element** **2 Monitoring Device** **3 Infusion Device** **M Neurostimulator Lead** **Y Other Device**	**Z No Qualifier**

Table 3, is split into three rows; values of characters must all be selected from within the same row of the table. Rows 1 and 2 have the same body part (character 4) value of Ø Brain and the same qualifier value (character 7) of Z No Qualifier. However, the approach (character 5) values are not the same for these two rows, and there is one additional device (character 6) value in row 1 that is not included in row 2. As shown in row 1, body part value Brain (Ø) with device value Radioactive Element, Cesium-131 Collagen Implant (4) can only be used with approach value Open (Ø). In other words, code ØØHØ34Z would be invalid as the approach value 3 is only applicable to row 2 and the device value 4 is only applicable to row 1. It would be inappropriate to build a code for body part Ø if all of the values are not contained in its own row.

Note: In this manual, there are instances in which some tables due to length must be continued on the next page. Each section must be used separately and value selection must be made within the same row of the table.

Character Meanings

In each section, each character has a specific meaning, and this character meaning remains constant within that section. Character meaning tables have been provided at the beginning of each body system in the Medical and Surgical section (Ø) and the Obstetric section (1) to help the user identify the character members available within that section. These tables have purple headers, unlike the official code tables that have green headers and **SHOULD NOT** be used to build a PCS code. Following is an excerpt of a character meaning table.

Table 4: Rows from Central Nervous System and Cranial Nerves - Character Meanings Table

Operation–Character 3	Body Part–Character 4	Approach–Character 5	Device–Character 6	Qualifier–Character 7
1 Bypass	Ø Brain	Ø Open	Ø Drainage Device	Ø Nasopharynx
2 Change	1 Cerebral Meninges	3 Percutaneous	1 Radioactive Element	1 Mastoid Sinus
5 Destruction	2 Dura Mater	4 Percutaneous Endoscopic	2 Monitoring Device	2 Atrium
7 Dilation	3 Epidural Space, Intracranial	X External	3 Infusion Device	3 Blood Vessel
8 Division	4 Subdural Space, Intracranial		4 Radioactive Element, Cesium-131 Collagen Implant	4 Pleural Cavity
9 Drainage	5 Subarachnoid Space, Intracranial		7 Autologous Tissue Substitute	5 Intestine
B Excision	6 Cerebral Ventricle		J Synthetic Substitute	6 Peritoneal Cavity
C Extirpation	7 Cerebral Hemisphere		K Nonautologous Tissue Substitute	7 Urinary Tract
D Extraction	8 Basal Ganglia		M Neurostimulator Lead	8 Bone Marrow
F Fragmentation	9 Thalamus		Y Other Device	9 Fallopian Tube
H Insertion	A Hypothalamus		Z No Device	A Subgaleal space
J Inspection	B Pons			B Cerebral Cisterns

Sections

Procedures are divided into sections that identify the general type of procedure (e.g., Medical and Surgical, Obstetrics, Imaging). The first character of the procedure code always specifies the section.

The sections are listed below:

Medical and Surgical section

- Ø Medical and Surgical

Medical and Surgical-related sections

- 1 Obstetrics
- 2 Placement
- 3 Administration
- 4 Measurement and Monitoring
- 5 Extracorporeal or Systemic Assistance and Performance
- 6 Extracorporeal or Systemic Therapies
- 7 Osteopathic
- 8 Other Procedures
- 9 Chiropractic

Ancillary Sections

- B Imaging
- C Nuclear Medicine
- D Radiation Therapy
- F Physical Rehabilitation and Diagnostic Audiology
- G Mental Health
- H Substance Abuse Treatment

New Technology Section

- X New Technology

Medical and Surgical Section (Ø)

Character Meaning

The seven characters for Medical and Surgical procedures have the following meaning:

Character	Meaning
1	Section
2	Body System
3	Root Operation
4	Body Part
5	Approach
6	Device
7	Qualifier

The Medical and Surgical section constitutes the vast majority of procedures reported in an inpatient setting. Medical and Surgical procedure codes all have a first character value of Ø. The second character indicates the general body system (e.g., Mouth and Throat, Gastrointestinal). The third character indicates the root operation, or specific objective, of the procedure (e.g., Excision). The fourth character indicates the specific body part on which the procedure was performed (e.g., Tonsils, Duodenum). The fifth character indicates the approach used to reach the procedure site (e.g., Open). The sixth character indicates whether a device was left in place during the procedure (e.g., Synthetic Substitute). The seventh character is qualifier, which has a specific meaning for each root operation. For example, the qualifier can be used to identify the destination site of a *Bypass*. The first through fifth characters are always assigned a specific value, but the device (sixth character) and the qualifier (seventh character) are not applicable to all procedures. The value *Z* is used for the sixth and seventh characters to indicate that a specific device or qualifier does not apply to the procedure.

Section (Character 1)

Medical and Surgical procedure codes all have a first character value of *Ø*.

Body Systems (Character 2)

Body systems for Medical and Surgical section codes are specified in the second character.

Body Systems

- Ø Central Nervous System and Cranial Nerves
- 1 Peripheral Nervous System
- 2 Heart and Great Vessels
- 3 Upper Arteries
- 4 Lower Arteries
- 5 Upper Veins
- 6 Lower Veins
- 7 Lymphatic and Hemic Systems
- 8 Eye
- 9 Ear, Nose, Sinus
- B Respiratory System
- C Mouth and Throat
- D Gastrointestinal System
- F Hepatobiliary System and Pancreas
- G Endocrine System
- H Skin and Breast
- J Subcutaneous Tissue and Fascia
- K Muscles
- L Tendons
- M Bursae and Ligaments
- N Head and Facial Bones
- P Upper Bones
- Q Lower Bones
- R Upper Joints
- S Lower Joints
- T Urinary System
- U Female Reproductive System
- V Male Reproductive System
- W Anatomical Regions, General
- X Anatomical Regions, Upper Extremities
- Y Anatomical Regions, Lower Extremities

Root Operations (Character 3)

The root operation is specified in the third character. In the Medical and Surgical section there are 31 different root operations. The root operation identifies the objective of the procedure. Each root operation has a precise definition.

- *Alteration:* Modifying the natural anatomic structure of a body part without affecting the function of the body part
- *Bypass:* Altering the route of passage of the contents of a tubular body part
- *Change:* Taking out or off a device from a body part and putting back an identical or similar device in or on the same body part without cutting or puncturing the skin or a mucous membrane
- *Control:* Stopping, or attempting to stop, postprocedural or other acute bleeding
- *Creation:* Putting in or on biological or synthetic material to form a new body part that to the extent possible replicates the anatomic structure or function of an absent body part
- *Destruction:* Physical eradication of all or a portion of a body part by the direct use of energy, force, or a destructive agent
- *Detachment:* Cutting off all or a portion of the upper or lower extremities
- *Dilation:* Expanding an orifice or the lumen of a tubular body part
- *Division:* Cutting into a body part without draining fluids and/or gases from the body part in order to separate or transect a body part
- *Drainage:* Taking or letting out fluids and/or gases from a body part
- *Excision:* Cutting out or off, without replacement, a portion of a body part
- *Extirpation:* Taking or cutting out solid matter from a body part
- *Extraction:* Pulling or stripping out or off all or a portion of a body part by the use of force
- *Fragmentation:* Breaking solid matter in a body part into pieces
- *Fusion:* Joining together portions of an articular body part rendering the articular body part immobile
- *Insertion:* Putting in a nonbiological appliance that monitors, assists, performs, or prevents a physiological function but does not physically take the place of a body part
- *Inspection:* Visually and/or manually exploring a body part
- *Map:* Locating the route of passage of electrical impulses and/or locating functional areas in a body part
- *Occlusion:* Completely closing an orifice or lumen of a tubular body part
- *Reattachment:* Putting back in or on all or a portion of a separated body part to its normal location or other suitable location
- *Release:* Freeing a body part from an abnormal physical constraint by cutting or by use of force
- *Removal:* Taking out or off a device from a body part
- *Repair:* Restoring, to the extent possible, a body part to its normal anatomic structure and function
- *Replacement:* Putting in or on biological or synthetic material that physically takes the place and/or function of all or a portion of a body part
- *Reposition:* Moving to its normal location or other suitable location all or a portion of a body part
- *Resection:* Cutting out or off, without replacement, all of a body part
- *Restriction:* Partially closing an orifice or lumen of a tubular body part
- *Revision:* Correcting, to the extent possible, a portion of a malfunctioning device or the position of a displaced device
- *Supplement:* Putting in or on biological or synthetic material that physically reinforces and/or augments the function of a portion of a body part
- *Transfer:* Moving, without taking out, all or a portion of a body part to another location to take over the function of all or a portion of a body part
- *Transplantation:* Putting in or on all or a portion of a living body part taken from another individual or animal to physically take the place and/or function of all or a portion of a similar body part

The above definitions of root operations illustrate the precision of code values defined in the system. There is a clear distinction between each root operation.

A root operation specifies the objective of the procedure. The term *anastomosis* is not a root operation, because it is a means of joining and is always an integral part of another procedure (e.g., Bypass, Resection) with a specific objective. Similarly, *incision* is not a root operation, since it is always part of the objective of another procedure (e.g., Division, Drainage). The root operation *Repair* in the Medical and Surgical section functions as a "not elsewhere classified" option. *Repair* is used when the procedure performed is not one of the other specific root operations.

Appendix B provides additional explanation and representative examples of the Medical and Surgical root operations. Appendix C groups all root operations in the Medical and Surgical section into subcategories and provides an example of each root operation.

Body Part (Character 4)

The body part is specified in the fourth character. The body part indicates the specific anatomical site of the body system on which the procedure was performed (e.g., Duodenum). Tubular body parts are defined in ICD-10-PCS as those hollow body parts that provide a route of passage for solids, liquids, or gases. They include the cardiovascular system and body parts such as those contained in the gastrointestinal tract, genitourinary tract, biliary tract, and respiratory tract.

Approach (Character 5)

The technique used to reach the site of the procedure is specified in the fifth character. There are seven different approaches:

- *Open*: Cutting through the skin or mucous membrane and any other body layers necessary to expose the site of the procedure
- *Percutaneous*: Entry, by puncture or minor incision, of instrumentation through the skin or mucous membrane and any other body layers necessary to reach the site of the procedure
- *Percutaneous Endoscopic*: Entry, by puncture or minor incision, of instrumentation through the skin or mucous membrane and any other body layers necessary to reach and visualize the site of the procedure
- *Via Natural or Artificial Opening*: Entry of instrumentation through a natural or artificial external opening to reach the site of the procedure
- *Via Natural or Artificial Opening Endoscopic*: Entry of instrumentation through a natural or artificial external opening to reach and visualize the site of the procedure

- *Via Natural or Artificial Opening with Percutaneous Endoscopic Assistance:* Entry of instrumentation through a natural or artificial external opening and entry, by puncture or minor incision, of instrumentation through the skin or mucous membrane and any other body layers necessary to aid in the performance of the procedure
- *External*: Procedures performed directly on the skin or mucous membrane and procedures performed indirectly by the application of external force through the skin or mucous membrane

The approach comprises three components: the access location, method, and type of instrumentation.

Access location: For procedures performed on an internal body part, the access location specifies the external site through which the site of the procedure is reached. There are two general types of access locations: skin or mucous membranes, and external orifices. Every approach value except external includes one of these two access locations. The skin or mucous membrane can be cut or punctured to reach the procedure site. All open and percutaneous approach values use this access location. The site of a procedure can also be reached through an external opening. External openings can be natural (e.g., mouth) or artificial (e.g., colostomy stoma).

Method: For procedures performed on an internal body part, the method specifies how the external access location is entered. An open method specifies cutting through the skin or mucous membrane and any other intervening body layers necessary to expose the site of the procedure. An instrumentation method specifies the entry of instrumentation through the access location to the internal procedure site. Instrumentation can be introduced by puncture or minor incision, or through an external opening. The puncture or minor incision does not constitute an open approach because it does not expose the site of the procedure. An approach can define multiple methods. For example, *Via Natural or Artificial Opening with Percutaneous Endoscopic Assistance* includes both the initial entry of instrumentation to reach the site of the procedure, and the placement of additional percutaneous instrumentation into the body part to visualize and assist in the performance of the procedure.

Type of instrumentation: For procedures performed on an internal body part, instrumentation means that specialized equipment is used to perform the procedure. Instrumentation is used in all internal approaches other than the basic open approach. Instrumentation may or may not include the capacity to visualize the procedure site. For example, the instrumentation used to perform a sigmoidoscopy permits the internal site of the procedure to be visualized, while the instrumentation used to perform a needle biopsy of the liver does not. The term "endoscopic" as used in approach values refers to instrumentation that permits a site to be visualized.

Procedures performed directly on the skin or mucous membrane are identified by the external approach (e.g., skin excision). Procedures performed indirectly by the application of external force are also identified by the external approach (e.g., closed reduction of fracture).

Appendix A compares the components (access location, method, and type of instrumentation) of each approach and provides an example and illustration of each approach.

Device (Character 6)

The device is specified in the sixth character. There are four general types of devices:

- Biological or synthetic material that takes the place of all or a portion of a body part (e.g, skin graft, joint prosthesis).
- Biological or synthetic material that assists or prevents a physiological function (e.g., IUD).
- Therapeutic material that is not absorbed by, eliminated by, or incorporated into a body part (e.g., radioactive implant).
- Mechanical or electronic appliances used to assist, monitor, take the place of or prevent a physiological function (e.g., cardiac pacemaker, orthopedic pin).

Appendix F compares the general device types and provides examples of each.

While all devices can be removed, some cannot be removed without putting in another nonbiological appliance or body-part substitute.

When a specific device value is used to identify the device for a root operation, such as *Insertion* and that same device value is not an option for a more broad range root operation such as *Removal*, select the general device value. For example, in the body system Heart and Great Vessels, the specific device character for Cardiac Lead, Pacemaker in root operation *Insertion* is J. For the root operation *Removal*, the general device character M Cardiac Lead would be selected for the pacemaker lead.

ICD-10-PCS contains a PCS Device Aggregation Table (see appendix G) that crosswalks the *specific* device character values that have been created for specific root operations and specific body part character values to the *general* device character value that would be used for root operations that represent a broad range of procedures and general body part character values, such as Removal and Revision.

Instruments used to visualize the procedure site are specified in the approach, not the device, value.

If the objective of the procedure is to put in the device, then the root operation is *Insertion*. If the device is put in to meet an objective other than *Insertion*, then the root operation defining the underlying objective of the procedure is used, with the device specified in the device character. For example, if a procedure to replace the hip joint is performed, the root operation *Replacement* is coded, and the prosthetic device is specified in the device character. Materials that are incidental to a procedure such as clips, ligatures, and sutures are not specified in the device character. Because new devices can be developed, the value *Other Device* is provided as a temporary option for use until a specific device value is added to the system.

Qualifier (Character 7)

The qualifier is specified in the seventh character. The qualifier contains unique values for individual procedures. For example, the qualifier can be used to identify the destination site in a *Bypass*.

Medical and Surgical Section Principles

In developing the Medical and Surgical procedure codes, several specific principles were followed.

Composite Terms Are Not Root Operations

Composite terms such as colonoscopy, sigmoidectomy, or appendectomy do not describe root operations, but they do specify multiple components of a specific root operation. In ICD-10-PCS, the components of a procedure are defined separately by the characters making up the complete code. The only component of a procedure specified in the root operation is the objective of the procedure. With each complete code the underlying objective of the procedure is specified by the root operation (third character), the precise part is specified by the body part (fourth character), and the method used to reach and visualize the procedure site is specified by the approach (fifth character). While colonoscopy, sigmoidectomy, and appendectomy are included in the Index, they do not constitute root operations in the Tables section. The objective of colonoscopy is the visualization of the colon and the root operation (character 3) is *Inspection*. Character 4 specifies the body part, which in this case is part of the colon. These composite terms, like colonoscopy or appendectomy, are included as cross-reference only. The index provides the correct root operation reference. Examples of other types of composite terms not representative of root operations are *partial* sigmoidectomy, *total* hysterectomy, and *partial* hip replacement. Always refer to the correct root operation in the Index and Tables section.

Root Operation Based on Objective of Procedure

The root operation is based on the objective of the procedure, such as *Resection* of transverse colon or *Dilation* of an artery. The assignment of the root operation is based on the procedure actually performed, which may or may not have been the intended procedure. If the intended procedure is modified or discontinued (e.g., excision instead of resection is performed), the root operation is determined by the procedure actually performed. If the desired result is not attained after completing the procedure (i.e., the artery does not remain expanded after the dilation procedure), the root operation is still determined by the procedure actually performed.

Examples:

- Dilating the urethra is coded as *Dilation* since the objective of the procedure is to dilate the urethra. If dilation of the urethra includes putting in an intraluminal stent, the root operation remains *Dilation* and not *Insertion* of the intraluminal device because the underlying objective of the procedure is dilation of the urethra. The stent is identified by the intraluminal device value in the sixth character of the dilation procedure code.
- If the objective is solely to put a radioactive element in the urethra, then the procedure is coded to the root operation *Insertion*, with the radioactive element identified in the sixth character of the code.
- If the objective of the procedure is to correct a malfunctioning or displaced device, then the procedure is coded to the root operation *Revision*. In the root operation *Revision*, the original device being revised is identified in the device character. *Revision* is typically performed on mechanical appliances (e.g., pacemaker) or materials used in replacement procedures (e.g., synthetic substitute). Typical revision procedures include adjustment of pacemaker position and correction of malfunctioning knee prosthesis.

Combination Procedures Are Coded Separately

If multiple procedures as defined by distinct objectives are performed during an operative episode, then multiple codes are used. For example, obtaining the vein graft used for coronary bypass surgery is coded as a separate procedure from the bypass itself.

Redo of Procedures

The complete or partial redo of the original procedure is coded to the root operation that identifies the procedure performed rather than *Revision*.

Example:

> A complete redo of a hip replacement procedure that requires putting in a new prosthesis is coded to the root operation *Replacement* rather than *Revision*.

The correction of complications arising from the original procedure, other than device complications, is coded to the procedure performed. Correction of a malfunctioning or displaced device would be coded to the root operation *Revision*.

Example:

> A procedure to control hemorrhage arising from the original procedure is coded to *Control* rather than *Revision*.

Examples of Procedures Coded in the Medical Surgical Section

The following are examples of procedures from the Medical and Surgical section, coded in ICD-10-PCS.

- Suture of skin laceration, left lower arm: ØHQEXZZ

  Medical and Surgical section (Ø), body system *Skin and Breast* (H), root operation *Repair* (Q), body part *Skin, Left Lower Arm* (E), *External* Approach (X) *No device* (Z), and *No qualifier* (Z).

- Laparoscopic appendectomy: ØDTJ4ZZ

  Medical and Surgical section (Ø), body system *Gastrointestinal* (D), root operation *Resection* (T), body part *Appendix* (J), *Percutaneous Endoscopic* approach (4), No Device (Z), and No qualifier (Z).

- Sigmoidoscopy with biopsy: ØDBN8ZX

  Medical and Surgical section (Ø), body system *Gastrointestinal* (D), root operation *Excision* (B), body part *Sigmoid Colon* (N), *Via Natural or Artificial Opening Endoscopic* approach (8), *No Device* (Z), and with qualifier *Diagnostic* (X).

- Tracheostomy with tracheostomy tube: ØB11ØF4

  Medical and Surgical section (Ø), body system *Respiratory* (B), root operation *Bypass* (1), body part *Trachea* (1), *Open* approach (Ø), with *Tracheostomy Device* (F), and qualifier *Cutaneous* (4).

Obstetrics Section (1)

Character Meanings

The seven characters in the Obstetrics section have the same meaning as in the Medical and Surgical section.

Character	Meaning
1	Section
2	Body System
3	Root Operation
4	Body Part
5	Approach
6	Device
7	Qualifier

The Obstetrics section includes procedures performed on the products of conception only. Procedures on the pregnant female are coded in the Medical and Surgical section (e.g., episiotomy). The term "products of conception" refers to all physical components of a pregnancy, including the fetus, amnion, umbilical cord, and placenta. There is no differentiation of the products of conception based on gestational age.

Thus, the specification of the products of conception as a zygote, embryo or fetus, or the trimester of the pregnancy is not part of the procedure code but can be found in the diagnosis code.

Section (Character 1)

Obstetrics procedure codes have a first character value of *1*.

Body System (Character 2)

The second character value for body system is *Pregnancy*.

Root Operation (Character 3)

The root operations *Change, Drainage, Extraction, Insertion, Inspection, Removal, Repair, Reposition, Resection,* and *Transplantation* are used in the obstetrics section and have the same meaning as in the Medical and Surgical section.

The Obstetrics section also includes two additional root operations, *Abortion* and *Delivery*, defined below:

- *Abortion*: Artificially terminating a pregnancy
- *Delivery*: Assisting the passage of the products of conception from the genital canal

A cesarean section is not a separate root operation because the underlying objective is *Extraction* (i.e., pulling out all or a portion of a body part).

Body Part (Character 4)

The body part values in the obstetrics section are:

- *Products of conception*
- *Products of conception, retained*
- *Products of conception, ectopic*

Approach (Character 5)

The fifth character specifies approaches and is defined as are those in the Medical and Surgical section. In the case of an abortion procedure that uses a laminaria or an abortifacient, the approach is *Via Natural or Artificial Opening*.

Device (Character 6)

The sixth character is used for devices such as fetal monitoring electrodes.

Qualifier (Character 7)

Qualifier values are specific to the root operation and are used to capture details of the procedure, such as whether forceps or a vacuum were used during an Extraction, the type of fluid taken out during a Drainage procedure, or the products of conception body system that was repaired.

Placement Section (2)

Character Meanings

The seven characters in the Placement section have the following meaning:

Character	Meaning
1	Section
2	Body System
3	Root Operation
4	Body Region
5	Approach
6	Device
7	Qualifier

Placement section codes represent procedures for putting a device in or on a body region for the purpose of protection, immobilization, stretching, compression, or packing.

Section (Character 1)

Placement procedure codes have a first character value of *2*.

Body System (Character 2)

The second character contains two values specifying either *Anatomical Regions* or *Anatomical Orifices*.

Root Operation (Character 3)

The root operations in the Placement section include only those procedures that are performed without making an incision or a puncture. The root operations *Change* and *Removal* are in the Placement section and have the same meaning as in the Medical and Surgical section.

The Placement section also includes five additional root operations, defined as follows:

- *Compression*: Putting pressure on a body region
- *Dressing*: Putting material on a body region for protection
- *Immobilization*: Limiting or preventing motion of an external body region
- *Packing*: Putting material in a body region or orifice
- *Traction*: Exerting a pulling force on a body region in a distal direction

Body Region (Character 4)

The fourth character values are either body regions (e.g., *Upper Leg*) or natural orifices (e.g., *Ear*).

Approach (Character 5)

Since all placement procedures are performed directly on the skin or mucous membrane, or performed indirectly by applying external force through the skin or mucous membrane, the approach value is always *External*.

Device (Character 6)

The device character is always specified (except in the case of manual traction) and indicates the device placed during the procedure (e.g., cast, splint, bandage, etc.). Except for casts for fractures and dislocations, devices in the Placement section are off the shelf and do not require any extensive design, fabrication, or fitting. Placement of devices that require extensive design, fabrication, or fitting are coded in the Rehabilitation section.

Qualifier (Character 7)
The qualifier character is not specified in the Placement section; the qualifier value is always *No Qualifier*.

Administration Section (3)

Character Meanings
The seven characters in the Administration section have the following meaning:

Character	Meaning
1	Section
2	Body System
3	Root Operation
4	Body System/Region
5	Approach
6	Substance
7	Qualifier

Administration section codes represent procedures for putting in or on a therapeutic, prophylactic, protective, diagnostic, nutritional, or physiological substance. The section includes transfusions, infusions, and injections, along with other similar services such as irrigation and tattooing.

Section (Character 1)
Administration procedure codes have a first character value of *3*.

Body System (Character 2)
The body system character contains only three values: *Indwelling Device, Physiological Systems and Anatomical Regions,* or *Circulatory System*. The *Circulatory System* is used for transfusion procedures.

Root Operation (Character 3)
There are three root operations in the Administration section.

- *Introduction*: Putting in or on a therapeutic, diagnostic, nutritional, physiological, or prophylactic substance except blood or blood products
- *Irrigation*: Putting in or on a cleansing substance
- *Transfusion*: Putting in blood or blood products

Body/System Region (Character 4)
The fourth character specifies the body system/region. The fourth character identifies the site where the substance is administered, not the site where the substance administered takes effect. Sites include *Skin and Mucous Membranes, Subcutaneous Tissue,* and *Muscle*. These differentiate intradermal, subcutaneous, and intramuscular injections, respectively. Other sites include *Eye, Respiratory Tract, Peritoneal Cavity,* and *Epidural Space*.

The body systems/regions for arteries and veins are *Peripheral Artery, Central Artery, Peripheral Vein,* and *Central Vein*. The *Peripheral Artery* or *Vein* is typically used when a substance is introduced locally into an artery or vein. For example, chemotherapy is the introduction of an antineoplastic substance into a peripheral artery or vein by a percutaneous approach. In general, the substance introduced into a peripheral artery or vein has a systemic effect.

The *Central Artery* or *Vein* is typically used when the site where the substance is introduced is distant from the point of entry into the artery or vein. For example, the introduction of a substance directly at the site of a clot within an artery or vein using a catheter is coded as an introduction of a thrombolytic substance into a central artery or vein by a percutaneous approach. In general, the substance introduced into a central artery or vein has a local effect.

Approach (Character 5)
The fifth character specifies approaches as defined in the Medical and Surgical section. The approach for intradermal, subcutaneous, and intramuscular introductions (i.e., injections) is *Percutaneous*. If a catheter is placed to introduce a substance into an internal site within the circulatory system, then the approach is also *Percutaneous*. For example, if a catheter is used to introduce contrast directly into the heart for angiography, then the procedure would be coded as a percutaneous introduction of contrast into the heart.

Substance (Character 6)
The sixth character specifies the substance being introduced. Broad categories of substances are defined, such as anesthetic, contrast, dialysate, and blood products such as platelets.

Qualifier (Character 7)
The seventh character is a qualifier and is used to indicate whether the substance is *Autologous* or *Nonautologous*, or to further specify the substance.

Measurement and Monitoring Section (4)

Character Meanings
The seven characters in the Measurement and Monitoring section have the following meaning:

Character	Meaning
1	Section
2	Body System
3	Root Operation
4	Body System
5	Approach
6	Function/Device
7	Qualifier

Measurement and Monitoring section codes represent procedures for determining the level of a physiological or physical function.

Section (Character 1)
Measurement and Monitoring procedure codes have a first character value of *4*.

Body System (Character 2)
The second character values for body system are A, *Physiological Systems* or *B, Physiological Devices*.

Root Operation (Character 3)
There are two root operations in the Measurement and Monitoring section, as defined below:

- *Measurement*: Determining the level of a physiological or physical function at a point in time
- *Monitoring*: Determining the level of a physiological or physical function repetitively over a period of time

Body System (Character 4)
The fourth character specifies the specific body system measured or monitored.

Approach (Character 5)
The fifth character specifies approaches as defined in the Medical and Surgical section.

Function/Device (Character 6)
The sixth character specifies the physiological or physical function being measured or monitored. Examples of physiological or physical functions are *Conductivity, Metabolism, Pulse, Temperature,* and *Volume*. If a device used to perform the measurement or monitoring is inserted and left in, then insertion of the device is coded as a separate Medical and Surgical procedure.

Qualifier (Character 7)
The seventh character qualifier contains specific values as needed to further specify the body part (e.g., central, portal, pulmonary) or a variation of the procedure performed (e.g., ambulatory, stress). Examples of typical procedures coded in this section are EKG, EEG, and cardiac catheterization. An EKG is the measurement of cardiac electrical activity, while an EEG is the measurement of electrical activity of the central nervous system. A cardiac catheterization performed to measure the pressure in the heart is coded as the measurement of cardiac pressure by percutaneous approach.

Extracorporeal or Systemic Assistance and Performance Section (5)

Character Meanings
The seven characters in the Extracorporeal or Systemic Assistance and Performance section have the following meaning:

Character	Meaning
1	Section
2	Body System
3	Root Operation
4	Body System
5	Duration
6	Function
7	Qualifier

In Extracorporeal or Systemic Assistance and Performance procedures, equipment outside the body is used to assist or perform a physiological function. The section includes procedures performed in a critical care setting, such as mechanical ventilation and cardioversion; it also includes other services such as hyperbaric oxygen treatment and hemodialysis.

Section (Character 1)
Extracorporeal or Systemic Assistance and Performance procedure codes have a first character value of *5*.

Body System (Character 2)
The second character value for body system is A, *Physiological Systems*.

Root Operation (Character 3)
There are three root operations in the Extracorporeal or Systemic Assistance and Performance section, as defined below.

- *Assistance*: Taking over a portion of a physiological function by extracorporeal means
- *Performance*: Completely taking over a physiological function by extracorporeal means
- *Restoration*: Returning, or attempting to return, a physiological function to its natural state by extracorporeal means

The root operation *Restoration* contains a single procedure code that identifies extracorporeal cardioversion.

Body System (Character 4)
The fourth character specifies the body system (e.g., cardiac, respiratory) to which extracorporeal or systemic assistance or performance is applied.

Duration (Character 5)
The fifth character specifies the duration of the procedure.

Function (Character 6)
The sixth character specifies the physiological function assisted or performed (e.g., oxygenation, ventilation) during the procedure.

Qualifier (Character 7)
The seventh character qualifier specifies the type of equipment used, if any.

Extracorporeal or Systemic Therapies Section (6)

Character Meanings
The seven characters in the Extracorporeal or Systemic Therapies section have the following meaning:

Character	Meaning
1	Section
2	Body System
3	Root Operation
4	Body System
5	Duration
6	Qualifier
7	Qualifier

In extracorporeal or systemic therapy, equipment outside the body is used for a therapeutic purpose that does not involve the assistance or performance of a physiological function.

Section (Character 1)
Extracorporeal or Systemic Therapy procedure codes have a first character value of 6.

Body System (Character 2)
The second character value for body system is *Physiological Systems*.

Root Operation (Character 3)

There are 11 root operations in the Extracorporeal or Systemic Therapy section, as defined below.

- *Atmospheric Control*: Extracorporeal control of atmospheric pressure and composition
- *Decompression*: Extracorporeal elimination of undissolved gas from body fluids

  Coding note: The root operation *Decompression* involves only one type of procedure: treatment for decompression sickness (the bends) in a hyperbaric chamber.
- *Electromagnetic Therapy*: Extracorporeal treatment by electromagnetic rays
- *Hyperthermia*: Extracorporeal raising of body temperature

  Coding note: The term hyperthermia is used to describe both a temperature imbalance treatment and also as an adjunct radiation treatment for cancer. When treating the temperature imbalance, it is coded to this section; for the cancer treatment, it is coded in section *D Radiation Therapy.*
- *Hypothermia*: Extracorporeal lowering of body temperature
- *Perfusion*: Extracorporeal treatment by diffusion of therapeutic fluid
- *Pheresis*: Extracorporeal separation of blood products

  Coding note: Pheresis may be used for two main purposes: to treat diseases when too much of a blood component is produced (e.g., leukemia) and to remove a blood product such as platelets from a donor, for transfusion into another patient.
- *Phototherapy*: Extracorporeal treatment by light rays

  Coding note: Phototherapy involves using a machine that exposes the blood to light rays outside the body, recirculates it, and then returns it to the body.
- *Shock Wave Therapy*: Extracorporeal treatment by shock waves
- *Ultrasound Therapy*: Extracorporeal treatment by ultrasound
- *Ultraviolet Light Therapy*: Extracorporeal treatment by ultraviolet light

Body System (Character 4)

The fourth character specifies the body system on which the extracorporeal or systemic therapy is performed (e.g., skin, circulatory).

Duration (Character 5)

The fifth character specifies whether the procedure was performed once (single) or multiple times.

Qualifier (Character 6)

The sixth character for Extracorporeal or Systemic Therapies is *No Qualifier*, except for root operation Perfusion which has a sixth character qualifier of *Donor Organ*.

Qualifier (Character 7)

The seventh character qualifier is used in the root operation *Pheresis* to specify the blood component on which pheresis is performed and in the root operation *Ultrasound Therapy* to specify site of treatment.

Osteopathic Section (7)

Character Meanings

The seven characters in the Osteopathic section have the following meaning:

Character	Meaning
1	Section
2	Body System
3	Root Operation
4	Body Region
5	Approach
6	Method
7	Qualifier

Section (Character 1)

Osteopathic procedure codes have a first character value of *7*.

Body System (Character 2)

The body system character contains the value *Anatomical Regions*.

Root Operation (Character 3)

There is only one root operation in the Osteopathic section.

- *Treatment*: Manual treatment to eliminate or alleviate somatic dysfunction and related disorders

Body Region (Character 4)

The fourth character specifies the body region on which the osteopathic treatment is performed.

Approach (Character 5)

The approach for osteopathic treatment is always *External*.

Method (Character 6)

The sixth character specifies the method by which the treatment is accomplished.

Qualifier (Character 7)

The seventh character is not specified in the Osteopathic section and always has the value *None*.

Other Procedures Section (8)

Character Meanings

The seven characters in the Other Procedures section have the following meaning:

Character	Meaning
1	Section
2	Body System
3	Root Operation
4	Body Region
5	Approach
6	Method
7	Qualifier

The Other Procedures section includes acupuncture, suture removal, and in vitro fertilization.

Section (Character 1)
Other Procedure section codes have a first character value of *8*.

Body System (Character 2)
The second character values for body systems are *Physiological Systems and Anatomical Regions* and *Indwelling Device*.

Root Operation (Character 3)
The Other Procedures section has only one root operation, defined as follows:

- *Other Procedures*: Methodologies that attempt to remediate or cure a disorder or disease.

Body Region (Character 4)
The fourth character contains specified body-region values, and also the body-region value *None*.

Approach (Character 5)
The fifth character specifies approaches as defined in the Medical and Surgical section.

Method (Character 6)
The sixth character specifies the method (e.g., *Acupuncture, Therapeutic Massage*).

Qualifier (Character 7)
The seventh character is a qualifier and contains specific values as needed.

Chiropractic Section (9)

Character Meanings
The seven characters in the Chiropractic section have the following meaning:

Character	Meaning
1	Section
2	Body System
3	Root Operation
4	Body Region
5	Approach
6	Method
7	Qualifier

Section (Character 1)
Chiropractic section procedure codes have a first character value of *9*.

Body System (Character 2)
The second character value for body system is *Anatomical Regions*.

Root Operation (Character 3)
There is only one root operation in the *Chiropractic* section.

- *Manipulation:* Manual procedure that involves a directed thrust to move a joint past the physiological range of motion, without exceeding the anatomical limit.

Body Region (Character 4)
The fourth character specifies the body region on which the chiropractic manipulation is performed.

Approach (Character 5)
The approach for chiropractic manipulation is always *External*.

Method (Character 6)
The sixth character is the method by which the manipulation is accomplished.

Qualifier (Character 7)
The seventh character is not specified in the Chiropractic section and always has the value *None*.

Imaging Section (B)

Character Meanings
The seven characters in Imaging procedures have the following meaning:

Character	Meaning
1	Section
2	Body System
3	Type
4	Body Part
5	Contrast
6	Qualifier
7	Qualifier

Imaging procedures include plain radiography, fluoroscopy, CT, MRI, and ultrasound. Nuclear medicine procedures, including PET, uptakes, and scans, are in the nuclear medicine section. Therapeutic radiation procedure codes are in a separate radiation therapy section.

Section (Character 1)
Imaging procedure codes have a first character value of *B*.

Body System (Character 2)
In the Imaging section, the second character defines the body system, such as *Heart* or *Gastrointestinal System*.

Type (Character 3)
The third character defines the type of imaging procedure (e.g., MRI, ultrasound). The following list includes all types in the *Imaging* section with a definition of each type:

- *Computerized Tomography (CT Scan)*: Computer reformatted digital display of multiplanar images developed from the capture of multiple exposures of external ionizing radiation
- *Fluoroscopy*: Single plane or bi-plane real time display of an image developed from the capture of external ionizing radiation on a fluorescent screen. The image may also be stored by either digital or analog means
- *Magnetic Resonance Imaging (MRI)*: Computer reformatted digital display of multiplanar images developed from the capture of radiofrequency signals emitted by nuclei in a body site excited within a magnetic field
- *Other Imaging:* Other specified modality for visualizing a body part

- *Plain Radiography*: Planar display of an image developed from the capture of external ionizing radiation on photographic or photoconductive plate
- *Ultrasonography*: Real time display of images of anatomy or flow information developed from the capture of reflected and attenuated high frequency sound waves

Body Part (Character 4)
The fourth character defines the body part with different values for each body system (character 2) value.

Contrast (Character 5)
The fifth character specifies whether the contrast material used in the imaging procedure is *High Osmolar, Low Osmolar*, or *Other Contrast* when applicable.

Qualifier (Character 6)
The sixth character qualifier provides further detail regarding the nature of the substance or technologies used, such as *Unenhanced and Enhanced (contrast), Laser, or Intravascular Optical Coherence.*

Qualifier (Character 7)
The seventh character is a qualifier that may be used to specify certain procedural circumstances, the method by which the procedure was performed, or technologies utilized, such as *Intraoperative, Intravascular, or Transesophageal.*

Nuclear Medicine Section (C)

Character Meanings
The seven characters in the Nuclear Medicine section have the following meaning:

Character	Meaning
1	Section
2	Body System
3	Type
4	Body Part
5	Radionuclide
6	Qualifier
7	Qualifier

Nuclear Medicine is the introduction of radioactive material into the body to create an image, to diagnose and treat pathologic conditions, or to assess metabolic functions. The Nuclear Medicine section does not include the introduction of encapsulated radioactive material for the treatment of cancer. These procedures are included in the Radiation Therapy section.

Section (Character 1)
Nuclear Medicine procedure codes have a first character value of C.

Body System (Character 2)
The second character specifies the body system on which the nuclear medicine procedure is performed.

Type (Character 3)
The third character indicates the type of nuclear medicine procedure (e.g., planar imaging or nonimaging uptake). The following list includes the types of nuclear medicine procedures with a definition of each type.

- *Nonimaging Nuclear Medicine Assay:* Introduction of radioactive materials into the body for the study of body fluids and blood elements, by the detection of radioactive emissions
- *Nonimaging Nuclear Medicine Probe:* Introduction of radioactive materials into the body for the study of distribution and fate of certain substances by the detection of radioactive emissions; or alternatively, measurement of absorption of radioactive emissions from an external source
- *Nonimaging Nuclear Medicine Uptake:* Introduction of radioactive materials into the body for measurements of organ function, from the detection of radioactive emissions
- *Planar Nuclear Medicine Imaging*: Introduction of radioactive materials into the body for single-plane display of images developed from the capture of radioactive emissions
- *Positron Emission Tomography (PET) Imaging:* Introduction of radioactive materials into the body for three dimensional display of images developed from the simultaneous capture, 180 degrees apart, of radioactive emissions
- *Systemic Nuclear Medicine Therapy:* Introduction of unsealed radioactive materials into the body for treatment
- *Tomographic (Tomo) Nuclear Medicine Imaging*: Introduction of radioactive materials into the body for three dimensional display of images developed from the capture of radioactive emissions

Body Part (Character 4)
The fourth character indicates the body part or body region studied; with regional (e.g., *lower extremity veins*) and combination (e.g., *liver and spleen*) body parts commonly used.

Radionuclide (Character 5)
The fifth character specifies the radionuclide, the radiation source. The option *Other Radionuclide* is provided in the nuclear medicine section for newly approved radionuclides until they can be added to the coding system. If more than one radiopharmaceutical is given to perform the procedure, then more than one code is used.

Qualifier (Character 6 and 7)
The sixth and seventh characters are qualifiers but are not specified in the *Nuclear Medicine* section; the value is always *None.*

Radiation Therapy Section (D)

Character Meanings
The seven characters in the Radiation Therapy section have the following meaning:

Character	Meaning
1	Section
2	Body System
3	Modality
4	Treatment Site
5	Modality Qualifier
6	Isotope
7	Qualifier

Section (Character 1)

Radiation therapy procedure codes have a first character value of *D*.

Body System (Character 2)

The second character specifies the body system (e.g., central nervous system, musculoskeletal) irradiated.

Modality (Character 3)

The third character specifies the general modality used (e.g., beam radiation).

Treatment Site (Character 4)

The fourth character specifies the body part that is the focus of the radiation therapy.

Modality Qualifier (Character 5)

The fifth character further specifies the radiation modality used (e.g., photons, electrons).

Isotope (Character 6)

The sixth character specifies the isotopes introduced into the body, if applicable.

Qualifier (Character 7)

The seventh character may specify whether the procedure was performed intraoperatively.

Physical Rehabilitation and Diagnostic Audiology Section (F)

Character Meanings

The seven characters in the Physical Rehabilitation and Diagnostic Audiology section have the following meaning:

Character	Meaning
1	Section
2	Section Qualifier
3	Type
4	Body System/Region
5	Type Qualifier
6	Equipment
7	Qualifier

Physical rehabilitation procedures include physical therapy, occupational therapy, and speech-language pathology. Osteopathic procedures and chiropractic procedures are in separate sections.

Section (Character 1)

Physical Rehabilitation and Diagnostic Audiology procedure codes have a first character value of *F*.

Section Qualifier (Character 2)

The section qualifier *Rehabilitation* or *Diagnostic Audiology* is specified in the second character.

Type (Character 3)

The third character specifies the type. There are 14 different values, which can be classified into four basic types of rehabilitation and diagnostic audiology procedures, defined as follows:

Assessment: Includes a determination of the patient's diagnosis when appropriate, need for treatment, planning for treatment, periodic assessment, and documentation related to these activities

Assessments are further classified into more than 100 different tests or methods. The majority of these focus on the faculties of hearing and speech, but others focus on various aspects of body function, and on the patient's quality of life, such as muscle performance, neuromotor development, and reintegration skills.

- *Speech Assessment*: Measurement of speech and related functions
- *Motor and/or Nerve Function Assessment*: Measurement of motor, nerve, and related functions
- *Activities of Daily Living Assessment*: Measurement of functional level for activities of daily living
- *Hearing Assessment*: Measurement of hearing and related functions
- *Hearing Aid Assessment*: Measurement of the appropriateness and/or effectiveness of a hearing device
- *Vestibular Assessment*: Measurement of the vestibular system and related functions

Caregiver Training: Educating caregiver with the skills and knowledge used to interact with and assist the patient

Caregiver Training is divided into 18 different broad subjects taught to help a caregiver provide proper patient care.

- *Caregiver Training*: Training in activities to support patient's optimal level of function

Fitting(s): Design, fabrication, modification, selection, and/or application of splint, orthosis, prosthesis, hearing aids, and/or other rehabilitation device

The fifth character used in *Device Fitting* procedures describes the device being fitted rather than the method used to fit the device. Definitions of devices, when provided, are located in the definitions portion of the ICD-10-PCS tables and index, under section F, character 5.

- *Device Fitting*: Fitting of a device designed to facilitate or support achievement of a higher level of function

Treatment: Use of specific activities or methods to develop, improve, and/or restore the performance of necessary functions, compensate for dysfunction and/or minimize debilitation

Treatment procedures include swallowing dysfunction exercises, bathing and showering techniques, wound management, gait training, and a host of activities typically associated with rehabilitation.

- *Speech Treatment*: Application of techniques to improve, augment, or compensate for speech and related functional impairment
- *Motor Treatment*: Exercise or activities to increase or facilitate motor function
- *Activities of Daily Living Treatment*: Exercise or activities to facilitate functional competence for activities of daily living
- *Hearing Treatment*: Application of techniques to improve, augment, or compensate for hearing and related functional impairment

- *Cochlear Implant Treatment*: Application of techniques to improve the communication abilities of individuals with cochlear implant
- *Vestibular Treatment*: Application of techniques to improve, augment, or compensate for vestibular and related functional impairment

The type of treatment includes training as well as activities that restore function.

Body System/Region (Character 4)

The fourth character specifies the body region and/or system on which the procedure is performed.

Type Qualifier (Character 5)

The fifth character is a type qualifier that further specifies the procedure performed. Examples include therapy to improve the range of motion and training for bathing techniques. Refer to appendix J for definitions of these types of procedures.

Equipment (Character 6)

The sixth character specifies the equipment used. Specific equipment is not defined in the equipment value. Instead, broad categories of equipment are specified (e.g., aerobic endurance and conditioning, assistive/adaptive/supportive, etc.)

Qualifier (Character 7)

The seventh character is not specified in the Physical Rehabilitation and Diagnostic Audiology section and always has the value *None*.

Mental Health Section (G)

Character Meanings

The seven characters in the Mental Health section have the following meaning:

Character	Meaning
1	Section
2	Body System
3	Type
4	Qualifier
5	Qualifier
6	Qualifier
7	Qualifier

Section (Character 1)

Mental health procedure codes have a first character value of *G*.

Body System (Character 2)

The second character is used to identify the body system elsewhere in ICD-10-PCS. In this section it always has the value *None*.

Type (Character 3)

The third character specifies the procedure type, such as crisis intervention or counseling. There are 12 types of mental health procedures.

- *Psychological Tests:* The administration and interpretation of standardized psychological tests and measurement instruments for the assessment of psychological function
- *Crisis Intervention:* Treatment of a traumatized, acutely disturbed, or distressed individual for the purpose of short-term stabilization
- *Medication Management:* Monitoring and adjusting the use of medications for the treatment of a mental health disorder
- *Individual Psychotherapy:* Treatment of an individual with a mental health disorder by behavioral, cognitive, psychoanalytic, psychodynamic, or psychophysiological means to improve functioning or well-being
- *Counseling:* The application of psychological methods to treat an individual with normal developmental issues and psychological problems in order to increase function, improve well-being, alleviate distress, maladjustment, or resolve crises
- *Family Psychotherapy:* Treatment that includes one or more family members of an individual with a mental health disorder by behavioral, cognitive, psychoanalytic, psychodynamic, or psychophysiological means to improve functioning or well-being
- *Electroconvulsive Therapy:* The application of controlled electrical voltages to treat a mental health disorder
- *Biofeedback:* Provision of information from the monitoring and regulating of physiological processes in conjunction with cognitive-behavioral techniques to improve patient functioning or well-being
- *Hypnosis:* Induction of a state of heightened suggestibility by auditory, visual, and tactile techniques to elicit an emotional or behavioral response
- *Narcosynthesis:* Administration of intravenous barbiturates in order to release suppressed or repressed thoughts
- *Group Psychotherapy:* Treatment of two or more individuals with a mental health disorder by behavioral, cognitive, psychoanalytic, psychodynamic, or psychophysiological means to improve functioning or well-being
- *Light Therapy:* Application of specialized light treatments to improve functioning or well-being

Qualifier (Character 4)

The fourth character is a qualifier to indicate that counseling was educational or vocational or to indicate type of test or method of therapy.

Qualifier (Character 5, 6 and 7)

The fifth, sixth, and seventh characters are not specified and always have the value *None*.

Substance Abuse Treatment Section (H)

Character Meanings

The seven characters in the Substance Abuse Treatment section have the following meaning:

Character	Meaning
1	Section
2	Body System
3	Type
4	Qualifier
5	Qualifier
6	Qualifier
7	Qualifier

Section (Character 1)
Substance Abuse Treatment codes have a first character value of *H*.

Body System (Character 2)
The second character is used to identify the body system elsewhere in ICD-10-PCS. In this section, it always has the value *None*.

Type (Character 3)
The third character specifies the type of procedure. There are seven values classified in this section, as listed below:

- *Detoxification Services:* Detoxification from alcohol and/or drugs
- *Individual Counseling:* The application of psychological methods to treat an individual with addictive behavior
- *Group Counseling:* The application of psychological methods to treat two or more individuals with addictive behavior
- *Individual Psychotherapy:* Treatment of an individual with addictive behavior by behavioral, cognitive, psychoanalytic, psychodynamic, or psychophysiological means
- *Family Counseling:* The application of psychological methods that includes one or more family members to treat an individual with addictive behavior
- *Medication Management:* Monitoring and adjusting the use of replacement medications for the treatment of addiction
- *Pharmacotherapy:* The use of replacement medications for the treatment of addiction

Qualifier (Character 4)
The fourth character further specifies the procedure type. These qualifier values vary dependent upon the Root Type procedure (Character 3). Root type 2, *Detoxification Services* contains only the value Z, *None* and Root type 6, *Family Counseling* contains only the value 3, *Other Family Counseling*, whereas the remainder Root Type procedures include multiple possible values.

Qualifier (Character 5, 6 and 7)
The fifth through seventh characters are designated as qualifiers but are never specified, so they always have the value *None*.

New Technology Section (X)

General Information
Section X New Technology is a section added to ICD-10-PCS beginning October 1, 2015. The new section provides a place for codes that uniquely identify procedures requested via the New Technology Application Process or that capture other new technologies not currently classified in ICD-10-PCS.

Section X does not introduce any new coding concepts or unusual guidelines for correct coding. In fact, Section X codes maintain continuity with the other sections in ICD-10-PCS by using the same root operation and body part values as their closest counterparts in other sections of ICD-10-PCS. For example, the codes for the infusion of ceftazidime-avibactam, use the same root operation (Introduction) and body part values (Central Vein and Peripheral Vein) in section X as the infusion codes in section 3 Administration, which are their closest counterparts in the other sections of ICD-10-PCS.

Character Meanings
The seven characters in the new technology section have the following meaning:

Character	Meaning
1	Section
2	Body System
3	Root Operation
4	Body Part
5	Approach
6	Device/Substance/Technology
7	Qualifier

Section (Character 1)
New technology procedure codes have a first character value of *X*.

Body System (Character 2)
The second character values for body system combine the uses of body system, body region, and physiological system as specified in other sections in ICD-10-PCS.

Root Operation (Character 3)
The third character utilizes the same root operation values as their counterparts in other sections of ICD-10-PCS.

Body Part (Character 4)
The fourth character specifies the same body part values as their closest counterparts in other sections of ICD-10-PCS.

Approach (Character 5)
The fifth character specifies approaches as defined in the Medical and Surgical section.

Device/Substance/Technology (Character 6)
The sixth character specifies the key feature of the new technology procedure. It may be specified as a new device, a new substance, or other new technology. Examples of sixth character values are *blinatumomab antineoplastic immunotherapy, orbital atherectomy technology,* and *intraoperative knee replacement sensor*.

Qualifier (Character 7)
The seventh character qualifier is used exclusively to specify the new technology group, a number or letter that changes each year that new technology codes are added to the system. For example, Section X codes added for the first year have the seventh character value 1, *New Technology Group 1*, and the next year that Section X codes are added have the seventh character value 2, *New Technology Group 2*, and so on. Changing the seventh character value to a unique letter or number every year that there are new codes in the new technology section allows the ICD-10-PCS to "recycle" the values in the third, fourth, and sixth characters as needed.

New Technology Coding Instruction
Section X codes are standalone codes. They are not supplemental codes. Section X codes fully represent the specific procedure described in the code title, and do not require any additional codes from other sections of ICD-10-PCS. When section X contains a code title which describes a specific new technology procedure, only that X code is reported for the procedure. There is no need to report a broader, non-specific code in another section of ICD-10-PCS.

For example, code XWØ4321 Introduction of Ceftazidime-Avibactam Anti-infective into Central Vein, Percutaneous Approach, New Technology Group 1, would be reported to indicate that Ceftazidime-Avibactam Anti-infective was administered via central vein. A separate code from table 3EØ in the Administration section of ICD-10-PCS would not be reported in addition to this code. The X section code fully identifies the administration of the ceftazidime-avibactam antibiotic, and no additional code is needed.

The New Technology section codes are easily found by looking in the ICD-10-PCS Index or the Tables. In the Index, the name of the new technology device, substance or technology for a section X code is included as a main term. In addition, all codes in section X are listed under the main term New Technology. The new technology code index entry for ceftazidime-avibactam is shown below.

Ceftazidime-Avibactam Anti-infective XWØ

New Technology
Ceftazidime-Avibactam Anti-infective XWØ

ICD-10-PCS Index and Tabular Format

The *ICD-10-PCS: The Complete Official Code Set* is based on the official version of the International Classification of Diseases, 10th Revision, Procedure Classification System, issued by the U.S. Department of Health and Human Services, Centers for Medicare and Medicaid Services. This book is consistent with the content of the government's version of ICD-10-PCS and follows their official format.

Index

The Alphabetic Index can be used to locate the appropriate table containing all the information necessary to construct a procedure code, however, the PCS tables should always be consulted to find the most appropriate valid code. Users may choose a valid code directly from the tables—he or she need not consult the index before proceeding to the tables to complete the code.

Main Terms

The Alphabetic Index reflects the structure of the tables. Therefore, the index is organized as an alphabetic listing. The index:

- Is based on the value of the third character
- Contains common procedure terms
- Lists anatomic sites
- Uses device terms

The main terms in the Alphabetic Index are root operations, root procedure types, or common procedure names. In addition, anatomic sites from the Body Part Key and device terms from the Device Key have been added for ease of use.

Examples:

Resection (root operation)

Fluoroscopy (root type)

Prostatectomy (common procedure name)

Brachiocephalic artery (body part)

Bard® Dulex™ mesh (device)

The index provides at least the first three or four values of the code, and some entries may provide complete valid codes. However, the user should always consult the appropriate table to verify that the most appropriate valid code has been selected.

Root Operation and Procedure Type Main Terms

For the *Medical and Surgical* and related sections, the root operation values are used as main terms in the index. The subterms under the root operation main terms are body parts. For the Ancillary section of the tables, the main terms in the index are the general type of procedure performed.

Examples:

Biofeedback GZC9ZZZ
Destruction
Acetabulum
Left ØQ55
Right ØQ54
Adenoids ØC5Q
Ampulla of Vater ØF5C
Planar Nuclear Medicine Imaging
Abdomen CW1Ø

See Reference

The second type of term in the index uses common procedure names, such as "appendectomy" or "fundoplication." These common terms are listed as main terms with a "see" reference noting the PCS root operations that are possible valid code tables based on the objective of the procedure.

Examples:

Tendonectomy
see Excision, Tendons ØLB
see Resection, Tendons ØLT

Use Reference

The index also lists anatomic sites from the Body Part Key and device terms from the Device Key. These terms are listed with a "use" reference. The purpose of these references is to act as an additional reference to the terms located in the Appendix Keys. The term provided is the Body Part value or Device value to be selected when constructing a procedure code using the code tables. This type of index reference is not intended to direct the user to another term in the index, but to provide guidance regarding character value selection. Therefore, "use" references generally do not refer to specific valid code tables.

Examples:

CoAxia NeuroFlo catheter
use Intraluminal Device
Epitrochlear lymph node
use Lymphatic, Left Upper Extremity
use Lymphatic, Right Upper Extremity
SynCardia Total Artificial Heart
use Synthetic Substitute

Code Tables

ICD-10-PCS contains 17 sections of Code Tables organized by general type of procedure. The first three characters of a procedure code define each table. The tables consist of columns providing the possible last four characters of codes and rows providing valid values for each character. Within a PCS table, valid codes include all combinations of choices in characters 4 through 7 contained in the same row of the table. All seven characters must be specified to form a valid code.

There are three main sections of tables:

- Medical and Surgical section:
  - *Medical and Surgical* (Ø)
- Medical and Surgical-related sections:
  - *Obstetrics* (1)
  - *Placement* (2)
  - *Administration* (3)
  - *Measurement and Monitoring* (4)
  - *Extracorporeal or Systemic Assistance and Performance* (5)
  - *Extracorporeal or Systemic Therapies* (6)
  - *Osteopathic* (7)
  - *Other Procedures* (8)
  - *Chiropractic* (9)

- Ancillary sections:
  - — *Imaging* (B)
  - — *Nuclear Medicine* (C)
  - — *Radiation Therapy* (D)
  - — *Physical Rehabilitation and Diagnostic Audiology* (F)
  - — *Mental Health* (G)
  - — *Substance Abuse Treatment* (H)
- New Technology section:
  - — *New Technology* (X)

The first three character values define each table. The root operation or root type designated for each table is accompanied by its official definition.

Example:

Table ØØF provides codes for procedures on the central nervous system that involve breaking up of solid matter into pieces:

Character 1, Section	Ø: Medical and Surgical
Character 2, Body System	Ø: Central Nervous System and Cranial Nerves
Character 3, Root Operation	F: Fragmentation: Breaking solid matter in a body part into pieces

Tables are arranged numerically, then alphabetically.

When reviewing tables, the user should keep in mind that:

- Some tables may cover multiple pages in the code book—to ensure maximum clarity about character choices, valid entries do not split rows between pages. For instance, the entire table of valid characters completing a code beginning with 4A1 is split between two pages, but the split is between, not within, rows. This means that all the valid sixth and seventh characters for, say, body system *Arterial* (3) and approach *External* (X) are contained on one page.
- Individual entries may be listed in several horizontal "selection" lines.
- When a table is continued onto another page, a note to this effect has been added in red.

Body Part Definitions:

An exclusive Optum360 feature in the tables is the incorporation of the body part definitions provided in appendix E into the Medical and Surgical section (Ø) tables under their appropriate body part characters in the first column (character 4). This provides the user a direct reference to all anatomical descriptions, terms, and sites that could be coded to that particular body part value.

Paired body parts typically have values for the right and left side and in some cases a value for bilateral. These paired body parts often have the same list of inclusive body part definitions. When there are paired body parts with the same body part definitions, the first listed body part (usually the right side) contains the list of body part definitions while the second listed body part (usually the left side) contains a ***See*** instruction. This ***See*** instruction references the body part value that contains the body part definitions. In the table below, body part value P – Upper Eyelid, Left is followed by a ***See*** instruction that states ***See*** *N Upper Eyelid, Right*. All body part descriptions under value N also apply to body part value P.

Example:

Ø Medical and Surgical
8 Eye
M Reattachment **Definition: Putting back in or on all or a portion of a separated body part to its normal location or other suitable location**
Explanation: Vascular circulation and nervous pathways may or may not be reestablished

Body Part Character 4	Approach Character 5	Device Character 6	Qualifier Character 7
N Upper Eyelid, Right Lateral canthus Levator palpebrae superioris muscle Orbicularis oculi muscle Superior tarsal plate **P Upper Eyelid, Left** *See N Upper Eyelid, Right* **Q Lower Eyelid, Right** Inferior tarsal plate Medial canthus **R Lower Eyelid, Left** *See Q Lower Eyelid, Right*	**X External**	**Z No Device**	**Z No Qualifier**

ICD-10-PCS Additional Features

Use of Official Sources

Color-coding, symbol, and other annotations in this manual that identify coding and reimbursement issues are derived from various official federal government sources, including the *Federal Register*, volume 85, number 104, May 29, 2020 ("Hospital Inpatient Prospective Payment Systems for Acute Care Hospitals and the Long Term Care Hospital Prospective Payment System and Proposed Policy Changes and Fiscal Year 2021 Rates; Proposed Rule") and the proposed, version 38, MS-DRG Grouper software, Definitions Manual files and Medicare Code Editor (MCE) files published with the fiscal 2021 IPPS proposed rule. For the most current files related to IPPS, please refer to the following:

- FY2021 IPPS Final Rule https://www.cms.gov/Medicare/Medicare-Fee-for-Service-Payment/AcuteInpatientPPS/IPPS-Regulations-and-Notices
- FY2021 Final Version 38, MS-DRG Grouper software https://www.cms.gov/Medicare/Medicare-Fee-for-Service-Payment/AcuteInpatientPPS/MS-DRG-Classifications-and-Software

Table Notations

Many tables in ICD-10-PCS contain color or symbol annotations that may aid in code selection, provide clinical or coding information, or alert the coder to reimbursement issues affected by the PCS code assignment. These annotations are most often displayed on or next to a character 4 value. Some character 4 values may have more than one annotation.

Refer to the color/symbol legend at the bottom of each page in the tables section for an abridged description of each color and symbol.

Annotation Box

An annotation box has been appended to all tables that contain color-coding or symbol annotations. The color bar or symbol attached to a character 4 value is provided in the box, as well as a list of the valid PCS code(s) to which that edit applies. The box may also list conditional criteria that must be met to satisfy the edit.

For example, see Table ØØF. Four character 4 body part values have a gray color bar. In the annotation box below the table, the gray color bar is defined as "Non-OR," or a nonoperating room procedure edit. Following the Non-OR annotation are the PCS codes that are considered nonoperating room procedures from that row of Table ØØF.

Bracketed Code Notation

The use of bracketed codes is an efficient convention to provide all valid character value alternatives for a specific set of circumstances. The character values in the brackets correspond to the valid values for the character in the position the bracket appears.

Examples:

In the annotation box for Table ØØF the Noncovered Procedure edit (NC) applies to codes represented in the bracketed code ØØF[3,4,5,6]XZZ.

ØØF[3,4,5,6]XZZ Fragmentation in (Central Nervous System and Cranial Nerves), External Approach

The valid fourth character values (Body Part) that may be selected for this specific circumstance are as follows:

3 Epidural Space, Intracranial
4 Subdural Space, Intracranial
5 Subarachnoid Space, Intracranial
6 Cerebral Ventricle

The fragmentation of matter in the spinal canal, Body Part value U, is not included in the noncovered procedure code edits.

Color-Coding/Symbols

New and Revised Text

To highlight changes to the PCS tables for the current year, the new and revised text is provided in green font.

Medicare Code Edits

Medicare administrative contractors (MACs) and many payers use Medicare code edits to check the coding accuracy on claims. The coding edits provided in this manual Include only those directly related to ICD-10-PCS codes used for acute care hospital inpatient admissions. These edits are based on the proposed, version 38, Medicare Code Editor (MCE) files published with the fiscal 2021 IPPS proposed rule.

The PCS related Medicare code edits are listed below:

- Invalid procedure code
- *Sex conflict
- *Questionable obstetric admission
- *Noncovered procedure
- *Limited coverage procedure

Starred edits above that are related to PCS issues are identified in this manual by symbols as described below.

Sex Edit Symbols

The sex edit symbols below are used to detect inconsistencies between the patient's sex and the procedure. The symbols below most often appear to the right of the body part (character 4) value but may also be found to the right of the qualifier (character 7) value:

♂ Male procedure only

♀ Female procedure only

QA **Questionable Obstetric Admission**

An inpatient admission is considered questionable when a vaginal or cesarean delivery code is assigned without a corresponding secondary diagnosis code describing the outcome of delivery. Both a delivery (ICD-10-PCS) code and an outcome-of-delivery (ICD-10-CM) code must be present to avoid errors in MS-DRG assignment. This symbol is found only in the Obstetrics Section, appearing to the right of the body part (character 4) value.

NC **Noncovered Procedure**

Medicare does not cover all procedures. However, some noncovered procedures, due to the presence of certain diagnoses, are reimbursed.

LC **Limited Coverage**

For certain procedures whose medical complexity and serious nature incur extraordinary associated costs, Medicare limits coverage to a portion of the cost. The limited coverage edit indicates the type of limited coverage.

ICD-10 MS-DRG Definitions Manual Edits

An MS-DRG is assigned based on specific patient attributes, such as principal diagnosis, secondary diagnoses, procedures, and discharge status. The attributes (edits) provided in this manual include only those directly related to ICD-10-PCS codes used for acute care hospital inpatient admissions. These edits are based on the proposed, version 38, MS-DRG Grouper software and Definitions Manual published with the fiscal 2021 IPPS proposed rule.

Non-Operating Room Procedures Not Affecting MS-DRG Assignment

In the Medical and Surgical section (ØØ1-ØYW) and the Obstetric section (1Ø2-1ØY) tables **only,** ICD-10-PCS procedures codes that DO NOT affect MS-DRG assignment are identified by a **gray color bar** over the body part (character 4) value and are considered non-operating room (non-OR) procedures.

NOTE: The majority of the ICD-10-PCS codes in the Medical and Surgical-Related, Ancillary and New Technology section tables are non-operating room procedures that do not typically affect MS-DRG assignment. Only the Valid Operating Room and DRG Non-Operating Room procedures are highlighted in these sections, *see* Non-Operating Room Procedures Affecting MS-DRG Assignment and Valid OR Procedure description below.

Non-Operating Room Procedures Affecting MS-DRG Assignment

Some ICD-10-PCS procedure codes, although considered non-operating room procedures, may still affect MS-DRG assignment. In all sections of the ICD-10-PCS book, these procedures are identified by a **purple color bar** over the body part (character 4) value.

Valid OR Procedure

In the Medical and Surgical-Related (2WØ-9WB), Ancillary (BØØ-HZ9) and New Technology (X2A-XYØ) section tables **only,** any codes that are considered a valid operating room procedure are identified with a **blue color bar** over the body part (character 4) value and will affect MS-DRG assignment. All codes without a color bar (blue or purple) are considered non-operating room procedures.

Hospital-Acquired Condition Related Procedures

Procedures associated with hospital-acquired conditions (HAC) are identified with the **yellow color bar** over the body part (character 4) value. Appendix K provides each specific HAC category and its associated ICD-10-CM and ICD-10-PCS codes.

Combination Only

Some ICD-10-PCS procedure codes that describe non-operating room procedures can group to a specific MS-DRG but only when used in combination with certain other ICD-10-PCS procedure codes. Such codes are designated by a **red color bar** over the body part (character 4) value.

⊞ **Combination Member**

A combination member, which can be either a valid operating room procedure or a non-operating room procedure, is an ICD-10-PCS procedure code that can influence MS-DRG assignment either on its own or in combination with other specific ICD-10-PCS procedure codes. Combination member codes are designated by a plus sign (⊞) to the right of the body part (character 4) value.

Note: In the few instances when a code is both a combination member and a non-operating room procedure affecting the MS-DRG assignment, the body part (character 4) value will have a purple color bar and the combination member icon.

See Appendix L for Procedure Combinations

Under certain circumstances, more than one procedure code is needed in order to group to a specific MS-DRG. When codes within a table have been identified as a Combination Only (**red color bar**) or Combination Member (⊞) code, there is also a footnote instructing the coder to *see Appendix L*. Appendix L contains tables that identify the other procedure codes needed in the combination and the title and number of the MS-DRG to which the combination will group.

Other Table Notations

AHA Coding Clinic:

Official citations from AHA's *Coding Clinic for ICD-10-CM/PCS* have been provided at the beginning of each section, when applicable. Each specific citation is listed below a header identifying the table to which that particular *Coding Clinic* citation applies. The citations appear in purple type with the year, quarter, and page of the reference as well as the title of the question as it appears in that *Coding Clinic's* table of contents. *Coding Clinic* citations included in this edition have been updated through second quarter 2020.

Appendixes

The resources described below have been included as appendixes for *ICD-10-PCS The Complete Official Code Set*. These resources further instruct the coder on the appropriate application of the ICD-10-PCS code set.

Appendix A: Components of the Medical and Surgical Approach Definitions

This resource further defines the approach characters used in the Medical and Surgical (Ø) section. Complementing the detailed definition of the approach, additional information includes whether or not instrumentation is a part of the approach, the typical access location, the method used to initiate the approach, related procedural examples, and illustrations all of which will help the user determine the appropriate approach value.

Appendix B: Root Operation Definitions

This resource is a compilation of all root operations found in the Medical and Surgical-related sections (Ø-9) of this PCS manual. It provides a definition and in some cases a more detailed explanation of the root operation, to better reflect the purpose or objective. Examples of related procedure(s) may also be provided.

Appendix C: Comparison of Medical and Surgical Root Operations

The Medical and Surgical root operations are divided into groups that share similar attributes. These groups, and the root operations in each group, are listed in this resource along with information identifying the target of the root operation, the action used to perform the root operation, any clarification or further explanation on the objective of the root operation, and procedure examples.

Appendix D: Body Part Key

When an anatomical term or description is provided in the documentation but does not have a specific body part character within a table, the user can reference this resource to search for the anatomical description or site noted in the documentation to determine if there is a specific PCS body part character (character 4) to which the anatomical description or site could be coded.

Appendix E: Body Part Definitions

This resource is the reverse look-up of the Body Part Key. Each table in the Medical and Surgical section (Ø) of the PCS manual contains anatomical terms linked to a body part character or value, for example, in Table ØBB the Body Part (character 4) of 1 is Trachea. The body part Trachea may have anatomical structures or descriptions that may be used in procedure documentation instead of the term trachea. The Body Part Definitions list other anatomical structures or synonyms that are included in specific ICD-10-PCS body part values. According to the body part definitions, in the example above, cricoid cartilage is included in the Trachea (character 1) body part.

Appendix F: Device Classification

This resource provides an explanation of how a device is defined in the ICD-10-PCS classification along with two tables. The first table groups devices used in the ICD-10-PCS tables into general categories, including a definition of each device type and related examples. The second table provides definitions of transplant and grafting tissue types and associated terminology that may be found in the documentation.

Appendix G: Device Key and Aggregation Table

The Device Key helps users code the appropriate PCS sixth character for device. Devices are listed alphabetically by brand name or commonly used medical terminology and are translated to the appropriate PCS language or value. The key also reflects the body system where the device Is located. For example, a SAPIEN valve used for transaortic valve replacement translates to Zooplastic Tissue in Heart and Great Vessels.

The Aggregation Table crosswalks specific device character value definitions for specific root operations in a specific body system to the more general device character value to be used when the root operation covers a wide range of body parts and the device character represents an entire family of devices.

Appendix H: Device Definitions

This resource is a reverse look-up to the Device Key. The user may reference this resource to see all the specific devices that may be grouped to a particular device character (character 6).

Example:
The operative report states, "An internal fixation device was used to repair a fractured femur. Kirschner wire, bone screws and neutralization plate all used and left in the bone at the end of the procedure. "

Although PCS requires all devices left in the body to be coded and the operative report lists three different devices, a check in the device definitions shows that all of these devices are included in the PCS value "Internal Fixation Device" and require only one code.

Appendix I: Substance Key/Substance Definitions

The Substance Key lists substances by trade name or synonym and relates them to a PCS character in the Administration (3) or New Technology (X) section in the Substance (sixth character) or Qualifier (seventh character) column.

The Substance Definitions table is the reverse look-up of the substance key, relating all substance categories, the sixth- or seventh character values, to all trade name or synonyms that may be classified to that particular character.

Appendix J: Sections B-H Character Definitions

In each ancillary section (B-H) the characters in a particular column may have different meanings depending on which section the user is working from. This resource provides the values for the characters in these sections as well as a definition of the character value.

Appendix K: Hospital Acquired Conditions

Hospital acquired conditions (HACs) are conditions that are considered reasonably preventable when occurring during the hospital admission and may prevent a case from grouping to a higher-paying MS-DRG. In certain instances the HACs are conditional, requiring a specific ICD-10-CM diagnosis code in combination with a specific ICD-10-PCS procedure code. This resource identifies these conditional HACs, listing the diagnosis and procedure codes that, in combination, may trigger a HAC edit. All codes, ICD-10-CM and ICD-10-PCS, are listed with their full descriptions.

Appendix L: Procedure Combination Tables

The procedure combination tables provided in this resource illustrate certain procedure combinations that must occur in order to assign a specific MS-DRG.

Appendix M: Coding Exercises and Answers

This resource provides the coding exercises with answers, and in some cases a brief explanation as to the reason that particular code was used.

ICD-10-PCS Official Guidelines for Coding and Reporting 2021

Narrative changes appear in **bold** text.

The Centers for Medicare and Medicaid Services (CMS) and the National Center for Health Statistics (NCHS), two departments within the U.S. Federal Government's Department of Health and Human Services (DHHS) provide the following guidelines for coding and reporting using the International Classification of Diseases, 10th Revision, Procedure Coding System (ICD-10-PCS). These guidelines should be used as a companion document to the official version of the ICD-10-PCS as published on the CMS website. The ICD-10-PCS is a procedure classification published by the United States for classifying procedures performed in hospital inpatient health care settings.

These guidelines have been approved by the four organizations that make up the Cooperating Parties for the ICD-10-PCS: the American Hospital Association (AHA), the American Health Information Management Association (AHIMA), CMS, and NCHS.

These guidelines are a set of rules that have been developed to accompany and complement the official conventions and instructions provided within the ICD-10-PCS itself. They are intended to provide direction that is applicable in most circumstances. However, there may be unique circumstances where exceptions are applied. The instructions and conventions of the classification take precedence over guidelines. These guidelines are based on the coding and sequencing instructions in the Tables, Index and Definitions of ICD-10-PCS, but provide additional instruction. Adherence to these guidelines when assigning ICD-10-PCS procedure codes is required under the Health Insurance Portability and Accountability Act (HIPAA). The procedure codes have been adopted under HIPAA for hospital inpatient healthcare settings. A joint effort between the healthcare provider and the coder is essential to achieve complete and accurate documentation, code assignment, and reporting of diagnoses and procedures. These guidelines have been developed to assist both the healthcare provider and the coder in identifying those procedures that are to be reported. The importance of consistent, complete documentation in the medical record cannot be overemphasized. Without such documentation accurate coding cannot be achieved.

Conventions

A1. ICD-10-PCS codes are composed of seven characters. Each character is an axis of classification that specifies information about the procedure performed. Within a defined code range, a character specifies the same type of information in that axis of classification.

> *Example:*
> The fifth axis of classification specifies the approach in sections Ø through 4 and 7 through 9 of the system.

A2. One of 34 possible values can be assigned to each axis of classification in the seven-character code: they are the numbers Ø through 9 and the alphabet (except I and O because they are easily confused with the numbers 1 and Ø). The number of unique values used in an axis of classification differs as needed.

> *Example:*
> Where the fifth axis of classification specifies the approach, seven different approach values are currently used to specify the approach.

A3. The valid values for an axis of classification can be added to as needed.

> *Example:*
> If a significantly distinct type of device is used in a new procedure, a new device value can be added to the system.

A4. As with words in their context, the meaning of any single value is a combination of its axis of classification and any preceding values on which it may be dependent.

> *Example:*
> The meaning of a body part value in the Medical and Surgical section is always dependent on the body system value. The body part value Ø in the Central Nervous body system specifies Brain and the body part value Ø in the Peripheral Nervous body system specifies Cervical Plexus.

A5. As the system is expanded to become increasingly detailed, over time more values will depend on preceding values for their meaning.

> *Example:*
> In the Lower Joints body system, the device value 3 in the root operation Insertion specifies Infusion Device and the device value 3 in the root operation Replacement specifies Ceramic Synthetic Substitute.

A6. The purpose of the alphabetic index is to locate the appropriate table that contains all information necessary to construct a procedure code. The PCS Tables should always be consulted to find the most appropriate valid code.

A7. It is not required to consult the index first before proceeding to the tables to complete the code. A valid code may be chosen directly from the tables.

A8. All seven characters must be specified to be a valid code. If the documentation is incomplete for coding purposes, the physician should be queried for the necessary information.

A9. Within a PCS table, valid codes include all combinations of choices in characters 4 through 7 contained in the same row of the table. In the example below, ØJHT3VZ is a valid code, and ØJHW3VZ is *not* a valid code.

Section: **Ø** **Medical and Surgical**
Body System: **J** **Subcutaneous Tissue and Fascia**
Operation: **H** **Insertion** Putting in a nonbiological appliance that monitors, assists, performs, or prevents a physiological function but does not physically take the place of a body part

Body Part	Approach	Device	Qualifier
S Subcutaneous Tissue and Fascia, Head and Neck **V** Subcutaneous Tissue and Fascia, Upper Extremity **W** Subcutaneous Tissue and Fascia, Lower Extremity	**Ø** Open **3** Percutaneous	**1** Radioactive Element **3** Infusion Device **Y** Other Device	**Z** No Qualifier
T Subcutaneous Tissue and Fascia, Trunk	**Ø** Open **3** Percutaneous	**1** Radioactive Element **3** Infusion Device **V** Infusion Pump **Y** Other Device	**Z** No Qualifier

A10. "And," when used in a code description, means "and/or," except when used to describe a combination of multiple body parts for which separate values exist for each body part (e.g., Skin and Subcutaneous Tissue used as a qualifier, where there are separate body part values for "Skin" and "Subcutaneous Tissue").

Example:
Lower Arm and Wrist Muscle means lower arm and/or wrist muscle.

A11. Many of the terms used to construct PCS codes are defined within the system. It is the coder's responsibility to determine what the documentation in the medical record equates to in the PCS definitions. The physician is not expected to use the terms used in PCS code descriptions, nor is the coder required to query the physician when the correlation between the documentation and the defined PCS terms is clear.

Example:
When the physician documents "partial resection" the coder can independently correlate "partial resection" to the root operation Excision without querying the physician for clarification.

Medical and Surgical Section Guidelines (section Ø)

B2. Body System

General guidelines

B2.1a. The procedure codes in Anatomical Regions, General, Anatomical Regions, Upper Extremities and Anatomical Regions, Lower Extremities can be used when the procedure is performed on an anatomical region rather than a specific body part, or on the rare occasion when no information is available to support assignment of a code to a specific body part.

Examples:
Chest tube drainage of the pleural cavity is coded to the root operation Drainage found in the body system Anatomical Regions, General.

Suture repair of the abdominal wall is coded to the root operation Repair in the body system Anatomical Regions, General.

Amputation of the foot is coded to the root operation Detachment in the body system Anatomical Regions, Lower Extremities.

B2.1b. Where the general body part values "upper" and "lower" are provided as an option in the Upper Arteries, Lower Arteries, Upper Veins, Lower Veins, Muscles and Tendons body systems, "upper" or "lower" specifies body parts located above or below the diaphragm respectively.

Example:
Vein body parts above the diaphragm are found in the Upper Veins body system; vein body parts below the diaphragm are found in the Lower Veins body system.

B3. Root Operation

General guidelines

B3.1a. In order to determine the appropriate root operation, the full definition of the root operation as contained in the PCS Tables must be applied.

B3.1b. Components of a procedure specified in the root operation definition or explanation as integral to that root operation are not coded separately. Procedural steps necessary to reach the operative site and close the operative site, including anastomosis of a tubular body part, are also not coded separately.

Examples:
Resection of a joint as part of a joint replacement procedure is included in the root operation definition of Replacement and is not coded separately.

Laparotomy performed to reach the site of an open liver biopsy is not coded separately.

In a resection of sigmoid colon with anastomosis of descending colon to rectum, the anastomosis is not coded separately.

Multiple procedures

B3.2. During the same operative episode, multiple procedures are coded if:

a. The same root operation is performed on different body parts as defined by distinct values of the body part character.
   Examples:
   Diagnostic excision of liver and pancreas are coded separately.

   Excision of lesion in the ascending colon and excision of lesion in the transverse colon are coded separately.

b. The same root operation is repeated in multiple body parts, and those body parts are separate and distinct body parts classified to a single ICD-10-PCS body part value.
   Examples:
   Excision of the sartorius muscle and excision of the gracilis muscle are both included in the upper leg muscle body part value, and multiple procedures are coded.

   Extraction of multiple toenails are coded separately.

c. Multiple root operations with distinct objectives are performed on the same body part.
   Example:
   Destruction of sigmoid lesion and bypass of sigmoid colon are coded separately.

d. The intended root operation is attempted using one approach but is converted to a different approach.
   Example:
   Laparoscopic cholecystectomy converted to an open cholecystectomy is coded as percutaneous endoscopic Inspection and open Resection.

Discontinued or incomplete procedures

B3.3. If the intended procedure is discontinued or otherwise not completed, code the procedure to the root operation performed. If a procedure is discontinued before any other root operation is performed, code the root operation Inspection of the body part or anatomical region inspected.

Example:
A planned aortic valve replacement procedure is discontinued after the initial thoracotomy and before any incision is made in the heart muscle, when the patient becomes hemodynamically unstable. This procedure is coded as an open Inspection of the mediastinum.

Biopsy procedures

B3.4a. Biopsy procedures are coded using the root operations Excision, Extraction, or Drainage and the qualifier Diagnostic.

Examples:
Fine needle aspiration biopsy of fluid in the lung is coded to the root operation Drainage with the qualifier Diagnostic.

Biopsy of bone marrow is coded to the root operation Extraction with the qualifier Diagnostic.

Lymph node sampling for biopsy is coded to the root operation Excision with the qualifier Diagnostic.

Biopsy followed by more definitive treatment

B3.4b. If a diagnostic Excision, Extraction, or Drainage procedure (biopsy) is followed by a more definitive procedure, such as Destruction, Excision or Resection at the same procedure site, both the biopsy and the more definitive treatment are coded.

Example:
Biopsy of breast followed by partial mastectomy at the same procedure site, both the biopsy and the partial mastectomy procedure are coded.

Overlapping body layers

B3.5. If root operations such as Excision, Extraction, Repair or Inspection are performed on overlapping layers of the musculoskeletal system, the body part specifying the deepest layer is coded.

Example:
Excisional debridement that includes skin and subcutaneous tissue and muscle is coded to the muscle body part.

Bypass procedures

B3.6a. Bypass procedures are coded by identifying the body part bypassed "from" and the body part bypassed "to." The fourth character body part specifies the body part bypassed from, and the qualifier specifies the body part bypassed to.

Example:
Bypass from stomach to jejunum, stomach is the body part and jejunum is the qualifier.

B3.6b. Coronary artery bypass procedures are coded differently than other bypass procedures as described in the previous guideline. Rather than identifying the body part bypassed from, the body part identifies the number of coronary arteries bypassed to, and the qualifier specifies the vessel bypassed from.

Example:
Aortocoronary artery bypass of the left anterior descending coronary artery and the obtuse marginal coronary artery is classified in the body part axis of classification as two coronary arteries, and the qualifier specifies the aorta as the body part bypassed from.

B3.6c. If multiple coronary arteries are bypassed, a separate procedure is coded for each coronary artery that uses a different device and/or qualifier.

Example:
Aortocoronary artery bypass and internal mammary coronary artery bypass are coded separately.

Control vs. more definitive root operations

B3.7. The root operation Control is defined as, "Stopping, or attempting to stop, postprocedural or other acute bleeding." If an attempt to stop postprocedural or other acute bleeding is unsuccessful, and to stop the bleeding requires performing a more definitive root operation, such as Bypass, Detachment, Excision, Extraction, Reposition, Replacement, or Resection, then the more definitive root operation is coded instead of Control.

Example:
Resection of spleen to stop bleeding is coded to Resection instead of Control.

Excision vs. Resection

B3.8. PCS contains specific body parts for anatomical subdivisions of a body part, such as lobes of the lungs or liver and regions of the intestine. Resection of the specific body part is coded whenever all of the body part is cut out or off, rather than coding Excision of a less specific body part.

Example:
Left upper lung lobectomy is coded to Resection of Upper Lung Lobe, Left rather than Excision of Lung, Left.

Excision for graft

B3.9. If an autograft is obtained from a different procedure site in order to complete the objective of the procedure, a separate procedure is coded, except when the seventh character qualifier value in the ICD-10-PCS table fully specifies the site from which the autograft was obtained.

Examples:
Coronary bypass with excision of saphenous vein graft, excision of saphenous vein is coded separately.

Replacement of breast with autologous deep inferior epigastric artery perforator (DIEP) flap, excision of the DIEP flap is not coded separately. The seventh character qualifier value Deep Inferior Epigastric Artery Perforator Flap in the Replacement table fully specifies the site of the autograft harvest.

Fusion procedures of the spine

B3.10a. The body part coded for a spinal vertebral joint(s) rendered immobile by a spinal fusion procedure is classified by the level of the spine (e.g. thoracic). There are distinct body part values for a single vertebral joint and for multiple vertebral joints at each spinal level.

Example:
Body part values specify Lumbar Vertebral Joint, Lumbar Vertebral Joints, 2 or More and Lumbosacral Vertebral Joint.

B3.10b. If multiple vertebral joints are fused, a separate procedure is coded for each vertebral joint that uses a different device and/or qualifier.

Example:
Fusion of lumbar vertebral joint, posterior approach, anterior column and fusion of lumbar vertebral joint, posterior approach, posterior column are coded separately.

B3.10c. Combinations of devices and materials are often used on a vertebral joint to render the joint immobile. When combinations of devices are used on the same vertebral joint, the device value coded for the procedure is as follows:

- If an interbody fusion device is used to render the joint immobile **(containing bone graft or bone graft substitute)**, the procedure is coded with the device value Interbody Fusion Device
- If bone graft is the *only* device used to render the joint immobile, the procedure is coded with the device value Nonautologous Tissue Substitute or Autologous Tissue Substitute
- If a mixture of autologous and nonautologous bone graft (with or without biological or synthetic extenders or binders) is used to render the joint immobile, code the procedure with the device value Autologous Tissue Substitute

Examples:
Fusion of a vertebral joint using a cage style interbody fusion device containing morsellized bone graft is coded to the device Interbody Fusion Device.

Fusion of a vertebral joint using a bone dowel interbody fusion device made of cadaver bone and packed with a mixture of local morsellized bone and demineralized bone matrix is coded to the device Interbody Fusion Device.

Fusion of a vertebral joint using both autologous bone graft and bone bank bone graft is coded to the device Autologous Tissue Substitute.

Inspection procedures

B3.11a. Inspection of a body part(s) performed in order to achieve the objective of a procedure is not coded separately.

Example:
Fiberoptic bronchoscopy performed for irrigation of bronchus, only the irrigation procedure is coded.

B3.11b. If multiple tubular body parts are inspected, the most distal body part (the body part furthest from the starting point of the inspection) is coded. If multiple non-tubular body parts in a region are inspected, the body part that specifies the entire area inspected is coded.

Examples:
Cystoureteroscopy with inspection of bladder and ureters is coded to the ureter body part value.

Exploratory laparotomy with general inspection of abdominal contents is coded to the peritoneal cavity body part value.

B3.11c. When both an Inspection procedure and another procedure are performed on the same body part during the same episode, if the Inspection procedure is performed using a different approach than the other procedure, the Inspection procedure is coded separately.

Example:
Endoscopic Inspection of the duodenum is coded separately when open Excision of the duodenum is performed during the same procedural episode.

Occlusion vs. Restriction for vessel embolization procedures

B3.12. If the objective of an embolization procedure is to completely close a vessel, the root operation Occlusion is coded. If the objective of an embolization procedure is to narrow the lumen of a vessel, the root operation Restriction is coded.

Examples:
Tumor embolization is coded to the root operation Occlusion, because the objective of the procedure is to cut off the blood supply to the vessel.

Embolization of a cerebral aneurysm is coded to the root operation Restriction, because the objective of the procedure is not to close off the vessel entirely, but to narrow the lumen of the vessel at the site of the aneurysm where it is abnormally wide.

Release procedures

B3.13. In the root operation Release, the body part value coded is the body part being freed and not the tissue being manipulated or cut to free the body part.

Example:
Lysis of intestinal adhesions is coded to the specific intestine body part value.

Release vs. Division

B3.14. If the sole objective of the procedure is freeing a body part without cutting the body part, the root operation is Release. If the sole objective of the procedure is separating or transecting a body part, the root operation is Division.

Examples:
Freeing a nerve root from surrounding scar tissue to relieve pain is coded to the root operation Release.

Severing a nerve root to relieve pain is coded to the root operation Division.

Reposition for fracture treatment

B3.15. Reduction of a displaced fracture is coded to the root operation Reposition and the application of a cast or splint in conjunction with the Reposition procedure is not coded separately. Treatment of a nondisplaced fracture is coded to the procedure performed.

Examples:
Casting of a nondisplaced fracture is coded to the root operation Immobilization in the Placement section.

Putting a pin in a nondisplaced fracture is coded to the root operation Insertion.

Transplantation vs. Administration

B3.16. Putting in a mature and functioning living body part taken from another individual or animal is coded to the root operation Transplantation. Putting in autologous or nonautologous cells is coded to the Administration section.

Example:
Putting in autologous or nonautologous bone marrow, pancreatic islet cells or stem cells is coded to the Administration section.

Transfer procedures using multiple tissue layers

B3.17. The root operation Transfer contains qualifiers that can be used to specify when a transfer flap is composed of more than one tissue layer, such as a musculocutaneous flap. For procedures involving transfer of multiple tissue layers including skin, subcutaneous tissue, fascia or muscle, the procedure is coded to the body part value that describes the deepest tissue layer in the flap, and the qualifier can be used to describe the other tissue layer(s) in the transfer flap.

Example:
A musculocutaneous flap transfer is coded to the appropriate body part value in the body system Muscles, and the qualifier is used to describe the additional tissue layer(s) in the transfer flap.

Excision/Resection followed by replacement

B3.18. If an excision or resection of a body part is followed by a replacement procedure, code both procedures to identify each distinct objective, except when the excision or resection is considered integral and preparatory for the replacement procedure.

Examples:
Mastectomy followed by reconstruction, both resection and replacement of the breast are coded to fully capture the distinct objectives of the procedures performed.

Maxillectomy with obturator reconstruction, both excision and replacement of the maxilla are coded to fully capture the distinct objectives of the procedures performed.

Excisional debridement of tendon with skin graft, both the excision of the tendon and the replacement of the skin with a graft are coded to fully capture the distinct objectives of the procedures performed.

Esophagectomy followed by reconstruction with colonic interposition, both the resection and the transfer of the large intestine to function as the esophagus are coded to fully capture the distinct objectives of the procedures performed.

Examples:
Resection of a joint as part of a joint replacement procedure is considered integral and preparatory for the replacement of the joint and the resection is not coded separately.

Resection of a valve as part of a valve replacement procedure is considered integral and preparatory for the valve replacement and the resection is not coded separately.

B4. Body Part

General guidelines

B4.1a. If a procedure is performed on a portion of a body part that does not have a separate body part value, code the body part value corresponding to the whole body part.

Example:

A procedure performed on the alveolar process of the mandible is coded to the mandible body part.

B4.1b. If the prefix "peri" is combined with a body part to identify the site of the procedure, and the site of the procedure is not further specified, then the procedure is coded to the body part named. This guideline applies only when a more specific body part value is not available.

Examples:

A procedure site identified as perirenal is coded to the kidney body part when the site of the procedure is not further specified.

A procedure site described in the documentation as peri-urethral, and the documentation also indicates that it is the vulvar tissue and not the urethral tissue that is the site of the procedure, then the procedure is coded to the vulva body part.

A procedure site documented as involving the periosteum is coded to the corresponding bone body part.

B4.1c. If a procedure is performed on a continuous section of a tubular body part, code the body part value corresponding to the furthest anatomical site from the point of entry.

Example:

A procedure performed on a continuous section of artery from the femoral artery to the external iliac artery with the point of entry at the femoral artery is coded to the external iliac body part.

Branches of body parts

B4.2. Where a specific branch of a body part does not have its own body part value in PCS, the body part is typically coded to the closest proximal branch that has a specific body part value. In the cardiovascular body systems, if a general body part is available in the correct root operation table, and coding to a proximal branch would require assigning a code in a different body system, the procedure is coded using the general body part value.

Examples:

A procedure performed on the mandibular branch of the trigeminal nerve is coded to the trigeminal nerve body part value.

Occlusion of the bronchial artery is coded to the body part value Upper Artery in the body system Upper Arteries, and not to the body part value Thoracic Aorta, Descending in the body system Heart and Great Vessels.

Bilateral body part values

B4.3. Bilateral body part values are available for a limited number of body parts. If the identical procedure is performed on contralateral body parts, and a bilateral body part value exists for that body part, a single procedure is coded using the bilateral body part value. If no bilateral body part value exists, each procedure is coded separately using the appropriate body part value.

Examples:

The identical procedure performed on both fallopian tubes is coded once using the body part value Fallopian Tube, Bilateral.

The identical procedure performed on both knee joints is coded twice using the body part values Knee Joint, Right and Knee Joint, Left.

Coronary arteries

B4.4. The coronary arteries are classified as a single body part that is further specified by number of arteries treated. One procedure code specifying multiple arteries is used when the same procedure is performed, including the same device and qualifier values.

Examples:

Angioplasty of two distinct coronary arteries with placement of two stents is coded as Dilation of Coronary Artery, Two Arteries with Two Intraluminal Devices.

Angioplasty of two distinct coronary arteries, one with stent placed and one without, is coded separately as Dilation of Coronary Artery, One Artery with Intraluminal Device, and Dilation of Coronary Artery, One Artery with no device.

Tendons, ligaments, bursae and fascia near a joint

B4.5. Procedures performed on tendons, ligaments, bursae and fascia supporting a joint are coded to the body part in the respective body system that is the focus of the procedure. Procedures performed on joint structures themselves are coded to the body part in the joint body systems.

Examples:

Repair of the anterior cruciate ligament of the knee is coded to the knee bursa and ligament body part in the bursae and ligaments body system.

Knee arthroscopy with shaving of articular cartilage is coded to the knee joint body part in the Lower Joints body system.

Skin, subcutaneous tissue and fascia overlying a joint

B4.6. If a procedure is performed on the skin, subcutaneous tissue or fascia overlying a joint, the procedure is coded to the following body part:

- Shoulder is coded to Upper Arm
- Elbow is coded to Lower Arm
- Wrist is coded to Lower Arm
- Hip is coded to Upper Leg
- Knee is coded to Lower Leg
- Ankle is coded to Foot

Fingers and toes

B4.7. If a body system does not contain a separate body part value for fingers, procedures performed on the fingers are coded to the body part value for the hand. If a body system does not contain a separate body part value for toes, procedures performed on the toes are coded to the body part value for the foot.

Example:

Excision of finger muscle is coded to one of the hand muscle body part values in the Muscles body system.

Upper and lower intestinal tract

B4.8. In the Gastrointestinal body system, the general body part values Upper Intestinal Tract and Lower Intestinal Tract are provided as an option for the root operations Change, Inspection, Removal and Revision. Upper Intestinal Tract includes the portion of the gastrointestinal tract from the esophagus down to and including the duodenum, and Lower Intestinal Tract includes the portion of the gastrointestinal tract from the jejunum down to and including the rectum and anus.

Example:
In the root operation Change table, change of a device in the jejunum is coded using the body part Lower Intestinal Tract.

B5. Approach

Open approach with percutaneous endoscopic assistance

B5.2a. Procedures performed using the open approach with percutaneous endoscopic assistance are coded to the approach Open.

Example:
Laparoscopic-assisted sigmoidectomy is coded to the approach Open.

Percutaneous endoscopic approach with extension of incision

B5.2b. Procedures performed using the percutaneous endoscopic approach, with incision or extension of an incision to assist in the removal of all or a portion of a body part or to anastomose a tubular body part to complete the procedure, are coded to the approach value Percutaneous Endoscopic.

Examples:
Laparoscopic sigmoid colectomy with extension of stapling port for removal of specimen and direct anastomosis is coded to the approach value percutaneous endoscopic.

Laparoscopic nephrectomy with midline incision for removing the resected kidney is coded to the approach value percutaneous endoscopic.

Robotic-assisted laparoscopic prostatectomy with extension of incision for removal of the resected prostate is coded to the approach value percutaneous endoscopic.

External approach

B5.3a. Procedures performed within an orifice on structures that are visible without the aid of any instrumentation are coded to the approach External.

Example:
Resection of tonsils is coded to the approach External.

B5.3b. Procedures performed indirectly by the application of external force through the intervening body layers are coded to the approach External.

Example:
Closed reduction of fracture is coded to the approach External.

Percutaneous procedure via device

B5.4. Procedures performed percutaneously via a device placed for the procedure are coded to the approach Percutaneous.

Example:
Fragmentation of kidney stone performed via percutaneous nephrostomy is coded to the approach Percutaneous.

B6. Device

General guidelines

B6.1a. A device is coded only if a device remains after the procedure is completed. If no device remains, the device value No Device is coded. In limited root operations, the classification provides the qualifier values Temporary and Intraoperative, for specific procedures involving clinically significant devices, where the purpose of the device is to be utilized for a brief duration during the procedure or current inpatient stay. If a device that is intended to remain after the procedure is completed requires removal before the end of the operative episode in which it was inserted (for example, the device size is inadequate or a complication occurs), both the insertion and removal of the device should be coded.

B6.1b. Materials such as sutures, ligatures, radiological markers and temporary post-operative wound drains are considered integral to the performance of a procedure and are not coded as devices.

B6.1c. Procedures performed on a device only and not on a body part are specified in the root operations Change, Irrigation, Removal and Revision, and are coded to the procedure performed.

Example:
Irrigation of percutaneous nephrostomy tube is coded to the root operation Irrigation of indwelling device in the Administration section.

Drainage device

B6.2. A separate procedure to put in a drainage device is coded to the root operation Drainage with the device value Drainage Device.

Obstetric Section Guidelines (section 1)

C. Obstetrics Section

Products of conception

C1. Procedures performed on the products of conception are coded to the Obstetrics section. Procedures performed on the pregnant female other than the products of conception are coded to the appropriate root operation in the Medical and Surgical section.

Examples:
Amniocentesis is coded to the products of conception body part in the Obstetrics section.

Repair of obstetric urethral laceration is coded to the urethra body part in the Medical and Surgical section.

Procedures following delivery or abortion

C2. Procedures performed following a delivery or abortion for curettage of the endometrium or evacuation of retained products of conception are all coded in the Obstetrics section, to the root operation Extraction and the body part Products of Conception, Retained.

Diagnostic or therapeutic dilation and curettage performed during times other than the postpartum or post-abortion period are all coded in the Medical and Surgical section, to the root operation Extraction and the body part Endometrium.

Radiation Therapy Section Guidelines (section D)

D. Radiation Therapy Section

Brachytherapy

D1.a. Brachytherapy is coded to the modality Brachytherapy in the Radiation Therapy section. When a radioactive brachytherapy source is left in the body at the end of the procedure, it is coded separately to the root operation Insertion with the device value Radioactive Element.

Example:
Brachytherapy with implantation of a low dose rate brachytherapy source left in the body at the end of the procedure is coded to the applicable treatment site in section D, Radiation Therapy, with the modality Brachytherapy, the modality qualifier value Low Dose Rate, and the applicable isotope value and qualifier value. The implantation of the brachytherapy source is coded separately to the device value Radioactive Element in the appropriate Insertion

table of the Medical and Surgical section. The Radiation Therapy section code identifies the specific modality and isotope of the brachytherapy, and the root operation Insertion code identifies the implantation of the brachytherapy source that remains in the body at the end of the procedure.

Exception:

Implantation of Cesium-131 brachytherapy seeds embedded in a collagen matrix to the treatment site after resection of brain tumor is coded to the root operation Insertion with the device value Radioactive Element, Cesium-131 Collagen Implant. The procedure is coded to the root operation Insertion only, because the device value identifies both the implantation of the radioactive element and a specific brachytherapy isotope that is not included in the Radiation Therapy section tables.

D1.b. A separate procedure to place a temporary applicator for delivering the brachytherapy is coded to the root operation Insertion and the device value Other Device.

Examples:

Intrauterine brachytherapy applicator placed as a separate procedure from the brachytherapy procedure is coded to Insertion of Other Device, and the brachytherapy is coded separately using the modality Brachytherapy in the Radiation Therapy section.

Intrauterine brachytherapy applicator placed concomitantly with delivery of the brachytherapy dose is coded with a single code using the modality Brachytherapy in the Radiation Therapy section.

New Technology Section Guidelines (section X)

E. New Technology Section

General guidelines

E1.a. Section X codes fully represent the specific procedure described in the code title, and do not require additional codes from other sections of ICD-10-PCS. When section X contains a code title which fully describes a specific new technology procedure, and it is the only procedure performed, only the section X code is reported for the procedure. There is no need to report an additional code in another section of ICD-10-PCS.

Example:

XWØ4321 Introduction of Ceftazidime-Avibactam Anti-infective into Central Vein, Percutaneous Approach, New Technology Group 1, can be coded to indicate that Ceftazidime-Avibactam Anti-infective was administered via a central vein. A separate code from table 3EØ in the Administration section of ICD-10-PCS is not coded in addition to this code.

E1.b. When multiple procedures are performed, New Technology section X codes are coded following the multiple procedures guideline.

Examples:

Dual filter cerebral embolic filtration used during transcatheter aortic valve replacement (TAVR), X2A5312 Cerebral Embolic Filtration, Dual Filter in Innominate Artery and Left Common Carotid Artery, Percutaneous Approach, New Technology Group 2, is coded for the cerebral embolic filtration, along with an ICD-10-PCS code for the TAVR procedure.

Magnetically controlled growth rod (MCGR) placed during a spinal fusion procedure, a code from table XNS, Reposition of the Bones is coded for the MCGR, along with an ICD-10-PCS code for the spinal fusion procedure.

F. Selection of Principal Procedure

The following instructions should be applied in the selection of principal procedure and clarification on the importance of the relation to the principal diagnosis when more than one procedure is performed:

1. Procedure performed for definitive treatment of both principal diagnosis and secondary diagnosis
   a. Sequence procedure performed for definitive treatment most related to principal diagnosis as principal procedure.
2. Procedure performed for definitive treatment and diagnostic procedures performed for both principal diagnosis and secondary diagnosis.
   a. Sequence procedure performed for definitive treatment most related to principal diagnosis as principal procedure
3. A diagnostic procedure was performed for the principal diagnosis and a procedure is performed for definitive treatment of a secondary diagnosis.
   a. Sequence diagnostic procedure as principal procedure, since the procedure most related to the principal diagnosis takes precedence.
4. No procedures performed that are related to principal diagnosis; procedures performed for definitive treatment and diagnostic procedures were performed for secondary diagnosis
   a. Sequence procedure performed for definitive treatment of secondary diagnosis as principal procedure, since there are no procedures (definitive or nondefinitive treatment) related to principal diagnosis.

3f (Aortic) Bioprosthesis valve *use* Zooplastic Tissue in Heart and Great Vessels

Abdominal aortic plexus *use* Abdominal Sympathetic Nerve
Abdominal esophagus *use* Esophagus, Lower
Abdominohysterectomy *see* Resection, Uterus ØUT9
Abdominoplasty
- *see* Alteration, Abdominal Wall ØWØF
- *see* Repair, Abdominal Wall ØWQF
- *see* Supplement, Abdominal Wall ØWUF

Abductor hallucis muscle
- *use* Foot Muscle, Left
- *use* Foot Muscle, Right

AbioCor® Total Replacement Heart *use* Synthetic Substitute
Ablation
- *see* Control bleeding in
- *see* Destruction

Abortion
- Abortifacient 1ØAØ7ZX
- Laminaria 1ØAØ7ZW
- Products of Conception 1ØAØ
- Vacuum 1ØAØ7Z6

Abrasion *see* Extraction
Absolute Pro Vascular (OTW) Self-Expanding Stent System *use* Intraluminal Device
Accelerate PhenoTest™ BC XXE5XN6
Accessory cephalic vein
- *use* Cephalic Vein, Left
- *use* Cephalic Vein, Right

Accessory obturator nerve *use* Lumbar Plexus
Accessory phrenic nerve *use* Phrenic Nerve
Accessory spleen *use* Spleen
Acculink (RX) Carotid Stent System *use* Intraluminal Device
Acellular Hydrated Dermis *use* Nonautologous Tissue Substitute
Acetabular cup *use* Liner in Lower Joints
Acetabulectomy
- *see* Excision, Lower Bones ØQB
- *see* Resection, Lower Bones ØQT

Acetabulofemoral joint
- *use* Hip Joint, Left
- *use* Hip Joint, Right

Acetabuloplasty
- *see* Repair, Lower Bones ØQQ
- *see* Replacement, Lower Bones ØQR
- *see* Supplement, Lower Bones ØQU

Achilles tendon
- *use* Lower Leg Tendon, Left
- *use* Lower Leg Tendon, Right

Achillorrhaphy *see* Repair, Tendons ØLQ
Achillotenotomy, achillotomy
- *see* Division, Tendons ØL8
- *see* Drainage, Tendons ØL9

Acoustic Pulse Thrombolysis *see* Fragmentation, Artery
Acromioclavicular ligament
- *use* Shoulder Bursa and Ligament, Left
- *use* Shoulder Bursa and Ligament, Right

Acromion (process)
- *use* Scapula, Left
- *use* Scapula, Right

Acromionectomy
- *see* Excision, Upper Joints ØRB
- *see* Resection, Upper Joints ØRT

Acromioplasty
- *see* Repair, Upper Joints ØRQ
- *see* Replacement, Upper Joints ØRR
- *see* Supplement, Upper Joints ØRU

Activa PC neurostimulator *use* Stimulator Generator, Multiple Array in ØJH
Activa RC neurostimulator *use* Stimulator Generator, Multiple Array Rechargeable in ØJH
Activa SC neurostimulator *use* Stimulator Generator, Single Array in ØJH
Activities of Daily Living Assessment FØ2
Activities of Daily Living Treatment FØ8
ACUITY™ Steerable Lead
- *use* Cardiac Lead, Defibrillator in Ø2H
- *use* Cardiac Lead, Pacemaker in Ø2H

Acupuncture
- Breast
  - Anesthesia 8EØH3ØØ
  - No Qualifier 8EØH3ØZ
- Integumentary System
  - Anesthesia 8EØH3ØØ
  - No Qualifier 8EØH3ØZ

Adductor brevis muscle
- *use* Upper Leg Muscle, Left
- *use* Upper Leg Muscle, Right

Adductor hallucis muscle
- *use* Foot Muscle, Left
- *use* Foot Muscle, Right

Adductor longus muscle
- *use* Upper Leg Muscle, Left
- *use* Upper Leg Muscle, Right

Adductor magnus muscle
- *use* Upper Leg Muscle, Left
- *use* Upper Leg Muscle, Right

Adenohypophysis *use* Pituitary Gland
Adenoidectomy
- *see* Excision, Adenoids ØCBQ
- *see* Resection, Adenoids ØCTQ

Adenoidotomy *see* Drainage, Adenoids ØC9Q
Adhesiolysis *see* Release
Administration
- Blood products *see* Transfusion
- Other substance *see* Introduction of substance in or on

Adrenalectomy
- *see* Excision, Endocrine System ØGB
- *see* Resection, Endocrine System ØGT

Adrenalorrhaphy *see* Repair, Endocrine System ØGQ
Adrenalotomy *see* Drainage, Endocrine System ØG9
Advancement
- *see* Reposition
- *see* Transfer

Advisa (MRI) *use* Pacemaker, Dual Chamber in ØJH
AFX® Endovascular AAA System *use* Intraluminal Device
AIGISRx Antibacterial Envelope *use* Anti-Infective Envelope
Alar ligament of axis *use* Head and Neck Bursa and Ligament
Alfieri Stitch Valvuloplasty *see* Restriction, Valve, Mitral Ø2VG
Alimentation *see* Introduction of substance in or on
Alteration
- Abdominal Wall ØWØF
- Ankle Region
  - Left ØYØL
  - Right ØYØK
- Arm
  - Lower
    - Left ØXØF
    - Right ØXØD
  - Upper
    - Left ØXØ9
    - Right ØXØ8
- Axilla
  - Left ØXØ5
  - Right ØXØ4
- Back
  - Lower ØWØL
  - Upper ØWØK
- Breast
  - Bilateral ØHØV
  - Left ØHØU
  - Right ØHØT
- Buttock
  - Left ØYØ1
  - Right ØYØØ
- Chest Wall ØWØ8
- Ear
  - Bilateral Ø9Ø2
  - Left Ø9Ø1
  - Right Ø9ØØ
- Elbow Region
  - Left ØXØC
  - Right ØXØB
- Extremity
  - Lower
    - Left ØYØB
    - Right ØYØ9
  - Upper
    - Left ØXØ7
    - Right ØXØ6
- Eyelid
  - Lower
    - Left Ø8ØR
    - Right Ø8ØQ
  - Upper
    - Left Ø8ØP
    - Right Ø8ØN
- Face ØWØ2
- Head ØWØØ
- Jaw
  - Lower ØWØ5
  - Upper ØWØ4
- Knee Region
  - Left ØYØG
  - Right ØYØF
- Leg
  - Lower
    - Left ØYØJ
    - Right ØYØH
  - Upper
    - Left ØYØD
    - Right ØYØC
- Lip
  - Lower ØCØ1X
  - Upper ØCØØX
- Nasal Mucosa and Soft Tissue Ø9ØK
- Neck ØWØ6
- Perineum
  - Female ØWØN
  - Male ØWØM
- Shoulder Region
  - Left ØXØ3
  - Right ØXØ2
- Subcutaneous Tissue and Fascia
  - Abdomen ØJØ8
  - Back ØJØ7
  - Buttock ØJØ9
  - Chest ØJØ6
  - Face ØJØ1
  - Lower Arm
    - Left ØJØH
    - Right ØJØG
  - Lower Leg
    - Left ØJØP
    - Right ØJØN
  - Neck
    - Left ØJØ5
    - Right ØJØ4
  - Upper Arm
    - Left ØJØF
    - Right ØJØD
  - Upper Leg
    - Left ØJØM
    - Right ØJØL
- Wrist Region
  - Left ØXØH
  - Right ØXØG

Alveolar process of mandible
- *use* Mandible, Left
- *use* Mandible, Right

Alveolar process of maxilla *use* Maxilla
Alveolectomy
- *see* Excision, Head and Facial Bones ØNB
- *see* Resection, Head and Facial Bones ØNT

Alveoloplasty
- *see* Repair, Head and Facial Bones ØNQ
- *see* Replacement, Head and Facial Bones ØNR
- *see* Supplement, Head and Facial Bones ØNU

Alveolotomy
- *see* Division, Head and Facial Bones ØN8
- *see* Drainage, Head and Facial Bones ØN9

Ambulatory cardiac monitoring 4A12X45
Amniocentesis *see* Drainage, Products of Conception 1Ø9Ø
Amnioinfusion *see* Introduction of substance in or on, Products of Conception 3EØE
Amnioscopy 1ØJØ8ZZ
Amniotomy *see* Drainage, Products of Conception 1Ø9Ø
AMPLATZER® Muscular VSD Occluder *use* Synthetic Substitute
Amputation *see* Detachment
AMS 8ØØ® Urinary Control System *use* Artificial Sphincter in Urinary System
Anal orifice *use* Anus

Analog radiography *see* Plain Radiography
Analog radiology *see* Plain Radiography
Anastomosis *see* Bypass
Anatomical snuffbox
use Lower Arm and Wrist Muscle, Left
use Lower Arm and Wrist Muscle, Right
Andexanet Alfa, Factor Xa Inhibitor Reversal Agent
use Coagulation Factor Xa, Inactivated
Andexxa *use* Coagulation Factor Xa, Inactivated
AneuRx® AAA Advantage® *use* Intraluminal Device
Angiectomy
see Excision, Heart and Great Vessels Ø2B
see Excision, Lower Arteries Ø4B
see Excision, Lower Veins Ø6B
see Excision, Upper Arteries Ø3B
see Excision, Upper Veins Ø5B
Angiocardiography
Combined right and left heart *see* Fluoroscopy, Heart, Right and Left B216
Left Heart *see* Fluoroscopy, Heart, Left B215
Right Heart *see* Fluoroscopy, Heart, Right B214
SPY system intravascular fluorescence *see* Monitoring, Physiological Systems 4A1
Angiography
see Fluoroscopy, Heart B21
see Plain Radiography, Heart B2Ø
Angioplasty
see Dilation, Heart and Great Vessels Ø27
see Dilation, Lower Arteries Ø47
see Dilation, Upper Arteries Ø37
see Repair, Heart and Great Vessels Ø2Q
see Repair, Lower Arteries Ø4Q
see Repair, Upper Arteries Ø3Q
see Replacement, Heart and Great Vessels Ø2R
see Replacement, Lower Arteries Ø4R
see Replacement, Upper Arteries Ø3R
see Supplement, Heart and Great Vessels Ø2U
see Supplement, Lower Arteries Ø4U
see Supplement, Upper Arteries Ø3U
Angiorrhaphy
see Repair, Heart and Great Vessels Ø2Q
see Repair, Lower Arteries Ø4Q
see Repair, Upper Arteries Ø3Q
Angioscopy Ø2JY4ZZ, Ø3JY4ZZ, Ø4JY4ZZ
Angiotensin II *use* Synthetic Human Angiotensin II
Angiotripsy
see Occlusion, Lower Arteries Ø4L
see Occlusion, Upper Arteries Ø3L
Angular artery *use* Face Artery
Angular vein
use Face Vein, Left
use Face Vein, Right
Annular ligament
use Elbow Bursa and Ligament, Left
use Elbow Bursa and Ligament, Right
Annuloplasty
see Repair, Heart and Great Vessels Ø2Q
see Supplement, Heart and Great Vessels Ø2U
Annuloplasty ring *use* Synthetic Substitute
Anoplasty
see Repair, Anus ØDQQ
see Supplement, Anus ØDUQ
Anorectal junction *use* Rectum
Anoscopy ØDJD8ZZ
Ansa cervicalis *use* Cervical Plexus
Antabuse therapy HZ93ZZZ
Antebrachial fascia
use Subcutaneous Tissue and Fascia, Left Lower Arm
use Subcutaneous Tissue and Fascia, Right Lower Arm
Anterior cerebral artery *use* Intracranial Artery
Anterior cerebral vein *use* Intracranial Vein
Anterior choroidal artery *use* Intracranial Artery
Anterior circumflex humeral artery
use Axillary Artery, Left
use Axillary Artery, Right
Anterior communicating artery *use* Intracranial Artery
Anterior cruciate ligament (ACL)
use Knee Bursa and Ligament, Left
use Knee Bursa and Ligament, Right
Anterior crural nerve *use* Femoral Nerve
Anterior facial vein
use Face Vein, Left
use Face Vein, Right
Anterior intercostal artery
use Internal Mammary Artery, Left
use Internal Mammary Artery, Right
Anterior interosseous nerve *use* Median Nerve
Anterior lateral malleolar artery
use Anterior Tibial Artery, Left
use Anterior Tibial Artery, Right
Anterior lingual gland *use* Minor Salivary Gland
Anterior (pectoral) lymph node
use Lymphatic, Left Axillary
use Lymphatic, Right Axillary
Anterior medial malleolar artery
use Anterior Tibial Artery, Left
use Anterior Tibial Artery, Right
Anterior spinal artery
use Vertebral Artery, Left
use Vertebral Artery, Right
Anterior tibial recurrent artery
use Anterior Tibial Artery, Left
use Anterior Tibial Artery, Right
Anterior ulnar recurrent artery
use Ulnar Artery, Left
use Ulnar Artery, Right
Anterior vagal trunk *use* Vagus Nerve
Anterior vertebral muscle
use Neck Muscle, Left
use Neck Muscle, Right
Antibacterial Envelope (TYRX) (AIGISRx) *use* Anti-Infective Envelope
Antigen-free air conditioning *see* Atmospheric Control, Physiological Systems 6AØ
Antihelix
use External Ear, Bilateral
use External Ear, Left
use External Ear, Right
Antimicrobial envelope *use* Anti-Infective Envelope
Antitragus
use External Ear, Bilateral
use External Ear, Left
use External Ear, Right
Antrostomy *see* Drainage, Ear, Nose, Sinus Ø99
Antrotomy *see* Drainage, Ear, Nose, Sinus Ø99
Antrum of Highmore
use Maxillary Sinus, Left
use Maxillary Sinus, Right
Aortic annulus *use* Aortic Valve
Aortic arch *use* Thoracic Aorta, Ascending/Arch
Aortic intercostal artery *use* Upper Artery
Aortography
see Fluoroscopy, Lower Arteries B41
see Fluoroscopy, Upper Arteries B31
see Plain Radiography, Lower Arteries B4Ø
see Plain Radiography, Upper Arteries B3Ø
Aortoplasty
see Repair, Aorta, Abdominal Ø4QØ
see Repair, Aorta, Thoracic, Ascending/Arch Ø2QX
see Repair, Aorta, Thoracic, Descending Ø2QW
see Replacement, Aorta, Abdominal Ø4RØ
see Replacement, Aorta, Thoracic, Ascending/Arch Ø2RX
see Replacement, Aorta, Thoracic, Descending Ø2RW
see Supplement, Aorta, Abdominal Ø4UØ
see Supplement, Aorta, Thoracic, Ascending/Arch Ø2UX
see Supplement, Aorta, Thoracic, Descending Ø2UW
Apalutamide Antineoplastic XWØDXJ5
Apical (subclavicular) lymph node
use Lymphatic, Left Axillary
use Lymphatic, Right Axillary
Apneustic center *use* Pons
Appendectomy
see Excision, Appendix ØDBJ
see Resection, Appendix ØDTJ
Appendicolysis *see* Release, Appendix ØDNJ
Appendicotomy *see* Drainage, Appendix ØD9J
Application *see* Introduction of substance in or on
Aquablation therapy, prostate XV5Ø8A4
Aquapheresis 6A55ØZ3
Aqueduct of Sylvius *use* Cerebral Ventricle
Aqueous humour
use Anterior Chamber, Left
use Anterior Chamber, Right
Arachnoid mater, intracranial *use* Cerebral Meninges
Arachnoid mater, spinal *use* Spinal Meninges
Arcuate artery
use Foot Artery, Left
use Foot Artery, Right
Areola
use Nipple, Left
use Nipple, Right
AROM (artificial rupture of membranes) 1Ø9Ø7ZC
Arterial canal (duct) *use* Pulmonary Artery, Left
Arterial pulse tracing *see* Measurement, Arterial 4AØ3
Arteriectomy
see Excision, Heart and Great Vessels Ø2B
see Excision, Lower Arteries Ø4B
see Excision, Upper Arteries Ø3B
Arteriography
see Fluoroscopy, Heart B21
see Fluoroscopy, Lower Arteries B41
see Fluoroscopy, Upper Arteries B31
see Plain Radiography, Heart B2Ø
see Plain Radiography, Lower Arteries B4Ø
see Plain Radiography, Upper Arteries B3Ø
Arterioplasty
see Repair, Heart and Great Vessels Ø2Q
see Repair, Lower Arteries Ø4Q
see Repair, Upper Arteries Ø3Q
see Replacement, Heart and Great Vessels Ø2R
see Replacement, Lower Arteries Ø4R
see Replacement, Upper Arteries Ø3R
see Supplement, Heart and Great Vessels Ø2U
see Supplement, Lower Arteries Ø4U
see Supplement, Upper Arteries Ø3U
Arteriorrhaphy
see Repair, Heart and Great Vessels Ø2Q
see Repair, Lower Arteries Ø4Q
see Repair, Upper Arteries Ø3Q
Arterioscopy
see Inspection, Artery, Lower Ø4JY
see Inspection, Artery, Upper Ø3JY
see Inspection, Great Vessel Ø2JY
Arthrectomy
see Excision, Lower Joints ØSB
see Excision, Upper Joints ØRB
see Resection, Lower Joints ØST
see Resection, Upper Joints ØRT
Arthrocentesis
see Drainage, Lower Joints ØS9
see Drainage, Upper Joints ØR9
Arthrodesis
see Fusion, Lower Joints ØSG
see Fusion, Upper Joints ØRG
Arthrography
see Plain Radiography, Non-Axial Lower Bones BQØ
see Plain Radiography, Non-Axial Upper Bones BPØ
see Plain Radiography, Skull and Facial Bones BNØ
Arthrolysis
see Release, Lower Joints ØSN
see Release, Upper Joints ØRN
Arthropexy
see Repair, Lower Joints ØSQ
see Repair, Upper Joints ØRQ
see Reposition, Lower Joints ØSS
see Reposition, Upper Joints ØRS
Arthroplasty
see Repair, Lower Joints ØSQ
see Repair, Upper Joints ØRQ
see Replacement, Lower Joints ØSR
see Replacement, Upper Joints ØRR
see Supplement, Lower Joints ØSU
see Supplement, Upper Joints ØRU
Arthroplasty, radial head
see Replacement, Radius, Left ØPRJ
see Replacement, Radius, Right ØPRH
Arthroscopy
see Inspection, Lower Joints ØSJ
see Inspection, Upper Joints ØRJ
Arthrotomy
see Drainage, Lower Joints ØS9
see Drainage, Upper Joints ØR9
Articulating Spacer (Antibiotic) *use* Articulating Spacer in Lower Joints
Artificial anal sphincter (AAS) *use* Artificial Sphincter in Gastrointestinal System
Artificial bowel sphincter (neosphincter) *use* Artificial Sphincter in Gastrointestinal System
Artificial Sphincter
Insertion of device in
Anus ØDHQ

Subterms under main terms may continue to next column or page

Artificial Sphincter — *continued*
Insertion of device in — *continued*
Bladder ØTHB
Bladder Neck ØTHC
Urethra ØTHD
Removal of device from
Anus ØDPQ
Bladder ØTPB
Urethra ØTPD
Revision of device in
Anus ØDWQ
Bladder ØTWB
Urethra ØTWD
Artificial urinary sphincter (AUS) *use* Artificial Sphincter in Urinary System
Aryepiglottic fold *use* Larynx
Arytenoid cartilage *use* Larynx
Arytenoid muscle
use Neck Muscle, Left
use Neck Muscle, Right
Arytenoidectomy *see* Excision, Larynx ØCBS
Arytenoidopexy *see* Repair, Larynx ØCQS
Ascenda Intrathecal Catheter *use* Infusion Device
Ascending aorta *use* Thoracic Aorta, Ascending/Arch
Ascending palatine artery *use* Face Artery
Ascending pharyngeal artery
use External Carotid Artery, Left
use External Carotid Artery, Right
Aspiration, fine needle
Fluid or gas *see* Drainage
Tissue biopsy
see Excision
see Extraction
Assessment
Activities of daily living *see* Activities of Daily Living Assessment, Rehabilitation FØ2
Hearing *see* Hearing Assessment, Diagnostic Audiology F13
Hearing aid *see* Hearing Aid Assessment, Diagnostic Audiology F14
Intravascular perfusion, using indocyanine green (ICG) dye *see* Monitoring, Physiological Systems 4A1
Motor function *see* Motor Function Assessment, Rehabilitation FØ1
Nerve function *see* Motor Function Assessment, Rehabilitation FØ1
Speech *see* Speech Assessment, Rehabilitation FØØ
Vestibular *see* Vestibular Assessment, Diagnostic Audiology F15
Vocational *see* Activities of Daily Living Treatment, Rehabilitation FØ8
Assistance
Cardiac
Continuous
Balloon Pump 5AØ221Ø
Impeller Pump 5AØ221D
Other Pump 5AØ2216
Pulsatile Compression 5AØ2215
Intermittent
Balloon Pump 5AØ211Ø
Impeller Pump 5AØ211D
Other Pump 5AØ2116
Pulsatile Compression 5AØ2115
Circulatory
Continuous
Hyperbaric 5AØ5221
Supersaturated 5AØ522C
Intermittent
Hyperbaric 5AØ5121
Supersaturated 5AØ512C
Respiratory
24-96 Consecutive Hours
Continuous Negative Airway Pressure 5AØ9459
Continuous Positive Airway Pressure 5AØ9457
High Nasal Flow/Velocity 5AØ945A
Intermittent Negative Airway Pressure 5AØ945B
Intermittent Positive Airway Pressure 5AØ9458
No Qualifier 5AØ945Z
Continuous, Filtration 5AØ92ØZ
Greater than 96 Consecutive Hours
Continuous Negative Airway Pressure 5AØ9559
Assistance — *continued*
Respiratory — *continued*
Greater than 96 Consecutive Hours — *continued*
Continuous Positive Airway Pressure 5AØ9557
High Nasal Flow/Velocity 5AØ955A
Intermittent Negative Airway Pressure 5AØ955B
Intermittent Positive Airway Pressure 5AØ9558
No Qualifier 5AØ955Z
Less than 24 Consecutive Hours
Continuous Negative Airway Pressure 5AØ9359
Continuous Positive Airway Pressure 5AØ9357
High Nasal Flow/Velocity 5AØ935A
Intermittent Negative Airway Pressure 5AØ935B
Intermittent Positive Airway Pressure 5AØ9358
No Qualifier 5AØ935Z
Assurant (Cobalt) stent *use* Intraluminal Device
Atezolizumab Antineoplastic XWØ
Atherectomy
see Extirpation, Heart and Great Vessels Ø2C
see Extirpation, Lower Arteries Ø4C
see Extirpation, Upper Arteries Ø3C
Atlantoaxial joint *use* Cervical Vertebral Joint
Atmospheric Control 6AØZ
AtriClip LAA Exclusion System *use* Extraluminal Device
Atrioseptoplasty
see Repair, Heart and Great Vessels Ø2Q
see Replacement, Heart and Great Vessels Ø2R
see Supplement, Heart and Great Vessels Ø2U
Atrioventricular node *use* Conduction Mechanism
Atrium dextrum cordis *use* Atrium, Right
Atrium pulmonale *use* Atrium, Left
Attain Ability® lead Ø2H
use Cardiac Lead, Defibrillator in Ø2H
use Cardiac Lead, Pacemaker in Ø2H
Attain Starfix® (OTW) lead
use Cardiac Lead, Defibrillator in Ø2H
use Cardiac Lead, Pacemaker in Ø2H
Audiology, diagnostic
see Hearing Aid Assessment, Diagnostic Audiology F14
see Hearing Assessment, Diagnostic Audiology F13
see Vestibular Assessment, Diagnostic Audiology F15
Audiometry *see* Hearing Assessment, Diagnostic Audiology F13
Auditory tube
use Eustachian Tube, Left
use Eustachian Tube, Right
Auerbach's (myenteric) plexus *use* Abdominal Sympathetic Nerve
Auricle
use External Ear, Bilateral
use External Ear, Left
use External Ear, Right
Auricularis muscle *use* Head Muscle
Autograft *use* Autologous Tissue Substitute
Autologous artery graft
use Autologous Arterial Tissue in Heart and Great Vessels
use Autologous Arterial Tissue in Lower Arteries
use Autologous Arterial Tissue in Lower Veins
use Autologous Arterial Tissue in Upper Arteries
use Autologous Arterial Tissue in Upper Veins
Autologous vein graft
use Autologous Venous Tissue in Heart and Great Vessels
use Autologous Venous Tissue in Lower Arteries
use Autologous Venous Tissue in Lower Veins
use Autologous Venous Tissue in Upper Arteries
use Autologous Venous Tissue in Upper Veins
Autotransfusion *see* Transfusion
Autotransplant
Adrenal tissue *see* Reposition, Endocrine System ØGS
Kidney *see* Reposition, Urinary System ØTS
Pancreatic tissue *see* Reposition, Pancreas ØFSG
Autotransplant — *continued*
Parathyroid tissue *see* Reposition, Endocrine System ØGS
Thyroid tissue *see* Reposition, Endocrine System ØGS
Tooth *see* Reattachment, Mouth and Throat ØCM
Avulsion *see* Extraction
Axial Lumbar Interbody Fusion System *use* Interbody Fusion Device in Lower Joints
AxiaLIF® System *use* Interbody Fusion Device in Lower Joints
Axicabtagene Ciloeucel *use* Engineered Autologous Chimeric Antigen Receptor T-cell Immunotherapy
Axillary fascia
use Subcutaneous Tissue and Fascia, Left Upper Arm
use Subcutaneous Tissue and Fascia, Right Upper Arm
Axillary nerve *use* Brachial Plexus
AZEDRA® *use* Iobenguane I-131 Antineoplastic

B

BAK/C® Interbody Cervical Fusion System *use* Interbody Fusion Device in Upper Joints
BAL (bronchial alveolar lavage), diagnostic *see* Drainage, Respiratory System ØB9
Balanoplasty
see Repair, Penis ØVQS
see Supplement, Penis ØVUS
Balloon atrial septostomy (BAS) Ø2163Z7
Balloon Pump
Continuous, Output 5AØ221Ø
Intermittent, Output 5AØ211Ø
Bandage, Elastic *see* Compression
Banding
see Occlusion
see Restriction
Banding, esophageal varices *see* Occlusion, Vein, Esophageal Ø6L3
Banding, laparoscopic (adjustable) gastric
Initial procedure ØDV64CZ
Surgical correction *see* Revision of device in, Stomach ØDW6
Bard® Composix® Kugel® patch *use* Synthetic Substitute
Bard® Composix® (E/X) (LP) mesh *use* Synthetic Substitute
Bard® Dulex™ mesh *use* Synthetic Substitute
Bard® Ventralex™ Hernia Patch *use* Synthetic Substitute
Barium swallow *see* Fluoroscopy, Gastrointestinal System BD1
Baroreflex Activation Therapy® (BAT®)
use Stimulator Generator in Subcutaneous Tissue and Fascia
use Stimulator Lead in Upper Arteries
Barricaid® Annular Closure Device (ACD) *use* Synthetic Substitute
Bartholin's (greater vestibular) gland *use* Vestibular Gland
Basal (internal) cerebral vein *use* Intracranial Vein
Basal metabolic rate (BMR) *see* Measurement, Physiological Systems 4AØZ
Basal nuclei *use* Basal Ganglia
Base of Tongue *use* Pharynx
Basilar artery *use* Intracranial Artery
Basis pontis *use* Pons
Beam Radiation
Abdomen DWØ3
Intraoperative DWØ33ZØ
Adrenal Gland DGØ2
Intraoperative DGØ23ZØ
Bile Ducts DFØ2
Intraoperative DFØ23ZØ
Bladder DTØ2
Intraoperative DTØ23ZØ
Bone
Intraoperative DPØC3ZØ
Other DPØC
Bone Marrow D7ØØ
Intraoperative D7ØØ3ZØ
Brain DØØØ
Intraoperative DØØØ3ZØ
Brain Stem DØØ1
Intraoperative DØØ13ZØ

Beam Radiation — *continued*
Breast
Left DMØØ
Intraoperative DMØØ3ZØ
Right DMØ1
Intraoperative DMØ13ZØ
Bronchus DBØ1
Intraoperative DBØ13ZØ
Cervix DUØ1
Intraoperative DUØ13ZØ
Chest DWØ2
Intraoperative DWØ23ZØ
Chest Wall DBØ7
Intraoperative DBØ73ZØ
Colon DDØ5
Intraoperative DDØ53ZØ
Diaphragm DBØ8
Intraoperative DBØ83ZØ
Duodenum DDØ2
Intraoperative DDØ23ZØ
Ear D9ØØ
Intraoperative D9ØØ3ZØ
Esophagus DDØØ
Intraoperative DDØØ3ZØ
Eye D8ØØ
Intraoperative D8ØØ3ZØ
Femur DPØ9
Intraoperative DPØ93ZØ
Fibula DPØB
Intraoperative DPØB3ZØ
Gallbladder DFØ1
Intraoperative DFØ13ZØ
Gland
Adrenal DGØ2
Intraoperative DGØ23ZØ
Parathyroid DGØ4
Intraoperative DGØ43ZØ
Pituitary DGØØ
Intraoperative DGØØ3ZØ
Thyroid DGØ5
Intraoperative DGØ53ZØ
Glands
Intraoperative D9Ø63ZØ
Salivary D9Ø6
Head and Neck DWØ1
Intraoperative DWØ13ZØ
Hemibody DWØ4
Intraoperative DWØ43ZØ
Humerus DPØ6
Intraoperative DPØ63ZØ
Hypopharynx D9Ø3
Intraoperative D9Ø33ZØ
Ileum DDØ4
Intraoperative DDØ43ZØ
Jejunum DDØ3
Intraoperative DDØ33ZØ
Kidney DTØØ
Intraoperative DTØØ3ZØ
Larynx D9ØB
Intraoperative D9ØB3ZØ
Liver DFØØ
Intraoperative DFØØ3ZØ
Lung DBØ2
Intraoperative DBØ23ZØ
Lymphatics
Abdomen D7Ø6
Intraoperative D7Ø63ZØ
Axillary D7Ø4
Intraoperative D7Ø43ZØ
Inguinal D7Ø8
Intraoperative D7Ø83ZØ
Neck D7Ø3
Intraoperative D7Ø33ZØ
Pelvis D7Ø7
Intraoperative D7Ø73ZØ
Thorax D7Ø5
Intraoperative D7Ø53ZØ
Mandible DPØ3
Intraoperative DPØ33ZØ
Maxilla DPØ2
Intraoperative DPØ23ZØ
Mediastinum DBØ6
Intraoperative DBØ63ZØ
Mouth D9Ø4
Intraoperative D9Ø43ZØ
Nasopharynx D9ØD
Intraoperative D9ØD3ZØ
Neck and Head DWØ1
Intraoperative DWØ13ZØ

Beam Radiation — *continued*
Nerve
Intraoperative DØØ73ZØ
Peripheral DØØ7
Nose D9Ø1
Intraoperative D9Ø13ZØ
Oropharynx D9ØF
Intraoperative D9ØF3ZØ
Ovary DUØØ
Intraoperative DUØØ3ZØ
Palate
Hard D9Ø8
Intraoperative D9Ø83ZØ
Soft D9Ø9
Intraoperative D9Ø93ZØ
Pancreas DFØ3
Intraoperative DFØ33ZØ
Parathyroid Gland DGØ4
Intraoperative DGØ43ZØ
Pelvic Bones DPØ8
Intraoperative DPØ83ZØ
Pelvic Region DWØ6
Intraoperative DWØ63ZØ
Pineal Body DGØ1
Intraoperative DGØ13ZØ
Pituitary Gland DGØØ
Intraoperative DGØØ3ZØ
Pleura DBØ5
Intraoperative DBØ53ZØ
Prostate DVØØ
Intraoperative DVØØ3ZØ
Radius DPØ7
Intraoperative DPØ73ZØ
Rectum DDØ7
Intraoperative DDØ73ZØ
Rib DPØ5
Intraoperative DPØ53ZØ
Sinuses D9Ø7
Intraoperative D9Ø73ZØ
Skin
Abdomen DHØ8
Intraoperative DHØ83ZØ
Arm DHØ4
Intraoperative DHØ43ZØ
Back DHØ7
Intraoperative DHØ73ZØ
Buttock DHØ9
Intraoperative DHØ93ZØ
Chest DHØ6
Intraoperative DHØ63ZØ
Face DHØ2
Intraoperative DHØ23ZØ
Leg DHØB
Intraoperative DHØB3ZØ
Neck DHØ3
Intraoperative DHØ33ZØ
Skull DPØØ
Intraoperative DPØØ3ZØ
Spinal Cord DØØ6
Intraoperative DØØ63ZØ
Spleen D7Ø2
Intraoperative D7Ø23ZØ
Sternum DPØ4
Intraoperative DPØ43ZØ
Stomach DDØ1
Intraoperative DDØ13ZØ
Testis DVØ1
Intraoperative DVØ13ZØ
Thymus D7Ø1
Intraoperative D7Ø13ZØ
Thyroid Gland DGØ5
Intraoperative DGØ53ZØ
Tibia DPØB
Intraoperative DPØB3ZØ
Tongue D9Ø5
Intraoperative D9Ø53ZØ
Trachea DBØØ
Intraoperative DBØØ3ZØ
Ulna DPØ7
Intraoperative DPØ73ZØ
Ureter DTØ1
Intraoperative DTØ13ZØ
Urethra DTØ3
Intraoperative DTØ33ZØ
Uterus DUØ2
Intraoperative DUØ23ZØ
Whole Body DWØ5
Intraoperative DWØ53ZØ
Bedside swallow FØØZJWZ

Berlin Heart Ventricular Assist Device *use* Implantable Heart Assist System in Heart and Great Vessels
Bezlotoxumab Monoclonal Antibody XWØ
Biceps brachii muscle
use Upper Arm Muscle, Left
use Upper Arm Muscle, Right
Biceps femoris muscle
use Upper Leg Muscle, Left
use Upper Leg Muscle, Right
Bicipital aponeurosis
use Subcutaneous Tissue and Fascia, Left Lower Arm
use Subcutaneous Tissue and Fascia, Right Lower Arm
Bicuspid valve *use* Mitral Valve
Bili light therapy *see* Phototherapy, Skin 6A6Ø
Bioactive embolization coil(s) *use* Intraluminal Device, Bioactive in Upper Arteries
Biofeedback GZC9ZZZ
BioFire® FilmArray® Pneumonia Panel XXEBXQ6
Biopsy
see Drainage with qualifier Diagnostic
see Excision with qualifier Diagnostic
see Extraction with qualifier Diagnostic
BiPAP *see* Assistance, Respiratory 5AØ9
Bisection *see* Division
Biventricular external heart assist system *use* Short-term External Heart Assist System in Heart and Great Vessels
Blepharectomy
see Excision, Eye Ø8B
see Resection, Eye Ø8T
Blepharoplasty
see Repair, Eye Ø8Q
see Replacement, Eye Ø8R
see Reposition, Eye Ø8S
see Supplement, Eye Ø8U
Blepharorrhaphy *see* Repair, Eye Ø8Q
Blepharotomy *see* Drainage, Eye Ø89
Blinatumomab Antineoplastic Immunotherapy XWØ
Block, Nerve, anesthetic injection 3EØT3BZ
Blood glucose monitoring system *use* Monitoring Device
Blood pressure *see* Measurement, Arterial 4AØ3
BMR (basal metabolic rate) *see* Measurement, Physiological Systems 4AØZ
Body of femur
use Femoral Shaft, Left
use Femoral Shaft, Right
Body of fibula
use Fibula, Left
use Fibula, Right
Bone anchored hearing device
use Hearing Device, Bone Conduction in Ø9H
use Hearing Device in Head and Facial Bones
Bone bank bone graft *use* Nonautologous Tissue Substitute
Bone Growth Stimulator
Insertion of device in
Bone
Facial ØNHW
Lower ØQHY
Nasal ØNHB
Upper ØPHY
Skull ØNHØ
Removal of device from
Bone
Facial ØNPW
Lower ØQPY
Nasal ØNPB
Upper ØPPY
Skull ØNPØ
Revision of device in
Bone
Facial ØNWW
Lower ØQWY
Nasal ØNWB
Upper ØPWY
Skull ØNWØ
Bone marrow transplant *see* Transfusion, Circulatory 3Ø2
Bone morphogenetic protein 2 (BMP 2) *use* Recombinant Bone Morphogenetic Protein

Subterms under main terms may continue to next column or page

Bone screw (interlocking) (lag) (pedicle) (recessed)
use Internal Fixation Device in Head and Facial Bones
use Internal Fixation Device in Lower Bones
use Internal Fixation Device in Upper Bones
Bony labyrinth
use Inner Ear, Left
use Inner Ear, Right
Bony orbit
use Orbit, Left
use Orbit, Right
Bony vestibule
use Inner Ear, Left
use Inner Ear, Right
Botallo's duct *use* Pulmonary Artery, Left
Bovine pericardial valve *use* Zooplastic Tissue in Heart and Great Vessels
Bovine pericardium graft *use* Zooplastic Tissue in Heart and Great Vessels
BP (blood pressure) *see* Measurement, Arterial 4A03
Brachial (lateral) lymph node
use Lymphatic, Left Axillary
use Lymphatic, Right Axillary
Brachialis muscle
use Upper Arm Muscle, Left
use Upper Arm Muscle, Right
Brachiocephalic artery *use* Innominate Artery
Brachiocephalic trunk *use* Innominate Artery
Brachiocephalic vein
use Innominate Vein, Left
use Innominate Vein, Right
Brachioradialis muscle
use Lower Arm and Wrist Muscle, Left
use Lower Arm and Wrist Muscle, Right
Brachytherapy
Abdomen DW13
Adrenal Gland DG12
Back
Lower DW1LBB
Upper DW1KBB
Bile Ducts DF12
Bladder DT12
Bone Marrow D710
Brain D010
Brain Stem D011
Breast
Left DM10
Right DM11
Bronchus DB11
Cervix DU11
Chest DW12
Chest Wall DB17
Colon DD15
Cranial Cavity DW10BB
Diaphragm DB18
Duodenum DD12
Ear D910
Esophagus DD10
Extremity
Lower DW1YBB
Upper DW1XBB
Eye D810
Gallbladder DF11
Gastrointestinal Tract DW1PBB
Genitourinary Tract DW1RBB
Gland
Adrenal DG12
Parathyroid DG14
Pituitary DG10
Thyroid DG15
Glands, Salivary D916
Head and Neck DW11
Hypopharynx D913
Ileum DD14
Jejunum DD13
Kidney DT10
Larynx D91B
Liver DF10
Lung DB12
Lymphatics
Abdomen D716
Axillary D714
Inguinal D718
Neck D713
Pelvis D717
Thorax D715
Mediastinum DB16
Mouth D914

Brachytherapy — *continued*
Nasopharynx D91D
Neck and Head DW11
Nerve, Peripheral D017
Nose D911
Oropharynx D91F
Ovary DU10
Palate
Hard D918
Soft D919
Pancreas DF13
Parathyroid Gland DG14
Pelvic Region DW16
Pineal Body DG11
Pituitary Gland DG10
Pleura DB15
Prostate DV10
Rectum DD17
Respiratory Tract DW1QBB
Sinuses D917
Spinal Cord D016
Spleen D712
Stomach DD11
Testis DV11
Thymus D711
Thyroid Gland DG15
Tongue D915
Trachea DB10
Ureter DT11
Urethra DT13
Uterus DU12
Brachytherapy, CivaSheet®
see Brachytherapy with qualifier Unidirectional Source
see Insertion with device Radioactive Element
Brachytherapy seeds *use* Radioactive Element
Breast procedures, skin only *use* Skin, Chest
Brexanolone XW0
Brexucabtagene Autoleucel *use* Brexucabtagene Autoleucel Immunotherapy
Brexucabtagene Autoleucel Immunotherapy XW2
Broad ligament *use* Uterine Supporting Structure
Bronchial artery *use* Upper Artery
Bronchography
see Fluoroscopy, Respiratory System BB1
see Plain Radiography, Respiratory System BB0
Bronchoplasty
see Repair, Respiratory System 0BQ
see Supplement, Respiratory System 0BU
Bronchorrhaphy *see* Repair, Respiratory System 0BQ
Bronchoscopy 0BJ08ZZ
Bronchotomy *see* Drainage, Respiratory System 0B9
Bronchus Intermedius *use* Main Bronchus, Right
BRYAN® Cervical Disc System *use* Synthetic Substitute
Buccal gland *use* Buccal Mucosa
Buccinator lymph node *use* Lymphatic, Head
Buccinator muscle *use* Facial Muscle
Buckling, scleral with implant *see* Supplement, Eye 08U
Bulbospongiosus muscle *use* Perineum Muscle
Bulbourethral (Cowper's) gland *use* Urethra
Bundle of His *use* Conduction Mechanism
Bundle of Kent *use* Conduction Mechanism
Bunionectomy *see* Excision, Lower Bones 0QB
Bursectomy
see Excision, Bursae and Ligaments 0MB
see Resection, Bursae and Ligaments 0MT
Bursocentesis *see* Drainage, Bursae and Ligaments 0M9
Bursography
see Plain Radiography, Non-Axial Lower Bones BQ0
see Plain Radiography, Non-Axial Upper Bones BP0
Bursotomy
see Division, Bursae and Ligaments 0M8
see Drainage, Bursae and Ligaments 0M9
BVS 5000 Ventricular Assist Device *use* Short-term External Heart Assist System in Heart and Great Vessels
Bypass
Anterior Chamber
Left 08133
Right 08123
Aorta
Abdominal 0410
Thoracic
Ascending/Arch 021X
Descending 021W

Bypass — *continued*
Artery
Anterior Tibial
Left 041Q
Right 041P
Axillary
Left 03160
Right 03150
Brachial
Left 03180
Right 03170
Common Carotid
Left 031J0
Right 031H0
Common Iliac
Left 041D
Right 041C
Coronary
Four or More Arteries 0213
One Artery 0210
Three Arteries 0212
Two Arteries 0211
External Carotid
Left 031N0
Right 031M0
External Iliac
Left 041J
Right 041H
Femoral
Left 041L
Right 041K
Foot
Left 041W
Right 041V
Hepatic 0413
Innominate 03120
Internal Carotid
Left 031L0
Right 031K0
Internal Iliac
Left 041F
Right 041E
Intracranial 031G0
Peroneal
Left 041U
Right 041T
Popliteal
Left 041N
Right 041M
Posterior Tibial
Left 041S
Right 041R
Pulmonary
Left 021R
Right 021Q
Pulmonary Trunk 021P
Radial
Left 031C
Right 031B
Splenic 0414
Subclavian
Left 03140
Right 03130
Temporal
Left 031T0
Right 031S0
Ulnar
Left 031A
Right 0319
Atrium
Left 0217
Right 0216
Bladder 0T1B
Cavity, Cranial 0W110J
Cecum 0D1H
Cerebral Ventricle 0016
Colon
Ascending 0D1K
Descending 0D1M
Sigmoid 0D1N
Transverse 0D1L
Duct
Common Bile 0F19
Cystic 0F18
Hepatic
Common 0F17
Left 0F16
Right 0F15

Bypass — *continued*
Duct — *continued*
Lacrimal
Left Ø81Y
Right Ø81X
Pancreatic ØF1D
Accessory ØF1F
Duodenum ØD19
Ear
Left Ø91EØ
Right Ø91DØ
Esophagus ØD15
Lower ØD13
Middle ØD12
Upper ØD11
Fallopian Tube
Left ØU16
Right ØU15
Gallbladder ØF14
Ileum ØD1B
Intestine
Large ØD1E
Small ØD18
Jejunum ØD1A
Kidney Pelvis
Left ØT14
Right ØT13
Pancreas ØF1G
Pelvic Cavity ØW1J
Peritoneal Cavity ØW1G
Pleural Cavity
Left ØW1B
Right ØW19
Spinal Canal ØØ1U
Stomach ØD16
Trachea ØB11
Ureter
Left ØT17
Right ØT16
Ureters, Bilateral ØT18
Vas Deferens
Bilateral ØV1Q
Left ØV1P
Right ØV1N
Vein
Axillary
Left Ø518
Right Ø517
Azygos Ø51Ø
Basilic
Left Ø51C
Right Ø51B
Brachial
Left Ø51A
Right Ø519
Cephalic
Left Ø51F
Right Ø51D
Colic Ø617
Common Iliac
Left Ø61D
Right Ø61C
Esophageal Ø613
External Iliac
Left Ø61G
Right Ø61F
External Jugular
Left Ø51Q
Right Ø51P
Face
Left Ø51V
Right Ø51T
Femoral
Left Ø61N
Right Ø61M
Foot
Left Ø61V
Right Ø61T
Gastric Ø612
Hand
Left Ø51H
Right Ø51G
Hemiazygos Ø511
Hepatic Ø614
Hypogastric
Left Ø61J
Right Ø61H
Inferior Mesenteric Ø616

Bypass — *continued*
Vein — *continued*
Innominate
Left Ø514
Right Ø513
Internal Jugular
Left Ø51N
Right Ø51M
Intracranial Ø51L
Portal Ø618
Renal
Left Ø61B
Right Ø619
Saphenous
Left Ø61Q
Right Ø61P
Splenic Ø611
Subclavian
Left Ø516
Right Ø515
Superior Mesenteric Ø615
Vertebral
Left Ø51S
Right Ø51R
Vena Cava
Inferior Ø61Ø
Superior Ø21V
Ventricle
Left Ø21L
Right Ø21K
Bypass, cardiopulmonary 5A1221Z

C

Caesarean section *see* Extraction, Products of Conception 1ØDØ
Calcaneocuboid joint
use Tarsal Joint, Left
use Tarsal Joint, Right
Calcaneocuboid ligament
use Foot Bursa and Ligament, Left
use Foot Bursa and Ligament, Right
Calcaneofibular ligament
use Ankle Bursa and Ligament, Left
use Ankle Bursa and Ligament, Right
Calcaneus
use Tarsal, Left
use Tarsal, Right
Cannulation
see Bypass
see Dilation
see Drainage
see Irrigation
Canthorrhaphy *see* Repair, Eye Ø8Q
Canthotomy *see* Release, Eye Ø8N
Capitate bone
use Carpal, Left
use Carpal, Right
Caplacizumab XWØ
Capsulectomy, lens *see* Excision, Eye Ø8B
Capsulorrhaphy, joint
see Repair, Lower Joints ØSQ
see Repair, Upper Joints ØRQ
Cardia *use* Esophagogastric Junction
Cardiac contractility modulation lead *use* Cardiac Lead in Heart and Great Vessels
Cardiac event recorder *use* Monitoring Device
Cardiac Lead
Defibrillator
Atrium
Left Ø2H7
Right Ø2H6
Pericardium Ø2HN
Vein, Coronary Ø2H4
Ventricle
Left Ø2HL
Right Ø2HK
Insertion of device in
Atrium
Left Ø2H7
Right Ø2H6
Pericardium Ø2HN
Vein, Coronary Ø2H4
Ventricle
Left Ø2HL
Right Ø2HK

Cardiac Lead — *continued*
Pacemaker
Atrium
Left Ø2H7
Right Ø2H6
Pericardium Ø2HN
Vein, Coronary Ø2H4
Ventricle
Left Ø2HL
Right Ø2HK
Removal of device from, Heart Ø2PA
Revision of device in, Heart Ø2WA
Cardiac plexus *use* Thoracic Sympathetic Nerve
Cardiac Resynchronization Defibrillator Pulse Generator
Abdomen ØJH8
Chest ØJH6
Cardiac Resynchronization Pacemaker Pulse Generator
Abdomen ØJH8
Chest ØJH6
Cardiac resynchronization therapy (CRT) lead
use Cardiac Lead, Defibrillator in Ø2H
use Cardiac Lead, Pacemaker in Ø2H
Cardiac Rhythm Related Device
Insertion of device in
Abdomen ØJH8
Chest ØJH6
Removal of device from, Subcutaneous Tissue and Fascia, Trunk ØJPT
Revision of device in, Subcutaneous Tissue and Fascia, Trunk ØJWT
Cardiocentesis *see* Drainage, Pericardial Cavity ØW9D
Cardioesophageal junction *use* Esophagogastric Junction
Cardiolysis *see* Release, Heart and Great Vessels Ø2N
CardioMEMS® pressure sensor *use* Monitoring Device, Pressure Sensor in Ø2H
Cardiomyotomy *see* Division, Esophagogastric Junction ØD84
Cardioplegia *see* Introduction of substance in or on, Heart 3EØ8
Cardiorrhaphy *see* Repair, Heart and Great Vessels Ø2Q
Cardioversion 5A22Ø4Z
Caregiver Training FØFZ
Caroticotympanic artery
use Internal Carotid Artery, Left
use Internal Carotid Artery, Right
Carotid glomus
use Carotid Bodies, Bilateral
use Carotid Body, Left
use Carotid Body, Right
Carotid sinus
use Internal Carotid Artery, Left
use Internal Carotid Artery, Right
Carotid (artery) sinus (baroreceptor) lead *use* Stimulator Lead in Upper Arteries
Carotid sinus nerve *use* Glossopharyngeal Nerve
Carotid WALLSTENT® Monorail® Endoprosthesis
use Intraluminal Device
Carpectomy
see Excision, Upper Bones ØPB
see Resection, Upper Bones ØPT
Carpometacarpal ligament
use Hand Bursa and Ligament, Left
use Hand Bursa and Ligament, Right
Casting *see* Immobilization
CAT scan *see* Computerized Tomography (CT Scan)
Catheterization
see Dilation
see Drainage
see Insertion of device in
see Irrigation
Heart *see* Measurement, Cardiac 4AØ2
Umbilical vein, for infusion Ø6HØ33T
Cauda equina *use* Lumbar Spinal Cord
Cauterization
see Destruction
see Repair
Cavernous plexus *use* Head and Neck Sympathetic Nerve
CBMA (Concentrated Bone Marrow Aspirate) *use* Concentrated Bone Marrow Aspirate
CBMA (Concentrated Bone Marrow Aspirate) injection, intramuscular XKØ23Ø3
Cecectomy
see Excision, Cecum ØDBH

Cecectomy — *continued*
see Resection, Cecum ØDTH
Cecocolostomy
see Bypass, Gastrointestinal System ØD1
see Drainage, Gastrointestinal System ØD9
Cecopexy
see Repair, Cecum ØDQH
see Reposition, Cecum ØDSH
Cecoplication *see* Restriction, Cecum ØDVH
Cecorrhaphy *see* Repair, Cecum ØDQH
Cecostomy
see Bypass, Cecum ØD1H
see Drainage, Cecum ØD9H
Cecotomy *see* Drainage, Cecum ØD9H
Cefiderocol Anti-infective XWØ
Ceftazidime-Avibactam Anti-infective XWØ
Ceftolozane/Tazobactam Anti-infective XWØ
Celiac ganglion *use* Abdominal Sympathetic Nerve
Celiac lymph node *use* Lymphatic, Aortic
Celiac (solar) plexus *use* Abdominal Sympathetic Nerve
Celiac trunk *use* Celiac Artery
Central axillary lymph node
use Lymphatic, Left Axillary
use Lymphatic, Right Axillary
Central venous pressure *see* Measurement, Venous 4AØ4
Centrimag® Blood Pump *use* Short-term External Heart Assist System in Heart and Great Vessels
Cephalogram BNØØZZZ
Ceramic on ceramic bearing surface *use* Synthetic Substitute, Ceramic in ØSR
Cerclage *see* Restriction
Cerebral aqueduct (Sylvius) *use* Cerebral Ventricle
Cerebral Embolic Filtration
Dual Filter X2A5312
Extracorporeal Flow Reversal Circuit X2A
Single Deflection Filter X2A6325
Cerebrum *use* Brain
Cervical esophagus *use* Esophagus, Upper
Cervical facet joint
use Cervical Vertebral Joint
use Cervical Vertebral Joint, 2 or more
Cervical ganglion *use* Head and Neck Sympathetic Nerve
Cervical interspinous ligament *use* Head and Neck Bursa and Ligament
Cervical intertransverse ligament *use* Head and Neck Bursa and Ligament
Cervical Ligamentum Flavum *use* Head and Neck Bursa and Ligament
Cervical Lymph Node
use Lymphatic, Left Neck
use Lymphatic, Right Neck
Cervicectomy
see Excision, Cervix ØUBC
see Resection, Cervix ØUTC
Cervicothoracic facet joint *use* Cervicothoracic Vertebral Joint
Cesarean section *see* Extraction, Products of Conception 1ØDØ
Cesium-131 Collagen Implant *use* Radioactive Element, Cesium-131 Collagen Implant in ØØH
Change Device in
Abdominal Wall ØW2FX
Back
Lower ØW2LX
Upper ØW2KX
Bladder ØT2BX
Bone
Facial ØN2WX
Lower ØQ2YX
Nasal ØN2BX
Upper ØP2YX
Bone Marrow Ø72TX
Brain ØØ2ØX
Breast
Left ØH2UX
Right ØH2TX
Bursa and Ligament
Lower ØM2YX
Upper ØM2XX
Cavity, Cranial ØW21X
Chest Wall ØW28X
Cisterna Chyli Ø72LX
Diaphragm ØB2TX

Change Device in — *continued*
Duct
Hepatobiliary ØF2BX
Pancreatic ØF2DX
Ear
Left Ø92JX
Right Ø92HX
Epididymis and Spermatic Cord ØV2MX
Extremity
Lower
Left ØY2BX
Right ØY29X
Upper
Left ØX27X
Right ØX26X
Eye
Left Ø821X
Right Ø82ØX
Face ØW22X
Fallopian Tube ØU28X
Gallbladder ØF24X
Gland
Adrenal ØG25X
Endocrine ØG2SX
Pituitary ØG2ØX
Salivary ØC2AX
Head ØW2ØX
Intestinal Tract
Lower ØD2DXUZ
Upper ØD2ØXUZ
Jaw
Lower ØW25X
Upper ØW24X
Joint
Lower ØS2YX
Upper ØR2YX
Kidney ØT25X
Larynx ØC2SX
Liver ØF2ØX
Lung
Left ØB2LX
Right ØB2KX
Lymphatic Ø72NX
Thoracic Duct Ø72KX
Mediastinum ØW2CX
Mesentery ØD2VX
Mouth and Throat ØC2YX
Muscle
Lower ØK2YX
Upper ØK2XX
Nasal Mucosa and Soft Tissue Ø92KX
Neck ØW26X
Nerve
Cranial ØØ2EX
Peripheral Ø12YX
Omentum ØD2UX
Ovary ØU23X
Pancreas ØF2GX
Parathyroid Gland ØG2RX
Pelvic Cavity ØW2JX
Penis ØV2SX
Pericardial Cavity ØW2DX
Perineum
Female ØW2NX
Male ØW2MX
Peritoneal Cavity ØW2GX
Peritoneum ØD2WX
Pineal Body ØG21X
Pleura ØB2QX
Pleural Cavity
Left ØW2BX
Right ØW29X
Products of Conception 1Ø2Ø7
Prostate and Seminal Vesicles ØV24X
Retroperitoneum ØW2HX
Scrotum and Tunica Vaginalis ØV28X
Sinus Ø92YX
Skin ØH2PX
Skull ØN2ØX
Spinal Canal ØØ2UX
Spleen Ø72PX
Subcutaneous Tissue and Fascia
Head and Neck ØJ2SX
Lower Extremity ØJ2WX
Trunk ØJ2TX
Upper Extremity ØJ2VX
Tendon
Lower ØL2YX
Upper ØL2XX

Change Device in — *continued*
Testis ØV2DX
Thymus Ø72MX
Thyroid Gland ØG2KX
Trachea ØB21
Tracheobronchial Tree ØB2ØX
Ureter ØT29X
Urethra ØT2DX
Uterus and Cervix ØU2DXHZ
Vagina and Cul-de-sac ØU2HXGZ
Vas Deferens ØV2RX
Vulva ØU2MX
Change Device in or on
Abdominal Wall 2WØ3X
Anorectal 2YØ3X5Z
Arm
Lower
Left 2WØDX
Right 2WØCX
Upper
Left 2WØBX
Right 2WØAX
Back 2WØ5X
Chest Wall 2WØ4X
Ear 2YØ2X5Z
Extremity
Lower
Left 2WØMX
Right 2WØLX
Upper
Left 2WØ9X
Right 2WØ8X
Face 2WØ1X
Finger
Left 2WØKX
Right 2WØJX
Foot
Left 2WØTX
Right 2WØSX
Genital Tract, Female 2YØ4X5Z
Hand
Left 2WØFX
Right 2WØEX
Head 2WØØX
Inguinal Region
Left 2WØ7X
Right 2WØ6X
Leg
Lower
Left 2WØRX
Right 2WØQX
Upper
Left 2WØPX
Right 2WØNX
Mouth and Pharynx 2YØØX5Z
Nasal 2YØ1X5Z
Neck 2WØ2X
Thumb
Left 2WØHX
Right 2WØGX
Toe
Left 2WØVX
Right 2WØUX
Urethra 2YØ5X5Z
Chemoembolization *see* Introduction of substance in or on
Chemosurgery, Skin 3EØØXTZ
Chemothalamectomy *see* Destruction, Thalamus ØØ59
Chemotherapy, Infusion for Cancer *see* Introduction of substance in or on
Chest x-ray *see* Plain Radiography, Chest BWØ3
Chiropractic Manipulation
Abdomen 9WB9X
Cervical 9WB1X
Extremities
Lower 9WB6X
Upper 9WB7X
Head 9WBØX
Lumbar 9WB3X
Pelvis 9WB5X
Rib Cage 9WB8X
Sacrum 9WB4X
Thoracic 9WB2X
Choana *use* Nasopharynx
Cholangiogram
see Fluoroscopy, Hepatobiliary System and Pancreas BF1

Cholangiogram — *continued*
see Plain Radiography, Hepatobiliary System and Pancreas BFØ
Cholecystectomy
see Excision, Gallbladder ØFB4
see Resection, Gallbladder ØFT4
Cholecystojejunostomy
see Bypass, Hepatobiliary System and Pancreas ØF1
see Drainage, Hepatobiliary System and Pancreas ØF9
Cholecystopexy
see Repair, Gallbladder ØFQ4
see Reposition, Gallbladder ØFS4
Cholecystoscopy ØFJ44ZZ
Cholecystostomy
see Bypass, Gallbladder ØF14
see Drainage, Gallbladder ØF94
Cholecystotomy *see* Drainage, Gallbladder ØF94
Choledochectomy
see Excision, Hepatobiliary System and Pancreas ØFB
see Resection, Hepatobiliary System and Pancreas ØFT
Choledocholithotomy *see* Extirpation, Duct, Common Bile ØFC9
Choledochoplasty
see Repair, Hepatobiliary System and Pancreas ØFQ
see Replacement, Hepatobiliary System and Pancreas ØFR
see Supplement, Hepatobiliary System and Pancreas ØFU
Choledochoscopy ØFJB8ZZ
Choledochotomy *see* Drainage, Hepatobiliary System and Pancreas ØF9
Cholelithotomy *see* Extirpation, Hepatobiliary System and Pancreas ØFC
Chondrectomy
see Excision, Lower Joints ØSB
see Excision, Upper Joints ØRB
Knee *see* Excision, Lower Joints ØSB
Semilunar cartilage *see* Excision, Lower Joints ØSB
Chondroglossus muscle *use* Tongue, Palate, Pharynx Muscle
Chorda tympani *use* Facial Nerve
Chordotomy *see* Division, Central Nervous System and Cranial Nerves ØØ8
Choroid plexus *use* Cerebral Ventricle
Choroidectomy
see Excision, Eye Ø8B
see Resection, Eye Ø8T
Ciliary body
use Eye, Left
use Eye, Right
Ciliary ganglion *use* Head and Neck Sympathetic Nerve
Circle of Willis *use* Intracranial Artery
Circumcision ØVTTXZZ
Circumflex iliac artery
use Femoral Artery, Left
use Femoral Artery, Right
CivaSheet® *use* Radioactive Element
CivaSheet® Brachytherapy
see Brachytherapy with qualifier Unidirectional Source
see Insertion with device Radioactive Element
Clamp and rod internal fixation system (CRIF)
use Internal Fixation Device in Lower Bones
use Internal Fixation Device in Upper Bones
Clamping *see* Occlusion
Claustrum *use* Basal Ganglia
Claviculectomy
see Excision, Upper Bones ØPB
see Resection, Upper Bones ØPT
Claviculotomy
see Division, Upper Bones ØP8
see Drainage, Upper Bones ØP9
Clipping, aneurysm
see Occlusion using Extraluminal Device
see Restriction using Extraluminal Device
Clitorectomy, clitoridectomy
see Excision, Clitoris ØUBJ
see Resection, Clitoris ØUTJ
Clolar *use* Clofarabine
Closure
see Occlusion
see Repair
Clysis *see* Introduction of substance in or on
Coagulation *see* Destruction
Coagulation Factor Xa, Inactivated XWØ
Coagulation Factor Xa, (Recombinant) Inactivated
use Coagulation Factor Xa, Inactivated
COALESCE® radiolucent interbody fusion device
use Interbody Fusion Device, Radiolucent Porous in New Technology
CoAxia NeuroFlo catheter *use* Intraluminal Device
Cobalt/chromium head and polyethylene socket
use Synthetic Substitute, Metal on Polyethylene in ØSR
Cobalt/chromium head and socket *use* Synthetic Substitute, Metal in ØSR
Coccygeal body *use* Coccygeal Glomus
Coccygeus muscle
use Trunk Muscle, Left
use Trunk Muscle, Right
Cochlea
use Inner Ear, Left
use Inner Ear, Right
Cochlear implant (CI), multiple channel (electrode)
use Hearing Device, Multiple Channel Cochlear Prosthesis in Ø9H
Cochlear implant (CI), single channel (electrode)
use Hearing Device, Single Channel Cochlear Prosthesis in Ø9H
Cochlear Implant Treatment FØBZØ
Cochlear nerve *use* Acoustic Nerve
COGNIS® CRT-D *use* Cardiac Resynchronization Defibrillator Pulse Generator in ØJH
COHERE® radiolucent interbody fusion device *use* Interbody Fusion Device, Radiolucent Porous in New Technology
Colectomy
see Excision, Gastrointestinal System ØDB
see Resection, Gastrointestinal System ØDT
Collapse *see* Occlusion
Collection from
Breast, Breast Milk 8EØHX62
Indwelling Device
Circulatory System
Blood 8CØ2X6K
Other Fluid 8CØ2X6L
Nervous System
Cerebrospinal Fluid 8CØ1X6J
Other Fluid 8CØ1X6L
Integumentary System, Breast Milk 8EØHX62
Reproductive System, Male, Sperm 8EØVX63
Colocentesis *see* Drainage, Gastrointestinal System ØD9
Colofixation
see Repair, Gastrointestinal System ØDQ
see Reposition, Gastrointestinal System ØDS
Cololysis *see* Release, Gastrointestinal System ØDN
Colonic Z-Stent® *use* Intraluminal Device
Colonoscopy ØDJD8ZZ
Colopexy
see Repair, Gastrointestinal System ØDQ
see Reposition, Gastrointestinal System ØDS
Coloplication *see* Restriction, Gastrointestinal System ØDV
Coloproctectomy
see Excision, Gastrointestinal System ØDB
see Resection, Gastrointestinal System ØDT
Coloproctostomy
see Bypass, Gastrointestinal System ØD1
see Drainage, Gastrointestinal System ØD9
Colopuncture *see* Drainage, Gastrointestinal System ØD9
Colorrhaphy *see* Repair, Gastrointestinal System ØDQ
Colostomy
see Bypass, Gastrointestinal System ØD1
see Drainage, Gastrointestinal System ØD9
Colpectomy
see Excision, Vagina ØUBG
see Resection, Vagina ØUTG
Colpocentesis *see* Drainage, Vagina ØU9G
Colpopexy
see Repair, Vagina ØUQG
see Reposition, Vagina ØUSG
Colpoplasty
see Repair, Vagina ØUQG
see Supplement, Vagina ØUUG
Colporrhaphy *see* Repair, Vagina ØUQG
Colposcopy ØUJH8ZZ
Columella *use* Nasal Mucosa and Soft Tissue
Common digital vein
use Foot Vein, Left
use Foot Vein, Right
Common facial vein
use Face Vein, Left
use Face Vein, Right
Common fibular nerve *use* Peroneal Nerve
Common hepatic artery *use* Hepatic Artery
Common iliac (subaortic) lymph node *use* Lymphatic, Pelvis
Common interosseous artery
use Ulnar Artery, Left
use Ulnar Artery, Right
Common peroneal nerve *use* Peroneal Nerve
Complete (SE) stent *use* Intraluminal Device
Compression
see Restriction
Abdominal Wall 2W13X
Arm
Lower
Left 2W1DX
Right 2W1CX
Upper
Left 2W1BX
Right 2W1AX
Back 2W15X
Chest Wall 2W14X
Extremity
Lower
Left 2W1MX
Right 2W1LX
Upper
Left 2W19X
Right 2W18X
Face 2W11X
Finger
Left 2W1KX
Right 2W1JX
Foot
Left 2W1TX
Right 2W1SX
Hand
Left 2W1FX
Right 2W1EX
Head 2W1ØX
Inguinal Region
Left 2W17X
Right 2W16X
Leg
Lower
Left 2W1RX
Right 2W1QX
Upper
Left 2W1PX
Right 2W1NX
Neck 2W12X
Thumb
Left 2W1HX
Right 2W1GX
Toe
Left 2W1VX
Right 2W1UX
Computer Assisted Procedure
Extremity
Lower
No Qualifier 8EØYXBZ
With Computerized Tomography 8EØYXBG
With Fluoroscopy 8EØYXBF
With Magnetic Resonance Imaging 8EØYXBH
Upper
No Qualifier 8EØXXBZ
With Computerized Tomography 8EØXXBG
With Fluoroscopy 8EØXXBF
With Magnetic Resonance Imaging 8EØXXBH
Head and Neck Region
No Qualifier 8EØ9XBZ
With Computerized Tomography 8EØ9XBG
With Fluoroscopy 8EØ9XBF
With Magnetic Resonance Imaging 8EØ9XBH
Trunk Region
No Qualifier 8EØWXBZ
With Computerized Tomography 8EØWXBG
With Fluoroscopy 8EØWXBF
With Magnetic Resonance Imaging 8EØWXBH

Computerized Tomography (CT Scan)
- Abdomen BW2Ø
  - Chest and Pelvis BW25
- Abdomen and Chest BW24
- Abdomen and Pelvis BW21
- Airway, Trachea BB2F
- Ankle
  - Left BQ2H
  - Right BQ2G
- Aorta
  - Abdominal B42Ø
    - Intravascular Optical Coherence B42ØZ2Z
  - Thoracic B32Ø
    - Intravascular Optical Coherence B32ØZ2Z
- Arm
  - Left BP2F
  - Right BP2E
- Artery
  - Celiac B421
    - Intravascular Optical Coherence B421Z2Z
  - Common Carotid
    - Bilateral B325
    - Intravascular Optical Coherence B325Z2Z
  - Coronary
    - Bypass Graft
      - Intravascular Optical Coherence B223Z2Z
      - Multiple B223
    - Multiple B221
      - Intravascular Optical Coherence B221Z2Z
  - Internal Carotid
    - Bilateral B328
    - Intravascular Optical Coherence B328Z2Z
  - Intracranial B32R
    - Intravascular Optical Coherence B32RZ2Z
  - Lower Extremity
    - Bilateral B42H
      - Intravascular Optical Coherence B42HZ2Z
    - Left B42G
      - Intravascular Optical Coherence B42GZ2Z
    - Right B42F
      - Intravascular Optical Coherence B42FZ2Z
  - Pelvic B42C
    - Intravascular Optical Coherence B42CZ2Z
  - Pulmonary
    - Left B32T
      - Intravascular Optical Coherence B32TZ2Z
    - Right B32S
      - Intravascular Optical Coherence B32SZ2Z
  - Renal
    - Bilateral B428
      - Intravascular Optical Coherence B428Z2Z
    - Transplant B42M
      - Intravascular Optical Coherence B42MZ2Z
  - Superior Mesenteric B424
    - Intravascular Optical Coherence B424Z2Z
  - Vertebral
    - Bilateral B32G
    - Intravascular Optical Coherence B32GZ2Z
- Bladder BT2Ø
- Bone
  - Facial BN25
  - Temporal BN2F
- Brain BØ2Ø
- Calcaneus
  - Left BQ2K
  - Right BQ2J
- Cerebral Ventricle BØ28
- Chest, Abdomen and Pelvis BW25
- Chest and Abdomen BW24
- Cisterna BØ27

Computerized Tomography (CT Scan) — *continued*
- Clavicle
  - Left BP25
  - Right BP24
- Coccyx BR2F
- Colon BD24
- Ear B92Ø
- Elbow
  - Left BP2H
  - Right BP2G
- Extremity
  - Lower
    - Left BQ2S
    - Right BQ2R
  - Upper
    - Bilateral BP2V
    - Left BP2U
    - Right BP2T
- Eye
  - Bilateral B827
  - Left B826
  - Right B825
- Femur
  - Left BQ24
  - Right BQ23
- Fibula
  - Left BQ2C
  - Right BQ2B
- Finger
  - Left BP2S
  - Right BP2R
- Foot
  - Left BQ2M
  - Right BQ2L
- Forearm
  - Left BP2K
  - Right BP2J
- Gland
  - Adrenal, Bilateral BG22
  - Parathyroid BG23
  - Parotid, Bilateral B926
  - Salivary, Bilateral B92D
  - Submandibular, Bilateral B929
  - Thyroid BG24
- Hand
  - Left BP2P
  - Right BP2N
- Hands and Wrists, Bilateral BP2Q
- Head BW28
- Head and Neck BW29
- Heart
  - Intravascular Optical Coherence B226Z2Z
  - Right and Left B226
- Hepatobiliary System, All BF2C
- Hip
  - Left BQ21
  - Right BQ2Ø
- Humerus
  - Left BP2B
  - Right BP2A
- Intracranial Sinus B522
  - Intravascular Optical Coherence B522Z2Z
- Joint
  - Acromioclavicular, Bilateral BP23
  - Finger
    - Left BP2DZZZ
    - Right BP2CZZZ
  - Foot
    - Left BQ2Y
    - Right BQ2X
  - Hand
    - Left BP2DZZZ
    - Right BP2CZZZ
  - Sacroiliac BR2D
  - Sternoclavicular
    - Bilateral BP22
    - Left BP21
    - Right BP2Ø
  - Temporomandibular, Bilateral BN29
  - Toe
    - Left BQ2Y
    - Right BQ2X
- Kidney
  - Bilateral BT23
  - Left BT22
  - Right BT21
  - Transplant BT29
- Knee
  - Left BQ28

Computerized Tomography (CT Scan) — *continued*
- Knee — *continued*
  - Right BQ27
- Larynx B92J
- Leg
  - Left BQ2F
  - Right BQ2D
- Liver BF25
- Liver and Spleen BF26
- Lung, Bilateral BB24
- Mandible BN26
- Nasopharynx B92F
- Neck BW2F
- Neck and Head BW29
- Orbit, Bilateral BN23
- Oropharynx B92F
- Pancreas BF27
- Patella
  - Left BQ2W
  - Right BQ2V
- Pelvic Region BW2G
- Pelvis BR2C
  - Chest and Abdomen BW25
- Pelvis and Abdomen BW21
- Pituitary Gland BØ29
- Prostate BV23
- Ribs
  - Left BP2Y
  - Right BP2X
- Sacrum BR2F
- Scapula
  - Left BP27
  - Right BP26
- Sella Turcica BØ29
- Shoulder
  - Left BP29
  - Right BP28
- Sinus
  - Intracranial B522
    - Intravascular Optical Coherence B522Z2Z
  - Paranasal B922
- Skull BN2Ø
- Spinal Cord BØ2B
- Spine
  - Cervical BR2Ø
  - Lumbar BR29
  - Thoracic BR27
- Spleen and Liver BF26
- Thorax BP2W
- Tibia
  - Left BQ2C
  - Right BQ2B
- Toe
  - Left BQ2Q
  - Right BQ2P
- Trachea BB2F
- Tracheobronchial Tree
  - Bilateral BB29
  - Left BB28
  - Right BB27
- Vein
  - Pelvic (Iliac)
    - Left B52G
      - Intravascular Optical Coherence B52GZ2Z
    - Right B52F
      - Intravascular Optical Coherence B52FZ2Z
  - Pelvic (Iliac) Bilateral B52H
    - Intravascular Optical Coherence B52HZ2Z
  - Portal B52T
    - Intravascular Optical Coherence B52TZ2Z
  - Pulmonary
    - Bilateral B52S
      - Intravascular Optical Coherence B52SZ2Z
    - Left B52R
      - Intravascular Optical Coherence B52RZ2Z
    - Right B52Q
      - Intravascular Optical Coherence B52QZ2Z
  - Renal
    - Bilateral B52L
      - Intravascular Optical Coherence B52LZ2Z

Computerized Tomography (CT Scan) — *continued*
Vein — *continued*
Renal — *continued*
Left B52K
Intravascular Optical Coherence B52KZ2Z
Right B52J
Intravascular Optical Coherence B52JZ2Z
Spanchnic B52T
Intravascular Optical Coherence B52TZ2Z
Vena Cava
Inferior B529
Intravascular Optical Coherence B529Z2Z
Superior B528
Intravascular Optical Coherence B528Z2Z
Ventricle, Cerebral B028
Wrist
Left BP2M
Right BP2L
Concentrated Bone Marrow Aspirate (CBMA) injection, intramuscular XK02303
Concerto II CRT-D *use* Cardiac Resynchronization Defibrillator Pulse Generator in 0JH
Condylectomy
see Excision, Head and Facial Bones 0NB
see Excision, Lower Bones 0QB
see Excision, Upper Bones 0PB
Condyloid process
use Mandible, Left
use Mandible, Right
Condylotomy
see Division, Head and Facial Bones 0N8
see Division, Lower Bones 0Q8
see Division, Upper Bones 0P8
see Drainage, Head and Facial Bones 0N9
see Drainage, Lower Bones 0Q9
see Drainage, Upper Bones 0P9
Condylysis
see Release, Head and Facial Bones 0NN
see Release, Lower Bones 0QN
see Release, Upper Bones 0PN
Conization, cervix *see* Excision, Cervix 0UBC
Conjunctivoplasty
see Repair, Eye 08Q
see Replacement, Eye 08R
CONSERVE® PLUS Total Resurfacing Hip System *use* Resurfacing Device in Lower Joints
Construction
Auricle, ear *see* Replacement, Ear, Nose, Sinus 09R
Ileal conduit *see* Bypass, Urinary System 0T1
Consulta CRT-D *use* Cardiac Resynchronization Defibrillator Pulse Generator in 0JH
Consulta CRT-P *use* Cardiac Resynchronization Pacemaker Pulse Generator in 0JH
Contact Radiation
Abdomen DWY37ZZ
Adrenal Gland DGY27ZZ
Bile Ducts DFY27ZZ
Bladder DTY27ZZ
Bone, Other DPYC7ZZ
Brain D0Y07ZZ
Brain Stem D0Y17ZZ
Breast
Left DMY07ZZ
Right DMY17ZZ
Bronchus DBY17ZZ
Cervix DUY17ZZ
Chest DWY27ZZ
Chest Wall DBY77ZZ
Colon DDY57ZZ
Diaphragm DBY87ZZ
Duodenum DDY27ZZ
Ear D9Y07ZZ
Esophagus DDY07ZZ
Eye D8Y07ZZ
Femur DPY97ZZ
Fibula DPYB7ZZ
Gallbladder DFY17ZZ
Gland
Adrenal DGY27ZZ
Parathyroid DGY47ZZ
Pituitary DGY07ZZ
Thyroid DGY57ZZ
Glands, Salivary D9Y67ZZ

Contact Radiation — *continued*
Head and Neck DWY17ZZ
Hemibody DWY47ZZ
Humerus DPY67ZZ
Hypopharynx D9Y37ZZ
Ileum DDY47ZZ
Jejunum DDY37ZZ
Kidney DTY07ZZ
Larynx D9YB7ZZ
Liver DFY07ZZ
Lung DBY27ZZ
Mandible DPY37ZZ
Maxilla DPY27ZZ
Mediastinum DBY67ZZ
Mouth D9Y47ZZ
Nasopharynx D9YD7ZZ
Neck and Head DWY17ZZ
Nerve, Peripheral D0Y77ZZ
Nose D9Y17ZZ
Oropharynx D9YF7ZZ
Ovary DUY07ZZ
Palate
Hard D9Y87ZZ
Soft D9Y97ZZ
Pancreas DFY37ZZ
Parathyroid Gland DGY47ZZ
Pelvic Bones DPY87ZZ
Pelvic Region DWY67ZZ
Pineal Body DGY17ZZ
Pituitary Gland DGY07ZZ
Pleura DBY57ZZ
Prostate DVY07ZZ
Radius DPY77ZZ
Rectum DDY77ZZ
Rib DPY57ZZ
Sinuses D9Y77ZZ
Skin
Abdomen DHY87ZZ
Arm DHY47ZZ
Back DHY77ZZ
Buttock DHY97ZZ
Chest DHY67ZZ
Face DHY27ZZ
Leg DHYB7ZZ
Neck DHY37ZZ
Skull DPY07ZZ
Spinal Cord D0Y67ZZ
Sternum DPY47ZZ
Stomach DDY17ZZ
Testis DVY17ZZ
Thyroid Gland DGY57ZZ
Tibia DPYB7ZZ
Tongue D9Y57ZZ
Trachea DBY07ZZ
Ulna DPY77ZZ
Ureter DTY17ZZ
Urethra DTY37ZZ
Uterus DUY27ZZ
Whole Body DWY57ZZ
ContaCT software (Measurement of intracranial arterial flow) 4A03X5D
CONTAK RENEWAL® 3 RF (HE) CRT-D *use* Cardiac Resynchronization Defibrillator Pulse Generator in 0JH
Contegra Pulmonary Valved Conduit *use* Zooplastic Tissue in Heart and Great Vessels
CONTEPO™ *use* Fosfomycin Anti-Infective
Continuous Glucose Monitoring (CGM) device *use* Monitoring Device
Continuous Negative Airway Pressure
24-96 Consecutive Hours, Ventilation 5A09459
Greater than 96 Consecutive Hours, Ventilation 5A09559
Less than 24 Consecutive Hours, Ventilation 5A09359
Continuous Positive Airway Pressure
24-96 Consecutive Hours, Ventilation 5A09457
Greater than 96 Consecutive Hours, Ventilation 5A09557
Less than 24 Consecutive Hours, Ventilation 5A09357
Continuous renal replacement therapy (CRRT) 5A1D90Z
Contraceptive Device
Change device in, Uterus and Cervix 0U2DXHZ
Insertion of device in
Cervix 0UHC

Contraceptive Device — *continued*
Insertion of device in — *continued*
Subcutaneous Tissue and Fascia
Abdomen 0JH8
Chest 0JH6
Lower Arm
Left 0JHH
Right 0JHG
Lower Leg
Left 0JHP
Right 0JHN
Upper Arm
Left 0JHF
Right 0JHD
Upper Leg
Left 0JHM
Right 0JHL
Uterus 0UH9
Removal of device from
Subcutaneous Tissue and Fascia
Lower Extremity 0JPW
Trunk 0JPT
Upper Extremity 0JPV
Uterus and Cervix 0UPD
Revision of device in
Subcutaneous Tissue and Fascia
Lower Extremity 0JWW
Trunk 0JWT
Upper Extremity 0JWV
Uterus and Cervix 0UWD
Contractility Modulation Device
Abdomen 0JH8
Chest 0JH6
Control bleeding in
Abdominal Wall 0W3F
Ankle Region
Left 0Y3L
Right 0Y3K
Arm
Lower
Left 0X3F
Right 0X3D
Upper
Left 0X39
Right 0X38
Axilla
Left 0X35
Right 0X34
Back
Lower 0W3L
Upper 0W3K
Buttock
Left 0Y31
Right 0Y30
Cavity, Cranial 0W31
Chest Wall 0W38
Elbow Region
Left 0X3C
Right 0X3B
Extremity
Lower
Left 0Y3B
Right 0Y39
Upper
Left 0X37
Right 0X36
Face 0W32
Femoral Region
Left 0Y38
Right 0Y37
Foot
Left 0Y3N
Right 0Y3M
Gastrointestinal Tract 0W3P
Genitourinary Tract 0W3R
Hand
Left 0X3K
Right 0X3J
Head 0W30
Inguinal Region
Left 0Y36
Right 0Y35
Jaw
Lower 0W35
Upper 0W34
Knee Region
Left 0Y3G
Right 0Y3F

Control bleeding in — *continued*
Leg
Lower
Left ØY3J
Right ØY3H
Upper
Left ØY3D
Right ØY3C
Mediastinum ØW3C
Nasal Mucosa and Soft Tissue Ø93K
Neck ØW36
Oral Cavity and Throat ØW33
Pelvic Cavity ØW3J
Pericardial Cavity ØW3D
Perineum
Female ØW3N
Male ØW3M
Peritoneal Cavity ØW3G
Pleural Cavity
Left ØW3B
Right ØW39
Respiratory Tract ØW3Q
Retroperitoneum ØW3H
Shoulder Region
Left ØX33
Right ØX32
Wrist Region
Left ØX3H
Right ØX3G
Control, Epistaxis *see* Control bleeding in, Nasal Mucosa and Soft Tissue Ø93K
Conus arteriosus *use* Ventricle, Right
Conus medullaris *use* Lumbar Spinal Cord
Conversion
Cardiac rhythm 5A22Ø4Z
Gastrostomy to jejunostomy feeding device *see* Insertion of device in, Jejunum ØDHA
Cook Biodesign® Fistula Plug(s) *use* Nonautologous Tissue Substitute
Cook Biodesign® Hernia Graft(s) *use* Nonautologous Tissue Substitute
Cook Biodesign® Layered Graft(s) *use* Nonautologous Tissue Substitute
Cook Zenaprom™ Layered Graft(s) *use* Nonautologous Tissue Substitute
Cook Zenith AAA Endovascular Graft *use* Intraluminal Device
Cook Zenith® Fenestrated AAA Endovascular Graft
use Intraluminal Device, Branched or Fenestrated, One or Two Arteries in Ø4V
use Intraluminal Device, Branched or Fenestrated, Three or More Arteries in Ø4V
Coracoacromial ligament
use Shoulder Bursa and Ligament, Left
use Shoulder Bursa and Ligament, Right
Coracobrachialis muscle
use Upper Arm Muscle, Left
use Upper Arm Muscle, Right
Coracoclavicular ligament
use Shoulder Bursa and Ligament, Left
use Shoulder Bursa and Ligament, Right
Coracohumeral ligament
use Shoulder Bursa and Ligament, Left
use Shoulder Bursa and Ligament, Right
Coracoid process
use Scapula, Left
use Scapula, Right
Cordotomy *see* Division, Central Nervous System and Cranial Nerves ØØ8
Core needle biopsy *see* Excision with qualifier Diagnostic
CoreValve transcatheter aortic valve *use* Zooplastic Tissue in Heart and Great Vessels
Cormet Hip Resurfacing System *use* Resurfacing Device in Lower Joints
Corniculate cartilage *use* Larynx
CoRoent® XL *use* Interbody Fusion Device in Lower Joints
Coronary arteriography
see Fluoroscopy, Heart B21
see Plain Radiography, Heart B2Ø
Corox (OTW) Bipolar Lead
use Cardiac Lead, Defibrillator in Ø2H
use Cardiac Lead, Pacemaker in Ø2H
Corpus callosum *use* Brain
Corpus cavernosum *use* Penis
Corpus spongiosum *use* Penis
Corpus striatum *use* Basal Ganglia
Corrugator supercilii muscle *use* Facial Muscle
Cortical strip neurostimulator lead *use* Neurostimulator Lead in Central Nervous System and Cranial Nerves
Corvia IASD® *use* Synthetic Substitute
Costatectomy
see Excision, Upper Bones ØPB
see Resection, Upper Bones ØPT
Costectomy
see Excision, Upper Bones ØPB
see Resection, Upper Bones ØPT
Costocervical trunk
use Subclavian Artery, Left
use Subclavian Artery, Right
Costochondrectomy
see Excision, Upper Bones ØPB
see Resection, Upper Bones ØPT
Costoclavicular ligament
use Shoulder Bursa and Ligament, Left
use Shoulder Bursa and Ligament, Right
Costosternoplasty
see Repair, Upper Bones ØPQ
see Replacement, Upper Bones ØPR
see Supplement, Upper Bones ØPU
Costotomy
see Division, Upper Bones ØP8
see Drainage, Upper Bones ØP9
Costotransverse joint *use* Thoracic Vertebral Joint
Costotransverse ligament *use* Rib(s) Bursa and Ligament
Costovertebral joint *use* Thoracic Vertebral Joint
Costoxiphoid ligament *use* Sternum Bursa and Ligament
Counseling
Family, for substance abuse, Other Family Counseling HZ63ZZZ
Group
12-Step HZ43ZZZ
Behavioral HZ41ZZZ
Cognitive HZ4ØZZZ
Cognitive-Behavioral HZ42ZZZ
Confrontational HZ48ZZZ
Continuing Care HZ49ZZZ
Infectious Disease
Post-Test HZ4CZZZ
Pre-Test HZ4CZZZ
Interpersonal HZ44ZZZ
Motivational Enhancement HZ47ZZZ
Psychoeducation HZ46ZZZ
Spiritual HZ4BZZZ
Vocational HZ45ZZZ
Individual
12-Step HZ33ZZZ
Behavioral HZ31ZZZ
Cognitive HZ3ØZZZ
Cognitive-Behavioral HZ32ZZZ
Confrontational HZ38ZZZ
Continuing Care HZ39ZZZ
Infectious Disease
Post-Test HZ3CZZZ
Pre-Test HZ3CZZZ
Interpersonal HZ34ZZZ
Motivational Enhancement HZ37ZZZ
Psychoeducation HZ36ZZZ
Spiritual HZ3BZZZ
Vocational HZ35ZZZ
Mental Health Services
Educational GZ6ØZZZ
Other Counseling GZ63ZZZ
Vocational GZ61ZZZ
Countershock, cardiac 5A22Ø4Z
Cowper's (bulbourethral) gland *use* Urethra
CPAP (continuous positive airway pressure) *see* Assistance, Respiratory 5AØ9
Craniectomy
see Excision, Head and Facial Bones ØNB
see Resection, Head and Facial Bones ØNT
Cranioplasty
see Repair, Head and Facial Bones ØNQ
see Replacement, Head and Facial Bones ØNR
see Supplement, Head and Facial Bones ØNU
Craniotomy
see Division, Head and Facial Bones ØN8
see Drainage, Central Nervous System and Cranial Nerves ØØ9
see Drainage, Head and Facial Bones ØN9
Creation
Perineum
Female ØW4NØ
Male ØW4MØ
Valve
Aortic Ø24FØ
Mitral Ø24GØ
Tricuspid Ø24JØ
Cremaster muscle *use* Perineum Muscle
Cribriform plate
use Ethmoid Bone, Left
use Ethmoid Bone, Right
Cricoid cartilage *use* Trachea
Cricoidectomy *see* Excision, Larynx ØCBS
Cricothyroid artery
use Thyroid Artery, Left
use Thyroid Artery, Right
Cricothyroid muscle
use Neck Muscle, Left
use Neck Muscle, Right
Crisis Intervention GZ2ZZZZ
CRRT (Continuous renal replacement therapy) 5A1D9ØZ
Crural fascia
use Subcutaneous Tissue and Fascia, Left Upper Leg
use Subcutaneous Tissue and Fascia, Right Upper Leg
Crushing, nerve
Cranial *see* Destruction, Central Nervous System and Cranial Nerves ØØ5
Peripheral *see* Destruction, Peripheral Nervous System Ø15
Cryoablation *see* Destruction
Cryotherapy *see* Destruction
Cryptorchidectomy
see Excision, Male Reproductive System ØVB
see Resection, Male Reproductive System ØVT
Cryptorchiectomy
see Excision, Male Reproductive System ØVB
see Resection, Male Reproductive System ØVT
Cryptotomy
see Division, Gastrointestinal System ØD8
see Drainage, Gastrointestinal System ØD9
CT scan *see* Computerized Tomography (CT Scan)
CT sialogram *see* Computerized Tomography (CT Scan), Ear, Nose, Mouth and Throat B92
Cubital lymph node
use Lymphatic, Left Upper Extremity
use Lymphatic, Right Upper Extremity
Cubital nerve *use* Ulnar Nerve
Cuboid bone
use Tarsal, Left
use Tarsal, Right
Cuboideonavicular joint
use Tarsal Joint, Left
use Tarsal Joint, Right
Culdocentesis *see* Drainage, Cul-de-sac ØU9F
Culdoplasty
see Repair, Cul-de-sac ØUQF
see Supplement, Cul-de-sac ØUUF
Culdoscopy ØUJH8ZZ
Culdotomy *see* Drainage, Cul-de-sac ØU9F
Culmen *use* Cerebellum
Cultured epidermal cell autograft *use* Autologous Tissue Substitute
Cuneiform cartilage *use* Larynx
Cuneonavicular joint
use Joint, Tarsal, Left
use Joint, Tarsal, Right
Cuneonavicular ligament
use Foot Bursa and Ligament, Left
use Foot Bursa and Ligament, Right
Curettage
see Excision
see Extraction
Cutaneous (transverse) cervical nerve *use* Cervical Plexus
CVP (central venous pressure) *see* Measurement, Venous 4AØ4
Cyclodiathermy *see* Destruction, Eye Ø85
Cyclophotocoagulation *see* Destruction, Eye Ø85
CYPHER® Stent *use* Intraluminal Device, Drug-eluting in Heart and Great Vessels
Cystectomy
see Excision, Bladder ØTBB
see Resection, Bladder ØTTB

Cystocele repair *see* Repair, Subcutaneous Tissue and Fascia, Pelvic Region ØJQC
Cystography
- *see* Fluoroscopy, Urinary System BT1
- *see* Plain Radiography, Urinary System BTØ

Cystolithotomy *see* Extirpation, Bladder ØTCB
Cystopexy
- *see* Repair, Bladder ØTQB
- *see* Reposition, Bladder ØTSB

Cystoplasty
- *see* Repair, Bladder ØTQB
- *see* Replacement, Bladder ØTRB
- *see* Supplement, Bladder ØTUB

Cystorrhaphy *see* Repair, Bladder ØTQB
Cystoscopy ØTJB8ZZ
Cystostomy *see* Bypass, Bladder ØT1B
Cystostomy tube *use* Drainage Device
Cystotomy *see* Drainage, Bladder ØT9B
Cystourethrography
- *see* Fluoroscopy, Urinary System BT1
- *see* Plain Radiography, Urinary System BTØ

Cystourethroplasty
- *see* Repair, Urinary System ØTQ
- *see* Replacement, Urinary System ØTR
- *see* Supplement, Urinary System ØTU

Cytarabine and Daunorubicin Liposome Antineoplastic XWØ

D

DBS lead *use* Neurostimulator Lead in Central Nervous System and Cranial Nerves
DeBakey Left Ventricular Assist Device *use* Implantable Heart Assist System in Heart and Great Vessels
Debridement
- Excisional *see* Excision
- Non-excisional *see* Extraction

Decompression, Circulatory 6A15
Decortication, lung
- *see* Extirpation, Respiratory System ØBC
- *see* Release, Respiratory System ØBN

Deep brain neurostimulator lead *use* Neurostimulator Lead in Central Nervous System and Cranial Nerves
Deep cervical fascia
- *use* Subcutaneous Tissue and Fascia, Left Neck
- *use* Subcutaneous Tissue and Fascia, Right Neck

Deep cervical vein
- *use* Vertebral Vein, Left
- *use* Vertebral Vein, Right

Deep circumflex iliac artery
- *use* External Iliac Artery, Left
- *use* External Iliac Artery, Right

Deep facial vein
- *use* Face Vein, Left
- *use* Face Vein, Right

Deep femoral artery
- *use* Femoral Artery, Left
- *use* Femoral Artery, Right

Deep femoral (profunda femoris) vein
- *use* Femoral Vein, Left
- *use* Femoral Vein, Right

Deep Inferior Epigastric Artery Perforator Flap
- Replacement
  - Bilateral ØHRVØ77
  - Left ØHRUØ77
  - Right ØHRTØ77
- Transfer
  - Left ØKXG
  - Right ØKXF

Deep palmar arch
- *use* Hand Artery, Left
- *use* Hand Artery, Right

Deep transverse perineal muscle *use* Perineum Muscle
Deferential artery
- *use* Internal Iliac Artery, Left
- *use* Internal Iliac Artery, Right

Defibrillator Generator
- Abdomen ØJH8
- Chest ØJH6

Defibrotide Sodium Anticoagulant XWØ
Defitelio *use* Defibrotide Sodium Anticoagulant
Delivery
- Cesarean *see* Extraction, Products of Conception 1ØDØ
- Forceps *see* Extraction, Products of Conception 1ØDØ
- Manually assisted 1ØEØXZZ
- Products of Conception 1ØEØXZZ
- Vacuum assisted *see* Extraction, Products of Conception 1ØDØ

Delta frame external fixator
- *use* External Fixation Device, Hybrid in ØPH
- *use* External Fixation Device, Hybrid in ØPS
- *use* External Fixation Device, Hybrid in ØQH
- *use* External Fixation Device, Hybrid in ØQS

Delta III Reverse shoulder prosthesis *use* Synthetic Substitute, Reverse Ball and Socket in ØRR
Deltoid fascia
- *use* Subcutaneous Tissue and Fascia, Left Upper Arm
- *use* Subcutaneous Tissue and Fascia, Right Upper Arm

Deltoid ligament
- *use* Ankle Bursa and Ligament, Left
- *use* Ankle Bursa and Ligament, Right

Deltoid muscle
- *use* Shoulder Muscle, Left
- *use* Shoulder Muscle, Right

Deltopectoral (infraclavicular) lymph node
- *use* Lymphatic, Left Upper Extremity
- *use* Lymphatic, Right Upper Extremity

Denervation
- Cranial nerve *see* Destruction, Central Nervous System and Cranial Nerves ØØ5
- Peripheral nerve *see* Destruction, Peripheral Nervous System Ø15

Dens *use* Cervical Vertebra
Densitometry
- Plain Radiography
  - Femur
    - Left BQØ4ZZ1
    - Right BQØ3ZZ1
  - Hip
    - Left BQØ1ZZ1
    - Right BQØØZZ1
  - Spine
    - Cervical BRØØZZ1
    - Lumbar BRØ9ZZ1
    - Thoracic BRØ7ZZ1
    - Whole BRØGZZ1
- Ultrasonography
  - Elbow
    - Left BP4HZZ1
    - Right BP4GZZ1
  - Hand
    - Left BP4PZZ1
    - Right BP4NZZ1
  - Shoulder
    - Left BP49ZZ1
    - Right BP48ZZ1
  - Wrist
    - Left BP4MZZ1
    - Right BP4LZZ1

Denticulate (dentate) ligament *use* Spinal Meninges
Depressor anguli oris muscle *use* Facial Muscle
Depressor labii inferioris muscle *use* Facial Muscle
Depressor septi nasi muscle *use* Facial Muscle
Depressor supercilii muscle *use* Facial Muscle
Dermabrasion *see* Extraction, Skin and Breast ØHD
Dermis *use* Skin
Descending genicular artery
- *use* Femoral Artery, Left
- *use* Femoral Artery, Right

Destruction
- Acetabulum
  - Left ØQ55
  - Right ØQ54
- Adenoids ØC5Q
- Ampulla of Vater ØF5C
- Anal Sphincter ØD5R
- Anterior Chamber
  - Left Ø8533ZZ
  - Right Ø8523ZZ
- Anus ØD5Q
- Aorta
  - Abdominal
  - Thoracic
    - Ascending/Arch Ø25X
    - Descending Ø25W

Destruction — *continued*
- Aortic Body ØG5D
- Appendix ØD5J
- Artery
  - Anterior Tibial
    - Left Ø45Q
    - Right Ø45P
  - Axillary
    - Left Ø356
    - Right Ø355
  - Brachial
    - Left Ø358
    - Right Ø357
  - Celiac Ø451
  - Colic
    - Left Ø457
    - Middle Ø458
    - Right Ø456
  - Common Carotid
    - Left Ø35J
    - Right Ø35H
  - Common Iliac
    - Left Ø45D
    - Right Ø45C
  - External Carotid
    - Left Ø35N
    - Right Ø35M
  - External Iliac
    - Left Ø45J
    - Right Ø45H
  - Face Ø35R
  - Femoral
    - Left Ø45L
    - Right Ø45K
  - Foot
    - Left Ø45W
    - Right Ø45V
  - Gastric Ø452
  - Hand
    - Left Ø35F
    - Right Ø35D
  - Hepatic Ø453
  - Inferior Mesenteric Ø45B
  - Innominate Ø352
  - Internal Carotid
    - Left Ø35L
    - Right Ø35K
  - Internal Iliac
    - Left Ø45F
    - Right Ø45E
  - Internal Mammary
    - Left Ø351
    - Right Ø35Ø
  - Intracranial Ø35G
  - Lower Ø45Y
  - Peroneal
    - Left Ø45U
    - Right Ø45T
  - Popliteal
    - Left Ø45N
    - Right Ø45M
  - Posterior Tibial
    - Left Ø45S
    - Right Ø45R
  - Pulmonary
    - Left Ø25R
    - Right Ø25Q
  - Pulmonary Trunk Ø25P
  - Radial
    - Left Ø35C
    - Right Ø35B
  - Renal
    - Left Ø45A
    - Right Ø459
  - Splenic Ø454
  - Subclavian
    - Left Ø354
    - Right Ø353
  - Superior Mesenteric Ø455
  - Temporal
    - Left Ø35T
    - Right Ø35S
  - Thyroid
    - Left Ø35V
    - Right Ø35U
  - Ulnar
    - Left Ø35A
    - Right Ø359
  - Upper Ø35Y

Subterms under main terms may continue to next column or page

Destruction — *continued*
Artery — *continued*
Vertebral
Left Ø35Q
Right Ø35P
Atrium
Left Ø257
Right Ø256
Auditory Ossicle
Left Ø95A
Right Ø959
Basal Ganglia Ø058
Bladder ØT5B
Bladder Neck ØT5C
Bone
Ethmoid
Left ØN5G
Right ØN5F
Frontal ØN51
Hyoid ØN5X
Lacrimal
Left ØN5J
Right ØN5H
Nasal ØN5B
Occipital ØN57
Palatine
Left ØN5L
Right ØN5K
Parietal
Left ØN54
Right ØN53
Pelvic
Left ØQ53
Right ØQ52
Sphenoid ØN5C
Temporal
Left ØN56
Right ØN55
Zygomatic
Left ØN5N
Right ØN5M
Brain Ø05Ø
Breast
Bilateral ØH5V
Left ØH5U
Right ØH5T
Bronchus
Lingula ØB59
Lower Lobe
Left ØB5B
Right ØB56
Main
Left ØB57
Right ØB53
Middle Lobe, Right ØB55
Upper Lobe
Left ØB58
Right ØB54
Buccal Mucosa ØC54
Bursa and Ligament
Abdomen
Left ØM5J
Right ØM5H
Ankle
Left ØM5R
Right ØM5Q
Elbow
Left ØM54
Right ØM53
Foot
Left ØM5T
Right ØM5S
Hand
Left ØM58
Right ØM57
Head and Neck ØM5Ø
Hip
Left ØM5M
Right ØM5L
Knee
Left ØM5P
Right ØM5N
Lower Extremity
Left ØM5W
Right ØM5V
Perineum ØM5K
Rib(s) ØM5G
Shoulder
Left ØM52

Destruction — *continued*
Bursa and Ligament — *continued*
Shoulder — *continued*
Right ØM51
Spine
Lower ØM5D
Upper ØM5C
Sternum ØM5F
Upper Extremity
Left ØM5B
Right ØM59
Wrist
Left ØM56
Right ØM55
Carina ØB52
Carotid Bodies, Bilateral ØG58
Carotid Body
Left ØG56
Right ØG57
Carpal
Left ØP5N
Right ØP5M
Cecum ØD5H
Cerebellum Ø05C
Cerebral Hemisphere Ø057
Cerebral Meninges Ø051
Cerebral Ventricle Ø056
Cervix ØU5C
Chordae Tendineae Ø259
Choroid
Left Ø85B
Right Ø85A
Cisterna Chyli Ø75L
Clavicle
Left ØP5B
Right ØP59
Clitoris ØU5J
Coccygeal Glomus ØG5B
Coccyx ØQ5S
Colon
Ascending ØD5K
Descending ØD5M
Sigmoid ØD5N
Transverse ØD5L
Conduction Mechanism Ø258
Conjunctiva
Left Ø85TXZZ
Right Ø85SXZZ
Cord
Bilateral ØV5H
Left ØV5G
Right ØV5F
Cornea
Left Ø859XZZ
Right Ø858XZZ
Cul-de-sac ØU5F
Diaphragm ØB5T
Disc
Cervical Vertebral ØR53
Cervicothoracic Vertebral ØR55
Lumbar Vertebral ØS52
Lumbosacral ØS54
Thoracic Vertebral ØR59
Thoracolumbar Vertebral ØR5B
Duct
Common Bile ØF59
Cystic ØF58
Hepatic
Common ØF57
Left ØF56
Right ØF55
Lacrimal
Left Ø85Y
Right Ø85X
Pancreatic ØF5D
Accessory ØF5F
Parotid
Left ØC5C
Right ØC5B
Duodenum ØD59
Dura Mater Ø052
Ear
External
Left Ø951
Right Ø95Ø
External Auditory Canal
Left Ø954
Right Ø953

Destruction — *continued*
Ear — *continued*
Inner
Left Ø95E
Right Ø95D
Middle
Left Ø956
Right Ø955
Endometrium ØU5B
Epididymis
Bilateral ØV5L
Left ØV5K
Right ØV5J
Epiglottis ØC5R
Esophagogastric Junction ØD54
Esophagus ØD55
Lower ØD53
Middle ØD52
Upper ØD51
Eustachian Tube
Left Ø95G
Right Ø95F
Eye
Left Ø851XZZ
Right Ø85ØXZZ
Eyelid
Lower
Left Ø85R
Right Ø85Q
Upper
Left Ø85P
Right Ø85N
Fallopian Tube
Left ØU56
Right ØU55
Fallopian Tubes, Bilateral ØU57
Femoral Shaft
Left ØQ59
Right ØQ58
Femur
Lower
Left ØQ5C
Right ØQ5B
Upper
Left ØQ57
Right ØQ56
Fibula
Left ØQ5K
Right ØQ5J
Finger Nail ØH5QXZZ
Gallbladder ØF54
Gingiva
Lower ØC56
Upper ØC55
Gland
Adrenal
Bilateral ØG54
Left ØG52
Right ØG53
Lacrimal
Left Ø85W
Right Ø85V
Minor Salivary ØC5J
Parotid
Left ØC59
Right ØC58
Pituitary ØG5Ø
Sublingual
Left ØC5F
Right ØC5D
Submaxillary
Left ØC5H
Right ØC5G
Vestibular ØU5L
Glenoid Cavity
Left ØP58
Right ØP57
Glomus Jugulare ØG5C
Humeral Head
Left ØP5D
Right ØP5C
Humeral Shaft
Left ØP5G
Right ØP5F
Hymen ØU5K
Hypothalamus Ø05A
Ileocecal Valve ØD5C
Ileum ØD5B

- Destruction — *continued*
  - Intestine
    - Large ØD5E
      - Left ØD5G
      - Right ØD5F
    - Small ØD58
  - Iris
    - Left Ø85D3ZZ
    - Right Ø85C3ZZ
  - Jejunum ØD5A
  - Joint
    - Acromioclavicular
      - Left ØR5H
      - Right ØR5G
    - Ankle
      - Left ØS5G
      - Right ØS5F
    - Carpal
      - Left ØR5R
      - Right ØR5Q
    - Carpometacarpal
      - Left ØR5T
      - Right ØR5S
    - Cervical Vertebral ØR51
    - Cervicothoracic Vertebral ØR54
    - Coccygeal ØS56
    - Elbow
      - Left ØR5M
      - Right ØR5L
    - Finger Phalangeal
      - Left ØR5X
      - Right ØR5W
    - Hip
      - Left ØS5B
      - Right ØS59
    - Knee
      - Left ØS5D
      - Right ØS5C
    - Lumbar Vertebral ØS5Ø
    - Lumbosacral ØS53
    - Metacarpophalangeal
      - Left ØR5V
      - Right ØR5U
    - Metatarsal-Phalangeal
      - Left ØS5N
      - Right ØS5M
    - Occipital-cervical ØR5Ø
    - Sacrococcygeal ØS55
    - Sacroiliac
      - Left ØS58
      - Right ØS57
    - Shoulder
      - Left ØR5K
      - Right ØR5J
    - Sternoclavicular
      - Left ØR5F
      - Right ØR5E
    - Tarsal
      - Left ØS5J
      - Right ØS5H
    - Tarsometatarsal
      - Left ØS5L
      - Right ØS5K
    - Temporomandibular
      - Left ØR5D
      - Right ØR5C
    - Thoracic Vertebral ØR56
    - Thoracolumbar Vertebral ØR5A
    - Toe Phalangeal
      - Left ØS5Q
      - Right ØS5P
    - Wrist
      - Left ØR5P
      - Right ØR5N
  - Kidney
    - Left ØT51
    - Right ØT5Ø
  - Kidney Pelvis
    - Left ØT54
    - Right ØT53
  - Larynx ØC5S
  - Lens
    - Left Ø85K3ZZ
    - Right Ø85J3ZZ
  - Lip
    - Lower ØC51
    - Upper ØC5Ø
  - Liver ØF5Ø
    - Left Lobe ØF52

- Destruction — *continued*
  - Liver — *continued*
    - Right Lobe ØF51
  - Lung
    - Bilateral ØB5M
    - Left ØB5L
    - Lower Lobe
      - Left ØB5J
      - Right ØB5F
    - Middle Lobe, Right ØB5D
    - Right ØB5K
    - Upper Lobe
      - Left ØB5G
      - Right ØB5C
  - Lung Lingula ØB5H
  - Lymphatic
    - Aortic Ø75D
    - Axillary
      - Left Ø756
      - Right Ø755
    - Head Ø75Ø
    - Inguinal
      - Left Ø75J
      - Right Ø75H
    - Internal Mammary
      - Left Ø759
      - Right Ø758
    - Lower Extremity
      - Left Ø75G
      - Right Ø75F
    - Mesenteric Ø75B
    - Neck
      - Left Ø752
      - Right Ø751
    - Pelvis Ø75C
    - Thoracic Duct Ø75K
    - Thorax Ø757
    - Upper Extremity
      - Left Ø754
      - Right Ø753
  - Mandible
    - Left ØN5V
    - Right ØN5T
  - Maxilla ØN5R
  - Medulla Oblongata ØØ5D
  - Mesentery ØD5V
  - Metacarpal
    - Left ØP5Q
    - Right ØP5P
  - Metatarsal
    - Left ØQ5P
    - Right ØQ5N
  - Muscle
    - Abdomen
      - Left ØK5L
      - Right ØK5K
    - Extraocular
      - Left Ø85M
      - Right Ø85L
    - Facial ØK51
    - Foot
      - Left ØK5W
      - Right ØK5V
    - Hand
      - Left ØK5D
      - Right ØK5C
    - Head ØK5Ø
    - Hip
      - Left ØK5P
      - Right ØK5N
    - Lower Arm and Wrist
      - Left ØK5B
      - Right ØK59
    - Lower Leg
      - Left ØK5T
      - Right ØK5S
    - Neck
      - Left ØK53
      - Right ØK52
    - Papillary Ø25D
    - Perineum ØK5M
    - Shoulder
      - Left ØK56
      - Right ØK55
    - Thorax
      - Left ØK5J
      - Right ØK5H
    - Tongue, Palate, Pharynx ØK54

- Destruction — *continued*
  - Muscle — *continued*
    - Trunk
      - Left ØK5G
      - Right ØK5F
    - Upper Arm
      - Left ØK58
      - Right ØK57
    - Upper Leg
      - Left ØK5R
      - Right ØK5Q
  - Nasal Mucosa and Soft Tissue Ø95K
  - Nasopharynx Ø95N
  - Nerve
    - Abdominal Sympathetic Ø15M
    - Abducens ØØ5L
    - Accessory ØØ5R
    - Acoustic ØØ5N
    - Brachial Plexus Ø153
    - Cervical Ø151
    - Cervical Plexus Ø15Ø
    - Facial ØØ5M
    - Femoral Ø15D
    - Glossopharyngeal ØØ5P
    - Head and Neck Sympathetic Ø15K
    - Hypoglossal ØØ5S
    - Lumbar Ø15B
    - Lumbar Plexus Ø159
    - Lumbar Sympathetic Ø15N
    - Lumbosacral Plexus Ø15A
    - Median Ø155
    - Oculomotor ØØ5H
    - Olfactory ØØ5F
    - Optic ØØ5G
    - Peroneal Ø15H
    - Phrenic Ø152
    - Pudendal Ø15C
    - Radial Ø156
    - Sacral Ø15R
    - Sacral Plexus Ø15Q
    - Sacral Sympathetic Ø15P
    - Sciatic Ø15F
    - Thoracic Ø158
    - Thoracic Sympathetic Ø15L
    - Tibial Ø15G
    - Trigeminal ØØ5K
    - Trochlear ØØ5J
    - Ulnar Ø154
    - Vagus ØØ5Q
  - Nipple
    - Left ØH5X
    - Right ØH5W
  - Omentum ØD5U
  - Orbit
    - Left ØN5Q
    - Right ØN5P
  - Ovary
    - Bilateral ØU52
    - Left ØU51
    - Right ØU5Ø
  - Palate
    - Hard ØC52
    - Soft ØC53
  - Pancreas ØF5G
  - Para-aortic Body ØG59
  - Paraganglion Extremity ØG5F
  - Parathyroid Gland ØG5R
    - Inferior
      - Left ØG5P
      - Right ØG5N
    - Multiple ØG5Q
    - Superior
      - Left ØG5M
      - Right ØG5L
  - Patella
    - Left ØQ5F
    - Right ØQ5D
  - Penis ØV5S
  - Pericardium Ø25N
  - Peritoneum ØD5W
  - Phalanx
    - Finger
      - Left ØP5V
      - Right ØP5T
    - Thumb
      - Left ØP5S
      - Right ØP5R
    - Toe
      - Left ØQ5R

Destruction — *continued*
- Phalanx — *continued*
  - Toe — *continued*
    - Right ØQ5Q
- Pharynx ØC5M
- Pineal Body ØG51
- Pleura
  - Left ØB5P
  - Right ØB5N
- Pons ØØ5B
- Prepuce ØV5T
- Prostate ØV5Ø
  - Robotic Waterjet Ablation XV5Ø8A4
- Radius
  - Left ØP5J
  - Right ØP5H
- Rectum ØD5P
- Retina
  - Left Ø85F3ZZ
  - Right Ø85E3ZZ
- Retinal Vessel
  - Left Ø85H3ZZ
  - Right Ø85G3ZZ
- Ribs
  - 1 to 2 ØP51
  - 3 or More ØP52
- Sacrum ØQ51
- Scapula
  - Left ØP56
  - Right ØP55
- Sclera
  - Left Ø857XZZ
  - Right Ø856XZZ
- Scrotum ØV55
- Septum
  - Atrial Ø255
  - Nasal Ø95M
  - Ventricular Ø25M
- Sinus
  - Accessory Ø95P
  - Ethmoid
    - Left Ø95V
    - Right Ø95U
  - Frontal
    - Left Ø95T
    - Right Ø95S
  - Mastoid
    - Left Ø95C
    - Right Ø95B
  - Maxillary
    - Left Ø95R
    - Right Ø95Q
  - Sphenoid
    - Left Ø95X
    - Right Ø95W
- Skin
  - Abdomen ØH57XZ
  - Back ØH56XZ
  - Buttock ØH58XZ
  - Chest ØH55XZ
  - Ear
    - Left ØH53XZ
    - Right ØH52XZ
  - Face ØH51XZ
  - Foot
    - Left ØH5NXZ
    - Right ØH5MXZ
  - Hand
    - Left ØH5GXZ
    - Right ØH5FXZ
  - Inguinal ØH5AXZ
  - Lower Arm
    - Left ØH5EXZ
    - Right ØH5DXZ
  - Lower Leg
    - Left ØH5LXZ
    - Right ØH5KXZ
  - Neck ØH54XZ
  - Perineum ØH59XZ
  - Scalp ØH5ØXZ
  - Upper Arm
    - Left ØH5CXZ
    - Right ØH5BXZ
  - Upper Leg
    - Left ØH5JXZ
    - Right ØH5HXZ
- Skull ØN5Ø
- Spinal Cord
  - Cervical ØØ5W

Destruction — *continued*
- Spinal Cord — *continued*
  - Lumbar ØØ5Y
  - Thoracic ØØ5X
- Spinal Meninges ØØ5T
- Spleen Ø75P
- Sternum ØP5Ø
- Stomach ØD56
  - Pylorus ØD57
- Subcutaneous Tissue and Fascia
  - Abdomen ØJ58
  - Back ØJ57
  - Buttock ØJ59
  - Chest ØJ56
  - Face ØJ51
  - Foot
    - Left ØJ5R
    - Right ØJ5Q
  - Hand
    - Left ØJ5K
    - Right ØJ5J
  - Lower Arm
    - Left ØJ5H
    - Right ØJ5G
  - Lower Leg
    - Left ØJ5P
    - Right ØJ5N
  - Neck
    - Left ØJ55
    - Right ØJ54
  - Pelvic Region ØJ5C
  - Perineum ØJ5B
  - Scalp ØJ5Ø
  - Upper Arm
    - Left ØJ5F
    - Right ØJ5D
  - Upper Leg
    - Left ØJ5M
    - Right ØJ5L
- Tarsal
  - Left ØQ5M
  - Right ØQ5L
- Tendon
  - Abdomen
    - Left ØL5G
    - Right ØL5F
  - Ankle
    - Left ØL5T
    - Right ØL5S
  - Foot
    - Left ØL5W
    - Right ØL5V
  - Hand
    - Left ØL58
    - Right ØL57
  - Head and Neck ØL5Ø
  - Hip
    - Left ØL5K
    - Right ØL5J
  - Knee
    - Left ØL5R
    - Right ØL5Q
  - Lower Arm and Wrist
    - Left ØL56
    - Right ØL55
  - Lower Leg
    - Left ØL5P
    - Right ØL5N
  - Perineum ØL5H
  - Shoulder
    - Left ØL52
    - Right ØL51
  - Thorax
    - Left ØL5D
    - Right ØL5C
  - Trunk
    - Left ØL5B
    - Right ØL59
  - Upper Arm
    - Left ØL54
    - Right ØL53
  - Upper Leg
    - Left ØL5M
    - Right ØL5L
- Testis
  - Bilateral ØV5C
  - Left ØV5B
  - Right ØV59
- Thalamus ØØ59

Destruction — *continued*
- Thymus Ø75M
- Thyroid Gland ØG5K
  - Left Lobe ØG5G
  - Right Lobe ØG5H
- Tibia
  - Left ØQ5H
  - Right ØQ5G
- Toe Nail ØH5RXZZ
- Tongue ØC57
- Tonsils ØC5P
- Tooth
  - Lower ØC5X
  - Upper ØC5W
- Trachea ØB51
- Tunica Vaginalis
  - Left ØV57
  - Right ØV56
- Turbinate, Nasal Ø95L
- Tympanic Membrane
  - Left Ø958
  - Right Ø957
- Ulna
  - Left ØP5L
  - Right ØP5K
- Ureter
  - Left ØT57
  - Right ØT56
- Urethra ØT5D
- Uterine Supporting Structure ØU54
- Uterus ØU59
- Uvula ØC5N
- Vagina ØU5G
- Valve
  - Aortic Ø25F
  - Mitral Ø25G
  - Pulmonary Ø25H
  - Tricuspid Ø25J
- Vas Deferens
  - Bilateral ØV5Q
  - Left ØV5P
  - Right ØV5N
- Vein
  - Axillary
    - Left Ø558
    - Right Ø557
  - Azygos Ø55Ø
  - Basilic
    - Left Ø55C
    - Right Ø55B
  - Brachial
    - Left Ø55A
    - Right Ø559
  - Cephalic
    - Left Ø55F
    - Right Ø55D
  - Colic Ø657
  - Common Iliac
    - Left Ø65D
    - Right Ø65C
  - Coronary Ø254
  - Esophageal Ø653
  - External Iliac
    - Left Ø65G
    - Right Ø65F
  - External Jugular
    - Left Ø55Q
    - Right Ø55P
  - Face
    - Left Ø55V
    - Right Ø55T
  - Femoral
    - Left Ø65N
    - Right Ø65M
  - Foot
    - Left Ø65V
    - Right Ø65T
  - Gastric Ø652
  - Hand
    - Left Ø55H
    - Right Ø55G
  - Hemiazygos Ø551
  - Hepatic Ø654
  - Hypogastric
    - Left Ø65J
    - Right Ø65H
  - Inferior Mesenteric Ø656
  - Innominate
    - Left Ø554

Index

Destruction — Destruction

Destruction — *continued*
Vein — *continued*
Innominate — *continued*
Right Ø553
Internal Jugular
Left Ø55N
Right Ø55M
Intracranial Ø55L
Lower Ø65Y
Portal Ø658
Pulmonary
Left Ø25T
Right Ø25S
Renal
Left Ø65B
Right Ø659
Saphenous
Left Ø65Q
Right Ø65P
Splenic Ø651
Subclavian
Left Ø556
Right Ø555
Superior Mesenteric Ø655
Upper Ø55Y
Vertebral
Left Ø55S
Right Ø55R
Vena Cava
Inferior Ø65Ø
Superior Ø25V
Ventricle
Left Ø25L
Right Ø25K
Vertebra
Cervical ØP53
Lumbar ØQ5Ø
Thoracic ØP54
Vesicle
Bilateral ØV53
Left ØV52
Right ØV51
Vitreous
Left Ø8553ZZ
Right Ø8543ZZ
Vocal Cord
Left ØC5V
Right ØC5T
Vulva ØU5M
Detachment
Arm
Lower
Left ØX6FØZ
Right ØX6DØZ
Upper
Left ØX69ØZ
Right ØX68ØZ
Elbow Region
Left ØX6CØZZ
Right ØX6BØZZ
Femoral Region
Left ØY68ØZZ
Right ØY67ØZZ
Finger
Index
Left ØX6PØZ
Right ØX6NØZ
Little
Left ØX6WØZ
Right ØX6VØZ
Middle
Left ØX6RØZ
Right ØX6QØZ
Ring
Left ØX6TØZ
Right ØX6SØZ
Foot
Left ØY6NØZ
Right ØY6MØZ
Forequarter
Left ØX61ØZZ
Right ØX6ØØZZ
Hand
Left ØX6KØZ
Right ØX6JØZ
Hindquarter
Bilateral ØY64ØZZ
Left ØY63ØZZ
Right ØY62ØZZ
Detachment — *continued*
Knee Region
Left ØY6GØZZ
Right ØY6FØZZ
Leg
Lower
Left ØY6JØZ
Right ØY6HØZ
Upper
Left ØY6DØZ
Right ØY6CØZ
Shoulder Region
Left ØX63ØZZ
Right ØX62ØZZ
Thumb
Left ØX6MØZ
Right ØX6LØZ
Toe
1st
Left ØY6QØZ
Right ØY6PØZ
2nd
Left ØY6SØZ
Right ØY6RØZ
3rd
Left ØY6UØZ
Right ØY6TØZ
4th
Left ØY6WØZ
Right ØY6VØZ
5th
Left ØY6YØZ
Right ØY6XØZ
Determination, Mental status GZ14ZZZ
Detorsion
see Release
see Reposition
Detoxification Services, for substance abuse HZ2ZZZZ
Device Fitting FØDZ
Diagnostic Audiology *see* Audiology, Diagnostic
Diagnostic imaging *see* Imaging, Diagnostic
Diagnostic radiology *see* Imaging, Diagnostic
Dialysis
Hemodialysis *see* Performance, Urinary 5A1D
Peritoneal 3E1M39Z
Diaphragma sellae *use* Dura Mater
Diaphragmatic pacemaker generator *use* Stimulator Generator in Subcutaneous Tissue and Fascia
Diaphragmatic Pacemaker Lead
Insertion of device in, Diaphragm ØBHT
Removal of device from, Diaphragm ØBPT
Revision of device in, Diaphragm ØBWT
Digital radiography, plain *see* Plain Radiography
Dilation
Ampulla of Vater ØF7C
Anus ØD7Q
Aorta
Abdominal
Thoracic
Ascending/Arch Ø27X
Descending Ø27W
Artery
Anterior Tibial
Left Ø47Q
Sustained Release Drug-eluting Intraluminal Device X27Q385
Four or More X27Q3C5
Three X27Q3B5
Two X27Q395
Right Ø47P
Sustained Release Drug-eluting Intraluminal Device X27P385
Four or More X27P3C5
Three X27P3B5
Two X27P395
Axillary
Left Ø376
Right Ø375
Brachial
Left Ø378
Right Ø377
Celiac Ø471
Colic
Left Ø477
Middle Ø478
Dilation — *continued*
Artery — *continued*
Colic — *continued*
Right Ø476
Common Carotid
Left Ø37J
Right Ø37H
Common Iliac
Left Ø47D
Right Ø47C
Coronary
Four or More Arteries Ø273
One Artery Ø27Ø
Three Arteries Ø272
Two Arteries Ø271
External Carotid
Left Ø37N
Right Ø37M
External Iliac
Left Ø47J
Right Ø47H
Face Ø37R
Femoral
Left Ø47L
Sustained Release Drug-eluting Intraluminal Device X27J385
Four or More X27J3C5
Three X27J3B5
Two X27J395
Right Ø47K
Sustained Release Drug-eluting Intraluminal Device X27H385
Four or More X27H3C5
Three X27H3B5
Two X27H395
Foot
Left Ø47W
Right Ø47V
Gastric Ø472
Hand
Left Ø37F
Right Ø37D
Hepatic Ø473
Inferior Mesenteric Ø47B
Innominate Ø372
Internal Carotid
Left Ø37L
Right Ø37K
Internal Iliac
Left Ø47F
Right Ø47E
Internal Mammary
Left Ø371
Right Ø37Ø
Intracranial Ø37G
Lower Ø47Y
Peroneal
Left Ø47U
Sustained Release Drug-eluting Intraluminal Device X27U385
Four or More X27U3C5
Three X27U3B5
Two X27U395
Right Ø47T
Sustained Release Drug-eluting Intraluminal Device X27T385
Four or More X27T3C5
Three X27T3B5
Two X27T395
Popliteal
Left Ø47N
Left Distal
Sustained Release Drug-eluting Intraluminal Device X27N385
Four or More X27N3C5
Three X27N3B5
Two X27N395
Left Proximal
Sustained Release Drug-eluting Intraluminal Device X27L385
Four or More X27L3C5
Three X27L3B5
Two X27L395

- **Dilation** — *continued*
  - Artery — *continued*
    - Popliteal — *continued*
      - Right Ø47M
      - Right Distal
        - Sustained Release Drug-eluting Intraluminal Device X27M385
          - Four or More X27M3C5
          - Three X27M3B5
          - Two X27M395
      - Right Proximal
        - Sustained Release Drug-eluting Intraluminal Device X27K385
          - Four or More X27K3C5
          - Three X27K3B5
          - Two X27K395
    - Posterior Tibial
      - Left Ø47S
        - Sustained Release Drug-eluting Intraluminal Device X27S385
          - Four or More X27S3C5
          - Three X27S3B5
          - Two X27S395
      - Right Ø47R
        - Sustained Release Drug-eluting Intraluminal Device X27R385
          - Four or More X27R3C5
          - Three X27R3B5
          - Two X27R395
    - Pulmonary
      - Left Ø27R
      - Right Ø27Q
    - Pulmonary Trunk Ø27P
    - Radial
      - Left Ø37C
      - Right Ø37B
    - Renal
      - Left Ø47A
      - Right Ø479
    - Splenic Ø474
    - Subclavian
      - Left Ø374
      - Right Ø373
    - Superior Mesenterlc Ø475
    - Temporal
      - Left Ø37T
      - Right Ø37S
    - Thyroid
      - Left Ø37V
      - Right Ø37U
    - Ulnar
      - Left Ø37A
      - Right Ø379
    - Upper Ø37Y
    - Vertebral
      - Left Ø37Q
      - Right Ø37P
  - Bladder ØT7B
  - Bladder Neck ØT7C
  - Bronchus
    - Lingula ØB79
    - Lower Lobe
      - Left ØB7B
      - Right ØB76
    - Main
      - Left ØB77
      - Right ØB73
    - Middle Lobe, Right ØB75
    - Upper Lobe
      - Left ØB78
      - Right ØB74
  - Carina ØB72
  - Cecum ØD7H
  - Cerebral Ventricle ØØ76
  - Cervix ØU7C
  - Colon
    - Ascending ØD7K
    - Descending ØD7M
    - Sigmoid ØD7N
    - Transverse ØD7L
  - Duct
    - Common Bile ØF79
    - Cystic ØF78
    - Hepatic
      - Common ØF77

- **Dilation** — *continued*
  - Duct — *continued*
    - Hepatic — *continued*
      - Left ØF76
      - Right ØF75
    - Lacrimal
      - Left Ø87Y
      - Right Ø87X
    - Pancreatic ØF7D
      - Accessory ØF7F
    - Parotid
      - Left ØC7C
      - Right ØC7B
  - Duodenum ØD79
  - Esophagogastric Junction ØD74
  - Esophagus ØD75
    - Lower ØD73
    - Middle ØD72
    - Upper ØD71
  - Eustachian Tube
    - Left Ø97G
    - Right Ø97F
  - Fallopian Tube
    - Left ØU76
    - Right ØU75
  - Fallopian Tubes, Bilateral ØU77
  - Hymen ØU7K
  - Ileocecal Valve ØD7C
  - Ileum ØD7B
  - Intestine
    - Large ØD7E
      - Left ØD7G
      - Right ØD7F
    - Small ØD78
  - Jejunum ØD7A
  - Kidney Pelvis
    - Left ØT74
    - Right ØT73
  - Larynx ØC7S
  - Pharynx ØC7M
  - Rectum ØD7P
  - Stomach ØD76
    - Pylorus ØD77
  - Trachea ØB71
  - Ureter
    - Left ØT77
    - Right ØT76
  - Ureters, Bilateral ØT78
  - Urethra ØT7D
  - Uterus ØU79
  - Vagina ØU7G
  - Valve
    - Aortic Ø27F
    - Mitral Ø27G
    - Pulmonary Ø27H
    - Tricuspid Ø27J
  - Vas Deferens
    - Bilateral ØV7Q
    - Left ØV7P
    - Right ØV7N
  - Vein
    - Axillary
      - Left Ø578
      - Right Ø577
    - Azygos Ø57Ø
    - Basilic
      - Left Ø57C
      - Right Ø57B
    - Brachial
      - Left Ø57A
      - Right Ø579
    - Cephalic
      - Left Ø57F
      - Right Ø57D
    - Colic Ø677
    - Common Iliac
      - Left Ø67D
      - Right Ø67C
    - Esophageal Ø673
    - External Iliac
      - Left Ø67G
      - Right Ø67F
    - External Jugular
      - Left Ø57Q
      - Right Ø57P
    - Face
      - Left Ø57V
      - Right Ø57T

- **Dilation** — *continued*
  - Vein — *continued*
    - Femoral
      - Left Ø67N
      - Right Ø67M
    - Foot
      - Left Ø67V
      - Right Ø67T
    - Gastric Ø672
    - Hand
      - Left Ø57H
      - Right Ø57G
    - Hemiazygos Ø571
    - Hepatic Ø674
    - Hypogastric
      - Left Ø67J
      - Right Ø67H
    - Inferior Mesenteric Ø676
    - Innominate
      - Left Ø574
      - Right Ø573
    - Internal Jugular
      - Left Ø57N
      - Right Ø57M
    - Intracranial Ø57L
    - Lower Ø67Y
    - Portal Ø678
    - Pulmonary
      - Left Ø27T
      - Right Ø27S
    - Renal
      - Left Ø67B
      - Right Ø679
    - Saphenous
      - Left Ø67Q
      - Right Ø67P
    - Splenic Ø671
    - Subclavian
      - Left Ø576
      - Right Ø575
    - Superior Mesenteric Ø675
    - Upper Ø57Y
    - Vertebral
      - Left Ø57S
      - Right Ø57R
  - Vena Cava
    - Inferior Ø67Ø
    - Superior Ø27V
  - Ventricle
    - Left Ø27L
    - Right Ø27K
- **Direct Lateral Interbody Fusion (DLIF) device** *use* Interbody Fusion Device in Lower Joints
- **Disarticulation** *see* Detachment
- **Discectomy, diskectomy**
  - *see* Excision, Lower Joints ØSB
  - *see* Excision, Upper Joints ØRB
  - *see* Resection, Lower Joints ØST
  - *see* Resection, Upper Joints ØRT
- **Discography**
  - *see* Fluoroscopy, Axial Skeleton, Except Skull and Facial Bones BR1
  - *see* Plain Radiography, Axial Skeleton, Except Skull and Facial Bones BRØ
- **Dismembered pyeloplasty** *see* Repair, Kidney Pelvis
- **Distal humerus**
  - *use* Humeral Shaft, Left
  - *use* Humeral Shaft, Right
- **Distal humerus, involving joint**
  - *use* Elbow Joint, Left
  - *use* Elbow Joint, Right
- **Distal radioulnar joint**
  - *use* Wrist Joint, Left
  - *use* Wrist Joint, Right
- **Diversion** *see* Bypass
- **Diverticulectomy** *see* Excision, Gastrointestinal System ØDB
- **Division**
  - Acetabulum
    - Left ØQ85
    - Right ØQ84
  - Anal Sphincter ØD8R
  - Basal Ganglia ØØ88
  - Bladder Neck ØT8C
  - Bone
    - Ethmoid
      - Left ØN8G
      - Right ØN8F

Division — *continued*
Bone — *continued*
Frontal ØN81
Hyoid ØN8X
Lacrimal
Left ØN8J
Right ØN8H
Nasal ØN8B
Occipital ØN87
Palatine
Left ØN8L
Right ØN8K
Parietal
Left ØN84
Right ØN83
Pelvic
Left ØQ83
Right ØQ82
Sphenoid ØN8C
Temporal
Left ØN86
Right ØN85
Zygomatic
Left ØN8N
Right ØN8M
Brain ØØ8Ø
Bursa and Ligament
Abdomen
Left ØM8J
Right ØM8H
Ankle
Left ØM8R
Right ØM8Q
Elbow
Left ØM84
Right ØM83
Foot
Left ØM8T
Right ØM8S
Hand
Left ØM88
Right ØM87
Head and Neck ØM8Ø
Hip
Left ØM8M
Right ØM8L
Knee
Left ØM8P
Right ØM8N
Lower Extremity
Left ØM8W
Right ØM8V
Perineum ØM8K
Rib(s) ØM8G
Shoulder
Left ØM82
Right ØM81
Spine
Lower ØM8D
Upper ØM8C
Sternum ØM8F
Upper Extremity
Left ØM8B
Right ØM89
Wrist
Left ØM86
Right ØM85
Carpal
Left ØP8N
Right ØP8M
Cerebral Hemisphere ØØ87
Chordae Tendineae Ø289
Clavicle
Left ØP8B
Right ØP89
Coccyx ØQ8S
Conduction Mechanism Ø288
Esophagogastric Junction ØD84
Femoral Shaft
Left ØQ89
Right ØQ88
Femur
Lower
Left ØQ8C
Right ØQ8B
Upper
Left ØQ87
Right ØQ86

Division — *continued*
Fibula
Left ØQ8K
Right ØQ8J
Gland, Pituitary ØG8Ø
Glenoid Cavity
Left ØP88
Right ØP87
Humeral Head
Left ØP8D
Right ØP8C
Humeral Shaft
Left ØP8G
Right ØP8F
Hymen ØU8K
Kidneys, Bilateral ØT82
Mandible
Left ØN8V
Right ØN8T
Maxilla ØN8R
Metacarpal
Left ØP8Q
Right ØP8P
Metatarsal
Left ØQ8P
Right ØQ8N
Muscle
Abdomen
Left ØK8L
Right ØK8K
Facial ØK81
Foot
Left ØK8W
Right ØK8V
Hand
Left ØK8D
Right ØK8C
Head ØK8Ø
Hip
Left ØK8P
Right ØK8N
Lower Arm and Wrist
Left ØK8B
Right ØK89
Lower Leg
Left ØK8T
Right ØK8S
Neck
Left ØK83
Right ØK82
Papillary Ø28D
Perineum ØK8M
Shoulder
Left ØK86
Right ØK85
Thorax
Left ØK8J
Right ØK8H
Tongue, Palate, Pharynx ØK84
Trunk
Left ØK8G
Right ØK8F
Upper Arm
Left ØK88
Right ØK87
Upper Leg
Left ØK8R
Right ØK8Q
Nerve
Abdominal Sympathetic Ø18M
Abducens ØØ8L
Accessory ØØ8R
Acoustic ØØ8N
Brachial Plexus Ø183
Cervical Ø181
Cervical Plexus Ø18Ø
Facial ØØ8M
Femoral Ø18D
Glossopharyngeal ØØ8P
Head and Neck Sympathetic Ø18K
Hypoglossal ØØ8S
Lumbar Ø18B
Lumbar Plexus Ø189
Lumbar Sympathetic Ø18N
Lumbosacral Plexus Ø18A
Median Ø185
Oculomotor ØØ8H
Olfactory ØØ8F
Optic ØØ8G

Division — *continued*
Nerve — *continued*
Peroneal Ø18H
Phrenic Ø182
Pudendal Ø18C
Radial Ø186
Sacral Ø18R
Sacral Plexus Ø18Q
Sacral Sympathetic Ø18P
Sciatic Ø18F
Thoracic Ø188
Thoracic Sympathetic Ø18L
Tibial Ø18G
Trigeminal ØØ8K
Trochlear ØØ8J
Ulnar Ø184
Vagus ØØ8Q
Orbit
Left ØN8Q
Right ØN8P
Ovary
Bilateral ØU82
Left ØU81
Right ØU8Ø
Pancreas ØF8G
Patella
Left ØQ8F
Right ØQ8D
Perineum, Female ØW8NXZZ
Phalanx
Finger
Left ØP8V
Right ØP8T
Thumb
Left ØP8S
Right ØP8R
Toe
Left ØQ8R
Right ØQ8Q
Radius
Left ØP8J
Right ØP8H
Ribs
1 to 2 ØP81
3 or More ØP82
Sacrum ØQ81
Scapula
Left ØP86
Right ØP85
Skin
Abdomen ØH87XZZ
Back ØH86XZZ
Buttock ØH88XZZ
Chest ØH85XZZ
Ear
Left ØH83XZZ
Right ØH82XZZ
Face ØH81XZZ
Foot
Left ØH8NXZZ
Right ØH8MXZZ
Hand
Left ØH8GXZZ
Right ØH8FXZZ
Inguinal ØH8AXZZ
Lower Arm
Left ØH8EXZZ
Right ØH8DXZZ
Lower Leg
Left ØH8LXZZ
Right ØH8KXZZ
Neck ØH84XZZ
Perineum ØH89XZZ
Scalp ØH8ØXZZ
Upper Arm
Left ØH8CXZZ
Right ØH8BXZZ
Upper Leg
Left ØH8JXZZ
Right ØH8HXZZ
Skull ØN8Ø
Spinal Cord
Cervical ØØ8W
Lumbar ØØ8Y
Thoracic ØØ8X
Sternum ØP8Ø
Stomach, Pylorus ØD87
Subcutaneous Tissue and Fascia
Abdomen ØJ88

Division — *continued*
Subcutaneous Tissue and Fascia — *continued*
Back ØJ87
Buttock ØJ89
Chest ØJ86
Face ØJ81
Foot
Left ØJ8R
Right ØJ8Q
Hand
Left ØJ8K
Right ØJ8J
Head and Neck ØJ8S
Lower Arm
Left ØJ8H
Right ØJ8G
Lower Extremity ØJ8W
Lower Leg
Left ØJ8P
Right ØJ8N
Neck
Left ØJ85
Right ØJ84
Pelvic Region ØJ8C
Perineum ØJ8B
Scalp ØJ8Ø
Trunk ØJ8T
Upper Arm
Left ØJ8F
Right ØJ8D
Upper Extremity ØJ8V
Upper Leg
Left ØJ8M
Right ØJ8L
Tarsal
Left ØQ8M
Right ØQ8L
Tendon
Abdomen
Left ØL8G
Right ØL8F
Ankle
Left ØL8T
Right ØL8S
Foot
Left ØL8W
Right ØL8V
Hand
Left ØL88
Right ØL87
Head and Neck ØL8Ø
Hip
Left ØL8K
Right ØL8J
Knee
Left ØL8R
Right ØL8Q
Lower Arm and Wrist
Left ØL86
Right ØL85
Lower Leg
Left ØL8P
Right ØL8N
Perineum ØL8H
Shoulder
Left ØL82
Right ØL81
Thorax
Left ØL8D
Right ØL8C
Trunk
Left ØL8B
Right ØL89
Upper Arm
Left ØL84
Right ØL83
Upper Leg
Left ØL8M
Right ØL8L
Thyroid Gland Isthmus ØG8J
Tibia
Left ØQ8H
Right ØQ8G
Turbinate, Nasal Ø98L
Ulna
Left ØP8L
Right ØP8K
Uterine Supporting Structure ØU84

Division — *continued*
Vertebra
Cervical ØP83
Lumbar ØQ8Ø
Thoracic ØP84
Doppler study *see* Ultrasonography
Dorsal digital nerve *use* Radial Nerve
Dorsal metacarpal vein
use Hand Vein, Left
use Hand Vein, Right
Dorsal metatarsal artery
use Foot Artery, Left
use Foot Artery, Right
Dorsal metatarsal vein
use Foot Vein, Left
use Foot Vein, Right
Dorsal scapular artery
use Subclavian Artery, Left
use Subclavian Artery, Right
Dorsal scapular nerve *use* Brachial Plexus
Dorsal venous arch
use Foot Vein, Left
use Foot Vein, Right
Dorsalis pedis artery
use Anterior Tibial Artery, Left
use Anterior Tibial Artery, Right
DownStream® System 5AØ512C, 5AØ522C
Drainage
Abdominal Wall ØW9F
Acetabulum
Left ØQ95
Right ØQ94
Adenoids ØC9Q
Ampulla of Vater ØF9C
Anal Sphincter ØD9R
Ankle Region
Left ØY9L
Right ØY9K
Anterior Chamber
Left Ø893
Right Ø892
Anus ØD9Q
Aorta, Abdominal Ø49Ø
Aortic Body ØG9D
Appendix ØD9J
Arm
Lower
Left ØX9F
Right ØX9D
Upper
Left ØX99
Right ØX98
Artery
Anterior Tibial
Left Ø49Q
Right Ø49P
Axillary
Left Ø396
Right Ø395
Brachial
Left Ø398
Right Ø397
Celiac Ø491
Colic
Left Ø497
Middle Ø498
Right Ø496
Common Carotid
Left Ø39J
Right Ø39H
Common Iliac
Left Ø49D
Right Ø49C
External Carotid
Left Ø39N
Right Ø39M
External Iliac
Left Ø49J
Right Ø49H
Face Ø39R
Femoral
Left Ø49L
Right Ø49K
Foot
Left Ø49W
Right Ø49V
Gastric Ø492

Drainage — *continued*
Artery — *continued*
Hand
Left Ø39F
Right Ø39D
Hepatic Ø493
Inferior Mesenteric Ø49B
Innominate Ø392
Internal Carotid
Left Ø39L
Right Ø39K
Internal Iliac
Left Ø49F
Right Ø49E
Internal Mammary
Left Ø391
Right Ø39Ø
Intracranial Ø39G
Lower Ø49Y
Peroneal
Left Ø49U
Right Ø49T
Popliteal
Left Ø49N
Right Ø49M
Posterior Tibial
Left Ø49S
Right Ø49R
Radial
Left Ø39C
Right Ø39B
Renal
Left Ø49A
Right Ø499
Splenic Ø494
Subclavian
Left Ø394
Right Ø393
Superior Mesenteric Ø495
Temporal
Left Ø39T
Right Ø39S
Thyroid
Left Ø39V
Right Ø39U
Ulnar
Left Ø39A
Right Ø399
Upper Ø39Y
Vertebral
Left Ø39Q
Right Ø39P
Auditory Ossicle
Left Ø99A
Right Ø999
Axilla
Left ØX95
Right ØX94
Back
Lower ØW9L
Upper ØW9K
Basal Ganglia ØØ98
Bladder ØT9B
Bladder Neck ØT9C
Bone
Ethmoid
Left ØN9G
Right ØN9F
Frontal ØN91
Hyoid ØN9X
Lacrimal
Left ØN9J
Right ØN9H
Nasal ØN9B
Occipital ØN97
Palatine
Left ØN9L
Right ØN9K
Parietal
Left ØN94
Right ØN93
Pelvic
Left ØQ93
Right ØQ92
Sphenoid ØN9C
Temporal
Left ØN96
Right ØN95

Drainage — *continued*
Bone — *continued*
Zygomatic
Left ØN9N
Right ØN9M
Bone Marrow Ø79T
Brain ØØ9Ø
Breast
Bilateral ØH9V
Left ØH9U
Right ØH9T
Bronchus
Lingula ØB99
Lower Lobe
Left ØB9B
Right ØB96
Main
Left ØB97
Right ØB93
Middle Lobe, Right ØB95
Upper Lobe
Left ØB98
Right ØB94
Buccal Mucosa ØC94
Bursa and Ligament
Abdomen
Left ØM9J
Right ØM9H
Ankle
Left ØM9R
Right ØM9Q
Elbow
Left ØM94
Right ØM93
Foot
Left ØM9T
Right ØM9S
Hand
Left ØM98
Right ØM97
Head and Neck ØM9Ø
Hip
Left ØM9M
Right ØM9L
Knee
Left ØM9P
Right ØM9N
Lower Extremity
Left ØM9W
Right ØM9V
Perineum ØM9K
Rib(s) ØM9G
Shoulder
Left ØM92
Right ØM91
Spine
Lower ØM9D
Upper ØM9C
Sternum ØM9F
Upper Extremity
Left ØM9B
Right ØM99
Wrist
Left ØM96
Right ØM95
Buttock
Left ØY91
Right ØY9Ø
Carina ØB92
Carotid Bodies, Bilateral ØG98
Carotid Body
Left ØG96
Right ØG97
Carpal
Left ØP9N
Right ØP9M
Cavity, Cranial ØW91
Cecum ØD9H
Cerebellum ØØ9C
Cerebral Hemisphere ØØ97
Cerebral Meninges ØØ91
Cerebral Ventricle ØØ96
Cervix ØU9C
Chest Wall ØW98
Choroid
Left Ø89B
Right Ø89A
Cisterna Chyli Ø79L

Drainage — *continued*
Clavicle
Left ØP9B
Right ØP99
Clitoris ØU9J
Coccygeal Glomus ØG9B
Coccyx ØQ9S
Colon
Ascending ØD9K
Descending ØD9M
Sigmoid ØD9N
Transverse ØD9L
Conjunctiva
Left Ø89T
Right Ø89S
Cord
Bilateral ØV9H
Left ØV9G
Right ØV9F
Cornea
Left Ø899
Right Ø898
Cul-de-sac ØU9F
Diaphragm ØB9T
Disc
Cervical Vertebral ØR93
Cervicothoracic Vertebral ØR95
Lumbar Vertebral ØS92
Lumbosacral ØS94
Thoracic Vertebral ØR99
Thoracolumbar Vertebral ØR9B
Duct
Common Bile ØF99
Cystic ØF98
Hepatic
Common ØF97
Left ØF96
Right ØF95
Lacrimal
Left Ø89Y
Right Ø89X
Pancreatic ØF9D
Accessory ØF9F
Parotid
Left ØC9C
Right ØC9B
Duodenum ØD99
Dura Mater ØØ92
Ear
External
Left Ø991
Right Ø99Ø
External Auditory Canal
Left Ø994
Right Ø993
Inner
Left Ø99E
Right Ø99D
Middle
Left Ø996
Right Ø995
Elbow Region
Left ØX9C
Right ØX9B
Epididymis
Bilateral ØV9L
Left ØV9K
Right ØV9J
Epidural Space, Intracranial ØØ93
Epiglottis ØC9R
Esophagogastric Junction ØD94
Esophagus ØD95
Lower ØD93
Middle ØD92
Upper ØD91
Eustachian Tube
Left Ø99G
Right Ø99F
Extremity
Lower
Left ØY9B
Right ØY99
Upper
Left ØX97
Right ØX96
Eye
Left Ø891
Right Ø89Ø

Drainage — *continued*
Eyelid
Lower
Left Ø89R
Right Ø89Q
Upper
Left Ø89P
Right Ø89N
Face ØW92
Fallopian Tube
Left ØU96
Right ØU95
Fallopian Tubes, Bilateral ØU97
Femoral Region
Left ØY98
Right ØY97
Femoral Shaft
Left ØQ99
Right ØQ98
Femur
Lower
Left ØQ9C
Right ØQ9B
Upper
Left ØQ97
Right ØQ96
Fibula
Left ØQ9K
Right ØQ9J
Finger Nail ØH9Q
Foot
Left ØY9N
Right ØY9M
Gallbladder ØF94
Gingiva
Lower ØC96
Upper ØC95
Gland
Adrenal
Bilateral ØG94
Left ØG92
Right ØG93
Lacrimal
Left Ø89W
Right Ø89V
Minor Salivary ØC9J
Parotid
Left ØC99
Right ØC98
Pituitary ØG9Ø
Sublingual
Left ØC9F
Right ØC9D
Submaxillary
Left ØC9H
Right ØC9G
Vestibular ØU9L
Glenoid Cavity
Left ØP98
Right ØP97
Glomus Jugulare ØG9C
Hand
Left ØX9K
Right ØX9J
Head ØW9Ø
Humeral Head
Left ØP9D
Right ØP9C
Humeral Shaft
Left ØP9G
Right ØP9F
Hymen ØU9K
Hypothalamus ØØ9A
Ileocecal Valve ØD9C
Ileum ØD9B
Inguinal Region
Left ØY96
Right ØY95
Intestine
Large ØD9E
Left ØD9G
Right ØD9F
Small ØD98
Iris
Left Ø89D
Right Ø89C
Jaw
Lower ØW95
Upper ØW94

Drainage — *continued*
Jejunum ØD9A
Joint
Acromioclavicular
Left ØR9H
Right ØR9G
Ankle
Left ØS9G
Right ØS9F
Carpal
Left ØR9R
Right ØR9Q
Carpometacarpal
Left ØR9T
Right ØR9S
Cervical Vertebral ØR91
Cervicothoracic Vertebral ØR94
Coccygeal ØS96
Elbow
Left ØR9M
Right ØR9L
Finger Phalangeal
Left ØR9X
Right ØR9W
Hip
Left ØS9B
Right ØS99
Knee
Left ØS9D
Right ØS9C
Lumbar Vertebral ØS9Ø
Lumbosacral ØS93
Metacarpophalangeal
Left ØR9V
Right ØR9U
Metatarsal-Phalangeal
Left ØS9N
Right ØS9M
Occipital-cervical ØR9Ø
Sacrococcygeal ØS95
Sacroiliac
Left ØS98
Right ØS97
Shoulder
Left ØR9K
Right ØR9J
Sternoclavicular
Left ØR9F
Right ØR9E
Tarsal
Left ØS9J
Right ØS9H
Tarsometatarsal
Left ØS9L
Right ØS9K
Temporomandibular
Left ØR9D
Right ØR9C
Thoracic Vertebral ØR96
Thoracolumbar Vertebral ØR9A
Toe Phalangeal
Left ØS9Q
Right ØS9P
Wrist
Left ØR9P
Right ØR9N
Kidney
Left ØT91
Right ØT9Ø
Kidney Pelvis
Left ØT94
Right ØT93
Knee Region
Left ØY9G
Right ØY9F
Larynx ØC9S
Leg
Lower
Left ØY9J
Right ØY9H
Upper
Left ØY9D
Right ØY9C
Lens
Left Ø89K
Right Ø89J
Lip
Lower ØC91
Upper ØC9Ø

Drainage — *continued*
Liver ØF9Ø
Left Lobe ØF92
Right Lobe ØF91
Lung
Bilateral ØB9M
Left ØB9L
Lower Lobe
Left ØB9J
Right ØB9F
Middle Lobe, Right ØB9D
Right ØB9K
Upper Lobe
Left ØB9G
Right ØB9C
Lung Lingula ØB9H
Lymphatic
Aortic Ø79D
Axillary
Left Ø796
Right Ø795
Head Ø79Ø
Inguinal
Left Ø79J
Right Ø79H
Internal Mammary
Left Ø799
Right Ø798
Lower Extremity
Left Ø79G
Right Ø79F
Mesenteric Ø79B
Neck
Left Ø792
Right Ø791
Pelvis Ø79C
Thoracic Duct Ø79K
Thorax Ø797
Upper Extremity
Left Ø794
Right Ø793
Mandible
Left ØN9V
Right ØN9T
Maxilla ØN9R
Mediastinum ØW9C
Medulla Oblongata ØØ9D
Mesentery ØD9V
Metacarpal
Left ØP9Q
Right ØP9P
Metatarsal
Left ØQ9P
Right ØQ9N
Muscle
Abdomen
Left ØK9L
Right ØK9K
Extraocular
Left Ø89M
Right Ø89L
Facial ØK91
Foot
Left ØK9W
Right ØK9V
Hand
Left ØK9D
Right ØK9C
Head ØK9Ø
Hip
Left ØK9P
Right ØK9N
Lower Arm and Wrist
Left ØK9B
Right ØK99
Lower Leg
Left ØK9T
Right ØK9S
Neck
Left ØK93
Right ØK92
Perineum ØK9M
Shoulder
Left ØK96
Right ØK95
Thorax
Left ØK9J
Right ØK9H
Tongue, Palate, Pharynx ØK94

Drainage — *continued*
Muscle — *continued*
Trunk
Left ØK9G
Right ØK9F
Upper Arm
Left ØK98
Right ØK97
Upper Leg
Left ØK9R
Right ØK9Q
Nasal Mucosa and Soft Tissue Ø99K
Nasopharynx Ø99N
Neck ØW96
Nerve
Abdominal Sympathetic Ø19M
Abducens ØØ9L
Accessory ØØ9R
Acoustic ØØ9N
Brachial Plexus Ø193
Cervical Ø191
Cervical Plexus Ø19Ø
Facial ØØ9M
Femoral Ø19D
Glossopharyngeal ØØ9P
Head and Neck Sympathetic Ø19K
Hypoglossal ØØ9S
Lumbar Ø19B
Lumbar Plexus Ø199
Lumbar Sympathetic Ø19N
Lumbosacral Plexus Ø19A
Median Ø195
Oculomotor ØØ9H
Olfactory ØØ9F
Optic ØØ9G
Peroneal Ø19H
Phrenic Ø192
Pudendal Ø19C
Radial Ø196
Sacral Ø19R
Sacral Plexus Ø19Q
Sacral Sympathetic Ø19P
Sciatic Ø19F
Thoracic Ø198
Thoracic Sympathetic Ø19L
Tibial Ø19G
Trigeminal ØØ9K
Trochlear ØØ9J
Ulnar Ø194
Vagus ØØ9Q
Nipple
Left ØH9X
Right ØH9W
Omentum ØD9U
Oral Cavity and Throat ØW93
Orbit
Left ØN9Q
Right ØN9P
Ovary
Bilateral ØU92
Left ØU91
Right ØU9Ø
Palate
Hard ØC92
Soft ØC93
Pancreas ØF9G
Para-aortic Body ØG99
Paraganglion Extremity ØG9F
Parathyroid Gland ØG9R
Inferior
Left ØG9P
Right ØG9N
Multiple ØG9Q
Superior
Left ØG9M
Right ØG9L
Patella
Left ØQ9F
Right ØQ9D
Pelvic Cavity ØW9J
Penis ØV9S
Pericardial Cavity ØW9D
Perineum
Female ØW9N
Male ØW9M
Peritoneal Cavity ØW9G
Peritoneum ØD9W

Drainage — *continued*
Phalanx
Finger
Left ØP9V
Right ØP9T
Thumb
Left ØP9S
Right ØP9R
Toe
Left ØQ9R
Right ØQ9Q
Pharynx ØC9M
Pineal Body ØG91
Pleura
Left ØB9P
Right ØB9N
Pleural Cavity
Left ØW9B
Right ØW99
Pons ØØ9B
Prepuce ØV9T
Products of Conception
Amniotic Fluid
Diagnostic 1Ø9Ø
Therapeutic 1Ø9Ø
Fetal Blood 1Ø9Ø
Fetal Cerebrospinal Fluid 1Ø9Ø
Fetal Fluid, Other 1Ø9Ø
Fluid, Other 1Ø9Ø
Prostate ØV9Ø
Radius
Left ØP9J
Right ØP9H
Rectum ØD9P
Retina
Left Ø89F
Right Ø89E
Retinal Vessel
Left Ø89H
Right Ø89G
Retroperitoneum ØW9H
Ribs
1 to 2 ØP91
3 or More ØP92
Sacrum ØQ91
Scapula
Left ØP96
Right ØP95
Sclera
Left Ø897
Right Ø896
Scrotum ØV95
Septum, Nasal Ø99M
Shoulder Region
Left ØX93
Right ØX92
Sinus
Accessory Ø99P
Ethmoid
Left Ø99V
Right Ø99U
Frontal
Left Ø99T
Right Ø99S
Mastoid
Left Ø99C
Right Ø99B
Maxillary
Left Ø99R
Right Ø99Q
Sphenoid
Left Ø99X
Right Ø99W
Skin
Abdomen ØH97
Back ØH96
Buttock ØH98
Chest ØH95
Ear
Left ØH93
Right ØH92
Face ØH91
Foot
Left ØH9N
Right ØH9M
Hand
Left ØH9G
Right ØH9F
Inguinal ØH9A

Drainage — *continued*
Skin — *continued*
Lower Arm
Left ØH9E
Right ØH9D
Lower Leg
Left ØH9L
Right ØH9K
Neck ØH94
Perineum ØH99
Scalp ØH9Ø
Upper Arm
Left ØH9C
Right ØH9B
Upper Leg
Left ØH9J
Right ØH9H
Skull ØN9Ø
Spinal Canal ØØ9U
Spinal Cord
Cervical ØØ9W
Lumbar ØØ9Y
Thoracic ØØ9X
Spinal Meninges ØØ9T
Spleen Ø79P
Sternum ØP9Ø
Stomach ØD96
Pylorus ØD97
Subarachnoid Space, Intracranial ØØ95
Subcutaneous Tissue and Fascia
Abdomen ØJ98
Back ØJ97
Buttock ØJ99
Chest ØJ96
Face ØJ91
Foot
Left ØJ9R
Right ØJ9Q
Hand
Left ØJ9K
Right ØJ9J
Lower Arm
Left ØJ9H
Right ØJ9G
Lower Leg
Left ØJ9P
Right ØJ9N
Neck
Left ØJ95
Right ØJ94
Pelvic Region ØJ9C
Perineum ØJ9B
Scalp ØJ9Ø
Upper Arm
Left ØJ9F
Right ØJ9D
Upper Leg
Left ØJ9M
Right ØJ9L
Subdural Space, Intracranial ØØ94
Tarsal
Left ØQ9M
Right ØQ9L
Tendon
Abdomen
Left ØL9G
Right ØL9F
Ankle
Left ØL9T
Right ØL9S
Foot
Left ØL9W
Right ØL9V
Hand
Left ØL98
Right ØL97
Head and Neck ØL9Ø
Hip
Left ØL9K
Right ØL9J
Knee
Left ØL9R
Right ØL9Q
Lower Arm and Wrist
Left ØL96
Right ØL95
Lower Leg
Left ØL9P
Right ØL9N

Drainage — *continued*
Tendon — *continued*
Perineum ØL9H
Shoulder
Left ØL92
Right ØL91
Thorax
Left ØL9D
Right ØL9C
Trunk
Left ØL9B
Right ØL99
Upper Arm
Left ØL94
Right ØL93
Upper Leg
Left ØL9M
Right ØL9L
Testis
Bilateral ØV9C
Left ØV9B
Right ØV99
Thalamus ØØ99
Thymus Ø79M
Thyroid Gland ØG9K
Left Lobe ØG9G
Right Lobe ØG9H
Tibia
Left ØQ9H
Right ØQ9G
Toe Nail ØH9R
Tongue ØC97
Tonsils ØC9P
Tooth
Lower ØC9X
Upper ØC9W
Trachea ØB91
Tunica Vaginalis
Left ØV97
Right ØV96
Turbinate, Nasal Ø99L
Tympanic Membrane
Left Ø998
Right Ø997
Ulna
Left ØP9L
Right ØP9K
Ureter
Left ØT97
Right ØT96
Ureters, Bilateral ØT98
Urethra ØT9D
Uterine Supporting Structure ØU94
Uterus ØU99
Uvula ØC9N
Vagina ØU9G
Vas Deferens
Bilateral ØV9Q
Left ØV9P
Right ØV9N
Vein
Axillary
Left Ø598
Right Ø597
Azygos Ø59Ø
Basilic
Left Ø59C
Right Ø59B
Brachial
Left Ø59A
Right Ø599
Cephalic
Left Ø59F
Right Ø59D
Colic Ø697
Common Iliac
Left Ø69D
Right Ø69C
Esophageal Ø693
External Iliac
Left Ø69G
Right Ø69F
External Jugular
Left Ø59Q
Right Ø59P
Face
Left Ø59V
Right Ø59T

Drainage — *continued*
Vein — *continued*
Femoral
Left Ø69N
Right Ø69M
Foot
Left Ø69V
Right Ø69T
Gastric Ø692
Hand
Left Ø59H
Right Ø59G
Hemiazygos Ø591
Hepatic Ø694
Hypogastric
Left Ø69J
Right Ø69H
Inferior Mesenteric Ø696
Innominate
Left Ø594
Right Ø593
Internal Jugular
Left Ø59N
Right Ø59M
Intracranial Ø59L
Lower Ø69Y
Portal Ø698
Renal
Left Ø69B
Right Ø699
Saphenous
Left Ø69Q
Right Ø69P
Splenic Ø691
Subclavian
Left Ø596
Right Ø595
Superior Mesenteric Ø695
Upper Ø59Y
Vertebral
Left Ø59S
Right Ø59R
Vena Cava, Inferior Ø69Ø
Vertebra
Cervical ØP93
Lumbar ØQ9Ø
Thoracic ØP94
Vesicle
Bilateral ØV93
Left ØV92
Right ØV91
Vitreous
Left Ø895
Right Ø894
Vocal Cord
Left ØC9V
Right ØC9T
Vulva ØU9M
Wrist Region
Left ØX9H
Right ØX9G
Dressing
Abdominal Wall 2W23X4Z
Arm
Lower
Left 2W2DX4Z
Right 2W2CX4Z
Upper
Left 2W2BX4Z
Right 2W2AX4Z
Back 2W25X4Z
Chest Wall 2W24X4Z
Extremity
Lower
Left 2W2MX4Z
Right 2W2LX4Z
Upper
Left 2W29X4Z
Right 2W28X4Z
Face 2W21X4Z
Finger
Left 2W2KX4Z
Right 2W2JX4Z
Foot
Left 2W2TX4Z
Right 2W2SX4Z
Hand
Left 2W2FX4Z
Right 2W2EX4Z
Dressing — *continued*
Head 2W2ØX4Z
Inguinal Region
Left 2W27X4Z
Right 2W26X4Z
Leg
Lower
Left 2W2RX4Z
Right 2W2QX4Z
Upper
Left 2W2PX4Z
Right 2W2NX4Z
Neck 2W22X4Z
Thumb
Left 2W2HX4Z
Right 2W2GX4Z
Toe
Left 2W2VX4Z
Right 2W2UX4Z
Driver stent (RX) (OTW) *use* Intraluminal Device
Drotrecogin alfa, infusion *see* Introduction of Recombinant Human-activated Protein C
Duct of Santorini *use* Pancreatic Duct, Accessory
Duct of Wirsung *use* Pancreatic Duct
Ductogram, mammary *see* Plain Radiography, Skin, Subcutaneous Tissue and Breast BHØ
Ductography, mammary *see* Plain Radiography, Skin, Subcutaneous Tissue and Breast BHØ
Ductus deferens
use Vas Deferens
use Vas Deferens, Bilateral
use Vas Deferens, Left
use Vas Deferens, Right
Duodenal ampulla *use* Ampulla of Vater
Duodenectomy
see Excision, Duodenum ØDB9
see Resection, Duodenum ØDT9
Duodenocholedochotomy *see* Drainage, Gallbladder ØF94
Duodenocystostomy
see Bypass, Gallbladder ØF14
see Drainage, Gallbladder ØF94
Duodenoenterostomy
see Bypass, Gastrointestinal System ØD1
see Drainage, Gastrointestinal System ØD9
Duodenojejunal flexure *use* Jejunum
Duodenolysis *see* Release, Duodenum ØDN9
Duodenorrhaphy *see* Repair, Duodenum ØDQ9
Duodenostomy
see Bypass, Duodenum ØD19
see Drainage, Duodenum ØD99
Duodenotomy *see* Drainage, Duodenum ØD99
Dura mater, intracranial *use* Dura Mater
Dura mater, spinal *use* Spinal Meninges
DuraGraft® Endothelial Damage Inhibitor *use* Endothelial Damage Inhibitor
DuraHeart Left Ventricular Assist System *use* Implantable Heart Assist System in Heart and Great Vessels
Dural venous sinus *use* Intracranial Vein
Durata® Defibrillation Lead *use* Cardiac Lead, Defibrillator in Ø2H
Durvalumab Antineoplastic XWØ
DynaNail Mini®
use Internal Fixation Device, Sustained Compression in ØRG
use Internal Fixation Device, Sustained Compression in ØSG
DynaNail®
use Internal Fixation Device, Sustained Compression in ØRG
use Internal Fixation Device, Sustained Compression in ØSG
Dynesys® Dynamic Stabilization System
use Spinal Stabilization Device, Pedicle-Based in ØRH
use Spinal Stabilization Device, Pedicle-Based in ØSH

E

Earlobe
use Ear, External, Bilateral
use Ear, External, Left
use Ear, External, Right
ECCO2R (Extracorporeal Carbon Dioxide Removal) 5AØ92ØZ
Echocardiogram *see* Ultrasonography, Heart B24
Echography *see* Ultrasonography
EchoTip® Insight™ Portosystemic Pressure Gradient Measurement System 4AØ44B2
ECMO *see* Performance, Circulatory 5A15
ECMO, intraoperative *see* Performance, Circulatory 5A15A
Eculizumab XWØ
EDWARDS INTUITY Elite valve system *use* Zooplastic Tissue, Rapid Deployment Technique in New Technology
EEG (electroencephalogram) *see* Measurement, Central Nervous 4AØØ
EGD (esophagogastroduodenoscopy) ØDJØ8ZZ
Eighth cranial nerve *use* Acoustic Nerve
Ejaculatory duct
use Vas Deferens
use Vas Deferens, Bilateral
use Vas Deferens, Left
use Vas Deferens, Right
EKG (electrocardiogram) *see* Measurement, Cardiac 4AØ2
EKOS™ EkoSonic® Endovascular System *see* Fragmentation, Artery
Eladocagene exuparvovec XWØQ316
Electrical bone growth stimulator (EBGS)
use Bone Growth Stimulator in Head and Facial Bones
use Bone Growth Stimulator in Lower Bones
use Bone Growth Stimulator in Upper Bones
Electrical muscle stimulation (EMS) lead *use* Stimulator Lead in Muscles
Electrocautery
Destruction *see* Destruction
Repair *see* Repair
Electroconvulsive Therapy
Bilateral-Multiple Seizure GZB3ZZZ
Bilateral-Single Seizure GZB2ZZZ
Electroconvulsive Therapy, Other GZB4ZZZ
Unilateral-Multiple Seizure GZB1ZZZ
Unilateral-Single Seizure GZBØZZZ
Electroencephalogram (EEG) *see* Measurement, Central Nervous 4AØØ
Electromagnetic Therapy
Central Nervous 6A22
Urinary 6A21
Electronic muscle stimulator lead *use* Stimulator Lead in Muscles
Electrophysiologic stimulation (EPS) *see* Measurement, Cardiac 4AØ2
Electroshock therapy *see* Electroconvulsive Therapy
Elevation, bone fragments, skull *see* Reposition, Head and Facial Bones ØNS
Eleventh cranial nerve *use* Accessory Nerve
Ellipsys® vascular access system
Radial Artery, Left Ø31C3ZF
Radial Artery, Right Ø31B3ZF
Ulnar Artery, Left Ø31A3ZF
Ulnar Artery, Right Ø3193ZF
E-Luminexx™ (Biliary) (Vascular) Stent *use* Intraluminal Device
Eluvia™ Drug-Eluting Vascular Stent System
use Intraluminal Device, Sustained Release Drug-eluting in New Technology
use Intraluminal Device, Sustained Release Drug-eluting, Two in New Technology
use Intraluminal Device, Sustained Release Drug-eluting, Three in New Technology
use Intraluminal Device, Sustained Release Drug-eluting, Four or More in New Technology
ELZONRIS™ *use* Tagraxofusp-erzs Antineoplastic
Embolectomy *see* Extirpation
Embolization
see Occlusion
see Restriction
Embolization coil(s) *use* Intraluminal Device
EMG (electromyogram) *see* Measurement, Musculoskeletal 4AØF
Encephalon *use* Brain
Endarterectomy
see Extirpation, Lower Arteries Ø4C
see Extirpation, Upper Arteries Ø3C
Endeavor® (III) (IV) (Sprint) Zotarolimus-eluting Coronary Stent System *use* Intraluminal Device, Drug-eluting in Heart and Great Vessels

EndoAVF procedure
Radial Artery, Left Ø31C3ZF
Radial Artery, Right Ø31B3ZF
Ulnar Artery, Left Ø31A3ZF
Ulnar Artery, Right Ø3193ZF
Endologix® AFX Endovascular AAA System *use* Intraluminal Device
EndoSure® sensor *use* Monitoring Device, Pressure Sensor in Ø2H
ENDOTAK RELIANCE® (G) Defibrillation Lead *use* Cardiac Lead, Defibrillator in Ø2H
Endothelial damage inhibitor, applied to vein graft XYØVX83
Endotracheal tube (cuffed) (double-lumen) *use* Intraluminal Device, Endotracheal Airway in Respiratory System
Endovascular fistula creation
Radial Artery, Left Ø31C3ZF
Radial Artery, Right Ø31B3ZF
Ulnar Artery, Left Ø31A3ZF
Ulnar Artery, Right Ø3193ZF
Endurant® Endovascular Stent Graft *use* Intraluminal Device
Endurant® II AAA stent graft system *use* Intraluminal Device
Engineered Autologous Chimeric Antigen Receptor T-cell Immunotherapy XWØ
Enlargement
see Dilation
see Repair
EnRhythm *use* Pacemaker, Dual Chamber in ØJH
ENROUTE® Transcarotid Neuroprotection System
see New Technology, Cardiovascular System X2A
Enterorrhaphy *see* Repair, Gastrointestinal System ØDQ
Enterra gastric neurostimulator *use* Stimulator Generator, Multiple Array in ØJH
Enucleation
Eyeball *see* Resection, Eye Ø8T
Eyeball with prosthetic implant *see* Replacement, Eye Ø8R
Ependyma *use* Cerebral Ventricle
Epicel® cultured epidermal autograft *use* Autologous Tissue Substitute
Epic™ Stented Tissue Valve (aortic) *use* Zooplastic Tissue in Heart and Great Vessels
Epidermis *use* Skin
Epididymectomy
see Excision, Male Reproductive System ØVB
see Resection, Male Reproductive System ØVT
Epididymoplasty
see Repair, Male Reproductive System ØVQ
see Supplement, Male Reproductive System ØVU
Epididymorrhaphy *see* Repair, Male Reproductive System ØVQ
Epididymotomy *see* Drainage, Male Reproductive System ØV9
Epidural space, spinal *use* Spinal Canal
Epiphysiodesis
see Insertion of device in, Lower Bones ØQH
see Insertion of device in, Upper Bones ØPH
see Repair, Lower Bones ØQQ
see Repair, Upper Bones ØPQ
Epiploic foramen *use* Peritoneum
Epiretinal Visual Prosthesis
Left Ø8H1Ø5Z
Right Ø8HØØ5Z
Episiorrhaphy *see* Repair, Perineum, Female ØWQN
Episiotomy *see* Division, Perineum, Female ØW8N
Epithalamus *use* Thalamus
Epitrochlear lymph node
use Lymphatic, Left Upper Extremity
use Lymphatic, Right Upper Extremity
EPS (electrophysiologic stimulation) *see* Measurement, Cardiac 4AØ2
Eptifibatide, infusion *see* Introduction of Platelet Inhibitor
ERCP (endoscopic retrograde cholangiopancreatography) *see* Fluoroscopy, Hepatobiliary System and Pancreas BF1
Erdafitinib Antineoplastic XWØDXL5
Erector spinae muscle
use Trunk Muscle, Left
use Trunk Muscle, Right
ERLEADA™ *use* Apalutamide Antineoplastic
Esketamine Hydrochloride XWØ97M5
Esophageal artery *use* Upper Artery
Esophageal obturator airway (EOA) *use* Intraluminal Device, Airway in Gastrointestinal System
Esophageal plexus *use* Thoracic Sympathetic Nerve
Esophagectomy
see Excision, Gastrointestinal System ØDB
see Resection, Gastrointestinal System ØDT
Esophagocoloplasty
see Repair, Gastrointestinal System ØDQ
see Supplement, Gastrointestinal System ØDU
Esophagoenterostomy
see Bypass, Gastrointestinal System ØD1
see Drainage, Gastrointestinal System ØD9
Esophagoesophagostomy
see Bypass, Gastrointestinal System ØD1
see Drainage, Gastrointestinal System ØD9
Esophagogastrectomy
see Excision, Gastrointestinal System ØDB
see Resection, Gastrointestinal System ØDT
Esophagogastroduodenoscopy (EGD) ØDJØ8ZZ
Esophagogastroplasty
see Repair, Gastrointestinal System ØDQ
see Supplement, Gastrointestinal System ØDU
Esophagogastroscopy ØDJ68ZZ
Esophagogastrostomy
see Bypass, Gastrointestinal System ØD1
see Drainage, Gastrointestinal System ØD9
Esophagojejunoplasty *see* Supplement, Gastrointestinal System ØDU
Esophagojejunostomy
see Bypass, Gastrointestinal System ØD1
see Drainage, Gastrointestinal System ØD9
Esophagomyotomy *see* Division, Esophagogastric Junction ØD84
Esophagoplasty
see Repair, Gastrointestinal System ØDQ
see Replacement, Esophagus ØDR5
see Supplement, Gastrointestinal System ØDU
Esophagoplication *see* Restriction, Gastrointestinal System ØDV
Esophagorrhaphy *see* Repair, Gastrointestinal System ØDQ
Esophagoscopy ØDJØ8ZZ
Esophagotomy *see* Drainage, Gastrointestinal System ØD9
Esteem® implantable hearing system *use* Hearing Device in Ear, Nose, Sinus
ESWL (extracorporeal shock wave lithotripsy) *see* Fragmentation
Ethmoidal air cell
use Ethmoid Sinus, Left
use Ethmoid Sinus, Right
Ethmoidectomy
see Excision, Ear, Nose, Sinus Ø9B
see Excision, Head and Facial Bones ØNB
see Resection, Ear, Nose, Sinus Ø9T
see Resection, Head and Facial Bones ØNT
Ethmoidotomy *see* Drainage, Ear, Nose, Sinus Ø99
Evacuation
Hematoma *see* Extirpation
Other Fluid *see* Drainage
Evera (XT) (S) (DR/VR) *use* Defibrillator Generator in ØJH
Everolimus-eluting coronary stent *use* Intraluminal Device, Drug-eluting in Heart and Great Vessels
Evisceration
Eyeball *see* Resection, Eye Ø8T
Eyeball with prosthetic implant *see* Replacement, Eye Ø8R
Examination *see* Inspection
Exchange *see* Change device in
Excision
Abdominal Wall ØWBF
Acetabulum
Left ØQB5
Right ØQB4
Adenoids ØCBQ
Ampulla of Vater ØFBC
Anal Sphincter ØDBR
Ankle Region
Left ØYBL
Right ØYBK
Anus ØDBQ
Aorta
Abdominal
Thoracic
Ascending/Arch Ø2BX
Descending Ø2BW
Excision — *continued*
Aortic Body ØGBD
Appendix ØDBJ
Arm
Lower
Left ØXBF
Right ØXBD
Upper
Left ØXB9
Right ØXB8
Artery
Anterior Tibial
Left Ø4BQ
Right Ø4BP
Axillary
Left Ø3B6
Right Ø3B5
Brachial
Left Ø3B8
Right Ø3B7
Celiac Ø4B1
Colic
Left Ø4B7
Middle Ø4B8
Right Ø4B6
Common Carotid
Left Ø3BJ
Right Ø3BH
Common Iliac
Left Ø4BD
Right Ø4BC
External Carotid
Left Ø3BN
Right Ø3BM
External Iliac
Left Ø4BJ
Right Ø4BH
Face Ø3BR
Femoral
Left Ø4BL
Right Ø4BK
Foot
Left Ø4BW
Right Ø4BV
Gastric Ø4B2
Hand
Left Ø3BF
Right Ø3BD
Hepatic Ø4B3
Inferior Mesenteric Ø4BB
Innominate Ø3B2
Internal Carotid
Left Ø3BL
Right Ø3BK
Internal Iliac
Left Ø4BF
Right Ø4BE
Internal Mammary
Left Ø3B1
Right Ø3BØ
Intracranial Ø3BG
Lower Ø4BY
Peroneal
Left Ø4BU
Right Ø4BT
Popliteal
Left Ø4BN
Right Ø4BM
Posterior Tibial
Left Ø4BS
Right Ø4BR
Pulmonary
Left Ø2BR
Right Ø2BQ
Pulmonary Trunk Ø2BP
Radial
Left Ø3BC
Right Ø3BB
Renal
Left Ø4BA
Right Ø4B9
Splenic Ø4B4
Subclavian
Left Ø3B4
Right Ø3B3
Superior Mesenteric Ø4B5
Temporal
Left Ø3BT
Right Ø3BS

- **Excision** — *continued*
  - Artery — *continued*
    - Thyroid
      - Left Ø3BV
      - Right Ø3BU
    - Ulnar
      - Left Ø3BA
      - Right Ø3B9
    - Upper Ø3BY
    - Vertebral
      - Left Ø3BQ
      - Right Ø3BP
  - Atrium
    - Left Ø2B7
    - Right Ø2B6
  - Auditory Ossicle
    - Left Ø9BA
    - Right Ø9B9
  - Axilla
    - Left ØXB5
    - Right ØXB4
  - Back
    - Lower ØWBL
    - Upper ØWBK
  - Basal Ganglia ØØB8
  - Bladder ØTBB
  - Bladder Neck ØTBC
  - Bone
    - Ethmoid
      - Left ØNBG
      - Right ØNBF
    - Frontal ØNB1
    - Hyoid ØNBX
    - Lacrimal
      - Left ØNBJ
      - Right ØNBH
    - Nasal ØNBB
    - Occipital ØNB7
    - Palatine
      - Left ØNBL
      - Right ØNBK
    - Parietal
      - Left ØNB4
      - Right ØNB3
    - Pelvic
      - Left ØQB3
      - Right ØQB2
    - Sphenoid ØNBC
    - Temporal
      - Left ØNB6
      - Right ØNB5
    - Zygomatic
      - Left ØNBN
      - Right ØNBM
  - Brain ØØBØ
  - Breast
    - Bilateral ØHBV
    - Left ØHBU
    - Right ØHBT
    - Supernumerary ØHBY
  - Bronchus
    - Lingula ØBB9
    - Lower Lobe
      - Left ØBBB
      - Right ØBB6
    - Main
      - Left ØBB7
      - Right ØBB3
    - Middle Lobe, Right ØBB5
    - Upper Lobe
      - Left ØBB8
      - Right ØBB4
  - Buccal Mucosa ØCB4
  - Bursa and Ligament
    - Abdomen
      - Left ØMBJ
      - Right ØMBH
    - Ankle
      - Left ØMBR
      - Right ØMBQ
    - Elbow
      - Left ØMB4
      - Right ØMB3
    - Foot
      - Left ØMBT
      - Right ØMBS
    - Hand
      - Left ØMB8
      - Right ØMB7
- **Excision** — *continued*
  - Bursa and Ligament — *continued*
    - Head and Neck ØMBØ
    - Hip
      - Left ØMBM
      - Right ØMBL
    - Knee
      - Left ØMBP
      - Right ØMBN
    - Lower Extremity
      - Left ØMBW
      - Right ØMBV
    - Perineum ØMBK
    - Rib(s) ØMBG
    - Shoulder
      - Left ØMB2
      - Right ØMB1
    - Spine
      - Lower ØMBD
      - Upper ØMBC
    - Sternum ØMBF
    - Upper Extremity
      - Left ØMBB
      - Right ØMB9
    - Wrist
      - Left ØMB6
      - Right ØMB5
  - Buttock
    - Left ØYB1
    - Right ØYBØ
  - Carina ØBB2
  - Carotid Bodies, Bilateral ØGB8
  - Carotid Body
    - Left ØGB6
    - Right ØGB7
  - Carpal
    - Left ØPBN
    - Right ØPBM
  - Cecum ØDBH
  - Cerebellum ØØBC
  - Cerebral Hemisphere ØØB7
  - Cerebral Meninges ØØB1
  - Cerebral Ventricle ØØB6
  - Cervix ØUBC
  - Chest Wall ØWB8
  - Chordae Tendineae Ø2B9
  - Choroid
    - Left Ø8BB
    - Right Ø8BA
  - Cisterna Chyli Ø7BL
  - Clavicle
    - Left ØPBB
    - Right ØPB9
  - Clitoris ØUBJ
  - Coccygeal Glomus ØGBB
  - Coccyx ØQBS
  - Colon
    - Ascending ØDBK
    - Descending ØDBM
    - Sigmoid ØDBN
    - Transverse ØDBL
  - Conduction Mechanism Ø2B8
  - Conjunctiva
    - Left Ø8BTXZ
    - Right Ø8BSXZ
  - Cord
    - Bilateral ØVBH
    - Left ØVBG
    - Right ØVBF
  - Cornea
    - Left Ø8B9XZ
    - Right Ø8B8XZ
  - Cul-de-sac ØUBF
  - Diaphragm ØBBT
  - Disc
    - Cervical Vertebral ØRB3
    - Cervicothoracic Vertebral ØRB5
    - Lumbar Vertebral ØSB2
    - Lumbosacral ØSB4
    - Thoracic Vertebral ØRB9
    - Thoracolumbar Vertebral ØRBB
  - Duct
    - Common Bile ØFB9
    - Cystic ØFB8
    - Hepatic
      - Common ØFB7
      - Left ØFB6
      - Right ØFB5
- **Excision** — *continued*
  - Duct — *continued*
    - Lacrimal
      - Left Ø8BY
      - Right Ø8BX
    - Pancreatic ØFBD
      - Accessory ØFBF
    - Parotid
      - Left ØCBC
      - Right ØCBB
  - Duodenum ØDB9
  - Dura Mater ØØB2
  - Ear
    - External
      - Left Ø9B1
      - Right Ø9BØ
    - External Auditory Canal
      - Left Ø9B4
      - Right Ø9B3
    - Inner
      - Left Ø9BE
      - Right Ø9BD
    - Middle
      - Left Ø9B6
      - Right Ø9B5
  - Elbow Region
    - Left ØXBC
    - Right ØXBB
  - Epididymis
    - Bilateral ØVBL
    - Left ØVBK
    - Right ØVBJ
  - Epiglottis ØCBR
  - Esophagogastric Junction ØDB4
  - Esophagus ØDB5
    - Lower ØDB3
    - Middle ØDB2
    - Upper ØDB1
  - Eustachian Tube
    - Left Ø9BG
    - Right Ø9BF
  - Extremity
    - Lower
      - Left ØYBB
      - Right ØYB9
    - Upper
      - Left ØXB7
      - Right ØXB6
  - Eye
    - Left Ø8B1
    - Right Ø8BØ
  - Eyelid
    - Lower
      - Left Ø8BR
      - Right Ø8BQ
    - Upper
      - Left Ø8BP
      - Right Ø8BN
  - Face ØWB2
  - Fallopian Tube
    - Left ØUB6
    - Right ØUB5
  - Fallopian Tubes, Bilateral ØUB7
  - Femoral Region
    - Left ØYB8
    - Right ØYB7
  - Femoral Shaft
    - Left ØQB9
    - Right ØQB8
  - Femur
    - Lower
      - Left ØQBC
      - Right ØQBB
    - Upper
      - Left ØQB7
      - Right ØQB6
  - Fibula
    - Left ØQBK
    - Right ØQBJ
  - Finger Nail ØHBQXZ
  - Floor of mouth *see* Excision, Oral Cavity and Throat ØWB3
  - Foot
    - Left ØYBN
    - Right ØYBM
  - Gallbladder ØFB4
  - Gingiva
    - Lower ØCB6
    - Upper ØCB5

Excision — *continued*
Gland
Adrenal
Bilateral ØGB4
Left ØGB2
Right ØGB3
Lacrimal
Left Ø8BW
Right Ø8BV
Minor Salivary ØCBJ
Parotid
Left ØCB9
Right ØCB8
Pituitary ØGBØ
Sublingual
Left ØCBF
Right ØCBD
Submaxillary
Left ØCBH
Right ØCBG
Vestibular ØUBL
Glenoid Cavity
Left ØPB8
Right ØPB7
Glomus Jugulare ØGBC
Hand
Left ØXBK
Right ØXBJ
Head ØWBØ
Humeral Head
Left ØPBD
Right ØPBC
Humeral Shaft
Left ØPBG
Right ØPBF
Hymen ØUBK
Hypothalamus ØØBA
Ileocecal Valve ØDBC
Ileum ØDBB
Inguinal Region
Left ØYB6
Right ØYB5
Intestine
Large ØDBE
Left ØDBG
Right ØDBF
Small ØDB8
Iris
Left Ø8BD3Z
Right Ø8BC3Z
Jaw
Lower ØWB5
Upper ØWB4
Jejunum ØDBA
Joint
Acromioclavicular
Left ØRBH
Right ØRBG
Ankle
Left ØSBG
Right ØSBF
Carpal
Left ØRBR
Right ØRBQ
Carpometacarpal
Left ØRBT
Right ØRBS
Cervical Vertebral ØRB1
Cervicothoracic Vertebral ØRB4
Coccygeal ØSB6
Elbow
Left ØRBM
Right ØRBL
Finger Phalangeal
Left ØRBX
Right ØRBW
Hip
Left ØSBB
Right ØSB9
Knee
Left ØSBD
Right ØSBC
Lumbar Vertebral ØSBØ
Lumbosacral ØSB3
Metacarpophalangeal
Left ØRBV
Right ØRBU
Metatarsal-Phalangeal
Left ØSBN

Excision — *continued*
Joint — *continued*
Metatarsal-Phalangeal — *continued*
Right ØSBM
Occipital-cervical ØRBØ
Sacrococcygeal ØSB5
Sacroiliac
Left ØSB8
Right ØSB7
Shoulder
Left ØRBK
Right ØRBJ
Sternoclavicular
Left ØRBF
Right ØRBE
Tarsal
Left ØSBJ
Right ØSBH
Tarsometatarsal
Left ØSBL
Right ØSBK
Temporomandibular
Left ØRBD
Right ØRBC
Thoracic Vertebral ØRB6
Thoracolumbar Vertebral ØRBA
Toe Phalangeal
Left ØSBQ
Right ØSBP
Wrist
Left ØRBP
Right ØRBN
Kidney
Left ØTB1
Right ØTBØ
Kidney Pelvis
Left ØTB4
Right ØTB3
Knee Region
Left ØYBG
Right ØYBF
Larynx ØCBS
Leg
Lower
Left ØYBJ
Right ØYBH
Upper
Left ØYBD
Right ØYBC
Lens
Left Ø8BK3Z
Right Ø8BJ3Z
Lip
Lower ØCB1
Upper ØCBØ
Liver ØFBØ
Left Lobe ØFB2
Right Lobe ØFB1
Lung
Bilateral ØBBM
Left ØBBL
Lower Lobe
Left ØBBJ
Right ØBBF
Middle Lobe, Right ØBBD
Right ØBBK
Upper Lobe
Left ØBBG
Right ØBBC
Lung Lingula ØBBH
Lymphatic
Aortic Ø7BD
Axillary
Left Ø7B6
Right Ø7B5
Head Ø7BØ
Inguinal
Left Ø7BJ
Right Ø7BH
Internal Mammary
Left Ø7B9
Right Ø7B8
Lower Extremity
Left Ø7BG
Right Ø7BF
Mesenteric Ø7BB
Neck
Left Ø7B2
Right Ø7B1

Excision — *continued*
Lymphatic — *continued*
Pelvis Ø7BC
Thoracic Duct Ø7BK
Thorax Ø7B7
Upper Extremity
Left Ø7B4
Right Ø7B3
Mandible
Left ØNBV
Right ØNBT
Maxilla ØNBR
Mediastinum ØWBC
Medulla Oblongata ØØBD
Mesentery ØDBV
Metacarpal
Left ØPBQ
Right ØPBP
Metatarsal
Left ØQBP
Right ØQBN
Muscle
Abdomen
Left ØKBL
Right ØKBK
Extraocular
Left Ø8BM
Right Ø8BL
Facial ØKB1
Foot
Left ØKBW
Right ØKBV
Hand
Left ØKBD
Right ØKBC
Head ØKBØ
Hip
Left ØKBP
Right ØKBN
Lower Arm and Wrist
Left ØKBB
Right ØKB9
Lower Leg
Left ØKBT
Right ØKBS
Neck
Left ØKB3
Right ØKB2
Papillary Ø2BD
Perineum ØKBM
Shoulder
Left ØKB6
Right ØKB5
Thorax
Left ØKBJ
Right ØKBH
Tongue, Palate, Pharynx ØKB4
Trunk
Left ØKBG
Right ØKBF
Upper Arm
Left ØKB8
Right ØKB7
Upper Leg
Left ØKBR
Right ØKBQ
Nasal Mucosa and Soft Tissue Ø9BK
Nasopharynx Ø9BN
Neck ØWB6
Nerve
Abdominal Sympathetic Ø1BM
Abducens ØØBL
Accessory ØØBR
Acoustic ØØBN
Brachial Plexus Ø1B3
Cervical Ø1B1
Cervical Plexus Ø1BØ
Facial ØØBM
Femoral Ø1BD
Glossopharyngeal ØØBP
Head and Neck Sympathetic Ø1BK
Hypoglossal ØØBS
Lumbar Ø1BB
Lumbar Plexus Ø1B9
Lumbar Sympathetic Ø1BN
Lumbosacral Plexus Ø1BA
Median Ø1B5
Oculomotor ØØBH
Olfactory ØØBF

Excision — *continued*
Nerve — *continued*
Optic ØØBG
Peroneal Ø1BH
Phrenic Ø1B2
Pudendal Ø1BC
Radial Ø1B6
Sacral Ø1BR
Sacral Plexus Ø1BQ
Sacral Sympathetic Ø1BP
Sciatic Ø1BF
Thoracic Ø1B8
Thoracic Sympathetic Ø1BL
Tibial Ø1BG
Trigeminal ØØBK
Trochlear ØØBJ
Ulnar Ø1B4
Vagus ØØBQ
Nipple
Left ØHBX
Right ØHBW
Omentum ØDBU
Oral Cavity and Throat ØWB3
Orbit
Left ØNBQ
Right ØNBP
Ovary
Bilateral ØUB2
Left ØUB1
Right ØUBØ
Palate
Hard ØCB2
Soft ØCB3
Pancreas ØFBG
Para-aortic Body ØGB9
Paraganglion Extremity ØGBF
Parathyroid Gland ØGBR
Inferior
Left ØGBP
Right ØGBN
Multiple ØGBQ
Superior
Left ØGBM
Right ØGBL
Patella
Left ØQBF
Right ØQBD
Penis ØVBS
Pericardium Ø2BN
Perineum
Female ØWBN
Male ØWBM
Peritoneum ØDBW
Phalanx
Finger
Left ØPBV
Right ØPBT
Thumb
Left ØPBS
Right ØPBR
Toe
Left ØQBR
Right ØQBQ
Pharynx ØCBM
Pineal Body ØGB1
Pleura
Left ØBBP
Right ØBBN
Pons ØØBB
Prepuce ØVBT
Prostate ØVBØ
Radius
Left ØPBJ
Right ØPBH
Rectum ØDBP
Retina
Left Ø8BF3Z
Right Ø8BE3Z
Retroperitoneum ØWBH
Ribs
1 to 2 ØPB1
3 or More ØPB2
Sacrum ØQB1
Scapula
Left ØPB6
Right ØPB5
Sclera
Left Ø8B7XZ
Right Ø8B6XZ

Excision — *continued*
Scrotum ØVB5
Septum
Atrial Ø2B5
Nasal Ø9BM
Ventricular Ø2BM
Shoulder Region
Left ØXB3
Right ØXB2
Sinus
Accessory Ø9BP
Ethmoid
Left Ø9BV
Right Ø9BU
Frontal
Left Ø9BT
Right Ø9BS
Mastoid
Left Ø9BC
Right Ø9BB
Maxillary
Left Ø9BR
Right Ø9BQ
Sphenoid
Left Ø9BX
Right Ø9BW
Skin
Abdomen ØHB7XZ
Back ØHB6XZ
Buttock ØHB8XZ
Chest ØHB5XZ
Ear
Left ØHB3XZ
Right ØHB2XZ
Face ØHB1XZ
Foot
Left ØHBNXZ
Right ØHBMXZ
Hand
Left ØHBGXZ
Right ØHBFXZ
Inguinal ØHBAXZ
Lower Arm
Left ØHBEXZ
Right ØHBDXZ
Lower Leg
Left ØHBLXZ
Right ØHBKXZ
Neck ØHB4XZ
Perineum ØHB9XZ
Scalp ØHBØXZ
Upper Arm
Left ØHBCXZ
Right ØHBBXZ
Upper Leg
Left ØHBJXZ
Right ØHBHXZ
Skull ØNBØ
Spinal Cord
Cervical ØØBW
Lumbar ØØBY
Thoracic ØØBX
Spinal Meninges ØØBT
Spleen Ø7BP
Sternum ØPBØ
Stomach ØDB6
Pylorus ØDB7
Subcutaneous Tissue and Fascia
Abdomen ØJB8
Back ØJB7
Buttock ØJB9
Chest ØJB6
Face ØJB1
Foot
Left ØJBR
Right ØJBQ
Hand
Left ØJBK
Right ØJBJ
Lower Arm
Left ØJBH
Right ØJBG
Lower Leg
Left ØJBP
Right ØJBN
Neck
Left ØJB5
Right ØJB4
Pelvic Region ØJBC

Excision — *continued*
Subcutaneous Tissue and Fascia — *continued*
Perineum ØJBB
Scalp ØJBØ
Upper Arm
Left ØJBF
Right ØJBD
Upper Leg
Left ØJBM
Right ØJBL
Tarsal
Left ØQBM
Right ØQBL
Tendon
Abdomen
Left ØLBG
Right ØLBF
Ankle
Left ØLBT
Right ØLBS
Foot
Left ØLBW
Right ØLBV
Hand
Left ØLB8
Right ØLB7
Head and Neck ØLBØ
Hip
Left ØLBK
Right ØLBJ
Knee
Left ØLBR
Right ØLBQ
Lower Arm and Wrist
Left ØLB6
Right ØLB5
Lower Leg
Left ØLBP
Right ØLBN
Perineum ØLBH
Shoulder
Left ØLB2
Right ØLB1
Thorax
Left ØLBD
Right ØLBC
Trunk
Left ØLBB
Right ØLB9
Upper Arm
Left ØLB4
Right ØLB3
Upper Leg
Left ØLBM
Right ØLBL
Testis
Bilateral ØVBC
Left ØVBB
Right ØVB9
Thalamus ØØB9
Thymus Ø7BM
Thyroid Gland
Left Lobe ØGBG
Right Lobe ØGBH
Thyroid Gland Isthmus ØGBJ
Tibia
Left ØQBH
Right ØQBG
Toe Nail ØHBRXZ
Tongue ØCB7
Tonsils ØCBP
Tooth
Lower ØCBX
Upper ØCBW
Trachea ØBB1
Tunica Vaginalis
Left ØVB7
Right ØVB6
Turbinate, Nasal Ø9BL
Tympanic Membrane
Left Ø9B8
Right Ø9B7
Ulna
Left ØPBL
Right ØPBK
Ureter
Left ØTB7
Right ØTB6
Urethra ØTBD

Subterms under main terms may continue to next column or page

Excision — *continued*
Uterine Supporting Structure ØUB4
Uterus ØUB9
Uvula ØCBN
Vagina ØUBG
Valve
Aortic Ø2BF
Mitral Ø2BG
Pulmonary Ø2BH
Tricuspid Ø2BJ
Vas Deferens
Bilateral ØVBQ
Left ØVBP
Right ØVBN
Vein
Axillary
Left Ø5B8
Right Ø5B7
Azygos Ø5BØ
Basilic
Left Ø5BC
Right Ø5BB
Brachial
Left Ø5BA
Right Ø5B9
Cephalic
Left Ø5BF
Right Ø5BD
Colic Ø6B7
Common Iliac
Left Ø6BD
Right Ø6BC
Coronary Ø2B4
Esophageal Ø6B3
External Iliac
Left Ø6BG
Right Ø6BF
External Jugular
Left Ø5BQ
Right Ø5BP
Face
Left Ø5BV
Right Ø5BT
Femoral
Left Ø6BN
Right Ø6BM
Foot
Left Ø6BV
Right Ø6BT
Gastric Ø6B2
Hand
Left Ø5BH
Right Ø5BG
Hemiazygos Ø5B1
Hepatic Ø6B4
Hypogastric
Left Ø6BJ
Right Ø6BH
Inferior Mesenteric Ø6B6
Innominate
Left Ø5B4
Right Ø5B3
Internal Jugular
Left Ø5BN
Right Ø5BM
Intracranial Ø5BL
Lower Ø6BY
Portal Ø6B8
Pulmonary
Left Ø2BT
Right Ø2BS
Renal
Left Ø6BB
Right Ø6B9
Saphenous
Left Ø6BQ
Right Ø6BP
Splenic Ø6B1
Subclavian
Left Ø5B6
Right Ø5B5
Superior Mesenteric Ø6B5
Upper Ø5BY
Vertebral
Left Ø5BS
Right Ø5BR
Vena Cava
Inferior Ø6BØ
Superior Ø2BV

Excision — *continued*
Ventricle
Left Ø2BL
Right Ø2BK
Vertebra
Cervical ØPB3
Lumbar ØQBØ
Thoracic ØPB4
Vesicle
Bilateral ØVB3
Left ØVB2
Right ØVB1
Vitreous
Left Ø8B53Z
Right Ø8B43Z
Vocal Cord
Left ØCBV
Right ØCBT
Vulva ØUBM
Wrist Region
Left ØXBH
Right ØXBG
EXCLUDER® AAA Endoprosthesis
use Intraluminal Device
use Intraluminal Device, Branched or Fenestrated, One or Two Arteries in Ø4V
use Intraluminal Device, Branched or Fenestrated, Three or More Arteries in Ø4V
EXCLUDER® IBE Endoprosthesis *use* Intraluminal Device, Branched or Fenestrated, One or Two Arteries in Ø4V
Exclusion, Left atrial appendage (LAA) *see* Occlusion, Atrium, Left Ø2L7
Exercise, rehabilitation *see* Motor Treatment, Rehabilitation FØ7
Exploration *see* Inspection
Express® Biliary SD Monorail® Premounted Stent System *use* Intraluminal Device
Express® (LD) Premounted Stent System *use* Intraluminal Device
Express® SD Renal Monorail® Premounted Stent System *use* Intraluminal Device
Ex-PRESS™ mini glaucoma shunt *use* Synthetic Substitute
Extensor carpi radialis muscle
use Lower Arm and Wrist Muscle, Left
use Lower Arm and Wrist Muscle, Right
Extensor carpi ulnaris muscle
use Lower Arm and Wrist Muscle, Left
use Lower Arm and Wrist Muscle, Right
Extensor digitorum brevis muscle
use Foot Muscle, Left
use Foot Muscle, Right
Extensor digitorum longus muscle
use Lower Leg Muscle, Left
use Lower Leg Muscle, Right
Extensor hallucis brevis muscle
use Foot Muscle, Left
use Foot Muscle, Right
Extensor hallucis longus muscle
use Lower Leg Muscle, Left
use Lower Leg Muscle, Right
External anal sphincter *use* Anal Sphincter
External auditory meatus
use External Auditory Canal, Left
use External Auditory Canal, Right
External fixator
use External Fixation Device in Head and Facial Bones
use External Fixation Device in Lower Bones
use External Fixation Device in Lower Joints
use External Fixation Device in Upper Bones
use External Fixation Device in Upper Joints
External maxillary artery *use* Face Artery
External naris *use* Nasal Mucosa and Soft Tissue
External oblique aponeurosis *use* Subcutaneous Tissue and Fascia, Trunk
External oblique muscle
use Abdomen Muscle, Left
use Abdomen Muscle, Right
External popliteal nerve *use* Peroneal Nerve
External pudendal artery
use Femoral Artery, Left
use Femoral Artery, Right
External pudendal vein
use Saphenous Vein, Left
use Saphenous Vein, Right

External urethral sphincter *use* Urethra
Extirpation
Acetabulum
Left ØQC5
Right ØQC4
Adenoids ØCCQ
Ampulla of Vater ØFCC
Anal Sphincter ØDCR
Anterior Chamber
Left Ø8C3
Right Ø8C2
Anus ØDCQ
Aorta
Abdominal Ø4CØ
Thoracic
Ascending/Arch Ø2CX
Descending Ø2CW
Aortic Body ØGCD
Appendix ØDCJ
Artery
Anterior Tibial
Left Ø4CQ
Right Ø4CP
Axillary
Left Ø3C6
Right Ø3C5
Brachial
Left Ø3C8
Right Ø3C7
Celiac Ø4C1
Colic
Left Ø4C7
Middle Ø4C8
Right Ø4C6
Common Carotid
Left Ø3CJ
Right Ø3CH
Common Iliac
Left Ø4CD
Right Ø4CC
Coronary
Four or More Arteries Ø2C3
One Artery Ø2CØ
Three Arteries Ø2C2
Two Arteries Ø2C1
External Carotid
Left Ø3CN
Right Ø3CM
External Iliac
Left Ø4CJ
Right Ø4CH
Face Ø3CR
Femoral
Left Ø4CL
Right Ø4CK
Foot
Left Ø4CW
Right Ø4CV
Gastric Ø4C2
Hand
Left Ø3CF
Right Ø3CD
Hepatic Ø4C3
Inferior Mesenteric Ø4CB
Innominate Ø3C2
Internal Carotid
Left Ø3CL
Right Ø3CK
Internal Iliac
Left Ø4CF
Right Ø4CE
Internal Mammary
Left Ø3C1
Right Ø3CØ
Intracranial Ø3CG
Lower Ø4CY
Peroneal
Left Ø4CU
Right Ø4CT
Popliteal
Left Ø4CN
Right Ø4CM
Posterior Tibial
Left Ø4CS
Right Ø4CR
Pulmonary
Left Ø2CR
Right Ø2CQ
Pulmonary Trunk Ø2CP

Extirpation — *continued*
Artery — *continued*
Radial
Left Ø3CC
Right Ø3CB
Renal
Left Ø4CA
Right Ø4C9
Splenic Ø4C4
Subclavian
Left Ø3C4
Right Ø3C3
Superior Mesenteric Ø4C5
Temporal
Left Ø3CT
Right Ø3CS
Thyroid
Left Ø3CV
Right Ø3CU
Ulnar
Left Ø3CA
Right Ø3C9
Upper Ø3CY
Vertebral
Left Ø3CQ
Right Ø3CP
Atrium
Left Ø2C7
Right Ø2C6
Auditory Ossicle
Left Ø9CA
Right Ø9C9
Basal Ganglia ØØC8
Bladder ØTCB
Bladder Neck ØTCC
Bone
Ethmoid
Left ØNCG
Right ØNCF
Frontal ØNC1
Hyoid ØNCX
Lacrimal
Left ØNCJ
Right ØNCH
Nasal ØNCB
Occipital ØNC7
Palatine
Left ØNCL
Right ØNCK
Parietal
Left ØNC4
Right ØNC3
Pelvic
Left ØQC3
Right ØQC2
Sphenoid ØNCC
Temporal
Left ØNC6
Right ØNC5
Zygomatic
Left ØNCN
Right ØNCM
Brain ØØCØ
Breast
Bilateral ØHCV
Left ØHCU
Right ØHCT
Bronchus
Lingula ØBC9
Lower Lobe
Left ØBCB
Right ØBC6
Main
Left ØBC7
Right ØBC3
Middle Lobe, Right ØBC5
Upper Lobe
Left ØBC8
Right ØBC4
Buccal Mucosa ØCC4
Bursa and Ligament
Abdomen
Left ØMCJ
Right ØMCH
Ankle
Left ØMCR
Right ØMCQ
Elbow
Left ØMC4

Extirpation — *continued*
Bursa and Ligament — *continued*
Elbow — *continued*
Right ØMC3
Foot
Left ØMCT
Right ØMCS
Hand
Left ØMC8
Right ØMC7
Head and Neck ØMCØ
Hip
Left ØMCM
Right ØMCL
Knee
Left ØMCP
Right ØMCN
Lower Extremity
Left ØMCW
Right ØMCV
Perineum ØMCK
Rib(s) ØMCG
Shoulder
Left ØMC2
Right ØMC1
Spine
Lower ØMCD
Upper ØMCC
Sternum ØMCF
Upper Extremity
Left ØMCB
Right ØMC9
Wrist
Left ØMC6
Right ØMC5
Carina ØBC2
Carotid Bodies, Bilateral ØGC8
Carotid Body
Left ØGC6
Right ØGC7
Carpal
Left ØPCN
Right ØPCM
Cavity, Cranial ØWC1
Cecum ØDCH
Cerebellum ØØCC
Cerebral Hemisphere ØØC7
Cerebral Meninges ØØC1
Cerebral Ventricle ØØC6
Cervix ØUCC
Chordae Tendineae Ø2C9
Choroid
Left Ø8CB
Right Ø8CA
Cisterna Chyli Ø7CL
Clavicle
Left ØPCB
Right ØPC9
Clitoris ØUCJ
Coccygeal Glomus ØGCB
Coccyx ØQCS
Colon
Ascending ØDCK
Descending ØDCM
Sigmoid ØDCN
Transverse ØDCL
Conduction Mechanism Ø2C8
Conjunctiva
Left Ø8CTXZZ
Right Ø8CSXZZ
Cord
Bilateral ØVCH
Left ØVCG
Right ØVCF
Cornea
Left Ø8C9XZZ
Right Ø8C8XZZ
Cul-de-sac ØUCF
Diaphragm ØBCT
Disc
Cervical Vertebral ØRC3
Cervicothoracic Vertebral ØRC5
Lumbar Vertebral ØSC2
Lumbosacral ØSC4
Thoracic Vertebral ØRC9
Thoracolumbar Vertebral ØRCB
Duct
Common Bile ØFC9
Cystic ØFC8

Extirpation — *continued*
Duct — *continued*
Hepatic
Common ØFC7
Left ØFC6
Right ØFC5
Lacrimal
Left Ø8CY
Right Ø8CX
Pancreatic ØFCD
Accessory ØFCF
Parotid
Left ØCCC
Right ØCCB
Duodenum ØDC9
Dura Mater ØØC2
Ear
External
Left Ø9C1
Right Ø9CØ
External Auditory Canal
Left Ø9C4
Right Ø9C3
Inner
Left Ø9CE
Right Ø9CD
Middle
Left Ø9C6
Right Ø9C5
Endometrium ØUCB
Epididymis
Bilateral ØVCL
Left ØVCK
Right ØVCJ
Epidural Space, Intracranial ØØC3
Epiglottis ØCCR
Esophagogastric Junction ØDC4
Esophagus ØDC5
Lower ØDC3
Middle ØDC2
Upper ØDC1
Eustachian Tube
Left Ø9CG
Right Ø9CF
Eye
Left Ø8C1XZZ
Right Ø8CØXZZ
Eyelid
Lower
Left Ø8CR
Right Ø8CQ
Upper
Left Ø8CP
Right Ø8CN
Fallopian Tube
Left ØUC6
Right ØUC5
Fallopian Tubes, Bilateral ØUC7
Femoral Shaft
Left ØQC9
Right ØQC8
Femur
Lower
Left ØQCC
Right ØQCB
Upper
Left ØQC7
Right ØQC6
Fibula
Left ØQCK
Right ØQCJ
Finger Nail ØHCQXZZ
Gallbladder ØFC4
Gastrointestinal Tract ØWCP
Genitourinary Tract ØWCR
Gingiva
Lower ØCC6
Upper ØCC5
Gland
Adrenal
Bilateral ØGC4
Left ØGC2
Right ØGC3
Lacrimal
Left Ø8CW
Right Ø8CV
Minor Salivary ØCCJ
Parotid
Left ØCC9

Extirpation — *continued*
Gland — *continued*
Parotid — *continued*
Right ØCC8
Pituitary ØGCØ
Sublingual
Left ØCCF
Right ØCCD
Submaxillary
Left ØCCH
Right ØCCG
Vestibular ØUCL
Glenoid Cavity
Left ØPC8
Right ØPC7
Glomus Jugulare ØGCC
Humeral Head
Left ØPCD
Right ØPCC
Humeral Shaft
Left ØPCG
Right ØPCF
Hymen ØUCK
Hypothalamus ØØCA
Ileocecal Valve ØDCC
Ileum ØDCB
Intestine
Large ØDCE
Left ØDCG
Right ØDCF
Small ØDC8
Iris
Left Ø8CD
Right Ø8CC
Jaw
Lower ØWC5
Upper ØWC4
Jejunum ØDCA
Joint
Acromioclavicular
Left ØRCH
Right ØRCG
Ankle
Left ØSCG
Right ØSCF
Carpal
Left ØRCR
Right ØRCQ
Carpometacarpal
Left ØRCT
Right ØRCS
Cervical Vertebral ØRC1
Cervicothoracic Vertebral ØRC4
Coccygeal ØSC6
Elbow
Left ØRCM
Right ØRCL
Finger Phalangeal
Left ØRCX
Right ØRCW
Hip
Left ØSCB
Right ØSC9
Knee
Left ØSCD
Right ØSCC
Lumbar Vertebral ØSCØ
Lumbosacral ØSC3
Metacarpophalangeal
Left ØRCV
Right ØRCU
Metatarsal-Phalangeal
Left ØSCN
Right ØSCM
Occipital-cervical ØRCØ
Sacrococcygeal ØSC5
Sacroiliac
Left ØSC8
Right ØSC7
Shoulder
Left ØRCK
Right ØRCJ
Sternoclavicular
Left ØRCF
Right ØRCE
Tarsal
Left ØSCJ
Right ØSCH

Extirpation — *continued*
Joint — *continued*
Tarsometatarsal
Left ØSCL
Right ØSCK
Temporomandibular
Left ØRCD
Right ØRCC
Thoracic Vertebral ØRC6
Thoracolumbar Vertebral ØRCA
Toe Phalangeal
Left ØSCQ
Right ØSCP
Wrist
Left ØRCP
Right ØRCN
Kidney
Left ØTC1
Right ØTCØ
Kidney Pelvis
Left ØTC4
Right ØTC3
Larynx ØCCS
Lens
Left Ø8CK
Right Ø8CJ
Lip
Lower ØCC1
Upper ØCCØ
Liver ØFCØ
Left Lobe ØFC2
Right Lobe ØFC1
Lung
Bilateral ØBCM
Left ØBCL
Lower Lobe
Left ØBCJ
Right ØBCF
Middle Lobe, Right ØBCD
Right ØBCK
Upper Lobe
Left ØBCG
Right ØBCC
Lung Lingula ØBCH
Lymphatic
Aortic Ø7CD
Axillary
Left Ø7C6
Right Ø7C5
Head Ø7CØ
Inguinal
Left Ø7CJ
Right Ø7CH
Internal Mammary
Left Ø7C9
Right Ø7C8
Lower Extremity
Left Ø7CG
Right Ø7CF
Mesenteric Ø7CB
Neck
Left Ø7C2
Right Ø7C1
Pelvis Ø7CC
Thoracic Duct Ø7CK
Thorax Ø7C7
Upper Extremity
Left Ø7C4
Right Ø7C3
Mandible
Left ØNCV
Right ØNCT
Maxilla ØNCR
Mediastinum ØWCC
Medulla Oblongata ØØCD
Mesentery ØDCV
Metacarpal
Left ØPCQ
Right ØPCP
Metatarsal
Left ØQCP
Right ØQCN
Muscle
Abdomen
Left ØKCL
Right ØKCK
Extraocular
Left Ø8CM
Right Ø8CL

Extirpation — *continued*
Muscle — *continued*
Facial ØKC1
Foot
Left ØKCW
Right ØKCV
Hand
Left ØKCD
Right ØKCC
Head ØKCØ
Hip
Left ØKCP
Right ØKCN
Lower Arm and Wrist
Left ØKCB
Right ØKC9
Lower Leg
Left ØKCT
Right ØKCS
Neck
Left ØKC3
Right ØKC2
Papillary Ø2CD
Perineum ØKCM
Shoulder
Left ØKC6
Right ØKC5
Thorax
Left ØKCJ
Right ØKCH
Tongue, Palate, Pharynx ØKC4
Trunk
Left ØKCG
Right ØKCF
Upper Arm
Left ØKC8
Right ØKC7
Upper Leg
Left ØKCR
Right ØKCQ
Nasal Mucosa and Soft Tissue Ø9CK
Nasopharynx Ø9CN
Nerve
Abdominal Sympathetic Ø1CM
Abducens ØØCL
Accessory ØØCR
Acoustic ØØCN
Brachial Plexus Ø1C3
Cervical Ø1C1
Cervical Plexus Ø1CØ
Facial ØØCM
Femoral Ø1CD
Glossopharyngeal ØØCP
Head and Neck Sympathetic Ø1CK
Hypoglossal ØØCS
Lumbar Ø1CB
Lumbar Plexus Ø1C9
Lumbar Sympathetic Ø1CN
Lumbosacral Plexus Ø1CA
Median Ø1C5
Oculomotor ØØCH
Olfactory ØØCF
Optic ØØCG
Peroneal Ø1CH
Phrenic Ø1C2
Pudendal Ø1CC
Radial Ø1C6
Sacral Ø1CR
Sacral Plexus Ø1CQ
Sacral Sympathetic Ø1CP
Sciatic Ø1CF
Thoracic Ø1C8
Thoracic Sympathetic Ø1CL
Tibial Ø1CG
Trigeminal ØØCK
Trochlear ØØCJ
Ulnar Ø1C4
Vagus ØØCQ
Nipple
Left ØHCX
Right ØHCW
Omentum ØDCU
Oral Cavity and Throat ØWC3
Orbit
Left ØNCQ
Right ØNCP
Orbital Atherectomy Technology X2C
Ovary
Bilateral ØUC2

Subterms under main terms may continue to next column or page

Extirpation — *continued*
Ovary — *continued*
Left ØUC1
Right ØUCØ
Palate
Hard ØCC2
Soft ØCC3
Pancreas ØFCG
Para-aortic Body ØGC9
Paraganglion Extremity ØGCF
Parathyroid Gland ØGCR
Inferior
Left ØGCP
Right ØGCN
Multiple ØGCQ
Superior
Left ØGCM
Right ØGCL
Patella
Left ØQCF
Right ØQCD
Pelvic Cavity ØWCJ
Penis ØVCS
Pericardial Cavity ØWCD
Pericardium Ø2CN
Peritoneal Cavity ØWCG
Peritoneum ØDCW
Phalanx
Finger
Left ØPCV
Right ØPCT
Thumb
Left ØPCS
Right ØPCR
Toe
Left ØQCR
Right ØQCQ
Pharynx ØCCM
Pineal Body ØGC1
Pleura
Left ØBCP
Right ØBCN
Pleural Cavity
Left ØWCB
Right ØWC9
Pons ØØCB
Prepuce ØVCT
Prostate ØVCØ
Radius
Left ØPCJ
Right ØPCH
Rectum ØDCP
Respiratory Tract ØWCQ
Retina
Left Ø8CF
Right Ø8CE
Retinal Vessel
Left Ø8CH
Right Ø8CG
Retroperitoneum ØWCH
Ribs
1 to 2 ØPC1
3 or More ØPC2
Sacrum ØQC1
Scapula
Left ØPC6
Right ØPC5
Sclera
Left Ø8C7XZZ
Right Ø8C6XZZ
Scrotum ØVC5
Septum
Atrial Ø2C5
Nasal Ø9CM
Ventricular Ø2CM
Sinus
Accessory Ø9CP
Ethmoid
Left Ø9CV
Right Ø9CU
Frontal
Left Ø9CT
Right Ø9CS
Mastoid
Left Ø9CC
Right Ø9CB
Maxillary
Left Ø9CR
Right Ø9CQ

Extirpation — *continued*
Sinus — *continued*
Sphenoid
Left Ø9CX
Right Ø9CW
Skin
Abdomen ØHC7XZZ
Back ØHC6XZZ
Buttock ØHC8XZZ
Chest ØHC5XZZ
Ear
Left ØHC3XZZ
Right ØHC2XZZ
Face ØHC1XZZ
Foot
Left ØHCNXZZ
Right ØHCMXZZ
Hand
Left ØHCGXZZ
Right ØHCFXZZ
Inguinal ØHCAXZZ
Lower Arm
Left ØHCEXZZ
Right ØHCDXZZ
Lower Leg
Left ØHCLXZZ
Right ØHCKXZZ
Neck ØHC4XZZ
Perineum ØHC9XZZ
Scalp ØHCØXZZ
Upper Arm
Left ØHCCXZZ
Right ØHCBXZZ
Upper Leg
Left ØHCJXZZ
Right ØHCHXZZ
Spinal Canal ØØCU
Spinal Cord
Cervical ØØCW
Lumbar ØØCY
Thoracic ØØCX
Spinal Meninges ØØCT
Spleen Ø7CP
Sternum ØPCØ
Stomach ØDC6
Pylorus ØDC7
Subarachnoid Space, Intracranial ØØC5
Subcutaneous Tissue and Fascia
Abdomen ØJC8
Back ØJC7
Buttock ØJC9
Chest ØJC6
Face ØJC1
Foot
Left ØJCR
Right ØJCQ
Hand
Left ØJCK
Right ØJCJ
Lower Arm
Left ØJCH
Right ØJCG
Lower Leg
Left ØJCP
Right ØJCN
Neck
Left ØJC5
Right ØJC4
Pelvic Region ØJCC
Perineum ØJCB
Scalp ØJCØ
Upper Arm
Left ØJCF
Right ØJCD
Upper Leg
Left ØJCM
Right ØJCL
Subdural Space, Intracranial ØØC4
Tarsal
Left ØQCM
Right ØQCL
Tendon
Abdomen
Left ØLCG
Right ØLCF
Ankle
Left ØLCT
Right ØLCS

Extirpation — *continued*
Tendon — *continued*
Foot
Left ØLCW
Right ØLCV
Hand
Left ØLC8
Right ØLC7
Head and Neck ØLCØ
Hip
Left ØLCK
Right ØLCJ
Knee
Left ØLCR
Right ØLCQ
Lower Arm and Wrist
Left ØLC6
Right ØLC5
Lower Leg
Left ØLCP
Right ØLCN
Perineum ØLCH
Shoulder
Left ØLC2
Right ØLC1
Thorax
Left ØLCD
Right ØLCC
Trunk
Left ØLCB
Right ØLC9
Upper Arm
Left ØLC4
Right ØLC3
Upper Leg
Left ØLCM
Right ØLCL
Testis
Bilateral ØVCC
Left ØVCB
Right ØVC9
Thalamus ØØC9
Thymus Ø7CM
Thyroid Gland ØGCK
Left Lobe ØGCG
Right Lobe ØGCH
Tibia
Left ØQCH
Right ØQCG
Toe Nail ØHCRXZZ
Tongue ØCC7
Tonsils ØCCP
Tooth
Lower ØCCX
Upper ØCCW
Trachea ØBC1
Tunica Vaginalis
Left ØVC7
Right ØVC6
Turbinate, Nasal Ø9CL
Tympanic Membrane
Left Ø9C8
Right Ø9C7
Ulna
Left ØPCL
Right ØPCK
Ureter
Left ØTC7
Right ØTC6
Urethra ØTCD
Uterine Supporting Structure ØUC4
Uterus ØUC9
Uvula ØCCN
Vagina ØUCG
Valve
Aortic Ø2CF
Mitral Ø2CG
Pulmonary Ø2CH
Tricuspid Ø2CJ
Vas Deferens
Bilateral ØVCQ
Left ØVCP
Right ØVCN
Vein
Axillary
Left Ø5C8
Right Ø5C7
Azygos Ø5CØ

Extirpation — *continued*
Vein — *continued*
Basilic
Left Ø5CC
Right Ø5CB
Brachial
Left Ø5CA
Right Ø5C9
Cephalic
Left Ø5CF
Right Ø5CD
Colic Ø6C7
Common Iliac
Left Ø6CD
Right Ø6CC
Coronary Ø2C4
Esophageal Ø6C3
External Iliac
Left Ø6CG
Right Ø6CF
External Jugular
Left Ø5CQ
Right Ø5CP
Face
Left Ø5CV
Right Ø5CT
Femoral
Left Ø6CN
Right Ø6CM
Foot
Left Ø6CV
Right Ø6CT
Gastric Ø6C2
Hand
Left Ø5CH
Right Ø5CG
Hemiazygos Ø5C1
Hepatic Ø6C4
Hypogastric
Left Ø6CJ
Right Ø6CH
Inferior Mesenteric Ø6C6
Innominate
Left Ø5C4
Right Ø5C3
Internal Jugular
Left Ø5CN
Right Ø5CM
Intracranial Ø5CL
Lower Ø6CY
Portal Ø6C8
Pulmonary
Left Ø2CT
Right Ø2CS
Renal
Left Ø6CB
Right Ø6C9
Saphenous
Left Ø6CQ
Right Ø6CP
Splenic Ø6C1
Subclavian
Left Ø5C6
Right Ø5C5
Superior Mesenteric Ø6C5
Upper Ø5CY
Vertebral
Left Ø5CS
Right Ø5CR
Vena Cava
Inferior Ø6CØ
Superior Ø2CV
Ventricle
Left Ø2CL
Right Ø2CK
Vertebra
Cervical ØPC3
Lumbar ØQCØ
Thoracic ØPC4
Vesicle
Bilateral ØVC3
Left ØVC2
Right ØVC1
Vitreous
Left Ø8C5
Right Ø8C4
Vocal Cord
Left ØCCV
Right ØCCT

Extirpation — *continued*
Vulva ØUCM
Extracorporeal Carbon Dioxide Removal (ECCO2R) 5AØ92ØZ
Extracorporeal shock wave lithotripsy *see* Fragmentation
Extracranial-intracranial bypass (EC-IC) *see* Bypass, Upper Arteries Ø31
Extraction
Acetabulum
Left ØQD5ØZZ
Right ØQD4ØZZ
Ampulla of Vater ØFDC
Anus ØDDQ
Appendix ØDDJ
Auditory Ossicle
Left Ø9DAØZZ
Right Ø9D9ØZZ
Bone
Ethmoid
Left ØNDGØZZ
Right ØNDFØZZ
Frontal ØND1ØZZ
Hyoid ØNDXØZZ
Lacrimal
Left ØNDJØZZ
Right ØNDHØZZ
Nasal ØNDBØZZ
Occipital ØND7ØZZ
Palatine
Left ØNDLØZZ
Right ØNDKØZZ
Parietal
Left ØND4ØZZ
Right ØND3ØZZ
Pelvic
Left ØQD3ØZZ
Right ØQD2ØZZ
Sphenoid ØNDCØZZ
Temporal
Left ØND6ØZZ
Right ØND5ØZZ
Zygomatic
Left ØNDNØZZ
Right ØNDMØZZ
Bone Marrow
Iliac Ø7DR
Sternum Ø7DQ
Vertebral Ø7DS
Breast
Bilateral ØHDVØZZ
Left ØHDUØZZ
Right ØHDTØZZ
Supernumerary ØHDYØZZ
Bronchus
Lingula ØBD9
Lower Lobe
Left ØBDB
Right ØBD6
Main
Left ØBD7
Right ØBD3
Middle Lobe, Right ØBD5
Upper Lobe
Left ØBD8
Right ØBD4
Bursa and Ligament
Abdomen
Left ØMDJ
Right ØMDH
Ankle
Left ØMDR
Right ØMDQ
Elbow
Left ØMD4
Right ØMD3
Foot
Left ØMDT
Right ØMDS
Hand
Left ØMD8
Right ØMD7
Head and Neck ØMDØ
Hip
Left ØMDM
Right ØMDL
Knee
Left ØMDP
Right ØMDN

Extraction — *continued*
Bursa and Ligament — *continued*
Lower Extremity
Left ØMDW
Right ØMDV
Perineum ØMDK
Rib(s) ØMDG
Shoulder
Left ØMD2
Right ØMD1
Spine
Lower ØMDD
Upper ØMDC
Sternum ØMDF
Upper Extremity
Left ØMDB
Right ØMD9
Wrist
Left ØMD6
Right ØMD5
Carina ØBD2
Carpal
Left ØPDNØZZ
Right ØPDMØZZ
Cecum ØDDH
Cerebral Meninges ØØD1
Cisterna Chyli Ø7DL
Clavicle
Left ØPDBØZZ
Right ØPD9ØZZ
Coccyx ØQDSØZZ
Colon
Ascending ØDDK
Descending ØDDM
Sigmoid ØDDN
Transverse ØDDL
Cornea
Left Ø8D9XZ
Right Ø8D8XZ
Duct
Common Bile ØFD9
Cystic ØFD8
Hepatic
Common ØFD7
Left ØFD6
Right ØFD5
Pancreatic ØFDD
Accessory ØFDF
Duodenum ØDD9
Dura Mater ØØD2
Endometrium ØUDB
Esophagogastric Junction ØDD4
Esophagus ØDD5
Lower ØDD3
Middle ØDD2
Upper ØDD1
Femoral Shaft
Left ØQD9ØZZ
Right ØQD8ØZZ
Femur
Lower
Left ØQDCØZZ
Right ØQDBØZZ
Upper
Left ØQD7ØZZ
Right ØQD6ØZZ
Fibula
Left ØQDKØZZ
Right ØQDJØZZ
Finger Nail ØHDQXZZ
Gallbladder ØFD4
Glenoid Cavity
Left ØPD8ØZZ
Right ØPD7ØZZ
Hair ØHDSXZZ
Humeral Head
Left ØPDDØZZ
Right ØPDCØZZ
Humeral Shaft
Left ØPDGØZZ
Right ØPDFØZZ
Ileocecal Valve ØDDC
Ileum ØDDB
Intestine
Large ØDDE
Left ØDDG
Right ØDDF
Small ØDD8
Jejunum ØDDA

Extraction — *continued*
Kidney
Left ØTD1
Right ØTDØ
Lens
Left Ø8DK3ZZ
Right Ø8DJ3ZZ
Liver ØFDØ
Left Lobe ØFD2
Right Lobe ØFD1
Lung
Bilateral ØBDM
Left ØBDL
Lower Lobe
Left ØBDJ
Right ØBDF
Middle Lobe, Right ØBDD
Right ØBDK
Upper Lobe
Left ØBDG
Right ØBDC
Lung Lingula ØBDH
Lymphatic
Aortic Ø7DD
Axillary
Left Ø7D6
Right Ø7D5
Head Ø7DØ
Inguinal
Left Ø7DJ
Right Ø7DH
Internal Mammary
Left Ø7D9
Right Ø7D8
Lower Extremity
Left Ø7DG
Right Ø7DF
Mesenteric Ø7DB
Neck
Left Ø7D2
Right Ø7D1
Pelvis Ø7DC
Thoracic Duct Ø7DK
Thorax Ø7D7
Upper Extremity
Left Ø7D4
Right Ø7D3
Mandible
Left ØNDVØZZ
Right ØNDTØZZ
Maxilla ØNDRØZZ
Metacarpal
Left ØPDQØZZ
Right ØPDPØZZ
Metatarsal
Left ØQDPØZZ
Right ØQDNØZZ
Muscle
Abdomen
Left ØKDLØZZ
Right ØKDKØZZ
Facial ØKD1ØZZ
Foot
Left ØKDWØZZ
Right ØKDVØZZ
Hand
Left ØKDDØZZ
Right ØKDCØZZ
Head ØKDØØZZ
Hip
Left ØKDPØZZ
Right ØKDNØZZ
Lower Arm and Wrist
Left ØKDBØZZ
Right ØKD9ØZZ
Lower Leg
Left ØKDTØZZ
Right ØKDSØZZ
Neck
Left ØKD3ØZZ
Right ØKD2ØZZ
Perineum ØKDMØZZ
Shoulder
Left ØKD6ØZZ
Right ØKD5ØZZ
Thorax
Left ØKDJØZZ
Right ØKDHØZZ
Tongue, Palate, Pharynx ØKD4ØZZ

Extraction — *continued*
Muscle — *continued*
Trunk
Left ØKDGØZZ
Right ØKDFØZZ
Upper Arm
Left ØKD8ØZZ
Right ØKD7ØZZ
Upper Leg
Left ØKDRØZZ
Right ØKDQØZZ
Nerve
Abdominal Sympathetic Ø1DM
Abducens ØØDL
Accessory ØØDR
Acoustic ØØDN
Brachial Plexus Ø1D3
Cervical Ø1D1
Cervical Plexus Ø1DØ
Facial ØØDM
Femoral Ø1DD
Glossopharyngeal ØØDP
Head and Neck Sympathetic Ø1DK
Hypoglossal ØØDS
Lumbar Ø1DB
Lumbar Plexus Ø1D9
Lumbar Sympathetic Ø1DN
Lumbosacral Plexus Ø1DA
Median Ø1D5
Oculomotor ØØDH
Olfactory ØØDF
Optic ØØDG
Peroneal Ø1DH
Phrenic Ø1D2
Pudendal Ø1DC
Radial Ø1D6
Sacral Ø1DR
Sacral Plexus Ø1DQ
Sacral Sympathetic Ø1DP
Sciatic Ø1DF
Thoracic Ø1D8
Thoracic Sympathetic Ø1DL
Tibial Ø1DG
Trigeminal ØØDK
Trochlear ØØDJ
Ulnar Ø1D4
Vagus ØØDQ
Orbit
Left ØNDQØZZ
Right ØNDPØZZ
Ova ØUDN
Pancreas ØFDG
Patella
Left ØQDFØZZ
Right ØQDDØZZ
Phalanx
Finger
Left ØPDVØZZ
Right ØPDTØZZ
Thumb
Left ØPDSØZZ
Right ØPDRØZZ
Toe
Left ØQDRØZZ
Right ØQDQØZZ
Pleura
Left ØBDP
Right ØBDN
Products of Conception
Ectopic 1ØD2
Extraperitoneal 1ØDØØZ2
High 1ØDØØZØ
High Forceps 1ØDØ7Z5
Internal Version 1ØDØ7Z7
Low 1ØDØØZ1
Low Forceps 1ØDØ7Z3
Mid Forceps 1ØDØ7Z4
Other 1ØDØ7Z8
Retained 1ØD1
Vacuum 1ØDØ7Z6
Radius
Left ØPDJØZZ
Right ØPDHØZZ
Rectum ØDDP
Ribs
1 to 2 ØPD1ØZZ
3 or More ØPD2ØZZ
Sacrum ØQD1ØZZ

Extraction — *continued*
Scapula
Left ØPD6ØZZ
Right ØPD5ØZZ
Septum, Nasal Ø9DM
Sinus
Accessory Ø9DP
Ethmoid
Left Ø9DV
Right Ø9DU
Frontal
Left Ø9DT
Right Ø9DS
Mastoid
Left Ø9DC
Right Ø9DB
Maxillary
Left Ø9DR
Right Ø9DQ
Sphenoid
Left Ø9DX
Right Ø9DW
Skin
Abdomen ØHD7XZZ
Back ØHD6XZZ
Buttock ØHD8XZZ
Chest ØHD5XZZ
Ear
Left ØHD3XZZ
Right ØHD2XZZ
Face ØHD1XZZ
Foot
Left ØHDNXZZ
Right ØHDMXZZ
Hand
Left ØHDGXZZ
Right ØHDFXZZ
Inguinal ØHDAXZZ
Lower Arm
Left ØHDEXZZ
Right ØHDDXZZ
Lower Leg
Left ØHDLXZZ
Right ØHDKXZZ
Neck ØHD4XZZ
Perineum ØHD9XZZ
Scalp ØHDØXZZ
Upper Arm
Left ØHDCXZZ
Right ØHDBXZZ
Upper Leg
Left ØHDJXZZ
Right ØHDHXZZ
Skull ØNDØØZZ
Spinal Meninges ØØDT
Spleen Ø7DP
Sternum ØPDØØZZ
Stomach ØDD6
Pylorus ØDD7
Subcutaneous Tissue and Fascia
Abdomen ØJD8
Back ØJD7
Buttock ØJD9
Chest ØJD6
Face ØJD1
Foot
Left ØJDR
Right ØJDQ
Hand
Left ØJDK
Right ØJDJ
Lower Arm
Left ØJDH
Right ØJDG
Lower Leg
Left ØJDP
Right ØJDN
Neck
Left ØJD5
Right ØJD4
Pelvic Region ØJDC
Perineum ØJDB
Scalp ØJDØ
Upper Arm
Left ØJDF
Right ØJDD
Upper Leg
Left ØJDM
Right ØJDL

Extraction — *continued*
Tarsal
Left ØQDMØZZ
Right ØQDLØZZ
Tendon
Abdomen
Left ØLDGØZZ
Right ØLDFØZZ
Ankle
Left ØLDTØZZ
Right ØLDSØZZ
Foot
Left ØLDWØZZ
Right ØLDVØZZ
Hand
Left ØLD8ØZZ
Right ØLD7ØZZ
Head and Neck ØLDØØZZ
Hip
Left ØLDKØZZ
Right ØLDJØZZ
Knee
Left ØLDRØZZ
Right ØLDQØZZ
Lower Arm and Wrist
Left ØLD6ØZZ
Right ØLD5ØZZ
Lower Leg
Left ØLDPØZZ
Right ØLDNØZZ
Perineum ØLDHØZZ
Shoulder
Left ØLD2ØZZ
Right ØLD1ØZZ
Thorax
Left ØLDDØZZ
Right ØLDCØZZ
Trunk
Left ØLDBØZZ
Right ØLD9ØZZ
Upper Arm
Left ØLD4ØZZ
Right ØLD3ØZZ
Upper Leg
Left ØLDMØZZ
Right ØLDLØZZ
Thymus Ø7DM
Tibia
Left ØQDHØZZ
Right ØQDGØZZ
Toe Nail ØHDRXZZ
Tooth
Lower ØCDXXZ
Upper ØCDWXZ
Trachea ØBD1
Turbinate, Nasal Ø9DL
Tympanic Membrane
Left Ø9D8
Right Ø9D7
Ulna
Left ØPDLØZZ
Right ØPDKØZZ
Vein
Basilic
Left Ø5DC
Right Ø5DB
Brachial
Left Ø5DA
Right Ø5D9
Cephalic
Left Ø5DF
Right Ø5DD
Femoral
Left Ø6DN
Right Ø6DM
Foot
Left Ø6DV
Right Ø6DT
Hand
Left Ø5DH
Right Ø5DG
Lower Ø6DY
Saphenous
Left Ø6DQ
Right Ø6DP
Upper Ø5DY
Vertebra
Cervical ØPD3ØZZ
Lumbar ØQDØØZZ

Extraction — *continued*
Vertebra — *continued*
Thoracic ØPD4ØZZ
Vocal Cord
Left ØCDV
Right ØCDT
Extradural space, intracranial *use* Epidural Space, Intracranial
Extradural space, spinal *use* Spinal Canal
EXtreme Lateral Interbody Fusion (XLIF) device *use* Interbody Fusion Device in Lower Joints

F

Face lift *see* Alteration, Face ØWØ2
Facet replacement spinal stabilization device
use Spinal Stabilization Device, Facet Replacement in ØRH
use Spinal Stabilization Device, Facet Replacement in ØSH
Facial artery *use* Face Artery
Factor Xa Inhibitor Reversal Agent, Andexanet Alfa *use* Coagulation Factor Xa, Inactivated
False vocal cord *use* Larynx
Falx cerebri *use* Dura Mater
Fascia lata
use Subcutaneous Tissue and Fascia, Left Upper Leg
use Subcutaneous Tissue and Fascia, Right Upper Leg
Fasciaplasty, fascioplasty
see Repair, Subcutaneous Tissue and Fascia ØJQ
see Replacement, Subcutaneous Tissue and Fascia ØJR
Fasciectomy *see* Excision, Subcutaneous Tissue and Fascia ØJB
Fasciorrhaphy *see* Repair, Subcutaneous Tissue and Fascia ØJQ
Fasciotomy
see Division, Subcutaneous Tissue and Fascia ØJ8
see Drainage, Subcutaneous Tissue and Fascia ØJ9
see Release
Feeding Device
Change device in
Lower ØD2DXUZ
Upper ØD2ØXUZ
Insertion of device in
Duodenum ØDH9
Esophagus ØDH5
Ileum ØDHB
Intestine, Small ØDH8
Jejunum ØDHA
Stomach ØDH6
Removal of device from
Esophagus ØDP5
Intestinal Tract
Lower ØDPD
Upper ØDPØ
Stomach ØDP6
Revision of device in
Intestinal Tract
Lower ØDWD
Upper ØDWØ
Stomach ØDW6
Femoral head
use Upper Femur, Left
use Upper Femur, Right
Femoral lymph node
use Lymphatic, Left Lower Extremity
use Lymphatic, Right Lower Extremity
Femoropatellar joint
use Knee Joint, Left
use Knee Joint, Left, Tibial Surface
use Knee Joint, Right
use Knee Joint, Right, Femoral Surface
Femorotibial joint
use Knee Joint, Left
use Knee Joint, Left, Tibial Surface
use Knee Joint, Right
use Knee Joint, Right, Tibial Surface
FETROJA® *use* Cefiderocol Anti-infective
FGS (fluorescence-guided surgery) *see* Fluorescence Guided Procedure
Fibular artery
use Peroneal Artery, Left
use Peroneal Artery, Right
Fibularis brevis muscle
use Lower Leg Muscle, Left
use Lower Leg Muscle, Right
Fibularis longus muscle
use Lower Leg Muscle, Left
use Lower Leg Muscle, Right
Fifth cranial nerve *use* Trigeminal Nerve
Filum terminale *use* Spinal Meninges
Fimbriectomy
see Excision, Female Reproductive System ØUB
see Resection, Female Reproductive System ØUT
Fine needle aspiration
Fluid or gas *see* Drainage
Tissue biopsy
see Excision
see Extraction
First cranial nerve *use* Olfactory Nerve
First intercostal nerve *use* Brachial Plexus
Fistulization
see Bypass
see Drainage
see Repair
Fitting
Arch bars, for fracture reduction *see* Reposition, Mouth and Throat ØCS
Arch bars, for immobilization *see* Immobilization, Face 2W31
Artificial limb *see* Device Fitting, Rehabilitation FØD
Hearing aid *see* Device Fitting, Rehabilitation FØD
Ocular prosthesis FØDZ8UZ
Prosthesis, limb *see* Device Fitting, Rehabilitation FØD
Prosthesis, ocular FØDZ8UZ
Fixation, bone
External, with fracture reduction *see* Reposition
External, without fracture reduction *see* Insertion
Internal, with fracture reduction *see* Reposition
Internal, without fracture reduction *see* Insertion
FLAIR® Endovascular Stent Graft *use* Intraluminal Device
Flexible Composite Mesh *use* Synthetic Substitute
Flexor carpi radialis muscle
use Lower Arm and Wrist Muscle, Left
use Lower Arm and Wrist Muscle, Right
Flexor carpi ulnaris muscle
use Lower Arm and Wrist Muscle, Left
use Lower Arm and Wrist Muscle, Right
Flexor digitorum brevis muscle
use Foot Muscle, Left
use Foot Muscle, Right
Flexor digitorum longus muscle
use Lower Leg Muscle, Left
use Lower Leg Muscle, Right
Flexor hallucis brevis muscle
use Foot Muscle, Left
use Foot Muscle, Right
Flexor hallucis longus muscle
use Lower Leg Muscle, Left
use Lower Leg Muscle, Right
Flexor pollicis longus muscle
use Lower Arm and Wrist Muscle, Left
use Lower Arm and Wrist Muscle, Right
Flow Diverter embolization device *use* Intraluminal Device, Flow Diverter in Ø3V
Fluorescence Guided Procedure
Extremity
Lower 8EØY
Upper 8EØX
Head and Neck Region 8EØ9
Aminolevulinic Acid 8EØ9ØEM
No Qualifier 8EØ9ØEZ
Trunk Region 8EØW
Fluorescent Pyrazine, Kidney XT25XE5
Fluoroscopy
Abdomen and Pelvis BW11
Airway, Upper BB1DZZZ
Ankle
Left BQ1H
Right BQ1G
Aorta
Abdominal B41Ø
Laser, Intraoperative B41Ø
Thoracic B31Ø
Laser, Intraoperative B31Ø
Thoraco-Abdominal B31P
Laser, Intraoperative B31P

Subterms under main terms may continue to next column or page

Fluoroscopy — *continued*
Aorta and Bilateral Lower Extremity Arteries B41D
Laser, Intraoperative B41D
Arm
Left BP1FZZZ
Right BP1EZZZ
Artery
Brachiocephalic-Subclavian
Laser, Intraoperative B311
Right B311
Bronchial B31L
Laser, Intraoperative B31L
Bypass Graft, Other B21F
Cervico-Cerebral Arch B31Q
Laser, Intraoperative B31Q
Common Carotid
Bilateral B315
Laser, Intraoperative B315
Left B314
Laser, Intraoperative B314
Right B313
Laser, Intraoperative B313
Coronary
Bypass Graft
Multiple B213
Laser, Intraoperative B213
Single B212
Laser, Intraoperative B212
Multiple B211
Laser, Intraoperative B211
Single B21Ø
Laser, Intraoperative B21Ø
External Carotid
Bilateral B31C
Laser, Intraoperative B31C
Left B31B
Laser, Intraoperative B31B
Right B319
Laser, Intraoperative B319
Hepatic B412
Laser, Intraoperative B412
Inferior Mesenteric B415
Laser, Intraoperative B415
Intercostal B31L
Laser, Intraoperative B31L
Internal Carotid
Bilateral B318
Laser, Intraoperative B318
Left B317
Laser, Intraoperative B317
Right B316
Laser, Intraoperative B316
Internal Mammary Bypass Graft
Left B218
Right B217
Intra-Abdominal
Laser, Intraoperative B41B
Other B41B
Intracranial B31R
Laser, Intraoperative B31R
Lower
Laser, Intraoperative B41J
Other B41J
Lower Extremity
Bilateral and Aorta B41D
Laser, Intraoperative B41D
Left B41G
Laser, Intraoperative B41G
Right B41F
Laser, Intraoperative B41F
Lumbar B419
Laser, Intraoperative B419
Pelvic B41C
Laser, Intraoperative B41C
Pulmonary
Left B31T
Laser, Intraoperative B31T
Right B31S
Laser, Intraoperative B31S
Pulmonary Trunk B31U
Laser, Intraoperative B31U
Renal
Bilateral B418
Laser, Intraoperative B418
Left B417
Laser, Intraoperative B417
Right B416
Laser, Intraoperative B416
Spinal B31M

Fluoroscopy — *continued*
Artery — *continued*
Spinal — *continued*
Laser, Intraoperative B31M
Splenic B413
Laser, Intraoperative B413
Subclavian
Laser, Intraoperative B312
Left B312
Superior Mesenteric B414
Laser, Intraoperative B414
Upper
Laser, Intraoperative B31N
Other B31N
Upper Extremity
Bilateral B31K
Laser, Intraoperative B31K
Left B31J
Laser, Intraoperative B31J
Right B31H
Laser, Intraoperative B31H
Vertebral
Bilateral B31G
Laser, Intraoperative B31G
Left B31F
Laser, Intraoperative B31F
Right B31D
Laser, Intraoperative B31D
Bile Duct BF1Ø
Pancreatic Duct and Gallbladder BF14
Bile Duct and Gallbladder BF13
Biliary Duct BF11
Bladder BT1Ø
Kidney and Ureter BT14
Left BT1F
Right BT1D
Bladder and Urethra BT1B
Bowel, Small BD1
Calcaneus
Left BQ1KZZZ
Right BQ1JZZZ
Clavicle
Left BP15ZZZ
Right BP14ZZZ
Coccyx BR1F
Colon BD14
Corpora Cavernosa BV1Ø
Dialysis Fistula B51W
Dialysis Shunt B51W
Diaphragm BB16ZZZ
Disc
Cervical BR11
Lumbar BR13
Thoracic BR12
Duodenum BD19
Elbow
Left BP1H
Right BP1G
Epiglottis B91G
Esophagus BD11
Extremity
Lower BW1C
Upper BW1J
Facet Joint
Cervical BR14
Lumbar BR16
Thoracic BR15
Fallopian Tube
Bilateral BU12
Left BU11
Right BU1Ø
Fallopian Tube and Uterus BU18
Femur
Left BQ14ZZZ
Right BQ13ZZZ
Finger
Left BP1SZZZ
Right BP1RZZZ
Foot
Left BQ1MZZZ
Right BQ1LZZZ
Forearm
Left BP1KZZZ
Right BP1JZZZ
Gallbladder BF12
Bile Duct and Pancreatic Duct BF14
Gallbladder and Bile Duct BF13
Gastrointestinal, Upper BD1

Fluoroscopy — *continued*
Hand
Left BP1PZZZ
Right BP1NZZZ
Head and Neck BW19
Heart
Left B215
Right B214
Right and Left B216
Hip
Left BQ11
Right BQ1Ø
Humerus
Left BP1BZZZ
Right BP1AZZZ
Ileal Diversion Loop BT1C
Ileal Loop, Ureters and Kidney BT1G
Intracranial Sinus B512
Joint
Acromioclavicular, Bilateral BP13ZZZ
Finger
Left BP1D
Right BP1C
Foot
Left BQ1Y
Right BQ1X
Hand
Left BP1D
Right BP1C
Lumbosacral BR1B
Sacroiliac BR1D
Sternoclavicular
Bilateral BP12ZZZ
Left BP11ZZZ
Right BP1ØZZZ
Temporomandibular
Bilateral BN19
Left BN18
Right BN17
Thoracolumbar BR18
Toe
Left BQ1Y
Right BQ1X
Kidney
Bilateral BT13
Ileal Loop and Ureter BT1G
Left BT12
Right BT11
Ureter and Bladder BT14
Left BT1F
Right BT1D
Knee
Left BQ18
Right BQ17
Larynx B91J
Leg
Left BQ1FZZZ
Right BQ1DZZZ
Lung
Bilateral BB14ZZZ
Left BB13ZZZ
Right BB12ZZZ
Mediastinum BB1CZZZ
Mouth BD1B
Neck and Head BW19
Oropharynx BD1B
Pancreatic Duct BF1
Gallbladder and Bile Buct BF14
Patella
Left BQ1WZZZ
Right BQ1VZZZ
Pelvis BR1C
Pelvis and Abdomen BW11
Pharynix B91G
Ribs
Left BP1YZZZ
Right BP1XZZZ
Sacrum BR1F
Scapula
Left BP17ZZZ
Right BP16ZZZ
Shoulder
Left BP19
Right BP18
Sinus, Intracranial B512
Spinal Cord BØ1B
Spine
Cervical BR1Ø
Lumbar BR19

Fluoroscopy — *continued*
Spine — *continued*
Thoracic BR17
Whole BR1G
Sternum BR1H
Stomach BD12
Toe
Left BQ1QZZZ
Right BQ1PZZZ
Tracheobronchial Tree
Bilateral BB19YZZ
Left BB18YZZ
Right BB17YZZ
Ureter
Ileal Loop and Kidney BT1G
Kidney and Bladder BT14
Left BT1F
Right BT1D
Left BT17
Right BT16
Urethra BT15
Urethra and Bladder BT1B
Uterus BU16
Uterus and Fallopian Tube BU18
Vagina BU19
Vasa Vasorum BV18
Vein
Cerebellar B511
Cerebral B511
Epidural B510
Jugular
Bilateral B515
Left B514
Right B513
Lower Extremity
Bilateral B51D
Left B51C
Right B51B
Other B51V
Pelvic (Iliac)
Left B51G
Right B51F
Pelvic (Iliac) Bilateral B51H
Portal B51T
Pulmonary
Bilateral B51S
Left B51R
Right B51Q
Renal
Bilateral B51L
Left B51K
Right B51J
Spanchnic B51T
Subclavian
Left B517
Right B516
Upper Extremity
Bilateral B51P
Left B51N
Right B51M
Vena Cava
Inferior B519
Superior B518
Wrist
Left BP1M
Right BP1L
Fluoroscopy, laser intraoperative
see Fluoroscopy, Heart B21
see Fluoroscopy, Lower Arteries B41
see Fluoroscopy, Upper Arteries B31
Flushing *see* Irrigation
Foley catheter *use* Drainage Device
Fontan completion procedure Stage II *see* Bypass, Vena Cava, Inferior 0610
Foramen magnum *use* Occipital Bone
Foramen of Monro (intraventricular) *use* Cerebral Ventricle
Foreskin *use* Prepuce
Formula™ Balloon-Expandable Renal Stent System *use* Intraluminal Device
Fosfomycin Anti-infective XW0
Fosfomycin injection *use* Fosfomycin Anti-infective
Fossa of Rosenmuller *use* Nasopharynx
Fourth cranial nerve *use* Trochlear Nerve
Fourth ventricle *use* Cerebral Ventricle
Fovea
use Retina, Left
use Retina, Right

Fragmentation
Ampulla of Vater 0FFC
Anus 0DFQ
Appendix 0DFJ
Artery
Anterior Tibial
Left 04FQ3Z
Right 04FP3Z
Axillary
Left 03F63Z
Right 03F53Z
Brachial
Left 03F83Z
Right 03F73Z
Common Iliac
Left 04FD3Z
Right 04FC3Z
External Iliac
Left 04FJ3Z
Right 04FH3Z
Femoral
Left 04FL3Z
Right 04FK3Z
Innominate 03F23Z
Internal Iliac
Left 04FF3Z
Right 04FE3Z
Lower 04FY3Z
Peroneal
Left 04FU3Z
Right 04FT3Z
Popliteal
Left 04FN3Z
Right 04FM3Z
Posterior Tibial
Left 04FS3Z
Right 04FR3Z
Pulmonary
Left 02FR3Z
Right 02FQ3Z
Pulmonary Trunk 02FP3Z
Radial
Left 03FC3Z
Right 03FB3Z
Subclavian
Left 03F43Z
Right 03F33Z
Ulnar
Left 03FA3Z
Right 03F93Z
Upper 03FY3Z
Bladder 0TFB
Bladder Neck 0TFC
Bronchus
Lingula 0BF9
Lower Lobe
Left 0BFB
Right 0BF6
Main
Left 0BF7
Right 0BF3
Middle Lobe, Right 0BF5
Upper Lobe
Left 0BF8
Right 0BF4
Carina 0BF2
Cavity, Cranial 0WF1
Cecum 0DFH
Cerebral Ventricle 00F6
Colon
Ascending 0DFK
Descending 0DFM
Sigmoid 0DFN
Transverse 0DFL
Duct
Common Bile 0FF9
Cystic 0FF8
Hepatic
Common 0FF7
Left 0FF6
Right 0FF5
Pancreatic 0FFD
Accessory 0FFF
Parotid
Left 0CFC
Right 0CFB
Duodenum 0DF9
Epidural Space, Intracranial 00F3
Esophagus 0DF5

Fragmentation — *continued*
Fallopian Tube
Left 0UF6
Right 0UF5
Fallopian Tubes, Bilateral 0UF7
Gallbladder 0FF4
Gastrointestinal Tract 0WFP
Genitourinary Tract 0WFR
Ileum 0DFB
Intestine
Large 0DFE
Left 0DFG
Right 0DFF
Small 0DF8
Jejunum 0DFA
Kidney Pelvis
Left 0TF4
Right 0TF3
Mediastinum 0WFC
Oral Cavity and Throat 0WF3
Pelvic Cavity 0WFJ
Pericardial Cavity 0WFD
Pericardium 02FN
Peritoneal Cavity 0WFG
Pleural Cavity
Left 0WFB
Right 0WF9
Rectum 0DFP
Respiratory Tract 0WFQ
Spinal Canal 00FU
Stomach 0DF6
Subarachnoid Space, Intracranial 00F5
Subdural Space, Intracranial 00F4
Trachea 0BF1
Ureter
Left 0TF7
Right 0TF6
Urethra 0TFD
Uterus 0UF9
Vein
Axillary
Left 05F83Z
Right 05F73Z
Basilic
Left 05FC3Z
Right 05FB3Z
Brachial
Left 05FA3Z
Right 05F93Z
Cephalic
Left 05FF3Z
Right 05FD3Z
Common Iliac
Left 06FD3Z
Right 06FC3Z
External Iliac
Left 06FG3Z
Right 06FF3Z
Femoral
Left 06FN3Z
Right 06FM3Z
Hypogastric
Left 06FJ3Z
Right 06FH3Z
Innominate
Left 05F43Z
Right 05F33Z
Lower 06FY3Z
Pulmonary
Left 02FT3Z
Right 02FS3Z
Saphenous
Left 06FQ3Z
Right 06FP3Z
Subclavian
Left 05F63Z
Right 05F53Z
Upper 05FY3Z
Vitreous
Left 08F5
Right 08F4
Fragmentation, Ultrasonic *see* Fragmentation, Artery
Freestyle (Stentless) Aortic Root Bioprosthesis *use* Zooplastic Tissue in Heart and Great Vessels
Frenectomy
see Excision, Mouth and Throat 0CB
see Resection, Mouth and Throat 0CT

Frenoplasty, frenuloplasty
see Repair, Mouth and Throat ØCQ
see Replacement, Mouth and Throat ØCR
see Supplement, Mouth and Throat ØCU
Frenotomy
see Drainage, Mouth and Throat ØC9
see Release, Mouth and Throat ØCN
Frenulotomy
see Drainage, Mouth and Throat ØC9
see Release, Mouth and Throat ØCN
Frenulum labii inferioris *use* Lower Lip
Frenulum labii superioris *use* Upper Lip
Frenulum linguae *use* Tongue
Frenulumectomy
see Excision, Mouth and Throat ØCB
see Resection, Mouth and Throat ØCT
Frontal lobe *use* Cerebral Hemisphere
Frontal vein
use Face Vein, Left
use Face Vein, Right
Fulguration *see* Destruction
Fundoplication, gastroesophageal *see* Restriction, Esophagogastric Junction ØDV4
Fundus uteri *use* Uterus
Fusion
Acromioclavicular
Left ØRGH
Right ØRGG
Ankle
Left ØSGG
Right ØSGF
Carpal
Left ØRGR
Right ØRGQ
Carpometacarpal
Left ØRGT
Right ØRGS
Cervical Vertebral ØRG1
2 or more ØRG2
Interbody Fusion Device
Nanotextured Surface XRG2Ø92
Radiolucent Porous XRG2ØF3
Interbody Fusion Device
Nanotextured Surface XRG1Ø92
Radiolucent Porous XRG1ØF3
Cervicothoracic Vertebral ØRG4
Interbody Fusion Device
Nanotextured Surface XRG4Ø92
Radiolucent Porous XRG4ØF3
Coccygeal ØSG6
Elbow
Left ØRGM
Right ØRGL
Finger Phalangeal
Left ØRGX
Right ØRGW
Hip
Left ØSGB
Right ØSG9
Knee
Left ØSGD
Right ØSGC
Lumbar Vertebral ØSGØ
2 or more ØSG1
Interbody Fusion Device
Nanotextured Surface XRGCØ92
Radiolucent Porous XRGCØF3
Interbody Fusion Device
Nanotextured Surface XRGBØ92
Radiolucent Porous XRGBØF3
Lumbosacral ØSG3
Interbody Fusion Device
Nanotextured Surface XRGDØ92
Radiolucent Porous XRGDØF3
Metacarpophalangeal
Left ØRGV
Right ØRGU
Metatarsal-Phalangeal
Left ØSGN
Right ØSGM
Occipital-cervical ØRGØ
Interbody Fusion Device
Nanotextured Surface XRGØØ92
Radiolucent Porous XRGØØF3
Sacrococcygeal ØSG5
Sacroiliac
Left ØSG8
Right ØSG7

Fusion — *continued*
Shoulder
Left ØRGK
Right ØRGJ
Sternoclavicular
Left ØRGF
Right ØRGE
Tarsal
Left ØSGJ
Right ØSGH
Tarsometatarsal
Left ØSGL
Right ØSGK
Temporomandibular
Left ØRGD
Right ØRGC
Thoracic Vertebral ØRG6
2 to 7 ØRG7
Interbody Fusion Device
Nanotextured Surface XRG7Ø92
Radiolucent Porous XRG7ØF3
8 or more ØRG8
Interbody Fusion Device
Nanotextured Surface XRG8Ø92
Radiolucent Porous XRG8ØF3
Interbody Fusion Device
Nanotextured Surface XRG6Ø92
Radiolucent Porous XRG6ØF3
Thoracolumbar Vertebral ØRGA
Interbody Fusion Device
Nanotextured Surface XRGAØ92
Radiolucent Porous XRGAØF3
Toe Phalangeal
Left ØSGQ
Right ØSGP
Wrist
Left ØRGP
Right ØRGN
Fusion screw (compression) (lag) (locking)
use Internal Fixation Device in Lower Joints
use Internal Fixation Device in Upper Joints

G

Gait training *see* Motor Treatment, Rehabilitation FØ7
Galea aponeurotica *use* Subcutaneous Tissue and Fascia, Scalp
GammaTile™ *use* Radioactive Element, Cesium-131 Collagen Implant in ØØH
Ganglion impar (ganglion of Walther) *use* Sacral Sympathetic Nerve
Ganglionectomy
Destruction of lesion *see* Destruction
Excision of lesion *see* Excision
Gasserian ganglion *use* Trigeminal Nerve
Gastrectomy
Partial *see* Excision, Stomach ØDB6
Total *see* Resection, Stomach ØDT6
Vertical (sleeve) *see* Excision, Stomach ØDB6
Gastric electrical stimulation (GES) lead *use* Stimulator Lead in Gastrointestinal System
Gastric lymph node *use* Lymphatic, Aortic
Gastric pacemaker lead *use* Stimulator Lead in Gastrointestinal System
Gastric plexus *use* Abdominal Sympathetic Nerve
Gastrocnemius muscle
use Lower Leg Muscle, Left
use Lower Leg Muscle, Right
Gastrocolic ligament *use* Omentum
Gastrocolic omentum *use* Omentum
Gastrocolostomy
see Bypass, Gastrointestinal System ØD1
see Drainage, Gastrointestinal System ØD9
Gastroduodenal artery *use* Hepatic Artery
Gastroduodenectomy
see Excision, Gastrointestinal System ØDB
see Resection, Gastrointestinal System ØDT
Gastroduodenoscopy ØDJØ8ZZ
Gastroenteroplasty
see Repair, Gastrointestinal System ØDQ
see Supplement, Gastrointestinal System ØDU
Gastroenterostomy
see Bypass, Gastrointestinal System ØD1
see Drainage, Gastrointestinal System ØD9
Gastroesophageal (GE) junction *use* Esophagogastric Junction

Gastrogastrostomy
see Bypass, Stomach ØD16
see Drainage, Stomach ØD96
Gastrohepatic omentum *use* Omentum
Gastrojejunostomy
see Bypass, Stomach ØD16
see Drainage, Stomach ØD96
Gastrolysis *see* Release, Stomach ØDN6
Gastropexy
see Repair, Stomach ØDQ6
see Reposition, Stomach ØDS6
Gastrophrenic ligament *use* Omentum
Gastroplasty
see Repair, Stomach ØDQ6
see Supplement, Stomach ØDU6
Gastroplication *see* Restriction, Stomach ØDV6
Gastropylorectomy *see* Excision, Gastrointestinal System ØDB
Gastrorrhaphy *see* Repair, Stomach ØDQ6
Gastroscopy ØDJ68ZZ
Gastrosplenic ligament *use* Omentum
Gastrostomy
see Bypass, Stomach ØD16
see Drainage, Stomach ØD96
Gastrotomy *see* Drainage, Stomach ØD96
Gemellus muscle
use Hip Muscle, Left
use Hip Muscle, Right
Geniculate ganglion *use* Facial Nerve
Geniculate nucleus *use* Thalamus
Genioglossus muscle *use* Tongue, Palate, Pharynx Muscle
Genioplasty *see* Alteration, Jaw, Lower ØWØ5
Genitofemoral nerve *use* Lumbar Plexus
GIAPREZA™ *use* Synthetic Human Angiotensin II
Gilteritinib Antineoplastic XWØDXV5
Gingivectomy *see* Excision, Mouth and Throat ØCB
Gingivoplasty
see Repair, Mouth and Throat ØCQ
see Replacement, Mouth and Throat ØCR
see Supplement, Mouth and Throat ØCU
Glans penis *use* Prepuce
Glenohumeral joint
use Shoulder Joint, Left
use Shoulder Joint, Right
Glenohumeral ligament
use Shoulder Bursa and Ligament, Left
use Shoulder Bursa and Ligament, Right
Glenoid fossa (of scapula)
use Glenoid Cavity, Left
use Glenoid Cavity, Right
Glenoid ligament (labrum)
use Shoulder Joint, Left
use Shoulder Joint, Right
Globus pallidus *use* Basal Ganglia
Glomectomy
see Excision, Endocrine System ØGB
see Resection, Endocrine System ØGT
Glossectomy
see Excision, Tongue ØCB7
see Resection, Tongue ØCT7
Glossoepiglottic fold *use* Epiglottis
Glossopexy
see Repair, Tongue ØCQ7
see Reposition, Tongue ØCS7
Glossoplasty
see Repair, Tongue ØCQ7
see Replacement, Tongue ØCR7
see Supplement, Tongue ØCU7
Glossorrhaphy *see* Repair, Tongue ØCQ7
Glossotomy *see* Drainage, Tongue ØC97
Glottis *use* Larynx
Gluteal Artery Perforator Flap
Replacement
Bilateral ØHRVØ79
Left ØHRUØ79
Right ØHRTØ79
Transfer
Left ØKXG
Right ØKXF
Gluteal lymph node *use* Lymphatic, Pelvis
Gluteal vein
use Hypogastric Vein, Left
use Hypogastric Vein, Right
Gluteus maximus muscle
use Hip Muscle, Left

Gluteus maximus muscle — *continued*
use Hip Muscle, Right
Gluteus medius muscle
use Hip Muscle, Left
use Hip Muscle, Right
Gluteus minimus muscle
use Hip Muscle, Left
use Hip Muscle, Right
GORE EXCLUDER® AAA Endoprosthesis
use Intraluminal Device
use Intraluminal Device, Branched or Fenestrated, One or Two Arteries in Ø4V
use Intraluminal Device, Branched or Fenestrated, Three or More Arteries in Ø4V
GORE EXCLUDER® IBE Endoprosthesis *use* Intraluminal Device, Branched or Fenestrated, One or Two Arteries in Ø4V
GORE TAG® Thoracic Endoprosthesis *use* Intraluminal Device
GORE® DUALMESH® *use* Synthetic Substitute
Gracilis muscle
use Upper Leg Muscle, Left
use Upper Leg Muscle, Right
Graft
see Replacement
see Supplement
Great auricular nerve *use* Cervical Plexus
Great cerebral vein *use* Intracranial Vein
Great(er) saphenous vein
use Saphenous Vein, Left
use Saphenous Vein, Right
Greater alar cartilage *use* Nasal Mucosa and Soft Tissue
Greater occipital nerve *use* Cervical Nerve
Greater Omentum *use* Omentum
Greater splanchnic nerve *use* Thoracic Sympathetic Nerve
Greater superficial petrosal nerve *use* Facial Nerve
Greater trochanter
use Upper Femur, Left
use Upper Femur, Right
Greater tuberosity
use Humeral Head, Left
use Humeral Head, Right
Greater vestibular (Bartholin's) gland *use* Vestibular Gland
Greater wing *use* Sphenoid Bone
Guedel airway *use* Intraluminal Device, Airway in Mouth and Throat
Guidance, catheter placement
EKG *see* Measurement, Physiological Systems 4AØ
Fluoroscopy *see* Fluoroscopy, Veins B51
Ultrasound *see* Ultrasonography, Veins B54

H

Hallux
use 1st Toe, Left
use 1st Toe, Right
Hamate bone
use Carpal, Left
use Carpal, Right
Hancock Bioprosthesis (aortic) (mitral) valve *use* Zooplastic Tissue in Heart and Great Vessels
Hancock Bioprosthetic Valved Conduit *use* Zooplastic Tissue in Heart and Great Vessels
Harvesting, stem cells *see* Pheresis, Circulatory 6A55
Head of fibula
use Fibula, Left
use Fibula, Right
Hearing Aid Assessment F14Z
Hearing Assessment F13Z
Hearing Device
Bone Conduction
Left Ø9HE
Right Ø9HD
Insertion of device in
Left ØNH6
Right ØNH5
Multiple Channel Cochlear Prosthesis
Left Ø9HE
Right Ø9HD
Removal of device from, Skull ØNPØ
Revision of device in, Skull ØNWØ
Single Channel Cochlear Prosthesis
Left Ø9HE
Hearing Device — *continued*
Single Channel Cochlear Prosthesis — *continued*
Right Ø9HD
Hearing Treatment FØ9Z
Heart Assist System
Implantable
Insertion of device in, Heart Ø2HA
Removal of device from, Heart Ø2PA
Revision of device in, Heart Ø2WA
Short-term External
Insertion of device in, Heart Ø2HA
Removal of device from, Heart Ø2PA
Revision of device in, Heart Ø2WA
HeartMate 3™ LVAS *use* Implantable Heart Assist System in Heart and Great Vessels
HeartMate II® Left Ventricular Assist Device (LVAD) *use* Implantable Heart Assist System in Heart and Great Vessels
HeartMate XVE® Left Ventricular Assist Device (LVAD) *use* Implantable Heart Assist System in Heart and Great Vessels
HeartMate® implantable heart assist system *see* Insertion of device in, Heart Ø2HA
Helix
use Ear, External, Bilateral
use Ear, External, Left
use Ear, External, Right
Hematopoietic cell transplant (HCT) *see* Transfusion, Circulatory 3Ø2
Hemicolectomy *see* Resection, Gastrointestinal System ØDT
Hemicystectomy *see* Excision, Urinary System ØTB
Hemigastrectomy *see* Excision, Gastrointestinal System ØDB
Hemiglossectomy *see* Excision, Mouth and Throat ØCB
Hemilaminectomy
see Excision, Lower Bones ØQB
see Excision, Upper Bones ØPB
Hemilaminotomy
see Drainage, Lower Bones ØQ9
see Drainage, Upper Bones ØP9
see Excision, Lower Bones ØQB
see Excision, Upper Bones ØPB
see Release, Central Nervous System and Cranial Nerves ØØN
see Release, Lower Bones ØQN
see Release, Peripheral Nervous System Ø1N
see Release, Upper Bones ØPN
Hemilaryngectomy *see* Excision, Larynx ØCBS
Hemimandibulectomy *see* Excision, Head and Facial Bones ØNB
Hemimaxillectomy *see* Excision, Head and Facial Bones ØNB
Hemipylorectomy *see* Excision, Gastrointestinal System ØDB
Hemispherectomy
see Excision, Central Nervous System and Cranial Nerves ØØB
see Resection, Central Nervous System and Cranial Nerves ØØT
Hemithyroidectomy
see Excision, Endocrine System ØGB
see Resection, Endocrine System ØGT
Hemodialysis *see* Performance, Urinary 5A1D
Hemolung® Respiratory Assist System (RAS) 5AØ92ØZ
Hemospray® Endoscopic Hemostat *use* Mineral-based Topical Hemostatic Agent
Hepatectomy
see Excision, Hepatobiliary System and Pancreas ØFB
see Resection, Hepatobiliary System and Pancreas ØFT
Hepatic artery proper *use* Hepatic Artery
Hepatic flexure *use* Transverse Colon
Hepatic lymph node *use* Lymphatic, Aortic
Hepatic plexus *use* Abdominal Sympathetic Nerve
Hepatic portal vein *use* Portal Vein
Hepaticoduodenostomy
see Bypass, Hepatobiliary System and Pancreas ØF1
see Drainage, Hepatobiliary System and Pancreas ØF9
Hepaticotomy *see* Drainage, Hepatobiliary System and Pancreas ØF9
Hepatocholedochostomy *see* Drainage, Duct, Common Bile ØF99
Hepatogastric ligament *use* Omentum
Hepatopancreatic ampulla *use* Ampulla of Vater
Hepatopexy
see Repair, Hepatobiliary System and Pancreas ØFQ
see Reposition, Hepatobiliary System and Pancreas ØFS
Hepatorrhaphy *see* Repair, Hepatobiliary System and Pancreas ØFQ
Hepatotomy *see* Drainage, Hepatobiliary System and Pancreas ØF9
Herculink (RX) Elite Renal Stent System *use* Intraluminal Device
Herniorrhaphy
see Repair, Anatomical Regions, General ØWQ
see Repair, Anatomical Regions, Lower Extremities ØYQ
With synthetic substitute
see Supplement, Anatomical Regions, General ØWU
see Supplement, Anatomical Regions, Lower Extremities ØYU
Hip (joint) liner *use* Liner in Lower Joints
HIPEC (hyperthermic intraperitoneal chemotherapy) 3EØM3ØY
Holter monitoring 4A12X45
Holter valve ventricular shunt *use* Synthetic Substitute
Human angiotensin II, synthetic *use* Synthetic Human Angiotensin II
Humeroradial joint
use Elbow Joint, Left
use Elbow Joint, Right
Humeroulnar joint
use Elbow Joint, Left
use Elbow Joint, Right
Humerus, distal
use Humeral Shaft, Left
use Humeral Shaft, Right
Hydrocelectomy *see* Excision, Male Reproductive System ØVB
Hydrotherapy
Assisted exercise in pool *see* Motor Treatment, Rehabilitation FØ7
Whirlpool *see* Activities of Daily Living Treatment, Rehabilitation FØ8
Hymenectomy
see Excision, Hymen ØUBK
see Resection, Hymen ØUTK
Hymenoplasty
see Repair, Hymen ØUQK
see Supplement, Hymen ØUUK
Hymenorrhaphy *see* Repair, Hymen ØUQK
Hymenotomy
see Division, Hymen ØU8K
see Drainage, Hymen ØU9K
Hyoglossus muscle *use* Tongue, Palate, Pharynx Muscle
Hyoid artery
use Thyroid Artery, Left
use Thyroid Artery, Right
Hyperalimentation *see* Introduction of substance in or on
Hyperbaric oxygenation
Decompression sickness treatment *see* Decompression, Circulatory 6A15
Wound treatment *see* Assistance, Circulatory 5AØ5
Hyperthermia
Radiation Therapy
Abdomen DWY38ZZ
Adrenal Gland DGY28ZZ
Bile Ducts DFY28ZZ
Bladder DTY28ZZ
Bone Marrow D7YØ8ZZ
Bone, Other DPYC8ZZ
Brain DØYØ8ZZ
Brain Stem DØY18ZZ
Breast
Left DMYØ8ZZ
Right DMY18ZZ
Bronchus DBY18ZZ
Cervix DUY18ZZ
Chest DWY28ZZ
Chest Wall DBY78ZZ
Colon DDY58ZZ
Diaphragm DBY88ZZ
Duodenum DDY28ZZ
Ear D9YØ8ZZ

Hyperthermia — *continued*
Radiation Therapy — *continued*
Esophagus DDY08ZZ
Eye D8Y08ZZ
Femur DPY98ZZ
Fibula DPYB8ZZ
Gallbladder DFY18ZZ
Gland
Adrenal DGY28ZZ
Parathyroid DGY48ZZ
Pituitary DGY08ZZ
Thyroid DGY58ZZ
Glands, Salivary D9Y68ZZ
Head and Neck DWY18ZZ
Hemibody DWY48ZZ
Humerus DPY68ZZ
Hypopharynx D9Y38ZZ
Ileum DDY48ZZ
Jejunum DDY38ZZ
Kidney DTY08ZZ
Larynx D9YB8ZZ
Liver DFY08ZZ
Lung DBY28ZZ
Lymphatics
Abdomen D7Y68ZZ
Axillary D7Y48ZZ
Inguinal D7Y88ZZ
Neck D7Y38ZZ
Pelvis D7Y78ZZ
Thorax D7Y58ZZ
Mandible DPY38ZZ
Maxilla DPY28ZZ
Mediastinum DBY68ZZ
Mouth D9Y48ZZ
Nasopharynx D9YD8ZZ
Neck and Head DWY18ZZ
Nerve, Peripheral D0Y78ZZ
Nose D9Y18ZZ
Oropharynx D9YF8ZZ
Ovary DUY08ZZ
Palate
Hard D9Y88ZZ
Soft D9Y98ZZ
Pancreas DFY38ZZ
Parathyroid Gland DGY48ZZ
Pelvic Bones DPY88ZZ
Pelvic Region DWY68ZZ
Pineal Body DGY18ZZ
Pituitary Gland DGY08ZZ
Pleura DBY58ZZ
Prostate DVY08ZZ
Radius DPY78ZZ
Rectum DDY78ZZ
Rib DPY58ZZ
Sinuses D9Y78ZZ
Skin
Abdomen DHY88ZZ
Arm DHY48ZZ
Back DHY78ZZ
Buttock DHY98ZZ
Chest DHY68ZZ
Face DHY28ZZ
Leg DHYB8ZZ
Neck DHY38ZZ
Skull DPY08ZZ
Spinal Cord D0Y68ZZ
Spleen D7Y28ZZ
Sternum DPY48ZZ
Stomach DDY18ZZ
Testis DVY18ZZ
Thymus D7Y18ZZ
Thyroid Gland DGY58ZZ
Tibia DPYB8ZZ
Tongue D9Y58ZZ
Trachea DBY08ZZ
Ulna DPY78ZZ
Ureter DTY18ZZ
Urethra DTY38ZZ
Uterus DUY28ZZ
Whole Body DWY58ZZ
Whole Body 6A3Z
Hyperthermic intraperitoneal chemotherapy (HIPEC) 3E0M30Y
Hypnosis GZFZZZZ
Hypogastric artery
use Internal Iliac Artery, Left
use Internal Iliac Artery, Right
Hypopharynx *use* Pharynx
Hypophysectomy
see Excision, Gland, Pituitary 0GB0
see Resection, Gland, Pituitary 0GT0
Hypophysis *use* Pituitary Gland
Hypothalamotomy *see* Destruction, Thalamus 0059
Hypothenar muscle
use Hand Muscle, Left
use Hand Muscle, Right
Hypothermia, Whole Body 6A4Z
Hysterectomy
Supracervical *see* Resection, Uterus 0UT9
Total *see* Resection, Uterus 0UT9
Hysterolysis *see* Release, Uterus 0UN9
Hysteropexy
see Repair, Uterus 0UQ9
see Reposition, Uterus 0US9
Hysteroplasty *see* Repair, Uterus 0UQ9
Hysterorrhaphy *see* Repair, Uterus 0UQ9
Hysteroscopy 0UJD8ZZ
Hysterotomy *see* Drainage, Uterus 0U99
Hysterotrachelectomy
see Resection, Cervix 0UTC
see Resection, Uterus 0UT9
Hysterotracheloplasty *see* Repair, Uterus 0UQ9
Hysterotrachelorrhaphy *see* Repair, Uterus 0UQ9

I

IABP (Intra-aortic balloon pump) *see* Assistance, Cardiac 5A02
IAEMT (Intraoperative anesthetic effect monitoring and titration) *see* Monitoring, Central Nervous 4A10
IASD® (InterAtrial Shunt Device), Corvia *use* Synthetic Substitute
Idarucizumab, Dabigatran Reversal Agent XW0
IHD (Intermittent hemodialysis) 5A1D70Z
Ileal artery *use* Superior Mesenteric Artery
Ileectomy
see Excision, Ileum 0DBB
see Resection, Ileum 0DTB
Ileocolic artery *use* Superior Mesenteric Artery
Ileocolic vein *use* Colic Vein
Ileopexy
see Repair, Ileum 0DQB
see Reposition, Ileum 0DSB
Ileorrhaphy *see* Repair, Ileum 0DQB
Ileoscopy 0DJD8ZZ
Ileostomy
see Bypass, Ileum 0D1B
see Drainage, Ileum 0D9B
Ileotomy *see* Drainage, Ileum 0D9B
Ileoureterostomy *see* Bypass, Urinary System 0T1
Iliac crest
use Pelvic Bone, Left
use Pelvic Bone, Right
Iliac fascia
use Subcutaneous Tissue and Fascia, Left Upper Leg
use Subcutaneous Tissue and Fascia, Right Upper Leg
Iliac lymph node *use* Lymphatic, Pelvis
Iliacus muscle
use Hip Muscle, Left
use Hip Muscle, Right
Iliofemoral ligament
use Hip Bursa and Ligament, Left
use Hip Bursa and Ligament, Right
Iliohypogastric nerve *use* Lumbar Plexus
Ilioinguinal nerve *use* Lumbar Plexus
Iliolumbar artery
use Internal Iliac Artery, Left
use Internal Iliac Artery, Right
Iliolumbar ligament *use* Lower Spine Bursa and Ligament
Iliotibial tract (band)
use Subcutaneous Tissue and Fascia, Left Upper Leg
use Subcutaneous Tissue and Fascia, Right Upper Leg
Ilium
use Pelvic Bone, Left
use Pelvic Bone, Right
Ilizarov external fixator
use External Fixation Device, Ring in 0PH
use External Fixation Device, Ring in 0PS
Ilizarov external fixator — *continued*
use External Fixation Device, Ring in 0QH
use External Fixation Device, Ring in 0QS
Ilizarov-Vecklich device
use External Fixation Device, Limb Lengthening in 0PH
use External Fixation Device, Limb Lengthening in 0QH
Imaging, diagnostic
see Computerized Tomography (CT Scan)
see Fluoroscopy
see Magnetic Resonance Imaging (MRI)
see Plain Radiography
see Ultrasonography
IMFINZI® *use* Durvalumab Antineoplastic
Imipenem-cilastatin-relebactam Anti-infective XW0
IMI/REL *use* Imipenem-cilastatin-relebactam Anti-infective
Immobilization
Abdominal Wall 2W33X
Arm
Lower
Left 2W3DX
Right 2W3CX
Upper
Left 2W3BX
Right 2W3AX
Back 2W35X
Chest Wall 2W34X
Extremity
Lower
Left 2W3MX
Right 2W3LX
Upper
Left 2W39X
Right 2W38X
Face 2W31X
Finger
Left 2W3KX
Right 2W3JX
Foot
Left 2W3TX
Right 2W3SX
Hand
Left 2W3FX
Right 2W3EX
Head 2W30X
Inguinal Region
Left 2W37X
Right 2W36X
Leg
Lower
Left 2W3RX
Right 2W3QX
Upper
Left 2W3PX
Right 2W3NX
Neck 2W32X
Thumb
Left 2W3HX
Right 2W3GX
Toe
Left 2W3VX
Right 2W3UX
Immunization *see* Introduction of Serum, Toxoid, and Vaccine
Immunotherapy *see* Introduction of Immunotherapeutic Substance
Immunotherapy, antineoplastic
Interferon *see* Introduction of Low-dose Interleukin-2
Interleukin-2, high-dose *see* Introduction of High-dose Interleukin-2
Interleukin-2, low-dose *see* Introduction of Low-dose Interleukin-2
Monoclonal antibody *see* Introduction of Monoclonal Antibody
Proleukin, high-dose *see* Introduction of High-dose Interleukin-2
Proleukin, low-dose *see* Introduction of Low-dose Interleukin-2
Impella® heart pump *use* Short-term External Heart Assist System in Heart and Great Vessels
Impeller Pump
Continuous, Output 5A0221D
Intermittent, Output 5A0211D

Implantable cardioverter-defibrillator (ICD) *use* Defibrillator Generator in ØJH
Implantable drug infusion pump (anti-spasmodic) (chemotherapy) (pain) *use* Infusion Device, Pump in Subcutaneous Tissue and Fascia
Implantable glucose monitoring device *use* Monitoring Device
Implantable hemodynamic monitor (IHM) *use* Monitoring Device, Hemodynamic in ØJH
Implantable hemodynamic monitoring system (IHMS) *use* Monitoring Device, Hemodynamic in ØJH
Implantable Miniature Telescope™ (IMT) *use* Synthetic Substitute, Intraocular Telescope in Ø8R
Implantation
see Insertion
see Replacement
Implanted (venous)(access) port *use* Vascular Access Device, Totally Implantable in Subcutaneous Tissue and Fascia
IMV (intermittent mandatory ventilation) *see* Assistance, Respiratory 5AØ9
In Vitro Fertilization 8EØZXY1
Incision, abscess *see* Drainage
Incudectomy
see Excision, Ear, Nose, Sinus Ø9B
see Resection, Ear, Nose, Sinus Ø9T
Incudopexy
see Repair, Ear, Nose, Sinus Ø9Q
see Reposition, Ear, Nose, Sinus Ø9S
Incus
use Auditory Ossicle, Left
use Auditory Ossicle, Right
Induction of labor
Artificial rupture of membranes *see* Drainage, Pregnancy 1Ø9
Oxytocin *see* Introduction of Hormone
InDura, intrathecal catheter (1P) (spinal) *use* Infusion Device
Inferior cardiac nerve *use* Thoracic Sympathetic Nerve
Inferior cerebellar vein *use* Intracranial Vein
Inferior cerebral vein *use* Intracranial Vein
Inferior epigastric artery
use External Iliac Artery, Left
use External Iliac Artery, Right
Inferior epigastric lymph node *use* Lymphatic, Pelvis
Inferior genicular artery
use Popliteal Artery, Left
use Popliteal Artery, Right
Inferior gluteal artery
use Internal Iliac Artery, Left
use Internal Iliac Artery, Right
Inferior gluteal nerve *use* Sacral Plexus
Inferior hypogastric plexus *use* Abdominal Sympathetic Nerve
Inferior labial artery *use* Face Artery
Inferior longitudinal muscle *use* Tongue, Palate, Pharynx Muscle
Inferior mesenteric ganglion *use* Abdominal Sympathetic Nerve
Inferior mesenteric lymph node *use* Lymphatic, Mesenteric
Inferior mesenteric plexus *use* Abdominal Sympathetic Nerve
Inferior oblique muscle
use Extraocular Muscle, Left
use Extraocular Muscle, Right
Inferior pancreaticoduodenal artery *use* Superior Mesenteric Artery
Inferior phrenic artery *use* Abdominal Aorta
Inferior rectus muscle
use Extraocular Muscle, Left
use Extraocular Muscle, Right
Inferior suprarenal artery
use Renal Artery, Left
use Renal Artery, Right
Inferior tarsal plate
use Lower Eyelid, Left
use Lower Eyelid, Right
Inferior thyroid vein
use Innominate Vein, Left
use Innominate Vein, Right
Inferior tibiofibular joint
use Ankle Joint, Left
use Ankle Joint, Right
Inferior turbinate *use* Nasal Turbinate
Inferior ulnar collateral artery
use Brachial Artery, Left
use Brachial Artery, Right
Inferior vesical artery
use Internal Iliac Artery, Left
use Internal Iliac Artery, Right
Infraauricular lymph node *use* Lymphatic, Head
Infraclavicular (deltopectoral) lymph node
use Lymphatic, Left Upper Extremity
use Lymphatic, Right Upper Extremity
Infrahyoid muscle
use Neck Muscle, Left
use Neck Muscle, Right
Infraparotid lymph node *use* Lymphatic, Head
Infraspinatus fascia
use Subcutaneous Tissue and Fascia, Left Upper Arm
use Subcutaneous Tissue and Fascia, Right Upper Arm
Infraspinatus muscle
use Shoulder Muscle, Left
use Shoulder Muscle, Right
Infundibulopelvic ligament *use* Uterine Supporting Structure
Infusion *see* Introduction of substance in or on
Infusion Device, Pump
Insertion of device in
Abdomen ØJH8
Back ØJH7
Chest ØJH6
Lower Arm
Left ØJHH
Right ØJHG
Lower Leg
Left ØJHP
Right ØJHN
Trunk ØJHT
Upper Arm
Left ØJHF
Right ØJHD
Upper Leg
Left ØJHM
Right ØJHL
Removal of device from
Lower Extremity ØJPW
Trunk ØJPT
Upper Extremity ØJPV
Revision of device in
Lower Extremity ØJWW
Trunk ØJWT
Upper Extremity ØJWV
Infusion, glucarpidase
Central Vein 3EØ43GQ
Peripheral Vein 3EØ33GQ
Inguinal canal
use Inguinal Region, Bilateral
use Inguinal Region, Left
use Inguinal Region, Right
Inguinal triangle
use Inguinal Region, Bilateral
use Inguinal Region, Left
use Inguinal Region, Right
Injection *see* Introduction of substance in or on
Injection, Concentrated Bone Marrow Aspirate (CBMA), intramuscular XKØ23Ø3
Injection reservoir, port *use* Vascular Access Device, Totally Implantable in Subcutaneous TIssue and Fascia
Injection reservoir, pump *use* Infusion Device, Pump in Subcutaneous Tissue and Fascia
Insemination, artificial 3EØP7LZ
Insertion
Antimicrobial envelope *see* Introduction of Anti-infective
Aqueous drainage shunt
see Bypass, Eye Ø81
see Drainage, Eye Ø89
Products of Conception 1ØHØ
Spinal Stabilization Device
see Insertion of device in, Lower Joints ØSH
see Insertion of device in, Upper Joints ØRH
Insertion of device in
Abdominal Wall ØWHF
Acetabulum
Left ØQH5
Right ØQH4
Anal Sphincter ØDHR
Insertion of device in — *continued*
Ankle Region
Left ØYHL
Right ØYHK
Anus ØDHQ
Aorta
Abdominal Ø4HØ
Thoracic
Ascending/Arch Ø2HX
Descending Ø2HW
Arm
Lower
Left ØXHF
Right ØXHD
Upper
Left ØXH9
Right ØXH8
Artery
Anterior Tibial
Left Ø4HQ
Right Ø4HP
Axillary
Left Ø3H6
Right Ø3H5
Brachial
Left Ø3H8
Right Ø3H7
Celiac Ø4H1
Colic
Left Ø4H7
Middle Ø4H8
Right Ø4H6
Common Carotid
Left Ø3HJ
Right Ø3HH
Common Iliac
Left Ø4HD
Right Ø4HC
Coronary
Four or More Arteries Ø2H3
One Artery Ø2HØ
Three Arteries Ø2H2
Two Arteries Ø2H1
External Carotid
Left Ø3HN
Right Ø3HM
External Iliac
Left Ø4HJ
Right Ø4HH
Face Ø3HR
Femoral
Left Ø4HL
Right Ø4HK
Foot
Left Ø4HW
Right Ø4HV
Gastric Ø4H2
Hand
Left Ø3HF
Right Ø3HD
Hepatic Ø4H3
Inferior Mesenteric Ø4HB
Innominate Ø3H2
Internal Carotid
Left Ø3HL
Right Ø3HK
Internal Iliac
Left Ø4HF
Right Ø4HE
Internal Mammary
Left Ø3H1
Right Ø3HØ
Intracranial Ø3HG
Lower Ø4HY
Peroneal
Left Ø4HU
Right Ø4HT
Popliteal
Left Ø4HN
Right Ø4HM
Posterior Tibial
Left Ø4HS
Right Ø4HR
Pulmonary
Left Ø2HR
Right Ø2HQ
Pulmonary Trunk Ø2HP
Radial
Left Ø3HC

Insertion of device in — *continued*
- Artery — *continued*
  - Radial — *continued*
    - Right Ø3HB
  - Renal
    - Left Ø4HA
    - Right Ø4H9
  - Splenic Ø4H4
  - Subclavian
    - Left Ø3H4
    - Right Ø3H3
  - Superior Mesenteric Ø4H5
  - Temporal
    - Left Ø3HT
    - Right Ø3HS
  - Thyroid
    - Left Ø3HV
    - Right Ø3HU
  - Ulnar
    - Left Ø3HA
    - Right Ø3H9
  - Upper Ø3HY
  - Vertebral
    - Left Ø3HQ
    - Right Ø3HP
- Atrium
  - Left Ø2H7
  - Right Ø2H6
- Axilla
  - Left ØXH5
  - Right ØXH4
- Back
  - Lower ØWHL
  - Upper ØWHK
- Bladder ØTHB
- Bladder Neck ØTHC
- Bone
  - Ethmoid
    - Left ØNHG
    - Right ØNHF
  - Facial ØNHW
  - Frontal ØNH1
  - Hyoid ØNHX
  - Lacrimal
    - Left ØNHJ
    - Right ØNHH
  - Lower ØQHY
  - Nasal ØNHB
  - Occipital ØNH7
  - Palatine
    - Left ØNHL
    - Right ØNHK
  - Parietal
    - Left ØNH4
    - Right ØNH3
  - Pelvic
    - Left ØQH3
    - Right ØQH2
  - Sphenoid ØNHC
  - Temporal
    - Left ØNH6
    - Right ØNH5
  - Upper ØPHY
  - Zygomatic
    - Left ØNHN
    - Right ØNHM
- Bone Marrow Ø7HT
- Brain ØØHØ
- Breast
  - Bilateral ØHHV
  - Left ØHHU
  - Right ØHHT
- Bronchus
  - Lingula ØBH9
  - Lower Lobe
    - Left ØBHB
    - Right ØBH6
  - Main
    - Left ØBH7
    - Right ØBH3
  - Middle Lobe, Right ØBH5
  - Upper Lobe
    - Left ØBH8
    - Right ØBH4
- Bursa and Ligament
  - Lower ØMHY
  - Upper ØMHX
- Buttock
  - Left ØYH1

Insertion of device in — *continued*
- Buttock — *continued*
  - Right ØYHØ
- Carpal
  - Left ØPHN
  - Right ØPHM
- Cavity, Cranial ØWH1
- Cerebral Ventricle ØØH6
- Cervix ØUHC
- Chest Wall ØWH8
- Cisterna Chyli Ø7HL
- Clavicle
  - Left ØPHB
  - Right ØPH9
- Coccyx ØQHS
- Cul-de-sac ØUHF
- Diaphragm ØBHT
- Disc
  - Cervical Vertebral ØRH3
  - Cervicothoracic Vertebral ØRH5
  - Lumbar Vertebral ØSH2
  - Lumbosacral ØSH4
  - Thoracic Vertebral ØRH9
  - Thoracolumbar Vertebral ØRHB
- Duct
  - Hepatobiliary ØFHB
  - Pancreatic ØFHD
- Duodenum ØDH9
- Ear
  - Inner
    - Left Ø9HE
    - Right Ø9HD
  - Left Ø9HJ
  - Right Ø9HH
- Elbow Region
  - Left ØXHC
  - Right ØXHB
- Epididymis and Spermatic Cord ØVHM
- Esophagus ØDH5
- Extremity
  - Lower
    - Left ØYHB
    - Right ØYH9
  - Upper
    - Left ØXH7
    - Right ØXH6
- Eye
  - Left Ø8H1
  - Right Ø8HØ
- Face ØWH2
- Fallopian Tube ØUH8
- Femoral Region
  - Left ØYH8
  - Right ØYH7
- Femoral Shaft
  - Left ØQH9
  - Right ØQH8
- Femur
  - Lower
    - Left ØQHC
    - Right ØQHB
  - Upper
    - Left ØQH7
    - Right ØQH6
- Fibula
  - Left ØQHK
  - Right ØQHJ
- Foot
  - Left ØYHN
  - Right ØYHM
- Gallbladder ØFH4
- Gastrointestinal Tract ØWHP
- Genitourinary Tract ØWHR
- Gland
  - Endocrine ØGHS
  - Salivary ØCHA
- Glenoid Cavity
  - Left ØPH8
  - Right ØPH7
- Hand
  - Left ØXHK
  - Right ØXHJ
- Head ØWHØ
- Heart Ø2HA
- Humeral Head
  - Left ØPHD
  - Right ØPHC
- Humeral Shaft
  - Left ØPHG

Insertion of device in — *continued*
- Humeral Shaft — *continued*
  - Right ØPHF
- Ileum ØDHB
- Inguinal Region
  - Left ØYH6
  - Right ØYH5
- Intestinal Tract
  - Lower ØDHD
  - Upper ØDHØ
- Intestine
  - Large ØDHE
  - Small ØDH8
- Jaw
  - Lower ØWH5
  - Upper ØWH4
- Jejunum ØDHA
- Joint
  - Acromioclavicular
    - Left ØRHH
    - Right ØRHG
  - Ankle
    - Left ØSHG
    - Right ØSHF
  - Carpal
    - Left ØRHR
    - Right ØRHQ
  - Carpometacarpal
    - Left ØRHT
    - Right ØRHS
  - Cervical Vertebral ØRH1
  - Cervicothoracic Vertebral ØRH4
  - Coccygeal ØSH6
  - Elbow
    - Left ØRHM
    - Right ØRHL
  - Finger Phalangeal
    - Left ØRHX
    - Right ØRHW
  - Hip
    - Left ØSHB
    - Right ØSH9
  - Knee
    - Left ØSHD
    - Right ØSHC
  - Lumbar Vertebral ØSHØ
  - Lumbosacral ØSH3
  - Metacarpophalangeal
    - Left ØRHV
    - Right ØRHU
  - Metatarsal-Phalangeal
    - Left ØSHN
    - Right ØSHM
  - Occipital-cervical ØRHØ
  - Sacrococcygeal ØSH5
  - Sacroiliac
    - Left ØSH8
    - Right ØSH7
  - Shoulder
    - Left ØRHK
    - Right ØRHJ
  - Sternoclavicular
    - Left ØRHF
    - Right ØRHE
  - Tarsal
    - Left ØSHJ
    - Right ØSHH
  - Tarsometatarsal
    - Left ØSHL
    - Right ØSHK
  - Temporomandibular
    - Left ØRHD
    - Right ØRHC
  - Thoracic Vertebral ØRH6
  - Thoracolumbar Vertebral ØRHA
  - Toe Phalangeal
    - Left ØSHQ
    - Right ØSHP
  - Wrist
    - Left ØRHP
    - Right ØRHN
- Kidney ØTH5
- Knee Region
  - Left ØYHG
  - Right ØYHF
- Larynx ØCHS
- Leg
  - Lower
    - Left ØYHJ

Insertion of device in — continued
Leg — continued
Lower — continued
Right ØYHH
Upper
Left ØYHD
Right ØYHC
Liver ØFHØ
Left Lobe ØFH2
Right Lobe ØFH1
Lung
Left ØBHL
Right ØBHK
Lymphatic Ø7HN
Thoracic Duct Ø7HK
Mandible
Left ØNHV
Right ØNHT
Maxilla ØNHR
Mediastinum ØWHC
Metacarpal
Left ØPHQ
Right ØPHP
Metatarsal
Left ØQHP
Right ØQHN
Mouth and Throat ØCHY
Muscle
Lower ØKHY
Upper ØKHX
Nasal Mucosa and Soft Tissue Ø9HK
Nasopharynx Ø9HN
Neck ØWH6
Nerve
Cranial ØØHE
Peripheral Ø1HY
Nipple
Left ØHHX
Right ØHHW
Oral Cavity and Throat ØWH3
Orbit
Left ØNHQ
Right ØNHP
Ovary ØUH3
Pancreas ØFHG
Patella
Left ØQHF
Right ØQHD
Pelvic Cavity ØWHJ
Penis ØVHS
Pericardial Cavity ØWHD
Pericardium Ø2HN
Perineum
Female ØWHN
Male ØWHM
Peritoneal Cavity ØWHG
Phalanx
Finger
Left ØPHV
Right ØPHT
Thumb
Left ØPHS
Right ØPHR
Toe
Left ØQHR
Right ØQHQ
Pleura ØBHQ
Pleural Cavity
Left ØWHB
Right ØWH9
Prostate ØVHØ
Prostate and Seminal Vesicles ØVH4
Radius
Left ØPHJ
Right ØPHH
Rectum ØDHP
Respiratory Tract ØWHQ
Retroperitoneum ØWHH
Ribs
1 to 2 ØPH1
3 or More ØPH2
Sacrum ØQH1
Scapula
Left ØPH6
Right ØPH5
Scrotum and Tunica Vaginalis ØVH8
Shoulder Region
Left ØXH3
Right ØXH2

Insertion of device in — continued
Sinus Ø9HY
Skin ØHHPXYZ
Skull ØNHØ
Spinal Canal ØØHU
Spinal Cord ØØHV
Spleen Ø7HP
Sternum ØPHØ
Stomach ØDH6
Subcutaneous Tissue and Fascia
Abdomen ØJH8
Back ØJH7
Buttock ØJH9
Chest ØJH6
Face ØJH1
Foot
Left ØJHR
Right ØJHQ
Hand
Left ØJHK
Right ØJHJ
Head and Neck ØJHS
Lower Arm
Left ØJHH
Right ØJHG
Lower Extremity ØJHW
Lower Leg
Left ØJHP
Right ØJHN
Neck
Left ØJH5
Right ØJH4
Pelvic Region ØJHC
Perineum ØJHB
Scalp ØJHØ
Trunk ØJHT
Upper Arm
Left ØJHF
Right ØJHD
Upper Extremity ØJHV
Upper Leg
Left ØJHM
Right ØJHL
Tarsal
Left ØQHM
Right ØQHL
Tendon
Lower ØLHY
Upper ØLHX
Testis ØVHD
Thymus Ø7HM
Tibia
Left ØQHH
Right ØQHG
Tongue ØCH7
Trachea ØBH1
Tracheobronchial Tree ØBHØ
Ulna
Left ØPHL
Right ØPHK
Ureter ØTH9
Urethra ØTHD
Uterus ØUH9
Uterus and Cervix ØUHD
Vagina ØUHG
Vagina and Cul-de-sac ØUHH
Vas Deferens ØVHR
Vein
Axillary
Left Ø5H8
Right Ø5H7
Azygos Ø5HØ
Basilic
Left Ø5HC
Right Ø5HB
Brachial
Left Ø5HA
Right Ø5H9
Cephalic
Left Ø5HF
Right Ø5HD
Colic Ø6H7
Common Iliac
Left Ø6HD
Right Ø6HC
Coronary Ø2H4
Esophageal Ø6H3
External Iliac
Left Ø6HG

Insertion of device in — continued
Vein — continued
External Iliac — continued
Right Ø6HF
External Jugular
Left Ø5HQ
Right Ø5HP
Face
Left Ø5HV
Right Ø5HT
Femoral
Left Ø6HN
Right Ø6HM
Foot
Left Ø6HV
Right Ø6HT
Gastric Ø6H2
Hand
Left Ø5HH
Right Ø5HG
Hemiazygos Ø5H1
Hepatic Ø6H4
Hypogastric
Left Ø6HJ
Right Ø6HH
Inferior Mesenteric Ø6H6
Innominate
Left Ø5H4
Right Ø5H3
Internal Jugular
Left Ø5HN
Right Ø5HM
Intracranial Ø5HL
Lower Ø6HY
Portal Ø6H8
Pulmonary
Left Ø2HT
Right Ø2HS
Renal
Left Ø6HB
Right Ø6H9
Saphenous
Left Ø6HQ
Right Ø6HP
Splenic Ø6H1
Subclavian
Left Ø5H6
Right Ø5H5
Superior Mesenteric Ø6H5
Upper Ø5HY
Vertebral
Left Ø5HS
Right Ø5HR
Vena Cava
Inferior Ø6HØ
Superior Ø2HV
Ventricle
Left Ø2HL
Right Ø2HK
Vertebra
Cervical ØPH3
Lumbar ØQHØ
Thoracic ØPH4
Wrist Region
Left ØXHH
Right ØXHG
Inspection
Abdominal Wall ØWJF
Ankle Region
Left ØYJL
Right ØYJK
Arm
Lower
Left ØXJF
Right ØXJD
Upper
Left ØXJ9
Right ØXJ8
Artery
Lower Ø4JY
Upper Ø3JY
Axilla
Left ØXJ5
Right ØXJ4
Back
Lower ØWJL
Upper ØWJK
Bladder ØTJB

Inspection — *continued*
Bone
Facial ØNJW
Lower ØQJY
Nasal ØNJB
Upper ØPJY
Bone Marrow Ø7JT
Brain ØØJØ
Breast
Left ØHJU
Right ØHJT
Bursa and Ligament
Lower ØMJY
Upper ØMJX
Buttock
Left ØYJ1
Right ØYJØ
Cavity, Cranial ØWJ1
Chest Wall ØWJ8
Cisterna Chyli Ø7JL
Diaphragm ØBJT
Disc
Cervical Vertebral ØRJ3
Cervicothoracic Vertebral ØRJ5
Lumbar Vertebral ØSJ2
Lumbosacral ØSJ4
Thoracic Vertebral ØRJ9
Thoracolumbar Vertebral ØRJB
Duct
Hepatobiliary ØFJB
Pancreatic ØFJD
Ear
Inner
Left Ø9JE
Right Ø9JD
Left Ø9JJ
Right Ø9JH
Elbow Region
Left ØXJC
Right ØXJB
Epididymis and Spermatic Cord ØVJM
Extremity
Lower
Left ØYJB
Right ØYJ9
Upper
Left ØXJ7
Right ØXJ6
Eye
Left Ø8J1XZZ
Right Ø8JØXZZ
Face ØWJ2
Fallopian Tube ØUJ8
Femoral Region
Bilateral ØYJE
Left ØYJ8
Right ØYJ7
Finger Nail ØHJQXZZ
Foot
Left ØYJN
Right ØYJM
Gallbladder ØFJ4
Gastrointestinal Tract ØWJP
Genitourinary Tract ØWJR
Gland
Adrenal ØGJ5
Endocrine ØGJS
Pituitary ØGJØ
Salivary ØCJA
Great Vessel Ø2JY
Hand
Left ØXJK
Right ØXJJ
Head ØWJØ
Heart Ø2JA
Inguinal Region
Bilateral ØYJA
Left ØYJ6
Right ØYJ5
Intestinal Tract
Lower ØDJD
Upper ØDJØ
Jaw
Lower ØWJ5
Upper ØWJ4
Joint
Acromioclavicular
Left ØRJH
Right ØRJG

Inspection — *continued*
Joint — *continued*
Ankle
Left ØSJG
Right ØSJF
Carpal
Left ØRJR
Right ØRJQ
Carpometacarpal
Left ØRJT
Right ØRJS
Cervical Vertebral ØRJ1
Cervicothoracic Vertebral ØRJ4
Coccygeal ØSJ6
Elbow
Left ØRJM
Right ØRJL
Finger Phalangeal
Left ØRJX
Right ØRJW
Hip
Left ØSJB
Right ØSJ9
Knee
Left ØSJD
Right ØSJC
Lumbar Vertebral ØSJØ
Lumbosacral ØSJ3
Metacarpophalangeal
Left ØRJV
Right ØRJU
Metatarsal-Phalangeal
Left ØSJN
Right ØSJM
Occipital-cervical ØRJØ
Sacrococcygeal ØSJ5
Sacroiliac
Left ØSJ8
Right ØSJ7
Shoulder
Left ØRJK
Right ØRJJ
Sternoclavicular
Left ØRJF
Right ØRJE
Tarsal
Left ØSJJ
Right ØSJH
Tarsometatarsal
Left ØSJL
Right ØSJK
Temporomandibular
Left ØRJD
Right ØRJC
Thoracic Vertebral ØRJ6
Thoracolumbar Vertebral ØRJA
Toe Phalangeal
Left ØSJQ
Right ØSJP
Wrist
Left ØRJP
Right ØRJN
Kidney ØTJ5
Knee Region
Left ØYJG
Right ØYJF
Larynx ØCJS
Leg
Lower
Left ØYJJ
Right ØYJH
Upper
Left ØYJD
Right ØYJC
Lens
Left Ø8JKXZZ
Right Ø8JJXZZ
Liver ØFJØ
Lung
Left ØBJL
Right ØBJK
Lymphatic Ø7JN
Thoracic Duct Ø7JK
Mediastinum ØWJC
Mesentery ØDJV
Mouth and Throat ØCJY
Muscle
Extraocular
Left Ø8JM

Inspection — *continued*
Muscle — *continued*
Extraocular — *continued*
Right Ø8JL
Lower ØKJY
Upper ØKJX
Nasal Mucosa and Soft Tissue Ø9JK
Neck ØWJ6
Nerve
Cranial ØØJE
Peripheral Ø1JY
Omentum ØDJU
Oral Cavity and Throat ØWJ3
Ovary ØUJ3
Pancreas ØFJG
Parathyroid Gland ØGJR
Pelvic Cavity ØWJJ
Penis ØVJS
Pericardial Cavity ØWJD
Perineum
Female ØWJN
Male ØWJM
Peritoneal Cavity ØWJG
Peritoneum ØDJW
Pineal Body ØGJ1
Pleura ØBJQ
Pleural Cavity
Left ØWJB
Right ØWJ9
Products of Conception 1ØJØ
Ectopic 1ØJ2
Retained 1ØJ1
Prostate and Seminal Vesicles ØVJ4
Respiratory Tract ØWJQ
Retroperitoneum ØWJH
Scrotum and Tunica Vaginalis ØVJ8
Shoulder Region
Left ØXJ3
Right ØXJ2
Sinus Ø9JY
Skin ØHJPXZZ
Skull ØNJØ
Spinal Canal ØØJU
Spinal Cord ØØJV
Spleen Ø7JP
Stomach ØDJ6
Subcutaneous Tissue and Fascia
Head and Neck ØJJS
Lower Extremity ØJJW
Trunk ØJJT
Upper Extremity ØJJV
Tendon
Lower ØLJY
Upper ØLJX
Testis ØVJD
Thymus Ø7JM
Thyroid Gland ØGJK
Toe Nail ØHJRXZZ
Trachea ØBJ1
Tracheobronchial Tree ØBJØ
Tympanic Membrane
Left Ø9J8
Right Ø9J7
Ureter ØTJ9
Urethra ØTJD
Uterus and Cervix ØUJD
Vagina and Cul-de-sac ØUJH
Vas Deferens ØVJR
Vein
Lower Ø6JY
Upper Ø5JY
Vulva ØUJM
Wrist Region
Left ØXJH
Right ØXJG
Instillation *see* Introduction of substance in or on
Insufflation *see* Introduction of substance in or on
Interatrial septum *use* Atrial Septum
InterAtrial Shunt Device IASD®, Corvia *use* Synthetic Substitute
Interbody fusion (spine) cage
use Interbody Fusion Device in Lower Joints
use Interbody Fusion Device in Upper Joints
Interbody Fusion Device
Nanotextured Surface
Cervical Vertebral XRG1Ø92
2 or more XRG2Ø92
Cervicothoracic Vertebral XRG4Ø92

Interbody Fusion Device — *continued*
Nanotextured Surface — *continued*
Lumbar Vertebral XRGBØ92
2 or more XRGCØ92
Lumbosacral XRGDØ92
Occipital-cervical XRGØØ92
Thoracic Vertebral XRG6Ø92
2 to 7 XRG7Ø92
8 or more XRG8Ø92
Thoracolumbar Vertebral XRGAØ92
Radiolucent Porous
Cervical Vertebral XRG1ØF3
2 or more XRG2ØF3
Cervicothoracic Vertebral XRG4ØF3
Lumbar Vertebral XRGBØF3
2 or more XRGCØF3
Lumbosacral XRGDØF3
Occipital-cervical XRGØØF3
Thoracic Vertebral XRG6ØF3
2 to 7 XRG7ØF3
8 or more XRG8ØF3
Thoracolumbar Vertebral XRGAØF3
Intercarpal joint
use Carpal Joint, Left
use Carpal Joint, Right
Intercarpal ligament
use Hand Bursa and Ligament, Left
use Hand Bursa and Ligament, Right
Interclavicular ligament
use Shoulder Bursa and Ligament, Left
use Shoulder Bursa and Ligament, Right
Intercostal lymph node *use* Lymphatic, Thorax
Intercostal muscle
use Thorax Muscle, Left
use Thorax Muscle, Right
Intercostal nerve *use* Thoracic Nerve
Intercostobrachial nerve *use* Thoracic Nerve
Intercuneiform joint
use Tarsal Joint, Left
use Tarsal Joint, Right
Intercuneiform ligament
use Foot Bursa and Ligament, Left
use Foot Bursa and Ligament, Right
Intermediate bronchus *use* Main Bronchus, Right
Intermediate cuneiform bone
use Tarsal, Left
use Tarsal, Right
Intermittent hemodialysis (IHD) 5A1D7ØZ
Intermittent mandatory ventilation *see* Assistance, Respiratory 5AØ9
Intermittent Negative Airway Pressure
24-96 Consecutive Hours, Ventilation 5AØ945B
Greater than 96 Consecutive Hours, Ventilation 5AØ955B
Less than 24 Consecutive Hours, Ventilation 5AØ935B
Intermittent Positive Airway Pressure
24-96 Consecutive Hours, Ventilation 5AØ9458
Greater than 96 Consecutive Hours, Ventilation 5AØ9558
Less than 24 Consecutive Hours, Ventilation 5AØ9358
Intermittent positive pressure breathing *see* Assistance, Respiratory 5AØ9
Internal anal sphincter *use* Anal Sphincter
Internal carotid artery, intracranial portion *use* Intracranial Artery
Internal carotid plexus *use* Head and Neck Sympathetic Nerve
Internal (basal) cerebral vein *use* Intracranial Vein
Internal iliac vein
use Hypogastric Vein, Left
use Hypogastric Vein, Right
Internal maxillary artery
use External Carotid Artery, Left
use External Carotid Artery, Right
Internal naris *use* Nasal Mucosa and Soft Tissue
Internal oblique muscle
use Abdomen Muscle, Left
use Abdomen Muscle, Right
Internal pudendal artery
use Internal Iliac Artery, Left
use Internal Iliac Artery, Right
Internal pudendal vein
use Hypogastric Vein, Left
use Hypogastric Vein, Right
Internal thoracic artery
use Internal Mammary Artery, Left
use Internal Mammary Artery, Right
use Subclavian Artery, Left
use Subclavian Artery, Right
Internal urethral sphincter *use* Urethra
Interphalangeal (IP) joint
use Finger Phalangeal Joint, Left
use Finger Phalangeal Joint, Right
use Toe Phalangeal Joint, Left
use Toe Phalangeal Joint, Right
Interphalangeal ligament
use Foot Bursa and Ligament, Left
use Foot Bursa and Ligament, Right
use Hand Bursa and Ligament, Left
use Hand Bursa and Ligament, Right
Interrogation, cardiac rhythm related device
Interrogation only *see* Measurement, Cardiac 4BØ2
With cardiac function testing *see* Measurement, Cardiac 4AØ2
Interruption *see* Occlusion
Interspinalis muscle
use Trunk Muscle, Left
use Trunk Muscle, Right
Interspinous ligament, cervical *use* Head and Neck Bursa and Ligament
Interspinous ligament, lumbar *use* Lower Spine Bursa and Ligament
Interspinous ligament, thoracic *use* Upper Spine Bursa and Ligament
Interspinous process spinal stabilization device
use Spinal Stabilization Device, Interspinous Process in ØRH
use Spinal Stabilization Device, Interspinous Process in ØSH
InterStim® Therapy lead *use* Neurostimulator Lead in Peripheral Nervous System
InterStim® Therapy neurostimulator *use* Stimulator Generator, Single Array in ØJH
Intertransversarius muscle
use Trunk Muscle, Left
use Trunk Muscle, Right
Intertransverse ligament, cervical *use* Head and Neck Bursa and Ligament
Intertransverse ligament, lumbar *use* Lower Spine Bursa and Ligament
Intertransverse ligament, thoracic *use* Upper Spine Bursa and Ligament
Interventricular foramen (Monro) *use* Cerebral Ventricle
Interventricular septum *use* Ventricular Septum
Intestinal lymphatic trunk *use* Cisterna Chyli
Intraluminal Device
Airway
Esophagus ØDH5
Mouth and Throat ØCHY
Nasopharynx Ø9HN
Bioactive
Occlusion
Common Carotid
Left Ø3LJ
Right Ø3LH
External Carotid
Left Ø3LN
Right Ø3LM
Internal Carotid
Left Ø3LL
Right Ø3LK
Intracranial Ø3LG
Vertebral
Left Ø3LQ
Right Ø3LP
Restriction
Common Carotid
Left Ø3VJ
Right Ø3VH
External Carotid
Left Ø3VN
Right Ø3VM
Internal Carotid
Left Ø3VL
Right Ø3VK
Intracranial Ø3VG
Vertebral
Left Ø3VQ
Right Ø3VP
Intraluminal Device — *continued*
Endobronchial Valve
Lingula ØBH9
Lower Lobe
Left ØBHB
Right ØBH6
Main
Left ØBH7
Right ØBH3
Middle Lobe, Right ØBH5
Upper Lobe
Left ØBH8
Right ØBH4
Endotracheal Airway
Change device in, Trachea ØB21XEZ
Insertion of device in, Trachea ØBH1
Pessary
Change device in, Vagina and Cul-de-sac ØU2HXGZ
Insertion of device in
Cul-de-sac ØUHF
Vagina ØUHG
Intramedullary (IM) rod (nail)
use Internal Fixation Device, Intramedullary in Lower Bones
use Internal Fixation Device, Intramedullary in Upper Bones
Intramedullary skeletal kinetic distractor (ISKD)
use Internal Fixation Device, Intramedullary in Lower Bones
use Internal Fixation Device, Intramedullary in Upper Bones
Intraocular Telescope
Left Ø8RK3ØZ
Right Ø8RJ3ØZ
Intraoperative Knee Replacement Sensor XR2
Intraoperative Radiation Therapy (IORT)
Anus DDY8CZZ
Bile Ducts DFY2CZZ
Bladder DTY2CZZ
Brain DØYØCZZ
Brain Stem DØY1CZZ
Cervix DUY1CZZ
Colon DDY5CZZ
Duodenum DDY2CZZ
Gallbladder DFY1CZZ
Ileum DDY4CZZ
Jejunum DDY3CZZ
Kidney DTYØCZZ
Larynx D9YBCZZ
Liver DFYØCZZ
Mouth D9Y4CZZ
Nasopharynx D9YDCZZ
Nerve, Peripheral DØY7CZZ
Ovary DUYØCZZ
Pancreas DFY3CZZ
Pharynx D9YCCZZ
Prostate DVYØCZZ
Rectum DDY7CZZ
Spinal Cord DØY6CZZ
Stomach DDY1CZZ
Ureter DTY1CZZ
Urethra DTY3CZZ
Uterus DUY2CZZ
Intra.OX 8EØ2XDZ
Intrauterine Device (IUD) *use* Contraceptive Device in Female Reproductive System
Intravascular fluorescence angiography (IFA) *see* Monitoring, Physiological Systems 4A1
Intravascular Lithotripsy (IVL) *see* Fragmentation
Intravascular ultrasound assisted thrombolysis *see* Fragmentation, Artery
Introduction of substance in or on
Artery
Central 3EØ6
Analgesics 3EØ6
Anesthetic, Intracirculatory 3EØ6
Antiarrhythmic 3EØ6
Anti-infective 3EØ6
Anti-inflammatory 3EØ6
Antineoplastic 3EØ6
Destructive Agent 3EØ6
Diagnostic Substance, Other 3EØ6
Electrolytic Substance 3EØ6
Hormone 3EØ6
Hypnotics 3EØ6
Immunotherapeutic 3EØ6
Nutritional Substance 3EØ6

Subterms under main terms may continue to next column or page

Introduction of substance in or on — *continued*
- Artery — *continued*
  - Central — *continued*
    - Platelet Inhibitor 3EØ6
    - Radioactive Substance 3EØ6
    - Sedatives 3EØ6
    - Serum 3EØ6
    - Thrombolytic 3EØ6
    - Toxoid 3EØ6
    - Vaccine 3EØ6
    - Vasopressor 3EØ6
    - Water Balance Substance 3EØ6
  - Coronary 3EØ7
    - Diagnostic Substance, Other 3EØ7
    - Platelet Inhibitor 3EØ7
    - Thrombolytic 3EØ7
  - Peripheral 3EØ5
    - Analgesics 3EØ5
    - Anesthetic, Intracirculatory 3EØ5
    - Antiarrhythmic 3EØ5
    - Anti-infective 3EØ5
    - Anti-inflammatory 3EØ5
    - Antineoplastic 3EØ5
    - Destructive Agent 3EØ5
    - Diagnostic Substance, Other 3EØ5
    - Electrolytic Substance 3EØ5
    - Hormone 3EØ5
    - Hypnotics 3EØ5
    - Immunotherapeutic 3EØ5
    - Nutritional Substance 3EØ5
    - Platelet Inhibitor 3EØ5
    - Radioactive Substance 3EØ5
    - Sedatives 3EØ5
    - Serum 3EØ5
    - Thrombolytic 3EØ5
    - Toxoid 3EØ5
    - Vaccine 3EØ5
    - Vasopressor 3EØ5
    - Water Balance Substance 3EØ5
- Biliary Tract 3EØJ
  - Analgesics 3EØJ
  - Anesthetic Agent 3EØJ
  - Anti-infective 3EØJ
  - Anti-inflammatory 3EØJ
  - Antineoplastic 3EØJ
  - Destructive Agent 3EØJ
  - Diagnostic Substance, Other 3EØJ
  - Electrolytic Substance 3EØJ
  - Gas 3EØJ
  - Hypnotics 3EØJ
  - Islet Cells, Pancreatic 3EØJ
  - Nutritional Substance 3EØJ
  - Radioactive Substance 3EØJ
  - Sedatives 3EØJ
  - Water Balance Substance 3EØJ
- Bone 3EØV
  - Analgesics 3EØV3NZ
  - Anesthetic Agent 3EØV3BZ
  - Anti-infective 3EØV32
  - Anti-inflammatory 3EØV33Z
  - Antineoplastic 3EØV3Ø
  - Destructive Agent 3EØV3TZ
  - Diagnostic Substance, Other 3EØV3KZ
  - Electrolytic Substance 3EØV37Z
  - Hypnotics 3EØV3NZ
  - Nutritional Substance 3EØV36Z
  - Radioactive Substance 3EØV3HZ
  - Sedatives 3EØV3NZ
  - Water Balance Substance 3EØV37Z
- Bone Marrow 3EØA3GC
  - Antineoplastic 3EØA3Ø
- Brain 3EØQ
  - Analgesics 3EØQ
  - Anesthetic Agent 3EØQ
  - Anti-infective 3EØQ
  - Anti-inflammatory 3EØQ
  - Antineoplastic 3EØQ
  - Destructive Agent 3EØQ
  - Diagnostic Substance, Other 3EØQ
  - Electrolytic Substance 3EØQ
  - Gas 3EØQ
  - Hypnotics 3EØQ
  - Nutritional Substance 3EØQ
  - Radioactive Substance 3EØQ
  - Sedatives 3EØQ
  - Stem Cells
    - Embryonic 3EØQ
    - Somatic 3EØQ
  - Water Balance Substance 3EØQ

Introduction of substance in or on — *continued*
- Cranial Cavity 3EØQ
  - Analgesics 3EØQ
  - Anesthetic Agent 3EØQ
  - Anti-infective 3EØQ
  - Anti-inflammatory 3EØQ
  - Antineoplastic 3EØQ
  - Destructive Agent 3EØQ
  - Diagnostic Substance, Other 3EØQ
  - Electrolytic Substance 3EØQ
  - Gas 3EØQ
  - Hypnotics 3EØQ
  - Nutritional Substance 3EØQ
  - Radioactive Substance 3EØQ
  - Sedatives 3EØQ
  - Stem Cells
    - Embryonic 3EØQ
    - Somatic 3EØQ
  - Water Balance Substance 3EØQ
- Ear 3EØB
  - Analgesics 3EØB
  - Anesthetic Agent 3EØB
  - Anti-infective 3EØB
  - Anti-inflammatory 3EØB
  - Antineoplastic 3EØB
  - Destructive Agent 3EØB
  - Diagnostic Substance, Other 3EØB
  - Hypnotics 3EØB
  - Radioactive Substance 3EØB
  - Sedatives 3EØB
- Epidural Space 3EØS3GC
  - Analgesics 3EØS3NZ
  - Anesthetic Agent 3EØS3BZ
  - Anti-infective 3EØS32
  - Anti-inflammatory 3EØS33Z
  - Antineoplastic 3EØS3Ø
  - Destructive Agent 3EØS3TZ
  - Diagnostic Substance, Other 3EØS3KZ
  - Electrolytic Substance 3EØS37Z
  - Gas 3EØS
  - Hypnotics 3EØS3NZ
  - Nutritional Substance 3EØS36Z
  - Radioactive Substance 3EØS3HZ
  - Sedatives 3EØS3NZ
  - Water Balance Substance 3EØS37Z
- Eye 3EØC
  - Analgesics 3EØC
  - Anesthetic Agent 3EØC
  - Anti-infective 3EØC
  - Anti-inflammatory 3EØC
  - Antineoplastic 3EØC
  - Destructive Agent 3EØC
  - Diagnostic Substance, Other 3EØC
  - Gas 3EØC
  - Hypnotics 3EØC
  - Pigment 3EØC
  - Radioactive Substance 3EØC
  - Sedatives 3EØC
- Gastrointestinal Tract
  - Lower 3EØH
    - Analgesics 3EØH
    - Anesthetic Agent 3EØH
    - Anti-infective 3EØH
    - Anti-inflammatory 3EØH
    - Antineoplastic 3EØH
    - Destructive Agent 3EØH
    - Diagnostic Substance, Other 3EØH
    - Electrolytic Substance 3EØH
    - Gas 3EØH
    - Hypnotics 3EØH
    - Nutritional Substance 3EØH
    - Radioactive Substance 3EØH
    - Sedatives 3EØH
    - Water Balance Substance 3EØH
  - Upper 3EØG
    - Analgesics 3EØG
    - Anesthetic Agent 3EØG
    - Anti-infective 3EØG
    - Anti-inflammatory 3EØG
    - Antineoplastic 3EØG
    - Destructive Agent 3EØG
    - Diagnostic Substance, Other 3EØG
    - Electrolytic Substance 3EØG
    - Gas 3EØG
    - Hypnotics 3EØG
    - Nutritional Substance 3EØG
    - Radioactive Substance 3EØG
    - Sedatives 3EØG
    - Water Balance Substance 3EØG

Introduction of substance in or on — *continued*
- Genitourinary Tract 3EØK
  - Analgesics 3EØK
  - Anesthetic Agent 3EØK
  - Anti-infective 3EØK
  - Anti-inflammatory 3EØK
  - Antineoplastic 3EØK
  - Destructive Agent 3EØK
  - Diagnostic Substance, Other 3EØK
  - Electrolytic Substance 3EØK
  - Gas 3EØK
  - Hypnotics 3EØK
  - Nutritional Substance 3EØK
  - Radioactive Substance 3EØK
  - Sedatives 3EØK
  - Water Balance Substance 3EØK
- Heart 3EØ8
  - Diagnostic Substance, Other 3EØ8
  - Platelet Inhibitor 3EØ8
  - Thrombolytic 3EØ8
- Joint 3EØU
  - Analgesics 3EØU3NZ
  - Anesthetic Agent 3EØU3BZ
  - Anti-infective 3EØU
  - Anti-inflammatory 3EØU33Z
  - Antineoplastic 3EØU3Ø
  - Destructive Agent 3EØU3TZ
  - Diagnostic Substance, Other 3EØU3KZ
  - Electrolytic Substance 3EØU37Z
  - Gas 3EØU3SF
  - Hypnotics 3EØU3NZ
  - Nutritional Substance 3EØU36Z
  - Radioactive Substance 3EØU3HZ
  - Sedatives 3EØU3NZ
  - Water Balance Substance 3EØU37Z
- Lymphatic 3EØW3GC
  - Analgesics 3EØW3NZ
  - Anesthetic Agent 3EØW3BZ
  - Anti-infective 3EØW32
  - Anti-inflammatory 3EØW33Z
  - Antineoplastic 3EØW3Ø
  - Destructive Agent 3EØW3TZ
  - Diagnostic Substance, Other 3EØW3KZ
  - Electrolytic Substance 3EØW37Z
  - Hypnotics 3EØW3NZ
  - Nutritional Substance 3EØW36Z
  - Radioactive Substance 3EØW3HZ
  - Sedatives 3EØW3NZ
  - Water Balance Substance 3EØW37Z
- Mouth 3EØD
  - Analgesics 3EØD
  - Anesthetic Agent 3EØD
  - Antiarrhythmic 3EØD
  - Anti-infective 3EØD
  - Anti-inflammatory 3EØD
  - Antineoplastic 3EØD
  - Destructive Agent 3EØD
  - Diagnostic Substance, Other 3EØD
  - Electrolytic Substance 3EØD
  - Hypnotics 3EØD
  - Nutritional Substance 3EØD
  - Radioactive Substance 3EØD
  - Sedatives 3EØD
  - Serum 3EØD
  - Toxoid 3EØD
  - Vaccine 3EØD
  - Water Balance Substance 3EØD
- Mucous Membrane 3EØØXGC
  - Analgesics 3EØØXNZ
  - Anesthetic Agent 3EØØXBZ
  - Anti-infective 3EØØX2
  - Anti-inflammatory 3EØØX3Z
  - Antineoplastic 3EØØXØ
  - Destructive Agent 3EØØXTZ
  - Diagnostic Substance, Other 3EØØXKZ
  - Hypnotics 3EØØXNZ
  - Pigment 3EØØXMZ
  - Sedatives 3EØØXNZ
  - Serum 3EØØX4Z
  - Toxoid 3EØØX4Z
  - Vaccine 3EØØX4Z
- Muscle 3EØ23GC
  - Analgesics 3EØ23NZ
  - Anesthetic Agent 3EØ23BZ
  - Anti-infective 3EØ232
  - Anti-inflammatory 3EØ233Z
  - Antineoplastic 3EØ23Ø
  - Destructive Agent 3EØ23TZ
  - Diagnostic Substance, Other 3EØ23KZ

Introduction of substance in or on — *continued*
- Muscle — *continued*
  - Electrolytic Substance 3EØ237Z
  - Hypnotics 3EØ23NZ
  - Nutritional Substance 3EØ236Z
  - Radioactive Substance 3EØ23HZ
  - Sedatives 3EØ23NZ
  - Serum 3EØ234Z
  - Toxoid 3EØ234Z
  - Vaccine 3EØ234Z
  - Water Balance Substance 3EØ237Z
- Nerve
  - Cranial 3EØX3GC
    - Anesthetic Agent 3EØX3BZ
    - Anti-inflammatory 3EØX33Z
    - Destructive Agent 3EØX3TZ
  - Peripheral 3EØT3GC
    - Anesthetic Agent 3EØT3BZ
    - Anti-inflammatory 3EØT33Z
    - Destructive Agent 3EØT3TZ
  - Plexus 3EØT3GC
    - Anesthetic Agent 3EØT3BZ
    - Anti-inflammatory 3EØT33Z
    - Destructive Agent 3EØT3TZ
- Nose 3EØ9
  - Analgesics 3EØ9
  - Anesthetic Agent 3EØ9
  - Anti-infective 3EØ9
  - Anti-inflammatory 3EØ9
  - Antineoplastic 3EØ9
  - Destructive Agent 3EØ9
  - Diagnostic Substance, Other 3EØ9
  - Hypnotics 3EØ9
  - Radioactive Substance 3EØ9
  - Sedatives 3EØ9
  - Serum 3EØ9
  - Toxoid 3EØ9
  - Vaccine 3EØ9
- Pancreatic Tract 3EØJ
  - Analgesics 3EØJ
  - Anesthetic Agent 3EØJ
  - Anti-infective 3EØJ
  - Anti-inflammatory 3EØJ
  - Antineoplastic 3EØJ
  - Destructive Agent 3EØJ
  - Diagnostic Substance, Other 3EØJ
  - Electrolytic Substance 3EØJ
  - Gas 3EØJ
  - Hypnotics 3EØJ
  - Islet Cells, Pancreatic 3EØJ
  - Nutritional Substance 3EØJ
  - Radioactive Substance 3EØJ
  - Sedatives 3EØJ
  - Water Balance Substance 3EØJ
- Pericardial Cavity 3EØY
  - Analgesics 3EØY3NZ
  - Anesthetic Agent 3EØY3BZ
  - Anti-infective 3EØY32
  - Anti-inflammatory 3EØY33Z
  - Antineoplastic 3EØY
  - Destructive Agent 3EØY3TZ
  - Diagnostic Substance, Other 3EØY3KZ
  - Electrolytic Substance 3EØY37Z
  - Gas 3EØY
  - Hypnotics 3EØY3NZ
  - Nutritional Substance 3EØY36Z
  - Radioactive Substance 3EØY3HZ
  - Sedatives 3EØY3NZ
  - Water Balance Substance 3EØY37Z
- Peritoneal Cavity 3EØM
  - Adhesion Barrier 3EØM
  - Analgesics 3EØM3NZ
  - Anesthetic Agent 3EØM3BZ
  - Anti-infective 3EØM32
  - Anti-inflammatory 3EØM33Z
  - Antineoplastic 3EØM
  - Destructive Agent 3EØM3TZ
  - Diagnostic Substance, Other 3EØM3KZ
  - Electrolytic Substance 3EØM37Z
  - Gas 3EØM
  - Hypnotics 3EØM3NZ
  - Nutritional Substance 3EØM36Z
  - Radioactive Substance 3EØM3HZ
  - Sedatives 3EØM3NZ
  - Water Balance Substance 3EØM37Z
- Pharynx 3EØD
  - Analgesics 3EØD
  - Anesthetic Agent 3EØD
  - Antiarrhythmic 3EØD

Introduction of substance in or on — *continued*
- Pharynx — *continued*
  - Anti-infective 3EØD
  - Anti-inflammatory 3EØD
  - Antineoplastic 3EØD
  - Destructive Agent 3EØD
  - Diagnostic Substance, Other 3EØD
  - Electrolytic Substance 3EØD
  - Hypnotics 3EØD
  - Nutritional Substance 3EØD
  - Radioactive Substance 3EØD
  - Sedatives 3EØD
  - Serum 3EØD
  - Toxoid 3EØD
  - Vaccine 3EØD
  - Water Balance Substance 3EØD
- Pleural Cavity 3EØL
  - Adhesion Barrier 3EØL
  - Analgesics 3EØL3NZ
  - Anesthetic Agent 3EØL3BZ
  - Anti-infective 3EØL32
  - Anti-inflammatory 3EØL33Z
  - Antineoplastic 3EØL
  - Destructive Agent 3EØL3TZ
  - Diagnostic Substance, Other 3EØL3KZ
  - Electrolytic Substance 3EØL37Z
  - Gas 3EØL
  - Hypnotics 3EØL3NZ
  - Nutritional Substance 3EØL36Z
  - Radioactive Substance 3EØL3HZ
  - Sedatives 3EØL3NZ
  - Water Balance Substance 3EØL37Z
- Products of Conception 3EØE
  - Analgesics 3EØE
  - Anesthetic Agent 3EØE
  - Anti-infective 3EØE
  - Anti-inflammatory 3EØE
  - Antineoplastic 3EØE
  - Destructive Agent 3EØE
  - Diagnostic Substance, Other 3EØE
  - Electrolytic Substance 3EØE
  - Gas 3EØE
  - Hypnotics 3EØE
  - Nutritional Substance 3EØE
  - Radioactive Substance 3EØE
  - Sedatives 3EØE
  - Water Balance Substance 3EØE
- Reproductive
  - Female 3EØP
    - Adhesion Barrier 3EØP
    - Analgesics 3EØP
    - Anesthetic Agent 3EØP
    - Anti-infective 3EØP
    - Anti-inflammatory 3EØP
    - Antineoplastic 3EØP
    - Destructive Agent 3EØP
    - Diagnostic Substance, Other 3EØP
    - Electrolytic Substance 3EØP
    - Gas 3EØP
    - Hormone 3EØP
    - Hypnotics 3EØP
    - Nutritional Substance 3EØP
    - Ovum, Fertilized 3EØP
    - Radioactive Substance 3EØP
    - Sedatives 3EØP
    - Sperm 3EØP
    - Water Balance Substance 3EØP
  - Male 3EØN
    - Analgesics 3EØN
    - Anesthetic Agent 3EØN
    - Anti-infective 3EØN
    - Anti-inflammatory 3EØN
    - Antineoplastic 3EØN
    - Destructive Agent 3EØN
    - Diagnostic Substance, Other 3EØN
    - Electrolytic Substance 3EØN
    - Gas 3EØN
    - Hypnotics 3EØN
    - Nutritional Substance 3EØN
    - Radioactive Substance 3EØN
    - Sedatives 3EØN
    - Water Balance Substance 3EØN
- Respiratory Tract 3EØF
  - Analgesics 3EØF
  - Anesthetic Agent 3EØF
  - Anti-infective 3EØF
  - Anti-inflammatory 3EØF
  - Antineoplastic 3EØF
  - Destructive Agent 3EØF

Introduction of substance in or on — *continued*
- Respiratory Tract — *continued*
  - Diagnostic Substance, Other 3EØF
  - Electrolytic Substance 3EØF
  - Gas 3EØF
  - Hypnotics 3EØF
  - Nutritional Substance 3EØF
  - Radioactive Substance 3EØF
  - Sedatives 3EØF
  - Water Balance Substance 3EØF
- Skin 3EØØXGC
  - Analgesics 3EØØXNZ
  - Anesthetic Agent 3EØØXBZ
  - Anti-infective 3EØØX2
  - Anti-inflammatory 3EØØX3Z
  - Antineoplastic 3EØØXØ
  - Destructive Agent 3EØØXTZ
  - Diagnostic Substance, Other 3EØØXKZ
  - Hypnotics 3EØØXNZ
  - Pigment 3EØØXMZ
  - Sedatives 3EØØXNZ
  - Serum 3EØØX4Z
  - Toxoid 3EØØX4Z
  - Vaccine 3EØØX4Z
- Spinal Canal 3EØR3GC
  - Analgesics 3EØR3NZ
  - Anesthetic Agent 3EØR3BZ
  - Anti-infective 3EØR32
  - Anti-inflammatory 3EØR33Z
  - Antineoplastic 3EØR3Ø
  - Destructive Agent 3EØR3TZ
  - Diagnostic Substance, Other 3EØR3KZ
  - Electrolytic Substance 3EØR37Z
  - Gas 3EØR
  - Hypnotics 3EØR3NZ
  - Nutritional Substance 3EØR36Z
  - Radioactive Substance 3EØR3HZ
  - Sedatives 3EØR3NZ
  - Stem Cells
    - Embryonic 3EØR
    - Somatic 3EØR
  - Water Balance Substance 3EØR37Z
- Subcutaneous Tissue 3EØ13GC
  - Analgesics 3EØ13NZ
  - Anesthetic Agent 3EØ13BZ
  - Anti-infective 3EØ1
  - Anti-inflammatory 3EØ133Z
  - Antineoplastic 3EØ13Ø
  - Destructive Agent 3EØ13TZ
  - Diagnostic Substance, Other 3EØ13KZ
  - Electrolytic Substance 3EØ137Z
  - Hormone 3EØ13V
  - Hypnotics 3EØ13NZ
  - Nutritional Substance 3EØ136Z
  - Radioactive Substance 3EØ13HZ
  - Sedatives 3EØ13NZ
  - Serum 3EØ134Z
  - Toxoid 3EØ134Z
  - Vaccine 3EØ134Z
  - Water Balance Substance 3EØ137Z
- Vein
  - Central 3EØ4
    - Analgesics 3EØ4
    - Anesthetic, Intracirculatory 3EØ4
    - Antiarrhythmic 3EØ4
    - Anti-infective 3EØ4
    - Anti-inflammatory 3EØ4
    - Antineoplastic 3EØ4
    - Destructive Agent 3EØ4
    - Diagnostic Substance, Other 3EØ4
    - Electrolytic Substance 3EØ4
    - Hormone 3EØ4
    - Hypnotics 3EØ4
    - Immunotherapeutic 3EØ4
    - Nutritional Substance 3EØ4
    - Platelet Inhibitor 3EØ4
    - Radioactive Substance 3EØ4
    - Sedatives 3EØ4
    - Serum 3EØ4
    - Thrombolytic 3EØ4
    - Toxoid 3EØ4
    - Vaccine 3EØ4
    - Vasopressor 3EØ4
    - Water Balance Substance 3EØ4
  - Peripheral 3EØ3
    - Analgesics 3EØ3
    - Anesthetic, Intracirculatory 3EØ3
    - Antiarrhythmic 3EØ3
    - Anti-infective 3EØ3

Introduction of substance in or on — *continued*
Vein — *continued*
Peripheral — *continued*
Anti-inflammatory 3EØ3
Antineoplastic 3EØ3
Destructive Agent 3EØ3
Diagnostic Substance, Other 3EØ3
Electrolytic Substance 3EØ3
Hormone 3EØ3
Hypnotics 3EØ3
Immunotherapeutic 3EØ3
Islet Cells, Pancreatic 3EØ3
Nutritional Substance 3EØ3
Platelet Inhibitor 3EØ3
Radioactive Substance 3EØ3
Sedatives 3EØ3
Serum 3EØ3
Thrombolytic 3EØ3
Toxoid 3EØ3
Vaccine 3EØ3
Vasopressor 3EØ3
Water Balance Substance 3EØ3
Intubation
Airway
see Insertion of device in, Esophagus ØDH5
see Insertion of device in, Mouth and Throat ØCHY
see Insertion of device in, Trachea ØBH1
Drainage device *see* Drainage
Feeding Device *see* Insertion of device in, Gastrointestinal System ØDH
INTUITY Elite valve system, EDWARDS *use* Zooplastic Tissue, Rapid Deployment Technique in New Technology
Iobenguane I-131 Antineoplastic XWØ
Iobenguane I-131, High Specific Activity (HSA) *use* Iobenguane I-131 Antineoplastic
IPPB (intermittent positive pressure breathing) *see* Assistance, Respiratory 5AØ9
IRE (Irreversible Electroporation) *see* Destruction, Hepatobiliary System and Pancreas ØF5
Iridectomy
see Excision, Eye Ø8B
see Resection, Eye Ø8T
Iridoplasty
see Repair, Eye Ø8Q
see Replacement, Eye Ø8R
see Supplement, Eye Ø8U
Iridotomy *see* Drainage, Eye Ø89
Irreversible Electroporation (IRE) *see* Destruction, Hepatobiliary System and Pancreas ØF5
Irrigation
Biliary Tract, Irrigating Substance 3E1J
Brain, Irrigating Substance 3E1Q38Z
Cranial Cavity, Irrigating Substance 3E1Q38Z
Ear, Irrigating Substance 3E1B
Epidural Space, Irrigating Substance 3E1S38Z
Eye, Irrigating Substance 3E1C
Gastrointestinal Tract
Lower, Irrigating Substance 3E1H
Upper, Irrigating Substance 3E1G
Genitourinary Tract, Irrigating Substance 3E1K
Irrigating Substance 3C1ZX8Z
Joint, Irrigating Substance 3E1U
Mucous Membrane, Irrigating Substance 3E1Ø
Nose, Irrigating Substance 3E19
Pancreatic Tract, Irrigating Substance 3E1J
Pericardial Cavity, Irrigating Substance 3E1Y38Z
Peritoneal Cavity
Dialysate 3E1M39Z
Irrigating Substance 3E1M38Z
Pleural Cavity, Irrigating Substance 3E1L38Z
Reproductive
Female, Irrigating Substance 3E1P
Male, Irrigating Substance 3E1N
Respiratory Tract, Irrigating Substance 3E1F
Skin, Irrigating Substance 3E1Ø
Spinal Canal, Irrigating Substance 3E1R38Z
Isavuconazole Anti-infective XWØ
Ischiatic nerve *use* Sciatic Nerve
Ischiocavernosus muscle *use* Perineum Muscle
Ischiofemoral ligament
use Hip Bursa and Ligament, Left
use Hip Bursa and Ligament, Right
Ischium
use Pelvic Bone, Left
use Pelvic Bone, Right
Isolation 8EØZXY6
Isotope Administration, Whole Body DWY5G
Itrel (3) (4) neurostimulator *use* Stimulator Generator, Single Array in ØJH

J

Jakafi® *use* Ruxolitinib
Jejunal artery *use* Superior Mesenteric Artery
Jejunectomy
see Excision, Jejunum ØDBA
see Resection, Jejunum ØDTA
Jejunocolostomy
see Bypass, Gastrointestinal System ØD1
see Drainage, Gastrointestinal System ØD9
Jejunopexy
see Repair, Jejunum ØDQA
see Reposition, Jejunum ØDSA
Jejunostomy
see Bypass, Jejunum ØD1A
see Drainage, Jejunum ØD9A
Jejunotomy *see* Drainage, Jejunum ØD9A
Joint fixation plate
use Internal Fixation Device in Lower Joints
use Internal Fixation Device in Upper Joints
Joint liner (insert) *use* Liner in Lower Joints
Joint spacer (antibiotic)
use Spacer in Lower Joints
use Spacer in Upper Joints
Jugular body *use* Glomus Jugulare
Jugular lymph node
use Lymphatic, Left Neck
use Lymphatic, Right Neck

Kappa *use* Pacemaker, Dual Chamber in ØJH
Kcentra *use* 4-Factor Prothrombin Complex Concentrate
Keratectomy, kerectomy
see Excision, Eye Ø8B
see Resection, Eye Ø8T
Keratocentesis *see* Drainage, Eye Ø89
Keratoplasty
see Repair, Eye Ø8Q
see Replacement, Eye Ø8R
see Supplement, Eye Ø8U
Keratotomy
see Drainage, Eye Ø89
see Repair, Eye Ø8Q
Keystone Heart TriGuard 3™ CEPD (cerebral embolic protection device) X2A6325
Kirschner wire (K-wire)
use Internal Fixation Device in Head and Facial Bones
use Internal Fixation Device in Lower Bones
use Internal Fixation Device in Lower Joints
use Internal Fixation Device in Upper Bones
use Internal Fixation Device in Upper Joints
Knee (implant) insert *use* Liner in Lower Joints
KUB x-ray *see* Plain Radiography, Kidney, Ureter and Bladder BTØ4
Kuntscher nail
use Internal Fixation Device, Intramedullary in Lower Bones
use Internal Fixation Device, Intramedullary in Upper Bones
KYMRIAH *use* Engineered Autologous Chimeric Antigen Receptor T-cell Immunotherapy

L

Labia majora *use* Vulva
Labia minora *use* Vulva
Labial gland
use Lower Lip
use Upper Lip
Labiectomy
see Excision, Female Reproductive System ØUB
see Resection, Female Reproductive System ØUT
Lacrimal canaliculus
use Lacrimal Duct, Left
use Lacrimal Duct, Right
Lacrimal punctum
use Lacrimal Duct, Left
Lacrimal punctum — *continued*
use Lacrimal Duct, Right
Lacrimal sac
use Lacrimal Duct, Left
use Lacrimal Duct, Right
LAGB (laparoscopic adjustable gastric banding)
Initial procedure ØDV64CZ
Surgical correction *see* Revision of device in, Stomach ØDW6
Laminectomy
see Excision, Lower Bones ØQB
see Excision, Upper Bones ØPB
see Release, Central Nervous System and Cranial Nerves ØØN
see Release, Peripheral Nervous System Ø1N
Laminotomy
see Drainage, Lower Bones ØQ9
see Drainage, Upper Bones ØP9
see Excision, Lower Bones ØQB
see Excision, Upper Bones ØPB
see Release, Central Nervous System and Cranial Nerves ØØN
see Release, Lower Bones ØQN
see Release, Peripheral Nervous System Ø1N
see Release, Upper Bones ØPN
Laparoscopic-assisted transanal pull-through
see Excision, Gastrointestinal System ØDB
see Resection, Gastrointestinal System ØDT
Laparoscopy *see* Inspection
Laparotomy
Drainage *see* Drainage, Peritoneal Cavity ØW9G
Exploratory *see* Inspection, Peritoneal Cavity ØWJG
LAP-BAND® Adjustable Gastric Banding System *use* Extraluminal Device
Laryngectomy
see Excision, Larynx ØCBS
see Resection, Larynx ØCTS
Laryngocentesis *see* Drainage, Larynx ØC9S
Laryngogram *see* Fluoroscopy, Larynx B91J
Laryngopexy *see* Repair, Larynx ØCQS
Laryngopharynx *use* Pharynx
Laryngoplasty
see Repair, Larynx ØCQS
see Replacement, Larynx ØCRS
see Supplement, Larynx ØCUS
Laryngorrhaphy *see* Repair, Larynx ØCQS
Laryngoscopy ØCJS8ZZ
Laryngotomy *see* Drainage, Larynx ØC9S
Laser Interstitial Thermal Therapy
Adrenal Gland DGY2KZZ
Anus DDY8KZZ
Bile Ducts DFY2KZZ
Brain DØYØKZZ
Brain Stem DØY1KZZ
Breast
Left DMYØKZZ
Right DMY1KZZ
Bronchus DBY1KZZ
Chest Wall DBY7KZZ
Colon DDY5KZZ
Diaphragm DBY8KZZ
Duodenum DDY2KZZ
Esophagus DDYØKZZ
Gallbladder DFY1KZZ
Gland
Adrenal DGY2KZZ
Parathyroid DGY4KZZ
Pituitary DGYØKZZ
Thyroid DGY5KZZ
Ileum DDY4KZZ
Jejunum DDY3KZZ
Liver DFYØKZZ
Lung DBY2KZZ
Mediastinum DBY6KZZ
Nerve, Peripheral DØY7KZZ
Pancreas DFY3KZZ
Parathyroid Gland DGY4KZZ
Pineal Body DGY1KZZ
Pituitary Gland DGYØKZZ
Pleura DBY5KZZ
Prostate DVYØKZZ
Rectum DDY7KZZ
Spinal Cord DØY6KZZ
Stomach DDY1KZZ
Thyroid Gland DGY5KZZ
Trachea DBYØKZZ

Lateral canthus
use Upper Eyelid, Left
use Upper Eyelid, Right
Lateral collateral ligament (LCL)
use Knee Bursa and Ligament, Left
use Knee Bursa and Ligament, Right
Lateral condyle of femur
use Lower Femur, Left
use Lower Femur, Right
Lateral condyle of tibia
use Tibia, Left
use Tibia, Right
Lateral cuneiform bone
use Tarsal, Left
use Tarsal, Right
Lateral epicondyle of femur
use Lower Femur, Left
use Lower Femur, Right
Lateral epicondyle of humerus
use Humeral Shaft, Left
use Humeral Shaft, Right
Lateral femoral cutaneous nerve *use* Lumbar Plexus
Lateral (brachial) lymph node
use Lymphatic, Left Axillary
use Lymphatic, Right Axillary
Lateral malleolus
use Fibula, Left
use Fibula, Right
Lateral meniscus
use Knee Joint, Left
use Knee Joint, Right
Lateral nasal cartilage *use* Nasal Mucosa and Soft Tissue
Lateral plantar artery
use Foot Artery, Left
use Foot Artery, Right
Lateral plantar nerve *use* Tibial Nerve
Lateral rectus muscle
use Extraocular Muscle, Left
use Extraocular Muscle, Right
Lateral sacral artery
use Internal Iliac Artery, Left
use Internal Iliac Artery, Right
Lateral sacral vein
use Hypogastric Vein, Left
use Hypogastric Vein, Right
Lateral sural cutaneous nerve *use* Peroneal Nerve
Lateral tarsal artery
use Foot Artery, Left
use Foot Artery, Right
Lateral temporomandibular ligament *use* Head and Neck Bursa and Ligament
Lateral thoracic artery
use Axillary Artery, Left
use Axillary Artery, Right
Latissimus dorsi muscle
use Trunk Muscle, Left
use Trunk Muscle, Right
Latissimus Dorsi Myocutaneous Flap
Replacement
Bilateral ØHRVØ75
Left ØHRUØ75
Right ØHRTØ75
Transfer
Left ØKXG
Right ØKXF
Lavage
see Irrigation
Bronchial alveolar, diagnostic *see* Drainage, Respiratory System ØB9
Least splanchnic nerve *use* Thoracic Sympathetic Nerve
Lefamulin Anti-infective XWØ
Left ascending lumbar vein *use* Hemiazygos Vein
Left atrioventricular valve *use* Mitral Valve
Left auricular appendix *use* Atrium, Left
Left colic vein *use* Colic Vein
Left coronary sulcus *use* Heart, Left
Left gastric artery *use* Gastric Artery
Left gastroepiploic artery *use* Splenic Artery
Left gastroepiploic vein *use* Splenic Vein
Left inferior phrenic vein *use* Renal Vein, Left
Left inferior pulmonary vein *use* Pulmonary Vein, Left
Left jugular trunk *use* Thoracic Duct
Left lateral ventricle *use* Cerebral Ventricle
Left ovarian vein *use* Renal Vein, Left
Left second lumbar vein *use* Renal Vein, Left
Left subclavian trunk *use* Thoracic Duct
Left subcostal vein *use* Hemiazygos Vein
Left superior pulmonary vein *use* Pulmonary Vein, Left
Left suprarenal vein *use* Renal Vein, Left
Left testicular vein *use* Renal Vein, Left
Lengthening
Bone, with device *see* Insertion of Limb Lengthening Device
Muscle, by incision *see* Division, Muscles ØK8
Tendon, by incision *see* Division, Tendons ØL8
Leptomeninges, intracranial *use* Cerebral Meninges
Leptomeninges, spinal *use* Spinal Meninges
Lesser alar cartilage *use* Nasal Mucosa and Soft Tissue
Lesser occipital nerve *use* Cervical Plexus
Lesser Omentum *use* Omentum
Lesser saphenous vein
use Saphenous Vein, Left
use Saphenous Vein, Right
Lesser splanchnic nerve *use* Thoracic Sympathetic Nerve
Lesser trochanter
use Upper Femur, Left
use Upper Femur, Right
Lesser tuberosity
use Humeral Head, Left
use Humeral Head, Right
Lesser wing *use* Sphenoid Bone
Leukopheresis, therapeutic *see* Pheresis, Circulatory 6A55
Levator anguli oris muscle *use* Facial Muscle
Levator ani muscle *use* Perineum Muscle
Levator labii superioris alaeque nasi muscle *use* Facial Muscle
Levator labii superioris muscle *use* Facial Muscle
Levator palpebrae superioris muscle
use Upper Eyelid, Left
use Upper Eyelid, Right
Levator scapulae muscle
use Neck Muscle, Left
use Neck Muscle, Right
Levator veli palatini muscle *use* Tongue, Palate, Pharynx Muscle
Levatores costarum muscle
use Thorax Muscle, Left
use Thorax Muscle, Right
LifeStent® (Flexstar) (XL) Vascular Stent System *use* Intraluminal Device
Ligament of head of fibula
use Knee Bursa and Ligament, Left
use Knee Bursa and Ligament, Right
Ligament of the lateral malleolus
use Ankle Bursa and Ligament, Left
use Ankle Bursa and Ligament, Right
Ligamentum flavum, cervical *use* Head and Neck Bursa and Ligament
Ligamentum flavum, lumbar *use* Lower Spine Bursa and Ligament
Ligamentum flavum, thoracic *use* Upper Spine Bursa and Ligament
Ligation *see* Occlusion
Ligation, hemorrhoid *see* Occlusion, Lower Veins, Hemorrhoidal Plexus
Light Therapy GZJZZZZ
Liner
Removal of device from
Hip
Left ØSPBØ9Z
Right ØSP9Ø9Z
Knee
Left ØSPDØ9Z
Right ØSPCØ9Z
Revision of device in
Hip
Left ØSWBØ9Z
Right ØSW9Ø9Z
Knee
Left ØSWDØ9Z
Right ØSWCØ9Z
Supplement
Hip
Left ØSUBØ9Z
Acetabular Surface ØSUEØ9Z
Femoral Surface ØSUSØ9Z
Right ØSU9Ø9Z
Liner — *continued*
Supplement — *continued*
Hip — *continued*
Right — *continued*
Acetabular Surface ØSUAØ9Z
Femoral Surface ØSURØ9Z
Knee
Left ØSUDØ9
Femoral Surface ØSUUØ9Z
Tibial Surface ØSUWØ9Z
Right ØSUCØ9
Femoral Surface ØSUTØ9Z
Tibial Surface ØSUVØ9Z
Lingual artery
use External Carotid Artery, Left
use External Carotid Artery, Right
Lingual tonsil *use* Pharynx
Lingulectomy, lung
see Excision, Lung Lingula ØBBH
see Resection, Lung Lingula ØBTH
Lisocabtagene Maraleucel *use* Lisocabtagene Maraleucel Immunotherapy
Lisocabtagene Maraleucel Immunotherapy XW2
Lithoplasty *see* Fragmentation
Lithotripsy
see Fragmentation
With removal of fragments *see* Extirpation
LITT (laser interstitial thermal therapy) *see* Laser Interstitial Thermal Therapy
LIVIAN™ CRT-D *use* Cardiac Resynchronization Defibrillator Pulse Generator in ØJH
Lobectomy
see Excision, Central Nervous System and Cranial Nerves ØØB
see Excision, Endocrine System ØGB
see Excision, Hepatobiliary System and Pancreas ØFB
see Excision, Respiratory System ØBB
see Resection, Endocrine System ØGT
see Resection, Hepatobiliary System and Pancreas ØFT
see Resection, Respiratory System ØBT
Lobotomy *see* Division, Brain ØØ8Ø
Localization
see Imaging
see Map
Locus ceruleus *use* Pons
Long thoracic nerve *use* Brachial Plexus
Loop ileostomy *see* Bypass, Ileum ØD1B
Loop recorder, implantable *use* Monitoring Device
Lower GI series *see* Fluoroscopy, Colon BD14
Lower Respiratory Fluid Nucleic Acid-base Microbial Detection XXEBXQ6
Lumbar artery *use* Abdominal Aorta
Lumbar facet joint *use* Lumbar Vertebral Joint
Lumbar ganglion *use* Lumbar Sympathetic Nerve
Lumbar lymph node *use* Lymphatic, Aortic
Lumbar lymphatic trunk *use* Cisterna Chyli
Lumbar splanchnic nerve *use* Lumbar Sympathetic Nerve
Lumbosacral facet joint *use* Lumbosacral Joint
Lumbosacral trunk *use* Lumbar Nerve
Lumpectomy *see* Excision
Lunate bone
use Carpal, Left
use Carpal, Right
Lunotriquetral ligament
use Hand Bursa and Ligament, Left
use Hand Bursa and Ligament, Right
Lymphadenectomy
see Excision, Lymphatic and Hemic Systems Ø7B
see Resection, Lymphatic and Hemic Systems Ø7T
Lymphadenotomy *see* Drainage, Lymphatic and Hemic Systems Ø79
Lymphangiectomy
see Excision, Lymphatic and Hemic Systems Ø7B
see Resection, Lymphatic and Hemic Systems Ø7T
Lymphangiogram *see* Plain Radiography, Lymphatic System B7Ø
Lymphangioplasty
see Repair, Lymphatic and Hemic Systems Ø7Q
see Supplement, Lymphatic and Hemic Systems Ø7U
Lymphangiorrhaphy *see* Repair, Lymphatic and Hemic Systems Ø7Q
Lymphangiotomy *see* Drainage, Lymphatic and Hemic Systems Ø79

Lysis *see* Release

M

Macula
use Retina, Left
use Retina, Right
MAGEC® Spinal Bracing and Distraction System
use Magnetically Controlled Growth Rod(s) in New Technology
Magnet extraction, ocular foreign body *see* Extirpation, Eye Ø8C
Magnetic Resonance Imaging (MRI)
Abdomen BW3Ø
Ankle
Left BQ3H
Right BQ3G
Aorta
Abdominal B43Ø
Thoracic B33Ø
Arm
Left BP3F
Right BP3E
Artery
Celiac B431
Cervico-Cerebral Arch B33Q
Common Carotid, Bilateral B335
Coronary
Bypass Graft, Multiple B233
Multiple B231
Internal Carotid, Bilateral B338
Intracranial B33R
Lower Extremity
Bilateral B43H
Left B43G
Right B43F
Pelvic B43C
Renal, Bilateral B438
Spinal B33M
Superior Mesenteric B434
Upper Extremity
Bilateral B33K
Left B33J
Right B33H
Vertebral, Bilateral B33G
Bladder BT3Ø
Brachial Plexus BW3P
Brain BØ3Ø
Breast
Bilateral BH32
Left BH31
Right BH3Ø
Calcaneus
Left BQ3K
Right BQ3J
Chest BW33Y
Coccyx BR3F
Connective Tissue
Lower Extremity BL31
Upper Extremity BL3Ø
Corpora Cavernosa BV3Ø
Disc
Cervical BR31
Lumbar BR33
Thoracic BR32
Ear B93Ø
Elbow
Left BP3H
Right BP3G
Eye
Bilateral B837
Left B836
Right B835
Femur
Left BQ34
Right BQ33
Fetal Abdomen BY33
Fetal Extremity BY35
Fetal Head BY3Ø
Fetal Heart BY31
Fetal Spine BY34
Fetal Thorax BY32
Fetus, Whole BY36
Foot
Left BQ3M
Right BQ3L
Forearm
Left BP3K

Magnetic Resonance Imaging (MRI) — *continued*
Forearm — *continued*
Right BP3J
Gland
Adrenal, Bilateral BG32
Parathyroid BG33
Parotid, Bilateral B936
Salivary, Bilateral B93D
Submandibular, Bilateral B939
Thyroid BG34
Head BW38
Heart, Right and Left B236
Hip
Left BQ31
Right BQ3Ø
Intracranial Sinus B532
Joint
Finger
Left BP3D
Right BP3C
Hand
Left BP3D
Right BP3C
Temporomandibular, Bilateral BN39
Kidney
Bilateral BT33
Left BT32
Right BT31
Transplant BT39
Knee
Left BQ38
Right BQ37
Larynx B93J
Leg
Left BQ3F
Right BQ3D
Liver BF35
Liver and Spleen BF36
Lung Apices BB3G
Nasopharynx B93F
Neck BW3F
Nerve
Acoustic BØ3C
Brachial Plexus BW3P
Oropharynx B93F
Ovary
Bilateral BU35
Left BU34
Right BU33
Ovary and Uterus BU3C
Pancreas BF37
Patella
Left BQ3W
Right BQ3V
Pelvic Region BW3G
Pelvis BR3C
Pituitary Gland BØ39
Plexus, Brachial BW3P
Prostate BV33
Retroperitoneum BW3H
Sacrum BR3F
Scrotum BV34
Sella Turcica BØ39
Shoulder
Left BP39
Right BP38
Sinus
Intracranial B532
Paranasal B932
Spinal Cord BØ3B
Spine
Cervical BR3Ø
Lumbar BR39
Thoracic BR37
Spleen and Liver BF36
Subcutaneous Tissue
Abdomen BH3H
Extremity
Lower BH3J
Upper BH3F
Head BH3D
Neck BH3D
Pelvis BH3H
Thorax BH3G
Tendon
Lower Extremity BL33
Upper Extremity BL32
Testicle
Bilateral BV37

Magnetic Resonance Imaging (MRI) — *continued*
Testicle — *continued*
Left BV36
Right BV35
Toe
Left BQ3Q
Right BQ3P
Uterus BU36
Pregnant BU3B
Uterus and Ovary BU3C
Vagina BU39
Vein
Cerebellar B531
Cerebral B531
Jugular, Bilateral B535
Lower Extremity
Bilateral B53D
Left B53C
Right B53B
Other B53V
Pelvic (Iliac) Bilateral B53H
Portal B53T
Pulmonary, Bilateral B53S
Renal, Bilateral B53L
Spanchnic B53T
Upper Extremity
Bilateral B53P
Left B53N
Right B53M
Vena Cava
Inferior B539
Superior B538
Wrist
Left BP3M
Right BP3L
Magnetically Controlled Growth Rod(s)
Cervical XNS3
Lumbar XNSØ
Thoracic XNS4
Magnetic-guided radiofrequency endovascular fistula
Radial Artery, Left Ø31C3ZF
Radial Artery, Right Ø31B3ZF
Ulnar Artery, Left Ø31A3ZF
Ulnar Artery, Right Ø3193ZF
Malleotomy *see* Drainage, Ear, Nose, Sinus Ø99
Malleus
use Auditory Ossicle, Left
use Auditory Ossicle, Right
Mammaplasty, mammoplasty
see Alteration, Skin and Breast ØHØ
see Repair, Skin and Breast ØHQ
see Replacement, Skin and Breast ØHR
see Supplement, Skin and Breast ØHU
Mammary duct
use Breast, Bilateral
use Breast, Left
use Breast, Right
Mammary gland
use Breast, Bilateral
use Breast, Left
use Breast, Right
Mammectomy
see Excision, Skin and Breast ØHB
see Resection, Skin and Breast ØHT
Mammillary body *use* Hypothalamus
Mammography *see* Plain Radiography, Skin, Subcutaneous Tissue and Breast BHØ
Mammotomy *see* Drainage, Skin and Breast ØH9
Mandibular nerve *use* Trigeminal Nerve
Mandibular notch
use Mandible, Left
use Mandible, Right
Mandibulectomy
see Excision, Head and Facial Bones ØNB
see Resection, Head and Facial Bones ØNT
Manipulation
Adhesions *see* Release
Chiropractic *see* Chiropractic Manipulation
Manual removal, retained placenta *see* Extraction, Products of Conception, Retained 1ØD1
Manubrium *use* Sternum
Map
Basal Ganglia ØØK8
Brain ØØKØ
Cerebellum ØØKC
Cerebral Hemisphere ØØK7

Map — *continued*
Conduction Mechanism Ø2K8
Hypothalamus ØØKA
Medulla Oblongata ØØKD
Pons ØØKB
Thalamus ØØK9
Mapping
Doppler ultrasound *see* Ultrasonography
Electrocardiogram only *see* Measurement, Cardiac 4AØ2
Mark IV Breathing Pacemaker System *use* Stimulator Generator in Subcutaneous Tissue and Fascia
Marsupialization
see Drainage
see Excision
Massage, cardiac
External 5A12Ø12
Open Ø2QAØZZ
Masseter muscle *use* Head Muscle
Masseteric fascia *use* Subcutaneous Tissue and Fascia, Face
Mastectomy
see Excision, Skin and Breast ØHB
see Resection, Skin and Breast ØHT
Mastoid air cells
use Mastoid Sinus, Left
use Mastoid Sinus, Right
Mastoid (postauricular) lymph node
use Lymphatic, Left Neck
use Lymphatic, Right Neck
Mastoid process
use Temporal Bone, Left
use Temporal Bone, Right
Mastoidectomy
see Excision, Ear, Nose, Sinus Ø9B
see Resection, Ear, Nose, Sinus Ø9T
Mastoidotomy *see* Drainage, Ear, Nose, Sinus Ø99
Mastopexy
see Repair, Skin and Breast ØHQ
see Reposition, Skin and Breast ØHS
Mastorrhaphy *see* Repair, Skin and Breast ØHQ
Mastotomy *see* Drainage, Skin and Breast ØH9
Maxillary artery
use External Carotid Artery, Left
use External Carotid Artery, Right
Maxillary nerve *use* Trigeminal Nerve
Maximo II DR (VR) *use* Defibrillator Generator in ØJH
Maximo II DR CRT-D *use* Cardiac Resynchronization Defibrillator Pulse Generator in ØJH
Measurement
Arterial
Flow
Coronary 4AØ3
Intracranial 4AØ3X5D
Peripheral 4AØ3
Pulmonary 4AØ3
Pressure
Coronary 4AØ3
Peripheral 4AØ3
Pulmonary 4AØ3
Thoracic, Other 4AØ3
Pulse
Coronary 4AØ3
Peripheral 4AØ3
Pulmonary 4AØ3
Saturation, Peripheral 4AØ3
Sound, Peripheral 4AØ3
Biliary
Flow 4AØC
Pressure 4AØC
Cardiac
Action Currents 4AØ2
Defibrillator 4BØ2XTZ
Electrical Activity 4AØ2
Guidance 4AØ2X4A
No Qualifier 4AØ2X4Z
Output 4AØ2
Pacemaker 4BØ2XSZ
Rate 4AØ2
Rhythm 4AØ2
Sampling and Pressure
Bilateral 4AØ2
Left Heart 4AØ2
Right Heart 4AØ2
Sound 4AØ2
Total Activity, Stress 4AØ2XM4
Central Nervous
Conductivity 4AØØ

Measurement — *continued*
Central Nervous — *continued*
Electrical Activity 4AØØ
Pressure 4AØØØBZ
Intracranial 4AØØ
Saturation, Intracranial 4AØØ
Stimulator 4BØØXVZ
Temperature, Intracranial 4AØØ
Circulatory, Volume 4AØ5XLZ
Gastrointestinal
Motility 4AØB
Pressure 4AØB
Secretion 4AØB
Lower Respiratory Fluid Nucleic Acid-base Microbial Detection XXEBXQ6
Lymphatic
Flow 4AØ6
Pressure 4AØ6
Metabolism 4AØZ
Musculoskeletal
Contractility 4AØF
Pressure 4AØF3BE
Stimulator 4BØFXVZ
Olfactory, Acuity 4AØ8XØZ
Peripheral Nervous
Conductivity
Motor 4AØ1
Sensory 4AØ1
Electrical Activity 4AØ1
Stimulator 4BØ1XVZ
Positive Blood Culture Fluorescence Hybridization for Organism Identification, Concentration and Susceptibility XXE5XN6
Products of Conception
Cardiac
Electrical Activity 4AØH
Rate 4AØH
Rhythm 4AØH
Sound 4AØH
Nervous
Conductivity 4AØJ
Electrical Activity 4AØJ
Pressure 4AØJ
Respiratory
Capacity 4AØ9
Flow 4AØ9
Pacemaker 4BØ9XSZ
Rate 4AØ9
Resistance 4AØ9
Total Activity 4AØ9
Volume 4AØ9
Sleep 4AØZXQZ
Temperature 4AØZ
Urinary
Contractility 4AØD
Flow 4AØD
Pressure 4AØD
Resistance 4AØD
Volume 4AØD
Venous
Flow
Central 4AØ4
Peripheral 4AØ4
Portal 4AØ4
Pulmonary 4AØ4
Pressure
Central 4AØ4
Peripheral 4AØ4
Portal 4AØ4
Pulmonary 4AØ4
Pulse
Central 4AØ4
Peripheral 4AØ4
Portal 4AØ4
Pulmonary 4AØ4
Saturation, Peripheral 4AØ4
Visual
Acuity 4AØ7XØZ
Mobility 4AØ7X7Z
Pressure 4AØ7XBZ
Whole Blood Nucleic Acid-base Microbial Detection XXE5XM5
Meatoplasty, urethra *see* Repair, Urethra ØTQD
Meatotomy *see* Drainage, Urinary System ØT9
Mechanical ventilation *see* Performance, Respiratory 5A19
Medial canthus
use Lower Eyelid, Left
use Lower Eyelid, Right

Medial collateral ligament (MCL)
use Knee Bursa and Ligament, Left
use Knee Bursa and Ligament, Right
Medial condyle of femur
use Lower Femur, Left
use Lower Femur, Right
Medial condyle of tibia
use Tibia, Left
use Tibia, Right
Medial cuneiform bone
use Tarsal, Left
use Tarsal, Right
Medial epicondyle of femur
use Lower Femur, Left
use Lower Femur, Right
Medial epicondyle of humerus
use Humeral Shaft, Left
use Humeral Shaft, Right
Medial malleolus
use Tibia, Left
use Tibia, Right
Medial meniscus
use Knee Joint, Left
use Knee Joint, Right
Medial plantar artery
use Foot Artery, Left
use Foot Artery, Right
Medial plantar nerve *use* Tibial Nerve
Medial popliteal nerve *use* Tibial Nerve
Medial rectus muscle
use Extraocular Muscle, Left
use Extraocular Muscle, Right
Medial sural cutaneous nerve *use* Tibial Nerve
Median antebrachial vein
use Basilic Vein, Left
use Basilic Vein, Right
Median cubital vein
use Basilic Vein, Left
use Basilic Vein, Right
Median sacral artery *use* Abdominal Aorta
Mediastinal cavity *use* Mediastinum
Mediastinal lymph node *use* Lymphatic, Thorax
Mediastinal space *use* Mediastinum
Mediastinoscopy ØWJC4ZZ
Medication Management GZ3ZZZZ
for substance abuse
Antabuse HZ83ZZZ
Bupropion HZ87ZZZ
Clonidine HZ86ZZZ
Levo-alpha-acetyl-methadol (LAAM) HZ82ZZZ
Methadone Maintenance HZ81ZZZ
Naloxone HZ85ZZZ
Naltrexone HZ84ZZZ
Nicotine Replacement HZ8ØZZZ
Other Replacement Medication HZ89ZZZ
Psychiatric Medication HZ88ZZZ
Meditation 8EØZXY5
Medtronic Endurant® II AAA stent graft system *use* Intraluminal Device
Meissner's (submucous) plexus *use* Abdominal Sympathetic Nerve
Melody® transcatheter pulmonary valve *use* Zooplastic Tissue in Heart and Great Vessels
Membranous urethra *use* Urethra
Meningeorrhaphy
see Repair, Cerebral Meninges ØØQ1
see Repair, Spinal Meninges ØØQT
Meniscectomy, knee
see Excision, Joint, Knee, Left ØSBD
see Excision, Joint, Knee, Right ØSBC
Mental foramen
use Mandible, Left
use Mandible, Right
Mentalis muscle *use* Facial Muscle
Mentoplasty *see* Alteration, Jaw, Lower ØWØ5
Meropenem-vaborbactam Anti-infective XWØ
Mesenterectomy *see* Excision, Mesentery ØDBV
Mesenteriorrhaphy, mesenterorrhaphy *see* Repair, Mesentery ØDQV
Mesenteriplication *see* Repair, Mesentery ØDQV
Mesoappendix *use* Mesentery
Mesocolon *use* Mesentery
Metacarpal ligament
use Hand Bursa and Ligament, Left
use Hand Bursa and Ligament, Right

Metacarpophalangeal ligament
use Hand Bursa and Ligament, Left
use Hand Bursa and Ligament, Right
Metal on metal bearing surface *use* Synthetic Substitute, Metal in ØSR
Metatarsal ligament
use Foot Bursa and Ligament, Left
use Foot Bursa and Ligament, Right
Metatarsectomy
see Excision, Lower Bones ØQB
see Resection, Lower Bones ØQT
Metatarsophalangeal (MTP) joint
use Metatarsal-Phalangeal Joint, Left
use Metatarsal-Phalangeal Joint, Right
Metatarsophalangeal ligament
use Foot Bursa and Ligament, Left
use Foot Bursa and Ligament, Right
Metathalamus *use* Thalamus
Micro-Driver stent (RX) (OTW) *use* Intraluminal Device
MicroMed HeartAssist *use* Implantable Heart Assist System in Heart and Great Vessels
Micrus CERECYTE Microcoil *use* Intraluminal Device, Bioactive in Upper Arteries
Midcarpal joint
use Carpal Joint, Left
use Carpal Joint, Right
Middle cardiac nerve *use* Thoracic Sympathetic Nerve
Middle cerebral artery *use* Intracranial Artery
Middle cerebral vein *use* Intracranial Vein
Middle colic vein *use* Colic Vein
Middle genicular artery
use Popliteal Artery, Left
use Popliteal Artery, Right
Middle hemorrhoidal vein
use Hypogastric Vein, Left
use Hypogastric Vein, Right
Middle rectal artery
use Internal Iliac Artery, Left
use Internal Iliac Artery, Right
Middle suprarenal artery *use* Abdominal Aorta
Middle temporal artery
use Temporal Artery, Left
use Temporal Artery, Right
Middle turbinate *use* Nasal Turbinate
Mineral-based Topical Hemostatic Agent XWØ
MIRODERM™ Biologic Wound Matrix *use* Skin Substitute, Porcine Liver Derived in New Technology
MitraClip valve repair system *use* Synthetic Substitute
Mitral annulus *use* Mitral Valve
Mitroflow® Aortic Pericardial Heart Valve *use* Zooplastic Tissue in Heart and Great Vessels
Mobilization, adhesions *see* Release
Molar gland *use* Buccal Mucosa
MolecuLight i:X® wound imaging *see* Other Imaging, Anatomical Regions BW5
Monitoring
Arterial
Flow
Coronary 4A13
Peripheral 4A13
Pulmonary 4A13
Pressure
Coronary 4A13
Peripheral 4A13
Pulmonary 4A13
Pulse
Coronary 4A13
Peripheral 4A13
Pulmonary 4A13
Saturation, Peripheral 4A13
Sound, Peripheral 4A13
Cardiac
Electrical Activity 4A12
Ambulatory 4A12X45
No Qualifier 4A12X4Z
Output 4A12
Rate 4A12
Rhythm 4A12
Sound 4A12
Total Activity, Stress 4A12XM4
Vascular Perfusion, Indocyanine Green Dye 4A12XSH
Central Nervous
Conductivity 4A1Ø
Electrical Activity
Intraoperative 4A1Ø
Monitoring — *continued*
Central Nervous — *continued*
Electrical Activity — *continued*
No Qualifier 4A1Ø
Pressure 4A1ØØBZ
Intracranial 4A1Ø
Saturation, Intracranial 4A1Ø
Temperature, Intracranial 4A1Ø
Gastrointestinal
Motility 4A1B
Pressure 4A1B
Secretion 4A1B
Vascular Perfusion, Indocyanine Green Dye 4A1BXSH
Intraoperative Knee Replacement Sensor XR2
Kidney, Fluorescent Pyrazine XT25XE5
Lymphatic
Flow
Indocyanine Green Dye 4A16
No Qualifier 4A16
Pressure 4A16
Peripheral Nervous
Conductivity
Motor 4A11
Sensory 4A11
Electrical Activity
Intraoperative 4A11
No Qualifier 4A11
Products of Conception
Cardiac
Electrical Activity 4A1H
Rate 4A1H
Rhythm 4A1H
Sound 4A1H
Nervous
Conductivity 4A1J
Electrical Activity 4A1J
Pressure 4A1J
Respiratory
Capacity 4A19
Flow 4A19
Rate 4A19
Resistance 4A19
Volume 4A19
Skin and Breast, Vascular Perfusion, Indocyanine Green Dye 4A1GXSH
Sleep 4A1ZXQZ
Temperature 4A1Z
Urinary
Contractility 4A1D
Flow 4A1D
Pressure 4A1D
Resistance 4A1D
Volume 4A1D
Venous
Flow
Central 4A14
Peripheral 4A14
Portal 4A14
Pulmonary 4A14
Pressure
Central 4A14
Peripheral 4A14
Portal 4A14
Pulmonary 4A14
Pulse
Central 4A14
Peripheral 4A14
Portal 4A14
Pulmonary 4A14
Saturation
Central 4A14
Portal 4A14
Pulmonary 4A14
Monitoring Device, Hemodynamic
Abdomen ØJH8
Chest ØJH6
Mosaic Bioprosthesis (aortic) (mitral) valve *use* Zooplastic Tissue in Heart and Great Vessels
Motor Function Assessment FØ1
Motor Treatment FØ7
MR Angiography
see Magnetic Resonance Imaging (MRI), Heart B23
see Magnetic Resonance Imaging (MRI), Lower Arteries B43
see Magnetic Resonance Imaging (MRI), Upper Arteries B33
MULTI-LINK (VISION) (MINI-VISION) (ULTRA) Coronary Stent System *use* Intraluminal Device
Multiple sleep latency test 4AØZXQZ
Musculocutaneous nerve *use* Brachial Plexus
Musculopexy
see Repair, Muscles ØKQ
see Reposition, Muscles ØKS
Musculophrenic artery
use Internal Mammary Artery, Left
use Internal Mammary Artery, Right
Musculoplasty
see Repair, Muscles ØKQ
see Supplement, Muscles ØKU
Musculorrhaphy *see* Repair, Muscles ØKQ
Musculospiral nerve *use* Radial Nerve
Myectomy
see Excision, Muscles ØKB
see Resection, Muscles ØKT
Myelencephalon *use* Medulla Oblongata
Myelogram
CT *see* Computerized Tomography (CT Scan), Central Nervous System BØ2
MRI *see* Magnetic Resonance Imaging (MRI), Central Nervous System BØ3
Myenteric (Auerbach's) plexus *use* Abdominal Sympathetic Nerve
Myocardial Bridge Release *see* Release, Artery, Coronary
Myomectomy *see* Excision, Female Reproductive System ØUB
Myometrium *use* Uterus
Myopexy
see Repair, Muscles ØKQ
see Reposition, Muscles ØKS
Myoplasty
see Repair, Muscles ØKQ
see Supplement, Muscles ØKU
Myorrhaphy *see* Repair, Muscles ØKQ
Myoscopy *see* Inspection, Muscles ØKJ
Myotomy
see Division, Muscles ØK8
see Drainage, Muscles ØK9
Myringectomy
see Excision, Ear, Nose, Sinus Ø9B
see Resection, Ear, Nose, Sinus Ø9T
Myringoplasty
see Repair, Ear, Nose, Sinus Ø9Q
see Replacement, Ear, Nose, Sinus Ø9R
see Supplement, Ear, Nose, Sinus Ø9U
Myringostomy *see* Drainage, Ear, Nose, Sinus Ø99
Myringotomy *see* Drainage, Ear, Nose, Sinus Ø99

N

NA-1 (Nerinitide) *use* Nerinitide
Nail bed
use Finger Nail
use Toe Nail
Nail plate
use Finger Nail
use Toe Nail
nanoLOCK™ interbody fusion device *use* Interbody Fusion Device, Nanotextured Surface in New Technology
Narcosynthesis GZGZZZZ
Nasal cavity *use* Nasal Mucosa and Soft Tissue
Nasal concha *use* Nasal Turbinate
Nasalis muscle *use* Facial Muscle
Nasolacrimal duct
use Lacrimal Duct, Left
use Lacrimal Duct, Right
Nasopharyngeal airway (NPA) *use* Intraluminal Device, Airway in Ear, Nose, Sinus
Navicular bone
use Tarsal, Left
use Tarsal, Right
Near Infrared Spectroscopy, Circulatory System 8EØ2
Neck of femur
use Upper Femur, Left
use Upper Femur, Right
Neck of humerus (anatomical) (surgical)
use Humeral Head, Left
use Humeral Head, Right
Nephrectomy
see Excision, Urinary System ØTB

Nephrectomy — *continued*
see Resection, Urinary System ØTT
Nephrolithotomy *see* Extirpation, Urinary System ØTC
Nephrolysis *see* Release, Urinary System ØTN
Nephropexy
see Repair, Urinary System ØTQ
see Reposition, Urinary System ØTS
Nephroplasty
see Repair, Urinary System ØTQ
see Supplement, Urinary System ØTU
Nephropyeloureterostomy
see Bypass, Urinary System ØT1
see Drainage, Urinary System ØT9
Nephrorrhaphy *see* Repair, Urinary System ØTQ
Nephroscopy, transurethral ØTJ58ZZ
Nephrostomy
see Bypass, Urinary System ØT1
see Drainage, Urinary System ØT9
Nephrotomography
see Fluoroscopy, Urinary System BT1
see Plain Radiography, Urinary System BTØ
Nephrotomy
see Division, Urinary System ØT8
see Drainage, Urinary System ØT9
Nerinitide XWØ
Nerve conduction study
see Measurement, Central Nervous 4AØØ
see Measurement, Peripheral Nervous 4AØ1
Nerve Function Assessment FØ1
Nerve to the stapedius *use* Facial Nerve
Nesiritide *use* Human B-Type Natriuretic Peptide
Neurectomy
see Excision, Central Nervous System and Cranial Nerves ØØB
see Excision, Peripheral Nervous System Ø1B
Neurexeresis
see Extraction, Central Nervous System and Cranial Nerves ØØD
see Extraction, Peripheral Nervous System Ø1D
Neurohypophysis *use* Pituitary Gland
Neurolysis
see Release, Central Nervous System and Cranial Nerves ØØN
see Release, Peripheral Nervous System Ø1N
Neuromuscular electrical stimulation (NEMS) lead
use Stimulator Lead in Muscles
Neurophysiologic monitoring *see* Monitoring, Central Nervous 4A1Ø
Neuroplasty
see Repair, Central Nervous System and Cranial Nerves ØØQ
see Repair, Peripheral Nervous System Ø1Q
see Supplement, Central Nervous System and Cranial Nerves ØØU
see Supplement, Peripheral Nervous System Ø1U
Neurorrhaphy
see Repair, Central Nervous System and Cranial Nerves ØØQ
see Repair, Peripheral Nervous System Ø1Q
Neurostimulator Generator
Insertion of device in, Skull ØNHØØNZ
Removal of device from, Skull ØNPØØNZ
Revision of device in, Skull ØNWØØNZ
Neurostimulator generator, multiple channel *use* Stimulator Generator, Multiple Array in ØJH
Neurostimulator generator, multiple channel rechargeable *use* Stimulator Generator, Multiple Array Rechargeable in ØJH
Neurostimulator generator, single channel *use* Stimulator Generator, Single Array in ØJH
Neurostimulator generator, single channel rechargeable *use* Stimulator Generator, Single Array Rechargeable in ØJH
Neurostimulator Lead
Insertion of device in
Brain ØØHØ
Cerebral Ventricle ØØH6
Nerve
Cranial ØØHE
Peripheral Ø1HY
Spinal Canal ØØHU
Spinal Cord ØØHV
Vein
Azygos Ø5HØ
Innominate
Left Ø5H4
Right Ø5H3
Neurostimulator Lead — *continued*
Removal of device from
Brain ØØPØ
Cerebral Ventricle ØØP6
Nerve
Cranial ØØPE
Peripheral Ø1PY
Spinal Canal ØØPU
Spinal Cord ØØPV
Vein
Azygos Ø5PØ
Innominate
Left Ø5P4
Right Ø5P3
Revision of device in
Brain ØØWØ
Cerebral Ventricle ØØW6
Nerve
Cranial ØØWE
Peripheral Ø1WY
Spinal Canal ØØWU
Spinal Cord ØØWV
Vein
Azygos Ø5WØ
Innominate
Left Ø5W4
Right Ø5W3
Neurotomy
see Division, Central Nervous System and Cranial Nerves ØØ8
see Division, Peripheral Nervous System Ø18
Neurotripsy
see Destruction, Central Nervous System and Cranial Nerves ØØ5
see Destruction, Peripheral Nervous System Ø15
Neutralization plate
use Internal Fixation Device in Head and Facial Bones
use Internal Fixation Device in Lower Bones
use Internal Fixation Device in Upper Bones
New Technology
Apalutamide Antineoplastic XWØDXJ5
Atezolizumab Antineoplastic XWØ
Bezlotoxumab Monoclonal Antibody XWØ
Blinatumomab Antineoplastic Immunotherapy XWØ
Brexanolone XWØ
Brexucabtagene Autoleucel Immunotherapy XW2
Caplacizumab XWØ
Cefiderocol Anti-infective XWØ
Ceftazidime-Avibactam Anti-infective XWØ
Ceftolozane/Tazobactam Anti-infective XWØ
Cerebral Embolic Filtration
Dual Filter X2A5312
Extracorporeal Flow Reversal Circuit X2A
Single Deflection Filter X2A6325
Coagulation Factor Xa, Inactivated XWØ
Concentrated Bone Marrow Aspirate XKØ23Ø3
Cytarabine and Daunorubicin Liposome Antineoplastic XWØ
Defibrotide Sodium Anticoagulant XWØ
Destruction, Prostate, Robotic Waterjet Ablation XV5Ø8A4
Dilation
Anterior Tibial
Left
Sustained Release Drug-eluting Intraluminal Device X27Q385
Four or More X27Q3C5
Three X27Q3B5
Two X27Q395
Right
Sustained Release Drug-eluting Intraluminal Device X27P385
Four or More X27P3C5
Three X27P3B5
Two X27P395
Femoral
Left
Sustained Release Drug-eluting Intraluminal Device X27J385
Four or More X27J3C5
Three X27J3B5
Two X27J395
New Technology — *continued*
Dilation — *continued*
Femoral — *continued*
Right
Sustained Release Drug-eluting Intraluminal Device X27H385
Four or More X27H3C5
Three X27H3B5
Two X27H395
Peroneal
Left
Sustained Release Drug-eluting Intraluminal Device X27U385
Four or More X27U3C5
Three X27U3B5
Two X27U395
Right
Sustained Release Drug-eluting Intraluminal Device X27T385
Four or More X27T3C5
Three X27T3B5
Two X27T395
Popliteal
Left Distal
Sustained Release Drug-eluting Intraluminal Device X27N385
Four or More X27N3C5
Three X27N3B5
Two X27N395
Left Proximal
Sustained Release Drug-eluting Intraluminal Device X27L385
Four or More X27L3C5
Three X27L3B5
Two X27L395
Right Distal
Sustained Release Drug-eluting Intraluminal Device X27M385
Four or More X27M3C5
Three X27M3B5
Two X27M395
Right Proximal
Sustained Release Drug-eluting Intraluminal Device X27K385
Four or More X27K3C5
Three X27K3B5
Two X27K395
Posterior Tibial
Left
Sustained Release Drug-eluting Intraluminal Device X27S385
Four or More X27S3C5
Three X27S3B5
Two X27S395
Right
Sustained Release Drug-eluting Intraluminal Device X27R385
Four or More X27R3C5
Three X27R3B5
Two X27R395
Durvalumab Antineoplastic XWØ
Eculizumab XWØ
Eladocagene exuparvovec XWØQ316
Endothelial Damage Inhibitor XYØVX83
Engineered Autologous Chimeric Antigen Receptor T-cell Immunotherapy XWØ
Erdafitinib Antineoplastic XWØDXL5
Esketamine Hydrochloride XWØ97M5
Fosfomycin Anti-infective XWØ
Fusion
Cervical Vertebral
2 or more
Nanotextured Surface XRG2Ø92
Radiolucent Porous XRG2ØF3
Interbody Fusion Device
Nanotextured Surface XRG1Ø92
Radiolucent Porous XRG1ØF3
Cervicothoracic Vertebral
Nanotextured Surface XRG4Ø92
Radiolucent Porous XRG4ØF3

New Technology — *continued*
Fusion — *continued*
Lumbar Vertebral
2 or more
Nanotextured Surface XRGC092
Radiolucent Porous XRGC0F3
Interbody Fusion Device
Nanotextured Surface XRGB092
Radiolucent Porous XRGB0F3
Lumbosacral
Nanotextured Surface XRGD092
Radiolucent Porous XRGD0F3
Occipital-cervical
Nanotextured Surface XRG0092
Radiolucent Porous XRG00F3
Thoracic Vertebral
2 to 7
Nanotextured Surface XRG7092
Radiolucent Porous XRG70F3
8 or more
Nanotextured Surface XRG8092
Radiolucent Porous XRG80F3
Interbody Fusion Device
Nanotextured Surface XRG6092
Radiolucent Porous XRG60F3
Thoracolumbar Vertebral
Nanotextured Surface XRGA092
Radiolucent Porous XRGA0F3
Gilteritinib Antineoplastic XW0DXV5
Idarucizumab, Dabigatran Reversal Agent XW0
Imipenem-cilastatin-relebactam Anti-infective XW0
Intraoperative Knee Replacement Sensor XR2
Iobenguane I-131 Antineoplastic XW0
Isavuconazole Anti-infective XW0
Kidney, Fluorescent Pyrazine XT25XE5
Lefamulin Anti-infective XW0
Lisocabtagene Maraleucel Immunotherapy XW2
Lower Respiratory Fluid Nucleic Acid-base Microbial Detection XXEBXQ6
Meropenem-vaborbactam Anti-infective XW0
Mineral-based Topical Hemostatic Agent XW0
Nerinitide XW0
Omadacycline Anti-infective XW0
Orbital Atherectomy Technology X2C
Other New Technology Therapeutic Substance XW0
Plazomicin Anti-infective XW0
Positive Blood Culture Fluorescence Hybridization for Organism Identification, Concentration and Susceptibility XXE5XN6
Replacement
Skin Substitute, Porcine Liver Derived XHRPXL2
Zooplastic Tissue, Rapid Deployment Technique X2RF
Reposition
Cervical, Magnetically Controlled Growth Rod(s) XNS3
Lumbar, Magnetically Controlled Growth Rod(s) XNS0
Thoracic, Magnetically Controlled Growth Rod(s) XNS4
Ruxolitinib XW0DXT5
Supplement
Lumbar, Mechanically Expandable (Paired) Synthetic Substitute XNU0356
Thoracic, Mechanically Expandable (Paired) Synthetic Substitute XNU4356
Synthetic Human Angiotensin II XW0
Tagraxofusp-erzs Antineoplastic XW0
Uridine Triacetate XW0DX82
Venetoclax Antineoplastic XW0DXR5
Whole Blood Nucleic Acid-base Microbial Detection XXE5XM5
Ninth cranial nerve *use* Glossopharyngeal Nerve
NIRS (Near Infrared Spectroscopy) *see* Physiological Systems and Anatomical Regions 8E0
Nitinol framed polymer mesh *use* Synthetic Substitute
Nonimaging Nuclear Medicine Assay
Bladder, Kidneys and Ureters CT63
Blood C763
Kidneys, Ureters and Bladder CT63
Lymphatics and Hematologic System C76YYZZ
Ureters, Kidneys and Bladder CT63
Urinary System CT6YYZZ
Nonimaging Nuclear Medicine Probe
Abdomen CW50
Nonimaging Nuclear Medicine Probe — *continued*
Abdomen and Chest CW54
Abdomen and Pelvis CW51
Brain C050
Central Nervous System C05YYZZ
Chest CW53
Chest and Abdomen CW54
Chest and Neck CW56
Extremity
Lower CP5PZZZ
Upper CP5NZZZ
Head and Neck CW5B
Heart C25YYZZ
Right and Left C256
Lymphatics
Head C75J
Head and Neck C755
Lower Extremity C75P
Neck C75K
Pelvic C75D
Trunk C75M
Upper Chest C75L
Upper Extremity C75N
Lymphatics and Hematologic System C75YYZZ
Musculoskeletal System, Other CP5YYZZ
Neck and Chest CW56
Neck and Head CW5B
Pelvic Region CW5J
Pelvis and Abdomen CW51
Spine CP55ZZZ
Nonimaging Nuclear Medicine Uptake
Endocrine System CG4YYZZ
Gland, Thyroid CG42
Non-tunneled central venous catheter *use* Infusion Device
Nostril *use* Nasal Mucosa and Soft Tissue
Novacor Left Ventricular Assist Device *use* Implantable Heart Assist System in Heart and Great Vessels
Novation® Ceramic AHS® (Articulation Hip System) *use* Synthetic Substitute, Ceramic in 0SR
Nuclear medicine
see Nonimaging Nuclear Medicine Assay
see Nonimaging Nuclear Medicine Probe
see Nonimaging Nuclear Medicine Uptake
see Planar Nuclear Medicine Imaging
see Positron Emission Tomographic (PET) Imaging
see Systemic Nuclear Medicine Therapy
see Tomographic (Tomo) Nuclear Medicine Imaging
Nuclear scintigraphy *see* Nuclear Medicine
Nutrition, concentrated substances
Enteral infusion 3E0G36Z
Parenteral (peripheral) infusion *see* Introduction of Nutritional Substance
NUZYRA™ *use* Omadacycline Anti-infective

O

Obliteration *see* Destruction
Obturator artery
use Internal Iliac Artery, Left
use Internal Iliac Artery, Right
Obturator lymph node *use* Lymphatic, Pelvis
Obturator muscle
use Hip Muscle, Left
use Hip Muscle, Right
Obturator nerve *use* Lumbar Plexus
Obturator vein
use Hypogastric Vein, Left
use Hypogastric Vein, Right
Obtuse margin *use* Heart, Left
Occipital artery
use External Carotid Artery, Left
use External Carotid Artery, Right
Occipital lobe *use* Cerebral Hemisphere
Occipital lymph node
use Lymphatic, Left Neck
use Lymphatic, Right Neck
Occipitofrontalis muscle *use* Facial Muscle
Occlusion
Ampulla of Vater 0FLC
Anus 0DLQ
Aorta
Abdominal 04L0
Thoracic, Descending 02LW3DJ
Occlusion — *continued*
Artery
Anterior Tibial
Left 04LQ
Right 04LP
Axillary
Left 03L6
Right 03L5
Brachial
Left 03L8
Right 03L7
Celiac 04L1
Colic
Left 04L7
Middle 04L8
Right 04L6
Common Carotid
Left 03LJ
Right 03LH
Common Iliac
Left 04LD
Right 04LC
External Carotid
Left 03LN
Right 03LM
External Iliac
Left 04LJ
Right 04LH
Face 03LR
Femoral
Left 04LL
Right 04LK
Foot
Left 04LW
Right 04LV
Gastric 04L2
Hand
Left 03LF
Right 03LD
Hepatic 04L3
Inferior Mesenteric 04LB
Innominate 03L2
Internal Carotid
Left 03LL
Right 03LK
Internal Iliac
Left 04LF
Right 04LE
Internal Mammary
Left 03L1
Right 03L0
Intracranial 03LG
Lower 04LY
Peroneal
Left 04LU
Right 04LT
Popliteal
Left 04LN
Right 04LM
Posterior Tibial
Left 04LS
Right 04LR
Pulmonary
Left 02LR
Right 02LQ
Pulmonary Trunk 02LP
Radial
Left 03LC
Right 03LB
Renal
Left 04LA
Right 04L9
Splenic 04L4
Subclavian
Left 03L4
Right 03L3
Superior Mesenteric 04L5
Temporal
Left 03LT
Right 03LS
Thyroid
Left 03LV
Right 03LU
Ulnar
Left 03LA
Right 03L9
Upper 03LY
Vertebral
Left 03LQ

Occlusion — *continued*
Artery — *continued*
Vertebral — *continued*
Right Ø3LP
Atrium, Left Ø2L7
Bladder ØTLB
Bladder Neck ØTLC
Bronchus
Lingula ØBL9
Lower Lobe
Left ØBLB
Right ØBL6
Main
Left ØBL7
Right ØBL3
Middle Lobe, Right ØBL5
Upper Lobe
Left ØBL8
Right ØBL4
Carina ØBL2
Cecum ØDLH
Cisterna Chyli Ø7LL
Colon
Ascending ØDLK
Descending ØDLM
Sigmoid ØDLN
Transverse ØDLL
Cord
Bilateral ØVLH
Left ØVLG
Right ØVLF
Cul-de-sac ØULF
Duct
Common Bile ØFL9
Cystic ØFL8
Hepatic
Common ØFL7
Left ØFL6
Right ØFL5
Lacrimal
Left Ø8LY
Right Ø8LX
Pancreatic ØFLD
Accessory ØFLF
Parotid
Left ØCLC
Right ØCLB
Duodenum ØDL9
Esophagogastric Junction ØDL4
Esophagus ØDL5
Lower ØDL3
Middle ØDL2
Upper ØDL1
Fallopian Tube
Left ØUL6
Right ØUL5
Fallopian Tubes, Bilateral ØUL7
Ileocecal Valve ØDLC
Ileum ØDLB
Intestine
Large ØDLE
Left ØDLG
Right ØDLF
Small ØDL8
Jejunum ØDLA
Kidney Pelvis
Left ØTL4
Right ØTL3
Left atrial appendage (LAA) *see* Occlusion, Atrium, Left Ø2L7
Lymphatic
Aortic Ø7LD
Axillary
Left Ø7L6
Right Ø7L5
Head Ø7LØ
Inguinal
Left Ø7LJ
Right Ø7LH
Internal Mammary
Left Ø7L9
Right Ø7L8
Lower Extremity
Left Ø7LG
Right Ø7LF
Mesenteric Ø7LB
Neck
Left Ø7L2
Right Ø7L1

Occlusion — *continued*
Lymphatic — *continued*
Pelvis Ø7LC
Thoracic Duct Ø7LK
Thorax Ø7L7
Upper Extremity
Left Ø7L4
Right Ø7L3
Rectum ØDLP
Stomach ØDL6
Pylorus ØDL7
Trachea ØBL1
Ureter
Left ØTL7
Right ØTL6
Urethra ØTLD
Vagina ØULG
Valve, Pulmonary Ø2LH
Vas Deferens
Bilateral ØVLQ
Left ØVLP
Right ØVLN
Vein
Axillary
Left Ø5L8
Right Ø5L7
Azygos Ø5LØ
Basilic
Left Ø5LC
Right Ø5LB
Brachial
Left Ø5LA
Right Ø5L9
Cephalic
Left Ø5LF
Right Ø5LD
Colic Ø6L7
Common Iliac
Left Ø6LD
Right Ø6LC
Esophageal Ø6L3
External Iliac
Left Ø6LG
Right Ø6LF
External Jugular
Left Ø5LQ
Right Ø5LP
Face
Left Ø5LV
Right Ø5LT
Femoral
Left Ø6LN
Right Ø6LM
Foot
Left Ø6LV
Right Ø6LT
Gastric Ø6L2
Hand
Left Ø5LH
Right Ø5LG
Hemiazygos Ø5L1
Hepatic Ø6L4
Hypogastric
Left Ø6LJ
Right Ø6LH
Inferior Mesenteric Ø6L6
Innominate
Left Ø5L4
Right Ø5L3
Internal Jugular
Left Ø5LN
Right Ø5LM
Intracranial Ø5LL
Lower Ø6LY
Portal Ø6L8
Pulmonary
Left Ø2LT
Right Ø2LS
Renal
Left Ø6LB
Right Ø6L9
Saphenous
Left Ø6LQ
Right Ø6LP
Splenic Ø6L1
Subclavian
Left Ø5L6
Right Ø5L5
Superior Mesenteric Ø6L5

Occlusion — *continued*
Vein — *continued*
Upper Ø5LY
Vertebral
Left Ø5LS
Right Ø5LR
Vena Cava
Inferior Ø6LØ
Superior Ø2LV
Occlusion, REBOA (resuscitative endovascular balloon occlusion of the aorta)
Ø2LW3DJ
Ø4LØ3DJ
Occupational therapy *see* Activities of Daily Living Treatment, Rehabilitation FØ8
Odentectomy
see Excision, Mouth and Throat ØCB
see Resection, Mouth and Throat ØCT
Odontoid process *use* Cervical Vertebra
Olecranon bursa
use Elbow Bursa and Ligament, Left
use Elbow Bursa and Ligament, Right
Olecranon process
use Ulna, Left
use Ulna, Right
Olfactory bulb *use* Olfactory Nerve
Omadacycline Anti-infective XWØ
Omentectomy, omentumectomy
see Excision, Gastrointestinal System ØDB
see Resection, Gastrointestinal System ØDT
Omentofixation *see* Repair, Gastrointestinal System ØDQ
Omentoplasty
see Repair, Gastrointestinal System ØDQ
see Replacement, Gastrointestinal System ØDR
see Supplement, Gastrointestinal System ØDU
Omentorrhaphy *see* Repair, Gastrointestinal System ØDQ
Omentotomy *see* Drainage, Gastrointestinal System ØD9
Omnilink Elite Vascular Balloon Expandable Stent System *use* Intraluminal Device
Onychectomy
see Excision, Skin and Breast ØHB
see Resection, Skin and Breast ØHT
Onychoplasty
see Repair, Skin and Breast ØHQ
see Replacement, Skin and Breast ØHR
Onychotomy *see* Drainage, Skin and Breast ØH9
Oophorectomy
see Excision, Female Reproductive System ØUB
see Resection, Female Reproductive System ØUT
Oophoropexy
see Repair, Female Reproductive System ØUQ
see Reposition, Female Reproductive System ØUS
Oophoroplasty
see Repair, Female Reproductive System ØUQ
see Supplement, Female Reproductive System ØUU
Oophororrhaphy *see* Repair, Female Reproductive System ØUQ
Oophorostomy *see* Drainage, Female Reproductive System ØU9
Oophorotomy
see Division, Female Reproductive System ØU8
see Drainage, Female Reproductive System ØU9
Oophorrhaphy *see* Repair, Female Reproductive System ØUQ
Open Pivot Aortic Valve Graft (AVG) *use* Synthetic Substitute
Open Pivot (mechanical) Valve *use* Synthetic Substitute
Ophthalmic artery *use* Intracranial Artery
Ophthalmic nerve *use* Trigeminal Nerve
Ophthalmic vein *use* Intracranial Vein
Opponensplasty
Tendon replacement *see* Replacement, Tendons ØLR
Tendon transfer *see* Transfer, Tendons ØLX
Optic chiasma *use* Optic Nerve
Optic disc
use Retina, Left
use Retina, Right
Optic foramen *use* Sphenoid Bone
Optical coherence tomography, intravascular *see* Computerized Tomography (CT Scan)
Optimizer™ III implantable pulse generator *use* Contractility Modulation Device in ØJH

Orbicularis oculi muscle
use Upper Eyelid, Left
use Upper Eyelid, Right
Orbicularis oris muscle *use* Facial Muscle
Orbital Atherectomy Technology X2C
Orbital fascia *use* Subcutaneous Tissue and Fascia, Face
Orbital portion of ethmoid bone
use Orbit, Left
use Orbit, Right
Orbital portion of frontal bone
use Orbit, Left
use Orbit, Right
Orbital portion of lacrimal bone
use Orbit, Left
use Orbit, Right
Orbital portion of maxilla
use Orbit, Left
use Orbit, Right
Orbital portion of palatine bone
use Orbit, Left
use Orbit, Right
Orbital portion of sphenoid bone
use Orbit, Left
use Orbit, Right
Orbital portion of zygomatic bone
use Orbit, Left
use Orbit, Right
Orchectomy, orchidectomy, orchiectomy
see Excision, Male Reproductive System ØVB
see Resection, Male Reproductive System ØVT
Orchidoplasty, orchioplasty
see Repair, Male Reproductive System ØVQ
see Replacement, Male Reproductive System ØVR
see Supplement, Male Reproductive System ØVU
Orchidorrhaphy, orchiorrhaphy *see* Repair, Male Reproductive System ØVQ
Orchidotomy, orchiotomy, orchotomy *see* Drainage, Male Reproductive System ØV9
Orchiopexy
see Repair, Male Reproductive System ØVQ
see Reposition, Male Reproductive System ØVS
Oropharyngeal airway (OPA) *use* Intraluminal Device, Airway in Mouth and Throat
Oropharynx *use* Pharynx
Ossiculectomy
see Excision, Ear, Nose, Sinus Ø9B
see Resection, Ear, Nose, Sinus Ø9T
Ossiculotomy *see* Drainage, Ear, Nose, Sinus Ø99
Ostectomy
see Excision, Head and Facial Bones ØNB
see Excision, Lower Bones ØQB
see Excision, Upper Bones ØPB
see Resection, Head and Facial Bones ØNT
see Resection, Lower Bones ØQT
see Resection, Upper Bones ØPT
Osteoclasis
see Division, Head and Facial Bones ØN8
see Division, Lower Bones ØQ8
see Division, Upper Bones ØP8
Osteolysis
see Release, Head and Facial Bones ØNN
see Release, Lower Bones ØQN
see Release, Upper Bones ØPN
Osteopathic Treatment
Abdomen 7WØ9X
Cervical 7WØ1X
Extremity
Lower 7WØ6X
Upper 7WØ7X
Head 7WØØX
Lumbar 7WØ3X
Pelvis 7WØ5X
Rib Cage 7WØ8X
Sacrum 7WØ4X
Thoracic 7WØ2X
Osteopexy
see Repair, Head and Facial Bones ØNQ
see Repair, Lower Bones ØQQ
see Repair, Upper Bones ØPQ
see Reposition, Head and Facial Bones ØNS
see Reposition, Lower Bones ØQS
see Reposition, Upper Bones ØPS
Osteoplasty
see Repair, Head and Facial Bones ØNQ
see Repair, Lower Bones ØQQ
Osteoplasty — *continued*
see Repair, Upper Bones ØPQ
see Replacement, Head and Facial Bones ØNR
see Replacement, Lower Bones ØQR
see Replacement, Upper Bones ØPR
see Supplement, Head and Facial Bones ØNU
see Supplement, Lower Bones ØQU
see Supplement, Upper Bones ØPU
Osteorrhaphy
see Repair, Head and Facial Bones ØNQ
see Repair, Lower Bones ØQQ
see Repair, Upper Bones ØPQ
Osteotomy, ostotomy
see Division, Head and Facial Bones ØN8
see Division, Lower Bones ØQ8
see Division, Upper Bones ØP8
see Drainage, Head and Facial Bones ØN9
see Drainage, Lower Bones ØQ9
see Drainage, Upper Bones ØP9
Other Imaging
Bile Duct and Gallbladder, Indocyanine Green Dye, Intraoperative BF532ØØ
Bile Duct, Indocyanine Green Dye, Intraoperative BF5Ø2ØØ
Extremity
Lower BW5CZ1Z
Upper BW5JZ1Z
Gallbladder and Bile Duct, Indocyanine Green Dye, Intraoperative BF532ØØ
Gallbladder, Indocyanine Green Dye, Intraoperative BF522ØØ
Head and Neck BW59Z1Z
Hepatobiliary System, All, Indocyanine Green Dye, Intraoperative BF5C2ØØ
Liver and Spleen, Indocyanine Green Dye, Intraoperative BF562ØØ
Liver, Indocyanine Green Dye, Intraoperative BF552ØØ
Neck and Head BW59Z1Z
Pancreas, Indocyanine Green Dye, Intraoperative BF572ØØ
Spleen and Liver, Indocyanine Green Dye, Intraoperative BF562ØØ
Trunk BW52Z1Z
Other New Technology Therapeutic Substance XWØ
Otic ganglion *use* Head and Neck Sympathetic Nerve
OTL-1Ø1 *use* Hematopoietic Stem/Progenitor Cells, Genetically Modified
Otoplasty
see Repair, Ear, Nose, Sinus Ø9Q
see Replacement, Ear, Nose, Sinus Ø9R
see Supplement, Ear, Nose, Sinus Ø9U
Otoscopy *see* Inspection, Ear, Nose, Sinus Ø9J
Oval window
use Middle Ear, Left
use Middle Ear, Right
Ovarian artery *use* Abdominal Aorta
Ovarian ligament *use* Uterine Supporting Structure
Ovariectomy
see Excision, Female Reproductive System ØUB
see Resection, Female Reproductive System ØUT
Ovariocentesis *see* Drainage, Female Reproductive System ØU9
Ovariopexy
see Repair, Female Reproductive System ØUQ
see Reposition, Female Reproductive System ØUS
Ovariotomy
see Division, Female Reproductive System ØU8
see Drainage, Female Reproductive System ØU9
Ovatio™ CRT-D *use* Cardiac Resynchronization Defibrillator Pulse Generator in ØJH
Oversewing
Gastrointestinal ulcer *see* Repair, Gastrointestinal System ØDQ
Pleural bleb *see* Repair, Respiratory System ØBQ
Oviduct
use Fallopian Tube, Left
use Fallopian Tube, Right
Oximetry, Fetal pulse 1ØHØ73Z
OXINIUM *use* Synthetic Substitute, Oxidized Zirconium on Polyethylene in ØSR
Oxygenation
Extracorporeal membrane (ECMO) *see* Performance, Circulatory 5A15
Hyperbaric *see* Assistance, Circulatory 5AØ5
Supersaturated *see* Assistance, Circulatory 5AØ5

P

Pacemaker
Dual Chamber
Abdomen ØJH8
Chest ØJH6
Intracardiac
Insertion of device in
Atrium
Left Ø2H7
Right Ø2H6
Vein, Coronary Ø2H4
Ventricle
Left Ø2HL
Right Ø2HK
Removal of device from, Heart Ø2PA
Revision of device in, Heart Ø2WA
Single Chamber
Abdomen ØJH8
Chest ØJH6
Single Chamber Rate Responsive
Abdomen ØJH8
Chest ØJH6
Packing
Abdominal Wall 2W43X5Z
Anorectal 2Y43X5Z
Arm
Lower
Left 2W4DX5Z
Right 2W4CX5Z
Upper
Left 2W4BX5Z
Right 2W4AX5Z
Back 2W45X5Z
Chest Wall 2W44X5Z
Ear 2Y42X5Z
Extremity
Lower
Left 2W4MX5Z
Right 2W4LX5Z
Upper
Left 2W49X5Z
Right 2W48X5Z
Face 2W41X5Z
Finger
Left 2W4KX5Z
Right 2W4JX5Z
Foot
Left 2W4TX5Z
Right 2W4SX5Z
Genital Tract, Female 2Y44X5Z
Hand
Left 2W4FX5Z
Right 2W4EX5Z
Head 2W4ØX5Z
Inguinal Region
Left 2W47X5Z
Right 2W46X5Z
Leg
Lower
Left 2W4RX5Z
Right 2W4QX5Z
Upper
Left 2W4PX5Z
Right 2W4NX5Z
Mouth and Pharynx 2Y4ØX5Z
Nasal 2Y41X5Z
Neck 2W42X5Z
Thumb
Left 2W4HX5Z
Right 2W4GX5Z
Toe
Left 2W4VX5Z
Right 2W4UX5Z
Urethra 2Y45X5Z
Paclitaxel-eluting coronary stent *use* Intraluminal Device, Drug-eluting in Heart and Great Vessels
Paclitaxel-eluting peripheral stent
use Intraluminal Device, Drug-eluting in Lower Arteries
use Intraluminal Device, Drug-eluting in Upper Arteries
Palatine gland *use* Buccal Mucosa
Palatine tonsil *use* Tonsils
Palatine uvula *use* Uvula
Palatoglossal muscle *use* Tongue, Palate, Pharynx Muscle

Palatopharyngeal muscle *use* Tongue, Palate, Pharynx Muscle
Palatoplasty
- *see* Repair, Mouth and Throat ØCQ
- *see* Replacement, Mouth and Throat ØCR
- *see* Supplement, Mouth and Throat ØCU

Palatorrhaphy *see* Repair, Mouth and Throat ØCQ
Palmar cutaneous nerve
- *use* Median Nerve
- *use* Radial Nerve

Palmar (volar) digital vein
- *use* Hand Vein, Left
- *use* Hand Vein, Right

Palmar fascia (aponeurosis)
- *use* Subcutaneous Tissue and Fascia, Left Hand
- *use* Subcutaneous Tissue and Fascia, Right Hand

Palmar interosseous muscle
- *use* Hand Muscle, Left
- *use* Hand Muscle, Right

Palmar (volar) metacarpal vein
- *use* Hand Vein, Left
- *use* Hand Vein, Right

Palmar ulnocarpal ligament
- *use* Wrist Bursa and Ligament, Left
- *use* Wrist Bursa and Ligament, Right

Palmaris longus muscle
- *use* Lower Arm and Wrist Muscle, Left
- *use* Lower Arm and Wrist Muscle, Right

Pancreatectomy
- *see* Excision, Pancreas ØFBG
- *see* Resection, Pancreas ØFTG

Pancreatic artery *use* Splenic Artery
Pancreatic plexus *use* Abdominal Sympathetic Nerve
Pancreatic vein *use* Splenic Vein
Pancreaticoduodenostomy *see* Bypass, Hepatobiliary System and Pancreas ØF1
Pancreaticosplenic lymph node *use* Lymphatic, Aortic
Pancreatogram, endoscopic retrograde *see* Fluoroscopy, Pancreatic Duct BF18
Pancreatolithotomy *see* Extirpation, Pancreas ØFCG
Pancreatotomy
- *see* Division, Pancreas ØF8G
- *see* Drainage, Pancreas ØF9G

Panniculectomy
- *see* Excision, Skin, Abdomen ØHB7
- *see* Excision, Subcutaneous Tissue and Fascia, Abdomen ØJB8

Paraaortic lymph node *use* Lymphatic, Aortic
Paracentesis
- Eye *see* Drainage, Eye Ø89
- Peritoneal Cavity *see* Drainage, Peritoneal Cavity ØW9G
- Tympanum *see* Drainage, Ear, Nose, Sinus Ø99

Pararectal lymph node *use* Lymphatic, Mesenteric
Parasternal lymph node *use* Lymphatic, Thorax
Parathyroidectomy
- *see* Excision, Endocrine System ØGB
- *see* Resection, Endocrine System ØGT

Paratracheal lymph node *use* Lymphatic, Thorax
Paraurethral (Skene's) gland *use* Vestibular Gland
Parenteral nutrition, total *see* Introduction of Nutritional Substance
Parietal lobe *use* Cerebral Hemisphere
Parotid lymph node *use* Lymphatic, Head
Parotid plexus *use* Facial Nerve
Parotidectomy
- *see* Excision, Mouth and Throat ØCB
- *see* Resection, Mouth and Throat ØCT

Pars flaccida
- *use* Tympanic Membrane, Left
- *use* Tympanic Membrane, Right

Partial joint replacement
- Hip *see* Replacement, Lower Joints ØSR
- Knee *see* Replacement, Lower Joints ØSR
- Shoulder *see* Replacement, Upper Joints ØRR

Partially absorbable mesh *use* Synthetic Substitute
Patch, blood, spinal 3EØR3GC
Patellapexy
- *see* Repair, Lower Bones ØQQ
- *see* Reposition, Lower Bones ØQS

Patellaplasty
- *see* Repair, Lower Bones ØQQ
- *see* Replacement, Lower Bones ØQR
- *see* Supplement, Lower Bones ØQU

Patellar ligament
- *use* Knee Bursa and Ligament, Left
- *use* Knee Bursa and Ligament, Right

Patellar tendon
- *use* Knee Tendon, Left
- *use* Knee Tendon, Right

Patellectomy
- *see* Excision, Lower Bones ØQB
- *see* Resection, Lower Bones ØQT

Patellofemoral joint
- *use* Knee Joint, Left
- *use* Knee Joint, Left, Femoral Surface
- *use* Knee Joint, Right
- *use* Knee Joint, Right, Femoral Surface

Pectineus muscle
- *use* Upper Leg Muscle, Left
- *use* Upper Leg Muscle, Right

Pectoral fascia *use* Subcutaneous Tissue and Fascia, Chest
Pectoral (anterior) lymph node
- *use* Lymphatic Left, Axillary
- *use* Lymphatic Right, Axillary

Pectoralis major muscle
- *use* Thorax Muscle, Left
- *use* Thorax Muscle, Right

Pectoralis minor muscle
- *use* Thorax Muscle, Left
- *use* Thorax Muscle, Right

Pedicle-based dynamic stabilization device
- *use* Spinal Stabilization Device, Pedicle-Based in ØSH
- *use* Spinal Stabilization Device, Pedicle-Based in ØRH

PEEP (positive end expiratory pressure) *see* Assistance, Respiratory 5AØ9
PEG (percutaneous endoscopic gastrostomy) ØDH63UZ
PEJ (percutaneous endoscopic jejunostomy) ØDHA3UZ
Pelvic splanchnic nerve
- *use* Abdominal Sympathetic Nerve
- *use* Sacral Sympathetic Nerve

Penectomy
- *see* Excision, Male Reproductive System ØVB
- *see* Resection, Male Reproductive System ØVT

Penile urethra *use* Urethra
Perceval sutureless valve *use* Zooplastic Tissue, Rapid Deployment Technique in New Technology
Percutaneous endoscopic gastrojejunostomy (PEG/J) tube *use* Feeding Device in Gastrointestinal System
Percutaneous endoscopic gastrostomy (PEG) tube
- *use* Feeding Device in Gastrointestinal System

Percutaneous nephrostomy catheter *use* Drainage Device
Percutaneous transluminal coronary angioplasty (PTCA) *see* Dilation, Heart and Great Vessels Ø27
Performance
- Biliary
  - Multiple, Filtration 5A1C6ØZ
  - Single, Filtration 5A1CØØZ
- Cardiac
  - Continuous
    - Output 5A1221Z
    - Pacing 5A1223Z
  - Intermittent, Pacing 5A1213Z
  - Single, Output, Manual 5A12Ø12
- Circulatory
  - Continuous
    - Central Membrane 5A1522F
    - Peripheral Veno-arterial Membrane 5A1522G
    - Peripheral Veno-venous Membrane 5A1522H
  - Intraoperative
    - Central Membrane 5A15A2F
    - Peripheral Veno-arterial Membrane 5A15A2G
    - Peripheral Veno-venous Membrane 5A15A2H
- Respiratory
  - 24-96 Consecutive Hours, Ventilation 5A1945Z
  - Greater than 96 Consecutive Hours, Ventilation 5A1955Z
  - Less than 24 Consecutive Hours, Ventilation 5A1935Z

Performance — *continued*
- Respiratory — *continued*
  - Single, Ventilation, Nonmechanical 5A19Ø54
- Urinary
  - Continuous, Greater than 18 hours per day, Filtration 5A1D9ØZ
  - Intermittent, Less than 6 Hours Per Day, Filtration 5A1D7ØZ
  - Prolonged Intermittent, 6-18 hours per day, Filtration 5A1D8ØZ

Perfusion *see* Introduction of substance in or on
Perfusion, donor organ
- Heart 6AB5ØBZ
- Kidney(s) 6ABTØBZ
- Liver 6ABFØBZ
- Lung(s) 6ABBØBZ

Pericardiectomy
- *see* Excision, Pericardium Ø2BN
- *see* Resection, Pericardium Ø2TN

Pericardiocentesis *see* Drainage, Pericardial Cavity ØW9D
Pericardiolysis *see* Release, Pericardium Ø2NN
Pericardiophrenic artery
- *use* Internal Mammary Artery, Left
- *use* Internal Mammary Artery, Right

Pericardioplasty
- *see* Repair, Pericardium Ø2QN
- *see* Replacement, Pericardium Ø2RN
- *see* Supplement, Pericardium Ø2UN

Pericardiorrhaphy *see* Repair, Pericardium Ø2QN
Pericardiostomy *see* Drainage, Pericardial Cavity ØW9D
Pericardiotomy *see* Drainage, Pericardial Cavity ØW9D
Perimetrium *use* Uterus
Peripheral Intravascular Lithotripsy (Peripheral IVL) *see* Fragmentation
Peripheral parenteral nutrition *see* Introduction of Nutritional Substance
Peripherally inserted central catheter (PICC) *use* Infusion Device
Peritoneal dialysis 3E1M39Z
Peritoneocentesis
- *see* Drainage, Peritoneal Cavity ØW9G
- *see* Drainage, Peritoneum ØD9W

Peritoneoplasty
- *see* Repair, Peritoneum ØDQW
- *see* Replacement, Peritoneum ØDRW
- *see* Supplement, Peritoneum ØDUW

Peritoneoscopy ØDJW4ZZ
Peritoneotomy *see* Drainage, Peritoneum ØD9W
Peritoneumectomy *see* Excision, Peritoneum ØDBW
Peroneus brevis muscle
- *use* Lower Leg Muscle, Left
- *use* Lower Leg Muscle, Right

Peroneus longus muscle
- *use* Lower Leg Muscle, Left
- *use* Lower Leg Muscle, Right

Pessary ring *use* Intraluminal Device, Pessary in Female Reproductive System
PET scan *see* Positron Emission Tomographic (PET) Imaging
Petrous part of temporal bone
- *use* Temporal Bone, Left
- *use* Temporal Bone, Right

Phacoemulsification, lens
- With IOL implant *see* Replacement, Eye Ø8R
- Without IOL implant *see* Extraction, Eye Ø8D

Phalangectomy
- *see* Excision, Lower Bones ØQB
- *see* Excision, Upper Bones ØPB
- *see* Resection, Lower Bones ØQT
- *see* Resection, Upper Bones ØPT

Phallectomy
- *see* Excision, Penis ØVBS
- *see* Resection, Penis ØVTS

Phalloplasty
- *see* Repair, Penis ØVQS
- *see* Supplement, Penis ØVUS

Phallotomy *see* Drainage, Penis ØV9S
Pharmacotherapy, for substance abuse
- Antabuse HZ93ZZZ
- Bupropion HZ97ZZZ
- Clonidine HZ96ZZZ
- Levo-alpha-acetyl-methadol (LAAM) HZ92ZZZ
- Methadone Maintenance HZ91ZZZ
- Naloxone HZ95ZZZ
- Naltrexone HZ94ZZZ
- Nicotine Replacement HZ9ØZZZ

Pharmacotherapy, for substance abuse — *continued*
Psychiatric Medication HZ98ZZZ
Replacement Medication, Other HZ99ZZZ
Pharyngeal constrictor muscle *use* Tongue, Palate, Pharynx Muscle
Pharyngeal plexus *use* Vagus Nerve
Pharyngeal recess *use* Nasopharynx
Pharyngeal tonsil *use* Adenoids
Pharyngogram *see* Fluoroscopy, Pharynix B91G
Pharyngoplasty
see Repair, Mouth and Throat ØCQ
see Replacement, Mouth and Throat ØCR
see Supplement, Mouth and Throat ØCU
Pharyngorrhaphy *see* Repair, Mouth and Throat ØCQ
Pharyngotomy *see* Drainage, Mouth and Throat ØC9
Pharyngotympanic tube
use Eustachian Tube, Left
use Eustachian Tube, Right
Pheresis
Erythrocytes 6A55
Leukocytes 6A55
Plasma 6A55
Platelets 6A55
Stem Cells
Cord Blood 6A55
Hematopoietic 6A55
Phlebectomy
see Excision, Lower Veins Ø6B
see Excision, Upper Veins Ø5B
see Extraction, Lower Veins Ø6D
see Extraction, Upper Veins Ø5D
Phlebography
see Plain Radiography, Veins B5Ø
Impedance 4AØ4X51
Phleborrhaphy
see Repair, Lower Veins Ø6Q
see Repair, Upper Veins Ø5Q
Phlebotomy
see Drainage, Lower Veins Ø69
see Drainage, Upper Veins Ø59
Photocoagulation
For Destruction *see* Destruction
For Repair *see* Repair
Photopheresis, therapeutic *see* Phototherapy, Circulatory 6A65
Phototherapy
Circulatory 6A65
Skin 6A6Ø
Ultraviolet light *see* Ultraviolet Light Therapy, Physiological Systems 6A8
Phrenectomy, phrenoneurectomy *see* Excision, Nerve, Phrenic Ø1B2
Phrenemphraxis *see* Destruction, Nerve, Phrenic Ø152
Phrenic nerve stimulator generator *use* Stimulator Generator in Subcutaneous Tissue and Fascia
Phrenic nerve stimulator lead *use* Diaphragmatic Pacemaker Lead in Respiratory System
Phreniclasis *see* Destruction, Nerve, Phrenic Ø152
Phrenicoexeresis *see* Extraction, Nerve, Phrenic Ø1D2
Phrenicotomy *see* Division, Nerve, Phrenic Ø182
Phrenicotripsy *see* Destruction, Nerve, Phrenic Ø152
Phrenoplasty
see Repair, Respiratory System ØBQ
see Supplement, Respiratory System ØBU
Phrenotomy *see* Drainage, Respiratory System ØB9
Physiatry *see* Motor Treatment, Rehabilitation FØ7
Physical medicine *see* Motor Treatment, Rehabilitation FØ7
Physical therapy *see* Motor Treatment, Rehabilitation FØ7
PHYSIOMESH™ Flexible Composite Mesh *use* Synthetic Substitute
Pia mater, intracranial *use* Cerebral Meninges
Pia mater, spinal *use* Spinal Meninges
Pinealectomy
see Excision, Pineal Body ØGB1
see Resection, Pineal Body ØGT1
Pinealoscopy ØGJ14ZZ
Pinealotomy *see* Drainage, Pineal Body ØG91
Pinna
use External Ear, Bilateral
use External Ear, Left
use External Ear, Right
Pipeline™ (Flex) embolization device *use* Intraluminal Device, Flow Diverter in Ø3V
Piriform recess (sinus) *use* Pharynx
Piriformis muscle
use Hip Muscle, Left
use Hip Muscle, Right
PIRRT (Prolonged intermittent renal replacement therapy) 5A1D8ØZ
Pisiform bone
use Carpal, Left
use Carpal, Right
Pisohamate ligament
use Hand Bursa and Ligament, Left
use Hand Bursa and Ligament, Right
Pisometacarpal ligament
use Hand Bursa and Ligament, Left
use Hand Bursa and Ligament, Right
Pituitectomy
see Excision, Gland, Pituitary ØGBØ
see Resection, Gland, Pituitary ØGTØ
Plain film radiology *see* Plain Radiography
Plain Radiography
Abdomen BWØØZZZ
Abdomen and Pelvis BWØ1ZZZ
Abdominal Lymphatic
Bilateral B7Ø1
Unilateral B7ØØ
Airway, Upper BBØDZZZ
Ankle
Left BQØH
Right BQØG
Aorta
Abdominal B4ØØ
Thoracic B3ØØ
Thoraco-Abdominal B3ØP
Aorta and Bilateral Lower Extremity Arteries B4ØD
Arch
Bilateral BNØDZZZ
Left BNØCZZZ
Right BNØBZZZ
Arm
Left BPØFZZZ
Right BPØEZZZ
Artery
Brachiocephalic-Subclavian, Right B3Ø1
Bronchial B3ØL
Bypass Graft, Other B2ØF
Cervico-Cerebral Arch B3ØQ
Common Carotid
Bilateral B3Ø5
Left B3Ø4
Right B3Ø3
Coronary
Bypass Graft
Multiple B2Ø3
Single B2Ø2
Multiple B2Ø1
Single B2ØØ
External Carotid
Bilateral B3ØC
Left B3ØB
Right B3Ø9
Hepatic B4Ø2
Inferior Mesenteric B4Ø5
Intercostal B3ØL
Internal Carotid
Bilateral B3Ø8
Left B3Ø7
Right B3Ø6
Internal Mammary Bypass Graft
Left B2Ø8
Right B2Ø7
Intra-Abdominal, Other B4ØB
Intracranial B3ØR
Lower Extremity
Bilateral and Aorta B4ØD
Left B4ØG
Right B4ØF
Lower, Other B4ØJ
Lumbar B4Ø9
Pelvic B4ØC
Pulmonary
Left B3ØT
Right B3ØS
Renal
Bilateral B4Ø8
Left B4Ø7
Right B4Ø6
Transplant B4ØM
Spinal B3ØM
Splenic B4Ø3
Plain Radiography — *continued*
Artery — *continued*
Subclavian, Left B3Ø2
Superior Mesenteric B4Ø4
Upper Extremity
Bilateral B3ØK
Left B3ØJ
Right B3ØH
Upper, Other B3ØN
Vertebral
Bilateral B3ØG
Left B3ØF
Right B3ØD
Bile Duct BFØØ
Bile Duct and Gallbladder BFØ3
Bladder BTØØ
Kidney and Ureter BTØ4
Bladder and Urethra BTØB
Bone
Facial BNØ5ZZZ
Nasal BNØ4ZZZ
Bones, Long, All BWØBZZZ
Breast
Bilateral BHØ2ZZZ
Left BHØ1ZZZ
Right BHØØZZZ
Calcaneus
Left BQØKZZZ
Right BQØJZZZ
Chest BWØ3ZZZ
Clavicle
Left BPØ5ZZZ
Right BPØ4ZZZ
Coccyx BRØFZZZ
Corpora Cavernosa BVØØ
Dialysis Fistula B5ØW
Dialysis Shunt B5ØW
Disc
Cervical BRØ1
Lumbar BRØ3
Thoracic BRØ2
Duct
Lacrimal
Bilateral B8Ø2
Left B8Ø1
Right B8ØØ
Mammary
Multiple
Left BHØ6
Right BHØ5
Single
Left BHØ4
Right BHØ3
Elbow
Left BPØH
Right BPØG
Epididymis
Left BVØ2
Right BVØ1
Extremity
Lower BWØCZZZ
Upper BWØJZZZ
Eye
Bilateral B8Ø7ZZZ
Left B8Ø6ZZZ
Right B8Ø5ZZZ
Facet Joint
Cervical BRØ4
Lumbar BRØ6
Thoracic BRØ5
Fallopian Tube
Bilateral BUØ2
Left BUØ1
Right BUØØ
Fallopian Tube and Uterus BUØ8
Femur
Left, Densitometry BQØ4ZZ1
Right, Densitometry BQØ3ZZ1
Finger
Left BPØSZZZ
Right BPØRZZZ
Foot
Left BQØMZZZ
Right BQØLZZZ
Forearm
Left BPØKZZZ
Right BPØJZZZ
Gallbladder and Bile Duct BFØ3

Plain Radiography — *continued*
Gland
Parotid
Bilateral B906
Left B905
Right B904
Salivary
Bilateral B90D
Left B90C
Right B90B
Submandibular
Bilateral B909
Left B908
Right B907
Hand
Left BP0PZZZ
Right BP0NZZZ
Heart
Left B205
Right B204
Right and Left B206
Hepatobiliary System, All BF0C
Hip
Left BQ01
Densitometry BQ01ZZ1
Right BQ00
Densitometry BQ00ZZ1
Humerus
Left BP0BZZZ
Right BP0AZZZ
Ileal Diversion Loop BT0C
Intracranial Sinus B502
Joint
Acromioclavicular, Bilateral BP03ZZZ
Finger
Left BP0D
Right BP0C
Foot
Left BQ0Y
Right BQ0X
Hand
Left BP0D
Right BP0C
Lumbosacral BR0BZZZ
Sacroiliac BR0D
Sternoclavicular
Bilateral BP02ZZZ
Left BP01ZZZ
Right BP00ZZZ
Temporomandibular
Bilateral BN09
Left BN08
Right BN07
Thoracolumbar BR08ZZZ
Toe
Left BQ0Y
Right BQ0X
Kidney
Bilateral BT03
Left BT02
Right BT01
Ureter and Bladder BT04
Knee
Left BQ08
Right BQ07
Leg
Left BQ0FZZZ
Right BQ0DZZZ
Lymphatic
Head B704
Lower Extremity
Bilateral B70B
Left B709
Right B708
Neck B704
Pelvic B70C
Upper Extremity
Bilateral B707
Left B706
Right B705
Mandible BN06ZZZ
Mastoid B90HZZZ
Nasopharynx B90FZZZ
Optic Foramina
Left B804ZZZ
Right B803ZZZ
Orbit
Bilateral BN03ZZZ
Left BN02ZZZ

Plain Radiography — *continued*
Orbit — *continued*
Right BN01ZZZ
Oropharynx B90FZZZ
Patella
Left BQ0WZZZ
Right BQ0VZZZ
Pelvis BR0CZZZ
Pelvis and Abdomen BW01ZZZ
Prostate BV03
Retroperitoneal Lymphatic
Bilateral B701
Unilateral B700
Ribs
Left BP0YZZZ
Right BP0XZZZ
Sacrum BR0FZZZ
Scapula
Left BP07ZZZ
Right BP06ZZZ
Shoulder
Left BP09
Right BP08
Sinus
Intracranial B502
Paranasal B902ZZZ
Skull BN00ZZZ
Spinal Cord B00B
Spine
Cervical, Densitometry BR00ZZ1
Lumbar, Densitometry BR09ZZ1
Thoracic, Densitometry BR07ZZ1
Whole, Densitometry BR0GZZ1
Sternum BR0HZZZ
Teeth
All BN0JZZZ
Multiple BN0HZZZ
Testicle
Left BV06
Right BV05
Toe
Left BQ0QZZZ
Right BQ0PZZZ
Tooth, Single BN0GZZZ
Tracheobronchial Tree
Bilateral BB09YZZ
Left BB08YZZ
Right BB07YZZ
Ureter
Bilateral BT08
Kidney and Bladder BT04
Left BT07
Right BT06
Urethra BT05
Urethra and Bladder BT0B
Uterus BU06
Uterus and Fallopian Tube BU08
Vagina BU09
Vasa Vasorum BV08
Vein
Cerebellar B501
Cerebral B501
Epidural B500
Jugular
Bilateral B505
Left B504
Right B503
Lower Extremity
Bilateral B50D
Left B50C
Right B50B
Other B50V
Pelvic (Iliac)
Left B50G
Right B50F
Pelvic (Iliac) Bilateral B50H
Portal B50T
Pulmonary
Bilateral B50S
Left B50R
Right B50Q
Renal
Bilateral B50L
Left B50K
Right B50J
Spanchnic B50T
Subclavian
Left B507
Right B506

Plain Radiography — *continued*
Vein — *continued*
Upper Extremity
Bilateral B50P
Left B50N
Right B50M
Vena Cava
Inferior B509
Superior B508
Whole Body BW0KZZZ
Infant BW0MZZZ
Whole Skeleton BW0LZZZ
Wrist
Left BP0M
Right BP0L

Planar Nuclear Medicine Imaging
Abdomen CW10
Abdomen and Chest CW14
Abdomen and Pelvis CW11
Anatomical Region, Other CW1ZZZZ
Anatomical Regions, Multiple CW1YYZZ
Bladder and Ureters CT1H
Bladder, Kidneys and Ureters CT13
Blood C713
Bone Marrow C710
Brain C010
Breast CH1YYZZ
Bilateral CH12
Left CH11
Right CH10
Bronchi and Lungs CB12
Central Nervous System C01YYZZ
Cerebrospinal Fluid C015
Chest CW13
Chest and Abdomen CW14
Chest and Neck CW16
Digestive System CD1YYZZ
Ducts, Lacrimal, Bilateral C819
Ear, Nose, Mouth and Throat C91YYZZ
Endocrine System CG1YYZZ
Extremity
Lower CW1D
Bilateral CP1F
Left CP1D
Right CP1C
Upper CW1M
Bilateral CP1B
Left CP19
Right CP18
Eye C81YYZZ
Gallbladder CF14
Gastrointestinal Tract CD17
Upper CD15
Gland
Adrenal, Bilateral CG14
Parathyroid CG11
Thyroid CG12
Glands, Salivary, Bilateral C91B
Head and Neck CW1B
Heart C21YYZZ
Right and Left C216
Hepatobiliary System, All CF1C
Hepatobiliary System and Pancreas CF1YYZZ
Kidneys, Ureters and Bladder CT13
Liver CF15
Liver and Spleen CF16
Lungs and Bronchi CB12
Lymphatics
Head C71J
Head and Neck C715
Lower Extremity C71P
Neck C71K
Pelvic C71D
Trunk C71M
Upper Chest C71L
Upper Extremity C71N
Lymphatics and Hematologic System C71YYZZ
Musculoskeletal System
All CP1Z
Other CP1YYZZ
Myocardium C21G
Neck and Chest CW16
Neck and Head CW1B
Pancreas and Hepatobiliary System CF1YYZZ
Pelvic Region CW1J
Pelvis CP16
Pelvis and Abdomen CW11
Pelvis and Spine CP17
Reproductive System, Male CV1YYZZ

Planar Nuclear Medicine Imaging — *continued*
Respiratory System CB1YYZZ
Skin CH1YYZZ
Skull CP11
Spine CP15
Spine and Pelvis CP17
Spleen C712
Spleen and Liver CF16
Subcutaneous Tissue CH1YYZZ
Testicles, Bilateral CV19
Thorax CP14
Ureters and Bladder CT1H
Ureters, Kidneys and Bladder CT13
Urinary System CT1YYZZ
Veins C51YYZZ
Central C51R
Lower Extremity
Bilateral C51D
Left C51C
Right C51B
Upper Extremity
Bilateral C51Q
Left C51P
Right C51N
Whole Body CW1N
Plantar digital vein
use Foot Vein, Left
use Foot Vein, Right
Plantar fascia (aponeurosis)
use Subcutaneous Tissue and Fascia, Left Foot
use Subcutaneous Tissue and Fascia, Right Foot
Plantar metatarsal vein
use Foot Vein, Left
use Foot Vein, Right
Plantar venous arch
use Foot Vein, Left
use Foot Vein, Right
Plaque Radiation
Abdomen DWY3FZZ
Adrenal Gland DGY2FZZ
Anus DDY8FZZ
Bile Ducts DFY2FZZ
Bladder DTY2FZZ
Bone Marrow D7YØFZZ
Bone, Other DPYCFZZ
Brain DØYØFZZ
Brain Stem DØY1FZZ
Breast
Left DMYØFZZ
Right DMY1FZZ
Bronchus DBY1FZZ
Cervix DUY1FZZ
Chest DWY2FZZ
Chest Wall DBY7FZZ
Colon DDY5FZZ
Diaphragm DBY8FZZ
Duodenum DDY2FZZ
Ear D9YØFZZ
Esophagus DDYØFZZ
Eye D8YØFZZ
Femur DPY9FZZ
Fibula DPYBFZZ
Gallbladder DFY1FZZ
Gland
Adrenal DGY2FZZ
Parathyroid DGY4FZZ
Pituitary DGYØFZZ
Thyroid DGY5FZZ
Glands, Salivary D9Y6FZZ
Head and Neck DWY1FZZ
Hemibody DWY4FZZ
Humerus DPY6FZZ
Ileum DDY4FZZ
Jejunum DDY3FZZ
Kidney DTYØFZZ
Larynx D9YBFZZ
Liver DFYØFZZ
Lung DBY2FZZ
Lymphatics
Abdomen D7Y6FZZ
Axillary D7Y4FZZ
Inguinal D7Y8FZZ
Neck D7Y3FZZ
Pelvis D7Y7FZZ
Thorax D7Y5FZZ
Mandible DPY3FZZ
Maxilla DPY2FZZ
Mediastinum DBY6FZZ

Plaque Radiation — *continued*
Mouth D9Y4FZZ
Nasopharynx D9YDFZZ
Neck and Head DWY1FZZ
Nerve, Peripheral DØY7FZZ
Nose D9Y1FZZ
Ovary DUYØFZZ
Palate
Hard D9Y8FZZ
Soft D9Y9FZZ
Pancreas DFY3FZZ
Parathyroid Gland DGY4FZZ
Pelvic Bones DPY8FZZ
Pelvic Region DWY6FZZ
Pharynx D9YCFZZ
Pineal Body DGY1FZZ
Pituitary Gland DGYØFZZ
Pleura DBY5FZZ
Prostate DVYØFZZ
Radius DPY7FZZ
Rectum DDY7FZZ
Rib DPY5FZZ
Sinuses D9Y7FZZ
Skin
Abdomen DHY8FZZ
Arm DHY4FZZ
Back DHY7FZZ
Buttock DHY9FZZ
Chest DHY6FZZ
Face DHY2FZZ
Foot DHYCFZZ
Hand DHY5FZZ
Leg DHYBFZZ
Neck DHY3FZZ
Skull DPYØFZZ
Spinal Cord DØY6FZZ
Spleen D7Y2FZZ
Sternum DPY4FZZ
Stomach DDY1FZZ
Testis DVY1FZZ
Thymus D7Y1FZZ
Thyroid Gland DGY5FZZ
Tibia DPYBFZZ
Tongue D9Y5FZZ
Trachea DBYØFZZ
Ulna DPY7FZZ
Ureter DTY1FZZ
Urethra DTY3FZZ
Uterus DUY2FZZ
Whole Body DWY5FZZ
Plasmapheresis, therapeutic *see* Pheresis, Physiological Systems 6A5
Plateletpheresis, therapeutic *see* Pheresis, Physiological Systems 6A5
Platysma muscle
use Neck Muscle, Left
use Neck Muscle, Right
Plazomicin Anti-infective XWØ
Pleurectomy
see Excision, Respiratory System ØBB
see Resection, Respiratory System ØBT
Pleurocentesis *see* Drainage, Anatomical Regions, General ØW9
Pleurodesis, pleurosclerosis
Chemical injection *see* Introduction of Substance in or on, Pleural Cavity 3EØL
Surgical *see* Destruction, Respiratory System ØB5
Pleurolysis *see* Release, Respiratory System ØBN
Pleuroscopy ØBJQ4ZZ
Pleurotomy *see* Drainage, Respiratory System ØB9
Plica semilunaris
use Conjunctiva, Left
use Conjunctiva, Right
Plication *see* Restriction
Pneumectomy
see Excision, Respiratory System ØBB
see Resection, Respiratory System ØBT
Pneumocentesis *see* Drainage, Respiratory System ØB9
Pneumogastric nerve *use* Vagus Nerve
Pneumolysis *see* Release, Respiratory System ØBN
Pneumonectomy *see* Resection, Respiratory System ØBT
Pneumonolysis *see* Release, Respiratory System ØBN
Pneumonopexy
see Repair, Respiratory System ØBQ
see Reposition, Respiratory System ØBS

Pneumonorrhaphy *see* Repair, Respiratory System ØBQ
Pneumonotomy *see* Drainage, Respiratory System ØB9
Pneumotaxic center *use* Pons
Pneumotomy *see* Drainage, Respiratory System ØB9
Pollicization *see* Transfer, Anatomical Regions, Upper Extremities ØXX
Polyethylene socket *use* Synthetic Substitute, Polyethylene in ØSR
Polymethylmethacrylate (PMMA) *use* Synthetic Substitute
Polypectomy, gastrointestinal *see* Excision, Gastrointestinal System ØDB
Polypropylene mesh *use* Synthetic Substitute
Polysomnogram 4A1ZXQZ
Pontine tegmentum *use* Pons
Popliteal ligament
use Knee Bursa and Ligament, Left
use Knee Bursa and Ligament, Right
Popliteal lymph node
use Lymphatic, Left Lower Extremity
use Lymphatic, Right Lower Extremity
Popliteal vein
use Femoral Vein, Left
use Femoral Vein, Right
Popliteus muscle
use Lower Leg Muscle, Left
use Lower Leg Muscle, Right
Porcine (bioprosthetic) valve *use* Zooplastic Tissue in Heart and Great Vessels
Positive Blood Culture Fluorescence Hybridization for Organism Identification, Concentration and Susceptibility XXE5XN6
Positive end expiratory pressure *see* Performance, Respiratory 5A19
Positron Emission Tomographic (PET) Imaging
Brain CØ3Ø
Bronchi and Lungs CB32
Central Nervous System CØ3YYZZ
Heart C23YYZZ
Lungs and Bronchi CB32
Myocardium C23G
Respiratory System CB3YYZZ
Whole Body CW3NYZZ
Positron emission tomography *see* Positron Emission Tomographic (PET) Imaging
Postauricular (mastoid) lymph node
use Lymphatic, Left Neck
use Lymphatic, Right Neck
Postcava *use* Inferior Vena Cava
Posterior auricular artery
use External Carotid Artery, Left
use External Carotid Artery, Right
Posterior auricular nerve *use* Facial Nerve
Posterior auricular vein
use External Jugular Vein, Left
use External Jugular Vein, Right
Posterior cerebral artery *use* Intracranial Artery
Posterior chamber
use Eye, Left
use Eye, Right
Posterior circumflex humeral artery
use Axillary Artery, Left
use Axillary Artery, Right
Posterior communicating artery *use* Intracranial Artery
Posterior cruciate ligament (PCL)
use Knee Bursa and Ligament, Left
use Knee Bursa and Ligament, Right
Posterior facial (retromandibular) vein
use Face Vein, Left
use Face Vein, Right
Posterior femoral cutaneous nerve *use* Sacral Plexus
Posterior inferior cerebellar artery (PICA) *use* Intracranial Artery
Posterior interosseous nerve *use* Radial Nerve
Posterior labial nerve *use* Pudendal Nerve
Posterior (subscapular) lymph node
use Lymphatic, Left Axillary
use Lymphatic, Right Axillary
Posterior scrotal nerve *use* Pudendal Nerve
Posterior spinal artery
use Vertebral Artery, Left
use Vertebral Artery, Right
Posterior tibial recurrent artery
use Anterior Tibial Artery, Left
use Anterior Tibial Artery, Right

Posterior ulnar recurrent artery
  use Ulnar Artery, Left
  use Ulnar Artery, Right
Posterior vagal trunk *use* Vagus Nerve
PPN (peripheral parenteral nutrition) *see* Introduction of Nutritional Substance
Preauricular lymph node *use* Lymphatic, Head
Precava *use* Superior Vena Cava
PRECICE intramedullary limb lengthening system
  use Internal Fixation Device, Intramedullary Limb Lengthening in ØPH
  use Internal Fixation Device, Intramedullary Limb Lengthening in ØQH
Prepatellar bursa
  use Knee Bursa and Ligament, Left
  use Knee Bursa and Ligament, Right
Preputiotomy *see* Drainage, Male Reproductive System ØV9
Pressure support ventilation *see* Performance, Respiratory 5A19
PRESTIGE® Cervical Disc *use* Synthetic Substitute
Pretracheal fascia
  use Subcutaneous Tissue and Fascia, Left Neck
  use Subcutaneous Tissue and Fascia, Right Neck
Prevertebral fascia
  use Subcutaneous Tissue and Fascia, Left Neck
  use Subcutaneous Tissue and Fascia, Right Neck
PrimeAdvanced neurostimulator (SureScan) (MRI Safe) *use* Stimulator Generator, Multiple Array in ØJH
Princeps pollicis artery
  use Hand Artery, Left
  use Hand Artery, Right
Probing, duct
  Diagnostic *see* Inspection
  Dilation *see* Dilation
PROCEED™ Ventral Patch *use* Synthetic Substitute
Procerus muscle *use* Facial Muscle
Proctectomy
  see Excision, Rectum ØDBP
  see Resection, Rectum ØDTP
Proctoclysis *see* Introduction of substance in or on, Gastrointestinal Tract, Lower 3EØH
Proctocolectomy
  see Excision, Gastrointestinal System ØDB
  see Resection, Gastrointestinal System ØDT
Proctocolpoplasty
  see Repair, Gastrointestinal System ØDQ
  see Supplement, Gastrointestinal System ØDU
Proctoperineoplasty
  see Repair, Gastrointestinal System ØDQ
  see Supplement, Gastrointestinal System ØDU
Proctoperineorrhaphy *see* Repair, Gastrointestinal System ØDQ
Proctopexy
  see Repair, Rectum ØDQP
  see Reposition, Rectum ØDSP
Proctoplasty
  see Repair, Rectum ØDQP
  see Supplement, Rectum ØDUP
Proctorrhaphy *see* Repair, Rectum ØDQP
Proctoscopy ØDJD8ZZ
Proctosigmoidectomy
  see Excision, Gastrointestinal System ØDB
  see Resection, Gastrointestinal System ØDT
Proctosigmoidoscopy ØDJD8ZZ
Proctostomy *see* Drainage, Rectum ØD9P
Proctotomy *see* Drainage, Rectum ØD9P
Prodisc-C *use* Synthetic Substitute
Prodisc-L *use* Synthetic Substitute
Production, atrial septal defect *see* Excision, Septum, Atrial Ø2B5
Profunda brachii
  use Brachial Artery, Left
  use Brachial Artery, Right
Profunda femoris (deep femoral) vein
  use Femoral Vein, Left
  use Femoral Vein, Right
PROLENE Polypropylene Hernia System (PHS) *use* Synthetic Substitute
Prolonged intermittent renal replacement therapy (PIRRT) 5A1D80Z
Pronator quadratus muscle
  use Lower Arm and Wrist Muscle, Left
  use Lower Arm and Wrist Muscle, Right
Pronator teres muscle
  use Lower Arm and Wrist Muscle, Left
  use Lower Arm and Wrist Muscle, Right
Prostatectomy
  see Excision, Prostate ØVBØ
  see Resection, Prostate ØVTØ
Prostatic urethra *use* Urethra
Prostatomy, prostatotomy *see* Drainage, Prostate ØV9Ø
Protecta XT CRT-D *use* Cardiac Resynchronization Defibrillator Pulse Generator in ØJH
Protecta XT DR (XT VR) *use* Defibrillator Generator in ØJH
Protégé® RX Carotid Stent System *use* Intraluminal Device
Proximal radioulnar joint
  use Elbow Joint, Left
  use Elbow Joint, Right
Psoas muscle
  use Hip Muscle, Left
  use Hip Muscle, Right
PSV (pressure support ventilation) *see* Performance, Respiratory 5A19
Psychoanalysis GZ54ZZZ
Psychological Tests
  Cognitive Status GZ14ZZZ
  Developmental GZ1ØZZZ
  Intellectual and Psychoeducational GZ12ZZZ
  Neurobehavioral Status GZ14ZZZ
  Neuropsychological GZ13ZZZ
  Personality and Behavioral GZ11ZZZ
Psychotherapy
  Family, Mental Health Services GZ72ZZZ
  Group GZHZZZZ
    Mental Health Services GZHZZZZ
  Individual
    see Psychotherapy, Individual, Mental Health Services
    for substance abuse
      12-Step HZ53ZZZ
      Behavioral HZ51ZZZ
      Cognitive HZ5ØZZZ
      Cognitive-Behavioral HZ52ZZZ
      Confrontational HZ58ZZZ
      Interactive HZ55ZZZ
      Interpersonal HZ54ZZZ
      Motivational Enhancement HZ57ZZZ
      Psychoanalysis HZ5BZZZ
      Psychodynamic HZ5CZZZ
      Psychoeducation HZ56ZZZ
      Psychophysiological HZ5DZZZ
      Supportive HZ59ZZZ
    Mental Health Services
      Behavioral GZ51ZZZ
      Cognitive GZ52ZZZ
      Cognitive-Behavioral GZ58ZZZ
      Interactive GZ5ØZZZ
      Interpersonal GZ53ZZZ
      Psychoanalysis GZ54ZZZ
      Psychodynamic GZ55ZZZ
      Psychophysiological GZ59ZZZ
      Supportive GZ56ZZZ
PTCA (percutaneous transluminal coronary angioplasty) *see* Dilation, Heart and Great Vessels Ø27
Pterygoid muscle *use* Head Muscle
Pterygoid process *use* Sphenoid Bone
Pterygopalatine (sphenopalatine) ganglion *use* Head and Neck Sympathetic Nerve
Pubis
  use Pelvic Bone, Left
  use Pelvic Bone, Right
Pubofemoral ligament
  use Hip Bursa and Ligament, Left
  use Hip Bursa and Ligament, Right
Pudendal nerve *use* Sacral Plexus
Pull-through, laparoscopic-assisted transanal
  see Excision, Gastrointestinal System ØDB
  see Resection, Gastrointestinal System ØDT
Pull-through, rectal *see* Resection, Rectum ØDTP
Pulmoaortic canal *use* Pulmonary Artery, Left
Pulmonary annulus *use* Pulmonary Valve
Pulmonary artery wedge monitoring *see* Monitoring, Arterial 4A13
Pulmonary plexus
  use Thoracic Sympathetic Nerve
  use Vagus Nerve
Pulmonic valve *use* Pulmonary Valve
Pulpectomy *see* Excision, Mouth and Throat ØCB
Pulverization *see* Fragmentation
Pulvinar *use* Thalamus
Pump reservoir *use* Infusion Device, Pump in Subcutaneous Tissue and Fascia
Punch biopsy *see* Excision with qualifier Diagnostic
Puncture *see* Drainage
Puncture, lumbar *see* Drainage, Spinal Canal ØØ9U
Pyelography
  see Fluoroscopy, Urinary System BT1
  see Plain Radiography, Urinary System BTØ
Pyeloileostomy, urinary diversion *see* Bypass, Urinary System ØT1
Pyeloplasty
  see Repair, Urinary System ØTQ
  see Replacement, Urinary System ØTR
  see Supplement, Urinary System ØTU
Pyeloplasty, dismembered *see* Repair, Kidney Pelvis
Pyelorrhaphy *see* Repair, Urinary System ØTQ
Pyeloscopy ØTJ58ZZ
Pyelostomy
  see Bypass, Urinary System ØT1
  see Drainage, Urinary System ØT9
Pyelotomy *see* Drainage, Urinary System ØT9
Pylorectomy
  see Excision, Stomach, Pylorus ØDB7
  see Resection, Stomach, Pylorus ØDT7
Pyloric antrum *use* Stomach, Pylorus
Pyloric canal *use* Stomach, Pylorus
Pyloric sphincter *use* Stomach, Pylorus
Pylorodiosis *see* Dilation, Stomach, Pylorus ØD77
Pylorogastrectomy
  see Excision, Gastrointestinal System ØDB
  see Resection, Gastrointestinal System ØDT
Pyloroplasty
  see Repair, Stomach, Pylorus ØDQ7
  see Supplement, Stomach, Pylorus ØDU7
Pyloroscopy ØDJ68ZZ
Pylorotomy *see* Drainage, Stomach, Pylorus ØD97
Pyramidalis muscle
  use Abdomen Muscle, Left
  use Abdomen Muscle, Right

Quadrangular cartilage *use* Nasal Septum
Quadrant resection of breast *see* Excision, Skin and Breast ØHB
Quadrate lobe *use* Liver
Quadratus femoris muscle
  use Hip Muscle, Left
  use Hip Muscle, Right
Quadratus lumborum muscle
  use Trunk Muscle, Left
  use Trunk Muscle, Right
Quadratus plantae muscle
  use Foot Muscle, Left
  use Foot Muscle, Right
Quadriceps (femoris)
  use Upper Leg Muscle, Left
  use Upper Leg Muscle, Right
Quarantine 8EØZXY6

R

Radial collateral carpal ligament
  use Wrist Bursa and Ligament, Left
  use Wrist Bursa and Ligament, Right
Radial collateral ligament
  use Elbow Bursa and Ligament, Left
  use Elbow Bursa and Ligament, Right
Radial notch
  use Ulna, Left
  use Ulna, Right
Radial recurrent artery
  use Radial Artery, Left
  use Radial Artery, Right
Radial vein
  use Brachial Vein, Left
  use Brachial Vein, Right
Radialis indicis
  use Hand Artery, Left
  use Hand Artery, Right
Radiation Therapy
  see Beam Radiation

Radiation Therapy — *continued*
see Brachytherapy
see Stereotactic Radiosurgery
Radiation treatment *see* Radiation Therapy
Radiocarpal joint
use Wrist Joint, Left
use Wrist Joint, Right
Radiocarpal ligament
use Wrist Bursa and Ligament, Left
use Wrist Bursa and Ligament, Right
Radiography *see* Plain Radiography
Radiology, analog *see* Plain Radiography
Radiology, diagnostic *see* Imaging, Diagnostic
Radioulnar ligament
use Wrist Bursa and Ligament, Left
use Wrist Bursa and Ligament, Right
Range of motion testing *see* Motor Function Assessment, Rehabilitation F01
REALIZE® Adjustable Gastric Band *use* Extraluminal Device
Reattachment
Abdominal Wall 0WMF0ZZ
Ampulla of Vater 0FMC
Ankle Region
Left 0YML0ZZ
Right 0YMK0ZZ
Arm
Lower
Left 0XMF0ZZ
Right 0XMD0ZZ
Upper
Left 0XM90ZZ
Right 0XM80ZZ
Axilla
Left 0XM50ZZ
Right 0XM40ZZ
Back
Lower 0WML0ZZ
Upper 0WMK0ZZ
Bladder 0TMB
Bladder Neck 0TMC
Breast
Bilateral 0HMVXZZ
Left 0HMUXZZ
Right 0HMTXZZ
Bronchus
Lingula 0BM90ZZ
Lower Lobe
Left 0BMB0ZZ
Right 0BM60ZZ
Main
Left 0BM70ZZ
Right 0BM30ZZ
Middle Lobe, Right 0BM50ZZ
Upper Lobe
Left 0BM80ZZ
Right 0BM40ZZ
Bursa and Ligament
Abdomen
Left 0MMJ
Right 0MMH
Ankle
Left 0MMR
Right 0MMQ
Elbow
Left 0MM4
Right 0MM3
Foot
Left 0MMT
Right 0MMS
Hand
Left 0MM8
Right 0MM7
Head and Neck 0MM0
Hip
Left 0MMM
Right 0MML
Knee
Left 0MMP
Right 0MMN
Lower Extremity
Left 0MMW
Right 0MMV
Perineum 0MMK
Rib(s) 0MMG
Shoulder
Left 0MM2
Right 0MM1

Reattachment — *continued*
Bursa and Ligament — *continued*
Spine
Lower 0MMD
Upper 0MMC
Sternum 0MMF
Upper Extremity
Left 0MMB
Right 0MM9
Wrist
Left 0MM6
Right 0MM5
Buttock
Left 0YM10ZZ
Right 0YM00ZZ
Carina 0BM20ZZ
Cecum 0DMH
Cervix 0UMC
Chest Wall 0WM80ZZ
Clitoris 0UMJXZZ
Colon
Ascending 0DMK
Descending 0DMM
Sigmoid 0DMN
Transverse 0DML
Cord
Bilateral 0VMH
Left 0VMG
Right 0VMF
Cul-de-sac 0UMF
Diaphragm 0BMT0ZZ
Duct
Common Bile 0FM9
Cystic 0FM8
Hepatic
Common 0FM7
Left 0FM6
Right 0FM5
Pancreatic 0FMD
Accessory 0FMF
Duodenum 0DM9
Ear
Left 09M1XZZ
Right 09M0XZZ
Elbow Region
Left 0XMC0ZZ
Right 0XMB0ZZ
Esophagus 0DM5
Extremity
Lower
Left 0YMB0ZZ
Right 0YM90ZZ
Upper
Left 0XM70ZZ
Right 0XM60ZZ
Eyelid
Lower
Left 08MRXZZ
Right 08MQXZZ
Upper
Left 08MPXZZ
Right 08MNXZZ
Face 0WM20ZZ
Fallopian Tube
Left 0UM6
Right 0UM5
Fallopian Tubes, Bilateral 0UM7
Femoral Region
Left 0YM80ZZ
Right 0YM70ZZ
Finger
Index
Left 0XMP0ZZ
Right 0XMN0ZZ
Little
Left 0XMW0ZZ
Right 0XMV0ZZ
Middle
Left 0XMR0ZZ
Right 0XMQ0ZZ
Ring
Left 0XMT0ZZ
Right 0XMS0ZZ
Foot
Left 0YMN0ZZ
Right 0YMM0ZZ
Forequarter
Left 0XM10ZZ
Right 0XM00ZZ

Reattachment — *continued*
Gallbladder 0FM4
Gland
Left 0GM2
Right 0GM3
Hand
Left 0XMK0ZZ
Right 0XMJ0ZZ
Hindquarter
Bilateral 0YM40ZZ
Left 0YM30ZZ
Right 0YM20ZZ
Hymen 0UMK
Ileum 0DMB
Inguinal Region
Left 0YM60ZZ
Right 0YM50ZZ
Intestine
Large 0DME
Left 0DMG
Right 0DMF
Small 0DM8
Jaw
Lower 0WM50ZZ
Upper 0WM40ZZ
Jejunum 0DMA
Kidney
Left 0TM1
Right 0TM0
Kidney Pelvis
Left 0TM4
Right 0TM3
Kidneys, Bilateral 0TM2
Knee Region
Left 0YMG0ZZ
Right 0YMF0ZZ
Leg
Lower
Left 0YMJ0ZZ
Right 0YMH0ZZ
Upper
Left 0YMD0ZZ
Right 0YMC0ZZ
Lip
Lower 0CM10ZZ
Upper 0CM00ZZ
Liver 0FM0
Left Lobe 0FM2
Right Lobe 0FM1
Lung
Left 0BML0ZZ
Lower Lobe
Left 0BMJ0ZZ
Right 0BMF0ZZ
Middle Lobe, Right 0BMD0ZZ
Right 0BMK0ZZ
Upper Lobe
Left 0BMG0ZZ
Right 0BMC0ZZ
Lung Lingula 0BMH0ZZ
Muscle
Abdomen
Left 0KML
Right 0KMK
Facial 0KM1
Foot
Left 0KMW
Right 0KMV
Hand
Left 0KMD
Right 0KMC
Head 0KM0
Hip
Left 0KMP
Right 0KMN
Lower Arm and Wrist
Left 0KMB
Right 0KM9
Lower Leg
Left 0KMT
Right 0KMS
Neck
Left 0KM3
Right 0KM2
Perineum 0KMM
Shoulder
Left 0KM6
Right 0KM5

Reattachment — *continued*
Muscle — *continued*
Thorax
Left ØKMJ
Right ØKMH
Tongue, Palate, Pharynx ØKM4
Trunk
Left ØKMG
Right ØKMF
Upper Arm
Left ØKM8
Right ØKM7
Upper Leg
Left ØKMR
Right ØKMQ
Nasal Mucosa and Soft Tissue Ø9MKXZZ
Neck ØWM6ØZZ
Nipple
Left ØHMXXZZ
Right ØHMWXZZ
Ovary
Bilateral ØUM2
Left ØUM1
Right ØUMØ
Palate, Soft ØCM3ØZZ
Pancreas ØFMG
Parathyroid Gland ØGMR
Inferior
Left ØGMP
Right ØGMN
Multiple ØGMQ
Superior
Left ØGMM
Right ØGML
Penis ØVMSXZZ
Perineum
Female ØWMNØZZ
Male ØWMMØZZ
Rectum ØDMP
Scrotum ØVM5XZZ
Shoulder Region
Left ØXM3ØZZ
Right ØXM2ØZZ
Skin
Abdomen ØHM7XZZ
Back ØHM6XZZ
Buttock ØHM8XZZ
Chest ØHM5XZZ
Ear
Left ØHM3XZZ
Right ØHM2XZZ
Face ØHM1XZZ
Foot
Left ØHMNXZZ
Right ØHMMXZZ
Hand
Left ØHMGXZZ
Right ØHMFXZZ
Inguinal ØHMAXZZ
Lower Arm
Left ØHMEXZZ
Right ØHMDXZZ
Lower Leg
Left ØHMLXZZ
Right ØHMKXZZ
Neck ØHM4XZZ
Perineum ØHM9XZZ
Scalp ØHMØXZZ
Upper Arm
Left ØHMCXZZ
Right ØHMBXZZ
Upper Leg
Left ØHMJXZZ
Right ØHMHXZZ
Stomach ØDM6
Tendon
Abdomen
Left ØLMG
Right ØLMF
Ankle
Left ØLMT
Right ØLMS
Foot
Left ØLMW
Right ØLMV
Hand
Left ØLM8
Right ØLM7
Head and Neck ØLMØ

Reattachment — *continued*
Tendon — *continued*
Hip
Left ØLMK
Right ØLMJ
Knee
Left ØLMR
Right ØLMQ
Lower Arm and Wrist
Left ØLM6
Right ØLM5
Lower Leg
Left ØLMP
Right ØLMN
Perineum ØLMH
Shoulder
Left ØLM2
Right ØLM1
Thorax
Left ØLMD
Right ØLMC
Trunk
Left ØLMB
Right ØLM9
Upper Arm
Left ØLM4
Right ØLM3
Upper Leg
Left ØLMM
Right ØLML
Testis
Bilateral ØVMC
Left ØVMB
Right ØVM9
Thumb
Left ØXMMØZZ
Right ØXMLØZZ
Thyroid Gland
Left Lobe ØGMG
Right Lobe ØGMH
Toe
1st
Left ØYMQØZZ
Right ØYMPØZZ
2nd
Left ØYMSØZZ
Right ØYMRØZZ
3rd
Left ØYMUØZZ
Right ØYMTØZZ
4th
Left ØYMWØZZ
Right ØYMVØZZ
5th
Left ØYMYØZZ
Right ØYMXØZZ
Tongue ØCM7ØZZ
Tooth
Lower ØCMX
Upper ØCMW
Trachea ØBM1ØZZ
Tunica Vaginalis
Left ØVM7
Right ØVM6
Ureter
Left ØTM7
Right ØTM6
Ureters, Bilateral ØTM8
Urethra ØTMD
Uterine Supporting Structure ØUM4
Uterus ØUM9
Uvula ØCMNØZZ
Vagina ØUMG
Vulva ØUMMXZZ
Wrist Region
Left ØXMHØZZ
Right ØXMGØZZ
REBOA (resuscitative endovascular balloon occlusion of the aorta)
Ø2LW3DJ
Ø4LØ3DJ
Rebound HRD® (Hernia Repair Device) *use* Synthetic Substitute
RECELL® cell suspension autograft *see* Replacement, Skin and Breast ØHR
Recession
see Repair
see Reposition

Reclosure, disrupted abdominal wall ØWQFXZZ
Reconstruction
see Repair
see Replacement
see Supplement
Rectectomy
see Excision, Rectum ØDBP
see Resection, Rectum ØDTP
Rectocele repair *see* Repair, Subcutaneous Tissue and Fascia, Pelvic Region ØJQC
Rectopexy
see Repair, Gastrointestinal System ØDQ
see Reposition, Gastrointestinal System ØDS
Rectoplasty
see Repair, Gastrointestinal System ØDQ
see Supplement, Gastrointestinal System ØDU
Rectorrhaphy *see* Repair, Gastrointestinal System ØDQ
Rectoscopy ØDJD8ZZ
Rectosigmoid junction *use* Sigmoid Colon
Rectosigmoidectomy
see Excision, Gastrointestinal System ØDB
see Resection, Gastrointestinal System ØDT
Rectostomy *see* Drainage, Rectum ØD9P
Rectotomy *see* Drainage, Rectum ØD9P
Rectus abdominis muscle
use Abdomen Muscle, Left
use Abdomen Muscle, Right
Rectus femoris muscle
use Upper Leg Muscle, Left
use Upper Leg Muscle, Right
Recurrent laryngeal nerve *use* Vagus Nerve
Reduction
Dislocation *see* Reposition
Fracture *see* Reposition
Intussusception, intestinal *see* Reposition, Gastrointestinal System ØDS
Mammoplasty *see* Excision, Skin and Breast ØHB
Prolapse *see* Reposition
Torsion *see* Reposition
Volvulus, gastrointestinal *see* Reposition, Gastrointestinal System ØDS
Refusion *see* Fusion
Rehabilitation
see Activities of Daily Living Assessment, Rehabilitation FØ2
see Activities of Daily Living Treatment, Rehabilitation FØ8
see Caregiver Training, Rehabilitation FØF
see Cochlear Implant Treatment, Rehabilitation FØB
see Device Fitting, Rehabilitation FØD
see Hearing Treatment, Rehabilitation FØ9
see Motor Function Assessment, Rehabilitation FØ1
see Motor Treatment, Rehabilitation FØ7
see Speech Assessment, Rehabilitation FØØ
see Speech Treatment, Rehabilitation FØ6
see Vestibular Treatment, Rehabilitation FØC
Reimplantation
see Reattachment
see Reposition
see Transfer
Reinforcement
see Repair
see Supplement
Relaxation, scar tissue *see* Release
Release
Acetabulum
Left ØQN5
Right ØQN4
Adenoids ØCNQ
Ampulla of Vater ØFNC
Anal Sphincter ØDNR
Anterior Chamber
Left Ø8N33ZZ
Right Ø8N23ZZ
Anus ØDNQ
Aorta
Abdominal Ø4NØ
Thoracic
Ascending/Arch Ø2NX
Descending Ø2NW
Aortic Body ØGND
Appendix ØDNJ
Artery
Anterior Tibial
Left Ø4NQ

Release — *continued*
Artery — *continued*
Anterior Tibial — *continued*
Right Ø4NP
Axillary
Left Ø3N6
Right Ø3N5
Brachial
Left Ø3N8
Right Ø3N7
Celiac Ø4N1
Colic
Left Ø4N7
Middle Ø4N8
Right Ø4N6
Common Carotid
Left Ø3NJ
Right Ø3NH
Common Iliac
Left Ø4ND
Right Ø4NC
Coronary
Four or More Arteries Ø2N3
One Artery Ø2NØ
Three Arteries Ø2N2
Two Arteries Ø2N1
External Carotid
Left Ø3NN
Right Ø3NM
External Iliac
Left Ø4NJ
Right Ø4NH
Face Ø3NR
Femoral
Left Ø4NL
Right Ø4NK
Foot
Left Ø4NW
Right Ø4NV
Gastric Ø4N2
Hand
Left Ø3NF
Right Ø3ND
Hepatic Ø4N3
Inferior Mesenteric Ø4NB
Innominate Ø3N2
Internal Carotid
Left Ø3NL
Right Ø3NK
Internal Iliac
Left Ø4NF
Right Ø4NE
Internal Mammary
Left Ø3N1
Right Ø3NØ
Intracranial Ø3NG
Lower Ø4NY
Peroneal
Left Ø4NU
Right Ø4NT
Popliteal
Left Ø4NN
Right Ø4NM
Posterior Tibial
Left Ø4NS
Right Ø4NR
Pulmonary
Left Ø2NR
Right Ø2NQ
Pulmonary Trunk Ø2NP
Radial
Left Ø3NC
Right Ø3NB
Renal
Left Ø4NA
Right Ø4N9
Splenic Ø4N4
Subclavian
Left Ø3N4
Right Ø3N3
Superior Mesenteric Ø4N5
Temporal
Left Ø3NT
Right Ø3NS
Thyroid
Left Ø3NV
Right Ø3NU
Ulnar
Left Ø3NA

Release — *continued*
Artery — *continued*
Ulnar — *continued*
Right Ø3N9
Upper Ø3NY
Vertebral
Left Ø3NQ
Right Ø3NP
Atrium
Left Ø2N7
Right Ø2N6
Auditory Ossicle
Left Ø9NA
Right Ø9N9
Basal Ganglia ØØN8
Bladder ØTNB
Bladder Neck ØTNC
Bone
Ethmoid
Left ØNNG
Right ØNNF
Frontal ØNN1
Hyoid ØNNX
Lacrimal
Left ØNNJ
Right ØNNH
Nasal ØNNB
Occipital ØNN7
Palatine
Left ØNNL
Right ØNNK
Parietal
Left ØNN4
Right ØNN3
Pelvic
Left ØQN3
Right ØQN2
Sphenoid ØNNC
Temporal
Left ØNN6
Right ØNN5
Zygomatic
Left ØNNN
Right ØNNM
Brain ØØNØ
Breast
Bilateral ØHNV
Left ØHNU
Right ØHNT
Bronchus
Lingula ØBN9
Lower Lobe
Left ØBNB
Right ØBN6
Main
Left ØBN7
Right ØBN3
Middle Lobe, Right ØBN5
Upper Lobe
Left ØBN8
Right ØBN4
Buccal Mucosa ØCN4
Bursa and Ligament
Abdomen
Left ØMNJ
Right ØMNH
Ankle
Left ØMNR
Right ØMNQ
Elbow
Left ØMN4
Right ØMN3
Foot
Left ØMNT
Right ØMNS
Hand
Left ØMN8
Right ØMN7
Head and Neck ØMNØ
Hip
Left ØMNM
Right ØMNL
Knee
Left ØMNP
Right ØMNN
Lower Extremity
Left ØMNW
Right ØMNV
Perineum ØMNK

Release — *continued*
Bursa and Ligament — *continued*
Rib(s) ØMNG
Shoulder
Left ØMN2
Right ØMN1
Spine
Lower ØMND
Upper ØMNC
Sternum ØMNF
Upper Extremity
Left ØMNB
Right ØMN9
Wrist
Left ØMN6
Right ØMN5
Carina ØBN2
Carotid Bodies, Bilateral ØGN8
Carotid Body
Left ØGN6
Right ØGN7
Carpal
Left ØPNN
Right ØPNM
Cecum ØDNH
Cerebellum ØØNC
Cerebral Hemisphere ØØN7
Cerebral Meninges ØØN1
Cerebral Ventricle ØØN6
Cervix ØUNC
Chordae Tendineae Ø2N9
Choroid
Left Ø8NB
Right Ø8NA
Cisterna Chyli Ø7NL
Clavicle
Left ØPNB
Right ØPN9
Clitoris ØUNJ
Coccygeal Glomus ØGNB
Coccyx ØQNS
Colon
Ascending ØDNK
Descending ØDNM
Sigmoid ØDNN
Transverse ØDNL
Conduction Mechanism Ø2N8
Conjunctiva
Left Ø8NTXZZ
Right Ø8NSXZZ
Cord
Bilateral ØVNH
Left ØVNG
Right ØVNF
Cornea
Left Ø8N9XZZ
Right Ø8N8XZZ
Cul-de-sac ØUNF
Diaphragm ØBNT
Disc
Cervical Vertebral ØRN3
Cervicothoracic Vertebral ØRN5
Lumbar Vertebral ØSN2
Lumbosacral ØSN4
Thoracic Vertebral ØRN9
Thoracolumbar Vertebral ØRNB
Duct
Common Bile ØFN9
Cystic ØFN8
Hepatic
Common ØFN7
Left ØFN6
Right ØFN5
Lacrimal
Left Ø8NY
Right Ø8NX
Pancreatic ØFND
Accessory ØFNF
Parotid
Left ØCNC
Right ØCNB
Duodenum ØDN9
Dura Mater ØØN2
Ear
External
Left Ø9N1
Right Ø9NØ
External Auditory Canal
Left Ø9N4

Release — *continued*
Ear — *continued*
External Auditory Canal — *continued*
Right Ø9N3
Inner
Left Ø9NE
Right Ø9ND
Middle
Left Ø9N6
Right Ø9N5
Epididymis
Bilateral ØVNL
Left ØVNK
Right ØVNJ
Epiglottis ØCNR
Esophagogastric Junction ØDN4
Esophagus ØDN5
Lower ØDN3
Middle ØDN2
Upper ØDN1
Eustachian Tube
Left Ø9NG
Right Ø9NF
Eye
Left Ø8N1XZZ
Right Ø8NØXZZ
Eyelid
Lower
Left Ø8NR
Right Ø8NQ
Upper
Left Ø8NP
Right Ø8NN
Fallopian Tube
Left ØUN6
Right ØUN5
Fallopian Tubes, Bilateral ØUN7
Femoral Shaft
Left ØQN9
Right ØQN8
Femur
Lower
Left ØQNC
Right ØQNB
Upper
Left ØQN7
Right ØQN6
Fibula
Left ØQNK
Right ØQNJ
Finger Nail ØHNQXZZ
Gallbladder ØFN4
Gingiva
Lower ØCN6
Upper ØCN5
Gland
Adrenal
Bilateral ØGN4
Left ØGN2
Right ØGN3
Lacrimal
Left Ø8NW
Right Ø8NV
Minor Salivary ØCNJ
Parotid
Left ØCN9
Right ØCN8
Pituitary ØGNØ
Sublingual
Left ØCNF
Right ØCND
Submaxillary
Left ØCNH
Right ØCNG
Vestibular ØUNL
Glenoid Cavity
Left ØPN8
Right ØPN7
Glomus Jugulare ØGNC
Humeral Head
Left ØPND
Right ØPNC
Humeral Shaft
Left ØPNG
Right ØPNF
Hymen ØUNK
Hypothalamus ØØNA
Ileocecal Valve ØDNC
Ileum ØDNB

Release — *continued*
Intestine
Large ØDNE
Left ØDNG
Right ØDNF
Small ØDN8
Iris
Left Ø8ND3ZZ
Right Ø8NC3ZZ
Jejunum ØDNA
Joint
Acromioclavicular
Left ØRNH
Right ØRNG
Ankle
Left ØSNG
Right ØSNF
Carpal
Left ØRNR
Right ØRNQ
Carpometacarpal
Left ØRNT
Right ØRNS
Cervical Vertebral ØRN1
Cervicothoracic Vertebral ØRN4
Coccygeal ØSN6
Elbow
Left ØRNM
Right ØRNL
Finger Phalangeal
Left ØRNX
Right ØRNW
Hip
Left ØSNB
Right ØSN9
Knee
Left ØSND
Right ØSNC
Lumbar Vertebral ØSNØ
Lumbosacral ØSN3
Metacarpophalangeal
Left ØRNV
Right ØRNU
Metatarsal-Phalangeal
Left ØSNN
Right ØSNM
Occipital-cervical ØRNØ
Sacrococcygeal ØSN5
Sacroiliac
Left ØSN8
Right ØSN7
Shoulder
Left ØRNK
Right ØRNJ
Sternoclavicular
Left ØRNF
Right ØRNE
Tarsal
Left ØSNJ
Right ØSNH
Tarsometatarsal
Left ØSNL
Right ØSNK
Temporomandibular
Left ØRND
Right ØRNC
Thoracic Vertebral ØRN6
Thoracolumbar Vertebral ØRNA
Toe Phalangeal
Left ØSNQ
Right ØSNP
Wrist
Left ØRNP
Right ØRNN
Kidney
Left ØTN1
Right ØTNØ
Kidney Pelvis
Left ØTN4
Right ØTN3
Larynx ØCNS
Lens
Left Ø8NK3ZZ
Right Ø8NJ3ZZ
Lip
Lower ØCN1
Upper ØCNØ
Liver ØFNØ
Left Lobe ØFN2

Release — *continued*
Liver — *continued*
Right Lobe ØFN1
Lung
Bilateral ØBNM
Left ØBNL
Lower Lobe
Left ØBNJ
Right ØBNF
Middle Lobe, Right ØBND
Right ØBNK
Upper Lobe
Left ØBNG
Right ØBNC
Lung Lingula ØBNH
Lymphatic
Aortic Ø7ND
Axillary
Left Ø7N6
Right Ø7N5
Head Ø7NØ
Inguinal
Left Ø7NJ
Right Ø7NH
Internal Mammary
Left Ø7N9
Right Ø7N8
Lower Extremity
Left Ø7NG
Right Ø7NF
Mesenteric Ø7NB
Neck
Left Ø7N2
Right Ø7N1
Pelvis Ø7NC
Thoracic Duct Ø7NK
Thorax Ø7N7
Upper Extremity
Left Ø7N4
Right Ø7N3
Mandible
Left ØNNV
Right ØNNT
Maxilla ØNNR
Medulla Oblongata ØØND
Mesentery ØDNV
Metacarpal
Left ØPNQ
Right ØPNP
Metatarsal
Left ØQNP
Right ØQNN
Muscle
Abdomen
Left ØKNL
Right ØKNK
Extraocular
Left Ø8NM
Right Ø8NL
Facial ØKN1
Foot
Left ØKNW
Right ØKNV
Hand
Left ØKND
Right ØKNC
Head ØKNØ
Hip
Left ØKNP
Right ØKNN
Lower Arm and Wrist
Left ØKNB
Right ØKN9
Lower Leg
Left ØKNT
Right ØKNS
Neck
Left ØKN3
Right ØKN2
Papillary Ø2ND
Perineum ØKNM
Shoulder
Left ØKN6
Right ØKN5
Thorax
Left ØKNJ
Right ØKNH
Tongue, Palate, Pharynx ØKN4

Subterms under main terms may continue to next column or page

Release — *continued*
- Muscle — *continued*
  - Trunk
    - Left ØKNG
    - Right ØKNF
  - Upper Arm
    - Left ØKN8
    - Right ØKN7
  - Upper Leg
    - Left ØKNR
    - Right ØKNQ
- Myocardial Bridge *see* Release, Artery, Coronary
- Nasal Mucosa and Soft Tissue Ø9NK
- Nasopharynx Ø9NN
- Nerve
  - Abdominal Sympathetic Ø1NM
  - Abducens ØØNL
  - Accessory ØØNR
  - Acoustic ØØNN
  - Brachial Plexus Ø1N3
  - Cervical Ø1N1
  - Cervical Plexus Ø1NØ
  - Facial ØØNM
  - Femoral Ø1ND
  - Glossopharyngeal ØØNP
  - Head and Neck Sympathetic Ø1NK
  - Hypoglossal ØØNS
  - Lumbar Ø1NB
  - Lumbar Plexus Ø1N9
  - Lumbar Sympathetic Ø1NN
  - Lumbosacral Plexus Ø1NA
  - Median Ø1N5
  - Oculomotor ØØNH
  - Olfactory ØØNF
  - Optic ØØNG
  - Peroneal Ø1NH
  - Phrenic Ø1N2
  - Pudendal Ø1NC
  - Radial Ø1N6
  - Sacral Ø1NR
  - Sacral Plexus Ø1NQ
  - Sacral Sympathetic Ø1NP
  - Sciatic Ø1NF
  - Thoracic Ø1N8
  - Thoracic Sympathetic Ø1NL
  - Tibial Ø1NG
  - Trigeminal ØØNK
  - Trochlear ØØNJ
  - Ulnar Ø1N4
  - Vagus ØØNQ
- Nipple
  - Left ØHNX
  - Right ØHNW
- Omentum ØDNU
- Orbit
  - Left ØNNQ
  - Right ØNNP
- Ovary
  - Bilateral ØUN2
  - Left ØUN1
  - Right ØUNØ
- Palate
  - Hard ØCN2
  - Soft ØCN3
- Pancreas ØFNG
- Para-aortic Body ØGN9
- Paraganglion Extremity ØGNF
- Parathyroid Gland ØGNR
  - Inferior
    - Left ØGNP
    - Right ØGNN
  - Multiple ØGNQ
  - Superior
    - Left ØGNM
    - Right ØGNL
- Patella
  - Left ØQNF
  - Right ØQND
- Penis ØVNS
- Pericardium Ø2NN
- Peritoneum ØDNW
- Phalanx
  - Finger
    - Left ØPNV
    - Right ØPNT
  - Thumb
    - Left ØPNS
    - Right ØPNR

Release — *continued*
- Phalanx — *continued*
  - Toe
    - Left ØQNR
    - Right ØQNQ
- Pharynx ØCNM
- Pineal Body ØGN1
- Pleura
  - Left ØBNP
  - Right ØBNN
- Pons ØØNB
- Prepuce ØVNT
- Prostate ØVNØ
- Radius
  - Left ØPNJ
  - Right ØPNH
- Rectum ØDNP
- Retina
  - Left Ø8NF3ZZ
  - Right Ø8NE3ZZ
- Retinal Vessel
  - Left Ø8NH3ZZ
  - Right Ø8NG3ZZ
- Ribs
  - 1 to 2 ØPN1
  - 3 or More ØPN2
- Sacrum ØQN1
- Scapula
  - Left ØPN6
  - Right ØPN5
- Sclera
  - Left Ø8N7XZZ
  - Right Ø8N6XZZ
- Scrotum ØVN5
- Septum
  - Atrial Ø2N5
  - Nasal Ø9NM
  - Ventricular Ø2NM
- Sinus
  - Accessory Ø9NP
  - Ethmoid
    - Left Ø9NV
    - Right Ø9NU
  - Frontal
    - Left Ø9NT
    - Right Ø9NS
  - Mastoid
    - Left Ø9NC
    - Right Ø9NB
  - Maxillary
    - Left Ø9NR
    - Right Ø9NQ
  - Sphenoid
    - Left Ø9NX
    - Right Ø9NW
- Skin
  - Abdomen ØHN7XZZ
  - Back ØHN6XZZ
  - Buttock ØHN8XZZ
  - Chest ØHN5XZZ
  - Ear
    - Left ØHN3XZZ
    - Right ØHN2XZZ
  - Face ØHN1XZZ
  - Foot
    - Left ØHNNXZZ
    - Right ØHNMXZZ
  - Hand
    - Left ØHNGXZZ
    - Right ØHNFXZZ
  - Inguinal ØHNAXZZ
  - Lower Arm
    - Left ØHNEXZZ
    - Right ØHNDXZZ
  - Lower Leg
    - Left ØHNLXZZ
    - Right ØHNKXZZ
  - Neck ØHN4XZZ
  - Perineum ØHN9XZZ
  - Scalp ØHNØXZZ
  - Upper Arm
    - Left ØHNCXZZ
    - Right ØHNBXZZ
  - Upper Leg
    - Left ØHNJXZZ
    - Right ØHNHXZZ
- Spinal Cord
  - Cervical ØØNW
  - Lumbar ØØNY

Release — *continued*
- Spinal Cord — *continued*
  - Thoracic ØØNX
- Spinal Meninges ØØNT
- Spleen Ø7NP
- Sternum ØPNØ
- Stomach ØDN6
  - Pylorus ØDN7
- Subcutaneous Tissue and Fascia
  - Abdomen ØJN8
  - Back ØJN7
  - Buttock ØJN9
  - Chest ØJN6
  - Face ØJN1
  - Foot
    - Left ØJNR
    - Right ØJNQ
  - Hand
    - Left ØJNK
    - Right ØJNJ
  - Lower Arm
    - Left ØJNH
    - Right ØJNG
  - Lower Leg
    - Left ØJNP
    - Right ØJNN
  - Neck
    - Left ØJN5
    - Right ØJN4
  - Pelvic Region ØJNC
  - Perineum ØJNB
  - Scalp ØJNØ
  - Upper Arm
    - Left ØJNF
    - Right ØJND
  - Upper Leg
    - Left ØJNM
    - Right ØJNL
- Tarsal
  - Left ØQNM
  - Right ØQNL
- Tendon
  - Abdomen
    - Left ØLNG
    - Right ØLNF
  - Ankle
    - Left ØLNT
    - Right ØLNS
  - Foot
    - Left ØLNW
    - Right ØLNV
  - Hand
    - Left ØLN8
    - Right ØLN7
  - Head and Neck ØLNØ
  - Hip
    - Left ØLNK
    - Right ØLNJ
  - Knee
    - Left ØLNR
    - Right ØLNQ
  - Lower Arm and Wrist
    - Left ØLN6
    - Right ØLN5
  - Lower Leg
    - Left ØLNP
    - Right ØLNN
  - Perineum ØLNH
  - Shoulder
    - Left ØLN2
    - Right ØLN1
  - Thorax
    - Left ØLND
    - Right ØLNC
  - Trunk
    - Left ØLNB
    - Right ØLN9
  - Upper Arm
    - Left ØLN4
    - Right ØLN3
  - Upper Leg
    - Left ØLNM
    - Right ØLNL
- Testis
  - Bilateral ØVNC
  - Left ØVNB
  - Right ØVN9
- Thalamus ØØN9
- Thymus Ø7NM

Release — *continued*
Thyroid Gland ØGNK
Left Lobe ØGNG
Right Lobe ØGNH
Tibia
Left ØQNH
Right ØQNG
Toe Nail ØHNRXZZ
Tongue ØCN7
Tonsils ØCNP
Tooth
Lower ØCNX
Upper ØCNW
Trachea ØBN1
Tunica Vaginalis
Left ØVN7
Right ØVN6
Turbinate, Nasal Ø9NL
Tympanic Membrane
Left Ø9N8
Right Ø9N7
Ulna
Left ØPNL
Right ØPNK
Ureter
Left ØTN7
Right ØTN6
Urethra ØTND
Uterine Supporting Structure ØUN4
Uterus ØUN9
Uvula ØCNN
Vagina ØUNG
Valve
Aortic Ø2NF
Mitral Ø2NG
Pulmonary Ø2NH
Tricuspid Ø2NJ
Vas Deferens
Bilateral ØVNQ
Left ØVNP
Right ØVNN
Vein
Axillary
Left Ø5N8
Right Ø5N7
Azygos Ø5NØ
Basilic
Left Ø5NC
Right Ø5NB
Brachial
Left Ø5NA
Right Ø5N9
Cephalic
Left Ø5NF
Right Ø5ND
Colic Ø6N7
Common Iliac
Left Ø6ND
Right Ø6NC
Coronary Ø2N4
Esophageal Ø6N3
External Iliac
Left Ø6NG
Right Ø6NF
External Jugular
Left Ø5NQ
Right Ø5NP
Face
Left Ø5NV
Right Ø5NT
Femoral
Left Ø6NN
Right Ø6NM
Foot
Left Ø6NV
Right Ø6NT
Gastric Ø6N2
Hand
Left Ø5NH
Right Ø5NG
Hemiazygos Ø5N1
Hepatic Ø6N4
Hypogastric
Left Ø6NJ
Right Ø6NH
Inferior Mesenteric Ø6N6
Innominate
Left Ø5N4
Right Ø5N3

Release — *continued*
Vein — *continued*
Internal Jugular
Left Ø5NN
Right Ø5NM
Intracranial Ø5NL
Lower Ø6NY
Portal Ø6N8
Pulmonary
Left Ø2NT
Right Ø2NS
Renal
Left Ø6NB
Right Ø6N9
Saphenous
Left Ø6NQ
Right Ø6NP
Splenic Ø6N1
Subclavian
Left Ø5N6
Right Ø5N5
Superior Mesenteric Ø6N5
Upper Ø5NY
Vertebral
Left Ø5NS
Right Ø5NR
Vena Cava
Inferior Ø6NØ
Superior Ø2NV
Ventricle
Left Ø2NL
Right Ø2NK
Vertebra
Cervical ØPN3
Lumbar ØQNØ
Thoracic ØPN4
Vesicle
Bilateral ØVN3
Left ØVN2
Right ØVN1
Vitreous
Left Ø8N53ZZ
Right Ø8N43ZZ
Vocal Cord
Left ØCNV
Right ØCNT
Vulva ØUNM
Relocation *see* Reposition
Removal
Abdominal Wall 2W53X
Anorectal 2Y53X5Z
Arm
Lower
Left 2W5DX
Right 2W5CX
Upper
Left 2W5BX
Right 2W5AX
Back 2W55X
Chest Wall 2W54X
Ear 2Y52X5Z
Extremity
Lower
Left 2W5MX
Right 2W5LX
Upper
Left 2W59X
Right 2W58X
Face 2W51X
Finger
Left 2W5KX
Right 2W5JX
Foot
Left 2W5TX
Right 2W5SX
Genital Tract, Female 2Y54X5Z
Hand
Left 2W5FX
Right 2W5EX
Head 2W5ØX
Inguinal Region
Left 2W57X
Right 2W56X
Leg
Lower
Left 2W5RX
Right 2W5QX
Upper
Left 2W5PX

Removal — *continued*
Leg — *continued*
Upper — *continued*
Right 2W5NX
Mouth and Pharynx 2Y5ØX5Z
Nasal 2Y51X5Z
Neck 2W52X
Thumb
Left 2W5HX
Right 2W5GX
Toe
Left 2W5VX
Right 2W5UX
Urethra 2Y55X5Z
Removal of device from
Abdominal Wall ØWPF
Acetabulum
Left ØQP5
Right ØQP4
Anal Sphincter ØDPR
Anus ØDPQ
Artery
Lower Ø4PY
Upper Ø3PY
Back
Lower ØWPL
Upper ØWPK
Bladder ØTPB
Bone
Facial ØNPW
Lower ØQPY
Nasal ØNPB
Pelvic
Left ØQP3
Right ØQP2
Upper ØPPY
Bone Marrow Ø7PT
Brain ØØPØ
Breast
Left ØHPU
Right ØHPT
Bursa and Ligament
Lower ØMPY
Upper ØMPX
Carpal
Left ØPPN
Right ØPPM
Cavity, Cranial ØWP1
Cerebral Ventricle ØØP6
Chest Wall ØWP8
Cisterna Chyli Ø7PL
Clavicle
Left ØPPB
Right ØPP9
Coccyx ØQPS
Diaphragm ØBPT
Disc
Cervical Vertebral ØRP3
Cervicothoracic Vertebral ØRP5
Lumbar Vertebral ØSP2
Lumbosacral ØSP4
Thoracic Vertebral ØRP9
Thoracolumbar Vertebral ØRPB
Duct
Hepatobiliary ØFPB
Pancreatic ØFPD
Ear
Inner
Left Ø9PJ
Right Ø9PD
Left Ø9PJ
Right Ø9PH
Epididymis and Spermatic Cord ØVPM
Esophagus ØDP5
Extremity
Lower
Left ØYPB
Right ØYP9
Upper
Left ØXP7
Right ØXP6
Eye
Left Ø8P1
Right Ø8PØ
Face ØWP2
Fallopian Tube ØUP8
Femoral Shaft
Left ØQP9
Right ØQP8

Removal of device from — *continued*
Femur
Lower
Left ØQPC
Right ØQPB
Upper
Left ØQP7
Right ØQP6
Fibula
Left ØQPK
Right ØQPJ
Finger Nail ØHPQX
Gallbladder ØFP4
Gastrointestinal Tract ØWPP
Genitourinary Tract ØWPR
Gland
Adrenal ØGP5
Endocrine ØGPS
Pituitary ØGPØ
Salivary ØCPA
Glenoid Cavity
Left ØPP8
Right ØPP7
Great Vessel Ø2PY
Hair ØHPSX
Head ØWPØ
Heart Ø2PA
Humeral Head
Left ØPPD
Right ØPPC
Humeral Shaft
Left ØPPG
Right ØPPF
Intestinal Tract
Lower ØDPD
Upper ØDPØ
Jaw
Lower ØWP5
Upper ØWP4
Joint
Acromloclavicular
Left ØRPH
Right ØRPG
Ankle
Left ØSPG
Right ØSPF
Carpal
Left ØRPR
Right ØRPQ
Carpometacarpal
Left ØRPT
Right ØRPS
Cervical Vertebral ØRP1
Cervicothoracic Vertebral ØRP4
Coccygeal ØSP6
Elbow
Left ØRPM
Right ØRPL
Finger Phalangeal
Left ØRPX
Right ØRPW
Hip
Left ØSPB
Acetabular Surface ØSPE
Femoral Surface ØSPS
Right ØSP9
Acetabular Surface ØSPA
Femoral Surface ØSPR
Knee
Left ØSPD
Femoral Surface ØSPU
Tibial Surface ØSPW
Right ØSPC
Femoral Surface ØSPT
Tibial Surface ØSPV
Lumbar Vertebral ØSPØ
Lumbosacral ØSP3
Metacarpophalangeal
Left ØRPV
Right ØRPU
Metatarsal-Phalangeal
Left ØSPN
Right ØSPM
Occipital-cervical ØRPØ
Sacrococcygeal ØSP5
Sacroiliac
Left ØSP8
Right ØSP7

Removal of device from — *continued*
Joint — *continued*
Shoulder
Left ØRPK
Right ØRPJ
Sternoclavicular
Left ØRPF
Right ØRPE
Tarsal
Left ØSPJ
Right ØSPH
Tarsometatarsal
Left ØSPL
Right ØSPK
Temporomandibular
Left ØRPD
Right ØRPC
Thoracic Vertebral ØRP6
Thoracolumbar Vertebral ØRPA
Toe Phalangeal
Left ØSPQ
Right ØSPP
Wrist
Left ØRPP
Right ØRPN
Kidney ØTP5
Larynx ØCPS
Lens
Left Ø8PK3
Right Ø8PJ3
Liver ØFPØ
Lung
Left ØBPL
Right ØBPK
Lymphatic Ø7PN
Thoracic Duct Ø7PK
Mediastinum ØWPC
Mesentery ØDPV
Metacarpal
Left ØPPQ
Right ØPPP
Metatarsal
Left ØQPP
Right ØQPN
Mouth and Throat ØCPY
Muscle
Extraocular
Left Ø8PM
Right Ø8PL
Lower ØKPY
Upper ØKPX
Nasal Mucosa and Soft Tissue Ø9PK
Neck ØWP6
Nerve
Cranial ØØPE
Peripheral Ø1PY
Omentum ØDPU
Ovary ØUP3
Pancreas ØFPG
Parathyroid Gland ØGPR
Patella
Left ØQPF
Right ØQPD
Pelvic Cavity ØWPJ
Penis ØVPS
Pericardial Cavity ØWPD
Perineum
Female ØWPN
Male ØWPM
Peritoneal Cavity ØWPG
Peritoneum ØDPW
Phalanx
Finger
Left ØPPV
Right ØPPT
Thumb
Left ØPPS
Right ØPPR
Toe
Left ØQPR
Right ØQPQ
Pineal Body ØGP1
Pleura ØBPQ
Pleural Cavity
Left ØWPB
Right ØWP9
Products of Conception 1ØPØ
Prostate and Seminal Vesicles ØVP4

Removal of device from — *continued*
Radius
Left ØPPJ
Right ØPPH
Rectum ØDPP
Respiratory Tract ØWPQ
Retroperitoneum ØWPH
Ribs
1 to 2 ØPP1
3 or More ØPP2
Sacrum ØQP1
Scapula
Left ØPP6
Right ØPP5
Scrotum and Tunica Vaginalis ØVP8
Sinus Ø9PY
Skin ØHPPX
Skull ØNPØ
Spinal Canal ØØPU
Spinal Cord ØØPV
Spleen Ø7PP
Sternum ØPPØ
Stomach ØDP6
Subcutaneous Tissue and Fascia
Head and Neck ØJPS
Lower Extremity ØJPW
Trunk ØJPT
Upper Extremity ØJPV
Tarsal
Left ØQPM
Right ØQPL
Tendon
Lower ØLPY
Upper ØLPX
Testis ØVPD
Thymus Ø7PM
Thyroid Gland ØGPK
Tibia
Left ØQPH
Right ØQPG
Toe Nail ØHPRX
Trachea ØBP1
Tracheobronchial Tree ØBPØ
Tympanic Membrane
Left Ø9P8
Right Ø9P7
Ulna
Left ØPPL
Right ØPPK
Ureter ØTP9
Urethra ØTPD
Uterus and Cervix ØUPD
Vagina and Cul-de-sac ØUPH
Vas Deferens ØVPR
Vein
Azygos Ø5PØ
Innominate
Left Ø5P4
Right Ø5P3
Lower Ø6PY
Upper Ø5PY
Vertebra
Cervical ØPP3
Lumbar ØQPØ
Thoracic ØPP4
Vulva ØUPM

Renal calyx
use Kidney
use Kidney, Left
use Kidney, Right
use Kidneys, Bilateral

Renal capsule
use Kidney
use Kidney, Left
use Kidney, Right
use Kidneys, Bilateral

Renal cortex
use Kidney
use Kidney, Left
use Kidney, Right
use Kidneys, Bilateral

Renal dialysis *see* Performance, Urinary 5A1D
Renal nerve *use* Abdominal Sympathetic Nerve
Renal plexus *use* Abdominal Sympathetic Nerve

Renal segment
use Kidney
use Kidney, Left
use Kidney, Right

- **Renal segment** — *continued*
  - *use* Kidneys, Bilateral
- **Renal segmental artery**
  - *use* Renal Artery, Left
  - *use* Renal Artery, Right
- **Reopening, operative site**
  - Control of bleeding *see* Control bleeding in
  - Inspection only *see* Inspection
- **Repair**
  - Abdominal Wall ØWQF
  - Acetabulum
    - Left ØQQ5
    - Right ØQQ4
  - Adenoids ØCQQ
  - Ampulla of Vater ØFQC
  - Anal Sphincter ØDQR
  - Ankle Region
    - Left ØYQL
    - Right ØYQK
  - Anterior Chamber
    - Left Ø8Q33ZZ
    - Right Ø8Q23ZZ
  - Anus ØDQQ
  - Aorta
    - Abdominal Ø4QØ
    - Thoracic
      - Ascending/Arch Ø2QX
      - Descending Ø2QW
  - Aortic Body ØGQD
  - Appendix ØDQJ
  - Arm
    - Lower
      - Left ØXQF
      - Right ØXQD
    - Upper
      - Left ØXQ9
      - Right ØXQ8
  - Artery
    - Anterior Tibial
      - Left Ø4QQ
      - Right Ø4QP
    - Axillary
      - Left Ø3Q6
      - Right Ø3Q5
    - Brachial
      - Left Ø3Q8
      - Right Ø3Q7
    - Celiac Ø4Q1
    - Colic
      - Left Ø4Q7
      - Middle Ø4Q8
      - Right Ø4Q6
    - Common Carotid
      - Left Ø3QJ
      - Right Ø3QH
    - Common Iliac
      - Left Ø4QD
      - Right Ø4QC
    - Coronary
      - Four or More Arteries Ø2Q3
      - One Artery Ø2QØ
      - Three Arteries Ø2Q2
      - Two Arteries Ø2Q1
    - External Carotid
      - Left Ø3QN
      - Right Ø3QM
    - External Iliac
      - Left Ø4QJ
      - Right Ø4QH
    - Face Ø3QR
    - Femoral
      - Left Ø4QL
      - Right Ø4QK
    - Foot
      - Left Ø4QW
      - Right Ø4QV
    - Gastric Ø4Q2
    - Hand
      - Left Ø3QF
      - Right Ø3QD
    - Hepatic Ø4Q3
    - Inferior Mesenteric Ø4QB
    - Innominate Ø3Q2
    - Internal Carotid
      - Left Ø3QL
      - Right Ø3QK
    - Internal Iliac
      - Left Ø4QF

- **Repair** — *continued*
  - Artery — *continued*
    - Internal Iliac — *continued*
      - Right Ø4QE
    - Internal Mammary
      - Left Ø3Q1
      - Right Ø3QØ
    - Intracranial Ø3QG
    - Lower Ø4QY
    - Peroneal
      - Left Ø4QU
      - Right Ø4QT
    - Popliteal
      - Left Ø4QN
      - Right Ø4QM
    - Posterior Tibial
      - Left Ø4QS
      - Right Ø4QR
    - Pulmonary
      - Left Ø2QR
      - Right Ø2QQ
    - Pulmonary Trunk Ø2QP
    - Radial
      - Left Ø3QC
      - Right Ø3QB
    - Renal
      - Left Ø4QA
      - Right Ø4Q9
    - Splenic Ø4Q4
    - Subclavian
      - Left Ø3Q4
      - Right Ø3Q3
    - Superior Mesenteric Ø4Q5
    - Temporal
      - Left Ø3QT
      - Right Ø3QS
    - Thyroid
      - Left Ø3QV
      - Right Ø3QU
    - Ulnar
      - Left Ø3QA
      - Right Ø3Q9
    - Upper Ø3QY
    - Vertebral
      - Left Ø3QQ
      - Right Ø3QP
  - Atrium
    - Left Ø2Q7
    - Right Ø2Q6
  - Auditory Ossicle
    - Left Ø9QA
    - Right Ø9Q9
  - Axilla
    - Left ØXQ5
    - Right ØXQ4
  - Back
    - Lower ØWQL
    - Upper ØWQK
  - Basal Ganglia ØØQ8
  - Bladder ØTQB
  - Bladder Neck ØTQC
  - Bone
    - Ethmoid
      - Left ØNQG
      - Right ØNQF
    - Frontal ØNQ1
    - Hyoid ØNQX
    - Lacrimal
      - Left ØNQJ
      - Right ØNQH
    - Nasal ØNQB
    - Occipital ØNQ7
    - Palatine
      - Left ØNQL
      - Right ØNQK
    - Parietal
      - Left ØNQ4
      - Right ØNQ3
    - Pelvic
      - Left ØQQ3
      - Right ØQQ2
    - Sphenoid ØNQC
    - Temporal
      - Left ØNQ6
      - Right ØNQ5
    - Zygomatic
      - Left ØNQN
      - Right ØNQM
  - Brain ØØQØ

- **Repair** — *continued*
  - Breast
    - Bilateral ØHQV
    - Left ØHQU
    - Right ØHQT
    - Supernumerary ØHQY
  - Bronchus
    - Lingula ØBQ9
    - Lower Lobe
      - Left ØBQB
      - Right ØBQ6
    - Main
      - Left ØBQ7
      - Right ØBQ3
    - Middle Lobe, Right ØBQ5
    - Upper Lobe
      - Left ØBQ8
      - Right ØBQ4
  - Buccal Mucosa ØCQ4
  - Bursa and Ligament
    - Abdomen
      - Left ØMQJ
      - Right ØMQH
    - Ankle
      - Left ØMQR
      - Right ØMQQ
    - Elbow
      - Left ØMQ4
      - Right ØMQ3
    - Foot
      - Left ØMQT
      - Right ØMQS
    - Hand
      - Left ØMQ8
      - Right ØMQ7
    - Head and Neck ØMQØ
    - Hip
      - Left ØMQM
      - Right ØMQL
    - Knee
      - Left ØMQP
      - Right ØMQN
    - Lower Extremity
      - Left ØMQW
      - Right ØMQV
    - Perineum ØMQK
    - Rib(s) ØMQG
    - Shoulder
      - Left ØMQ2
      - Right ØMQ1
    - Spine
      - Lower ØMQD
      - Upper ØMQC
    - Sternum ØMQF
    - Upper Extremity
      - Left ØMQB
      - Right ØMQ9
    - Wrist
      - Left ØMQ6
      - Right ØMQ5
  - Buttock
    - Left ØYQ1
    - Right ØYQØ
  - Carina ØBQ2
  - Carotid Bodies, Bilateral ØGQ8
  - Carotid Body
    - Left ØGQ6
    - Right ØGQ7
  - Carpal
    - Left ØPQN
    - Right ØPQM
  - Cecum ØDQH
  - Cerebellum ØØQC
  - Cerebral Hemisphere ØØQ7
  - Cerebral Meninges ØØQ1
  - Cerebral Ventricle ØØQ6
  - Cervix ØUQC
  - Chest Wall ØWQ8
  - Chordae Tendineae Ø2Q9
  - Choroid
    - Left Ø8QB
    - Right Ø8QA
  - Cisterna Chyli Ø7QL
  - Clavicle
    - Left ØPQB
    - Right ØPQ9
  - Clitoris ØUQJ
  - Coccygeal Glomus ØGQB
  - Coccyx ØQQS

Repair — *continued*
Colon
Ascending ØDQK
Descending ØDQM
Sigmoid ØDQN
Transverse ØDQL
Conduction Mechanism Ø2Q8
Conjunctiva
Left Ø8QTXZZ
Right Ø8QSXZZ
Cord
Bilateral ØVQH
Left ØVQG
Right ØVQF
Cornea
Left Ø8Q9XZZ
Right Ø8Q8XZZ
Cul-de-sac ØUQF
Diaphragm ØBQT
Disc
Cervical Vertebral ØRQ3
Cervicothoracic Vertebral ØRQ5
Lumbar Vertebral ØSQ2
Lumbosacral ØSQ4
Thoracic Vertebral ØRQ9
Thoracolumbar Vertebral ØRQB
Duct
Common Bile ØFQ9
Cystic ØFQ8
Hepatic
Common ØFQ7
Left ØFQ6
Right ØFQ5
Lacrimal
Left Ø8QY
Right Ø8QX
Pancreatic ØFQD
Accessory ØFQF
Parotid
Left ØCQC
Right ØCQB
Duodenum ØDQ9
Dura Mater ØØQ2
Ear
External
Bilateral Ø9Q2
Left Ø9Q1
Right Ø9QØ
External Auditory Canal
Left Ø9Q4
Right Ø9Q3
Inner
Left Ø9QE
Right Ø9QD
Middle
Left Ø9Q6
Right Ø9Q5
Elbow Region
Left ØXQC
Right ØXQB
Epididymis
Bilateral ØVQL
Left ØVQK
Right ØVQJ
Epiglottis ØCQR
Esophagogastric Junction ØDQ4
Esophagus ØDQ5
Lower ØDQ3
Middle ØDQ2
Upper ØDQ1
Eustachian Tube
Left Ø9QG
Right Ø9QF
Extremity
Lower
Left ØYQB
Right ØYQ9
Upper
Left ØXQ7
Right ØXQ6
Eye
Left Ø8Q1XZZ
Right Ø8QØXZZ
Eyelid
Lower
Left Ø8QR
Right Ø8QQ
Upper
Left Ø8QP

Repair — *continued*
Eyelid — *continued*
Upper — *continued*
Right Ø8QN
Face ØWQ2
Fallopian Tube
Left ØUQ6
Right ØUQ5
Fallopian Tubes, Bilateral ØUQ7
Femoral Region
Bilateral ØYQE
Left ØYQ8
Right ØYQ7
Femoral Shaft
Left ØQQ9
Right ØQQ8
Femur
Lower
Left ØQQC
Right ØQQB
Upper
Left ØQQ7
Right ØQQ6
Fibula
Left ØQQK
Right ØQQJ
Finger
Index
Left ØXQP
Right ØXQN
Little
Left ØXQW
Right ØXQV
Middle
Left ØXQR
Right ØXQQ
Ring
Left ØXQT
Right ØXQS
Finger Nail ØHQQXZZ
Floor of mouth *see* Repair, Oral Cavity and Throat ØWQ3
Foot
Left ØYQN
Right ØYQM
Gallbladder ØFQ4
Gingiva
Lower ØCQ6
Upper ØCQ5
Gland
Adrenal
Bilateral ØGQ4
Left ØGQ2
Right ØGQ3
Lacrimal
Left Ø8QW
Right Ø8QV
Minor Salivary ØCQJ
Parotid
Left ØCQ9
Right ØCQ8
Pituitary ØGQØ
Sublingual
Left ØCQF
Right ØCQD
Submaxillary
Left ØCQH
Right ØCQG
Vestibular ØUQL
Glenoid Cavity
Left ØPQ8
Right ØPQ7
Glomus Jugulare ØGQC
Hand
Left ØXQK
Right ØXQJ
Head ØWQØ
Heart Ø2QA
Left Ø2QC
Right Ø2QB
Humeral Head
Left ØPQD
Right ØPQC
Humeral Shaft
Left ØPQG
Right ØPQF
Hymen ØUQK
Hypothalamus ØØQA
Ileocecal Valve ØDQC

Repair — *continued*
Ileum ØDQB
Inguinal Region
Bilateral ØYQA
Left ØYQ6
Right ØYQ5
Intestine
Large ØDQE
Left ØDQG
Right ØDQF
Small ØDQ8
Iris
Left Ø8QD3ZZ
Right Ø8QC3ZZ
Jaw
Lower ØWQ5
Upper ØWQ4
Jejunum ØDQA
Joint
Acromioclavicular
Left ØRQH
Right ØRQG
Ankle
Left ØSQG
Right ØSQF
Carpal
Left ØRQR
Right ØRQQ
Carpometacarpal
Left ØRQT
Right ØRQS
Cervical Vertebral ØRQ1
Cervicothoracic Vertebral ØRQ4
Coccygeal ØSQ6
Elbow
Left ØRQM
Right ØRQL
Finger Phalangeal
Left ØRQX
Right ØRQW
Hip
Left ØSQB
Right ØSQ9
Knee
Left ØSQD
Right ØSQC
Lumbar Vertebral ØSQØ
Lumbosacral ØSQ3
Metacarpophalangeal
Left ØRQV
Right ØRQU
Metatarsal-Phalangeal
Left ØSQN
Right ØSQM
Occipital-cervical ØRQØ
Sacrococcygeal ØSQ5
Sacroiliac
Left ØSQ8
Right ØSQ7
Shoulder
Left ØRQK
Right ØRQJ
Sternoclavicular
Left ØRQF
Right ØRQE
Tarsal
Left ØSQJ
Right ØSQH
Tarsometatarsal
Left ØSQL
Right ØSQK
Temporomandibular
Left ØRQD
Right ØRQC
Thoracic Vertebral ØRQ6
Thoracolumbar Vertebral ØRQA
Toe Phalangeal
Left ØSQQ
Right ØSQP
Wrist
Left ØRQP
Right ØRQN
Kidney
Left ØTQ1
Right ØTQØ
Kidney Pelvis
Left ØTQ4
Right ØTQ3

- **Repair** — *continued*
  - Knee Region
    - Left ØYQG
    - Right ØYQF
  - Larynx ØCQS
  - Leg
    - Lower
      - Left ØYQJ
      - Right ØYQH
    - Upper
      - Left ØYQD
      - Right ØYQC
  - Lens
    - Left Ø8QK3ZZ
    - Right Ø8QJ3ZZ
  - Lip
    - Lower ØCQ1
    - Upper ØCQØ
  - Liver ØFQØ
    - Left Lobe ØFQ2
    - Right Lobe ØFQ1
  - Lung
    - Bilateral ØBQM
    - Left ØBQL
    - Lower Lobe
      - Left ØBQJ
      - Right ØBQF
    - Middle Lobe, Right ØBQD
    - Right ØBQK
    - Upper Lobe
      - Left ØBQG
      - Right ØBQC
  - Lung Lingula ØBQH
  - Lymphatic
    - Aortic Ø7QD
    - Axillary
      - Left Ø7Q6
      - Right Ø7Q5
    - Head Ø7QØ
    - Inguinal
      - Left Ø7QJ
      - Right Ø7QH
    - Internal Mammary
      - Left Ø7Q9
      - Right Ø7Q8
    - Lower Extremity
      - Left Ø7QG
      - Right Ø7QF
    - Mesenteric Ø7QB
    - Neck
      - Left Ø7Q2
      - Right Ø7Q1
    - Pelvis Ø7QC
    - Thoracic Duct Ø7QK
    - Thorax Ø7Q7
    - Upper Extremity
      - Left Ø7Q4
      - Right Ø7Q3
  - Mandible
    - Left ØNQV
    - Right ØNQT
  - Maxilla ØNQR
  - Mediastinum ØWQC
  - Medulla Oblongata ØØQD
  - Mesentery ØDQV
  - Metacarpal
    - Left ØPQQ
    - Right ØPQP
  - Metatarsal
    - Left ØQQP
    - Right ØQQN
  - Muscle
    - Abdomen
      - Left ØKQL
      - Right ØKQK
    - Extraocular
      - Left Ø8QM
      - Right Ø8QL
    - Facial ØKQ1
    - Foot
      - Left ØKQW
      - Right ØKQV
    - Hand
      - Left ØKQD
      - Right ØKQC
    - Head ØKQØ
    - Hip
      - Left ØKQP
      - Right ØKQN

- **Repair** — *continued*
  - Muscle — *continued*
    - Lower Arm and Wrist
      - Left ØKQB
      - Right ØKQ9
    - Lower Leg
      - Left ØKQT
      - Right ØKQS
    - Neck
      - Left ØKQ3
      - Right ØKQ2
    - Papillary Ø2QD
    - Perineum ØKQM
    - Shoulder
      - Left ØKQ6
      - Right ØKQ5
    - Thorax
      - Left ØKQJ
      - Right ØKQH
    - Tongue, Palate, Pharynx ØKQ4
    - Trunk
      - Left ØKQG
      - Right ØKQF
    - Upper Arm
      - Left ØKQ8
      - Right ØKQ7
    - Upper Leg
      - Left ØKQR
      - Right ØKQQ
  - Nasal Mucosa and Soft Tissue Ø9QK
  - Nasopharynx Ø9QN
  - Neck ØWQ6
  - Nerve
    - Abdominal Sympathetic Ø1QM
    - Abducens ØØQL
    - Accessory ØØQR
    - Acoustic ØØQN
    - Brachial Plexus Ø1Q3
    - Cervical Ø1Q1
    - Cervical Plexus Ø1QØ
    - Facial ØØQM
    - Femoral Ø1QD
    - Glossopharyngeal ØØQP
    - Head and Neck Sympathetic Ø1QK
    - Hypoglossal ØØQS
    - Lumbar Ø1QB
    - Lumbar Plexus Ø1Q9
    - Lumbar Sympathetic Ø1QN
    - Lumbosacral Plexus Ø1QA
    - Median Ø1Q5
    - Oculomotor ØØQH
    - Olfactory ØØQF
    - Optic ØØQG
    - Peroneal Ø1QH
    - Phrenic Ø1Q2
    - Pudendal Ø1QC
    - Radial Ø1Q6
    - Sacral Ø1QR
    - Sacral Plexus Ø1QQ
    - Sacral Sympathetic Ø1QP
    - Sciatic Ø1QF
    - Thoracic Ø1Q8
    - Thoracic Sympathetic Ø1QL
    - Tibial Ø1QG
    - Trigeminal ØØQK
    - Trochlear ØØQJ
    - Ulnar Ø1Q4
    - Vagus ØØQQ
  - Nipple
    - Left ØHQX
    - Right ØHQW
  - Omentum ØDQU
  - Oral Cavity and Throat ØWQ3
  - Orbit
    - Left ØNQQ
    - Right ØNQP
  - Ovary
    - Bilateral ØUQ2
    - Left ØUQ1
    - Right ØUQØ
  - Palate
    - Hard ØCQ2
    - Soft ØCQ3
  - Pancreas ØFQG
  - Para-aortic Body ØGQ9
  - Paraganglion Extremity ØGQF
  - Parathyroid Gland ØGQR
    - Inferior
      - Left ØGQP

- **Repair** — *continued*
  - Parathyroid Gland — *continued*
    - Inferior — *continued*
      - Right ØGQN
    - Multiple ØGQQ
    - Superior
      - Left ØGQM
      - Right ØGQL
  - Patella
    - Left ØQQF
    - Right ØQQD
  - Penis ØVQS
  - Pericardium Ø2QN
  - Perineum
    - Female ØWQN
    - Male ØWQM
  - Peritoneum ØDQW
  - Phalanx
    - Finger
      - Left ØPQV
      - Right ØPQT
    - Thumb
      - Left ØPQS
      - Right ØPQR
    - Toe
      - Left ØQQR
      - Right ØQQQ
  - Pharynx ØCQM
  - Pineal Body ØGQ1
  - Pleura
    - Left ØBQP
    - Right ØBQN
  - Pons ØØQB
  - Prepuce ØVQT
  - Products of Conception 1ØQØ
  - Prostate ØVQØ
  - Radius
    - Left ØPQJ
    - Right ØPQH
  - Rectum ØDQP
  - Retina
    - Left Ø8QF3ZZ
    - Right Ø8QE3ZZ
  - Retinal Vessel
    - Left Ø8QH3ZZ
    - Right Ø8QG3ZZ
  - Ribs
    - 1 to 2 ØPQ1
    - 3 or More ØPQ2
  - Sacrum ØQQ1
  - Scapula
    - Left ØPQ6
    - Right ØPQ5
  - Sclera
    - Left Ø8Q7XZZ
    - Right Ø8Q6XZZ
  - Scrotum ØVQ5
  - Septum
    - Atrial Ø2Q5
    - Nasal Ø9QM
    - Ventricular Ø2QM
  - Shoulder Region
    - Left ØXQ3
    - Right ØXQ2
  - Sinus
    - Accessory Ø9QP
    - Ethmoid
      - Left Ø9QV
      - Right Ø9QU
    - Frontal
      - Left Ø9QT
      - Right Ø9QS
    - Mastoid
      - Left Ø9QC
      - Right Ø9QB
    - Maxillary
      - Left Ø9QR
      - Right Ø9QQ
    - Sphenoid
      - Left Ø9QX
      - Right Ø9QW
  - Skin
    - Abdomen ØHQ7XZZ
    - Back ØHQ6XZZ
    - Buttock ØHQ8XZZ
    - Chest ØHQ5XZZ
    - Ear
      - Left ØHQ3XZZ
      - Right ØHQ2XZZ

Repair — *continued*
Skin — *continued*
Face ØHQ1XZZ
Foot
Left ØHQNXZZ
Right ØHQMXZZ
Hand
Left ØHQGXZZ
Right ØHQFXZZ
Inguinal ØHQAXZZ
Lower Arm
Left ØHQEXZZ
Right ØHQDXZZ
Lower Leg
Left ØHQLXZZ
Right ØHQKXZZ
Neck ØHQ4XZZ
Perineum ØHQ9XZZ
Scalp ØHQØXZZ
Upper Arm
Left ØHQCXZZ
Right ØHQBXZZ
Upper Leg
Left ØHQJXZZ
Right ØHQHXZZ
Skull ØNQØ
Spinal Cord
Cervical ØØQW
Lumbar ØØQY
Thoracic ØØQX
Spinal Meninges ØØQT
Spleen Ø7QP
Sternum ØPQØ
Stomach ØDQ6
Pylorus ØDQ7
Subcutaneous Tissue and Fascia
Abdomen ØJQ8
Back ØJQ7
Buttock ØJQ9
Chest ØJQ6
Face ØJQ1
Foot
Left ØJQR
Right ØJQQ
Hand
Left ØJQK
Right ØJQJ
Lower Arm
Left ØJQH
Right ØJQG
Lower Leg
Left ØJQP
Right ØJQN
Neck
Left ØJQ5
Right ØJQ4
Pelvic Region ØJQC
Perineum ØJQB
Scalp ØJQØ
Upper Arm
Left ØJQF
Right ØJQD
Upper Leg
Left ØJQM
Right ØJQL
Tarsal
Left ØQQM
Right ØQQL
Tendon
Abdomen
Left ØLQG
Right ØLQF
Ankle
Left ØLQT
Right ØLQS
Foot
Left ØLQW
Right ØLQV
Hand
Left ØLQ8
Right ØLQ7
Head and Neck ØLQØ
Hip
Left ØLQK
Right ØLQJ
Knee
Left ØLQR
Right ØLQQ

Repair — *continued*
Tendon — *continued*
Lower Arm and Wrist
Left ØLQ6
Right ØLQ5
Lower Leg
Left ØLQP
Right ØLQN
Perineum ØLQH
Shoulder
Left ØLQ2
Right ØLQ1
Thorax
Left ØLQD
Right ØLQC
Trunk
Left ØLQB
Right ØLQ9
Upper Arm
Left ØLQ4
Right ØLQ3
Upper Leg
Left ØLQM
Right ØLQL
Testis
Bilateral ØVQC
Left ØVQB
Right ØVQ9
Thalamus ØØQ9
Thumb
Left ØXQM
Right ØXQL
Thymus Ø7QM
Thyroid Gland ØGQK
Left Lobe ØGQG
Right Lobe ØGQH
Thyroid Gland Isthmus ØGQJ
Tibia
Left ØQQH
Right ØQQG
Toe
1st
Left ØYQQ
Right ØYQP
2nd
Left ØYQS
Right ØYQR
3rd
Left ØYQU
Right ØYQT
4th
Left ØYQW
Right ØYQV
5th
Left ØYQY
Right ØYQX
Toe Nail ØHQRXZZ
Tongue ØCQ7
Tonsils ØCQP
Tooth
Lower ØCQX
Upper ØCQW
Trachea ØBQ1
Tunica Vaginalis
Left ØVQ7
Right ØVQ6
Turbinate, Nasal Ø9QL
Tympanic Membrane
Left Ø9Q8
Right Ø9Q7
Ulna
Left ØPQL
Right ØPQK
Ureter
Left ØTQ7
Right ØTQ6
Urethra ØTQD
Uterine Supporting Structure ØUQ4
Uterus ØUQ9
Uvula ØCQN
Vagina ØUQG
Valve
Aortic Ø2QF
Mitral Ø2QG
Pulmonary Ø2QH
Tricuspid Ø2QJ
Vas Deferens
Bilateral ØVQQ
Left ØVQP

Repair — *continued*
Vas Deferens — *continued*
Right ØVQN
Vein
Axillary
Left Ø5Q8
Right Ø5Q7
Azygos Ø5QØ
Basilic
Left Ø5QC
Right Ø5QB
Brachial
Left Ø5QA
Right Ø5Q9
Cephalic
Left Ø5QF
Right Ø5QD
Colic Ø6Q7
Common Iliac
Left Ø6QD
Right Ø6QC
Coronary Ø2Q4
Esophageal Ø6Q3
External Iliac
Left Ø6QG
Right Ø6QF
External Jugular
Left Ø5QQ
Right Ø5QP
Face
Left Ø5QV
Right Ø5QT
Femoral
Left Ø6QN
Right Ø6QM
Foot
Left Ø6QV
Right Ø6QT
Gastric Ø6Q2
Hand
Left Ø5QH
Right Ø5QG
Hemiazygos Ø5Q1
Hepatic Ø6Q4
Hypogastric
Left Ø6QJ
Right Ø6QH
Inferior Mesenteric Ø6Q6
Innominate
Left Ø5Q4
Right Ø5Q3
Internal Jugular
Left Ø5QN
Right Ø5QM
Intracranial Ø5QL
Lower Ø6QY
Portal Ø6Q8
Pulmonary
Left Ø2QT
Right Ø2QS
Renal
Left Ø6QB
Right Ø6Q9
Saphenous
Left Ø6QQ
Right Ø6QP
Splenic Ø6Q1
Subclavian
Left Ø5Q6
Right Ø5Q5
Superior Mesenteric Ø6Q5
Upper Ø5QY
Vertebral
Left Ø5QS
Right Ø5QR
Vena Cava
Inferior Ø6QØ
Superior Ø2QV
Ventricle
Left Ø2QL
Right Ø2QK
Vertebra
Cervical ØPQ3
Lumbar ØQQØ
Thoracic ØPQ4
Vesicle
Bilateral ØVQ3
Left ØVQ2
Right ØVQ1

Repair — *continued*
Vitreous
Left Ø8Q53ZZ
Right Ø8Q43ZZ
Vocal Cord
Left ØCQV
Right ØCQT
Vulva ØUQM
Wrist Region
Left ØXQH
Right ØXQG
Repair, obstetric laceration, periurethral ØUQMXZZ
Replacement
Acetabulum
Left ØQR5
Right ØQR4
Ampulla of Vater ØFRC
Anal Sphincter ØDRR
Aorta
Abdominal Ø4RØ
Thoracic
Ascending/Arch Ø2RX
Descending Ø2RW
Artery
Anterior Tibial
Left Ø4RQ
Right Ø4RP
Axillary
Left Ø3R6
Right Ø3R5
Brachial
Left Ø3R8
Right Ø3R7
Celiac Ø4R1
Colic
Left Ø4R7
Middle Ø4R8
Right Ø4R6
Common Carotid
Left Ø3RJ
Right Ø3RH
Common Iliac
Left Ø4RD
Right Ø4RC
External Carotid
Left Ø3RN
Right Ø3RM
External Iliac
Left Ø4RJ
Right Ø4RH
Face Ø3RR
Femoral
Left Ø4RL
Right Ø4RK
Foot
Left Ø4RW
Right Ø4RV
Gastric Ø4R2
Hand
Left Ø3RF
Right Ø3RD
Hepatic Ø4R3
Inferior Mesenteric Ø4RB
Innominate Ø3R2
Internal Carotid
Left Ø3RL
Right Ø3RK
Internal Iliac
Left Ø4RF
Right Ø4RE
Internal Mammary
Left Ø3R1
Right Ø3RØ
Intracranial Ø3RG
Lower Ø4RY
Peroneal
Left Ø4RU
Right Ø4RT
Popliteal
Left Ø4RN
Right Ø4RM
Posterior Tibial
Left Ø4RS
Right Ø4RR
Pulmonary
Left Ø2RR
Right Ø2RQ
Pulmonary Trunk Ø2RP

Replacement — *continued*
Artery — *continued*
Radial
Left Ø3RC
Right Ø3RB
Renal
Left Ø4RA
Right Ø4R9
Splenic Ø4R4
Subclavian
Left Ø3R4
Right Ø3R3
Superior Mesenteric Ø4R5
Temporal
Left Ø3RT
Right Ø3RS
Thyroid
Left Ø3RV
Right Ø3RU
Ulnar
Left Ø3RA
Right Ø3R9
Upper Ø3RY
Vertebral
Left Ø3RQ
Right Ø3RP
Atrium
Left Ø2R7
Right Ø2R6
Auditory Ossicle
Left Ø9RAØ
Right Ø9R9Ø
Bladder ØTRB
Bladder Neck ØTRC
Bone
Ethmoid
Left ØNRG
Right ØNRF
Frontal ØNR1
Hyoid ØNRX
Lacrimal
Left ØNRJ
Right ØNRH
Nasal ØNRB
Occipital ØNR7
Palatine
Left ØNRL
Right ØNRK
Parietal
Left ØNR4
Right ØNR3
Pelvic
Left ØQR3
Right ØQR2
Sphenoid ØNRC
Temporal
Left ØNR6
Right ØNR5
Zygomatic
Left ØNRN
Right ØNRM
Breast
Bilateral ØHRV
Left ØHRU
Right ØHRT
Bronchus
Lingula ØBR9
Lower Lobe
Left ØBRB
Right ØBR6
Main
Left ØBR7
Right ØBR3
Middle Lobe, Right ØBR5
Upper Lobe
Left ØBR8
Right ØBR4
Buccal Mucosa ØCR4
Bursa and Ligament
Abdomen
Left ØMRJ
Right ØMRH
Ankle
Left ØMRR
Right ØMRQ
Elbow
Left ØMR4
Right ØMR3

Replacement — *continued*
Bursa and Ligament — *continued*
Foot
Left ØMRT
Right ØMRS
Hand
Left ØMR8
Right ØMR7
Head and Neck ØMRØ
Hip
Left ØMRM
Right ØMRL
Knee
Left ØMRP
Right ØMRN
Lower Extremity
Left ØMRW
Right ØMRV
Perineum ØMRK
Rib(s) ØMRG
Shoulder
Left ØMR2
Right ØMR1
Spine
Lower ØMRD
Upper ØMRC
Sternum ØMRF
Upper Extremity
Left ØMRB
Right ØMR9
Wrist
Left ØMR6
Right ØMR5
Carina ØBR2
Carpal
Left ØPRN
Right ØPRM
Cerebral Meninges ØØR1
Cerebral Ventricle ØØR6
Chordae Tendineae Ø2R9
Choroid
Left Ø8RB
Right Ø8RA
Clavicle
Left ØPRB
Right ØPR9
Coccyx ØQRS
Conjunctiva
Left Ø8RTX
Right Ø8RSX
Cornea
Left Ø8R9
Right Ø8R8
Diaphragm ØBRT
Disc
Cervical Vertebral ØRR3Ø
Cervicothoracic Vertebral ØRR5Ø
Lumbar Vertebral ØSR2Ø
Lumbosacral ØSR4Ø
Thoracic Vertebral ØRR9Ø
Thoracolumbar Vertebral ØRRBØ
Duct
Common Bile ØFR9
Cystic ØFR8
Hepatic
Common ØFR7
Left ØFR6
Right ØFR5
Lacrimal
Left Ø8RY
Right Ø8RX
Pancreatic ØFRD
Accessory ØFRF
Parotid
Left ØCRC
Right ØCRB
Dura Mater ØØR2
Ear
External
Bilateral Ø9R2
Left Ø9R1
Right Ø9RØ
Inner
Left Ø9REØ
Right Ø9RDØ
Middle
Left Ø9R6Ø
Right Ø9R5Ø
Epiglottis ØCRR

Replacement — *continued*
Esophagus ØDR5
Eye
Left Ø8R1
Right Ø8RØ
Eyelid
Lower
Left Ø8RR
Right Ø8RQ
Upper
Left Ø8RP
Right Ø8RN
Femoral Shaft
Left ØQR9
Right ØQR8
Femur
Lower
Left ØQRC
Right ØQRB
Upper
Left ØQR7
Right ØQR6
Fibula
Left ØQRK
Right ØQRJ
Finger Nail ØHRQX
Gingiva
Lower ØCR6
Upper ØCR5
Glenoid Cavity
Left ØPR8
Right ØPR7
Hair ØHRSX
Humeral Head
Left ØPRD
Right ØPRC
Humeral Shaft
Left ØPRG
Right ØPRF
Iris
Left Ø8RD3
Right Ø8RC3
Joint
Acromioclavicular
Left ØRRHØ
Right ØRRGØ
Ankle
Left ØSRG
Right ØSRF
Carpal
Left ØRRRØ
Right ØRRQØ
Carpometacarpal
Left ØRRTØ
Right ØRRSØ
Cervical Vertebral ØRR1Ø
Cervicothoracic Vertebral ØRR4Ø
Coccygeal ØSR6Ø
Elbow
Left ØRRMØ
Right ØRRLØ
Finger Phalangeal
Left ØRRXØ
Right ØRRWØ
Hip
Left ØSRB
Acetabular Surface ØSRE
Femoral Surface ØSRS
Right ØSR9
Acetabular Surface ØSRA
Femoral Surface ØSRR
Knee
Left ØSRD
Femoral Surface ØSRU
Tibial Surface ØSRW
Right ØSRC
Femoral Surface ØSRT
Tibial Surface ØSRV
Lumbar Vertebral ØSRØØ
Lumbosacral ØSR3Ø
Metacarpophalangeal
Left ØRRVØ
Right ØRRUØ
Metatarsal-Phalangeal
Left ØSRNØ
Right ØSRMØ
Occipital-cervical ØRRØØ
Sacrococcygeal ØSR5Ø

Replacement — *continued*
Joint — *continued*
Sacroiliac
Left ØSR8Ø
Right ØSR7Ø
Shoulder
Left ØRRK
Right ØRRJ
Sternoclavicular
Left ØRRFØ
Right ØRREØ
Tarsal
Left ØSRJØ
Right ØSRHØ
Tarsometatarsal
Left ØSRLØ
Right ØSRKØ
Temporomandibular
Left ØRRDØ
Right ØRRCØ
Thoracic Vertebral ØRR6Ø
Thoracolumbar Vertebral ØRRAØ
Toe Phalangeal
Left ØSRQØ
Right ØSRPØ
Wrist
Left ØRRPØ
Right ØRRNØ
Kidney Pelvis
Left ØTR4
Right ØTR3
Larynx ØCRS
Lens
Left Ø8RK3ØZ
Right Ø8RJ3ØZ
Lip
Lower ØCR1
Upper ØCRØ
Mandible
Left ØNRV
Right ØNRT
Maxilla ØNRR
Mesentery ØDRV
Metacarpal
Left ØPRQ
Right ØPRP
Metatarsal
Left ØQRP
Right ØQRN
Muscle
Abdomen
Left ØKRL
Right ØKRK
Facial ØKR1
Foot
Left ØKRW
Right ØKRV
Hand
Left ØKRD
Right ØKRC
Head ØKRØ
Hip
Left ØKRP
Right ØKRN
Lower Arm and Wrist
Left ØKRB
Right ØKR9
Lower Leg
Left ØKRT
Right ØKRS
Neck
Left ØKR3
Right ØKR2
Papillary Ø2RD
Perineum ØKRM
Shoulder
Left ØKR6
Right ØKR5
Thorax
Left ØKRJ
Right ØKRH
Tongue, Palate, Pharynx ØKR4
Trunk
Left ØKRG
Right ØKRF
Upper Arm
Left ØKR8
Right ØKR7

Replacement — *continued*
Muscle — *continued*
Upper Leg
Left ØKRR
Right ØKRQ
Nasal Mucosa and Soft Tissue Ø9RK
Nasopharynx Ø9RN
Nerve
Abducens ØØRL
Accessory ØØRR
Acoustic ØØRN
Cervical Ø1R1
Facial ØØRM
Femoral Ø1RD
Glossopharyngeal ØØRP
Hypoglossal ØØRS
Lumbar Ø1RB
Median Ø1R5
Oculomotor ØØRH
Olfactory ØØRF
Optic ØØRG
Peroneal Ø1RH
Phrenic Ø1R2
Pudendal Ø1RC
Radial Ø1R6
Sacral Ø1RR
Sciatic Ø1RF
Thoracic Ø1R8
Tibial Ø1RG
Trigeminal ØØRK
Trochlear ØØRJ
Ulnar Ø1R4
Vagus ØØRQ
Nipple
Left ØHRX
Right ØHRW
Omentum ØDRU
Orbit
Left ØNRQ
Right ØNRP
Palate
Hard ØCR2
Soft ØCR3
Patella
Left ØQRF
Right ØQRD
Pericardium Ø2RN
Peritoneum ØDRW
Phalanx
Finger
Left ØPRV
Right ØPRT
Thumb
Left ØPRS
Right ØPRR
Toe
Left ØQRR
Right ØQRQ
Pharynx ØCRM
Radius
Left ØPRJ
Right ØPRH
Retinal Vessel
Left Ø8RH3
Right Ø8RG3
Ribs
1 to 2 ØPR1
3 or More ØPR2
Sacrum ØQR1
Scapula
Left ØPR6
Right ØPR5
Sclera
Left Ø8R7X
Right Ø8R6X
Septum
Atrial Ø2R5
Nasal Ø9RM
Ventricular Ø2RM
Skin
Abdomen ØHR7
Back ØHR6
Buttock ØHR8
Chest ØHR5
Ear
Left ØHR3
Right ØHR2
Face ØHR1

Replacement — *continued*
Skin — *continued*
Foot
Left ØHRN
Right ØHRM
Hand
Left ØHRG
Right ØHRF
Inguinal ØHRA
Lower Arm
Left ØHRE
Right ØHRD
Lower Leg
Left ØHRL
Right ØHRK
Neck ØHR4
Perineum ØHR9
Scalp ØHRØ
Upper Arm
Left ØHRC
Right ØHRB
Upper Leg
Left ØHRJ
Right ØHRH
Skin Substitute, Porcine Liver Derived XHRPXL2
Skull ØNRØ
Spinal Meninges ØØRT
Sternum ØPRØ
Subcutaneous Tissue and Fascia
Abdomen ØJR8
Back ØJR7
Buttock ØJR9
Chest ØJR6
Face ØJR1
Foot
Left ØJRR
Right ØJRQ
Hand
Left ØJRK
Right ØJRJ
Lower Arm
Left ØJRH
Right ØJRG
Lower Leg
Left ØJRP
Right ØJRN
Neck
Left ØJR5
Right ØJR4
Pelvic Region ØJRC
Perineum ØJRB
Scalp ØJRØ
Upper Arm
Left ØJRF
Right ØJRD
Upper Leg
Left ØJRM
Right ØJRL
Tarsal
Left ØQRM
Right ØQRL
Tendon
Abdomen
Left ØLRG
Right ØLRF
Ankle
Left ØLRT
Right ØLRS
Foot
Left ØLRW
Right ØLRV
Hand
Left ØLR8
Right ØLR7
Head and Neck ØLRØ
Hip
Left ØLRK
Right ØLRJ
Knee
Left ØLRR
Right ØLRQ
Lower Arm and Wrist
Left ØLR6
Right ØLR5
Lower Leg
Left ØLRP
Right ØLRN
Perineum ØLRH

Replacement — *continued*
Tendon — *continued*
Shoulder
Left ØLR2
Right ØLR1
Thorax
Left ØLRD
Right ØLRC
Trunk
Left ØLRB
Right ØLR9
Upper Arm
Left ØLR4
Right ØLR3
Upper Leg
Left ØLRM
Right ØLRL
Testis
Bilateral ØVRCØJZ
Left ØVRBØJZ
Right ØVR9ØJZ
Thumb
Left ØXRM
Right ØXRL
Tibia
Left ØQRH
Right ØQRG
Toe Nail ØHRRX
Tongue ØCR7
Tooth
Lower ØCRX
Upper ØCRW
Trachea ØBR1
Turbinate, Nasal Ø9RL
Tympanic Membrane
Left Ø9R8
Right Ø9R7
Ulna
Left ØPRL
Right ØPRK
Ureter
Left ØTR7
Right ØTR6
Urethra ØTRD
Uvula ØCRN
Valve
Aortic Ø2RF
Mitral Ø2RG
Pulmonary Ø2RH
Tricuspid Ø2RJ
Vein
Axillary
Left Ø5R8
Right Ø5R7
Azygos Ø5RØ
Basilic
Left Ø5RC
Right Ø5RB
Brachial
Left Ø5RA
Right Ø5R9
Cephalic
Left Ø5RF
Right Ø5RD
Colic Ø6R7
Common Iliac
Left Ø6RD
Right Ø6RC
Esophageal Ø6R3
External Iliac
Left Ø6RG
Right Ø6RF
External Jugular
Left Ø5RQ
Right Ø5RP
Face
Left Ø5RV
Right Ø5RT
Femoral
Left Ø6RN
Right Ø6RM
Foot
Left Ø6RV
Right Ø6RT
Gastric Ø6R2
Hand
Left Ø5RH
Right Ø5RG
Hemiazygos Ø5R1

Replacement — *continued*
Vein — *continued*
Hepatic Ø6R4
Hypogastric
Left Ø6RJ
Right Ø6RH
Inferior Mesenteric Ø6R6
Innominate
Left Ø5R4
Right Ø5R3
Internal Jugular
Left Ø5RN
Right Ø5RM
Intracranial Ø5RL
Lower Ø6RY
Portal Ø6R8
Pulmonary
Left Ø2RT
Right Ø2RS
Renal
Left Ø6RB
Right Ø6R9
Saphenous
Left Ø6RQ
Right Ø6RP
Splenic Ø6R1
Subclavian
Left Ø5R6
Right Ø5R5
Superior Mesenteric Ø6R5
Upper Ø5RY
Vertebral
Left Ø5RS
Right Ø5RR
Vena Cava
Inferior Ø6RØ
Superior Ø2RV
Ventricle
Left Ø2RL
Right Ø2RK
Vertebra
Cervical ØPR3
Lumbar ØQRØ
Thoracic ØPR4
Vitreous
Left Ø8R53
Right Ø8R43
Vocal Cord
Left ØCRV
Right ØCRT
Zooplastic Tissue, Rapid Deployment Technique X2RF
Replacement, hip
Partial or total *see* Replacement, Lower Joints ØSR
Resurfacing only *see* Supplement, Lower Joints ØSU
Replantation *see* Reposition
Replantation, scalp *see* Reattachment, Skin, Scalp ØHMØ
Reposition
Acetabulum
Left ØQS5
Right ØQS4
Ampulla of Vater ØFSC
Anus ØDSQ
Aorta
Abdominal Ø4SØ
Thoracic
Ascending/Arch Ø2SXØZZ
Descending Ø2SWØZZ
Artery
Anterior Tibial
Left Ø4SQ
Right Ø4SP
Axillary
Left Ø3S6
Right Ø3S5
Brachial
Left Ø3S8
Right Ø3S7
Celiac Ø4S1
Colic
Left Ø4S7
Middle Ø4S8
Right Ø4S6
Common Carotid
Left Ø3SJ
Right Ø3SH

Reposition — *continued*
- Artery — *continued*
  - Common Iliac
    - Left Ø4SD
    - Right Ø4SC
  - Coronary
    - One Artery Ø2SØØZZ
    - Two Arteries Ø2S1ØZZ
  - External Carotid
    - Left Ø3SN
    - Right Ø3SM
  - External Iliac
    - Left Ø4SJ
    - Right Ø4SH
  - Face Ø3SR
  - Femoral
    - Left Ø4SL
    - Right Ø4SK
  - Foot
    - Left Ø4SW
    - Right Ø4SV
  - Gastric Ø4S2
  - Hand
    - Left Ø3SF
    - Right Ø3SD
  - Hepatic Ø4S3
  - Inferior Mesenteric Ø4SB
  - Innominate Ø3S2
  - Internal Carotid
    - Left Ø3SL
    - Right Ø3SK
  - Internal Iliac
    - Left Ø4SF
    - Right Ø4SE
  - Internal Mammary
    - Left Ø3S1
    - Right Ø3SØ
  - Intracranial Ø3SG
  - Lower Ø4SY
  - Peroneal
    - Left Ø4SU
    - Right Ø4ST
  - Popliteal
    - Left Ø4SN
    - Right Ø4SM
  - Posterior Tibial
    - Left Ø4SS
    - Right Ø4SR
  - Pulmonary
    - Left Ø2SRØZZ
    - Right Ø2SQØZZ
  - Pulmonary Trunk Ø2SPØZZ
  - Radial
    - Left Ø3SC
    - Right Ø3SB
  - Renal
    - Left Ø4SA
    - Right Ø4S9
  - Splenic Ø4S4
  - Subclavian
    - Left Ø3S4
    - Right Ø3S3
  - Superior Mesenteric Ø4S5
  - Temporal
    - Left Ø3ST
    - Right Ø3SS
  - Thyroid
    - Left Ø3SV
    - Right Ø3SU
  - Ulnar
    - Left Ø3SA
    - Right Ø3S9
  - Upper Ø3SY
  - Vertebral
    - Left Ø3SQ
    - Right Ø3SP
- Auditory Ossicle
  - Left Ø9SA
  - Right Ø9S9
- Bladder ØTSB
- Bladder Neck ØTSC
- Bone
  - Ethmoid
    - Left ØNSG
    - Right ØNSF
  - Frontal ØNS1
  - Hyoid ØNSX
  - Lacrimal
    - Left ØNSJ

Reposition — *continued*
- Bone — *continued*
  - Lacrimal — *continued*
    - Right ØNSH
  - Nasal ØNSB
  - Occipital ØNS7
  - Palatine
    - Left ØNSL
    - Right ØNSK
  - Parietal
    - Left ØNS4
    - Right ØNS3
  - Pelvic
    - Left ØQS3
    - Right ØQS2
  - Sphenoid ØNSC
  - Temporal
    - Left ØNS6
    - Right ØNS5
  - Zygomatic
    - Left ØNSN
    - Right ØNSM
- Breast
  - Bilateral ØHSVØZZ
  - Left ØHSUØZZ
  - Right ØHSTØZZ
- Bronchus
  - Lingula ØBS9ØZZ
  - Lower Lobe
    - Left ØBSBØZZ
    - Right ØBS6ØZZ
  - Main
    - Left ØBS7ØZZ
    - Right ØBS3ØZZ
  - Middle Lobe, Right ØBS5ØZZ
  - Upper Lobe
    - Left ØBS8ØZZ
    - Right ØBS4ØZZ
- Bursa and Ligament
  - Abdomen
    - Left ØMSJ
    - Right ØMSH
  - Ankle
    - Left ØMSR
    - Right ØMSQ
  - Elbow
    - Left ØMS4
    - Right ØMS3
  - Foot
    - Left ØMST
    - Right ØMSS
  - Hand
    - Left ØMS8
    - Right ØMS7
  - Head and Neck ØMSØ
  - Hip
    - Left ØMSM
    - Right ØMSL
  - Knee
    - Left ØMSP
    - Right ØMSN
  - Lower Extremity
    - Left ØMSW
    - Right ØMSV
  - Perineum ØMSK
  - Rib(s) ØMSG
  - Shoulder
    - Left ØMS2
    - Right ØMS1
  - Spine
    - Lower ØMSD
    - Upper ØMSC
  - Sternum ØMSF
  - Upper Extremity
    - Left ØMSB
    - Right ØMS9
  - Wrist
    - Left ØMS6
    - Right ØMS5
- Carina ØBS2ØZZ
- Carpal
  - Left ØPSN
  - Right ØPSM
- Cecum ØDSH
- Cervix ØUSC
- Clavicle
  - Left ØPSB
  - Right ØPS9
- Coccyx ØQSS

Reposition — *continued*
- Colon
  - Ascending ØDSK
  - Descending ØDSM
  - Sigmoid ØDSN
  - Transverse ØDSL
- Cord
  - Bilateral ØVSH
  - Left ØVSG
  - Right ØVSF
- Cul-de-sac ØUSF
- Diaphragm ØBSTØZZ
- Duct
  - Common Bile ØFS9
  - Cystic ØFS8
  - Hepatic
    - Common ØFS7
    - Left ØFS6
    - Right ØFS5
  - Lacrimal
    - Left Ø8SY
    - Right Ø8SX
  - Pancreatic ØFSD
    - Accessory ØFSF
  - Parotid
    - Left ØCSC
    - Right ØCSB
- Duodenum ØDS9
- Ear
  - Bilateral Ø9S2
  - Left Ø9S1
  - Right Ø9SØ
- Epiglottis ØCSR
- Esophagus ØDS5
- Eustachian Tube
  - Left Ø9SG
  - Right Ø9SF
- Eyelid
  - Lower
    - Left Ø8SR
    - Right Ø8SQ
  - Upper
    - Left Ø8SP
    - Right Ø8SN
- Fallopian Tube
  - Left ØUS6
  - Right ØUS5
- Fallopian Tubes, Bilateral ØUS7
- Femoral Shaft
  - Left ØQS9
  - Right ØQS8
- Femur
  - Lower
    - Left ØQSC
    - Right ØQSB
  - Upper
    - Left ØQS7
    - Right ØQS6
- Fibula
  - Left ØQSK
  - Right ØQSJ
- Gallbladder ØFS4
- Gland
  - Adrenal
    - Left ØGS2
    - Right ØGS3
  - Lacrimal
    - Left Ø8SW
    - Right Ø8SV
- Glenoid Cavity
  - Left ØPS8
  - Right ØPS7
- Hair ØHSSXZZ
- Humeral Head
  - Left ØPSD
  - Right ØPSC
- Humeral Shaft
  - Left ØPSG
  - Right ØPSF
- Ileum ØDSB
- Intestine
  - Large ØDSE
  - Small ØDS8
- Iris
  - Left Ø8SD3ZZ
  - Right Ø8SC3ZZ
- Jejunum ØDSA

Reposition — *continued*
Joint
Acromioclavicular
Left ØRSH
Right ØRSG
Ankle
Left ØSSG
Right ØSSF
Carpal
Left ØRSR
Right ØRSQ
Carpometacarpal
Left ØRST
Right ØRSS
Cervical Vertebral ØRS1
Cervicothoracic Vertebral ØRS4
Coccygeal ØSS6
Elbow
Left ØRSM
Right ØRSL
Finger Phalangeal
Left ØRSX
Right ØRSW
Hip
Left ØSSB
Right ØSS9
Knee
Left ØSSD
Right ØSSC
Lumbar Vertebral ØSSØ
Lumbosacral ØSS3
Metacarpophalangeal
Left ØRSV
Right ØRSU
Metatarsal-Phalangeal
Left ØSSN
Right ØSSM
Occipital-cervical ØRSØ
Sacrococcygeal ØSS5
Sacroiliac
Left ØSS8
Right ØSS7
Shoulder
Left ØRSK
Right ØRSJ
Sternoclavicular
Left ØRSF
Right ØRSE
Tarsal
Left ØSSJ
Right ØSSH
Tarsometatarsal
Left ØSSL
Right ØSSK
Temporomandibular
Left ØRSD
Right ØRSC
Thoracic Vertebral ØRS6
Thoracolumbar Vertebral ØRSA
Toe Phalangeal
Left ØSSQ
Right ØSSP
Wrist
Left ØRSP
Right ØRSN
Kidney
Left ØTS1
Right ØTSØ
Kidney Pelvis
Left ØTS4
Right ØTS3
Kidneys, Bilateral ØTS2
Lens
Left Ø8SK3ZZ
Right Ø8SJ3ZZ
Lip
Lower ØCS1
Upper ØCSØ
Liver ØFSØ
Lung
Left ØBSLØZZ
Lower Lobe
Left ØBSJØZZ
Right ØBSFØZZ
Middle Lobe, Right ØBSDØZZ
Right ØBSKØZZ
Upper Lobe
Left ØBSGØZZ
Right ØBSCØZZ

Reposition — *continued*
Lung Lingula ØBSHØZZ
Mandible
Left ØNSV
Right ØNST
Maxilla ØNSR
Metacarpal
Left ØPSQ
Right ØPSP
Metatarsal
Left ØQSP
Right ØQSN
Muscle
Abdomen
Left ØKSL
Right ØKSK
Extraocular
Left Ø8SM
Right Ø8SL
Facial ØKS1
Foot
Left ØKSW
Right ØKSV
Hand
Left ØKSD
Right ØKSC
Head ØKSØ
Hip
Left ØKSP
Right ØKSN
Lower Arm and Wrist
Left ØKSB
Right ØKS9
Lower Leg
Left ØKST
Right ØKSS
Neck
Left ØKS3
Right ØKS2
Perineum ØKSM
Shoulder
Left ØKS6
Right ØKS5
Thorax
Left ØKSJ
Right ØKSH
Tongue, Palate, Pharynx ØKS4
Trunk
Left ØKSG
Right ØKSF
Upper Arm
Left ØKS8
Right ØKS7
Upper Leg
Left ØKSR
Right ØKSQ
Nasal Mucosa and Soft Tissue Ø9SK
Nerve
Abducens ØØSL
Accessory ØØSR
Acoustic ØØSN
Brachial Plexus Ø1S3
Cervical Ø1S1
Cervical Plexus Ø1SØ
Facial ØØSM
Femoral Ø1SD
Glossopharyngeal ØØSP
Hypoglossal ØØSS
Lumbar Ø1SB
Lumbar Plexus Ø1S9
Lumbosacral Plexus Ø1SA
Median Ø1S5
Oculomotor ØØSH
Olfactory ØØSF
Optic ØØSG
Peroneal Ø1SH
Phrenic Ø1S2
Pudendal Ø1SC
Radial Ø1S6
Sacral Ø1SR
Sacral Plexus Ø1SQ
Sciatic Ø1SF
Thoracic Ø1S8
Tibial Ø1SG
Trigeminal ØØSK
Trochlear ØØSJ
Ulnar Ø1S4
Vagus ØØSQ

Reposition — *continued*
Nipple
Left ØHSXXZZ
Right ØHSWXZZ
Orbit
Left ØNSQ
Right ØNSP
Ovary
Bilateral ØUS2
Left ØUS1
Right ØUSØ
Palate
Hard ØCS2
Soft ØCS3
Pancreas ØFSG
Parathyroid Gland ØGSR
Inferior
Left ØGSP
Right ØGSN
Multiple ØGSQ
Superior
Left ØGSM
Right ØGSL
Patella
Left ØQSF
Right ØQSD
Phalanx
Finger
Left ØPSV
Right ØPST
Thumb
Left ØPSS
Right ØPSR
Toe
Left ØQSR
Right ØQSQ
Products of Conception 1ØSØ
Ectopic 1ØS2
Radius
Left ØPSJ
Right ØPSH
Rectum ØDSP
Retinal Vessel
Left Ø8SH3ZZ
Right Ø8SG3ZZ
Ribs
1 to 2 ØPS1
3 or More ØPS2
Sacrum ØQS1
Scapula
Left ØPS6
Right ØPS5
Septum, Nasal Ø9SM
Sesamoid Bone(s) 1st Toe
see Reposition, Metatarsal, Left ØQSP
see Reposition, Metatarsal, Right ØQSN
Skull ØNSØ
Spinal Cord
Cervical ØØSW
Lumbar ØØSY
Thoracic ØØSX
Spleen Ø7SPØZZ
Sternum ØPSØ
Stomach ØDS6
Tarsal
Left ØQSM
Right ØQSL
Tendon
Abdomen
Left ØLSG
Right ØLSF
Ankle
Left ØLST
Right ØLSS
Foot
Left ØLSW
Right ØLSV
Hand
Left ØLS8
Right ØLS7
Head and Neck ØLSØ
Hip
Left ØLSK
Right ØLSJ
Knee
Left ØLSR
Right ØLSQ
Lower Arm and Wrist
Left ØLS6

Reposition — *continued*
Tendon — *continued*
Lower Arm and Wrist — *continued*
Right ØLS5
Lower Leg
Left ØLSP
Right ØLSN
Perineum ØLSH
Shoulder
Left ØLS2
Right ØLS1
Thorax
Left ØLSD
Right ØLSC
Trunk
Left ØLSB
Right ØLS9
Upper Arm
Left ØLS4
Right ØLS3
Upper Leg
Left ØLSM
Right ØLSL
Testis
Bilateral ØVSC
Left ØVSB
Right ØVS9
Thymus Ø7SMØZZ
Thyroid Gland
Left Lobe ØGSG
Right Lobe ØGSH
Tibia
Left ØQSH
Right ØQSG
Tongue ØCS7
Tooth
Lower ØCSX
Upper ØCSW
Trachea ØBS1ØZZ
Turbinate, Nasal Ø9SL
Tympanic Membrane
Left Ø9S8
Right Ø9S7
Ulna
Left ØPSL
Right ØPSK
Ureter
Left ØTS7
Right ØTS6
Ureters, Bilateral ØTS8
Urethra ØTSD
Uterine Supporting Structure ØUS4
Uterus ØUS9
Uvula ØCSN
Vagina ØUSG
Vein
Axillary
Left Ø5S8
Right Ø5S7
Azygos Ø5SØ
Basilic
Left Ø5SC
Right Ø5SB
Brachial
Left Ø5SA
Right Ø5S9
Cephalic
Left Ø5SF
Right Ø5SD
Colic Ø6S7
Common Iliac
Left Ø6SD
Right Ø6SC
Esophageal Ø6S3
External Iliac
Left Ø6SG
Right Ø6SF
External Jugular
Left Ø5SQ
Right Ø5SP
Face
Left Ø5SV
Right Ø5ST
Femoral
Left Ø6SN
Right Ø6SM
Foot
Left Ø6SV
Right Ø6ST

Reposition — *continued*
Vein — *continued*
Gastric Ø6S2
Hand
Left Ø5SH
Right Ø5SG
Hemiazygos Ø5S1
Hepatic Ø6S4
Hypogastric
Left Ø6SJ
Right Ø6SH
Inferior Mesenteric Ø6S6
Innominate
Left Ø5S4
Right Ø5S3
Internal Jugular
Left Ø5SN
Right Ø5SM
Intracranial Ø5SL
Lower Ø6SY
Portal Ø6S8
Pulmonary
Left Ø2STØZZ
Right Ø2SSØZZ
Renal
Left Ø6SB
Right Ø6S9
Saphenous
Left Ø6SQ
Right Ø6SP
Splenic Ø6S1
Subclavian
Left Ø5S6
Right Ø5S5
Superior Mesenteric Ø6S5
Upper Ø5SY
Vertebral
Left Ø5SS
Right Ø5SR
Vena Cava
Inferior Ø6SØ
Superior Ø2SVØZZ
Vertebra
Cervical ØPS3
Magnetically Controlled Growth Rod(s) XNS3
Lumbar ØQSØ
Magnetically Controlled Growth Rod(s) XNSØ
Thoracic ØPS4
Magnetically Controlled Growth Rod(s) XNS4
Vocal Cord
Left ØCSV
Right ØCST

Resection
Acetabulum
Left ØQT5ØZZ
Right ØQT4ØZZ
Adenoids ØCTQ
Ampulla of Vater ØFTC
Anal Sphincter ØDTR
Anus ØDTQ
Aortic Body ØGTD
Appendix ØDTJ
Auditory Ossicle
Left Ø9TA
Right Ø9T9
Bladder ØTTB
Bladder Neck ØTTC
Bone
Ethmoid
Left ØNTGØZZ
Right ØNTFØZZ
Frontal ØNT1ØZZ
Hyoid ØNTXØZZ
Lacrimal
Left ØNTJØZZ
Right ØNTHØZZ
Nasal ØNTBØZZ
Occipital ØNT7ØZZ
Palatine
Left ØNTLØZZ
Right ØNTKØZZ
Parietal
Left ØNT4ØZZ
Right ØNT3ØZZ
Pelvic
Left ØQT3ØZZ

Resection — *continued*
Bone — *continued*
Pelvic — *continued*
Right ØQT2ØZZ
Sphenoid ØNTCØZZ
Temporal
Left ØNT6ØZZ
Right ØNT5ØZZ
Zygomatic
Left ØNTNØZZ
Right ØNTMØZZ
Breast
Bilateral ØHTVØZZ
Left ØHTUØZZ
Right ØHTTØZZ
Supernumerary ØHTYØZZ
Bronchus
Lingula ØBT9
Lower Lobe
Left ØBTB
Right ØBT6
Main
Left ØBT7
Right ØBT3
Middle Lobe, Right ØBT5
Upper Lobe
Left ØBT8
Right ØBT4
Bursa and Ligament
Abdomen
Left ØMTJ
Right ØMTH
Ankle
Left ØMTR
Right ØMTQ
Elbow
Left ØMT4
Right ØMT3
Foot
Left ØMTT
Right ØMTS
Hand
Left ØMT8
Right ØMT7
Head and Neck ØMTØ
Hip
Left ØMTM
Right ØMTL
Knee
Left ØMTP
Right ØMTN
Lower Extremity
Left ØMTW
Right ØMTV
Perineum ØMTK
Rib(s) ØMTG
Shoulder
Left ØMT2
Right ØMT1
Spine
Lower ØMTD
Upper ØMTC
Sternum ØMTF
Upper Extremity
Left ØMTB
Right ØMT9
Wrist
Left ØMT6
Right ØMT5
Carina ØBT2
Carotid Bodies, Bilateral ØGT8
Carotid Body
Left ØGT6
Right ØGT7
Carpal
Left ØPTNØZZ
Right ØPTMØZZ
Cecum ØDTH
Cerebral Hemisphere ØØT7
Cervix ØUTC
Chordae Tendineae Ø2T9
Cisterna Chyli Ø7TL
Clavicle
Left ØPTBØZZ
Right ØPT9ØZZ
Clitoris ØUTJ
Coccygeal Glomus ØGTB
Coccyx ØQTSØZZ

Resection — *continued*
Colon
Ascending ØDTK
Descending ØDTM
Sigmoid ØDTN
Transverse ØDTL
Conduction Mechanism Ø2T8
Cord
Bilateral ØVTH
Left ØVTG
Right ØVTF
Cornea
Left Ø8T9XZZ
Right Ø8T8XZZ
Cul-de-sac ØUTF
Diaphragm ØBTT
Disc
Cervical Vertebral ØRT3ØZZ
Cervicothoracic Vertebral ØRT5ØZZ
Lumbar Vertebral ØST2ØZZ
Lumbosacral ØST4ØZZ
Thoracic Vertebral ØRT9ØZZ
Thoracolumbar Vertebral ØRTBØZZ
Duct
Common Bile ØFT9
Cystic ØFT8
Hepatic
Common ØFT7
Left ØFT6
Right ØFT5
Lacrimal
Left Ø8TY
Right Ø8TX
Pancreatic ØFTD
Accessory ØFTF
Parotid
Left ØCTCØZZ
Right ØCTBØZZ
Duodenum ØDT9
Ear
External
Left Ø9T1
Right Ø9TØ
Inner
Left Ø9TE
Right Ø9TD
Middle
Left Ø9T6
Right Ø9T5
Epididymis
Bilateral ØVTL
Left ØVTK
Right ØVTJ
Epiglottis ØCTR
Esophagogastric Junction ØDT4
Esophagus ØDT5
Lower ØDT3
Middle ØDT2
Upper ØDT1
Eustachian Tube
Left Ø9TG
Right Ø9TF
Eye
Left Ø8T1XZZ
Right Ø8TØXZZ
Eyelid
Lower
Left Ø8TR
Right Ø8TQ
Upper
Left Ø8TP
Right Ø8TN
Fallopian Tube
Left ØUT6
Right ØUT5
Fallopian Tubes, Bilateral ØUT7
Femoral Shaft
Left ØQT9ØZZ
Right ØQT8ØZZ
Femur
Lower
Left ØQTCØZZ
Right ØQTBØZZ
Upper
Left ØQT7ØZZ
Right ØQT6ØZZ
Fibula
Left ØQTKØZZ
Right ØQTJØZZ

Resection — *continued*
Finger Nail ØHTQXZZ
Gallbladder ØFT4
Gland
Adrenal
Bilateral ØGT4
Left ØGT2
Right ØGT3
Lacrimal
Left Ø8TW
Right Ø8TV
Minor Salivary ØCTJØZZ
Parotid
Left ØCT9ØZZ
Right ØCT8ØZZ
Pituitary ØGTØ
Sublingual
Left ØCTFØZZ
Right ØCTDØZZ
Submaxillary
Left ØCTHØZZ
Right ØCTGØZZ
Vestibular ØUTL
Glenoid Cavity
Left ØPT8ØZZ
Right ØPT7ØZZ
Glomus Jugulare ØGTC
Humeral Head
Left ØPTDØZZ
Right ØPTCØZZ
Humeral Shaft
Left ØPTGØZZ
Right ØPTFØZZ
Hymen ØUTK
Ileocecal Valve ØDTC
Ileum ØDTB
Intestine
Large ØDTE
Left ØDTG
Right ØDTF
Small ØDT8
Iris
Left Ø8TD3ZZ
Right Ø8TC3ZZ
Jejunum ØDTA
Joint
Acromioclavicular
Left ØRTHØZZ
Right ØRTGØZZ
Ankle
Left ØSTGØZZ
Right ØSTFØZZ
Carpal
Left ØRTRØZZ
Right ØRTQØZZ
Carpometacarpal
Left ØRTTØZZ
Right ØRTSØZZ
Cervicothoracic Vertebral ØRT4ØZZ
Coccygeal ØST6ØZZ
Elbow
Left ØRTMØZZ
Right ØRTLØZZ
Finger Phalangeal
Left ØRTXØZZ
Right ØRTWØZZ
Hip
Left ØSTBØZZ
Right ØST9ØZZ
Knee
Left ØSTDØZZ
Right ØSTCØZZ
Metacarpophalangeal
Left ØRTVØZZ
Right ØRTUØZZ
Metatarsal-Phalangeal
Left ØSTNØZZ
Right ØSTMØZZ
Sacrococcygeal ØST5ØZZ
Sacroiliac
Left ØST8ØZZ
Right ØST7ØZZ
Shoulder
Left ØRTKØZZ
Right ØRTJØZZ
Sternoclavicular
Left ØRTFØZZ
Right ØRTEØZZ

Resection — *continued*
Joint — *continued*
Tarsal
Left ØSTJØZZ
Right ØSTHØZZ
Tarsometatarsal
Left ØSTLØZZ
Right ØSTKØZZ
Temporomandibular
Left ØRTDØZZ
Right ØRTCØZZ
Toe Phalangeal
Left ØSTQØZZ
Right ØSTPØZZ
Wrist
Left ØRTPØZZ
Right ØRTNØZZ
Kidney
Left ØTT1
Right ØTTØ
Kidney Pelvis
Left ØTT4
Right ØTT3
Kidneys, Bilateral ØTT2
Larynx ØCTS
Lens
Left Ø8TK3ZZ
Right Ø8TJ3ZZ
Lip
Lower ØCT1
Upper ØCTØ
Liver ØFTØ
Left Lobe ØFT2
Right Lobe ØFT1
Lung
Bilateral ØBTM
Left ØBTL
Lower Lobe
Left ØBTJ
Right ØBTF
Middle Lobe, Right ØBTD
Right ØBTK
Upper Lobe
Left ØBTG
Right ØBTC
Lung Lingula ØBTH
Lymphatic
Aortic Ø7TD
Axillary
Left Ø7T6
Right Ø7T5
Head Ø7TØ
Inguinal
Left Ø7TJ
Right Ø7TH
Internal Mammary
Left Ø7T9
Right Ø7T8
Lower Extremity
Left Ø7TG
Right Ø7TF
Mesenteric Ø7TB
Neck
Left Ø7T2
Right Ø7T1
Pelvis Ø7TC
Thoracic Duct Ø7TK
Thorax Ø7T7
Upper Extremity
Left Ø7T4
Right Ø7T3
Mandible
Left ØNTVØZZ
Right ØNTTØZZ
Maxilla ØNTRØZZ
Metacarpal
Left ØPTQØZZ
Right ØPTPØZZ
Metatarsal
Left ØQTPØZZ
Right ØQTNØZZ
Muscle
Abdomen
Left ØKTL
Right ØKTK
Extraocular
Left Ø8TM
Right Ø8TL
Facial ØKT1

Subterms under main terms may continue to next column or page

Resection — *continued*
Muscle — *continued*
Foot
Left ØKTW
Right ØKTV
Hand
Left ØKTD
Right ØKTC
Head ØKTØ
Hip
Left ØKTP
Right ØKTN
Lower Arm and Wrist
Left ØKTB
Right ØKT9
Lower Leg
Left ØKTT
Right ØKTS
Neck
Left ØKT3
Right ØKT2
Papillary Ø2TD
Perineum ØKTM
Shoulder
Left ØKT6
Right ØKT5
Thorax
Left ØKTJ
Right ØKTH
Tongue, Palate, Pharynx ØKT4
Trunk
Left ØKTG
Right ØKTF
Upper Arm
Left ØKT8
Right ØKT7
Upper Leg
Left ØKTR
Right ØKTQ
Nasal Mucosa and Soft Tissue Ø9TK
Nasopharynx Ø9TN
Nipple
Left ØHTXXZZ
Right ØHTWXZZ
Omentum ØDTU
Orbit
Left ØNTQØZZ
Right ØNTPØZZ
Ovary
Bilateral ØUT2
Left ØUT1
Right ØUTØ
Palate
Hard ØCT2
Soft ØCT3
Pancreas ØFTG
Para-aortic Body ØGT9
Paraganglion Extremity ØGTF
Parathyroid Gland ØGTR
Inferior
Left ØGTP
Right ØGTN
Multiple ØGTQ
Superior
Left ØGTM
Right ØGTL
Patella
Left ØQTFØZZ
Right ØQTDØZZ
Penis ØVTS
Pericardium Ø2TN
Phalanx
Finger
Left ØPTVØZZ
Right ØPTTØZZ
Thumb
Left ØPTSØZZ
Right ØPTRØZZ
Toe
Left ØQTRØZZ
Right ØQTQØZZ
Pharynx ØCTM
Pineal Body ØGT1
Prepuce ØVTT
Products of Conception, Ectopic 1ØT2
Prostate ØVTØ
Radius
Left ØPTJØZZ
Right ØPTHØZZ

Resection — *continued*
Rectum ØDTP
Ribs
1 to 2 ØPT1ØZZ
3 or More ØPT2ØZZ
Scapula
Left ØPT6ØZZ
Right ØPT5ØZZ
Scrotum ØVT5
Septum
Atrial Ø2T5
Nasal Ø9TM
Ventricular Ø2TM
Sinus
Accessory Ø9TP
Ethmoid
Left Ø9TV
Right Ø9TU
Frontal
Left Ø9TT
Right Ø9TS
Mastoid
Left Ø9TC
Right Ø9TB
Maxillary
Left Ø9TR
Right Ø9TQ
Sphenoid
Left Ø9TX
Right Ø9TW
Spleen Ø7TP
Sternum ØPTØØZZ
Stomach ØDT6
Pylorus ØDT7
Tarsal
Left ØQTMØZZ
Right ØQTLØZZ
Tendon
Abdomen
Left ØLTG
Right ØLTF
Ankle
Left ØLTT
Right ØLTS
Foot
Left ØLTW
Right ØLTV
Hand
Left ØLT8
Right ØLT7
Head and Neck ØLTØ
Hip
Left ØLTK
Right ØLTJ
Knee
Left ØLTR
Right ØLTQ
Lower Arm and Wrist
Left ØLT6
Right ØLT5
Lower Leg
Left ØLTP
Right ØLTN
Perineum ØLTH
Shoulder
Left ØLT2
Right ØLT1
Thorax
Left ØLTD
Right ØLTC
Trunk
Left ØLTB
Right ØLT9
Upper Arm
Left ØLT4
Right ØLT3
Upper Leg
Left ØLTM
Right ØLTL
Testis
Bilateral ØVTC
Left ØVTB
Right ØVT9
Thymus Ø7TM
Thyroid Gland ØGTK
Left Lobe ØGTG
Right Lobe ØGTH
Thyroid Gland Isthmus ØGTJ

Resection — *continued*
Tibia
Left ØQTHØZZ
Right ØQTGØZZ
Toe Nail ØHTRXZZ
Tongue ØCT7
Tonsils ØCTP
Tooth
Lower ØCTXØZ
Upper ØCTWØZ
Trachea ØBT1
Tunica Vaginalis
Left ØVT7
Right ØVT6
Turbinate, Nasal Ø9TL
Tympanic Membrane
Left Ø9T8
Right Ø9T7
Ulna
Left ØPTLØZZ
Right ØPTKØZZ
Ureter
Left ØTT7
Right ØTT6
Urethra ØTTD
Uterine Supporting Structure ØUT4
Uterus ØUT9
Uvula ØCTN
Vagina ØUTG
Valve, Pulmonary Ø2TH
Vas Deferens
Bilateral ØVTQ
Left ØVTP
Right ØVTN
Vesicle
Bilateral ØVT3
Left ØVT2
Right ØVT1
Vitreous
Left Ø8T53ZZ
Right Ø8T43ZZ
Vocal Cord
Left ØCTV
Right ØCTT
Vulva ØUTM
Resection, Left ventricular outflow tract obstruction (LVOT) *see* Dilation, Ventricle, Left Ø27L
Resection, Subaortic membrane (Left ventricular outflow tract obstruction) *see* Dilation, Ventricle, Left Ø27L
Restoration, Cardiac, Single, Rhythm 5A22Ø4Z
RestoreAdvanced neurostimulator (SureScan) (MRI Safe) *use* Stimulator Generator, Multiple Array Rechargeable in ØJH
RestoreSensor neurostimulator (SureScan) (MRI Safe) *use* Stimulator Generator, Multiple Array Rechargeable in ØJH
RestoreUltra neurostimulator (SureScan) (MRI Safe) *use* Stimulator Generator, Multiple Array Rechargeable in ØJH
Restriction
Ampulla of Vater ØFVC
Anus ØDVQ
Aorta
Abdominal Ø4VØ
Intraluminal Device, Branched or Fenestrated Ø4VØ
Thoracic
Ascending/Arch, Intraluminal Device, Branched or Fenestrated Ø2VX
Descending, Intraluminal Device, Branched or Fenestrated Ø2VW
Artery
Anterior Tibial
Left Ø4VQ
Right Ø4VP
Axillary
Left Ø3V6
Right Ø3V5
Brachial
Left Ø3V8
Right Ø3V7
Celiac Ø4V1
Colic
Left Ø4V7
Middle Ø4V8
Right Ø4V6

Restriction — *continued*
Artery — *continued*
Common Carotid
Left Ø3VJ
Right Ø3VH
Common Iliac
Left Ø4VD
Right Ø4VC
External Carotid
Left Ø3VN
Right Ø3VM
External Iliac
Left Ø4VJ
Right Ø4VH
Face Ø3VR
Femoral
Left Ø4VL
Right Ø4VK
Foot
Left Ø4VW
Right Ø4VV
Gastric Ø4V2
Hand
Left Ø3VF
Right Ø3VD
Hepatic Ø4V3
Inferior Mesenteric Ø4VB
Innominate Ø3V2
Internal Carotid
Left Ø3VL
Right Ø3VK
Internal Iliac
Left Ø4VF
Right Ø4VE
Internal Mammary
Left Ø3V1
Right Ø3VØ
Intracranial Ø3VG
Lower Ø4VY
Peroneal
Left Ø4VU
Right Ø4VT
Popliteal
Left Ø4VN
Right Ø4VM
Posterior Tibial
Left Ø4VS
Right Ø4VR
Pulmonary
Left Ø2VR
Right Ø2VQ
Pulmonary Trunk Ø2VP
Radial
Left Ø3VC
Right Ø3VB
Renal
Left Ø4VA
Right Ø4V9
Splenic Ø4V4
Subclavian
Left Ø3V4
Right Ø3V3
Superior Mesenteric Ø4V5
Temporal
Left Ø3VT
Right Ø3VS
Thyroid
Left Ø3VV
Right Ø3VU
Ulnar
Left Ø3VA
Right Ø3V9
Upper Ø3VY
Vertebral
Left Ø3VQ
Right Ø3VP
Bladder ØTVB
Bladder Neck ØTVC
Bronchus
Lingula ØBV9
Lower Lobe
Left ØBVB
Right ØBV6
Main
Left ØBV7
Right ØBV3
Middle Lobe, Right ØBV5
Upper Lobe
Left ØBV8

Restriction — *continued*
Bronchus — *continued*
Upper Lobe — *continued*
Right ØBV4
Carina ØBV2
Cecum ØDVH
Cervix ØUVC
Cisterna Chyli Ø7VL
Colon
Ascending ØDVK
Descending ØDVM
Sigmoid ØDVN
Transverse ØDVL
Duct
Common Bile ØFV9
Cystic ØFV8
Hepatic
Common ØFV7
Left ØFV6
Right ØFV5
Lacrimal
Left Ø8VY
Right Ø8VX
Pancreatic ØFVD
Accessory ØFVF
Parotid
Left ØCVC
Right ØCVB
Duodenum ØDV9
Esophagogastric Junction ØDV4
Esophagus ØDV5
Lower ØDV3
Middle ØDV2
Upper ØDV1
Heart Ø2VA
Ileocecal Valve ØDVC
Ileum ØDVB
Intestine
Large ØDVE
Left ØDVG
Right ØDVF
Small ØDV8
Jejunum ØDVA
Kidney Pelvis
Left ØTV4
Right ØTV3
Lymphatic
Aortic Ø7VD
Axillary
Left Ø7V6
Right Ø7V5
Head Ø7VØ
Inguinal
Left Ø7VJ
Right Ø7VH
Internal Mammary
Left Ø7V9
Right Ø7V8
Lower Extremity
Left Ø7VG
Right Ø7VF
Mesenteric Ø7VB
Neck
Left Ø7V2
Right Ø7V1
Pelvis Ø7VC
Thoracic Duct Ø7VK
Thorax Ø7V7
Upper Extremity
Left Ø7V4
Right Ø7V3
Rectum ØDVP
Stomach ØDV6
Pylorus ØDV7
Trachea ØBV1
Ureter
Left ØTV7
Right ØTV6
Urethra ØTVD
Valve, Mitral Ø2VG
Vein
Axillary
Left Ø5V8
Right Ø5V7
Azygos Ø5VØ
Basilic
Left Ø5VC
Right Ø5VB

Restriction — *continued*
Vein — *continued*
Brachial
Left Ø5VA
Right Ø5V9
Cephalic
Left Ø5VF
Right Ø5VD
Colic Ø6V7
Common Iliac
Left Ø6VD
Right Ø6VC
Esophageal Ø6V3
External Iliac
Left Ø6VG
Right Ø6VF
External Jugular
Left Ø5VQ
Right Ø5VP
Face
Left Ø5VV
Right Ø5VT
Femoral
Left Ø6VN
Right Ø6VM
Foot
Left Ø6VV
Right Ø6VT
Gastric Ø6V2
Hand
Left Ø5VH
Right Ø5VG
Hemiazygos Ø5V1
Hepatic Ø6V4
Hypogastric
Left Ø6VJ
Right Ø6VH
Inferior Mesenteric Ø6V6
Innominate
Left Ø5V4
Right Ø5V3
Internal Jugular
Left Ø5VN
Right Ø5VM
Intracranial Ø5VL
Lower Ø6VY
Portal Ø6V8
Pulmonary
Left Ø2VT
Right Ø2VS
Renal
Left Ø6VB
Right Ø6V9
Saphenous
Left Ø6VQ
Right Ø6VP
Splenic Ø6V1
Subclavian
Left Ø5V6
Right Ø5V5
Superior Mesenteric Ø6V5
Upper Ø5VY
Vertebral
Left Ø5VS
Right Ø5VR
Vena Cava
Inferior Ø6VØ
Superior Ø2VV
Resurfacing Device
Removal of device from
Left ØSPBØBZ
Right ØSP9ØBZ
Revision of device in
Left ØSWBØBZ
Right ØSW9ØBZ
Supplement
Left ØSUBØBZ
Acetabular Surface ØSUEØBZ
Femoral Surface ØSUSØBZ
Right ØSU9ØBZ
Acetabular Surface ØSUAØBZ
Femoral Surface ØSURØBZ
Resuscitation
Cardiopulmonary *see* Assistance, Cardiac 5AØ2
Cardioversion 5A22Ø4Z
Defibrillation 5A22Ø4Z
Endotracheal intubation *see* Insertion of device in, Trachea ØBH1
External chest compression 5A12Ø12

Resuscitation — *continued*
Pulmonary 5A19Ø54
Resuscitative endovascular balloon occlusion of the aorta (REBOA)
Ø2LW3DJ
Ø4LØ3DJ
Resuture, Heart valve prosthesis *see* Revision of device in, Heart and Great Vessels Ø2W
Retained placenta, manual removal *see* Extraction, Products of Conception, Retained 1ØD1
Retraining
Cardiac *see* Motor Treatment, Rehabilitation FØ7
Vocational *see* Activities of Daily Living Treatment, Rehabilitation FØ8
Retrogasserian rhizotomy *see* Division, Nerve, Trigeminal ØØ8K
Retroperitoneal cavity *use* Retroperitoneum
Retroperitoneal lymph node *use* Lymphatic, Aortic
Retroperitoneal space *use* Retroperitoneum
Retropharyngeal lymph node
use Lymphatic, Left Neck
use Lymphatic, Right Neck
Retropubic space *use* Pelvic Cavity
Reveal (LINQ) (DX) (XT) *use* Monitoring Device
Reverse total shoulder replacement *see* Replacement, Upper Joints ØRR
Reverse® Shoulder Prosthesis *use* Synthetic Substitute, Reverse Ball and Socket in ØRR
Revision
Correcting a portion of existing device *see* Revision of device in
Removal of device without replacement *see* Removal of device from
Replacement of existing device
see Removal of device from
see Root operation to place new device, e.g., Insertion, Replacement, Supplement
Revision of device in
Abdominal Wall ØWWF
Acetabulum
Left ØQW5
Right ØQW4
Anal Sphincter ØDWR
Anus ØDWQ
Artery
Lower Ø4WY
Upper Ø3WY
Auditory Ossicle
Left Ø9WA
Right Ø9W9
Back
Lower ØWWL
Upper ØWWK
Bladder ØTWB
Bone
Facial ØNWW
Lower ØQWY
Nasal ØNWB
Pelvic
Left ØQW3
Right ØQW2
Upper ØPWY
Bone Marrow Ø7WT
Brain ØØWØ
Breast
Left ØHWU
Right ØHWT
Bursa and Ligament
Lower ØMWY
Upper ØMWX
Carpal
Left ØPWN
Right ØPWM
Cavity, Cranial ØWW1
Cerebral Ventricle ØØW6
Chest Wall ØWW8
Cisterna Chyli Ø7WL
Clavicle
Left ØPWB
Right ØPW9
Coccyx ØQWS
Diaphragm ØBWT
Disc
Cervical Vertebral ØRW3
Cervicothoracic Vertebral ØRW5
Lumbar Vertebral ØSW2
Lumbosacral ØSW4
Thoracic Vertebral ØRW9

Revision of device in — *continued*
Disc — *continued*
Thoracolumbar Vertebral ØRWB
Duct
Hepatobiliary ØFWB
Pancreatic ØFWD
Ear
Inner
Left Ø9WE
Right Ø9WD
Left Ø9WJ
Right Ø9WH
Epididymis and Spermatic Cord ØVWM
Esophagus ØDW5
Extremity
Lower
Left ØYWB
Right ØYW9
Upper
Left ØXW7
Right ØXW6
Eye
Left Ø8W1
Right Ø8WØ
Face ØWW2
Fallopian Tube ØUW8
Femoral Shaft
Left ØQW9
Right ØQW8
Femur
Lower
Left ØQWC
Right ØQWB
Upper
Left ØQW7
Right ØQW6
Fibula
Left ØQWK
Right ØQWJ
Finger Nail ØHWQX
Gallbladder ØFW4
Gastrointestinal Tract ØWWP
Genitourinary Tract ØWWR
Gland
Adrenal ØGW5
Endocrine ØGWS
Pituitary ØGWØ
Salivary ØCWA
Glenoid Cavity
Left ØPW8
Right ØPW7
Great Vessel Ø2WY
Hair ØHWSX
Head ØWWØ
Heart Ø2WA
Humeral Head
Left ØPWD
Right ØPWC
Humeral Shaft
Left ØPWG
Right ØPWF
Intestinal Tract
Lower ØDWD
Upper ØDWØ
Intestine
Large ØDWE
Small ØDW8
Jaw
Lower ØWW5
Upper ØWW4
Joint
Acromioclavicular
Left ØRWH
Right ØRWG
Ankle
Left ØSWG
Right ØSWF
Carpal
Left ØRWR
Right ØRWQ
Carpometacarpal
Left ØRWT
Right ØRWS
Cervical Vertebral ØRW1
Cervicothoracic Vertebral ØRW4
Coccygeal ØSW6
Elbow
Left ØRWM
Right ØRWL

Revision of device in — *continued*
Joint — *continued*
Finger Phalangeal
Left ØRWX
Right ØRWW
Hip
Left ØSWB
Acetabular Surface ØSWE
Femoral Surface ØSWS
Right ØSW9
Acetabular Surface ØSWA
Femoral Surface ØSWR
Knee
Left ØSWD
Femoral Surface ØSWU
Tibial Surface ØSWW
Right ØSWC
Femoral Surface ØSWT
Tibial Surface ØSWV
Lumbar Vertebral ØSWØ
Lumbosacral ØSW3
Metacarpophalangeal
Left ØRWV
Right ØRWU
Metatarsal-Phalangeal
Left ØSWN
Right ØSWM
Occipital-cervical ØRWØ
Sacrococcygeal ØSW5
Sacroiliac
Left ØSW8
Right ØSW7
Shoulder
Left ØRWK
Right ØRWJ
Sternoclavicular
Left ØRWF
Right ØRWE
Tarsal
Left ØSWJ
Right ØSWH
Tarsometatarsal
Left ØSWL
Right ØSWK
Temporomandibular
Left ØRWD
Right ØRWC
Thoracic Vertebral ØRW6
Thoracolumbar Vertebral ØRWA
Toe Phalangeal
Left ØSWQ
Right ØSWP
Wrist
Left ØRWP
Right ØRWN
Kidney ØTW5
Larynx ØCWS
Lens
Left Ø8WK
Right Ø8WJ
Liver ØFWØ
Lung
Left ØBWL
Right ØBWK
Lymphatic Ø7WN
Thoracic Duct Ø7WK
Mediastinum ØWWC
Mesentery ØDWV
Metacarpal
Left ØPWQ
Right ØPWP
Metatarsal
Left ØQWP
Right ØQWN
Mouth and Throat ØCWY
Muscle
Extraocular
Left Ø8WM
Right Ø8WL
Lower ØKWY
Upper ØKWX
Nasal Mucosa and Soft Tissue Ø9WK
Neck ØWW6
Nerve
Cranial ØØWE
Peripheral Ø1WY
Omentum ØDWU
Ovary ØUW3
Pancreas ØFWG

Revision of device in — *continued*
Parathyroid Gland ØGWR
Patella
Left ØQWF
Right ØQWD
Pelvic Cavity ØWWJ
Penis ØVWS
Pericardial Cavity ØWWD
Perineum
Female ØWWN
Male ØWWM
Peritoneal Cavity ØWWG
Peritoneum ØDWW
Phalanx
Finger
Left ØPWV
Right ØPWT
Thumb
Left ØPWS
Right ØPWR
Toe
Left ØQWR
Right ØQWQ
Pineal Body ØGW1
Pleura ØBWQ
Pleural Cavity
Left ØWWB
Right ØWW9
Prostate and Seminal Vesicles ØVW4
Radius
Left ØPWJ
Right ØPWH
Respiratory Tract ØWWQ
Retroperitoneum ØWWH
Ribs
1 to 2 ØPW1
3 or More ØPW2
Sacrum ØQW1
Scapula
Left ØPW6
Right ØPW5
Scrotum and Tunica Vaginalis ØVW8
Septum
Atrial Ø2W5
Ventricular Ø2WM
Sinus Ø9WY
Skin ØHWPX
Skull ØNWØ
Spinal Canal ØØWU
Spinal Cord ØØWV
Spleen Ø7WP
Sternum ØPWØ
Stomach ØDW6
Subcutaneous Tissue and Fascia
Head and Neck ØJWS
Lower Extremity ØJWW
Trunk ØJWT
Upper Extremity ØJWV
Tarsal
Left ØQWM
Right ØQWL
Tendon
Lower ØLWY
Upper ØLWX
Testis ØVWD
Thymus Ø7WM
Thyroid Gland ØGWK
Tibia
Left ØQWH
Right ØQWG
Toe Nail ØHWRX
Trachea ØBW1
Tracheobronchial Tree ØBWØ
Tympanic Membrane
Left Ø9W8
Right Ø9W7
Ulna
Left ØPWL
Right ØPWK
Ureter ØTW9
Urethra ØTWD
Uterus and Cervix ØUWD
Vagina and Cul-de-sac ØUWH
Valve
Aortic Ø2WF
Mitral Ø2WG
Pulmonary Ø2WH
Tricuspid Ø2WJ
Vas Deferens ØVWR

Revision of device in — *continued*
Vein
Azygos Ø5WØ
Innominate
Left Ø5W4
Right Ø5W3
Lower Ø6WY
Upper Ø5WY
Vertebra
Cervical ØPW3
Lumbar ØQWØ
Thoracic ØPW4
Vulva ØUWM
Revo MRI™ SureScan® pacemaker *use* Pacemaker, Dual Chamber in ØJH
rhBMP-2 *use* Recombinant Bone Morphogenetic Protein
Rheos® System device *use* Stimulator Generator in Subcutaneous Tissue and Fascia
Rheos® System lead *use* Stimulator Lead in Upper Arteries
Rhinopharynx *use* Nasopharynx
Rhinoplasty
see Alteration, Nasal Mucosa and Soft Tissue Ø9ØK
see Repair, Nasal Mucosa and Soft Tissue Ø9QK
see Replacement, Nasal Mucosa and Soft Tissue Ø9RK
see Supplement, Nasal Mucosa and Soft Tissue Ø9UK
Rhinorrhaphy *see* Repair, Nasal Mucosa and Soft Tissue Ø9QK
Rhinoscopy Ø9JKXZZ
Rhizotomy
see Division, Central Nervous System and Cranial Nerves ØØ8
see Division, Peripheral Nervous System Ø18
Rhomboid major muscle
use Trunk Muscle, Left
use Trunk Muscle, Right
Rhomboid minor muscle
use Trunk Muscle, Left
use Trunk Muscle, Right
Rhythm electrocardiogram *see* Measurement, Cardiac 4AØ2
Rhytidectomy *see* Alteration, Face ØWØ2
Right ascending lumbar vein *use* Azygos Vein
Right atrioventricular valve *use* Tricuspid Valve
Right auricular appendix *use* Atrium, Right
Right colic vein *use* Colic Vein
Right coronary sulcus *use* Heart, Right
Right gastric artery *use* Gastric Artery
Right gastroepiploic vein *use* Superior Mesenteric Vein
Right inferior phrenic vein *use* Inferior Vena Cava
Right inferior pulmonary vein *use* Pulmonary Vein, Right
Right jugular trunk *use* Lymphatic, Right Neck
Right lateral ventricle *use* Cerebral Ventricle
Right lymphatic duct *use* Lymphatic, Right Neck
Right ovarian vein *use* Inferior Vena Cava
Right second lumbar vein *use* Inferior Vena Cava
Right subclavian trunk *use* Lymphatic, Right Neck
Right subcostal vein *use* Azygos Vein
Right superior pulmonary vein *use* Pulmonary Vein, Right
Right suprarenal vein *use* Inferior Vena Cava
Right testicular vein *use* Inferior Vena Cava
Rima glottidis *use* Larynx
Risorius muscle *use* Facial Muscle
RNS System lead *use* Neurostimulator Lead in Central Nervous System and Cranial Nerves
RNS system neurostimulator generator *use* Neurostimulator Generator in Head and Facial Bones
Robotic Assisted Procedure
Extremity
Lower 8EØY
Upper 8EØX
Head and Neck Region 8EØ9
Trunk Region 8EØW
Robotic Waterjet Ablation, Destruction, Prostate XV5Ø8A4
Rotation of fetal head
Forceps 1ØSØ7ZZ
Manual 1ØSØXZZ
Round ligament of uterus *use* Uterine Supporting Structure
Round window
use Inner Ear, Left
use Inner Ear, Right
Roux-en-Y operation
see Bypass, Gastrointestinal System ØD1
see Bypass, Hepatobiliary System and Pancreas ØF1
Rupture
Adhesions *see* Release
Fluid collection *see* Drainage
Ruxolitinib XWØDXT5

S

Sacral ganglion *use* Sacral Sympathetic Nerve
Sacral lymph node *use* Lymphatic, Pelvis
Sacral nerve modulation (SNM) lead *use* Stimulator Lead in Urinary System
Sacral neuromodulation lead *use* Stimulator Lead in Urinary System
Sacral splanchnic nerve *use* Sacral Sympathetic Nerve
Sacrectomy *see* Excision, Lower Bones ØQB
Sacrococcygeal ligament *use* Lower Spine Bursa and Ligament
Sacrococcygeal symphysis *use* Sacrococcygeal Joint
Sacroiliac ligament *use* Lower Spine Bursa and Ligament
Sacrospinous ligament *use* Lower Spine Bursa and Ligament
Sacrotuberous ligament *use* Lower Spine Bursa and Ligament
Salpingectomy
see Excision, Female Reproductive System ØUB
see Resection, Female Reproductive System ØUT
Salpingolysis *see* Release, Female Reproductive System ØUN
Salpingopexy
see Repair, Female Reproductive System ØUQ
see Reposition, Female Reproductive System ØUS
Salpingopharyngeus muscle *use* Tongue, Palate, Pharynx Muscle
Salpingoplasty
see Repair, Female Reproductive System ØUQ
see Supplement, Female Reproductive System ØUU
Salpingorrhaphy *see* Repair, Female Reproductive System ØUQ
Salpingoscopy ØUJ88ZZ
Salpingostomy *see* Drainage, Female Reproductive System ØU9
Salpingotomy *see* Drainage, Female Reproductive System ØU9
Salpinx
use Fallopian Tube, Left
use Fallopian Tube, Right
Saphenous nerve *use* Femoral Nerve
SAPIEN transcatheter aortic valve *use* Zooplastic Tissue in Heart and Great Vessels
Sartorius muscle
use Upper Leg Muscle, Left
use Upper Leg Muscle, Right
SAVAL below-the-knee (BTK) drug-eluting stent system
use Intraluminal Device, Sustained Release Drug-eluting in New Technology
use Intraluminal Device, Sustained Release Drug-eluting, Two in New Technology
use Intraluminal Device, Sustained Release Drug-eluting, Three in New Technology
use Intraluminal Device, Sustained Release Drug-eluting, Four or More in New Technology
Scalene muscle
use Neck Muscle, Left
use Neck Muscle, Right
Scan
Computerized Tomography (CT) *see* Computerized Tomography (CT Scan)
Radioisotope *see* Planar Nuclear Medicine Imaging
Scaphoid bone
use Carpal, Left
use Carpal, Right
Scapholunate ligament
use Wrist Bursa and Ligament, Left
use Wrist Bursa and Ligament, Right
Scaphotrapezium ligament
use Hand Bursa and Ligament, Left
use Hand Bursa and Ligament, Right

Scapulectomy
- *see* Excision, Upper Bones ØPB
- *see* Resection, Upper Bones ØPT

Scapulopexy
- *see* Repair, Upper Bones ØPQ
- *see* Reposition, Upper Bones ØPS

Scarpa's (vestibular) ganglion *use* Acoustic Nerve

Sclerectomy *see* Excision, Eye Ø8B

Sclerotherapy, mechanical *see* Destruction

Sclerotherapy, via injection of sclerosing agent *see* Introduction, Destructive Agent

Sclerotomy *see* Drainage, Eye Ø89

Scrotectomy
- *see* Excision, Male Reproductive System ØVB
- *see* Resection, Male Reproductive System ØVT

Scrotoplasty
- *see* Repair, Male Reproductive System ØVQ
- *see* Supplement, Male Reproductive System ØVU

Scrotorrhaphy *see* Repair, Male Reproductive System ØVQ

Scrototomy *see* Drainage, Male Reproductive System ØV9

Sebaceous gland *use* Skin

Second cranial nerve *use* Optic Nerve

Section, cesarean *see* Extraction, Pregnancy 1ØD

Secura (DR) (VR) *use* Defibrillator Generator in ØJH

Sella turcica *use* Sphenoid Bone

Semicircular canal
- *use* Inner Ear, Left
- *use* Inner Ear, Right

Semimembranosus muscle
- *use* Upper Leg Muscle, Left
- *use* Upper Leg Muscle, Right

Semitendinosus muscle
- *use* Upper Leg Muscle, Left
- *use* Upper Leg Muscle, Right

Sentinel™ Cerebral Protection System (CPS) X2A5312

Seprafilm *use* Adhesion Barrier

Septal cartilage *use* Nasal Septum

Septectomy
- *see* Excision, Ear, Nose, Sinus Ø9B
- *see* Excision, Heart and Great Vessels Ø2B
- *see* Resection, Ear, Nose, Sinus Ø9T
- *see* Resection, Heart and Great Vessels Ø2T

Septoplasty
- *see* Repair, Ear, Nose, Sinus Ø9Q
- *see* Repair, Heart and Great Vessels Ø2Q
- *see* Replacement, Ear, Nose, Sinus Ø9R
- *see* Replacement, Heart and Great Vessels Ø2R
- *see* Reposition, Ear, Nose, Sinus Ø9S
- *see* Supplement, Ear, Nose, Sinus Ø9U
- *see* Supplement, Heart and Great Vessels Ø2U

Septostomy, balloon atrial Ø2163Z7

Septotomy *see* Drainage, Ear, Nose, Sinus Ø99

Sequestrectomy, bone *see* Extirpation

Serratus anterior muscle
- *use* Thorax Muscle, Left
- *use* Thorax Muscle, Right

Serratus posterior muscle
- *use* Trunk Muscle, Left
- *use* Trunk Muscle, Right

Seventh cranial nerve *use* Facial Nerve

Shapshot_NIR 8EØ2XDZ

Sheffield hybrid external fixator
- *use* External Fixation Device, Hybrid in ØPH
- *use* External Fixation Device, Hybrid in ØPS
- *use* External Fixation Device, Hybrid in ØQH
- *use* External Fixation Device, Hybrid in ØQS

Sheffield ring external fixator
- *use* External Fixation Device, Ring in ØPH
- *use* External Fixation Device, Ring in ØPS
- *use* External Fixation Device, Ring in ØQH
- *use* External Fixation Device, Ring in ØQS

Shirodkar cervical cerclage ØUVC7ZZ

Shock Wave Therapy, Musculoskeletal 6A93

Shockwave Intravascular Lithotripsy (Shockwave IVL) *see* Fragmentation

Short gastric artery *use* Splenic Artery

Shortening
- *see* Excision
- *see* Repair
- *see* Reposition

Shunt creation *see* Bypass

Sialoadenectomy
- Complete *see* Resection, Mouth and Throat ØCT
- Partial *see* Excision, Mouth and Throat ØCB

Sialodochoplasty
- *see* Repair, Mouth and Throat ØCQ
- *see* Replacement, Mouth and Throat ØCR
- *see* Supplement, Mouth and Throat ØCU

Sialoectomy
- *see* Excision, Mouth and Throat ØCB
- *see* Resection, Mouth and Throat ØCT

Sialography *see* Plain Radiography, Ear, Nose, Mouth and Throat B9Ø

Sialolithotomy *see* Extirpation, Mouth and Throat ØCC

S-ICD™ lead *use* Subcutaneous Defibrillator Lead in Subcutaneous Tissue and Fascia

Sigmoid artery *use* Inferior Mesenteric Artery

Sigmoid flexure *use* Sigmoid Colon

Sigmoid vein *use* Inferior Mesenteric Vein

Sigmoidectomy
- *see* Excision, Gastrointestinal System ØDB
- *see* Resection, Gastrointestinal System ØDT

Sigmoidorrhaphy *see* Repair, Gastrointestinal System ØDQ

Sigmoidoscopy ØDJD8ZZ

Sigmoidotomy *see* Drainage, Gastrointestinal System ØD9

Single lead pacemaker (atrium) (ventricle) *use* Pacemaker, Single Chamber in ØJH

Single lead rate responsive pacemaker (atrium) (ventricle) *use* Pacemaker, Single Chamber Rate Responsive in ØJH

Sinoatrial node *use* Conduction Mechanism

Sinogram
- Abdominal Wall *see* Fluoroscopy, Abdomen and Pelvis BW11
- Chest Wall *see* Plain Radiography, Chest BWØ3
- Retroperitoneum *see* Fluoroscopy, Abdomen and Pelvis BW11

Sinus venosus *use* Atrium, Right

Sinusectomy
- *see* Excision, Ear, Nose, Sinus Ø9B
- *see* Resection, Ear, Nose, Sinus Ø9T

Sinusoscopy Ø9JY4ZZ

Sinusotomy *see* Drainage, Ear, Nose, Sinus Ø99

Sirolimus-eluting coronary stent *use* Intraluminal Device, Drug-eluting in Heart and Great Vessels

Sixth cranial nerve *use* Abducens Nerve

Size reduction, breast *see* Excision, Skin and Breast ØHB

SJM Biocor® Stented Valve System *use* Zooplastic Tissue in Heart and Great Vessels

Skene's (paraurethral) gland *use* Vestibular Gland

Skin Substitute, Porcine Liver Derived, Replacement XHRPXL2

Sling
- Fascial, orbicularis muscle (mouth) *see* Supplement, Muscle, Facial ØKU1
- Levator muscle, for urethral suspension *see* Reposition, Bladder Neck ØTSC
- Pubococcygeal, for urethral suspension *see* Reposition, Bladder Neck ØTSC
- Rectum *see* Reposition, Rectum ØDSP

Small bowel series *see* Fluoroscopy, Bowel, Small BD13

Small saphenous vein
- *use* Saphenous Vein, Left
- *use* Saphenous Vein, Right

Snapshot_NIR 8EØ2XDZ

Snaring, polyp, colon *see* Excision, Gastrointestinal System ØDB

Solar (celiac) plexus *use* Abdominal Sympathetic Nerve

Soleus muscle
- *use* Lower Leg Muscle, Left
- *use* Lower Leg Muscle, Right

Soliris® *use* Eculizumab

Spacer
- Insertion of device in
  - Disc
    - Lumbar Vertebral ØSH2
    - Lumbosacral ØSH4
  - Joint
    - Acromioclavicular
      - Left ØRHH
      - Right ØRHG
    - Ankle
      - Left ØSHG
      - Right ØSHF
    - Carpal
      - Left ØRHR
      - Right ØRHQ
    - Carpometacarpal
      - Left ØRHT
      - Right ØRHS
    - Cervical Vertebral ØRH1
    - Cervicothoracic Vertebral ØRH4
    - Coccygeal ØSH6
    - Elbow
      - Left ØRHM
      - Right ØRHL
    - Finger Phalangeal
      - Left ØRHX
      - Right ØRHW
    - Hip
      - Left ØSHB
      - Right ØSH9
    - Knee
      - Left ØSHD
      - Right ØSHC
    - Lumbar Vertebral ØSHØ
    - Lumbosacral ØSH3
    - Metacarpophalangeal
      - Left ØRHV
      - Right ØRHU
    - Metatarsal-Phalangeal
      - Left ØSHN
      - Right ØSHM
    - Occipital-cervical ØRHØ
    - Sacrococcygeal ØSH5
    - Sacroiliac
      - Left ØSH8
      - Right ØSH7
    - Shoulder
      - Left ØRHK
      - Right ØRHJ
    - Sternoclavicular
      - Left ØRHF
      - Right ØRHE
    - Tarsal
      - Left ØSHJ
      - Right ØSHH
    - Tarsometatarsal
      - Left ØSHL
      - Right ØSHK
    - Temporomandibular
      - Left ØRHD
      - Right ØRHC
    - Thoracic Vertebral ØRH6
    - Thoracolumbar Vertebral ØRHA
    - Toe Phalangeal
      - Left ØSHQ
      - Right ØSHP
    - Wrist
      - Left ØRHP
      - Right ØRHN
- Removal of device from
  - Acromioclavicular
    - Left ØRPH
    - Right ØRPG
  - Ankle
    - Left ØSPG
    - Right ØSPF
  - Carpal
    - Left ØRPR
    - Right ØRPQ
  - Carpometacarpal
    - Left ØRPT
    - Right ØRPS
  - Cervical Vertebral ØRP1
  - Cervicothoracic Vertebral ØRP4
  - Coccygeal ØSP6
  - Elbow
    - Left ØRPM
    - Right ØRPL
  - Finger Phalangeal
    - Left ØRPX
    - Right ØRPW
  - Hip
    - Left ØSPB
    - Right ØSP9
  - Knee
    - Left ØSPD
    - Right ØSPC
  - Lumbar Vertebral ØSPØ

Spacer — *continued*
Removal of device from — *continued*
Lumbosacral ØSP3
Metacarpophalangeal
Left ØRPV
Right ØRPU
Metatarsal-Phalangeal
Left ØSPN
Right ØSPM
Occipital-cervical ØRPØ
Sacrococcygeal ØSP5
Sacroiliac
Left ØSP8
Right ØSP7
Shoulder
Left ØRPK
Right ØRPJ
Sternoclavicular
Left ØRPF
Right ØRPE
Tarsal
Left ØSPJ
Right ØSPH
Tarsometatarsal
Left ØSPL
Right ØSPK
Temporomandibular
Left ØRPD
Right ØRPC
Thoracic Vertebral ØRP6
Thoracolumbar Vertebral ØRPA
Toe Phalangeal
Left ØSPQ
Right ØSPP
Wrist
Left ØRPP
Right ØRPN
Revision of device in
Acromioclavicular
Left ØRWH
Right ØRWG
Ankle
Left ØSWG
Right ØSWF
Carpal
Left ØRWR
Right ØRWQ
Carpometacarpal
Left ØRWT
Right ØRWS
Cervical Vertebral ØRW1
Cervicothoracic Vertebral ØRW4
Coccygeal ØSW6
Elbow
Left ØRWM
Right ØRWL
Finger Phalangeal
Left ØRWX
Right ØRWW
Hip
Left ØSWB
Right ØSW9
Knee
Left ØSWD
Right ØSWC
Lumbar Vertebral ØSWØ
Lumbosacral ØSW3
Metacarpophalangeal
Left ØRWV
Right ØRWU
Metatarsal-Phalangeal
Left ØSWN
Right ØSWM
Occipital-cervical ØRWØ
Sacrococcygeal ØSW5
Sacroiliac
Left ØSW8
Right ØSW7
Shoulder
Left ØRWK
Right ØRWJ
Sternoclavicular
Left ØRWF
Right ØRWE
Tarsal
Left ØSWJ
Right ØSWH
Tarsometatarsal
Left ØSWL

Spacer — *continued*
Revision of device in — *continued*
Tarsometatarsal — *continued*
Right ØSWK
Temporomandibular
Left ØRWD
Right ØRWC
Thoracic Vertebral ØRW6
Thoracolumbar Vertebral ØRWA
Toe Phalangeal
Left ØSWQ
Right ØSWP
Wrist
Left ØRWP
Right ØRWN
Spacer, Articulating (Antibiotic) *use* Articulating Spacer in Lower Joints
Spacer, Static (Antibiotic) *use* Spacer in Lower Joints
Spectroscopy
Intravascular Near Infrared 8EØ23DZ
Near Infrared *see* Physiological Systems and Anatomical Regions 8EØ
Speech Assessment FØØ
Speech therapy *see* Speech Treatment, Rehabilitation FØ6
Speech Treatment FØ6
Sphenoidectomy
see Excision, Ear, Nose, Sinus Ø9B
see Excision, Head and Facial Bones ØNB
see Resection, Ear, Nose, Sinus Ø9T
see Resection, Head and Facial Bones ØNT
Sphenoidotomy *see* Drainage, Ear, Nose, Sinus Ø99
Sphenomandibular ligament *use* Head and Neck Bursa and Ligament
Sphenopalatine (pterygopalatine) ganglion *use* Head and Neck Sympathetic Nerve
Sphincterorrhaphy, anal *see* Repair, Anal Sphincter ØDQR
Sphincterotomy, anal
see Division, Anal Sphincter ØD8R
see Drainage, Anal Sphincter ØD9R
Spinal cord neurostimulator lead *use* Neurostimulator Lead in Central Nervous System and Cranial Nerves
Spinal growth rods, magnetically controlled *use* Magnetically Controlled Growth Rod(s) in New Technology
Spinal nerve, cervical *use* Cervical Nerve
Spinal nerve, lumbar *use* Lumbar Nerve
Spinal nerve, sacral *use* Sacral Nerve
Spinal nerve, thoracic *use* Thoracic Nerve
Spinal Stabilization Device
Facet Replacement
Cervical Vertebral ØRH1
Cervicothoracic Vertebral ØRH4
Lumbar Vertebral ØSHØ
Lumbosacral ØSH3
Occipital-cervical ØRHØ
Thoracic Vertebral ØRH6
Thoracolumbar Vertebral ØRHA
Interspinous Process
Cervical Vertebral ØRH1
Cervicothoracic Vertebral ØRH4
Lumbar Vertebral ØSHØ
Lumbosacral ØSH3
Occipital-cervical ØRHØ
Thoracic Vertebral ØRH6
Thoracolumbar Vertebral ØRHA
Pedicle-Based
Cervical Vertebral ØRH1
Cervicothoracic Vertebral ØRH4
Lumbar Vertebral ØSHØ
Lumbosacral ØSH3
Occipital-cervical ØRHØ
Thoracic Vertebral ØRH6
Thoracolumbar Vertebral ØRHA
SpineJack® system *use* Synthetic Substitute, Mechanically Expandable (Paired) in New Technology
Spinous process
use Cervical Vertebra
use Lumbar Vertebra
use Thoracic Vertebra
Spiral ganglion *use* Acoustic Nerve
Spiration IBV™ Valve System *use* Intraluminal Device, Endobronchial Valve in Respiratory System
Splenectomy
see Excision, Lymphatic and Hemic Systems Ø7B
see Resection, Lymphatic and Hemic Systems Ø7T

Splenic flexure *use* Transverse Colon
Splenic plexus *use* Abdominal Sympathetic Nerve
Splenius capitis muscle *use* Head Muscle
Splenius cervicis muscle
use Neck Muscle, Left
use Neck Muscle, Right
Splenolysis *see* Release, Lymphatic and Hemic Systems Ø7N
Splenopexy
see Repair, Lymphatic and Hemic Systems Ø7Q
see Reposition, Lymphatic and Hemic Systems Ø7S
Splenoplasty *see* Repair, Lymphatic and Hemic Systems Ø7Q
Splenorrhaphy *see* Repair, Lymphatic and Hemic Systems Ø7Q
Splenotomy *see* Drainage, Lymphatic and Hemic Systems Ø79
Splinting, musculoskeletal *see* Immobilization, Anatomical Regions 2W3
SPRAVATO™ *use* Esketamine Hydrochloride
SPY PINPOINT fluorescence imaging system
see Monitoring, Physiological Systems 4A1
see Other Imaging, Hepatobiliary System and Pancreas BF5
SPY system intraoperative fluorescence cholangiography *see* Other Imaging, Hepatobiliary System and Pancreas BF5
SPY system intravascular fluorescence angiography *see* Monitoring, Physiological Systems 4A1
Stapedectomy
see Excision, Ear, Nose, Sinus Ø9B
see Resection, Ear, Nose, Sinus Ø9T
Stapediolysis *see* Release, Ear, Nose, Sinus Ø9N
Stapedioplasty
see Repair, Ear, Nose, Sinus Ø9Q
see Replacement, Ear, Nose, Sinus Ø9R
see Supplement, Ear, Nose, Sinus Ø9U
Stapedotomy *see* Drainage, Ear, Nose, Sinus Ø99
Stapes
use Auditory Ossicle, Left
use Auditory Ossicle, Right
Static Spacer (Antibiotic) *use* Spacer in Lower Joints
STELARA® *use* Other New Technology Therapeutic Substance
Stellate ganglion *use* Head and Neck Sympathetic Nerve
Stem cell transplant *see* Transfusion, Circulatory 3Ø2
Stensen's duct
use Parotid Duct, Left
use Parotid Duct, Right
Stent, intraluminal (cardiovascular) (gastrointestinal) (hepatobiliary) (urinary) *use* Intraluminal Device
Stent retriever thrombectomy *see* Extirpation, Upper Arteries Ø3C
Stented tissue valve *use* Zooplastic Tissue in Heart and Great Vessels
Stereotactic Radiosurgery
Abdomen DW23
Adrenal Gland DG22
Bile Ducts DF22
Bladder DT22
Bone Marrow D72Ø
Brain DØ2Ø
Brain Stem DØ21
Breast
Left DM2Ø
Right DM21
Bronchus DB21
Cervix DU21
Chest DW22
Chest Wall DB27
Colon DD25
Diaphragm DB28
Duodenum DD22
Ear D92Ø
Esophagus DD2Ø
Eye D82Ø
Gallbladder DF21
Gamma Beam
Abdomen DW23JZZ
Adrenal Gland DG22JZZ
Bile Ducts DF22JZZ
Bladder DT22JZZ
Bone Marrow D72ØJZZ
Brain DØ2ØJZZ
Brain Stem DØ21JZZ

Stereotactic Radiosurgery — *continued*
Gamma Beam — *continued*
Breast
Left DM20JZZ
Right DM21JZZ
Bronchus DB21JZZ
Cervix DU21JZZ
Chest DW22JZZ
Chest Wall DB27JZZ
Colon DD25JZZ
Diaphragm DB28JZZ
Duodenum DD22JZZ
Ear D920JZZ
Esophagus DD20JZZ
Eye D820JZZ
Gallbladder DF21JZZ
Gland
Adrenal DG22JZZ
Parathyroid DG24JZZ
Pituitary DG20JZZ
Thyroid DG25JZZ
Glands, Salivary D926JZZ
Head and Neck DW21JZZ
Ileum DD24JZZ
Jejunum DD23JZZ
Kidney DT20JZZ
Larynx D92BJZZ
Liver DF20JZZ
Lung DB22JZZ
Lymphatics
Abdomen D726JZZ
Axillary D724JZZ
Inguinal D728JZZ
Neck D723JZZ
Pelvis D727JZZ
Thorax D725JZZ
Mediastinum DB26JZZ
Mouth D924JZZ
Nasopharynx D92DJZZ
Neck and Head DW21JZZ
Nerve, Peripheral D027JZZ
Nose D921JZZ
Ovary DU20JZZ
Palate
Hard D928JZZ
Soft D929JZZ
Pancreas DF23JZZ
Parathyroid Gland DG24JZZ
Pelvic Region DW26JZZ
Pharynx D92CJZZ
Pineal Body DG21JZZ
Pituitary Gland DG20JZZ
Pleura DB25JZZ
Prostate DV20JZZ
Rectum DD27JZZ
Sinuses D927JZZ
Spinal Cord D026JZZ
Spleen D722JZZ
Stomach DD21JZZ
Testis DV21JZZ
Thymus D721JZZ
Thyroid Gland DG25JZZ
Tongue D925JZZ
Trachea DB20JZZ
Ureter DT21JZZ
Urethra DT23JZZ
Uterus DU22JZZ
Gland
Adrenal DG22
Parathyroid DG24
Pituitary DG20
Thyroid DG25
Glands, Salivary D926
Head and Neck DW21
Ileum DD24
Jejunum DD23
Kidney DT20
Larynx D92B
Liver DF20
Lung DB22
Lymphatics
Abdomen D726
Axillary D724
Inguinal D728
Neck D723
Pelvis D727
Thorax D725
Mediastinum DB26
Mouth D924

Stereotactic Radiosurgery — *continued*
Nasopharynx D92D
Neck and Head DW21
Nerve, Peripheral D027
Nose D921
Other Photon
Abdomen DW23DZZ
Adrenal Gland DG22DZZ
Bile Ducts DF22DZZ
Bladder DT22DZZ
Bone Marrow D720DZZ
Brain D020DZZ
Brain Stem D021DZZ
Breast
Left DM20DZZ
Right DM21DZZ
Bronchus DB21DZZ
Cervix DU21DZZ
Chest DW22DZZ
Chest Wall DB27DZZ
Colon DD25DZZ
Diaphragm DB28DZZ
Duodenum DD22DZZ
Ear D920DZZ
Esophagus DD20DZZ
Eye D820DZZ
Gallbladder DF21DZZ
Gland
Adrenal DG22DZZ
Parathyroid DG24DZZ
Pituitary DG20DZZ
Thyroid DG25DZZ
Glands, Salivary D926DZZ
Head and Neck DW21DZZ
Ileum DD24DZZ
Jejunum DD23DZZ
Kidney DT20DZZ
Larynx D92BDZZ
Liver DF20DZZ
Lung DB22DZZ
Lymphatics
Abdomen D726DZZ
Axillary D724DZZ
Inguinal D728DZZ
Neck D723DZZ
Pelvis D727DZZ
Thorax D725DZZ
Mediastinum DB26DZZ
Mouth D924DZZ
Nasopharynx D92DDZZ
Neck and Head DW21DZZ
Nerve, Peripheral D027DZZ
Nose D921DZZ
Ovary DU20DZZ
Palate
Hard D928DZZ
Soft D929DZZ
Pancreas DF23DZZ
Parathyroid Gland DG24DZZ
Pelvic Region DW26DZZ
Pharynx D92CDZZ
Pineal Body DG21DZZ
Pituitary Gland DG20DZZ
Pleura DB25DZZ
Prostate DV20DZZ
Rectum DD27DZZ
Sinuses D927DZZ
Spinal Cord D026DZZ
Spleen D722DZZ
Stomach DD21DZZ
Testis DV21DZZ
Thymus D721DZZ
Thyroid Gland DG25DZZ
Tongue D925DZZ
Trachea DB20DZZ
Ureter DT21DZZ
Urethra DT23DZZ
Uterus DU22DZZ
Ovary DU20
Palate
Hard D928
Soft D929
Pancreas DF23
Parathyroid Gland DG24
Particulate
Abdomen DW23HZZ
Adrenal Gland DG22HZZ
Bile Ducts DF22HZZ
Bladder DT22HZZ

Stereotactic Radiosurgery — *continued*
Particulate — *continued*
Bone Marrow D720HZZ
Brain D020HZZ
Brain Stem D021HZZ
Breast
Left DM20HZZ
Right DM21HZZ
Bronchus DB21HZZ
Cervix DU21HZZ
Chest DW22HZZ
Chest Wall DB27HZZ
Colon DD25HZZ
Diaphragm DB28HZZ
Duodenum DD22HZZ
Ear D920HZZ
Esophagus DD20HZZ
Eye D820HZZ
Gallbladder DF21HZZ
Gland
Adrenal DG22HZZ
Parathyroid DG24HZZ
Pituitary DG20HZZ
Thyroid DG25HZZ
Glands, Salivary D926HZZ
Head and Neck DW21HZZ
Ileum DD24HZZ
Jejunum DD23HZZ
Kidney DT20HZZ
Larynx D92BHZZ
Liver DF20HZZ
Lung DB22HZZ
Lymphatics
Abdomen D726HZZ
Axillary D724HZZ
Inguinal D728HZZ
Neck D723HZZ
Pelvis D727HZZ
Thorax D725HZZ
Mediastinum DB26HZZ
Mouth D924HZZ
Nasopharynx D92DHZZ
Neck and Head DW21HZZ
Nerve, Peripheral D027HZZ
Nose D921HZZ
Ovary DU20HZZ
Palate
Hard D928HZZ
Soft D929HZZ
Pancreas DF23HZZ
Parathyroid Gland DG24HZZ
Pelvic Region DW26HZZ
Pharynx D92CHZZ
Pineal Body DG21HZZ
Pituitary Gland DG20HZZ
Pleura DB25HZZ
Prostate DV20HZZ
Rectum DD27HZZ
Sinuses D927HZZ
Spinal Cord D026HZZ
Spleen D722HZZ
Stomach DD21HZZ
Testis DV21HZZ
Thymus D721HZZ
Thyroid Gland DG25HZZ
Tongue D925HZZ
Trachea DB20HZZ
Ureter DT21HZZ
Urethra DT23HZZ
Uterus DU22HZZ
Pelvic Region DW26
Pharynx D92C
Pineal Body DG21
Pituitary Gland DG20
Pleura DB25
Prostate DV20
Rectum DD27
Sinuses D927
Spinal Cord D026
Spleen D722
Stomach DD21
Testis DV21
Thymus D721
Thyroid Gland DG25
Tongue D925
Trachea DB20
Ureter DT21
Urethra DT23
Uterus DU22

Sternoclavicular ligament
use Shoulder Bursa and Ligament, Left
use Shoulder Bursa and Ligament, Right
Sternocleidomastoid artery
use Thyroid Artery, Left
use Thyroid Artery, Right
Sternocleidomastoid muscle
use Neck Muscle, Left
use Neck Muscle, Right
Sternocostal ligament *use* Sternum Bursa and Ligament
Sternotomy
see Division, Sternum ØP8Ø
see Drainage, Sternum ØP9Ø
Stimulation, cardiac
Cardioversion 5A22Ø4Z
Electrophysiologic testing *see* Measurement, Cardiac 4AØ2
Stimulator Generator
Insertion of device In
Abdomen ØJH8
Back ØJH7
Chest ØJH6
Multiple Array
Abdomen ØJH8
Back ØJH7
Chest ØJH6
Multiple Array Rechargeable
Abdomen ØJH8
Back ØJH7
Chest ØJH6
Removal of device from, Subcutaneous Tissue and Fascia, Trunk ØJPT
Revision of device in, Subcutaneous Tissue and Fascia, Trunk ØJWT
Single Array
Abdomen ØJH8
Back ØJH7
Chest ØJH6
Single Array Rechargeable
Abdomen ØJH8
Back ØJH7
Chest ØJH6
Stimulator Lead
Insertion of device in
Anal Sphincter ØDHR
Artery
Left Ø3HL
Right Ø3HK
Bladder ØTHB
Muscle
Lower ØKHY
Upper ØKHX
Stomach ØDH6
Ureter ØTH9
Removal of device from
Anal Sphincter ØDPR
Artery, Upper Ø3PY
Bladder ØTPB
Muscle
Lower ØKPY
Upper ØKPX
Stomach ØDP6
Ureter ØTP9
Revision of device in
Anal Sphincter ØDWR
Artery, Upper Ø3WY
Bladder ØTWB
Muscle
Lower ØKWY
Upper ØKWX
Stomach ØDW6
Ureter ØTW9
Stoma
Excision
Abdominal Wall ØWBFXZ2
Neck ØWB6XZ2
Repair
Abdominal Wall ØWQFXZ2
Neck ØWQ6XZ2
Stomatoplasty
see Repair, Mouth and Throat ØCQ
see Replacement, Mouth and Throat ØCR
see Supplement, Mouth and Throat ØCU
Stomatorrhaphy *see* Repair, Mouth and Throat ØCQ
Stratos LV *use* Cardiac Resynchronization Pacemaker Pulse Generator in ØJH
Stress test 4AØ2XM4, 4A12XM4
Stripping *see* Extraction
Study
Electrophysiologic stimulation, cardiac *see* Measurement, Cardiac 4AØ2
Ocular motility 4AØ7X7Z
Pulmonary airway flow measurement *see* Measurement, Respiratory 4AØ9
Visual acuity 4AØ7XØZ
Styloglossus muscle *use* Tongue, Palate, Pharynx Muscle
Stylomandibular ligament *use* Head and Neck Bursa and Ligament
Stylopharyngeus muscle *use* Tongue, Palate, Pharynx Muscle
Subacromial bursa
use Shoulder Bursa and Ligament, Left
use Shoulder Bursa and Ligament, Right
Subaortic (common iliac) lymph node *use* Lymphatic, Pelvis
Subarachnoid space, spinal *use* Spinal Canal
Subclavicular (apical) lymph node
use Lymphatic, Left Axillary
use Lymphatic, Right Axillary
Subclavius muscle
use Thorax Muscle, Left
use Thorax Muscle, Right
Subclavius nerve *use* Brachial Plexus
Subcostal artery *use* Upper Artery
Subcostal muscle
use Thorax Muscle, Left
use Thorax Muscle, Right
Subcostal nerve *use* Thoracic Nerve
Subcutaneous Defibrillator Lead
Insertion of device in, Subcutaneous Tissue and Fascia, Chest ØJH6
Removal of device from, Subcutaneous Tissue and Fascia, Trunk ØJPT
Revision of device in, Subcutaneous Tissue and Fascia, Trunk ØJWT
Subcutaneous injection reservoir, port *use* Vascular Access Device, Totally Implantable in Subcutaneous Tissue and Fascia
Subcutaneous injection reservoir, pump *use* Infusion Device, Pump in Subcutaneous Tissue and Fascia
Subdermal progesterone implant *use* Contraceptive Device in Subcutaneous Tissue and Fascia
Subdural space, spinal *use* Spinal Canal
Submandibular ganglion
use Facial Nerve
use Head and Neck Sympathetic Nerve
Submandibular gland
use Submaxillary Gland, Left
use Submaxillary Gland, Right
Submandibular lymph node *use* Lymphatic, Head
Submandibular space *use* Subcutaneous Tissue and Fascia, Face
Submaxillary ganglion *use* Head and Neck Sympathetic Nerve
Submaxillary lymph node *use* Lymphatic, Head
Submental artery *use* Face Artery
Submental lymph node *use* Lymphatic, Head
Submucous (Meissner's) plexus *use* Abdominal Sympathetic Nerve
Suboccipital nerve *use* Cervical Nerve
Suboccipital venous plexus
use Vertebral Vein, Left
use Vertebral Vein, Right
Subparotid lymph node *use* Lymphatic, Head
Subscapular aponeurosis
use Subcutaneous Tissue and Fascia, Left Upper Arm
use Subcutaneous Tissue and Fascia, Right Upper Arm
Subscapular artery
use Axillary Artery, Left
use Axillary Artery, Right
Subscapular (posterior) lymph node
use Lymphatic, Axillary, Left
use Lymphatic, Axillary, Right
Subscapularis muscle
use Shoulder Muscle, Left
use Shoulder Muscle, Right
Substance Abuse Treatment
Counseling
Family, for substance abuse, Other Family Counseling HZ63ZZZ
Substance Abuse Treatment — *continued*
Counseling — *continued*
Group
12-Step HZ43ZZZ
Behavioral HZ41ZZZ
Cognitive HZ4ØZZZ
Cognitive-Behavioral HZ42ZZZ
Confrontational HZ48ZZZ
Continuing Care HZ49ZZZ
Infectious Disease
Post-Test HZ4CZZZ
Pre-Test HZ4CZZZ
Interpersonal HZ44ZZZ
Motivational Enhancement HZ47ZZZ
Psychoeducation HZ46ZZZ
Spiritual HZ4BZZZ
Vocational HZ45ZZZ
Individual
12-Step HZ33ZZZ
Behavioral HZ31ZZZ
Cognitive HZ3ØZZZ
Cognitive-Behavioral HZ32ZZZ
Confrontational HZ38ZZZ
Continuing Care HZ39ZZZ
Infectious Disease
Post-Test HZ3CZZZ
Pre-Test HZ3CZZZ
Interpersonal HZ34ZZZ
Motivational Enhancement HZ37ZZZ
Psychoeducation HZ36ZZZ
Spiritual HZ3BZZZ
Vocational HZ35ZZZ
Detoxification Services, for substance abuse HZ2ZZZZ
Medication Management
Antabuse HZ83ZZZ
Bupropion HZ87ZZZ
Clonidine HZ86ZZZ
Levo-alpha-acetyl-methadol (LAAM) HZ82ZZZ
Methadone Maintenance HZ81ZZZ
Naloxone HZ85ZZZ
Naltrexone HZ84ZZZ
Nicotine Replacement HZ8ØZZZ
Other Replacement Medication HZ89ZZZ
Psychiatric Medication HZ88ZZZ
Pharmacotherapy
Antabuse HZ93ZZZ
Bupropion HZ97ZZZ
Clonidine HZ96ZZZ
Levo-alpha-acetyl-methadol (LAAM) HZ92ZZZ
Methadone Maintenance HZ91ZZZ
Naloxone HZ95ZZZ
Naltrexone HZ94ZZZ
Nicotine Replacement HZ9ØZZZ
Psychiatric Medication HZ98ZZZ
Replacement Medication, Other HZ99ZZZ
Psychotherapy
12-Step HZ53ZZZ
Behavioral HZ51ZZZ
Cognitive HZ5ØZZZ
Cognitive-Behavioral HZ52ZZZ
Confrontational HZ58ZZZ
Interactive HZ55ZZZ
Interpersonal HZ54ZZZ
Motivational Enhancement HZ57ZZZ
Psychoanalysis HZ5BZZZ
Psychodynamic HZ5CZZZ
Psychoeducation HZ56ZZZ
Psychophysiological HZ5DZZZ
Supportive HZ59ZZZ
Substantia nigra *use* Basal Ganglia
Subtalar (talocalcaneal) joint
use Tarsal Joint, Left
use Tarsal Joint, Right
Subtalar ligament
use Foot Bursa and Ligament, Left
use Foot Bursa and Ligament, Right
Subthalamic nucleus *use* Basal Ganglia
Suction curettage (D&C), nonobstetric *see* Extraction, Endometrium ØUDB
Suction curettage, obstetric post-delivery *see* Extraction, Products of Conception, Retained 1ØD1
Superficial circumflex iliac vein
use Saphenous Vein, Left
use Saphenous Vein, Right

Superficial epigastric artery
use Femoral Artery, Left
use Femoral Artery, Right
Superficial epigastric vein
use Saphenous Vein, Left
use Saphenous Vein, Right
Superficial Inferior Epigastric Artery Flap
Replacement
Bilateral ØHRVØ78
Left ØHRUØ78
Right ØHRTØ78
Transfer
Left ØKXG
Right ØKXF
Superficial palmar arch
use Hand Artery, Left
use Hand Artery, Right
Superficial palmar venous arch
use Hand Vein, Left
use Hand Vein, Right
Superficial temporal artery
use Temporal Artery, Left
use Temporal Artery, Right
Superficial transverse perineal muscle *use* Perineum Muscle
Superior cardiac nerve *use* Thoracic Sympathetic Nerve
Superior cerebellar vein *use* Intracranial Vein
Superior cerebral vein *use* Intracranial Vein
Superior clunic (cluneal) nerve *use* Lumbar Nerve
Superior epigastric artery
use Internal Mammary Artery, Left
use Internal Mammary Artery, Right
Superior genicular artery
use Popliteal Artery, Left
use Popliteal Artery, Right
Superior gluteal artery
use Internal Iliac Artery, Left
use Internal Iliac Artery, Right
Superior gluteal nerve *use* Lumbar Plexus
Superior hypogastric plexus *use* Abdominal Sympathetic Nerve
Superior labial artery *use* Face Artery
Superior laryngeal artery
use Thyroid Artery, Left
use Thyroid Artery, Right
Superior laryngeal nerve *use* Vagus Nerve
Superior longitudinal muscle *use* Tongue, Palate, Pharynx Muscle
Superior mesenteric ganglion *use* Abdominal Sympathetic Nerve
Superior mesenteric lymph node *use* Lymphatic, Mesenteric
Superior mesenteric plexus *use* Abdominal Sympathetic Nerve
Superior oblique muscle
use Extraocular Muscle, Left
use Extraocular Muscle, Right
Superior olivary nucleus *use* Pons
Superior rectal artery *use* Inferior Mesenteric Artery
Superior rectal vein *use* Inferior Mesenteric Vein
Superior rectus muscle
use Extraocular Muscle, Left
use Extraocular Muscle, Right
Superior tarsal plate
use Upper Eyelid, Left
use Upper Eyelid, Right
Superior thoracic artery
use Axillary Artery, Left
use Axillary Artery, Right
Superior thyroid artery
use External Carotid Artery, Left
use External Carotid Artery, Right
use Thyroid Artery, Left
use Thyroid Artery, Right
Superior turbinate *use* Nasal Turbinate
Superior ulnar collateral artery
use Brachial Artery, Left
use Brachial Artery, Right
Supersaturated Oxygen therapy 5AØ512C, 5AØ522C
Supplement
Abdominal Wall ØWUF
Acetabulum
Left ØQU5
Right ØQU4
Ampulla of Vater ØFUC
Anal Sphincter ØDUR
Supplement — *continued*
Ankle Region
Left ØYUL
Right ØYUK
Anus ØDUQ
Aorta
Abdominal Ø4UØ
Thoracic
Ascending/Arch Ø2UX
Descending Ø2UW
Arm
Lower
Left ØXUF
Right ØXUD
Upper
Left ØXU9
Right ØXU8
Artery
Anterior Tibial
Left Ø4UQ
Right Ø4UP
Axillary
Left Ø3U6
Right Ø3U5
Brachial
Left Ø3U8
Right Ø3U7
Celiac Ø4U1
Colic
Left Ø4U7
Middle Ø4U8
Right Ø4U6
Common Carotid
Left Ø3UJ
Right Ø3UH
Common Iliac
Left Ø4UD
Right Ø4UC
Coronary
Four or More Arteries Ø2U3
One Artery Ø2UØ
Three Arteries Ø2U2
Two Arteries Ø2U1
External Carotid
Left Ø3UN
Right Ø3UM
External Iliac
Left Ø4UJ
Right Ø4UH
Face Ø3UR
Femoral
Left Ø4UL
Right Ø4UK
Foot
Left Ø4UW
Right Ø4UV
Gastric Ø4U2
Hand
Left Ø3UF
Right Ø3UD
Hepatic Ø4U3
Inferior Mesenteric Ø4UB
Innominate Ø3U2
Internal Carotid
Left Ø3UL
Right Ø3UK
Internal Iliac
Left Ø4UF
Right Ø4UE
Internal Mammary
Left Ø3U1
Right Ø3UØ
Intracranial Ø3UG
Lower Ø4UY
Peroneal
Left Ø4UU
Right Ø4UT
Popliteal
Left Ø4UN
Right Ø4UM
Posterior Tibial
Left Ø4US
Right Ø4UR
Pulmonary
Left Ø2UR
Right Ø2UQ
Pulmonary Trunk Ø2UP
Radial
Left Ø3UC
Supplement — *continued*
Artery — *continued*
Radial — *continued*
Right Ø3UB
Renal
Left Ø4UA
Right Ø4U9
Splenic Ø4U4
Subclavian
Left Ø3U4
Right Ø3U3
Superior Mesenteric Ø4U5
Temporal
Left Ø3UT
Right Ø3US
Thyroid
Left Ø3UV
Right Ø3UU
Ulnar
Left Ø3UA
Right Ø3U9
Upper Ø3UY
Vertebral
Left Ø3UQ
Right Ø3UP
Atrium
Left Ø2U7
Right Ø2U6
Auditory Ossicle
Left Ø9UA
Right Ø9U9
Axilla
Left ØXU5
Right ØXU4
Back
Lower ØWUL
Upper ØWUK
Bladder ØTUB
Bladder Neck ØTUC
Bone
Ethmoid
Left ØNUG
Right ØNUF
Frontal ØNU1
Hyoid ØNUX
Lacrimal
Left ØNUJ
Right ØNUH
Nasal ØNUB
Occipital ØNU7
Palatine
Left ØNUL
Right ØNUK
Parietal
Left ØNU4
Right ØNU3
Pelvic
Left ØQU3
Right ØQU2
Sphenoid ØNUC
Temporal
Left ØNU6
Right ØNU5
Zygomatic
Left ØNUN
Right ØNUM
Breast
Bilateral ØHUV
Left ØHUU
Right ØHUT
Bronchus
Lingula ØBU9
Lower Lobe
Left ØBUB
Right ØBU6
Main
Left ØBU7
Right ØBU3
Middle Lobe, Right ØBU5
Upper Lobe
Left ØBU8
Right ØBU4
Buccal Mucosa ØCU4
Bursa and Ligament
Abdomen
Left ØMUJ
Right ØMUH
Ankle
Left ØMUR

- **Supplement** — *continued*
  - Bursa and Ligament — *continued*
    - Ankle — *continued*
      - Right ØMUQ
    - Elbow
      - Left ØMU4
      - Right ØMU3
    - Foot
      - Left ØMUT
      - Right ØMUS
    - Hand
      - Left ØMU8
      - Right ØMU7
    - Head and Neck ØMUØ
    - Hip
      - Left ØMUM
      - Right ØMUL
    - Knee
      - Left ØMUP
      - Right ØMUN
    - Lower Extremity
      - Left ØMUW
      - Right ØMUV
    - Perineum ØMUK
    - Rib(s) ØMUG
    - Shoulder
      - Left ØMU2
      - Right ØMU1
    - Spine
      - Lower ØMUD
      - Upper ØMUC
    - Sternum ØMUF
    - Upper Extremity
      - Left ØMUB
      - Right ØMU9
    - Wrist
      - Left ØMU6
      - Right ØMU5
  - Buttock
    - Left ØYU1
    - Right ØYUØ
  - Carina ØBU2
  - Carpal
    - Left ØPUN
    - Right ØPUM
  - Cecum ØDUH
  - Cerebral Meninges ØØU1
  - Cerebral Ventricle ØØU6
  - Chest Wall ØWU8
  - Chordae Tendineae Ø2U9
  - Cisterna Chyli Ø7UL
  - Clavicle
    - Left ØPUB
    - Right ØPU9
  - Clitoris ØUUJ
  - Coccyx ØQUS
  - Colon
    - Ascending ØDUK
    - Descending ØDUM
    - Sigmoid ØDUN
    - Transverse ØDUL
  - Cord
    - Bilateral ØVUH
    - Left ØVUG
    - Right ØVUF
  - Cornea
    - Left Ø8U9
    - Right Ø8U8
  - Cul-de-sac ØUUF
  - Diaphragm ØBUT
  - Disc
    - Cervical Vertebral ØRU3
    - Cervicothoracic Vertebral ØRU5
    - Lumbar Vertebral ØSU2
    - Lumbosacral ØSU4
    - Thoracic Vertebral ØRU9
    - Thoracolumbar Vertebral ØRUB
  - Duct
    - Common Bile ØFU9
    - Cystic ØFU8
    - Hepatic
      - Common ØFU7
      - Left ØFU6
      - Right ØFU5
    - Lacrimal
      - Left Ø8UY
      - Right Ø8UX
    - Pancreatic ØFUD
      - Accessory ØFUF

- **Supplement** — *continued*
  - Duodenum ØDU9
  - Dura Mater ØØU2
  - Ear
    - External
      - Bilateral Ø9U2
      - Left Ø9U1
      - Right Ø9UØ
    - Inner
      - Left Ø9UE
      - Right Ø9UD
    - Middle
      - Left Ø9U6
      - Right Ø9U5
  - Elbow Region
    - Left ØXUC
    - Right ØXUB
  - Epididymis
    - Bilateral ØVUL
    - Left ØVUK
    - Right ØVUJ
  - Epiglottis ØCUR
  - Esophagogastric Junction ØDU4
  - Esophagus ØDU5
    - Lower ØDU3
    - Middle ØDU2
    - Upper ØDU1
  - Extremity
    - Lower
      - Left ØYUB
      - Right ØYU9
    - Upper
      - Left ØXU7
      - Right ØXU6
  - Eye
    - Left Ø8U1
    - Right Ø8UØ
  - Eyelid
    - Lower
      - Left Ø8UR
      - Right Ø8UQ
    - Upper
      - Left Ø8UP
      - Right Ø8UN
  - Face ØWU2
  - Fallopian Tube
    - Left ØUU6
    - Right ØUU5
  - Fallopian Tubes, Bilateral ØUU7
  - Femoral Region
    - Bilateral ØYUE
    - Left ØYU8
    - Right ØYU7
  - Femoral Shaft
    - Left ØQU9
    - Right ØQU8
  - Femur
    - Lower
      - Left ØQUC
      - Right ØQUB
    - Upper
      - Left ØQU7
      - Right ØQU6
  - Fibula
    - Left ØQUK
    - Right ØQUJ
  - Finger
    - Index
      - Left ØXUP
      - Right ØXUN
    - Little
      - Left ØXUW
      - Right ØXUV
    - Middle
      - Left ØXUR
      - Right ØXUQ
    - Ring
      - Left ØXUT
      - Right ØXUS
  - Foot
    - Left ØYUN
    - Right ØYUM
  - Gingiva
    - Lower ØCU6
    - Upper ØCU5
  - Glenoid Cavity
    - Left ØPU8
    - Right ØPU7

- **Supplement** — *continued*
  - Hand
    - Left ØXUK
    - Right ØXUJ
  - Head ØWUØ
  - Heart Ø2UA
  - Humeral Head
    - Left ØPUD
    - Right ØPUC
  - Humeral Shaft
    - Left ØPUG
    - Right ØPUF
  - Hymen ØUUK
  - Ileocecal Valve ØDUC
  - Ileum ØDUB
  - Inguinal Region
    - Bilateral ØYUA
    - Left ØYU6
    - Right ØYU5
  - Intestine
    - Large ØDUE
      - Left ØDUG
      - Right ØDUF
    - Small ØDU8
  - Iris
    - Left Ø8UD
    - Right Ø8UC
  - Jaw
    - Lower ØWU5
    - Upper ØWU4
  - Jejunum ØDUA
  - Joint
    - Acromioclavicular
      - Left ØRUH
      - Right ØRUG
    - Ankle
      - Left ØSUG
      - Right ØSUF
    - Carpal
      - Left ØRUR
      - Right ØRUQ
    - Carpometacarpal
      - Left ØRUT
      - Right ØRUS
    - Cervical Vertebral ØRU1
    - Cervicothoracic Vertebral ØRU4
    - Coccygeal ØSU6
    - Elbow
      - Left ØRUM
      - Right ØRUL
    - Finger Phalangeal
      - Left ØRUX
      - Right ØRUW
    - Hip
      - Left ØSUB
        - Acetabular Surface ØSUE
        - Femoral Surface ØSUS
      - Right ØSU9
        - Acetabular Surface ØSUA
        - Femoral Surface ØSUR
    - Knee
      - Left ØSUD
        - Femoral Surface ØSUUØ9Z
        - Tibial Surface ØSUWØ9Z
      - Right ØSUC
        - Femoral Surface ØSUTØ9Z
        - Tibial Surface ØSUVØ9Z
    - Lumbar Vertebral ØSUØ
    - Lumbosacral ØSU3
    - Metacarpophalangeal
      - Left ØRUV
      - Right ØRUU
    - Metatarsal-Phalangeal
      - Left ØSUN
      - Right ØSUM
    - Occipital-cervical ØRUØ
    - Sacrococcygeal ØSU5
    - Sacroiliac
      - Left ØSU8
      - Right ØSU7
    - Shoulder
      - Left ØRUK
      - Right ØRUJ
    - Sternoclavicular
      - Left ØRUF
      - Right ØRUE
    - Tarsal
      - Left ØSUJ
      - Right ØSUH

Supplement — *continued*
- Joint — *continued*
  - Tarsometatarsal
    - Left ØSUL
    - Right ØSUK
  - Temporomandibular
    - Left ØRUD
    - Right ØRUC
  - Thoracic Vertebral ØRU6
  - Thoracolumbar Vertebral ØRUA
  - Toe Phalangeal
    - Left ØSUQ
    - Right ØSUP
  - Wrist
    - Left ØRUP
    - Right ØRUN
- Kidney Pelvis
  - Left ØTU4
  - Right ØTU3
- Knee Region
  - Left ØYUG
  - Right ØYUF
- Larynx ØCUS
- Leg
  - Lower
    - Left ØYUJ
    - Right ØYUH
  - Upper
    - Left ØYUD
    - Right ØYUC
- Lip
  - Lower ØCU1
  - Upper ØCUØ
- Lymphatic
  - Aortic Ø7UD
  - Axillary
    - Left Ø7U6
    - Right Ø7U5
  - Head Ø7UØ
  - Inguinal
    - Left Ø7UJ
    - Right Ø7UH
  - Internal Mammary
    - Left Ø7U9
    - Right Ø7U8
  - Lower Extremity
    - Left Ø7UG
    - Right Ø7UF
  - Mesenteric Ø7UB
  - Neck
    - Left Ø7U2
    - Right Ø7U1
  - Pelvis Ø7UC
  - Thoracic Duct Ø7UK
  - Thorax Ø7U7
  - Upper Extremity
    - Left Ø7U4
    - Right Ø7U3
- Mandible
  - Left ØNUV
  - Right ØNUT
- Maxilla ØNUR
- Mediastinum ØWUC
- Mesentery ØDUV
- Metacarpal
  - Left ØPUQ
  - Right ØPUP
- Metatarsal
  - Left ØQUP
  - Right ØQUN
- Muscle
  - Abdomen
    - Left ØKUL
    - Right ØKUK
  - Extraocular
    - Left Ø8UM
    - Right Ø8UL
  - Facial ØKU1
  - Foot
    - Left ØKUW
    - Right ØKUV
  - Hand
    - Left ØKUD
    - Right ØKUC
  - Head ØKUØ
  - Hip
    - Left ØKUP
    - Right ØKUN

Supplement — *continued*
- Muscle — *continued*
  - Lower Arm and Wrist
    - Left ØKUB
    - Right ØKU9
  - Lower Leg
    - Left ØKUT
    - Right ØKUS
  - Neck
    - Left ØKU3
    - Right ØKU2
  - Papillary Ø2UD
  - Perineum ØKUM
  - Shoulder
    - Left ØKU6
    - Right ØKU5
  - Thorax
    - Left ØKUJ
    - Right ØKUH
  - Tongue, Palate, Pharynx ØKU4
  - Trunk
    - Left ØKUG
    - Right ØKUF
  - Upper Arm
    - Left ØKU8
    - Right ØKU7
  - Upper Leg
    - Left ØKUR
    - Right ØKUQ
- Nasal Mucosa and Soft Tissue Ø9UK
- Nasopharynx Ø9UN
- Neck ØWU6
- Nerve
  - Abducens ØØUL
  - Accessory ØØUR
  - Acoustic ØØUN
  - Cervical Ø1U1
  - Facial ØØUM
  - Femoral Ø1UD
  - Glossopharyngeal ØØUP
  - Hypoglossal ØØUS
  - Lumbar Ø1UB
  - Median Ø1U5
  - Oculomotor ØØUH
  - Olfactory ØØUF
  - Optic ØØUG
  - Peroneal Ø1UH
  - Phrenic Ø1U2
  - Pudendal Ø1UC
  - Radial Ø1U6
  - Sacral Ø1UR
  - Sciatic Ø1UF
  - Thoracic Ø1U8
  - Tibial Ø1UG
  - Trigeminal ØØUK
  - Trochlear ØØUJ
  - Ulnar Ø1U4
  - Vagus ØØUQ
- Nipple
  - Left ØHUX
  - Right ØHUW
- Omentum ØDUU
- Orbit
  - Left ØNUQ
  - Right ØNUP
- Palate
  - Hard ØCU2
  - Soft ØCU3
- Patella
  - Left ØQUF
  - Right ØQUD
- Penis ØVUS
- Pericardium Ø2UN
- Perineum
  - Female ØWUN
  - Male ØWUM
- Peritoneum ØDUW
- Phalanx
  - Finger
    - Left ØPUV
    - Right ØPUT
  - Thumb
    - Left ØPUS
    - Right ØPUR
  - Toe
    - Left ØQUR
    - Right ØQUQ
- Pharynx ØCUM
- Prepuce ØVUT

Supplement — *continued*
- Radius
  - Left ØPUJ
  - Right ØPUH
- Rectum ØDUP
- Retina
  - Left Ø8UF
  - Right Ø8UE
- Retinal Vessel
  - Left Ø8UH
  - Right Ø8UG
- Ribs
  - 1 to 2 ØPU1
  - 3 or More ØPU2
- Sacrum ØQU1
- Scapula
  - Left ØPU6
  - Right ØPU5
- Scrotum ØVU5
- Septum
  - Atrial Ø2U5
  - Nasal Ø9UM
  - Ventricular Ø2UM
- Shoulder Region
  - Left ØXU3
  - Right ØXU2
- Sinus
  - Accessory Ø9UP
  - Ethmoid
    - Left Ø9UV
    - Right Ø9UU
  - Frontal
    - Left Ø9UT
    - Right Ø9US
  - Mastoid
    - Left Ø9UC
    - Right Ø9UB
  - Maxillary
    - Left Ø9UR
    - Right Ø9UQ
  - Sphenoid
    - Left Ø9UX
    - Right Ø9UW
- Skull ØNUØ
- Spinal Meninges ØØUT
- Sternum ØPUØ
- Stomach ØDU6
  - Pylorus ØDU7
- Subcutaneous Tissue and Fascia
  - Abdomen ØJU8
  - Back ØJU7
  - Buttock ØJU9
  - Chest ØJU6
  - Face ØJU1
  - Foot
    - Left ØJUR
    - Right ØJUQ
  - Hand
    - Left ØJUK
    - Right ØJUJ
  - Lower Arm
    - Left ØJUH
    - Right ØJUG
  - Lower Leg
    - Left ØJUP
    - Right ØJUN
  - Neck
    - Left ØJU5
    - Right ØJU4
  - Pelvic Region ØJUC
  - Perineum ØJUB
  - Scalp ØJUØ
  - Upper Arm
    - Left ØJUF
    - Right ØJUD
  - Upper Leg
    - Left ØJUM
    - Right ØJUL
- Tarsal
  - Left ØQUM
  - Right ØQUL
- Tendon
  - Abdomen
    - Left ØLUG
    - Right ØLUF
  - Ankle
    - Left ØLUT
    - Right ØLUS

Supplement — *continued*
Tendon — *continued*
Foot
Left ØLUW
Right ØLUV
Hand
Left ØLU8
Right ØLU7
Head and Neck ØLUØ
Hip
Left ØLUK
Right ØLUJ
Knee
Left ØLUR
Right ØLUQ
Lower Arm and Wrist
Left ØLU6
Right ØLU5
Lower Leg
Left ØLUP
Right ØLUN
Perineum ØLUH
Shoulder
Left ØLU2
Right ØLU1
Thorax
Left ØLUD
Right ØLUC
Trunk
Left ØLUB
Right ØLU9
Upper Arm
Left ØLU4
Right ØLU3
Upper Leg
Left ØLUM
Right ØLUL
Testis
Bilateral ØVUCØ
Left ØVUBØ
Right ØVU9Ø
Thumb
Left ØXUM
Right ØXUL
Tibia
Left ØQUH
Right ØQUG
Toe
1st
Left ØYUQ
Right ØYUP
2nd
Left ØYUS
Right ØYUR
3rd
Left ØYUU
Right ØYUT
4th
Left ØYUW
Right ØYUV
5th
Left ØYUY
Right ØYUX
Tongue ØCU7
Trachea ØBU1
Tunica Vaginalis
Left ØVU7
Right ØVU6
Turbinate, Nasal Ø9UL
Tympanic Membrane
Left Ø9U8
Right Ø9U7
Ulna
Left ØPUL
Right ØPUK
Ureter
Left ØTU7
Right ØTU6
Urethra ØTUD
Uterine Supporting Structure ØUU4
Uvula ØCUN
Vagina ØUUG
Valve
Aortic Ø2UF
Mitral Ø2UG
Pulmonary Ø2UH
Tricuspid Ø2UJ
Vas Deferens
Bilateral ØVUQ

Supplement — *continued*
Vas Deferens — *continued*
Left ØVUP
Right ØVUN
Vein
Axillary
Left Ø5U8
Right Ø5U7
Azygos Ø5UØ
Basilic
Left Ø5UC
Right Ø5UB
Brachial
Left Ø5UA
Right Ø5U9
Cephalic
Left Ø5UF
Right Ø5UD
Colic Ø6U7
Common Iliac
Left Ø6UD
Right Ø6UC
Esophageal Ø6U3
External Iliac
Left Ø6UG
Right Ø6UF
External Jugular
Left Ø5UQ
Right Ø5UP
Face
Left Ø5UV
Right Ø5UT
Femoral
Left Ø6UN
Right Ø6UM
Foot
Left Ø6UV
Right Ø6UT
Gastric Ø6U2
Hand
Left Ø5UH
Right Ø5UG
Hemiazygos Ø5U1
Hepatic Ø6U4
Hypogastric
Left Ø6UJ
Right Ø6UH
Inferior Mesenteric Ø6U6
Innominate
Left Ø5U4
Right Ø5U3
Internal Jugular
Left Ø5UN
Right Ø5UM
Intracranial Ø5UL
Lower Ø6UY
Portal Ø6U8
Pulmonary
Left Ø2UT
Right Ø2US
Renal
Left Ø6UB
Right Ø6U9
Saphenous
Left Ø6UQ
Right Ø6UP
Splenic Ø6U1
Subclavian
Left Ø5U6
Right Ø5U5
Superior Mesenteric Ø6U5
Upper Ø5UY
Vertebral
Left Ø5US
Right Ø5UR
Vena Cava
Inferior Ø6UØ
Superior Ø2UV
Ventricle
Left Ø2UL
Right Ø2UK
Vertebra
Cervical ØPU3
Lumbar ØQUØ
Mechanically Expandable (Paired) Synthetic Substitute XNUØ356
Thoracic ØPU4
Mechanically Expandable (Paired) Synthetic Substitute XNU4356

Supplement — *continued*
Vesicle
Bilateral ØVU3
Left ØVU2
Right ØVU1
Vocal Cord
Left ØCUV
Right ØCUT
Vulva ØUUM
Wrist Region
Left ØXUH
Right ØXUG
Supraclavicular (Virchow's) lymph node
use Lymphatic, Left Neck
use Lymphatic, Right Neck
Supraclavicular nerve *use* Cervical Plexus
Suprahyoid lymph node *use* Lymphatic, Head
Suprahyoid muscle
use Neck Muscle, Left
use Neck Muscle, Right
Suprainguinal lymph node *use* Lymphatic, Pelvis
Supraorbital vein
use Face Vein, Left
use Face Vein, Right
Suprarenal gland
use Adrenal Gland
use Adrenal Gland, Bilateral
use Adrenal Gland, Left
use Adrenal Gland, Right
Suprarenal plexus *use* Abdominal Sympathetic Nerve
Suprascapular nerve *use* Brachial Plexus
Supraspinatus fascia
use Subcutaneous Tissue and Fascia, Left Upper Arm
use Subcutaneous Tissue and Fascia, Right Upper Arm
Supraspinatus muscle
use Shoulder Muscle, Left
use Shoulder Muscle, Right
Supraspinous ligament
use Lower Spine Bursa and Ligament
use Upper Spine Bursa and Ligament
Suprasternal notch *use* Sternum
Supratrochlear lymph node
use Lymphatic, Left Upper Extremity
use Lymphatic, Right Upper Extremity
Sural artery
use Popliteal Artery, Left
use Popliteal Artery, Right
Surpass Streamline™ Flow Diverter *use* Intraluminal Device, Flow Diverter in Ø3V
Suspension
Bladder Neck *see* Reposition, Bladder Neck ØTSC
Kidney *see* Reposition, Urinary System ØTS
Urethra *see* Reposition, Urinary System ØTS
Urethrovesical *see* Reposition, Bladder Neck ØTSC
Uterus *see* Reposition, Uterus ØUS9
Vagina *see* Reposition, Vagina ØUSG
Sustained Release Drug-eluting Intraluminal Device
Dilation
Anterior Tibial
Left X27Q385
Right X27P385
Femoral
Left X27J385
Right X27H385
Peroneal
Left X27U385
Right X27T385
Popliteal
Left Distal X27N385
Left Proximal X27L385
Right Distal X27M385
Right Proximal X27K385
Posterior Tibial
Left X27S385
Right X27R385
Four or More
Anterior Tibial
Left X27Q3C5
Right X27P3C5
Femoral
Left X27J3C5
Right X27H3C5
Peroneal
Left X27U3C5

Subterms under main terms may continue to next column or page

Sustained Release Drug-eluting Intraluminal Device — *continued*
Four or More — *continued*
Peroneal — *continued*
Right X27T3C5
Popliteal
Left Distal X27N3C5
Left Proximal X27L3C5
Right Distal X27M3C5
Right Proximal X27K3C5
Posterior Tibial
Left X27S3C5
Right X27R3C5
Three
Anterior Tibial
Left X27Q3B5
Right X27P3B5
Femoral
Left X27J3B5
Right X27H3B5
Peroneal
Left X27U3B5
Right X27T3B5
Popliteal
Left Distal X27N3B5
Left Proximal X27L3B5
Right Distal X27M3B5
Right Proximal X27K3B5
Posterior Tibial
Left X27S3B5
Right X27R3B5
Two
Anterior Tibial
Left X27Q395
Right X27P395
Femoral
Left X27J395
Right X27H395
Peroneal
Left X27U395
Right X27T395
Popliteal
Left Distal X27N395
Left Proximal X27L395
Right Distal X27M395
Right Proximal X27K395
Posterior Tibial
Left X27S395
Right X27R395
Suture
Laceration repair *see* Repair
Ligation *see* Occlusion
Suture Removal
Extremity
Lower 8E0YXY8
Upper 8E0XXY8
Head and Neck Region 8E09XY8
Trunk Region 8E0WXY8
Sutureless valve, Perceval *use* Zooplastic Tissue, Rapid Deployment Technique in New Technology
Sweat gland *use* Skin
Sympathectomy *see* Excision, Peripheral Nervous System 01B
SynCardia Total Artificial Heart *use* Synthetic Substitute
Synchra CRT-P *use* Cardiac Resynchronization Pacemaker Pulse Generator in 0JH
SynchroMed pump *use* Infusion Device, Pump in Subcutaneous Tissue and Fascia
Synechiotomy, iris *see* Release, Eye 08N
Synovectomy
Lower joint *see* Excision, Lower Joints 0SB
Upper joint *see* Excision, Upper Joints 0RB
Synthetic Human Angiotensin II XW0
Systemic Nuclear Medicine Therapy
Abdomen CW70
Anatomical Regions, Multiple CW7YYZZ
Chest CW73
Thyroid CW7G
Whole Body CW7N

T

Tagraxofusp-erzs Antineoplastic XW0
Takedown
Arteriovenous shunt *see* Removal of device from, Upper Arteries 03P
Arteriovenous shunt, with creation of new shunt *see* Bypass, Upper Arteries 031
Stoma
see Excision
see Reposition
Talent® Converter *use* Intraluminal Device
Talent® Occluder *use* Intraluminal Device
Talent® Stent Graft (abdominal) (thoracic) *use* Intraluminal Device
Talocalcaneal (subtalar) joint
use Tarsal Joint, Left
use Tarsal Joint, Right
Talocalcaneal ligament
use Foot Bursa and Ligament, Left
use Foot Bursa and Ligament, Right
Talocalcaneonavicular joint
use Tarsal Joint, Left
use Tarsal Joint, Right
Talocalcaneonavicular ligament
use Foot Bursa and Ligament, Left
use Foot Bursa and Ligament, Right
Talocrural joint
use Ankle Joint, Left
use Joint, Ankle, Right
Talofibular ligament
use Ankle Bursa and Ligament, Left
use Ankle Bursa and Ligament, Right
Talus bone
use Tarsal, Left
use Tarsal, Right
TandemHeart® System *use* Short-term External Heart Assist System in Heart and Great Vessels
Tarsectomy
see Excision, Lower Bones 0QB
see Resection, Lower Bones 0QT
Tarsometatarsal ligament
use Foot Bursa and Ligament, Left
use Foot Bursa and Ligament, Right
Tarsorrhaphy *see* Repair, Eye 08Q
Tattooing
Cornea 3E0CXMZ
Skin *see* Introduction of substance in or on, Skin 3E00
TAXUS® Liberté® Paclitaxel-eluting Coronary Stent System *use* Intraluminal Device, Drug-eluting in Heart and Great Vessels
TBNA (transbronchial needle aspiration)
Fluid or gas *see* Drainage, Respiratory System 0B9
Tissue biopsy *see* Extraction, Respiratory System 0BD
TECENTRIQ® *use* Atezolizumab Antineoplastic
Telemetry 4A12X4Z
Ambulatory 4A12X45
Temperature gradient study 4A0ZXKZ
Temporal lobe *use* Cerebral Hemisphere
Temporalis muscle *use* Head Muscle
Temporoparietalis muscle *use* Head Muscle
Tendolysis *see* Release, Tendons 0LN
Tendonectomy
see Excision, Tendons 0LB
see Resection, Tendons 0LT
Tendonoplasty, tenoplasty
see Repair, Tendons 0LQ
see Replacement, Tendons 0LR
see Supplement, Tendons 0LU
Tendorrhaphy *see* Repair, Tendons 0LQ
Tendototomy
see Division, Tendons 0L8
see Drainage, Tendons 0L9
Tenectomy, tenonectomy
see Excision, Tendons 0LB
see Resection, Tendons 0LT
Tenolysis *see* Release, Tendons 0LN
Tenontorrhaphy *see* Repair, Tendons 0LQ
Tenontotomy
see Division, Tendons 0L8
see Drainage, Tendons 0L9
Tenorrhaphy *see* Repair, Tendons 0LQ
Tenosynovectomy
see Excision, Tendons 0LB
see Resection, Tendons 0LT
Tenotomy
see Division, Tendons 0L8
see Drainage, Tendons 0L9
Tensor fasciae latae muscle
use Hip Muscle, Left
use Hip Muscle, Right
Tensor veli palatini muscle *use* Tongue, Palate, Pharynx Muscle
Tenth cranial nerve *use* Vagus Nerve
Tentorium cerebelli *use* Dura Mater
Teres major muscle
use Shoulder Muscle, Left
use Shoulder Muscle, Right
Teres minor muscle
use Shoulder Muscle, Left
use Shoulder Muscle, Right
Termination of pregnancy
Aspiration curettage 10A07ZZ
Dilation and curettage 10A07ZZ
Hysterotomy 10A00ZZ
Intra-amniotic injection 10A03ZZ
Laminaria 10A07ZW
Vacuum 10A07Z6
Testectomy
see Excision, Male Reproductive System 0VB
see Resection, Male Reproductive System 0VT
Testicular artery *use* Abdominal Aorta
Testing
Glaucoma 4A07XBZ
Hearing *see* Hearing Assessment, Diagnostic Audiology F13
Mental health *see* Psychological Tests
Muscle function, electromyography (EMG) *see* Measurement, Musculoskeletal 4A0F
Muscle function, manual *see* Motor Function Assessment, Rehabilitation F01
Neurophysiologic monitoring, intra-operative *see* Monitoring, Physiological Systems 4A1
Range of motion *see* Motor Function Assessment, Rehabilitation F01
Vestibular function *see* Vestibular Assessment, Diagnostic Audiology F15
Thalamectomy *see* Excision, Thalamus 00B9
Thalamotomy *see* Drainage, Thalamus 0099
Thenar muscle
use Hand Muscle, Left
use Hand Muscle, Right
Therapeutic Massage
Musculoskeletal System 8E0KX1Z
Reproductive System
Prostate 8E0VX1C
Rectum 8E0VX1D
Therapeutic occlusion coil(s) *use* Intraluminal Device
Thermography 4A0ZXKZ
Thermotherapy, prostate *see* Destruction, Prostate 0V50
Third cranial nerve *use* Oculomotor Nerve
Third occipital nerve *use* Cervical Nerve
Third ventricle *use* Cerebral Ventricle
Thoracectomy *see* Excision, Anatomical Regions, General 0WB
Thoracentesis *see* Drainage, Anatomical Regions, General 0W9
Thoracic aortic plexus *use* Thoracic Sympathetic Nerve
Thoracic esophagus *use* Esophagus, Middle
Thoracic facet joint *use* Thoracic Vertebral Joint
Thoracic ganglion *use* Thoracic Sympathetic Nerve
Thoracoacromial artery
use Axillary Artery, Left
use Axillary Artery, Right
Thoracocentesis *see* Drainage, Anatomical Regions, General 0W9
Thoracolumbar facet joint *use* Thoracolumbar Vertebral Joint
Thoracoplasty
see Repair, Anatomical Regions, General 0WQ
see Supplement, Anatomical Regions, General 0WU
Thoracostomy, for lung collapse *see* Drainage, Respiratory System 0B9
Thoracostomy tube *use* Drainage Device
Thoracotomy *see* Drainage, Anatomical Regions, General 0W9
Thoratec IVAD (Implantable Ventricular Assist Device) *use* Implantable Heart Assist System in Heart and Great Vessels
Thoratec Paracorporeal Ventricular Assist Device *use* Short-term External Heart Assist System in Heart and Great Vessels
Thrombectomy *see* Extirpation

Thrombolysis, Ultrasound assisted *see* Fragmentation, Artery
Thymectomy
see Excision, Lymphatic and Hemic Systems 07B
see Resection, Lymphatic and Hemic Systems 07T
Thymopexy
see Repair, Lymphatic and Hemic Systems 07Q
see Reposition, Lymphatic and Hemic Systems 07S
Thymus gland *use* Thymus
Thyroarytenoid muscle
use Neck Muscle, Left
use Neck Muscle, Right
Thyrocervical trunk
use Thyroid Artery, Left
use Thyroid Artery, Right
Thyroid cartilage *use* Larynx
Thyroidectomy
see Excision, Endocrine System 0GB
see Resection, Endocrine System 0GT
Thyroidorrhaphy *see* Repair, Endocrine System 0GQ
Thyroidoscopy 0GJK4ZZ
Thyroidotomy *see* Drainage, Endocrine System 0G9
Tibial insert *use* Liner in Lower Joints
Tibialis anterior muscle
use Lower Leg Muscle, Left
use Lower Leg Muscle, Right
Tibialis posterior muscle
use Lower Leg Muscle, Left
use Lower Leg Muscle, Right
Tibiofemoral joint
use Knee Joint, Left
use Knee Joint, Right
use Knee Joint, Tibial Surface, Left
use Knee Joint, Tibial Surface, Right
Tibioperoneal trunk
use Popliteal Artery, Left
use Popliteal Artery, Right
Tisagenlecleucel *use* Engineered Autologous Chimeric Antigen Receptor T-cell Immunotherapy
Tissue bank graft *use* Nonautologous Tissue Substitute
Tissue expander (inflatable) (injectable)
use Tissue Expander in Skin and Breast
use Tissue Expander in Subcutaneous Tissue and Fascia
Tissue Expander
Insertion of device in
Breast
Bilateral 0HHV
Left 0HHU
Right 0HHT
Nipple
Left 0HHX
Right 0HHW
Subcutaneous Tissue and Fascia
Abdomen 0JH8
Back 0JH7
Buttock 0JH9
Chest 0JH6
Face 0JH1
Foot
Left 0JHR
Right 0JHQ
Hand
Left 0JHK
Right 0JHJ
Lower Arm
Left 0JHH
Right 0JHG
Lower Leg
Left 0JHP
Right 0JHN
Neck
Left 0JH5
Right 0JH4
Pelvic Region 0JHC
Perineum 0JHB
Scalp 0JH0
Upper Arm
Left 0JHF
Right 0JHD
Upper Leg
Left 0JHM
Right 0JHL
Removal of device from
Breast
Left 0HPU
Right 0HPT

Tissue Expander — *continued*
Removal of device from — *continued*
Subcutaneous Tissue and Fascia
Head and Neck 0JPS
Lower Extremity 0JPW
Trunk 0JPT
Upper Extremity 0JPV
Revision of device in
Breast
Left 0HWU
Right 0HWT
Subcutaneous Tissue and Fascia
Head and Neck 0JWS
Lower Extremity 0JWW
Trunk 0JWT
Upper Extremity 0JWV
Tissue Plasminogen Activator (tPA) (r-tPA) *use* Other Thrombolytic
Titanium Sternal Fixation System (TSFS)
use Internal Fixation Device, Rigid Plate in 0PS
use Internal Fixation Device, Rigid Plate in 0PH
Tomographic (Tomo) Nuclear Medicine Imaging
Abdomen CW20
Abdomen and Chest CW24
Abdomen and Pelvis CW21
Anatomical Regions, Multiple CW2YYZZ
Bladder, Kidneys and Ureters CT23
Brain C020
Breast CH2YYZZ
Bilateral CH22
Left CH21
Right CH20
Bronchi and Lungs CB22
Central Nervous System C02YYZZ
Cerebrospinal Fluid C025
Chest CW23
Chest and Abdomen CW24
Chest and Neck CW26
Digestive System CD2YYZZ
Endocrine System CG2YYZZ
Extremity
Lower CW2D
Bilateral CP2F
Left CP2D
Right CP2C
Upper CW2M
Bilateral CP2B
Left CP29
Right CP28
Gallbladder CF24
Gastrointestinal Tract CD27
Gland, Parathyroid CG21
Head and Neck CW2B
Heart C22YYZZ
Right and Left C226
Hepatobiliary System and Pancreas CF2YYZZ
Kidneys, Ureters and Bladder CT23
Liver CF25
Liver and Spleen CF26
Lungs and Bronchi CB22
Lymphatics and Hematologic System C72YYZZ
Musculoskeletal System, Other CP2YYZZ
Myocardium C22G
Neck and Chest CW26
Neck and Head CW2B
Pancreas and Hepatobiliary System CF2YYZZ
Pelvic Region CW2J
Pelvis CP26
Pelvis and Abdomen CW21
Pelvis and Spine CP27
Respiratory System CB2YYZZ
Skin CH2YYZZ
Skull CP21
Skull and Cervical Spine CP23
Spine
Cervical CP22
Cervical and Skull CP23
Lumbar CP2H
Thoracic CP2G
Thoracolumbar CP2J
Spine and Pelvis CP27
Spleen C722
Spleen and Liver CF26
Subcutaneous Tissue CH2YYZZ
Thorax CP24
Ureters, Kidneys and Bladder CT23
Urinary System CT2YYZZ
Tomography, computerized *see* Computerized Tomography (CT Scan)

Tongue, base of *use* Pharynx
Tonometry 4A07XBZ
Tonsillectomy
see Excision, Mouth and Throat 0CB
see Resection, Mouth and Throat 0CT
Tonsillotomy *see* Drainage, Mouth and Throat 0C9
Total Anomalous Pulmonary Venous Return (TAPVR) repair
see Bypass, Atrium, Left 0217
see Bypass, Vena Cava, Superior 021V
Total artificial (replacement) heart *use* Synthetic Substitute
Total parenteral nutrition (TPN) *see* Introduction of Nutritional Substance
Trachectomy
see Excision, Trachea 0BB1
see Resection, Trachea 0BT1
Trachelectomy
see Excision, Cervix 0UBC
see Resection, Cervix 0UTC
Trachelopexy
see Repair, Cervix 0UQC
see Reposition, Cervix 0USC
Tracheloplasty *see* Repair, Cervix 0UQC
Trachelorrhaphy *see* Repair, Cervix 0UQC
Trachelotomy *see* Drainage, Cervix 0U9C
Tracheobronchial lymph node *use* Lymphatic, Thorax
Tracheoesophageal fistulization 0B110D6
Tracheolysis *see* Release, Respiratory System 0BN
Tracheoplasty
see Repair, Respiratory System 0BQ
see Supplement, Respiratory System 0BU
Tracheorrhaphy *see* Repair, Respiratory System 0BQ
Tracheoscopy 0BJ18ZZ
Tracheostomy *see* Bypass, Respiratory System 0B1
Tracheostomy Device
Bypass, Trachea 0B11
Change device in, Trachea 0B21XFZ
Removal of device from, Trachea 0BP1
Revision of device in, Trachea 0BW1
Tracheostomy tube *use* Tracheostomy Device in Respiratory System
Tracheotomy *see* Drainage, Respiratory System 0B9
Traction
Abdominal Wall 2W63X
Arm
Lower
Left 2W6DX
Right 2W6CX
Upper
Left 2W6BX
Right 2W6AX
Back 2W65X
Chest Wall 2W64X
Extremity
Lower
Left 2W6MX
Right 2W6LX
Upper
Left 2W69X
Right 2W68X
Face 2W61X
Finger
Left 2W6KX
Right 2W6JX
Foot
Left 2W6TX
Right 2W6SX
Hand
Left 2W6FX
Right 2W6EX
Head 2W60X
Inguinal Region
Left 2W67X
Right 2W66X
Leg
Lower
Left 2W6RX
Right 2W6QX
Upper
Left 2W6PX
Right 2W6NX
Neck 2W62X
Thumb
Left 2W6HX
Right 2W6GX
Toe
Left 2W6VX

Traction — *continued*
Toe — *continued*
Right 2W6UX
Tractotomy *see* Division, Central Nervous System and Cranial Nerves ØØ8
Tragus
use External Ear, Bilateral
use External Ear, Left
use External Ear, Right
Training, caregiver *see* Caregiver Training
TRAM (transverse rectus abdominis myocutaneous) flap reconstruction
Free *see* Replacement, Skin and Breast ØHR
Pedicled *see* Transfer, Muscles ØKX
Transdermal Glomerular Filtration Rate (GFR) Measurement System XT25XE5
Transection *see* Division
Transfer
Buccal Mucosa ØCX4
Bursa and Ligament
Abdomen
Left ØMXJ
Right ØMXH
Ankle
Left ØMXR
Right ØMXQ
Elbow
Left ØMX4
Right ØMX3
Foot
Left ØMXT
Right ØMXS
Hand
Left ØMX8
Right ØMX7
Head and Neck ØMXØ
Hip
Left ØMXM
Right ØMXL
Knee
Left ØMXP
Right ØMXN
Lower Extremity
Left ØMXW
Right ØMXV
Perineum ØMXK
Rib(s) ØMXG
Shoulder
Left ØMX2
Right ØMX1
Spine
Lower ØMXD
Upper ØMXC
Sternum ØMXF
Upper Extremity
Left ØMXB
Right ØMX9
Wrist
Left ØMX6
Right ØMX5
Finger
Left ØXXPØZM
Right ØXXNØZL
Gingiva
Lower ØCX6
Upper ØCX5
Intestine
Large ØDXE
Small ØDX8
Lip
Lower ØCX1
Upper ØCXØ
Muscle
Abdomen
Left ØKXL
Right ØKXK
Extraocular
Left Ø8XM
Right Ø8XL
Facial ØKX1
Foot
Left ØKXW
Right ØKXV
Hand
Left ØKXD
Right ØKXC
Head ØKXØ

Transfer — *continued*
Muscle — *continued*
Hip
Left ØKXP
Right ØKXN
Lower Arm and Wrist
Left ØKXB
Right ØKX9
Lower Leg
Left ØKXT
Right ØKXS
Neck
Left ØKX3
Right ØKX2
Perineum ØKXM
Shoulder
Left ØKX6
Right ØKX5
Thorax
Left ØKXJ
Right ØKXH
Tongue, Palate, Pharynx ØKX4
Trunk
Left ØKXG
Right ØKXF
Upper Arm
Left ØKX8
Right ØKX7
Upper Leg
Left ØKXR
Right ØKXQ
Nerve
Abducens ØØXL
Accessory ØØXR
Acoustic ØØXN
Cervical Ø1X1
Facial ØØXM
Femoral Ø1XD
Glossopharyngeal ØØXP
Hypoglossal ØØXS
Lumbar Ø1XB
Median Ø1X5
Oculomotor ØØXH
Olfactory ØØXF
Optic ØØXG
Peroneal Ø1XH
Phrenic Ø1X2
Pudendal Ø1XC
Radial Ø1X6
Sciatic Ø1XF
Thoracic Ø1X8
Tibial Ø1XG
Trigeminal ØØXK
Trochlear ØØXJ
Ulnar Ø1X4
Vagus ØØXQ
Palate, Soft ØCX3
Prepuce ØVXT
Skin
Abdomen ØHX7XZZ
Back ØHX6XZZ
Buttock ØHX8XZZ
Chest ØHX5XZZ
Ear
Left ØHX3XZZ
Right ØHX2XZZ
Face ØHX1XZZ
Foot
Left ØHXNXZZ
Right ØHXMXZZ
Hand
Left ØHXGXZZ
Right ØHXFXZZ
Inguinal ØHXAXZZ
Lower Arm
Left ØHXEXZZ
Right ØHXDXZZ
Lower Leg
Left ØHXLXZZ
Right ØHXKXZZ
Neck ØHX4XZZ
Perineum ØHX9XZZ
Scalp ØHXØXZZ
Upper Arm
Left ØHXCXZZ
Right ØHXBXZZ
Upper Leg
Left ØHXJXZZ
Right ØHXHXZZ

Transfer — *continued*
Stomach ØDX6
Subcutaneous Tissue and Fascia
Abdomen ØJX8
Back ØJX7
Buttock ØJX9
Chest ØJX6
Face ØJX1
Foot
Left ØJXR
Right ØJXQ
Hand
Left ØJXK
Right ØJXJ
Lower Arm
Left ØJXH
Right ØJXG
Lower Leg
Left ØJXP
Right ØJXN
Neck
Left ØJX5
Right ØJX4
Pelvic Region ØJXC
Perineum ØJXB
Scalp ØJXØ
Upper Arm
Left ØJXF
Right ØJXD
Upper Leg
Left ØJXM
Right ØJXL
Tendon
Abdomen
Left ØLXG
Right ØLXF
Ankle
Left ØLXT
Right ØLXS
Foot
Left ØLXW
Right ØLXV
Hand
Left ØLX8
Right ØLX7
Head and Neck ØLXØ
Hip
Left ØLXK
Right ØLXJ
Knee
Left ØLXR
Right ØLXQ
Lower Arm and Wrist
Left ØLX6
Right ØLX5
Lower Leg
Left ØLXP
Right ØLXN
Perineum ØLXH
Shoulder
Left ØLX2
Right ØLX1
Thorax
Left ØLXD
Right ØLXC
Trunk
Left ØLXB
Right ØLX9
Upper Arm
Left ØLX4
Right ØLX3
Upper Leg
Left ØLXM
Right ØLXL
Tongue ØCX7
Transfusion
Immunotherapy *see* New Technology, Anatomical Regions XW2
Products of Conception
Antihemophilic Factors 3Ø27
Blood
Platelets 3Ø27
Red Cells 3Ø27
Frozen 3Ø27
White Cells 3Ø27
Whole 3Ø27
Factor IX 3Ø27
Fibrinogen 3Ø27
Globulin 3Ø27

Transfusion — *continued*
- Products of Conception — *continued*
  - Plasma
    - Fresh 3027
    - Frozen 3027
  - Plasma Cryoprecipitate 3027
  - Serum Albumin 3027
- Vein
  - 4-Factor Prothrombin Complex Concentrate 30280B1
  - Central
    - Antihemophilic Factors 3024
    - Blood
      - Platelets 3024
      - Red Cells 3024
        - Frozen 3024
      - White Cells 3024
      - Whole 3024
    - Bone Marrow 3024
    - Factor IX 3024
    - Fibrinogen 3024
    - Globulin 3024
    - Hematopoietic Stem/Progenitor Cells (HSPC), Genetically Modified 3024
    - Plasma
      - Fresh 3024
      - Frozen 3024
    - Plasma Cryoprecipitate 3024
    - Serum Albumin 3024
    - Stem Cells
      - Cord Blood 3024
      - Embryonic 3024
      - Hematopoietic 3024
      - T-cell Depleted Hematopoietic 3024
  - Peripheral
    - Antihemophilic Factors 3023
    - Blood
      - Platelets 3023
      - Red Cells 3023
        - Frozen 3023
      - White Cells 3023
      - Whole 3023
    - Bone Marrow 3023
    - Factor IX 3023
    - Fibrinogen 3023
    - Globulin 3023
    - Hematopoietic Stem/Progenitor Cells (HSPC), Genetically Modified 3023
    - Plasma
      - Fresh 3023
      - Frozen 3023
    - Plasma Cryoprecipitate 3023
    - Serum Albumin 3023
    - Stem Cells
      - Cord Blood 3023
      - Embryonic 3023
      - Hematopoietic 3023
      - T-cell Depleted Hematopoietic 3023

Transplant *see* Transplantation

Transplantation
- Bone marrow *see* Transfusion, Circulatory 302
- Esophagus ØDY5ØZ
- Face ØWY2ØZ
- Hand
  - Left ØXYKØZ
  - Right ØXYJØZ
- Heart Ø2YAØZ
- Hematopoietic cell *see* Transfusion, Circulatory 302
- Intestine
  - Large ØDYEØZ
  - Small ØDY8ØZ
- Kidney
  - Left ØTY1ØZ
  - Right ØTYØØZ
- Liver ØFYØØZ
- Lung
  - Bilateral ØBYMØZ
  - Left ØBYLØZ
  - Lower Lobe
    - Left ØBYJØZ
    - Right ØBYFØZ
  - Middle Lobe, Right ØBYDØZ
  - Right ØBYKØZ

Transplantation — *continued*
- Lung — *continued*
  - Upper Lobe
    - Left ØBYGØZ
    - Right ØBYCØZ
- Lung Lingula ØBYHØZ
- Ovary
  - Left ØUY1ØZ
  - Right ØUYØØZ
- Pancreas ØFYGØZ
- Penis ØVYSØZ
- Products of Conception 1ØYØ
- Scrotum ØVY5ØZ
- Spleen Ø7YPØZ
- Stem cell *see* Transfusion, Circulatory 3Ø2
- Stomach ØDY6ØZ
- Thymus Ø7YMØZ
- Uterus ØUY9ØZ

Transposition
- *see* Bypass
- *see* Reposition
- *see* Transfer

Transversalis fascia *use* Subcutaneous Tissue and Fascia, Trunk

Transverse acetabular ligament
- *use* Hip Bursa and Ligament, Left
- *use* Hip Bursa and Ligament, Right

Transverse (cutaneous) cervical nerve *use* Cervical Plexus

Transverse facial artery
- *use* Temporal Artery, Left
- *use* Temporal Artery, Right

Transverse foramen *use* Cervical Vertebra

Transverse humeral ligament
- *use* Shoulder Bursa and Ligament, Left
- *use* Shoulder Bursa and Ligament, Right

Transverse ligament of atlas *use* Head and Neck Bursa and Ligament

Transverse process
- *use* Cervical Vertebra
- *use* Lumbar Vertebra
- *use* Thoracic Vertebra

Transverse Rectus Abdominis Myocutaneous Flap
- Replacement
  - Bilateral ØHRVØ76
  - Left ØHRUØ76
  - Right ØHRTØ76
- Transfer
  - Left ØKXL
  - Right ØKXK

Transverse scapular ligament
- *use* Shoulder Bursa and Ligament, Left
- *use* Shoulder Bursa and Ligament, Right

Transverse thoracis muscle
- *use* Thorax Muscle, Left
- *use* Thorax Muscle, Right

Transversospinalis muscle
- *use* Trunk Muscle, Left
- *use* Trunk Muscle, Right

Transversus abdominis muscle
- *use* Abdomen Muscle, Left
- *use* Abdomen Muscle, Right

Trapezium bone
- *use* Carpal, Left
- *use* Carpal, Right

Trapezius muscle
- *use* Trunk Muscle, Left
- *use* Trunk Muscle, Right

Trapezoid bone
- *use* Carpal, Left
- *use* Carpal, Right

Triceps brachii muscle
- *use* Upper Arm Muscle, Left
- *use* Upper Arm Muscle, Right

Tricuspid annulus *use* Tricuspid Valve

Trifacial nerve *use* Trigeminal Nerve

Trifecta™ Valve (aortic) *use* Zooplastic Tissue in Heart and Great Vessels

Trigone of bladder *use* Bladder

TriGuard 3™ CEPD (cerebral embolic protection device) X2A6325

Trimming, excisional *see* Excision

Triquetral bone
- *use* Carpal, Left
- *use* Carpal, Right

Trochanteric bursa
- *use* Hip Bursa and Ligament, Left

Trochanteric bursa — *continued*
- *use* Hip Bursa and Ligament, Right

TUMT (transurethral microwave thermotherapy of prostate) ØV5Ø7ZZ

TUNA (transurethral needle ablation of prostate) ØV5Ø7ZZ

Tunneled central venous catheter *use* Vascular Access Device, Tunneled in Subcutaneous Tissue and Fascia

Tunneled spinal (intrathecal) catheter *use* Infusion Device

Turbinectomy
- *see* Excision, Ear, Nose, Sinus Ø9B
- *see* Resection, Ear, Nose, Sinus Ø9T

Turbinoplasty
- *see* Repair, Ear, Nose, Sinus Ø9Q
- *see* Replacement, Ear, Nose, Sinus Ø9R
- *see* Supplement, Ear, Nose, Sinus Ø9U

Turbinotomy
- *see* Division, Ear, Nose, Sinus Ø98
- *see* Drainage, Ear, Nose, Sinus Ø99

TURP (transurethral resection of prostate) ØVBØ7ZZ
- *see* Excision, Prostate ØVBØ
- *see* Resection, Prostate ØVTØ

Twelfth cranial nerve *use* Hypoglossal Nerve

Two lead pacemaker *use* Pacemaker, Dual Chamber in ØJH

Tympanic cavity
- *use* Middle Ear, Left
- *use* Middle Ear, Right

Tympanic nerve *use* Glossopharyngeal Nerve

Tympanic part of temoporal bone
- *use* Temporal Bone, Left
- *use* Temporal Bone, Right

Tympanogram *see* Hearing Assessment, Diagnostic Audiology F13

Tympanoplasty
- *see* Repair, Ear, Nose, Sinus Ø9Q
- *see* Replacement, Ear, Nose, Sinus Ø9R
- *see* Supplement, Ear, Nose, Sinus Ø9U

Tympanosympathectomy *see* Excision, Nerve, Head and Neck Sympathetic Ø1BK

Tympanotomy *see* Drainage, Ear, Nose, Sinus Ø99

TYRX Antibacterial Envelope *use* Anti-Infective Envelope

U

Ulnar collateral carpal ligament
- *use* Wrist Bursa and Ligament, Left
- *use* Wrist Bursa and Ligament, Right

Ulnar collateral ligament
- *use* Elbow Bursa and Ligament, Left
- *use* Elbow Bursa and Ligament, Right

Ulnar notch
- *use* Radius, Left
- *use* Radius, Right

Ulnar vein
- *use* Brachial Vein, Left
- *use* Brachial Vein, Right

Ultrafiltration
- Hemodialysis *see* Performance, Urinary 5A1D
- Therapeutic plasmapheresis *see* Pheresis, Circulatory 6A55

Ultraflex™ Precision Colonic Stent System *use* Intraluminal Device

ULTRAPRO Hernia System (UHS) *use* Synthetic Substitute

ULTRAPRO Partially Absorbable Lightweight Mesh *use* Synthetic Substitute

ULTRAPRO Plug *use* Synthetic Substitute

Ultrasonic osteogenic stimulator
- *use* Bone Growth Stimulator in Head and Facial Bones
- *use* Bone Growth Stimulator in Lower Bones
- *use* Bone Growth Stimulator in Upper Bones

Ultrasonography
- Abdomen BW4ØZZZ
- Abdomen and Pelvis BW41ZZZ
- Abdominal Wall BH49ZZZ
- Aorta
  - Abdominal, Intravascular B44ØZZ3
  - Thoracic, Intravascular B34ØZZ3
- Appendix BD48ZZZ

Ultrasonography — *continued*
Artery
Brachiocephalic-Subclavian, Right, Intravascular B341ZZ3
Celiac and Mesenteric, Intravascular B44KZZ3
Common Carotid
Bilateral, Intravascular B345ZZ3
Left, Intravascular B344ZZ3
Right, Intravascular B343ZZ3
Coronary
Multiple B241YZZ
Intravascular B241ZZ3
Transesophageal B241ZZ4
Single B240YZZ
Intravascular B240ZZ3
Transesophageal B240ZZ4
Femoral, Intravascular B44LZZ3
Inferior Mesenteric, Intravascular B445ZZ3
Internal Carotid
Bilateral, Intravascular B348ZZ3
Left, Intravascular B347ZZ3
Right, Intravascular B346ZZ3
Intra-Abdominal, Other, Intravascular B44BZZ3
Intracranial, Intravascular B34RZZ3
Lower Extremity
Bilateral, Intravascular B44HZZ3
Left, Intravascular B44GZZ3
Right, Intravascular B44FZZ3
Mesenteric and Celiac, Intravascular B44KZZ3
Ophthalmic, Intravascular B34VZZ3
Penile, Intravascular B44NZZ3
Pulmonary
Left, Intravascular B34TZZ3
Right, Intravascular B34SZZ3
Renal
Bilateral, Intravascular B448ZZ3
Left, Intravascular B447ZZ3
Right, Intravascular B446ZZ3
Subclavian, Left, Intravascular B342ZZ3
Superior Mesenteric, Intravascular B444ZZ3
Upper Extremity
Bilateral, Intravascular B34KZZ3
Left, Intravascular B34JZZ3
Right, Intravascular B34HZZ3
Bile Duct BF40ZZZ
Bile Duct and Gallbladder BF43ZZZ
Bladder BT40ZZZ
and Kidney BT4JZZZ
Brain B040ZZZ
Breast
Bilateral BH42ZZZ
Left BH41ZZZ
Right BH40ZZZ
Chest Wall BH4BZZZ
Coccyx BR4FZZZ
Connective Tissue
Lower Extremity BL41ZZZ
Upper Extremity BL40ZZZ
Duodenum BD49ZZZ
Elbow
Left, Densitometry BP4HZZ1
Right, Densitometry BP4GZZ1
Esophagus BD41ZZZ
Extremity
Lower BH48ZZZ
Upper BH47ZZZ
Eye
Bilateral B847ZZZ
Left B846ZZZ
Right B845ZZZ
Fallopian Tube
Bilateral BU42
Left BU41
Right BU40
Fetal Umbilical Cord BY47ZZZ
Fetus
First Trimester, Multiple Gestation BY4BZZZ
Second Trimester, Multiple Gestation BY4DZZZ
Single
First Trimester BY49ZZZ
Second Trimester BY4CZZZ
Third Trimester BY4FZZZ
Third Trimester, Multiple Gestation BY4GZZZ
Gallbladder BF42ZZZ
Gallbladder and Bile Duct BF43ZZZ
Gastrointestinal Tract BD47ZZZ

Ultrasonography — *continued*
Gland
Adrenal
Bilateral BG42ZZZ
Left BG41ZZZ
Right BG40ZZZ
Parathyroid BG43ZZZ
Thyroid BG44ZZZ
Hand
Left, Densitometry BP4PZZ1
Right, Densitometry BP4NZZ1
Head and Neck BH4CZZZ
Heart
Left B245YZZ
Intravascular B245ZZ3
Transesophageal B245ZZ4
Pediatric B24DYZZ
Intravascular B24DZZ3
Transesophageal B24DZZ4
Right B244YZZ
Intravascular B244ZZ3
Transesophageal B244ZZ4
Right and Left B246YZZ
Intravascular B246ZZ3
Transesophageal B246ZZ4
Heart with Aorta B24BYZZ
Intravascular B24BZZ3
Transesophageal B24BZZ4
Hepatobiliary System, All BF4CZZZ
Hip
Bilateral BQ42ZZZ
Left BQ41ZZZ
Right BQ40ZZZ
Kidney
and Bladder BT4JZZZ
Bilateral BT43ZZZ
Left BT42ZZZ
Right BT41ZZZ
Transplant BT49ZZZ
Knee
Bilateral BQ49ZZZ
Left BQ48ZZZ
Right BQ47ZZZ
Liver BF45ZZZ
Liver and Spleen BF46ZZZ
Mediastinum BB4CZZZ
Neck BW4FZZZ
Ovary
Bilateral BU45
Left BU44
Right BU43
Ovary and Uterus BU4C
Pancreas BF47ZZZ
Pelvic Region BW4GZZZ
Pelvis and Abdomen BW41ZZZ
Penis BV4BZZZ
Pericardium B24CYZZ
Intravascular B24CZZ3
Transesophageal B24CZZ4
Placenta BY48ZZZ
Pleura BB4BZZZ
Prostate and Seminal Vesicle BV49ZZZ
Rectum BD4CZZZ
Sacrum BR4FZZZ
Scrotum BV44ZZZ
Seminal Vesicle and Prostate BV49ZZZ
Shoulder
Left, Densitometry BP49ZZ1
Right, Densitometry BP48ZZ1
Spinal Cord B04BZZZ
Spine
Cervical BR40ZZZ
Lumbar BR49ZZZ
Thoracic BR47ZZZ
Spleen and Liver BF46ZZZ
Stomach BD42ZZZ
Tendon
Lower Extremity BL43ZZZ
Upper Extremity BL42ZZZ
Ureter
Bilateral BT48ZZZ
Left BT47ZZZ
Right BT46ZZZ
Urethra BT45ZZZ
Uterus BU46
Uterus and Ovary BU4C
Vein
Jugular
Left, Intravascular B544ZZ3

Ultrasonography — *continued*
Vein — *continued*
Jugular — *continued*
Right, Intravascular B543ZZ3
Lower Extremity
Bilateral, Intravascular B54DZZ3
Left, Intravascular B54CZZ3
Right, Intravascular B54BZZ3
Portal, Intravascular B54TZZ3
Renal
Bilateral, Intravascular B54LZZ3
Left, Intravascular B54KZZ3
Right, Intravascular B54JZZ3
Spanchnic, Intravascular B54TZZ3
Subclavian
Left, Intravascular B547ZZ3
Right, Intravascular B546ZZ3
Upper Extremity
Bilateral, Intravascular B54PZZ3
Left, Intravascular B54NZZ3
Right, Intravascular B54MZZ3
Vena Cava
Inferior, Intravascular B549ZZ3
Superior, Intravascular B548ZZ3
Wrist
Left, Densitometry BP4MZZ1
Right, Densitometry BP4LZZ1
Ultrasound bone healing system
use Bone Growth Stimulator in Head and Facial Bones
use Bone Growth Stimulator in Lower Bones
use Bone Growth Stimulator in Upper Bones
Ultrasound Therapy
Heart 6A75
No Qualifier 6A75
Vessels
Head and Neck 6A75
Other 6A75
Peripheral 6A75
Ultraviolet Light Therapy, Skin 6A80
Umbilical artery
use Internal Iliac Artery, Left
use Internal Iliac Artery, Right
use Lower Artery
Uniplanar external fixator
use External Fixation Device, Monoplanar in 0PH
use External Fixation Device, Monoplanar in 0PS
use External Fixation Device, Monoplanar in 0QH
use External Fixation Device, Monoplanar in 0QS
Upper GI series *see* Fluoroscopy, Gastrointestinal, Upper BD15
Ureteral orifice
use Ureter
use Ureter, Left
use Ureter, Right
use Ureters, Bilateral
Ureterectomy
see Excision, Urinary System 0TB
see Resection, Urinary System 0TT
Ureterocolostomy *see* Bypass, Urinary System 0T1
Ureterocystostomy *see* Bypass, Urinary System 0T1
Ureteroenterostomy *see* Bypass, Urinary System 0T1
Ureteroileostomy *see* Bypass, Urinary System 0T1
Ureterolithotomy *see* Extirpation, Urinary System 0TC
Ureterolysis *see* Release, Urinary System 0TN
Ureteroneocystostomy
see Bypass, Urinary System 0T1
see Reposition, Urinary System 0TS
Ureteropelvic junction (UPJ)
use Kidney Pelvis, Left
use Kidney Pelvis, Right
Ureteropexy
see Repair, Urinary System 0TQ
see Reposition, Urinary System 0TS
Ureteroplasty
see Repair, Urinary System 0TQ
see Replacement, Urinary System 0TR
see Supplement, Urinary System 0TU
Ureteroplication *see* Restriction, Urinary System 0TV
Ureteropyelography *see* Fluoroscopy, Urinary System BT1
Ureterorrhaphy *see* Repair, Urinary System 0TQ
Ureteroscopy 0TJ98ZZ
Ureterostomy
see Bypass, Urinary System 0T1
see Drainage, Urinary System 0T9
Ureterotomy *see* Drainage, Urinary System 0T9

Ureteroureterostomy *see* Bypass, Urinary System ØT1
Ureterovesical orifice
use Ureter
use Ureter, Left
use Ureter, Right
use Ureters, Bilateral
Urethral catheterization, indwelling ØT9B7ØZ
Urethrectomy
see Excision, Urethra ØTBD
see Resection, Urethra ØTTD
Urethrolithotomy *see* Extirpation, Urethra ØTCD
Urethrolysis *see* Release, Urethra ØTND
Urethropexy
see Repair, Urethra ØTQD
see Reposition, Urethra ØTSD
Urethroplasty
see Repair, Urethra ØTQD
see Replacement, Urethra ØTRD
see Supplement, Urethra ØTUD
Urethrorrhaphy *see* Repair, Urethra ØTQD
Urethroscopy ØTJD8ZZ
Urethrotomy *see* Drainage, Urethra ØT9D
Uridine Triacetate XWØDX82
Urinary incontinence stimulator lead *use* Stimulator Lead in Urinary System
Urography *see* Fluoroscopy, Urinary System BT1
Ustekinumab *use* Other New Technology Therapeutic Substance
Uterine Artery
use Internal Iliac Artery, Left
use Internal Iliac Artery, Right
Uterine artery embolization (UAE) *see* Occlusion, Lower Arteries Ø4L
Uterine cornu *use* Uterus
Uterine tube
use Fallopian Tube, Left
use Fallopian Tube, Right
Uterine vein
use Hypogastric Vein, Left
use Hypogastric Vein, Right
Uvulectomy
see Excision, Uvula ØCBN
see Resection, Uvula ØCTN
Uvulorrhaphy *see* Repair, Uvula ØCQN
Uvulotomy *see* Drainage, Uvula ØC9N

V

Vabomere™ *use* Meropenem-vaborbactam Anti-infective
Vaccination *see* Introduction of Serum, Toxoid, and Vaccine
Vacuum extraction, obstetric 1ØDØ7Z6
Vaginal artery
use Internal Iliac Artery, Left
use Internal Iliac Artery, Right
Vaginal pessary *use* Intraluminal Device, Pessary in Female Reproductive System
Vaginal vein
use Hypogastric Vein, Left
use Hypogastric Vein, Right
Vaginectomy
see Excision, Vagina ØUBG
see Resection, Vagina ØUTG
Vaginofixation
see Repair, Vagina ØUQG
see Reposition, Vagina ØUSG
Vaginoplasty
see Repair, Vagina ØUQG
see Supplement, Vagina ØUUG
Vaginorrhaphy *see* Repair, Vagina ØUQG
Vaginoscopy ØUJH8ZZ
Vaginotomy *see* Drainage, Female Reproductive System ØU9
Vagotomy *see* Division, Nerve, Vagus ØØ8Q
Valiant Thoracic Stent Graft *use* Intraluminal Device
Valvotomy, valvulotomy
see Division, Heart and Great Vessels Ø28
see Release, Heart and Great Vessels Ø2N
Valvuloplasty
see Repair, Heart and Great Vessels Ø2Q
see Replacement, Heart and Great Vessels Ø2R
see Supplement, Heart and Great Vessels Ø2U
Valvuloplasty, Alfieri Stitch *see* Restriction, Valve, Mitral Ø2VG
Vascular Access Device
Totally Implantable
Insertion of device in
Abdomen ØJH8
Chest ØJH6
Lower Arm
Left ØJHH
Right ØJHG
Lower Leg
Left ØJHP
Right ØJHN
Upper Arm
Left ØJHF
Right ØJHD
Upper Leg
Left ØJHM
Right ØJHL
Removal of device from
Lower Extremity ØJPW
Trunk ØJPT
Upper Extremity ØJPV
Revision of device in
Lower Extremity ØJWW
Trunk ØJWT
Upper Extremity ØJWV
Tunneled
Insertion of device in
Abdomen ØJH8
Chest ØJH6
Lower Arm
Left ØJHH
Right ØJHG
Lower Leg
Left ØJHP
Right ØJHN
Upper Arm
Left ØJHF
Right ØJHD
Upper Leg
Left ØJHM
Right ØJHL
Removal of device from
Lower Extremity ØJPW
Trunk ØJPT
Upper Extremity ØJPV
Revision of device in
Lower Extremity ØJWW
Trunk ØJWT
Upper Extremity ØJWV
Vasectomy *see* Excision, Male Reproductive System ØVB
Vasography
see Fluoroscopy, Male Reproductive System BV1
see Plain Radiography, Male Reproductive System BVØ
Vasoligation *see* Occlusion, Male Reproductive System ØVL
Vasorrhaphy *see* Repair, Male Reproductive System ØVQ
Vasostomy *see* Bypass, Male Reproductive System ØV1
Vasotomy
Drainage *see* Drainage, Male Reproductive System ØV9
With ligation *see* Occlusion, Male Reproductive System ØVL
Vasovasostomy *see* Repair, Male Reproductive System ØVQ
Vastus intermedius muscle
use Upper Leg Muscle, Left
use Upper Leg Muscle, Right
Vastus lateralis muscle
use Upper Leg Muscle, Left
use Upper Leg Muscle, Right
Vastus medialis muscle
use Upper Leg Muscle, Left
use Upper Leg Muscle, Right
VCG (vectorcardiogram) *see* Measurement, Cardiac 4AØ2
Vectra® Vascular Access Graft *use* Vascular Access Device, Tunneled in Subcutaneous Tissue and Fascia
Venclexta® *use* Venetoclax Antineoplastic
Venectomy
see Excision, Lower Veins Ø6B
see Excision, Upper Veins Ø5B
Venetoclax Antineoplastic XWØDXR5
Venography
see Fluoroscopy, Veins B51
Venography — *continued*
see Plain Radiography, Veins B5Ø
Venorrhaphy
see Repair, Lower Veins Ø6Q
see Repair, Upper Veins Ø5Q
Venotripsy
see Occlusion, Lower Veins Ø6L
see Occlusion, Upper Veins Ø5L
Ventricular fold *use* Larynx
Ventriculoatriostomy *see* Bypass, Central Nervous System and Cranial Nerves ØØ1
Ventriculocisternostomy *see* Bypass, Central Nervous System and Cranial Nerves ØØ1
Ventriculogram, cardiac
Combined left and right heart *see* Fluoroscopy, Heart, Right and Left B216
Left ventricle *see* Fluoroscopy, Heart, Left B215
Right ventricle *see* Fluoroscopy, Heart, Right B214
Ventriculopuncture, through previously implanted catheter 8CØ1X6J
Ventriculoscopy ØØJØ4ZZ
Ventriculostomy
External drainage *see* Drainage, Cerebral Ventricle ØØ96
Internal shunt *see* Bypass, Cerebral Ventricle ØØ16
Ventriculovenostomy *see* Bypass, Cerebral Ventricle ØØ16
Ventrio™ Hernia Patch *use* Synthetic Substitute
VEP (visual evoked potential) 4AØ7XØZ
Vermiform appendix *use* Appendix
Vermilion border
use Lower Lip
use Upper Lip
Versa *use* Pacemaker, Dual Chamber in ØJH
Version, obstetric
External 1ØSØXZZ
Internal 1ØSØ7ZZ
Vertebral arch
use Cervical Vertebra
use Lumbar Vertebra
use Thoracic Vertebra
Vertebral body
use Cervical Vertebra
use Lumbar Vertebra
use Thoracic Vertebra
Vertebral canal *use* Spinal Canal
Vertebral foramen
use Cervical Vertebra
use Lumbar Vertebra
use Thoracic Vertebra
Vertebral lamina
use Cervical Vertebra
use Lumbar Vertebra
use Thoracic Vertebra
Vertebral pedicle
use Cervical Vertebra
use Lumbar Vertebra
use Thoracic Vertebra
Vesical vein
use Hypogastric Vein, Left
use Hypogastric Vein, Right
Vesicotomy *see* Drainage, Urinary System ØT9
Vesiculectomy
see Excision, Male Reproductive System ØVB
see Resection, Male Reproductive System ØVT
Vesiculogram, seminal *see* Plain Radiography, Male Reproductive System BVØ
Vesiculotomy *see* Drainage, Male Reproductive System ØV9
Vestibular Assessment F15Z
Vestibular (Scarpa's) ganglion *use* Acoustic Nerve
Vestibular nerve *use* Acoustic Nerve
Vestibular Treatment FØC
Vestibulocochlear nerve *use* Acoustic Nerve
VH-IVUS (virtual histology intravascular ultrasound) *see* Ultrasonography, Heart B24
Virchow's (supraclavicular) lymph node
use Lymphatic, Left Neck
use Lymphatic, Right Neck
Virtuoso (II) (DR) (VR) *use* Defibrillator Generator in ØJH
Vistogard(R) *use* Uridine Triacetate
Vitrectomy
see Excision, Eye Ø8B
see Resection, Eye Ø8T

Subterms under main terms may continue to next column or page

Vitreous body
use Vitreous, Left
use Vitreous, Right
Viva (XT) (S) *use* Cardiac Resynchronization Defibrillator Pulse Generator in ØJH
Vocal fold
use Vocal Cord, Left
use Vocal Cord, Right
Vocational
Assessment *see* Activities of Daily Living Assessment, Rehabilitation FØ2
Retraining *see* Activities of Daily Living Treatment, Rehabilitation FØ8
Volar (palmar) digital vein
use Hand Vein, Left
use Hand Vein, Right
Volar (palmar) metacarpal vein
use Hand Vein, Left
use Hand Vein, Right
Vomer bone *use* Nasal Septum
Vomer of nasal septum *use* Nasal Bone
Voraxaze *use* Glucarpidase
Vulvectomy
see Excision, Female Reproductive System ØUB
see Resection, Female Reproductive System ØUT
V-Wave Interatrial Shunt System *use* Synthetic Substitute
VYXEOS™ *use* Cytarabine and Daunorubicin Liposome Antineoplastic

W

WALLSTENT® Endoprosthesis *use* Intraluminal Device
Washing *see* Irrigation
WavelinQ EndoAVF system
Radial Artery, Left Ø31C3ZF
Radial Artery, Right Ø31B3ZF
Ulnar Artery, Left Ø31A3ZF
WavelinQ EndoAVF system — *continued*
Ulnar Artery, Right Ø3193ZF
Wedge resection, pulmonary *see* Excision, Respiratory System ØBB
Whole Blood Nucleic Acid-base Microbial Detection XXE5XM5
Window *see* Drainage
Wiring, dental 2W31X9Z

Xact Carotid Stent System *use* Intraluminal Device
XENLETA™ *use* Lefamulin Anti-infective
Xenograft *use* Zooplastic Tissue in Heart and Great Vessels
XIENCE Everolimus Eluting Coronary Stent System
use Intraluminal Device, Drug-eluting in Heart and Great Vessels
Xiphoid process *use* Sternum
XLIF® System *use* Interbody Fusion Device in Lower Joints
XOSPATA® *use* Gilteritinib Antineoplastic
X-ray *see* Plain Radiography
X-STOP® Spacer
use Spinal Stabilization Device, Interspinous Process in ØRH
use Spinal Stabilization Device, Interspinous Process in ØSH

Yoga Therapy 8EØZXY4

Z

Z-plasty, skin for scar contracture *see* Release, Skin and Breast ØHN
Zenith AAA Endovascular Graft *use* Intraluminal Device
Zenith® Fenestrated AAA Endovascular Graft
use Intraluminal Device, Branched or Fenestrated, One or Two Arteries in Ø4V
use Intraluminal Device, Branched or Fenestrated, Three or More Arteries in Ø4V
Zenith Flex® AAA Endovascular Graft *use* Intraluminal Device
Zenith® Renu™ AAA Ancillary Graft *use* Intraluminal Device
Zenith TX2® TAA Endovascular Graft *use* Intraluminal Device
ZERBAXA® *use* Ceftolozane/Tazobactam Anti-infective
Zilver® PTX® (paclitaxel) Drug-Eluting Peripheral Stent
use Intraluminal Device, Drug-eluting in Lower Arteries
use Intraluminal Device, Drug-eluting in Upper Arteries
Zimmer® NexGen® LPS Mobile Bearing Knee *use* Synthetic Substitute
Zimmer® NexGen® LPS-Flex Mobile Knee *use* Synthetic Substitute
ZINPLAVA™ use Bezlotoxumab Monoclonal Antibody
Zonule of Zinn
use Lens, Left
use Lens, Right
Zooplastic Tissue, Rapid Deployment Technique, Replacement X2RF
Zotarolimus-eluting Coronary Stent *use* Intraluminal Device, Drug-eluting in Heart and Great Vessels
ZULRESSO™ use Brexanolone
Zygomatic process of frontal bone *use* Frontal Bone
Zygomatic process of temporal bone
use Temporal Bone, Left
use Temporal Bone, Right
Zygomaticus muscle *use* Facial Muscle
Zyvox *use* Oxazolidinones

ICD-10-PCS Tables

Central Nervous System and Cranial Nerves 001–00X

Character Meanings

This Character Meaning table is provided as a guide to assist the user in the identification of character members that may be found in this section of code tables. It **SHOULD NOT** be used to build a PCS code.

Operation–Character 3	Body Part–Character 4	Approach–Character 5	Device–Character 6	Qualifier–Character 7
1 Bypass	0 Brain	0 Open	0 Drainage Device	0 Nasopharynx
2 Change	1 Cerebral Meninges	3 Percutaneous	1 Radioactive Element	1 Mastoid Sinus
5 Destruction	2 Dura Mater	4 Percutaneous Endoscopic	2 Monitoring Device	2 Atrium
7 Dilation	3 Epidural Space, Intracranial	X External	3 Infusion Device	3 Blood Vessel
8 Division	4 Subdural Space, Intracranial		4 Radioactive Element, Cesium-131 Collagen Implant	4 Pleural Cavity
9 Drainage	5 Subarachnoid Space, Intracranial		7 Autologous Tissue Substitute	5 Intestine
B Excision	6 Cerebral Ventricle		J Synthetic Substitute	6 Peritoneal Cavity
C Extirpation	7 Cerebral Hemisphere		K Nonautologous Tissue Substitute	7 Urinary Tract
D Extraction	8 Basal Ganglia		M Neurostimulator Lead	8 Bone Marrow
F Fragmentation	9 Thalamus		Y Other Device	9 Fallopian Tube
H Insertion	A Hypothalamus		Z No Device	A Subgaleal Space
J Inspection	B Pons			B Cerebral Cisterns
K Map	C Cerebellum			F Olfactory Nerve
N Release	D Medulla Oblongata			G Optic Nerve
P Removal	E Cranial Nerve			H Oculomotor Nerve
Q Repair	F Olfactory Nerve			J Trochlear Nerve
R Replacement	G Optic Nerve			K Trigeminal Nerve
S Reposition	H Oculomotor Nerve			L Abducens Nerve
T Resection	J Trochlear Nerve			M Facial Nerve
U Supplement	K Trigeminal Nerve			N Acoustic Nerve
W Revision	L Abducens Nerve			P Glossopharyngeal Nerve
X Transfer	M Facial Nerve			Q Vagus Nerve
	N Acoustic Nerve			R Accessory Nerve
	P Glossopharyngeal Nerve			S Hypoglossal Nerve
	Q Vagus Nerve			X Diagnostic
	R Accessory Nerve			Z No Qualifier
	S Hypoglossal Nerve			
	T Spinal Meninges			
	U Spinal Canal			
	V Spinal Cord			
	W Cervical Spinal Cord			
	X Thoracic Spinal Cord			
	Y Lumbar Spinal Cord			

Central Nervous System and Cranial Nerves

AHA Coding Clinic for table ØØ1

2019, 4Q, 21-22 Cerebral ventricle bypass Qualifier
2018, 4Q, 86 Placement of lumboatrial shunt
2017, 4Q, 39-41 Dilation and bypass of cerebral ventricle
2015, 2Q, 9 Revision of ventriculoperitoneal (VP) shunt
2013, 2Q, 36 Insertion of ventriculoperitoneal shunt with laparoscopic assistance

AHA Coding Clinic for table ØØ7

2017, 4Q, 39-41 Dilation and bypass of cerebral ventricle

AHA Coding Clinic for table ØØ9

2018, 4Q, 85 Externalization of lumboatrial shunt
2017, 1Q, 50 Failed lumbar puncture
2015, 3Q, 10 Open evacuation of subdural hematoma
2015, 3Q, 11 Percutaneous drainage of subdural hematoma
2015, 3Q, 12 Subdural evacuation portal system (SEPS) placement
2015, 3Q, 12 Placement of ventriculostomy catheter via burr hole
2015, 2Q, 30 Drainage of syrinx
2015, 1Q, 31 Intrathecal chemotherapy
2014, 1Q, 8 Diagnostic lumbar tap
2014, 1Q, 8 Lumbar drainage port aspiration

AHA Coding Clinic for table ØØB

2017, 3Q, 17 Resection of schwannoma and placement of DuraGen and Lorenz cranial plating system
2016, 2Q, 12 Resection of malignant neoplasm of infratemporal fossa
2016, 2Q, 18 Amygdalohippocampectomy
2014, 4Q, 34 Resection of brain malignancy with implantation of chemotherapeutic wafer
2014, 3Q, 24 Repair of lipomyelomeningocele and tethered cord

AHA Coding Clinic for table ØØC

2019, 3Q, 4 Evacuation of subdural hematoma and control of bleeding artery
2019, 2Q, 36 Evacuation of hematoma using NICO Brainpath® technology
2017, 4Q, 48 New and revised body part values - Extirpation spinal canal
2016, 2Q, 29 Decompressive craniectomy with cryopreservation and storage of bone flap
2015, 3Q, 10 Open evacuation of subdural hematoma
2015, 3Q, 11 Percutaneous drainage of subdural hematoma
2015, 3Q, 13 Evacuation of intracerebral hematoma

AHA Coding Clinic for table ØØD

2015, 3Q, 13 Nonexcisional debridement of cranial wound with removal and replacement of hardware

AHA Coding Clinic for table ØØH

2020, 2Q, 15 Ommaya Reservoir with Ventricular Catheter Placement
2020, 2Q, 16 Ommaya Reservoir Placement for Cerebrospinal Fluid Infusion Therapy
2017, 4Q, 30-31 Radiotherapeutic brain implant
2017, 3Q, 13 Implantation of bilateral neurostimulator electrodes
2014, 3Q, 19 End of life replacement of Baclofen pump

AHA Coding Clinic for table ØØJ

2019, 2Q, 36 Evacuation of hematoma using NICO Brainpath® technology
2017, 1Q, 50 Failed lumbar puncture

AHA Coding Clinic for table ØØN

2019, 2Q, 19 Cervical spinal fusion, decompression and placement of interfacet stabilization device
2019, 1Q, 28 Decompressive laminectomy of both spinal cord and nerve roots
2018, 3Q, 30 Decompressive laminectomy (release of spinal cord versus release of spinal meninges)
2017, 3Q, 10 Repair of Chiari malformation
2017, 2Q, 23 Decompression of spinal cord and placement of instrumentation
2016, 2Q, 29 Decompressive craniectomy with cryopreservation and storage of bone flap
2015, 2Q, 20 Cervical laminoplasty
2015, 2Q, 21 Multiple decompressive cervical laminectomies
2015, 2Q, 34 Decompressive laminectomy
2014, 3Q, 24 Repair of lipomyelomeningocele and tethered cord

AHA Coding Clinic for table ØØP

2014, 3Q, 19 End of life replacement of Baclofen pump

AHA Coding Clinic for table ØØQ

2014, 3Q, 7 Hemi-cranioplasty for repair of cranial defect
2013, 3Q, 25 Fracture of frontal bone with repair and coagulation for hemostasis

AHA Coding Clinic for table ØØS

2014, 4Q, 35 Reimplantation of buccal nerve

AHA Coding Clinic for table ØØU

2018, 1Q, 9 Craniectomy with DuraGaurd placement
2017, 4Q, 62 Added and revised device values - Nerve substitutes
2017, 3Q, 10 Repair of Chiari malformation
2017, 3Q, 17 Resection of schwannoma and placement of DuraGen and Lorenz cranial plating system
2015, 4Q, 39 Dural patch graft
2014, 3Q, 24 Repair of lipomyelomeningocele and tethered cord

AHA Coding Clinic for table ØØW

2018, 4Q, 86 Placement of lumboatrial shunt

Brain

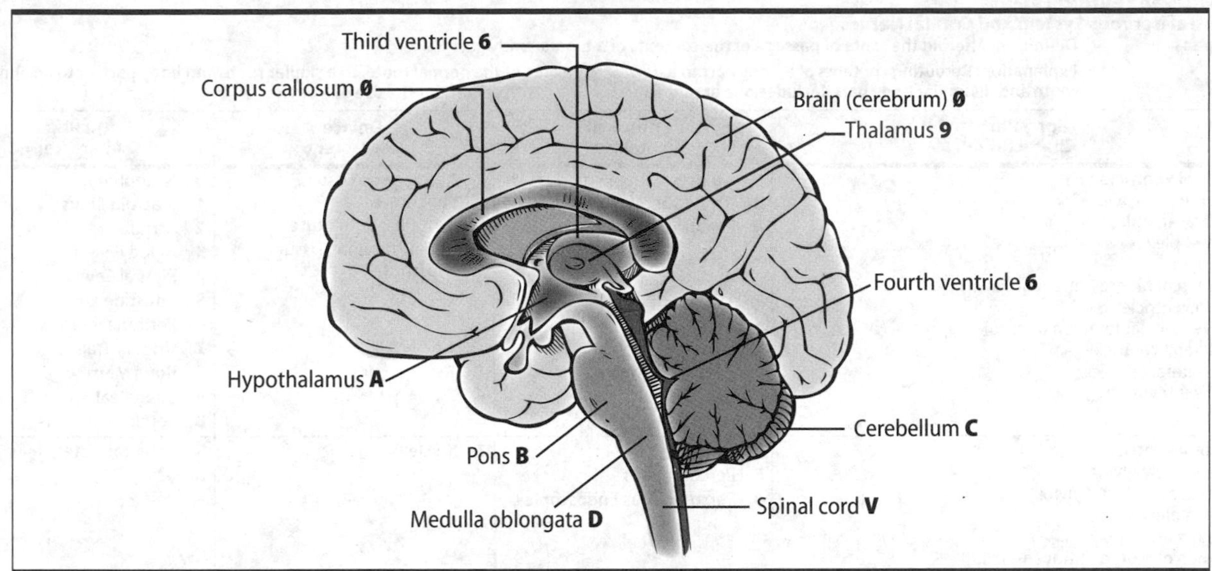

Cranial Nerves

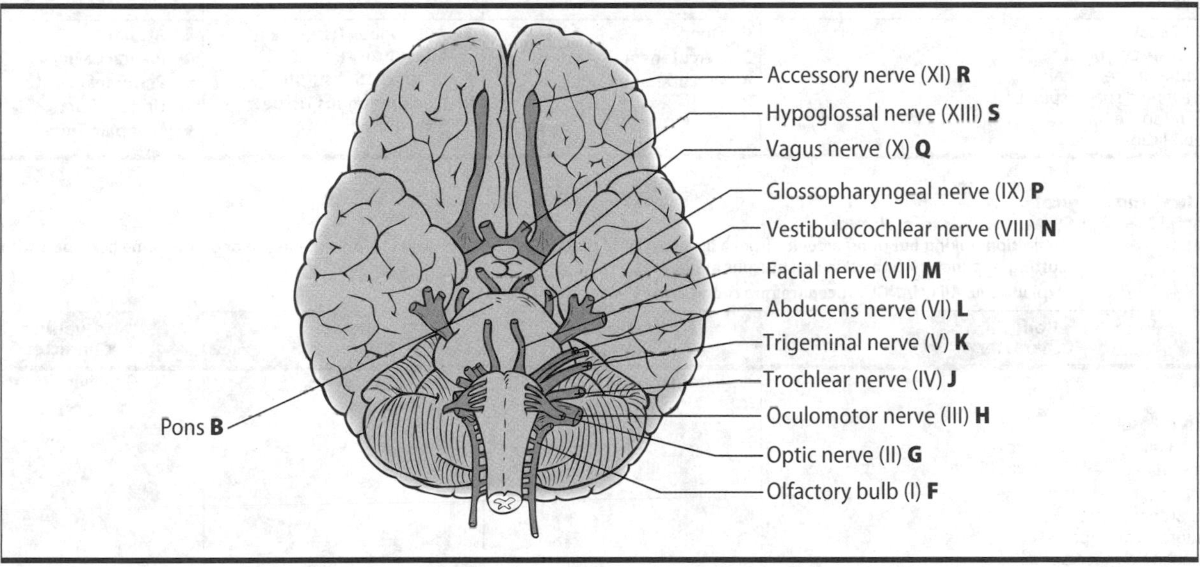

Ø Medical and Surgical
Ø Central Nervous System and Cranial Nerves
1 Bypass Definition: Altering the route of passage of the contents of a tubular body part

Explanation: Rerouting contents of a body part to a downstream area of the normal route, to a similar route and body part, or to an abnormal route and dissimilar body part. Includes one or more anastomoses, with or without the use of a device.

Body Part Character 4	Approach Character 5	Device Character 6	Qualifier Character 7
6 Cerebral Ventricle Aqueduct of Sylvius Cerebral aqueduct (Sylvius) Choroid plexus Ependyma Foramen of Monro (intraventricular) Fourth ventricle Interventricular foramen (Monro) Left lateral ventricle Right lateral ventricle Third ventricle	**Ø Open** **3 Percutaneous** **4 Percutaneous Endoscopic**	**7 Autologous Tissue Substitute** **J Synthetic Substitute** **K Nonautologous Tissue Substitute**	**Ø Nasopharynx** **1 Mastoid Sinus** **2 Atrium** **3 Blood Vessel** **4 Pleural Cavity** **5 Intestine** **6 Peritoneal Cavity** **7 Urinary Tract** **8 Bone Marrow** **A Subgaleal Space** **B Cerebral Cisterns**
6 Cerebral Ventricle Aqueduct of Sylvius Cerebral aqueduct (Sylvius) Choroid plexus Ependyma Foramen of Monro (intraventricular) Fourth ventricle Interventricular foramen (Monro) Left lateral ventricle Right lateral ventricle Third ventricle	**Ø Open** **3 Percutaneous** **4 Percutaneous Endoscopic**	**Z No Device**	**B Cerebral Cisterns**
U Spinal Canal Epidural space, spinal Extradural space, spinal Subarachnoid space, spinal Subdural space, spinal Vertebral canal	**Ø Open** **3 Percutaneous** **4 Percutaneous Endoscopic**	**7 Autologous Tissue Substitute** **J Synthetic Substitute** **K Nonautologous Tissue Substitute**	**2 Atrium** **4 Pleural Cavity** **6 Peritoneal Cavity** **7 Urinary Tract** **9 Fallopian Tube**

Ø Medical and Surgical
Ø Central Nervous System and Cranial Nerves
2 Change Definition: Taking out or off a device from a body part and putting back an identical or similar device in or on the same body part without cutting or puncturing the skin or a mucous membrane

Explanation: All CHANGE procedures are coded using the approach EXTERNAL

Body Part Character 4	Approach Character 5	Device Character 6	Qualifier Character 7
Ø Brain Cerebrum Corpus callosum Encephalon **E Cranial Nerve** **U Spinal Canal** Epidural space, spinal Extradural space, spinal Subarachnoid space, spinal Subdural space, spinal Vertebral canal	**X External**	**Ø Drainage Device** **Y Other Device**	**Z No Qualifier**

Non-OR All body part, approach, device, and qualifier values

Ø Medical and Surgical
Ø Central Nervous System and Cranial Nerves
5 Destruction Definition: Physical eradication of all or a portion of a body part by the direct use of energy, force, or a destructive agent
Explanation: None of the body part is physically taken out

Body Part Character 4		Approach Character 5	Device Character 6	Qualifier Character 7
Ø Brain Cerebrum Corpus callosum Encephalon **1 Cerebral Meninges** Arachnoid mater, intracranial Leptomeninges, intracranial Pia mater, intracranial **2 Dura Mater** Diaphragma sellae Dura mater, intracranial Falx cerebri Tentorium cerebelli **6 Cerebral Ventricle** Aqueduct of Sylvius Cerebral aqueduct (Sylvius) Choroid plexus Ependyma Foramen of Monro (intraventricular) Fourth ventricle Interventricular foramen (Monro) Left lateral ventricle Right lateral ventricle Third ventricle **7 Cerebral Hemisphere** Frontal lobe Occipital lobe Parietal lobe Temporal lobe **8 Basal Ganglia** Basal nuclei Claustrum Corpus striatum Globus pallidus Substantia nigra Subthalamic nucleus **9 Thalamus** Epithalamus Geniculate nucleus Metathalamus Pulvinar **A Hypothalamus** Mammillary body **B Pons** Apneustic center Basis pontis Locus ceruleus Pneumotaxic center Pontine tegmentum Superior olivary nucleus **C Cerebellum** Culmen **D Medulla Oblongata** Myelencephalon **F Olfactory Nerve** First cranial nerve Olfactory bulb **G Optic Nerve** Optic chiasma Second cranial nerve	**H Oculomotor Nerve** Third cranial nerve **J Trochlear Nerve** Fourth cranial nerve **K Trigeminal Nerve** Fifth cranial nerve Gasserian ganglion Mandibular nerve Maxillary nerve Ophthalmic nerve Trifacial nerve **L Abducens Nerve** Sixth cranial nerve **M Facial Nerve** Chorda tympani Geniculate ganglion Greater superficial petrosal nerve Nerve to the stapedius Parotid plexus Posterior auricular nerve Seventh cranial nerve Submandibular ganglion **N Acoustic Nerve** Cochlear nerve Eighth cranial nerve Scarpa's (vestibular) ganglion Spiral ganglion Vestibular (Scarpa's) ganglion Vestibular nerve Vestibulocochlear nerve **P Glossopharyngeal Nerve** Carotid sinus nerve Ninth cranial nerve Tympanic nerve **Q Vagus Nerve** Anterior vagal trunk Pharyngeal plexus Pneumogastric nerve Posterior vagal trunk Pulmonary plexus Recurrent laryngeal nerve Superior laryngeal nerve Tenth cranial nerve **R Accessory Nerve** Eleventh cranial nerve **S Hypoglossal Nerve** Twelfth cranial nerve **T Spinal Meninges** Arachnoid mater, spinal Denticulate (dentate) ligament Dura mater, spinal Filum terminale Leptomeninges, spinal Pia mater, spinal **W Cervical Spinal Cord** **X Thoracic Spinal Cord** **Y Lumbar Spinal Cord** Cauda equina Conus medullaris	**Ø Open** **3 Percutaneous** **4 Percutaneous Endoscopic**	**Z No Device**	**Z No Qualifier**

Non-OR ØØ5[F,G,H,J,K,L,M,N,P,Q,R,S][Ø,3,4]ZZ

Ø Medical and Surgical
Ø Central Nervous System and Cranial Nerves
7 Dilation Definition: Expanding an orifice or the lumen of a tubular body part

Explanation: The orifice can be a natural orifice or an artificially created orifice. Accomplished by stretching a tubular body part using intraluminal pressure or by cutting part of the orifice or wall of the tubular body part.

Body Part Character 4	Approach Character 5	Device Character 6	Qualifier Character 7
6 Cerebral Ventricle Aqueduct of Sylvius Cerebral aqueduct (Sylvius) Choroid plexus Ependyma Foramen of Monro (intraventricular) Fourth ventricle Interventricular foramen (Monro) Left lateral ventricle Right lateral ventricle Third ventricle	**Ø Open** **3 Percutaneous** **4 Percutaneous Endoscopic**	**Z No Device**	**Z No Qualifier**

Ø Medical and Surgical
Ø Central Nervous System and Cranial Nerves
8 Division Definition: Cutting into a body part, without draining fluids and/or gases from the body part, in order to separate or transect a body part

Explanation: All or a portion of the body part is separated into two or more portions

Body Part Character 4	Approach Character 5	Device Character 6	Qualifier Character 7
Ø Brain Cerebrum Corpus callosum Encephalon **7 Cerebral Hemisphere** Frontal lobe Occipital lobe Parietal lobe Temporal lobe **8 Basal Ganglia** Basal nuclei Claustrum Corpus striatum Globus pallidus Substantia nigra Subthalamic nucleus **F Olfactory Nerve** First cranial nerve Olfactory bulb **G Optic Nerve** Optic chiasma Second cranial nerve **H Oculomotor Nerve** Third cranial nerve **J Trochlear Nerve** Fourth cranial nerve **K Trigeminal Nerve** Fifth cranial nerve Gasserian ganglion Mandibular nerve Maxillary nerve Ophthalmic nerve Trifacial nerve **L Abducens Nerve** Sixth cranial nerve **M Facial Nerve** Chorda tympani Geniculate ganglion Greater superficial petrosal nerve Nerve to the stapedius Parotid plexus Posterior auricular nerve Seventh cranial nerve Submandibular ganglion **N Acoustic Nerve** Cochlear nerve Eighth cranial nerve Scarpa's (vestibular) ganglion Spiral ganglion Vestibular (Scarpa's) ganglion Vestibular nerve Vestibulocochlear nerve **P Glossopharyngeal Nerve** Carotid sinus nerve Ninth cranial nerve Tympanic nerve **Q Vagus Nerve** Anterior vagal trunk Pharyngeal plexus Pneumogastric nerve Posterior vagal trunk Pulmonary plexus Recurrent laryngeal nerve Superior laryngeal nerve Tenth cranial nerve **R Accessory Nerve** Eleventh cranial nerve **S Hypoglossal Nerve** Twelfth cranial nerve **W Cervical Spinal Cord** **X Thoracic Spinal Cord** **Y Lumbar Spinal Cord** Cauda equina Conus medullaris	**Ø Open** **3 Percutaneous** **4 Percutaneous Endoscopic**	**Z No Device**	**Z No Qualifier**

Ø Medical and Surgical
Ø Central Nervous System and Cranial Nerves
9 Drainage Definition: Taking or letting out fluids and/or gases from a body part
Explanation: The qualifier DIAGNOSTIC is used to identify drainage procedures that are biopsies

Body Part Character 4	Approach Character 5	Device Character 6	Qualifier Character 7
Ø Brain Cerebrum Corpus callosum Encephalon **1 Cerebral Meninges** Arachnoid mater, intracranial Leptomeninges, intracranial Pia mater, intracranial **2 Dura Mater** Diaphragma sellae Dura mater, intracranial Falx cerebri Tentorium cerebelli **3 Epidural Space, Intracranial** Extradural space, intracranial **4 Subdural Space, Intracranial** **5 Subarachnoid Space, Intracranial** **6 Cerebral Ventricle** Aqueduct of Sylvius Cerebral aqueduct (Sylvius) Choroid plexus Ependyma Foramen of Monro (intraventricular) Fourth ventricle Interventricular foramen (Monro) Left lateral ventricle Right lateral ventricle Third ventricle **7 Cerebral Hemisphere** Frontal lobe Occipital lobe Parietal lobe Temporal lobe **8 Basal Ganglia** Basal nuclei Claustrum Corpus striatum Globus pallidus Substantia nigra Subthalamic nucleus **9 Thalamus** Epithalamus Geniculate nucleus Metathalamus Pulvinar **A Hypothalamus** Mammillary body **B Pons** Apneustic center Basis pontis Locus ceruleus Pneumotaxic center Pontine tegmentum Superior olivary nucleus **C Cerebellum** Culmen **D Medulla Oblongata** Myelencephalon **F Olfactory Nerve** First cranial nerve Olfactory bulb **G Optic Nerve** Optic chiasma Second cranial nerve **H Oculomotor Nerve** Third cranial nerve **J Trochlear Nerve** Fourth cranial nerve **K Trigeminal Nerve** Fifth cranial nerve Gasserian ganglion Mandibular nerve Maxillary nerve Ophthalmic nerve Trifacial nerve **L Abducens Nerve** Sixth cranial nerve **M Facial Nerve** Chorda tympani Geniculate ganglion Greater superficial petrosal nerve Nerve to the stapedius Parotid plexus Posterior auricular nerve Seventh cranial nerve Submandibular ganglion **N Acoustic Nerve** Cochlear nerve Eighth cranial nerve Scarpa's (vestibular) ganglion Spiral ganglion Vestibular (Scarpa's) ganglion Vestibular nerve Vestibulocochlear nerve **P Glossopharyngeal Nerve** Carotid sinus nerve Ninth cranial nerve Tympanic nerve **Q Vagus Nerve** Anterior vagal trunk Pharyngeal plexus Pneumogastric nerve Posterior vagal trunk Pulmonary plexus Recurrent laryngeal nerve Superior laryngeal nerve Tenth cranial nerve **R Accessory Nerve** Eleventh cranial nerve **S Hypoglossal Nerve** Twelfth cranial nerve **T Spinal Meninges** Arachnoid mater, spinal Denticulate (dentate) ligament Dura mater, spinal Filum terminale Leptomeninges, spinal Pia mater, spinal **U Spinal Canal** Epidural space, spinal Extradural space, spinal Subarachnoid space, spinal Subdural space, spinal Vertebral canal **W Cervical Spinal Cord** **X Thoracic Spinal Cord** **Y Lumbar Spinal Cord** Cauda equina Conus medullaris	**Ø Open** **3 Percutaneous** **4 Percutaneous Endoscopic**	**Ø Drainage Device**	**Z No Qualifier**

Non-OR ØØ9[T,W,X,Y]3ØZ
Non-OR ØØ9U[3,4]ØZ

ØØ9 Continued on next page

0 Medical and Surgical
0 Central Nervous System and Cranial Nerves
9 Drainage Definition: Taking or letting out fluids and/or gases from a body part
Explanation: The qualifier DIAGNOSTIC is used to identify drainage procedures that are biopsies

009 Continued

Body Part Character 4		Approach Character 5	Device Character 6	Qualifier Character 7
0 **Brain** Cerebrum Corpus callosum Encephalon 1 **Cerebral Meninges** Arachnoid mater, intracranial Leptomeninges, intracranial Pia mater, intracranial 2 **Dura Mater** Diaphragma sellae Dura mater, intracranial Falx cerebri Tentorium cerebelli 3 **Epidural Space, Intracranial** Extradural space, intracranial 4 **Subdural Space, Intracranial** 5 **Subarachnoid Space, Intracranial** 6 **Cerebral Ventricle** Aqueduct of Sylvius Cerebral aqueduct (Sylvius) Choroid plexus Ependyma Foramen of Monro (intraventricular) Fourth ventricle Interventricular foramen (Monro) Left lateral ventricle Right lateral ventricle Third ventricle 7 **Cerebral Hemisphere** Frontal lobe Occipital lobe Parietal lobe Temporal lobe 8 **Basal Ganglia** Basal nuclei Claustrum Corpus striatum Globus pallidus Substantia nigra Subthalamic nucleus 9 **Thalamus** Epithalamus Geniculate nucleus Metathalamus Pulvinar A **Hypothalamus** Mammillary body B **Pons** Apneustic center Basis pontis Locus ceruleus Pneumotaxic center Pontine tegmentum Superior olivary nucleus C **Cerebellum** Culmen D **Medulla Oblongata** Myelencephalon F **Olfactory Nerve** First cranial nerve Olfactory bulb	G **Optic Nerve** Optic chiasma Second cranial nerve H **Oculomotor Nerve** Third cranial nerve J **Trochlear Nerve** Fourth cranial nerve K **Trigeminal Nerve** Fifth cranial nerve Gasserian ganglion Mandibular nerve Maxillary nerve Ophthalmic nerve Trifacial nerve L **Abducens Nerve** Sixth cranial nerve M **Facial Nerve** Chorda tympani Geniculate ganglion Greater superficial petrosal nerve Nerve to the stapedius Parotid plexus Posterior auricular nerve Seventh cranial nerve Submandibular ganglion N **Acoustic Nerve** Cochlear nerve Eighth cranial nerve Scarpa's (vestibular) ganglion Spiral ganglion Vestibular (Scarpa's) ganglion Vestibular nerve Vestibulocochlear nerve P **Glossopharyngeal Nerve** Carotid sinus nerve Ninth cranial nerve Tympanic nerve Q **Vagus Nerve** Anterior vagal trunk Pharyngeal plexus Pneumogastric nerve Posterior vagal trunk Pulmonary plexus Recurrent laryngeal nerve Superior laryngeal nerve Tenth cranial nerve R **Accessory Nerve** Eleventh cranial nerve S **Hypoglossal Nerve** Twelfth cranial nerve T **Spinal Meninges** Arachnoid mater, spinal Denticulate (dentate) ligament Dura mater, spinal Filum terminale Leptomeninges, spinal Pia mater, spinal U **Spinal Canal** Epidural space, spinal Extradural space, spinal Subarachnoid space, spinal Subdural space, spinal Vertebral canal W **Cervical Spinal Cord** X **Thoracic Spinal Cord** Y **Lumbar Spinal Cord** Cauda equina Conus medullaris	0 Open 3 Percutaneous 4 Percutaneous Endoscopic	Z No Device	X Diagnostic Z No Qualifier

Non-OR 009[0,1,2,3,4,5,6,7,8,9,A,B,C,D,F,G,H,J,K,L,M,N,P,Q,R,S][3,4]ZX
Non-OR 009[T,W,X,Y]3Z[X,Z]
Non-OR 009U[3,4]Z[X,Z]

Ø Medical and Surgical
Ø Central Nervous System and Cranial Nerves
B Excision Definition: Cutting out or off, without replacement, a portion of a body part
Explanation: The qualifier DIAGNOSTIC is used to identify excision procedures that are biopsies

Body Part Character 4	Approach Character 5	Device Character 6	Qualifier Character 7
Ø Brain Cerebrum Corpus callosum Encephalon **1 Cerebral Meninges** Arachnoid mater, intracranial Leptomeninges, intracranial Pia mater, intracranial **2 Dura Mater** Diaphragma sellae Dura mater, intracranial Falx cerebri Tentorium cerebelli **6 Cerebral Ventricle** Aqueduct of Sylvius Cerebral aqueduct (Sylvius) Choroid plexus Ependyma Foramen of Monro (intraventricular) Fourth ventricle Interventricular foramen (Monro) Left lateral ventricle Right lateral ventricle Third ventricle **7 Cerebral Hemisphere** Frontal lobe Occipital lobe Parietal lobe Temporal lobe **8 Basal Ganglia** Basal nuclei Claustrum Corpus striatum Globus pallidus Substantia nigra Subthalamic nucleus **9 Thalamus** Epithalamus Geniculate nucleus Metathalamus Pulvinar **A Hypothalamus** Mammillary body **B Pons** Apneustic center Basis pontis Locus ceruleus Pneumotaxic center Pontine tegmentum Superior olivary nucleus **C Cerebellum** Culmen **D Medulla Oblongata** Myelencephalon **F Olfactory Nerve** First cranial nerve Olfactory bulb **G Optic Nerve** Optic chiasma Second cranial nerve **H Oculomotor Nerve** Third cranial nerve **J Trochlear Nerve** Fourth cranial nerve **K Trigeminal Nerve** Fifth cranial nerve Gasserian ganglion Mandibular nerve Maxillary nerve Ophthalmic nerve Trifacial nerve **L Abducens Nerve** Sixth cranial nerve **M Facial Nerve** Chorda tympani Geniculate ganglion Greater superficial petrosal nerve Nerve to the stapedius Parotid plexus Posterior auricular nerve Seventh cranial nerve Submandibular ganglion **N Acoustic Nerve** Cochlear nerve Eighth cranial nerve Scarpa's (vestibular) ganglion Spiral ganglion Vestibular (Scarpa's) ganglion Vestibular nerve Vestibulocochlear nerve **P Glossopharyngeal Nerve** Carotid sinus nerve Ninth cranial nerve Tympanic nerve **Q Vagus Nerve** Anterior vagal trunk Pharyngeal plexus Pneumogastric nerve Posterior vagal trunk Pulmonary plexus Recurrent laryngeal nerve Superior laryngeal nerve Tenth cranial nerve **R Accessory Nerve** Eleventh cranial nerve **S Hypoglossal Nerve** Twelfth cranial nerve **T Spinal Meninges** Arachnoid mater, spinal Denticulate (dentate) ligament Dura mater, spinal Filum terminale Leptomeninges, spinal Pia mater, spinal **W Cervical Spinal Cord** **X Thoracic Spinal Cord** **Y Lumbar Spinal Cord** Cauda equina Conus medullaris	**Ø Open** **3 Percutaneous** **4 Percutaneous Endoscopic**	**Z No Device**	**X Diagnostic** **Z No Qualifier**

Non-OR ØØB[F,G,H,J,K,L,M,N,P,Q,R,S][3,4]ZX

Ø Medical and Surgical
Ø Central Nervous System and Cranial Nerves
C Extirpation Definition: Taking or cutting out solid matter from a body part

Explanation: The solid matter may be an abnormal byproduct of a biological function or a foreign body; it may be imbedded in a body part or in the lumen of a tubular body part. The solid matter may or may not have been previously broken into pieces.

Body Part Character 4	Approach Character 5	Device Character 6	Qualifier Character 7
Ø Brain Cerebrum Corpus callosum Encephalon **1 Cerebral Meninges** Arachnoid mater, intracranial Leptomeninges, intracranial Pia mater, intracranial **2 Dura Mater** Diaphragma sellae Dura mater, intracranial Falx cerebri Tentorium cerebelli **3 Epidural Space, Intracranial** Extradural space, intracranial **4 Subdural Space, Intracranial** **5 Subarachnoid Space, Intracranial** **6 Cerebral Ventricle** Aqueduct of Sylvius Cerebral aqueduct (Sylvius) Choroid plexus Ependyma Foramen of Monro (intraventricular) Fourth ventricle Interventricular foramen (Monro) Left lateral ventricle Right lateral ventricle Third ventricle **7 Cerebral Hemisphere** Frontal lobe Occipital lobe Parietal lobe Temporal lobe **8 Basal Ganglia** Basal nuclei Claustrum Corpus striatum Globus pallidus Substantia nigra Subthalamic nucleus **9 Thalamus** Epithalamus Geniculate nucleus Metathalamus Pulvinar **A Hypothalamus** Mammillary body **B Pons** Apneustic center Basis pontis Locus ceruleus Pneumotaxic center Pontine tegmentum Superior olivary nucleus **C Cerebellum** Culmen **D Medulla Oblongata** Myelencephalon **F Olfactory Nerve** First cranial nerve Olfactory bulb **G Optic Nerve** Optic chiasma Second cranial nerve **H Oculomotor Nerve** Third cranial nerve **J Trochlear Nerve** Fourth cranial nerve **K Trigeminal Nerve** Fifth cranial nerve Gasserian ganglion Mandibular nerve Maxillary nerve Ophthalmic nerve Trifacial nerve **L Abducens Nerve** Sixth cranial nerve **M Facial Nerve** Chorda tympani Geniculate ganglion Greater superficial petrosal nerve Nerve to the stapedius Parotid plexus Posterior auricular nerve Seventh cranial nerve Submandibular ganglion **N Acoustic Nerve** Cochlear nerve Eighth cranial nerve Scarpa's (vestibular) ganglion Spiral ganglion Vestibular (Scarpa's) ganglion Vestibular nerve Vestibulocochlear nerve **P Glossopharyngeal Nerve** Carotid sinus nerve Ninth cranial nerve Tympanic nerve **Q Vagus Nerve** Anterior vagal trunk Pharyngeal plexus Pneumogastric nerve Posterior vagal trunk Pulmonary plexus Recurrent laryngeal nerve Superior laryngeal nerve Tenth cranial nerve **R Accessory Nerve** Eleventh cranial nerve **S Hypoglossal Nerve** Twelfth cranial nerve **T Spinal Meninges** Arachnoid mater, spinal Denticulate (dentate) ligament Dura mater, spinal Filum terminale Leptomeninges, spinal Pia mater, spinal **U Spinal Canal** **W Cervical Spinal Cord** **X Thoracic Spinal Cord** **Y Lumbar Spinal Cord** Cauda equina Conus medullaris	**Ø Open** **3 Percutaneous** **4 Percutaneous Endoscopic**	**Z No Device**	**Z No Qualifier**

Ø Medical and Surgical
Ø Central Nervous System and Cranial Nerves
D Extraction Definition: Pulling or stripping out or off all or a portion of a body part by the use of force

Explanation: The qualifier DIAGNOSTIC is used to identify extraction procedures that are biopsies

Body Part Character 4	Approach Character 5	Device Character 6	Qualifier Character 7
1 Cerebral Meninges Arachnoid mater, intracranial Leptomeninges, intracranial Pia mater, intracranial **2 Dura Mater** Diaphragma sellae Dura mater, intracranial Falx cerebri Tentorium cerebelli **F Olfactory Nerve** First cranial nerve Olfactory bulb **G Optic Nerve** Optic chiasma Second cranial nerve **H Oculomotor Nerve** Third cranial nerve **J Trochlear Nerve** Fourth cranial nerve **K Trigeminal Nerve** Fifth cranial nerve Gasserian ganglion Mandibular nerve Maxillary nerve Ophthalmic nerve Trifacial nerve **L Abducens Nerve** Sixth cranial nerve **M Facial Nerve** Chorda tympani Geniculate ganglion Greater superficial petrosal nerve Nerve to the stapedius Parotid plexus Posterior auricular nerve Seventh cranial nerve Submandibular ganglion **N Acoustic Nerve** Cochlear nerve Eighth cranial nerve Scarpa's (vestibular) ganglion Spiral ganglion Vestibular (Scarpa's) ganglion Vestibular nerve Vestibulocochlear nerve **P Glossopharyngeal Nerve** Carotid sinus nerve Ninth cranial nerve Tympanic nerve **Q Vagus Nerve** Anterior vagal trunk Pharyngeal plexus Pneumogastric nerve Posterior vagal trunk Pulmonary plexus Recurrent laryngeal nerve Superior laryngeal nerve Tenth cranial nerve **R Accessory Nerve** Eleventh cranial nerve **S Hypoglossal Nerve** Twelfth cranial nerve **T Spinal Meninges** Arachnoid mater, spinal Denticulate (dentate) ligament Dura mater, spinal Filum terminale Leptomeninges, spinal Pia mater, spinal	**Ø Open** **3 Percutaneous** **4 Percutaneous Endoscopic**	**Z No Device**	**Z No Qualifier**

Ø Medical and Surgical
Ø Central Nervous System and Cranial Nerves
F Fragmentation Definition: Breaking solid matter in a body part into pieces

Explanation: Physical force (e.g., manual, ultrasonic) applied directly or indirectly is used to break the solid matter into pieces. The solid matter may be an abnormal byproduct of a biological function or a foreign body. The pieces of solid matter are not taken out.

Body Part Character 4	Approach Character 5	Device Character 6	Qualifier Character 7
3 Epidural Space, Intracranial NC Extradural space, intracranial **4 Subdural Space, Intracranial** NC **5 Subarachnoid Space, Intracranial** NC **6 Cerebral Ventricle** NC Aqueduct of Sylvius Cerebral aqueduct (Sylvius) Choroid plexus Ependyma Foramen of Monro (intraventricular) Fourth ventricle Interventricular foramen (Monro) Left lateral ventricle Right lateral ventricle Third ventricle **U Spinal Canal** Epidural space, spinal Extradural space, spinal Subarachnoid space, spinal Subdural space, spinal Vertebral canal	**Ø Open** **3 Percutaneous** **4 Percutaneous Endoscopic** **X External**	**Z No Device**	**Z No Qualifier**

Non-OR ØØF[3,4,5,6]XZZ
NC ØØF[3,4,5,6]XZZ

Ø Medical and Surgical
Ø Central Nervous System and Cranial Nerves
H Insertion Definition: Putting in a nonbiological appliance that monitors, assists, performs, or prevents a physiological function but does not physically take the place of a body part
Explanation: None

Body Part Character 4	Approach Character 5	Device Character 6	Qualifier Character 7
Ø Brain ⊞ Cerebrum Corpus callosum Encephalon	Ø Open	1 Radioactive Element 2 Monitoring Device 3 Infusion Device 4 Radioactive Element, Cesium-131 Collagen Implant M Neurostimulator Lead Y Other Device	Z No Qualifier
Ø Brain ⊞ Cerebrum Corpus callosum Encephalon	3 Percutaneous 4 Percutaneous Endoscopic	1 Radioactive Element 2 Monitoring Device 3 Infusion Device M Neurostimulator Lead Y Other Device	Z No Qualifier
6 Cerebral Ventricle ⊞ Aqueduct of Sylvius Cerebral aqueduct (Sylvius) Choroid plexus Ependyma Foramen of Monro (intraventricular) Fourth ventricle Interventricular foramen (Monro) Left lateral ventricle Right lateral ventricle Third ventricle E Cranial Nerve ⊞ U Spinal Canal ⊞ Epidural space, spinal Extradural space, spinal Subarachnoid space, spinal Subdural space, spinal Vertebral canal V Spinal Cord ⊞	Ø Open 3 Percutaneous 4 Percutaneous Endoscopic	1 Radioactive Element 2 Monitoring Device 3 Infusion Device M Neurostimulator Lead Y Other Device	Z No Qualifier

DRG Non-OR ØØHØØ4Z
Non-OR ØØH[E,U,V]32Z
Non-OR ØØH[E,U][3,4]YZ
Non-OR ØØH[U,V][Ø,3,4]3Z

See Appendix L for Procedure Combinations
⊞ ØØHØØMZ
⊞ ØØHØ[3,4]MZ
⊞ ØØH[6,E,U,V][Ø,3,4]MZ

Ø Medical and Surgical
Ø Central Nervous System and Cranial Nerves
J Inspection Definition: Visually and/or manually exploring a body part
Explanation: Visual exploration may be performed with or without optical instrumentation. Manual exploration may be performed directly or through intervening body layers.

Body Part Character 4	Approach Character 5	Device Character 6	Qualifier Character 7
Ø Brain Cerebrum Corpus callosum Encephalon E Cranial Nerve U Spinal Canal Epidural space, spinal Extradural space, spinal Subarachnoid space, spinal Subdural space, spinal Vertebral canal V Spinal Cord	Ø Open 3 Percutaneous 4 Percutaneous Endoscopic	Z No Device	Z No Qualifier

Non-OR ØØJ[Ø,E,U,V]3ZZ

Ø Medical and Surgical
Ø Central Nervous System and Cranial Nerves
K Map Definition: Locating the route of passage of electrical impulses and/or locating functional areas in a body part
Explanation: Applicable only to the cardiac conduction mechanism and the central nervous system

Body Part Character 4	Approach Character 5	Device Character 6	Qualifier Character 7
Ø Brain Cerebrum Corpus callosum Encephalon 7 Cerebral Hemisphere Frontal lobe Occipital lobe Parietal lobe Temporal lobe 8 Basal Ganglia Basal nuclei Claustrum Corpus striatum Globus pallidus Substantia nigra Subthalamic nucleus 9 Thalamus Epithalamus Geniculate nucleus Metathalamus Pulvinar A Hypothalamus Mammillary body B Pons Apneustic center Basis pontis Locus ceruleus Pneumotaxic center Pontine tegmentum Superior olivary nucleus C Cerebellum Culmen D Medulla Oblongata Myelencephalon	Ø Open 3 Percutaneous 4 Percutaneous Endoscopic	Z No Device	Z No Qualifier

Ø Medical and Surgical
Ø Central Nervous System and Cranial Nerves
N Release Definition: Freeing a body part from an abnormal physical constraint by cutting or by the use of force

Explanation: Some of the restraining tissue may be taken out but none of the body part is taken out

Body Part Character 4	Approach Character 5	Device Character 6	Qualifier Character 7
Ø Brain Cerebrum Corpus callosum Encephalon **1 Cerebral Meninges** Arachnoid mater, intracranial Leptomeninges, intracranial Pia mater, intracranial **2 Dura Mater** Diaphragma sellae Dura mater, intracranial Falx cerebri Tentorium cerebelli **6 Cerebral Ventricle** Aqueduct of Sylvius Cerebral aqueduct (Sylvius) Choroid plexus Ependyma Foramen of Monro (intraventricular) Fourth ventricle Interventricular foramen (Monro) Left lateral ventricle Right lateral ventricle Third ventricle **7 Cerebral Hemisphere** Frontal lobe Occipital lobe Parietal lobe Temporal lobe **8 Basal Ganglia** Basal nuclei Claustrum Corpus striatum Globus pallidus Substantia nigra Subthalamic nucleus **9 Thalamus** Epithalamus Geniculate nucleus Metathalamus Pulvinar **A Hypothalamus** Mammillary body **B Pons** Apneustic center Basis pontis Locus ceruleus Pneumotaxic center Pontine tegmentum Superior olivary nucleus **C Cerebellum** Culmen **D Medulla Oblongata** Myelencephalon **F Olfactory Nerve** First cranial nerve Olfactory bulb **G Optic Nerve** Optic chiasma Second cranial nerve **H Oculomotor Nerve** Third cranial nerve **J Trochlear Nerve** Fourth cranial nerve **K Trigeminal Nerve** Fifth cranial nerve Gasserian ganglion Mandibular nerve Maxillary nerve Ophthalmic nerve Trifacial nerve **L Abducens Nerve** Sixth cranial nerve **M Facial Nerve** Chorda tympani Geniculate ganglion Greater superficial petrosal nerve Nerve to the stapedius Parotid plexus Posterior auricular nerve Seventh cranial nerve Submandibular ganglion **N Acoustic Nerve** Cochlear nerve Eighth cranial nerve Scarpa's (vestibular) ganglion Spiral ganglion Vestibular (Scarpa's) ganglion Vestibular nerve Vestibulocochlear nerve **P Glossopharyngeal Nerve** Carotid sinus nerve Ninth cranial nerve Tympanic nerve **Q Vagus Nerve** Anterior vagal trunk Pharyngeal plexus Pneumogastric nerve Posterior vagal trunk Pulmonary plexus Recurrent laryngeal nerve Superior laryngeal nerve Tenth cranial nerve **R Accessory Nerve** Eleventh cranial nerve **S Hypoglossal Nerve** Twelfth cranial nerve **T Spinal Meninges** Arachnoid mater, spinal Denticulate (dentate) ligament Dura mater, spinal Filum terminale Leptomeninges, spinal Pia mater, spinal **W Cervical Spinal Cord** **X Thoracic Spinal Cord** **Y Lumbar Spinal Cord** Cauda equina Conus medullaris	**Ø Open** **3 Percutaneous** **4 Percutaneous Endoscopic**	**Z No Device**	**Z No Qualifier**

Ø Medical and Surgical
Ø Central Nervous System and Cranial Nerves
P Removal Definition: Taking out or off a device from a body part

Explanation: If a device is taken out and a similar device put in without cutting or puncturing the skin or mucous membrane, the procedure is coded to the root operation CHANGE. Otherwise, the procedure for taking out a device is coded to the root operation REMOVAL.

Body Part Character 4	Approach Character 5	Device Character 6	Qualifier Character 7
Ø Brain Cerebrum Corpus callosum Encephalon **V Spinal Cord**	**Ø Open** **3 Percutaneous** **4 Percutaneous Endoscopic**	**Ø Drainage Device** **2 Monitoring Device** **3 Infusion Device** **7 Autologous Tissue Substitute** **J Synthetic Substitute** **K Nonautologous Tissue Substitute** **M Neurostimulator Lead** **Y Other Device**	**Z No Qualifier**
Ø Brain Cerebrum Corpus callosum Encephalon **V Spinal Cord**	**X External**	**Ø Drainage Device** **2 Monitoring Device** **3 Infusion Device** **M Neurostimulator Lead**	**Z No Qualifier**
6 Cerebral Ventricle Aqueduct of Sylvius Cerebral aqueduct (Sylvius) Choroid plexus Ependyma Foramen of Monro (intraventricular) Fourth ventricle Interventricular foramen (Monro) Left lateral ventricle Right lateral ventricle Third ventricle **U Spinal Canal** Epidural space, spinal Extradural space, spinal Subarachnoid space, spinal Subdural space, spinal Vertebral canal	**Ø Open** **3 Percutaneous** **4 Percutaneous Endoscopic**	**Ø Drainage Device** **2 Monitoring Device** **3 Infusion Device** **J Synthetic Substitute** **M Neurostimulator Lead** **Y Other Device**	**Z No Qualifier**
6 Cerebral Ventricle Aqueduct of Sylvius Cerebral aqueduct (Sylvius) Choroid plexus Ependyma Foramen of Monro (intraventricular) Fourth ventricle Interventricular foramen (Monro) Left lateral ventricle Right lateral ventricle Third ventricle **U Spinal Canal** Epidural space, spinal Extradural space, spinal Subarachnoid space, spinal Subdural space, spinal Vertebral canal	**X External**	**Ø Drainage Device** **2 Monitoring Device** **3 Infusion Device** **M Neurostimulator Lead**	**Z No Qualifier**
E Cranial Nerve	**Ø Open** **3 Percutaneous** **4 Percutaneous Endoscopic**	**Ø Drainage Device** **2 Monitoring Device** **3 Infusion Device** **7 Autologous Tissue Substitute** **M Neurostimulator Lead** **Y Other Device**	**Z No Qualifier**
E Cranial Nerve	**X External**	**Ø Drainage Device** **2 Monitoring Device** **3 Infusion Device** **M Neurostimulator Lead**	**Z No Qualifier**

Non-OR ØØP[Ø,V]3[Ø,2,3]Z
Non-OR ØØP[Ø,V][3,4]YZ
Non-OR ØØP[Ø,V]X[Ø,2,3,M]Z
Non-OR ØØP[6,U]3[Ø,2,3]Z
Non-OR ØØP[6,U][3,4]YZ
Non-OR ØØP[6,U]X[Ø,2,3,M]Z
Non-OR ØØPE3[Ø,2,3]Z
Non-OR ØØPE[3,4]YZ
Non-OR ØØPEX[Ø,2,3,M]Z

Ø Medical and Surgical
Ø Central Nervous System and Cranial Nerves
Q Repair Definition: Restoring, to the extent possible, a body part to its normal anatomic structure and function
Explanation: Used only when the method to accomplish the repair is not one of the other root operations

Body Part Character 4	Approach Character 5	Device Character 6	Qualifier Character 7
Ø Brain Cerebrum Corpus callosum Encephalon **1 Cerebral Meninges** Arachnoid mater, intracranial Leptomeninges, intracranial Pia mater, intracranial **2 Dura Mater** Diaphragma sellae Dura mater, intracranial Falx cerebri Tentorium cerebelli **6 Cerebral Ventricle** Aqueduct of Sylvius Cerebral aqueduct (Sylvius) Choroid plexus Ependyma Foramen of Monro (intraventricular) Fourth ventricle Interventricular foramen (Monro) Left lateral ventricle Right lateral ventricle Third ventricle **7 Cerebral Hemisphere** Frontal lobe Occipital lobe Parietal lobe Temporal lobe **8 Basal Ganglia** Basal nuclei Claustrum Corpus striatum Globus pallidus Substantia nigra Subthalamic nucleus **9 Thalamus** Epithalamus Geniculate nucleus Metathalamus Pulvinar **A Hypothalamus** Mammillary body **B Pons** Apneustic center Basis pontis Locus ceruleus Pneumotaxic center Pontine tegmentum Superior olivary nucleus **C Cerebellum** Culmen **D Medulla Oblongata** Myelencephalon **F Olfactory Nerve** First cranial nerve Olfactory bulb **G Optic Nerve** Optic chiasma Second cranial nerve **H Oculomotor Nerve** Third cranial nerve **J Trochlear Nerve** Fourth cranial nerve **K Trigeminal Nerve** Fifth cranial nerve Gasserian ganglion Mandibular nerve Maxillary nerve Ophthalmic nerve Trifacial nerve **L Abducens Nerve** Sixth cranial nerve **M Facial Nerve** Chorda tympani Geniculate ganglion Greater superficial petrosal nerve Nerve to the stapedius Parotid plexus Posterior auricular nerve Seventh cranial nerve Submandibular ganglion **N Acoustic Nerve** Cochlear nerve Eighth cranial nerve Scarpa's (vestibular) ganglion Spiral ganglion Vestibular (Scarpa's) ganglion Vestibular nerve Vestibulocochlear nerve **P Glossopharyngeal Nerve** Carotid sinus nerve Ninth cranial nerve Tympanic nerve **Q Vagus Nerve** Anterior vagal trunk Pharyngeal plexus Pneumogastric nerve Posterior vagal trunk Pulmonary plexus Recurrent laryngeal nerve Superior laryngeal nerve Tenth cranial nerve **R Accessory Nerve** Eleventh cranial nerve **S Hypoglossal Nerve** Twelfth cranial nerve **T Spinal Meninges** Arachnoid mater, spinal Denticulate (dentate) ligament Dura mater, spinal Filum terminale Leptomeninges, spinal Pia mater, spinal **W Cervical Spinal Cord** **X Thoracic Spinal Cord** **Y Lumbar Spinal Cord** Cauda equina Conus medullaris	**Ø Open** **3 Percutaneous** **4 Percutaneous Endoscopic**	**Z No Device**	**Z No Qualifier**

Ø Medical and Surgical
Ø Central Nervous System and Cranial Nerves
R Replacement Definition: Putting in or on biological or synthetic material that physically takes the place and/or function of all or a portion of a body part

Explanation: The body part may have been taken out or replaced, or may be taken out, physically eradicated, or rendered nonfunctional during the REPLACEMENT procedure. A REMOVAL procedure is coded for taking out the device used in a previous replacement procedure.

Body Part Character 4	Approach Character 5	Device Character 6	Qualifier Character 7
1 Cerebral Meninges Arachnoid mater, intracranial Leptomeninges, intracranial Pia mater, intracranial **2 Dura Mater** Diaphragma sellae Dura mater, intracranial Falx cerebri Tentorium cerebelli **6 Cerebral Ventricle** Aqueduct of Sylvius Cerebral aqueduct (Sylvius) Choroid plexus Ependyma Foramen of Monro (intraventricular) Fourth ventricle Interventricular foramen (Monro) Left lateral ventricle Right lateral ventricle Third ventricle **F Olfactory Nerve** First cranial nerve Olfactory bulb **G Optic Nerve** Optic chiasma Second cranial nerve **H Oculomotor Nerve** Third cranial nerve **J Trochlear Nerve** Fourth cranial nerve **K Trigeminal Nerve** Fifth cranial nerve Gasserian ganglion Mandibular nerve Maxillary nerve Ophthalmic nerve Trifacial nerve **L Abducens Nerve** Sixth cranial nerve **M Facial Nerve** Chorda tympani Geniculate ganglion Greater superficial petrosal nerve Nerve to the stapedius Parotid plexus Posterior auricular nerve Seventh cranial nerve Submandibular ganglion **N Acoustic Nerve** Cochlear nerve Eighth cranial nerve Scarpa's (vestibular) ganglion Spiral ganglion Vestibular (Scarpa's) ganglion Vestibular nerve Vestibulocochlear nerve **P Glossopharyngeal Nerve** Carotid sinus nerve Ninth cranial nerve Tympanic nerve **Q Vagus Nerve** Anterior vagal trunk Pharyngeal plexus Pneumogastric nerve Posterior vagal trunk Pulmonary plexus Recurrent laryngeal nerve Superior laryngeal nerve Tenth cranial nerve **R Accessory Nerve** Eleventh cranial nerve **S Hypoglossal Nerve** Twelfth cranial nerve **T Spinal Meninges** Arachnoid mater, spinal Denticulate (dentate) ligament Dura mater, spinal Filum terminale Leptomeninges, spinal Pia mater, spinal	**Ø Open** **4 Percutaneous Endoscopic**	**7 Autologous Tissue Substitute** **J Synthetic Substitute** **K Nonautologous Tissue Substitute**	**Z No Qualifier**

Ø Medical and Surgical
Ø Central Nervous System and Cranial Nerves
S Reposition Definition: Moving to its normal location, or other suitable location, all or a portion of a body part

Explanation: The body part is moved to a new location from an abnormal location, or from a normal location where it is not functioning correctly. The body part may or may not be cut out or off to be moved to the new location.

Body Part Character 4	Approach Character 5	Device Character 6	Qualifier Character 7
F Olfactory Nerve First cranial nerve Olfactory bulb **G Optic Nerve** Optic chiasma Second cranial nerve **H Oculomotor Nerve** Third cranial nerve **J Trochlear Nerve** Fourth cranial nerve **K Trigeminal Nerve** Fifth cranial nerve Gasserian ganglion Mandibular nerve Maxillary nerve Ophthalmic nerve Trifacial nerve **L Abducens Nerve** Sixth cranial nerve **M Facial Nerve** Chorda tympani Geniculate ganglion Greater superficial petrosal nerve Nerve to the stapedius Parotid plexus Posterior auricular nerve Seventh cranial nerve Submandibular ganglion **N Acoustic Nerve** Cochlear nerve Eighth cranial nerve Scarpa's (vestibular) ganglion Spiral ganglion Vestibular (Scarpa's) ganglion Vestibular nerve Vestibulocochlear nerve **P Glossopharyngeal Nerve** Carotid sinus nerve Ninth cranial nerve Tympanic nerve **Q Vagus Nerve** Anterior vagal trunk Pharyngeal plexus Pneumogastric nerve Posterior vagal trunk Pulmonary plexus Recurrent laryngeal nerve Superior laryngeal nerve Tenth cranial nerve **R Accessory Nerve** Eleventh cranial nerve **S Hypoglossal Nerve** Twelfth cranial nerve **W Cervical Spinal Cord** **X Thoracic Spinal Cord** **Y Lumbar Spinal Cord** Cauda equina Conus medullaris	**Ø Open** **3 Percutaneous** **4 Percutaneous Endoscopic**	**Z No Device**	**Z No Qualifier**

Ø Medical and Surgical
Ø Central Nervous System and Cranial Nerves
T Resection Definition: Cutting out or off, without replacement, all of a body part

Explanation: None

Body Part Character 4	Approach Character 5	Device Character 6	Qualifier Character 7
7 Cerebral Hemisphere Frontal lobe Occipital lobe Parietal lobe Temporal lobe	**Ø Open** **3 Percutaneous** **4 Percutaneous Endoscopic**	**Z No Device**	**Z No Qualifier**

Ø Medical and Surgical
Ø Central Nervous System and Cranial Nerves
U Supplement Definition: Putting in or on biological or synthetic material that physically reinforces and/or augments the function of a portion of a body part

Explanation: The biological material is non-living, or is living and from the same individual. The body part may have been previously replaced, and the SUPPLEMENT procedure is performed to physically reinforce and/or augment the function of the replaced body part.

Body Part Character 4		Approach Character 5	Device Character 6	Qualifier Character 7
1 Cerebral Meninges Arachnoid mater, intracranial Leptomeninges, intracranial Pia mater, intracranial **2 Dura Mater** Diaphragma sellae Dura mater, intracranial Falx cerebri Tentorium cerebelli **6 Cerebral Ventricle** Aqueduct of Sylvius Cerebral aqueduct (Sylvius) Choroid plexus Ependyma Foramen of Monro (intraventricular) Fourth ventricle Interventricular foramen (Monro) Left lateral ventricle Right lateral ventricle Third ventricle **F Olfactory Nerve** First cranial nerve Olfactory bulb **G Optic Nerve** Optic chiasma Second cranial nerve **H Oculomotor Nerve** Third cranial nerve **J Trochlear Nerve** Fourth cranial nerve **K Trigeminal Nerve** Fifth cranial nerve Gasserian ganglion Mandibular nerve Maxillary nerve Ophthalmic nerve Trifacial nerve **L Abducens Nerve** Sixth cranial nerve	**M Facial Nerve** Chorda tympani Geniculate ganglion Greater superficial petrosal nerve Nerve to the stapedius Parotid plexus Posterior auricular nerve Seventh cranial nerve Submandibular ganglion **N Acoustic Nerve** Cochlear nerve Eighth cranial nerve Scarpa's (vestibular) ganglion Spiral ganglion Vestibular (Scarpa's) ganglion Vestibular nerve Vestibulocochlear nerve **P Glossopharyngeal Nerve** Carotid sinus nerve Ninth cranial nerve Tympanic nerve **Q Vagus Nerve** Anterior vagal trunk Pharyngeal plexus Pneumogastric nerve Posterior vagal trunk Pulmonary plexus Recurrent laryngeal nerve Superior laryngeal nerve Tenth cranial nerve **R Accessory Nerve** Eleventh cranial nerve **S Hypoglossal Nerve** Twelfth cranial nerve **T Spinal Meninges** Arachnoid mater, spinal Denticulate (dentate) ligament Dura mater, spinal Filum terminale Leptomeninges, spinal Pia mater, spinal	**Ø Open** **3 Percutaneous** **4 Percutaneous Endoscopic**	**7 Autologous Tissue Substitute** **J Synthetic Substitute** **K Nonautologous Tissue Substitute**	**Z No Qualifier**

Ø Medical and Surgical
Ø Central Nervous System and Cranial Nerves
W Revision Definition: Correcting, to the extent possible, a portion of a malfunctioning device or the position of a displaced device

Explanation: Revision can include correcting a malfunctioning or displaced device by taking out or putting in components of the device such as a screw or pin

Body Part Character 4	Approach Character 5	Device Character 6	Qualifier Character 7
Ø Brain Cerebrum Corpus callosum Encephalon V Spinal Cord	Ø Open 3 Percutaneous 4 Percutaneous Endoscopic	Ø Drainage Device 2 Monitoring Device 3 Infusion Device 7 Autologous Tissue Substitute J Synthetic Substitute K Nonautologous Tissue Substitute M Neurostimulator Lead Y Other Device	Z No Qualifier
Ø Brain Cerebrum Corpus callosum Encephalon V Spinal Cord	X External	Ø Drainage Device 2 Monitoring Device 3 Infusion Device 7 Autologous Tissue Substitute J Synthetic Substitute K Nonautologous Tissue Substitute M Neurostimulator Lead	Z No Qualifier
6 Cerebral Ventricle Aqueduct of Sylvius Cerebral aqueduct (Sylvius) Choroid plexus Ependyma Foramen of Monro (intraventricular) Fourth ventricle Interventricular foramen (Monro) Left lateral ventricle Right lateral ventricle Third ventricle U Spinal Canal Epidural space, spinal Extradural space, spinal Subarachnoid space, spinal Subdural space, spinal Vertebral canal	Ø Open 3 Percutaneous 4 Percutaneous Endoscopic	Ø Drainage Device 2 Monitoring Device 3 Infusion Device J Synthetic Substitute M Neurostimulator Lead Y Other Device	Z No Qualifier
6 Cerebral Ventricle Aqueduct of Sylvius Cerebral aqueduct (Sylvius) Choroid plexus Ependyma Foramen of Monro (intraventricular) Fourth ventricle Interventricular foramen (Monro) Left lateral ventricle Right lateral ventricle Third ventricle U Spinal Canal Epidural space, spinal Extradural space, spinal Subarachnoid space, spinal Subdural space, spinal Vertebral canal	X External	Ø Drainage Device 2 Monitoring Device 3 Infusion Device J Synthetic Substitute M Neurostimulator Lead	Z No Qualifier
E Cranial Nerve	Ø Open 3 Percutaneous 4 Percutaneous Endoscopic	Ø Drainage Device 2 Monitoring Device 3 Infusion Device 7 Autologous Tissue Substitute M Neurostimulator Lead Y Other Device	Z No Qualifier
E Cranial Nerve	X External	Ø Drainage Device 2 Monitoring Device 3 Infusion Device 7 Autologous Tissue Substitute M Neurostimulator Lead	Z No Qualifier

Non-OR ØØW[Ø,V][3,4]YZ
Non-OR ØØW[Ø,V]X[Ø,2,3,7,J,K,M]Z
Non-OR ØØW[6,U][3,4]YZ
Non-OR ØØW[6,U]X[Ø,2,3,J,M]Z
Non-OR ØØWE[3,4]YZ
Non-OR ØØWEX[Ø,2,3,7,M]Z

Ø Medical and Surgical
Ø Central Nervous System and Cranial Nerves
X Transfer Definition: Moving, without taking out, all or a portion of a body part to another location to take over the function of all or a portion of a body part
Explanation: The body part transferred remains connected to its vascular and nervous supply

Body Part Character 4	Approach Character 5	Device Character 6	Qualifier Character 7
F Olfactory Nerve First cranial nerve Olfactory bulb **G Optic Nerve** Optic chiasma Second cranial nerve **H Oculomotor Nerve** Third cranial nerve **J Trochlear Nerve** Fourth cranial nerve **K Trigeminal Nerve** Fifth cranial nerve Gasserian ganglion Mandibular nerve Maxillary nerve Ophthalmic nerve Trifacial nerve **L Abducens Nerve** Sixth cranial nerve **M Facial Nerve** Chorda tympani Geniculate ganglion Greater superficial petrosal nerve Nerve to the stapedius Parotid plexus Posterior auricular nerve Seventh cranial nerve Submandibular ganglion **N Acoustic Nerve** Cochlear nerve Eighth cranial nerve Scarpa's (vestibular) ganglion Spiral ganglion Vestibular (Scarpa's) ganglion Vestibular nerve Vestibulocochlear nerve **P Glossopharyngeal Nerve** Carotid sinus nerve Ninth cranial nerve Tympanic nerve **Q Vagus Nerve** Anterior vagal trunk Pharyngeal plexus Pneumogastric nerve Posterior vagal trunk Pulmonary plexus Recurrent laryngeal nerve Superior laryngeal nerve Tenth cranial nerve **R Accessory Nerve** Eleventh cranial nerve **S Hypoglossal Nerve** Twelfth cranial nerve	**Ø Open** **4 Percutaneous Endoscopic**	**Z No Device**	**F Olfactory Nerve** **G Optic Nerve** **H Oculomotor Nerve** **J Trochlear Nerve** **K Trigeminal Nerve** **L Abducens Nerve** **M Facial Nerve** **N Acoustic Nerve** **P Glossopharyngeal Nerve** **Q Vagus Nerve** **R Accessory Nerve** **S Hypoglossal Nerve**

Peripheral Nervous System Ø12–Ø1X

Character Meanings

This Character Meaning table is provided as a guide to assist the user in the identification of character members that may be found in this section of code tables. It **SHOULD NOT** be used to build a PCS code.

Operation–Character 3	Body Part–Character 4	Approach–Character 5	Device–Character 6	Qualifier–Character 7
2 Change	Ø Cervical Plexus	Ø Open	Ø Drainage Device	1 Cervical Nerve
5 Destruction	1 Cervical Nerve	3 Percutaneous	1 Radioactive Element	2 Phrenic Nerve
8 Division	2 Phrenic Nerve	4 Percutaneous Endoscopic	2 Monitoring Device	4 Ulnar Nerve
9 Drainage	3 Brachial Plexus	X External	7 Autologous Tissue Substitute	5 Median Nerve
B Excision	4 Ulnar Nerve		M Neurostimulator Lead	6 Radial Nerve
C Extirpation	5 Median Nerve		Y Other Device	8 Thoracic Nerve
D Extraction	6 Radial Nerve		Z No Device	B Lumbar Nerve
H Insertion	8 Thoracic Nerve			C Perineal Nerve
J Inspection	9 Lumbar Plexus			D Femoral Nerve
N Release	A Lumbosacral Plexus			F Sciatic Nerve
P Removal	B Lumbar Nerve			G Tibial Nerve
Q Repair	C Pudendal Nerve			H Peroneal Nerve
R Replacement	D Femoral Nerve			X Diagnostic
S Reposition	F Sciatic Nerve			Z No Qualifier
U Supplement	G Tibial Nerve			
W Revision	H Peroneal Nerve			
X Transfer	K Head and Neck Sympathetic Nerve			
	L Thoracic Sympathetic Nerve			
	M Abdominal Sympathetic Nerve			
	N Lumbar Sympathetic Nerve			
	P Sacral Sympathetic Nerve			
	Q Sacral Plexus			
	R Sacral Nerve			
	Y Peripheral Nerve			

AHA Coding Clinic for table Ø1B
2018, 2Q, 22 Excision of synovial cyst
2017, 2Q, 19 Thoracic outlet decompression with sympathectomy

AHA Coding Clinic for table Ø1N
2019, 1Q, 28 Decompressive laminectomy of both spinal cord and nerve roots
2018, 2Q, 22 Excision of synovial cyst
2017, 2Q, 19 Thoracic outlet decompression with sympathectomy
2016, 2Q, 16 Decompressive laminectomy/foraminotomy and lumbar discectomy
2016, 2Q, 17 Removal of longitudinal ligament to decompress cervical nerve root
2016, 2Q, 23 Thoracic outlet syndrome and release of brachial plexus
2015, 2Q, 34 Decompressive laminectomy
2014, 3Q, 33 Radial fracture treatment with open reduction internal fixation, and release of carpal ligament

AHA Coding Clinic for table Ø1Q
2019, 3Q, 32 Breast reconstruction with neurotization

AHA Coding Clinic for table Ø1U
2019, 3Q, 32 Breast reconstruction with neurotization
2017, 4Q, 62 Added and revised device values - Nerve substitutes

Median and Ulnar Nerves

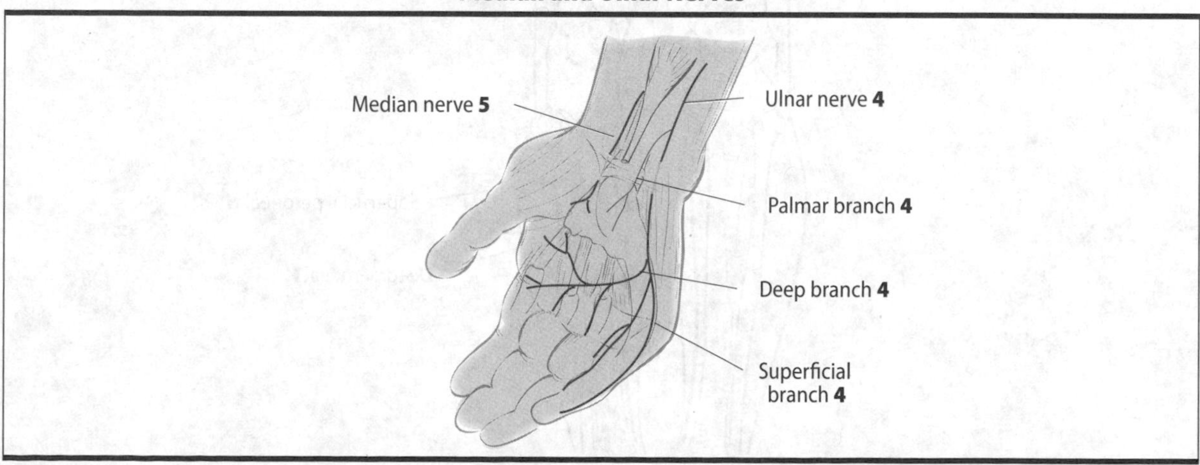

Peripheral Nervous System

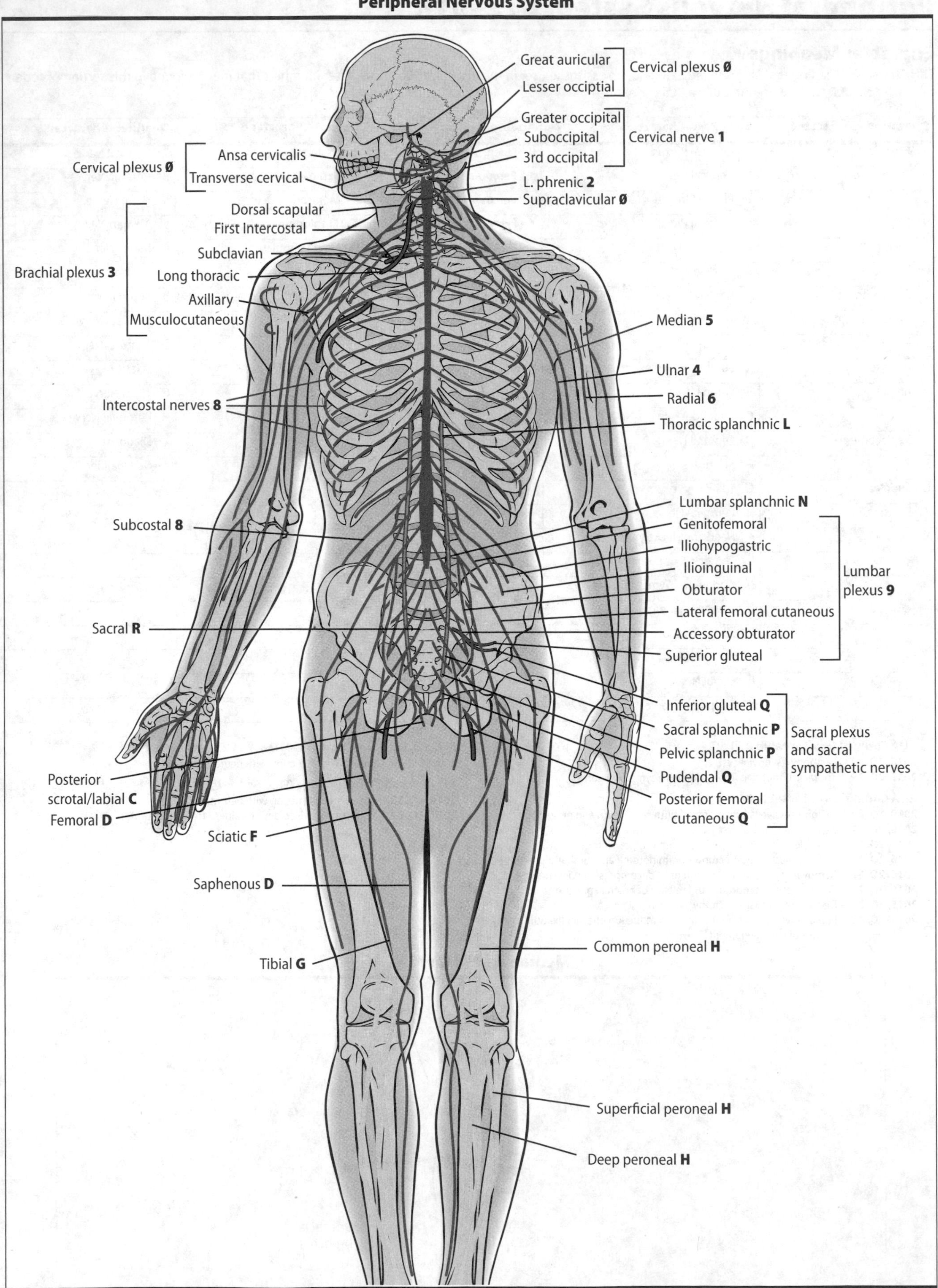

Ø Medical and Surgical
1 Peripheral Nervous System
2 Change Definition: Taking out or off a device from a body part and putting back an identical or similar device in or on the same body part without cutting or puncturing the skin or a mucous membrane

Explanation: All CHANGE procedures are coded using the approach EXTERNAL

Body Part Character 4	Approach Character 5	Device Character 6	Qualifier Character 7
Y Peripheral Nerve	X External	Ø Drainage Device Y Other Device	Z No Qualifier

Non-OR All body part, approach, device, and qualifier values

Ø Medical and Surgical
1 Peripheral Nervous System
5 Destruction Definition: Physical eradication of all or a portion of a body part by the direct use of energy, force, or a destructive agent

Explanation: None of the body part is physically taken out

Body Part Character 4	Approach Character 5	Device Character 6	Qualifier Character 7
Ø **Cervical Plexus** Ansa cervicalis Cutaneous (transverse) cervical nerve Great auricular nerve Lesser occipital nerve Supraclavicular nerve Transverse (cutaneous) cervical nerve 1 **Cervical Nerve** Greater occipital nerve Spinal nerve, cervical Suboccipital nerve Third occipital nerve 2 **Phrenic Nerve** Accessory phrenic nerve 3 **Brachial Plexus** Axillary nerve Dorsal scapular nerve First intercostal nerve Long thoracic nerve Musculocutaneous nerve Subclavius nerve Suprascapular nerve 4 **Ulnar Nerve** Cubital nerve 5 **Median Nerve** Anterior interosseous nerve Palmar cutaneous nerve 6 **Radial Nerve** Dorsal digital nerve Musculospiral nerve Palmar cutaneous nerve Posterior interosseous nerve 8 **Thoracic Nerve** Intercostal nerve Intercostobrachial nerve Spinal nerve, thoracic Subcostal nerve 9 **Lumbar Plexus** Accessory obturator nerve Genitofemoral nerve Iliohypogastric nerve Ilioinguinal nerve Lateral femoral cutaneous nerve Obturator nerve Superior gluteal nerve A **Lumbosacral Plexus** B **Lumbar Nerve** Lumbosacral trunk Spinal nerve, lumbar Superior clunic (cluneal) nerve C **Pudendal Nerve** Posterior labial nerve Posterior scrotal nerve D **Femoral Nerve** Anterior crural nerve Saphenous nerve F **Sciatic Nerve** Ischiatic nerve G **Tibial Nerve** Lateral plantar nerve Medial plantar nerve Medial popliteal nerve Medial sural cutaneous nerve H **Peroneal Nerve** Common fibular nerve Common peroneal nerve External popliteal nerve Lateral sural cutaneous nerve K **Head and Neck Sympathetic Nerve** Cavernous plexus Cervical ganglion Ciliary ganglion Internal carotid plexus Otic ganglion Pterygopalatine (sphenopalatine) ganglion Sphenopalatine (pterygopalatine) ganglion Stellate ganglion Submandibular ganglion Submaxillary ganglion L **Thoracic Sympathetic Nerve** Cardiac plexus Esophageal plexus Greater splanchnic nerve Inferior cardiac nerve Least splanchnic nerve Lesser splanchnic nerve Middle cardiac nerve Pulmonary plexus Superior cardiac nerve Thoracic aortic plexus Thoracic ganglion M **Abdominal Sympathetic Nerve** Abdominal aortic plexus Auerbach's (myenteric) plexus Celiac (solar) plexus Celiac ganglion Gastric plexus Hepatic plexus Inferior hypogastric plexus Inferior mesenteric ganglion Inferior mesenteric plexus Meissner's (submucous) plexus Myenteric (Auerbach's) plexus Pancreatic plexus Pelvic splanchnic nerve Renal nerve Renal plexus Solar (celiac) plexus Splenic plexus Submucous (Meissner's) plexus Superior hypogastric plexus Superior mesenteric ganglion Superior mesenteric plexus Suprarenal plexus N **Lumbar Sympathetic Nerve** Lumbar ganglion Lumbar splanchnic nerve P **Sacral Sympathetic Nerve** Ganglion impar (ganglion of Walther) Pelvic splanchnic nerve Sacral ganglion Sacral splanchnic nerve Q **Sacral Plexus** Inferior gluteal nerve Posterior femoral cutaneous nerve Pudendal nerve R **Sacral Nerve** Spinal nerve, sacral	Ø Open 3 Percutaneous 4 Percutaneous Endoscopic	Z No Device	Z No Qualifier

Non-OR Ø15[Ø,2,3,4,5,6,9,A,C,D,F,G,H,Q][Ø,3,4]ZZ Non-OR Ø15[1,8,B,R]3ZZ

Ø Medical and Surgical
1 Peripheral Nervous System
8 Division Definition: Cutting into a body part, without draining fluids and/or gases from the body part, in order to separate or transect a body part
Explanation: All or a portion of the body part is separated into two or more portions

Body Part Character 4	Approach Character 5	Device Character 6	Qualifier Character 7
Ø Cervical Plexus Ansa cervicalis Cutaneous (transverse) cervical nerve Great auricular nerve Lesser occipital nerve Supraclavicular nerve Transverse (cutaneous) cervical nerve **1 Cervical Nerve** Greater occipital nerve Spinal nerve, cervical Suboccipital nerve Third occipital nerve **2 Phrenic Nerve** Accessory phrenic nerve **3 Brachial Plexus** Axillary nerve Dorsal scapular nerve First intercostal nerve Long thoracic nerve Musculocutaneous nerve Subclavius nerve Suprascapular nerve **4 Ulnar Nerve** Cubital nerve **5 Median Nerve** Anterior interosseous nerve Palmar cutaneous nerve **6 Radial Nerve** Dorsal digital nerve Musculospiral nerve Palmar cutaneous nerve Posterior interosseous nerve **8 Thoracic Nerve** Intercostal nerve Intercostobrachial nerve Spinal nerve, thoracic Subcostal nerve **9 Lumbar Plexus** Accessory obturator nerve Genitofemoral nerve Iliohypogastric nerve Ilioinguinal nerve Lateral femoral cutaneous nerve Obturator nerve Superior gluteal nerve **A Lumbosacral Plexus** **B Lumbar Nerve** Lumbosacral trunk Spinal nerve, lumbar Superior clunic (cluneal) nerve **C Pudendal Nerve** Posterior labial nerve Posterior scrotal nerve **D Femoral Nerve** Anterior crural nerve Saphenous nerve **F Sciatic Nerve** Ischiatic nerve **G Tibial Nerve** Lateral plantar nerve Medial plantar nerve Medial popliteal nerve Medial sural cutaneous nerve **H Peroneal Nerve** Common fibular nerve Common peroneal nerve External popliteal nerve Lateral sural cutaneous nerve **K Head and Neck Sympathetic Nerve** Cavernous plexus Cervical ganglion Ciliary ganglion Internal carotid plexus Otic ganglion Pterygopalatine (sphenopalatine) ganglion Sphenopalatine (pterygopalatine) ganglion Stellate ganglion Submandibular ganglion Submaxillary ganglion **L Thoracic Sympathetic Nerve** Cardiac plexus Esophageal plexus Greater splanchnic nerve Inferior cardiac nerve Least splanchnic nerve Lesser splanchnic nerve Middle cardiac nerve Pulmonary plexus Superior cardiac nerve Thoracic aortic plexus Thoracic ganglion **M Abdominal Sympathetic Nerve** Abdominal aortic plexus Auerbach's (myenteric) plexus Celiac (solar) plexus Celiac ganglion Gastric plexus Hepatic plexus Inferior hypogastric plexus Inferior mesenteric ganglion Inferior mesenteric plexus Meissner's (submucous) plexus Myenteric (Auerbach's) plexus Pancreatic plexus Pelvic splanchnic nerve Renal nerve Renal plexus Solar (celiac) plexus Splenic plexus Submucous (Meissner's) plexus Superior hypogastric plexus Superior mesenteric ganglion Superior mesenteric plexus Suprarenal plexus **N Lumbar Sympathetic Nerve** Lumbar ganglion Lumbar splanchnic nerve **P Sacral Sympathetic Nerve** Ganglion impar (ganglion of Walther) Pelvic splanchnic nerve Sacral ganglion Sacral splanchnic nerve **Q Sacral Plexus** Inferior gluteal nerve Posterior femoral cutaneous nerve Pudendal nerve **R Sacral Nerve** Spinal nerve, sacral	**Ø Open** **3 Percutaneous** **4 Percutaneous Endoscopic**	**Z No Device**	**Z No Qualifier**

Ø Medical and Surgical
1 Peripheral Nervous System
9 Drainage Definition: Taking or letting out fluids and/or gases from a body part
Explanation: The qualifier DIAGNOSTIC is used to identify drainage procedures that are biopsies

Body Part Character 4		Approach Character 5	Device Character 6	Qualifier Character 7
Ø **Cervical Plexus** Ansa cervicalis Cutaneous (transverse) cervical nerve Great auricular nerve Lesser occipital nerve Supraclavicular nerve Transverse (cutaneous) cervical nerve 1 **Cervical Nerve** Greater occipital nerve Spinal nerve, cervical Suboccipital nerve Third occipital nerve 2 **Phrenic Nerve** Accessory phrenic nerve 3 **Brachial Plexus** Axillary nerve Dorsal scapular nerve First intercostal nerve Long thoracic nerve Musculocutaneous nerve Subclavius nerve Suprascapular nerve 4 **Ulnar Nerve** Cubital nerve 5 **Median Nerve** Anterior interosseous nerve Palmar cutaneous nerve 6 **Radial Nerve** Dorsal digital nerve Musculospiral nerve Palmar cutaneous nerve Posterior interosseous nerve 8 **Thoracic Nerve** Intercostal nerve Intercostobrachial nerve Spinal nerve, thoracic Subcostal nerve 9 **Lumbar Plexus** Accessory obturator nerve Genitofemoral nerve Iliohypogastric nerve Ilioinguinal nerve Lateral femoral cutaneous nerve Obturator nerve Superior gluteal nerve A **Lumbosacral Plexus** B **Lumbar Nerve** Lumbosacral trunk Spinal nerve, lumbar Superior clunic (cluneal) nerve C **Pudendal Nerve** Posterior labial nerve Posterior scrotal nerve D **Femoral Nerve** Anterior crural nerve Saphenous nerve F **Sciatic Nerve** Ischiatic nerve G **Tibial Nerve** Lateral plantar nerve Medial plantar nerve Medial popliteal nerve Medial sural cutaneous nerve	H **Peroneal Nerve** Common fibular nerve Common peroneal nerve External popliteal nerve Lateral sural cutaneous nerve K **Head and Neck Sympathetic Nerve** Cavernous plexus Cervical ganglion Ciliary ganglion Internal carotid plexus Otic ganglion Pterygopalatine (sphenopalatine) ganglion Sphenopalatine (pterygopalatine) ganglion Stellate ganglion Submandibular ganglion Submaxillary ganglion L **Thoracic Sympathetic Nerve** Cardiac plexus Esophageal plexus Greater splanchnic nerve Inferior cardiac nerve Least splanchnic nerve Lesser splanchnic nerve Middle cardiac nerve Pulmonary plexus Superior cardiac nerve Thoracic aortic plexus Thoracic ganglion M **Abdominal Sympathetic Nerve** Abdominal aortic plexus Auerbach's (myenteric) plexus Celiac (solar) plexus Celiac ganglion Gastric plexus Hepatic plexus Inferior hypogastric plexus Inferior mesenteric ganglion Inferior mesenteric plexus Meissner's (submucous) plexus Myenteric (Auerbach's) plexus Pancreatic plexus Pelvic splanchnic nerve Renal nerve Renal plexus Solar (celiac) plexus Splenic plexus Submucous (Meissner's) plexus Superior hypogastric plexus Superior mesenteric ganglion Superior mesenteric plexus Suprarenal plexus N **Lumbar Sympathetic Nerve** Lumbar ganglion Lumbar splanchnic nerve P **Sacral Sympathetic Nerve** Ganglion impar (ganglion of Walther) Pelvic splanchnic nerve Sacral ganglion Sacral splanchnic nerve Q **Sacral Plexus** Inferior gluteal nerve Posterior femoral cutaneous nerve Pudendal nerve R **Sacral Nerve** Spinal nerve, sacral	Ø Open 3 Percutaneous 4 Percutaneous Endoscopic	Ø Drainage Device	Z No Qualifier

Non-OR Ø19[Ø,1,2,3,4,5,6,8,9,A,B,C,D,F,G,H,K,L,M,N,P,Q,R]3ØZ

Ø19 Continued on next page

Ø19 Continued

Ø Medical and Surgical
1 Peripheral Nervous System
9 Drainage Definition: Taking or letting out fluids and/or gases from a body part
Explanation: The qualifier DIAGNOSTIC is used to identify drainage procedures that are biopsies

Body Part Character 4	Approach Character 5	Device Character 6	Qualifier Character 7
Ø Cervical Plexus Ansa cervicalis Cutaneous (transverse) cervical nerve Great auricular nerve Lesser occipital nerve Supraclavicular nerve Transverse (cutaneous) cervical nerve **1 Cervical Nerve** Greater occipital nerve Spinal nerve, cervical Suboccipital nerve Third occipital nerve **2 Phrenic Nerve** Accessory phrenic nerve **3 Brachial Plexus** Axillary nerve Dorsal scapular nerve First intercostal nerve Long thoracic nerve Musculocutaneous nerve Subclavius nerve Suprascapular nerve **4 Ulnar Nerve** Cubital nerve **5 Median Nerve** Anterior interosseous nerve Palmar cutaneous nerve **6 Radial Nerve** Dorsal digital nerve Musculospiral nerve Palmar cutaneous nerve Posterior interosseous nerve **8 Thoracic Nerve** Intercostal nerve Intercostobrachial nerve Spinal nerve, thoracic Subcostal nerve **9 Lumbar Plexus** Accessory obturator nerve Genitofemoral nerve Iliohypogastric nerve Ilioinguinal nerve Lateral femoral cutaneous nerve Obturator nerve Superior gluteal nerve **A Lumbosacral Plexus** **B Lumbar Nerve** Lumbosacral trunk Spinal nerve, lumbar Superior clunic (cluneal) nerve **C Pudendal Nerve** Posterior labial nerve Posterior scrotal nerve **D Femoral Nerve** Anterior crural nerve Saphenous nerve **F Sciatic Nerve** Ischiatic nerve **G Tibial Nerve** Lateral plantar nerve Medial plantar nerve Medial popliteal nerve Medial sural cutaneous nerve **H Peroneal Nerve** Common fibular nerve Common peroneal nerve External popliteal nerve Lateral sural cutaneous nerve **K Head and Neck Sympathetic Nerve** Cavernous plexus Cervical ganglion Ciliary ganglion Internal carotid plexus Otic ganglion Pterygopalatine (sphenopalatine) ganglion Sphenopalatine (pterygopalatine) ganglion Stellate ganglion Submandibular ganglion Submaxillary ganglion **L Thoracic Sympathetic Nerve** Cardiac plexus Esophageal plexus Greater splanchnic nerve Inferior cardiac nerve Least splanchnic nerve Lesser splanchnic nerve Middle cardiac nerve Pulmonary plexus Superior cardiac nerve Thoracic aortic plexus Thoracic ganglion **M Abdominal Sympathetic Nerve** Abdominal aortic plexus Auerbach's (myenteric) plexus Celiac (solar) plexus Celiac ganglion Gastric plexus Hepatic plexus Inferior hypogastric plexus Inferior mesenteric ganglion Inferior mesenteric plexus Meissner's (submucous) plexus Myenteric (Auerbach's) plexus Pancreatic plexus Pelvic splanchnic nerve Renal nerve Renal plexus Solar (celiac) plexus Splenic plexus Submucous (Meissner's) plexus Superior hypogastric plexus Superior mesenteric ganglion Superior mesenteric plexus Suprarenal plexus **N Lumbar Sympathetic Nerve** Lumbar ganglion Lumbar splanchnic nerve **P Sacral Sympathetic Nerve** Ganglion impar (ganglion of Walther) Pelvic splanchnic nerve Sacral ganglion Sacral splanchnic nerve **Q Sacral Plexus** Inferior gluteal nerve Posterior femoral cutaneous nerve Pudendal nerve **R Sacral Nerve** Spinal nerve, sacral	**Ø** Open **3** Percutaneous **4** Percutaneous Endoscopic	**Z** No Device	**X** Diagnostic **Z** No Qualifier

Non-OR Ø19[Ø,1,2,3,4,5,6,8,9,A,B,C,D,F,G,H,Q,R][3,4]ZX
Non-OR Ø19[Ø,1,2,3,4,5,6,8,9,A,B,C,D,F,G,H,K,L,M,N,P,Q,R]3ZZ

Ø Medical and Surgical
1 Peripheral Nervous System
B Excision Definition: Cutting out or off, without replacement, a portion of a body part

Explanation: The qualifier DIAGNOSTIC is used to identify excision procedures that are biopsies

Body Part Character 4	Approach Character 5	Device Character 6	Qualifier Character 7
Ø Cervical Plexus Ansa cervicalis Cutaneous (transverse) cervical nerve Great auricular nerve Lesser occipital nerve Supraclavicular nerve Transverse (cutaneous) cervical nerve **1 Cervical Nerve** Greater occipital nerve Spinal nerve, cervical Suboccipital nerve Third occipital nerve **2 Phrenic Nerve** Accessory phrenic nerve **3 Brachial Plexus** Axillary nerve Dorsal scapular nerve First intercostal nerve Long thoracic nerve Musculocutaneous nerve Subclavius nerve Suprascapular nerve **4 Ulnar Nerve** Cubital nerve **5 Median Nerve** Anterior interosseous nerve Palmar cutaneous nerve **6 Radial Nerve** Dorsal digital nerve Musculospiral nerve Palmar cutaneous nerve Posterior interosseous nerve **8 Thoracic Nerve** Intercostal nerve Intercostobrachial nerve Spinal nerve, thoracic Subcostal nerve **9 Lumbar Plexus** Accessory obturator nerve Genitofemoral nerve Iliohypogastric nerve Ilioinguinal nerve Lateral femoral cutaneous nerve Obturator nerve Superior gluteal nerve **A Lumbosacral Plexus** **B Lumbar Nerve** Lumbosacral trunk Spinal nerve, lumbar Superior clunic (cluneal) nerve **C Pudendal Nerve** Posterior labial nerve Posterior scrotal nerve **D Femoral Nerve** Anterior crural nerve Saphenous nerve **F Sciatic Nerve** Ischiatic nerve **G Tibial Nerve** Lateral plantar nerve Medial plantar nerve Medial popliteal nerve Medial sural cutaneous nerve **H Peroneal Nerve** Common fibular nerve Common peroneal nerve External popliteal nerve Lateral sural cutaneous nerve **K Head and Neck Sympathetic Nerve** Cavernous plexus Cervical ganglion Ciliary ganglion Internal carotid plexus Otic ganglion Pterygopalatine (sphenopalatine) ganglion Sphenopalatine (pterygopalatine) ganglion Stellate ganglion Submandibular ganglion Submaxillary ganglion **L Thoracic Sympathetic Nerve** Cardiac plexus Esophageal plexus Greater splanchnic nerve Inferior cardiac nerve Least splanchnic nerve Lesser splanchnic nerve Middle cardiac nerve Pulmonary plexus Superior cardiac nerve Thoracic aortic plexus Thoracic ganglion **M Abdominal Sympathetic Nerve** Abdominal aortic plexus Auerbach's (myenteric) plexus Celiac (solar) plexus Celiac ganglion Gastric plexus Hepatic plexus Inferior hypogastric plexus Inferior mesenteric ganglion Inferior mesenteric plexus Meissner's (submucous) plexus Myenteric (Auerbach's) plexus Pancreatic plexus Pelvic splanchnic nerve Renal nerve Renal plexus Solar (celiac) plexus Splenic plexus Submucous (Meissner's) plexus Superior hypogastric plexus Superior mesenteric ganglion Superior mesenteric plexus Suprarenal plexus **N Lumbar Sympathetic Nerve** Lumbar ganglion Lumbar splanchnic nerve **P Sacral Sympathetic Nerve** Ganglion impar (ganglion of Walther) Pelvic splanchnic nerve Sacral ganglion Sacral splanchnic nerve **Q Sacral Plexus** Inferior gluteal nerve Posterior femoral cutaneous nerve Pudendal nerve **R Sacral Nerve** Spinal nerve, sacral	**Ø Open** **3 Percutaneous** **4 Percutaneous Endoscopic**	**Z No Device**	**X Diagnostic** **Z No Qualifier**

Non-OR Ø1B[Ø,1,2,3,4,5,6,8,9,A,B,C,D,F,G,H,Q,R][3,4]ZX

Ø Medical and Surgical
1 Peripheral Nervous System
C Extirpation Definition: Taking or cutting out solid matter from a body part

Explanation: The solid matter may be an abnormal byproduct of a biological function or a foreign body; it may be imbedded in a body part or in the lumen of a tubular body part. The solid matter may or may not have been previously broken into pieces.

Body Part Character 4		Approach Character 5	Device Character 6	Qualifier Character 7
Ø Cervical Plexus Ansa cervicalis Cutaneous (transverse) cervical nerve Great auricular nerve Lesser occipital nerve Supraclavicular nerve Transverse (cutaneous) cervical nerve **1 Cervical Nerve** Greater occipital nerve Spinal nerve, cervical Suboccipital nerve Third occipital nerve **2 Phrenic Nerve** Accessory phrenic nerve **3 Brachial Plexus** Axillary nerve Dorsal scapular nerve First intercostal nerve Long thoracic nerve Musculocutaneous nerve Subclavius nerve Suprascapular nerve **4 Ulnar Nerve** Cubital nerve **5 Median Nerve** Anterior interosseous nerve Palmar cutaneous nerve **6 Radial Nerve** Dorsal digital nerve Musculospiral nerve Palmar cutaneous nerve Posterior interosseous nerve **8 Thoracic Nerve** Intercostal nerve Intercostobrachial nerve Spinal nerve, thoracic Subcostal nerve **9 Lumbar Plexus** Accessory obturator nerve Genitofemoral nerve Iliohypogastric nerve Ilioinguinal nerve Lateral femoral cutaneous nerve Obturator nerve Superior gluteal nerve **A Lumbosacral Plexus** **B Lumbar Nerve** Lumbosacral trunk Spinal nerve, lumbar Superior clunic (cluneal) nerve **C Pudendal Nerve** Posterior labial nerve Posterior scrotal nerve **D Femoral Nerve** Anterior crural nerve Saphenous nerve **F Sciatic Nerve** Ischiatic nerve **G Tibial Nerve** Lateral plantar nerve Medial plantar nerve Medial popliteal nerve Medial sural cutaneous nerve	**H Peroneal Nerve** Common fibular nerve Common peroneal nerve External popliteal nerve Lateral sural cutaneous nerve **K Head and Neck Sympathetic Nerve** Cavernous plexus Cervical ganglion Ciliary ganglion Internal carotid plexus Otic ganglion Pterygopalatine (sphenopalatine) ganglion Sphenopalatine (pterygopalatine) ganglion Stellate ganglion Submandibular ganglion Submaxillary ganglion **L Thoracic Sympathetic Nerve** Cardiac plexus Esophageal plexus Greater splanchnic nerve Inferior cardiac nerve Least splanchnic nerve Lesser splanchnic nerve Middle cardiac nerve Pulmonary plexus Superior cardiac nerve Thoracic aortic plexus Thoracic ganglion **M Abdominal Sympathetic Nerve** Abdominal aortic plexus Auerbach's (myenteric) plexus Celiac (solar) plexus Celiac ganglion Gastric plexus Hepatic plexus Inferior hypogastric plexus Inferior mesenteric ganglion Inferior mesenteric plexus Meissner's (submucous) plexus Myenteric (Auerbach's) plexus Pancreatic plexus Pelvic splanchnic nerve Renal nerve Renal plexus Solar (celiac) plexus Splenic plexus Submucous (Meissner's) plexus Superior hypogastric plexus Superior mesenteric ganglion Superior mesenteric plexus Suprarenal plexus **N Lumbar Sympathetic Nerve** Lumbar ganglion Lumbar splanchnic nerve **P Sacral Sympathetic Nerve** Ganglion impar (ganglion of Walther) Pelvic splanchnic nerve Sacral ganglion Sacral splanchnic nerve **Q Sacral Plexus** Inferior gluteal nerve Posterior femoral cutaneous nerve Pudendal nerve **R Sacral Nerve** Spinal nerve, sacral	**Ø Open** **3 Percutaneous** **4 Percutaneous Endoscopic**	**Z No Device**	**Z No Qualifier**

Ø Medical and Surgical
1 Peripheral Nervous System
D Extraction Definition: Pulling or stripping out or off all or a portion of a body part by the use of force
Explanation: The qualifier DIAGNOSTIC is used to identify extraction procedures that are biopsies

Body Part Character 4	Approach Character 5	Device Character 6	Qualifier Character 7
Ø Cervical Plexus Ansa cervicalis Cutaneous (transverse) cervical nerve Great auricular nerve Lesser occipital nerve Supraclavicular nerve Transverse (cutaneous) cervical nerve	**Ø Open** **3 Percutaneous** **4 Percutaneous Endoscopic**	**Z No Device**	**Z No Qualifier**
1 Cervical Nerve Greater occipital nerve Spinal nerve, cervical Suboccipital nerve Third occipital nerve			
2 Phrenic Nerve Accessory phrenic nerve			
3 Brachial Plexus Axillary nerve Dorsal scapular nerve First intercostal nerve Long thoracic nerve Musculocutaneous nerve Subclavius nerve Suprascapular nerve			
4 Ulnar Nerve Cubital nerve			
5 Median Nerve Anterior interosseous nerve Palmar cutaneous nerve			
6 Radial Nerve Dorsal digital nerve Musculospiral nerve Palmar cutaneous nerve Posterior interosseous nerve			
8 Thoracic Nerve Intercostal nerve Intercostobrachial nerve Spinal nerve, thoracic Subcostal nerve			
9 Lumbar Plexus Accessory obturator nerve Genitofemoral nerve Iliohypogastric nerve Ilioinguinal nerve Lateral femoral cutaneous nerve Obturator nerve Superior gluteal nerve			
A Lumbosacral Plexus			
B Lumbar Nerve Lumbosacral trunk Spinal nerve, lumbar Superior clunic (cluneal) nerve			
C Pudendal Nerve] Posterior labial nerve Posterior scrotal nerve			
D Femoral Nerve Anterior crural nerve Saphenous nerve			
F Sciatic Nerve Ischiatic nerve			
G Tibial Nerve Lateral plantar nerve Medial plantar nerve Medial popliteal nerve Medial sural cutaneous nerve			
H Peroneal Nerve Common fibular nerve Common peroneal nerve External popliteal nerve Lateral sural cutaneous nerve			
K Head and Neck Sympathetic Nerve Cavernous plexus Cervical ganglion Ciliary ganglion Internal carotid plexus Otic ganglion Pterygopalatine (sphenopalatine) ganglion Sphenopalatine (pterygopalatine) ganglion Stellate ganglion Submandibular ganglion Submaxillary ganglion			
L Thoracic Sympathetic Nerve Cardiac plexus Esophageal plexus Greater splanchnic nerve Inferior cardiac nerve Least splanchnic nerve Lesser splanchnic nerve Middle cardiac nerve Pulmonary plexus Superior cardiac nerve Thoracic aortic plexus Thoracic ganglion			
M Abdominal Sympathetic Nerve Abdominal aortic plexus Auerbach's (myenteric) plexus Celiac (solar) plexus Celiac ganglion Gastric plexus Hepatic plexus Inferior hypogastric plexus Inferior mesenteric ganglion Inferior mesenteric plexus Meissner's (submucous) plexus Myenteric (Auerbach's) plexus Pancreatic plexus Pelvic splanchnic nerve Renal nerve Renal plexus Solar (celiac) plexus Splenic plexus Submucous (Meissner's) plexus Superior hypogastric plexus Superior mesenteric ganglion Superior mesenteric plexus Suprarenal plexus			
N Lumbar Sympathetic Nerve Lumbar ganglion Lumbar splanchnic nerve			
P Sacral Sympathetic Nerve Ganglion impar (ganglion of Walther) Pelvic splanchnic nerve Sacral ganglion Sacral splanchnic nerve			
Q Sacral Plexus Inferior gluteal nerve Posterior femoral cutaneous nerve Pudendal nerve			
R Sacral Nerve Spinal nerve, sacral			

Ø Medical and Surgical
1 Peripheral Nervous System
H Insertion Definition: Putting in a nonbiological appliance that monitors, assists, performs, or prevents a physiological function but does not physically take the place of a body part

Explanation: None

Body Part Character 4	Approach Character 5	Device Character 6	Qualifier Character 7
Y Peripheral Nerve ⊞	Ø Open 3 Percutaneous 4 Percutaneous Endoscopic	1 Radioactive Element 2 Monitoring Device M Neurostimulator Lead Y Other Device	Z No Qualifier

Non-OR Ø1HY[3,4]YZ

See Appendix L for Procedure Combinations
⊞ Ø1HY[Ø,3,4]MZ

Ø Medical and Surgical
1 Peripheral Nervous System
J Inspection Definition: Visually and/or manually exploring a body part

Explanation: Visual exploration may be performed with or without optical instrumentation. Manual exploration may be performed directly or through intervening body layers.

Body Part Character 4	Approach Character 5	Device Character 6	Qualifier Character 7
Y Peripheral Nerve	Ø Open 3 Percutaneous 4 Percutaneous Endoscopic	Z No Device	Z No Qualifier

Non-OR Ø1JY3ZZ

Ø Medical and Surgical
1 Peripheral Nervous System
N Release Definition: Freeing a body part from an abnormal physical constraint by cutting or by the use of force
Explanation: Some of the restraining tissue may be taken out but none of the body part is taken out

Body Part Character 4		Approach Character 5	Device Character 6	Qualifier Character 7
Ø Cervical Plexus Ansa cervicalis Cutaneous (transverse) cervical nerve Great auricular nerve Lesser occipital nerve Supraclavicular nerve Transverse (cutaneous) cervical nerve **1 Cervical Nerve** Greater occipital nerve Spinal nerve, cervical Suboccipital nerve Third occipital nerve **2 Phrenic Nerve** Accessory phrenic nerve **3 Brachial Plexus** Axillary nerve Dorsal scapular nerve First intercostal nerve Long thoracic nerve Musculocutaneous nerve Subclavius nerve Suprascapular nerve **4 Ulnar Nerve** Cubital nerve **5 Median Nerve** Anterior interosseous nerve Palmar cutaneous nerve **6 Radial Nerve** Dorsal digital nerve Musculospiral nerve Palmar cutaneous nerve Posterior interosseous nerve **8 Thoracic Nerve** Intercostal nerve Intercostobrachial nerve Spinal nerve, thoracic Subcostal nerve **9 Lumbar Plexus** Accessory obturator nerve Genitofemoral nerve Iliohypogastric nerve Ilioinguinal nerve Lateral femoral cutaneous nerve Obturator nerve Superior gluteal nerve **A Lumbosacral Plexus** **B Lumbar Nerve** Lumbosacral trunk Spinal nerve, lumbar Superior clunic (cluneal) nerve **C Pudendal Nerve** Posterior labial nerve Posterior scrotal nerve **D Femoral Nerve** Anterior crural nerve Saphenous nerve **F Sciatic Nerve** Ischiatic nerve **G Tibial Nerve** Lateral plantar nerve Medial plantar nerve Medial popliteal nerve Medial sural cutaneous nerve	**H Peroneal Nerve** Common fibular nerve Common peroneal nerve External popliteal nerve Lateral sural cutaneous nerve **K Head and Neck Sympathetic Nerve** Cavernous plexus Cervical ganglion Ciliary ganglion Internal carotid plexus Otic ganglion Pterygopalatine (sphenopalatine) ganglion Sphenopalatine (pterygopalatine) ganglion Stellate ganglion Submandibular ganglion Submaxillary ganglion **L Thoracic Sympathetic Nerve** Cardiac plexus Esophageal plexus Greater splanchnic nerve Inferior cardiac nerve Least splanchnic nerve Lesser splanchnic nerve Middle cardiac nerve Pulmonary plexus Superior cardiac nerve Thoracic aortic plexus Thoracic ganglion **M Abdominal Sympathetic Nerve** Abdominal aortic plexus Auerbach's (myenteric) plexus Celiac (solar) plexus Celiac ganglion Gastric plexus Hepatic plexus Inferior hypogastric plexus Inferior mesenteric ganglion Inferior mesenteric plexus Meissner's (submucous) plexus Myenteric (Auerbach's) plexus Pancreatic plexus Pelvic splanchnic nerve Renal nerve Renal plexus Solar (celiac) plexus Splenic plexus Submucous (Meissner's) plexus Superior hypogastric plexus Superior mesenteric ganglion Superior mesenteric plexus Suprarenal plexus **N Lumbar Sympathetic Nerve** Lumbar ganglion Lumbar splanchnic nerve **P Sacral Sympathetic Nerve** Ganglion impar (ganglion of Walther) Pelvic splanchnic nerve Sacral ganglion Sacral splanchnic nerve **Q Sacral Plexus** Inferior gluteal nerve Posterior femoral cutaneous nerve Pudendal nerve **R Sacral Nerve** Spinal nerve, sacral	**Ø Open** **3 Percutaneous** **4 Percutaneous Endoscopic**	**Z No Device**	**Z No Qualifier**

Ø Medical and Surgical
1 Peripheral Nervous System
P Removal Definition: Taking out or off a device from a body part

Explanation: If a device is taken out and a similar device put in without cutting or puncturing the skin or mucous membrane, the procedure is coded to the root operation CHANGE. Otherwise, the procedure for taking out a device is coded to the root operation REMOVAL.

Body Part Character 4	Approach Character 5	Device Character 6	Qualifier Character 7
Y Peripheral Nerve	Ø Open 3 Percutaneous 4 Percutaneous Endoscopic	Ø Drainage Device 2 Monitoring Device 7 Autologous Tissue Substitute M Neurostimulator Lead Y Other Device	Z No Qualifier
Y Peripheral Nerve	X External	Ø Drainage Device 2 Monitoring Device M Neurostimulator Lead	Z No Qualifier

Non-OR Ø1PY3[Ø,2]Z
Non-OR Ø1PY[3,4]YZ
Non-OR Ø1PYX[Ø,2,M]Z

Ø Medical and Surgical
1 Peripheral Nervous System
Q Repair Definition: Restoring, to the extent possible, a body part to its normal anatomic structure and function
Explanation: Used only when the method to accomplish the repair is not one of the other root operations

Body Part Character 4		Approach Character 5	Device Character 6	Qualifier Character 7
Ø Cervical Plexus Ansa cervicalis Cutaneous (transverse) cervical nerve Great auricular nerve Lesser occipital nerve Supraclavicular nerve Transverse (cutaneous) cervical nerve **1 Cervical Nerve** Greater occipital nerve Spinal nerve, cervical Suboccipital nerve Third occipital nerve **2 Phrenic Nerve** Accessory phrenic nerve **3 Brachial Plexus** Axillary nerve Dorsal scapular nerve First intercostal nerve Long thoracic nerve Musculocutaneous nerve Subclavius nerve Suprascapular nerve **4 Ulnar Nerve** Cubital nerve **5 Median Nerve** Anterior interosseous nerve Palmar cutaneous nerve **6 Radial Nerve** Dorsal digital nerve Musculospiral nerve Palmar cutaneous nerve Posterior interosseous nerve **8 Thoracic Nerve** Intercostal nerve Intercostobrachial nerve Spinal nerve, thoracic Subcostal nerve **9 Lumbar Plexus** Accessory obturator nerve Genitofemoral nerve Iliohypogastric nerve Ilioinguinal nerve Lateral femoral cutaneous nerve Obturator nerve Superior gluteal nerve **A Lumbosacral Plexus** **B Lumbar Nerve** Lumbosacral trunk Spinal nerve, lumbar Superior clunic (cluneal) nerve **C Pudendal Nerve** Posterior labial nerve Posterior scrotal nerve **D Femoral Nerve** Anterior crural nerve Saphenous nerve **F Sciatic Nerve** Ischiatic nerve **G Tibial Nerve** Lateral plantar nerve Medial plantar nerve Medial popliteal nerve Medial sural cutaneous nerve	**H Peroneal Nerve** Common fibular nerve Common peroneal nerve External popliteal nerve Lateral sural cutaneous nerve **K Head and Neck Sympathetic Nerve** Cavernous plexus Cervical ganglion Ciliary ganglion Internal carotid plexus Otic ganglion Pterygopalatine (sphenopalatine) ganglion Sphenopalatine (pterygopalatine) ganglion Stellate ganglion Submandibular ganglion Submaxillary ganglion **L Thoracic Sympathetic Nerve** Cardiac plexus Esophageal plexus Greater splanchnic nerve Inferior cardiac nerve Least splanchnic nerve Lesser splanchnic nerve Middle cardiac nerve Pulmonary plexus Superior cardiac nerve Thoracic aortic plexus Thoracic ganglion **M Abdominal Sympathetic Nerve** Abdominal aortic plexus Auerbach's (myenteric) plexus Celiac (solar) plexus Celiac ganglion Gastric plexus Hepatic plexus Inferior hypogastric plexus Inferior mesenteric ganglion Inferior mesenteric plexus Meissner's (submucous) plexus Myenteric (Auerbach's) plexus Pancreatic plexus Pelvic splanchnic nerve Renal nerve Renal plexus Solar (celiac) plexus Splenic plexus Submucous (Meissner's) plexus Superior hypogastric plexus Superior mesenteric ganglion Superior mesenteric plexus Suprarenal plexus **N Lumbar Sympathetic Nerve** Lumbar ganglion Lumbar splanchnic nerve **P Sacral Sympathetic Nerve** Ganglion impar (ganglion of Walther) Pelvic splanchnic nerve Sacral ganglion Sacral splanchnic nerve **Q Sacral Plexus** Inferior gluteal nerve Posterior femoral cutaneous nerve Pudendal nerve **R Sacral Nerve** Spinal nerve, sacral	**Ø Open** **3 Percutaneous** **4 Percutaneous Endoscopic**	**Z No Device**	**Z No Qualifier**

Ø Medical and Surgical
1 Peripheral Nervous System
R Replacement Definition: Putting in or on biological or synthetic material that physically takes the place and/or function of all or a portion of a body part

Explanation: The body part may have been taken out or replaced, or may be taken out, physically eradicated, or rendered nonfunctional during the REPLACEMENT procedure. A REMOVAL procedure is coded for taking out the device used in a previous replacement procedure.

Body Part Character 4	Approach Character 5	Device Character 6	Qualifier Character 7
1 Cervical Nerve Greater occipital nerve Spinal nerve, cervical Suboccipital nerve Third occipital nerve **2 Phrenic Nerve** Accessory phrenic nerve **4 Ulnar Nerve** Cubital nerve **5 Median Nerve** Anterior interosseous nerve Palmar cutaneous nerve **6 Radial Nerve** Dorsal digital nerve Musculospiral nerve Palmar cutaneous nerve Posterior interosseous nerve **8 Thoracic Nerve** Intercostal nerve Intercostobrachial nerve Spinal nerve, thoracic Subcostal nerve **B Lumbar Nerve** Lumbosacral trunk Spinal nerve, lumbar Superior clunic (cluneal) nerve **C Pudendal Nerve** Posterior labial nerve Posterior scrotal nerve **D Femoral Nerve** Anterior crural nerve Saphenous nerve **F Sciatic Nerve** Ischiatic nerve **G Tibial Nerve** Lateral plantar nerve Medial plantar nerve Medial popliteal nerve Medial sural cutaneous nerve **H Peroneal Nerve** Common fibular nerve Common peroneal nerve External popliteal nerve Lateral sural cutaneous nerve **R Sacral Nerve** Spinal nerve, sacral	**Ø Open** **4 Percutaneous Endoscopic**	**7 Autologous Tissue Substitute** **J Synthetic Substitute** **K Nonautologous Tissue Substitute**	**Z No Qualifier**

Ø Medical and Surgical
1 Peripheral Nervous System
S Reposition Definition: Moving to its normal location, or other suitable location, all or a portion of a body part

Explanation: The body part is moved to a new location from an abnormal location, or from a normal location where it is not functioning correctly. The body part may or may not be cut out or off to be moved to the new location.

Body Part Character 4	Approach Character 5	Device Character 6	Qualifier Character 7
Ø Cervical Plexus Ansa cervicalis Cutaneous (transverse) cervical nerve Great auricular nerve Lesser occipital nerve Supraclavicular nerve Transverse (cutaneous) cervical nerve **1 Cervical Nerve** Greater occipital nerve Spinal nerve, cervical Suboccipital nerve Third occipital nerve **2 Phrenic Nerve** Accessory phrenic nerve **3 Brachial Plexus** Axillary nerve Dorsal scapular nerve First intercostal nerve Long thoracic nerve Musculocutaneous nerve Subclavius nerve Suprascapular nerve **4 Ulnar Nerve** Cubital nerve **5 Median Nerve** Anterior interosseous nerve Palmar cutaneous nerve **6 Radial Nerve** Dorsal digital nerve Musculospiral nerve Palmar cutaneous nerve Posterior interosseous nerve **8 Thoracic Nerve** Intercostal nerve Intercostobrachial nerve Spinal nerve, thoracic Subcostal nerve **9 Lumbar Plexus** Accessory obturator nerve Genitofemoral nerve Iliohypogastric nerve Ilioinguinal nerve Lateral femoral cutaneous nerve Obturator nerve Superior gluteal nerve **A Lumbosacral Plexus** **B Lumbar Nerve** Lumbosacral trunk Spinal nerve, lumbar Superior clunic (cluneal) nerve **C Pudendal Nerve** Posterior labial nerve Posterior scrotal nerve **D Femoral Nerve** Anterior crural nerve Saphenous nerve **F Sciatic Nerve** Ischiatic nerve **G Tibial Nerve** Lateral plantar nerve Medial plantar nerve Medial popliteal nerve Medial sural cutaneous nerve **H Peroneal Nerve** Common fibular nerve Common peroneal nerve External popliteal nerve Lateral sural cutaneous nerve **Q Sacral Plexus** Inferior gluteal nerve Posterior femoral cutaneous nerve Pudendal nerve **R Sacral Nerve** Spinal nerve, sacral	**Ø Open** **3 Percutaneous** **4 Percutaneous Endoscopic**	**Z No Device**	**Z No Qualifier**

Ø Medical and Surgical
1 Peripheral Nervous System
U Supplement Definition: Putting in or on biological or synthetic material that physically reinforces and/or augments the function of a portion of a body part

Explanation: The biological material is non-living, or is living and from the same individual. The body part may have been previously replaced, and the SUPPLEMENT procedure is performed to physically reinforce and/or augment the function of the replaced body part.

Body Part Character 4	Approach Character 5	Device Character 6	Qualifier Character 7
1 Cervical Nerve Greater occipital nerve Spinal nerve, cervical Suboccipital nerve Third occipital nerve **2 Phrenic Nerve** Accessory phrenic nerve **4 Ulnar Nerve** Cubital nerve **5 Median Nerve** Anterior interosseous nerve Palmar cutaneous nerve **6 Radial Nerve** Dorsal digital nerve Musculospiral nerve Palmar cutaneous nerve Posterior interosseous nerve **8 Thoracic Nerve** Intercostal nerve Intercostobrachial nerve Spinal nerve, thoracic Subcostal nerve **B Lumbar Nerve** Lumbosacral trunk Spinal nerve, lumbar Superior clunic (cluneal) nerve **C Pudendal Nerve** Posterior labial nerve Posterior scrotal nerve **D Femoral Nerve** Anterior crural nerve Saphenous nerve **F Sciatic Nerve** Ischiatic nerve **G Tibial Nerve** Lateral plantar nerve Medial plantar nerve Medial popliteal nerve Medial sural cutaneous nerve **H Peroneal Nerve** Common fibular nerve Common peroneal nerve External popliteal nerve Lateral sural cutaneous nerve **R Sacral Nerve** Spinal nerve, sacral	Ø Open 3 Percutaneous 4 Percutaneous Endoscopic	7 Autologous Tissue Substitute J Synthetic Substitute K Nonautologous Tissue Substitute	Z No Qualifier

Ø Medical and Surgical
1 Peripheral Nervous System
W Revision Definition: Correcting, to the extent possible, a portion of a malfunctioning device or the position of a displaced device

Explanation: Revision can include correcting a malfunctioning or displaced device by taking out or putting in components of the device such as a screw or pin

Body Part Character 4	Approach Character 5	Device Character 6	Qualifier Character 7
Y Peripheral Nerve	Ø Open 3 Percutaneous 4 Percutaneous Endoscopic	Ø Drainage Device 2 Monitoring Device 7 Autologous Tissue Substitute M Neurostimulator Lead Y Other Device	Z No Qualifier
Y Peripheral Nerve	X External	Ø Drainage Device 2 Monitoring Device 7 Autologous Tissue Substitute M Neurostimulator Lead	Z No Qualifier

Non-OR Ø1WY[3,4]YZ
Non-OR Ø1WYX[Ø,2,7,M]Z

Ø Medical and Surgical
1 Peripheral Nervous System
X Transfer Definition: Moving, without taking out, all or a portion of a body part to another location to take over the function of all or a portion of a body part
Explanation: The body part transferred remains connected to its vascular and nervous supply

Body Part Character 4	Approach Character 5	Device Character 6	Qualifier Character 7
1 Cervical Nerve Greater occipital nerve Spinal nerve, cervical Suboccipital nerve Third occipital nerve **2 Phrenic Nerve** Accessory phrenic nerve	**Ø Open** **4 Percutaneous Endoscopic**	**Z No Device**	**1 Cervical Nerve** **2 Phrenic Nerve**
4 Ulnar Nerve Cubital nerve **5 Median Nerve** Anterior interosseous nerve Palmar cutaneous nerve **6 Radial Nerve** Dorsal digital nerve Musculospiral nerve Palmar cutaneous nerve Posterior interosseous nerve	**Ø Open** **4 Percutaneous Endoscopic**	**Z No Device**	**4 Ulnar Nerve** **5 Median Nerve** **6 Radial Nerve**
8 Thoracic Nerve Intercostal nerve Intercostobrachial nerve Spinal nerve, thoracic Subcostal nerve	**Ø Open** **4 Percutaneous Endoscopic**	**Z No Device**	**8 Thoracic Nerve**
B Lumbar Nerve Lumbosacral trunk Spinal nerve, lumbar Superior clunic (cluneal) nerve **C Pudendal Nerve** Posterior labial nerve Posterior scrotal nerve	**Ø Open** **4 Percutaneous Endoscopic**	**Z No Device**	**B Lumbar Nerve** **C Perineal Nerve**
D Femoral Nerve Anterior crural nerve Saphenous nerve **F Sciatic Nerve** Ischiatic nerve **G Tibial Nerve** Lateral plantar nerve Medial plantar nerve Medial popliteal nerve Medial sural cutaneous nerve **H Peroneal Nerve** Common fibular nerve Common peroneal nerve External popliteal nerve Lateral sural cutaneous nerve	**Ø Open** **4 Percutaneous Endoscopic**	**Z No Device**	**D Femoral Nerve** **F Sciatic Nerve** **G Tibial Nerve** **H Peroneal Nerve**

Heart and Great Vessels Ø21–Ø2Y

Character Meanings

This Character Meaning table is provided as a guide to assist the user in the identification of character members that may be found in this section of code tables. It **SHOULD NOT** be used to build a PCS code.

Operation–Character 3	Body Part–Character 4	Approach–Character 5	Device–Character 6	Qualifier–Character 7
1 Bypass	Ø Coronary Artery, One Artery	Ø Open	Ø Monitoring Device, Pressure Sensor	Ø Allogeneic OR Ultrasonic
4 Creation	1 Coronary Artery, Two Arteries	3 Percutaneous	2 Monitoring Device	1 Syngeneic
5 Destruction	2 Coronary Artery, Three Arteries	4 Percutaneous Endoscopic	3 Infusion Device	2 Zooplastic OR Common Atrioventricular Valve
7 Dilation	3 Coronary Artery, Four or More Arteries	X External	4 Intraluminal Device, Drug-eluting	3 Coronary Artery
8 Division	4 Coronary Vein		5 Intraluminal Device, Drug-eluting, Two	4 Coronary Vein
B Excision	5 Atrial Septum		6 Intraluminal Device, Drug-eluting, Three	5 Coronary Circulation
C Extirpation	6 Atrium, Right		7 Intraluminal Device, Drug-eluting, Four or More OR Autologous Tissue Substitute	6 Bifurcation OR Atrium, Right
F Fragmentation	7 Atrium, Left		8 Zooplastic Tissue	7 Atrium, Left
H Insertion	8 Conduction Mechanism		9 Autologous Venous Tissue	8 Internal Mammary, Right
J Inspection	9 Chordae Tendineae		A Autologous Arterial Tissue	9 Internal Mammary, Left
K Map	A Heart		C Extraluminal Device	A Innominate Artery
L Occlusion	B Heart, Right		D Intraluminal Device	B Subclavian
N Release	C Heart, Left		E Intraluminal Device, Two OR Intraluminal Device, Branched or Fenestrated, One or Two Arteries	C Thoracic Artery
P Removal	D Papillary Muscle		F Intraluminal Device, Three OR Intraluminal Device, Branched or Fenestrated, Three or More Arteries	D Carotid
Q Repair	F Aortic Valve		G Intraluminal Device, Four or More	E Atrioventricular Valve, Left
R Replacement	G Mitral Valve		J Synthetic Substitute OR Cardiac Lead, Pacemaker	F Abdominal Artery
S Reposition	H Pulmonary Valve		K Nonautologous Tissue Substitute OR Cardiac Lead, Defibrillator	G Atrioventricular Valve, Right OR Axillary Artery
T Resection	J Tricuspid Valve		M Cardiac Lead	H Transapical OR Brachial Artery
U Supplement	K Ventricle, Right		N Intracardiac Pacemaker	J Truncal Valve OR Temporary OR Intraoperative
V Restriction	L Ventricle, Left		Q Implantable Heart Assist System	K Left Atrial Appendage
W Revision	M Ventricular Septum		R Short-term External Heart Assist System	P Pulmonary Trunk
Y Transplantation	N Pericardium		T Intraluminal Device, Radioactive	Q Pulmonary Artery, Right
	P Pulmonary Trunk		Y Other Device	R Pulmonary Artery, Left
	Q Pulmonary Artery, Right		Z No Device	S Pulmonary Vein, Right OR Biventricular
	R Pulmonary Artery, Left			T Pulmonary Vein, Left OR Ductus Arteriosus
	S Pulmonary Vein, Right			U Pulmonary Vein, Confluence
	T Pulmonary Vein, Left			V Lower Extremity Artery
	V Superior Vena Cava			W Aorta
	W Thoracic Aorta, Descending			X Diagnostic
	X Thoracic Aorta, Ascending/Arch			Z No Qualifier
	Y Great Vessel			

AHA Coding Clinic for table Ø21

2020, 1Q, 24 Pulmonary artery unifocalization
2020, 1Q, 37 Bypass of ascending aorta to brachiocephalic artery
2019, 4Q, 23 Bypass thoracic aorta to innominate artery
2019, 3Q, 30 Aortic aneurysm repair with debranching of common carotid and brachiocephalic arteries
2018, 4Q, 45-46 Descending thoracic aorta bypass
2018, 3Q, 8 Coronary artery bypass graft surgery (revision versus total redo)
2018, 3Q, 26 Coronary artery bypass graft surgery with endarterectomy
2017, 4Q, 56 Added approach values - Percutaneous heart valve procedures
2017, 1Q, 19 Norwood Sano procedure
2016, 4Q, 80-81 Thoracic aorta, ascending/arch and descending
2016, 4Q, 82-83 Coronary artery, number of arteries
2016, 4Q, 102-109 Correction of congenital heart defects
2016, 4Q, 144 Repair of atrial septal defect and anomalous pulmonary venous return
2016, 4Q, 145 Modified Warden procedure for repair of septal defect and right partial anomalous pulmonary venous return
2016, 1Q, 27 Aortocoronary bypass graft utilizing Y-graft
2015, 4Q, 22, 24 Congenital heart corrective procedures
2015, 3Q, 16 Revision of previous truncus arteriosus surgery with ventricle to pulmonary artery conduit
2014, 3Q, 3 Blalock-Taussig shunt procedure
2014, 3Q, 8 Coronary artery bypass graft utilizing internal mammary as pedicle graft
2014, 3Q, 20 MAZE procedure performed with coronary artery bypass graft
2014, 3Q, 29 Fontan completion procedure stage II
2014, 3Q, 30 Creation of conduit from right ventricle to pulmonary artery
2014, 1Q, 10 Repair of thoracic aortic aneurysm & coronary artery bypass graft
2013, 2Q, 37 Coronary artery release performed during coronary artery bypass graft

AHA Coding Clinic for table Ø24

2016, 4Q, 101 Root operation Creation
2016, 4Q, 102-109 Correction of congenital heart defects

AHA Coding Clinic for table Ø25

2020, 1Q, 32 Ablation convergent procedure (catheter-based and thoracoscopic ablations)
2018, 3Q, 27 Alcohol septal ablation
2016, 4Q, 80-81 Thoracic aorta, ascending/arch and descending
2016, 3Q, 43-44 Peri-pulmonary catheter ablation
2016, 3Q, 44-45 Maze procedure
2016, 2Q, 17 Photodynamic therapy for treatment of malignant mesothelioma
2014, 4Q, 47 Catheter ablation of peripulmonary veins
2014, 3Q, 19 Ablation of ventricular tachycardia with Impella® support
2014, 3Q, 20 MAZE procedure performed with coronary artery bypass graft
2013, 2Q, 38 Catheter ablation to treat atrial fibrillation

AHA Coding Clinic for table Ø27

2018, 3Q, 7 Coronary brachytherapy with angioplasty
2018, 3Q, 10 Disruption of perma-catheter fibrin sheath via angioplasty of superior vena cava
2018, 2Q, 24 Coronary artery bifurcation
2017, 4Q, 32-33 Corrective surgery of left ventricular outflow tract obstruction
2016, 4Q, 80-81 Thoracic aorta, ascending/arch and descending
2016, 4Q, 82-83 Coronary artery, number of arteries
2016, 4Q, 84-85 Coronary Artery, number of stents
2016, 4Q, 86-88 Coronary and peripheral artery bifurcation
2016, 1Q, 16 Pulmonary valvotomy and dilation of annulus
2015, 4Q, 13 New Section X codes—New Technology procedures
2015, 3Q, 9 Failed attempt to treat coronary artery occlusion
2015, 3Q, 10 Coronary angioplasty with unsuccessful stent insertion
2015, 3Q, 16 Revision of previous truncus arteriosus surgery with ventricle to pulmonary artery conduit
2015, 2Q, 3-5 Coronary artery intervention site
2014, 2Q, 4 Coronary angioplasty of bypassed vessel

AHA Coding Clinic for table Ø2B

2019, 3Q, 32 Endomyocardial biopsy and right heart catheterization
2019, 2Q, 20 Pericardiectomy for constrictive pericarditis
2017, 1Q, 38 Mitral valve repair and chordae tendineae transfer
2016, 4Q, 80-81 Thoracic aorta, ascending/arch and descending
2015, 2Q, 23 Annuloplasty ring

AHA Coding Clinic for table Ø2C

2019, 4Q, 25 Coronary artery to root operation Supplement
2018, 3Q, 26 Coronary artery bypass graft surgery with endarterectomy
2018, 2Q, 24 Coronary artery bifurcation
2017, 2Q, 23 Thrombectomy via Fogarty catheter
2016, 4Q, 80-81 Thoracic aorta, ascending/arch and descending
2016, 4Q, 82-83 Coronary artery, number of arteries
2016, 4Q, 86-87 Coronary and peripheral artery bifurcation
2016, 2Q, 24 Repair/decalcification of mitral valve
2016, 2Q, 25 Aortic valve surgery with excision of calcium deposits

AHA Coding Clinic for table Ø2H

2019, 4Q, 23-24 Coronary artery Body Part to root operation Insertion
2019, 3Q, 19 Insertion of left ventricular catheter
2019, 3Q, 23 Placement of pacemaker lead in Bundle of HIS
2019, 1Q, 24 Replacement of left ventricular assist device with retention of outflow graft
2018, 4Q, 94 Insertion and removal of failed Watchman™ device
2018, 2Q, 3-5 Intra-aortic balloon pump
2018, 2Q, 19 Pacing lead attached to automatic implantable cardioverter defibrillator
2017, 4Q, 42-45 Insertion of external heart assist devices
2017, 4Q, 63-64 Added and revised device values - Vascular access reservoir
2017, 4Q, 104 Placement of Watchman™ left atrial appendage device
2017, 3Q, 11 Placement of peripherally inserted central catheter using 3CG ECG technology
2017, 2Q, 24 Tunneled catheter versus totally implantable catheter
2017, 2Q, 26 Exchange of tunneled catheter
2017, 1Q, 10-11 External heart assist device
2016, 4Q, 80-81 Thoracic aorta, ascending/arch and descending
2016, 4Q, 95 Intracardiac pacemaker
2016, 4Q, 137-138 Heart assist device systems
2016, 2Q, 15 Removal and replacement of tunneled internal jugular catheter
2015, 4Q, 14 New Section X codes—New Technology procedures
2015, 4Q, 26-31 Vascular access devices
2015, 3Q, 35 Swan Ganz catheterization
2015, 2Q, 31 Leadless pacemaker insertion
2015, 2Q, 33 Totally implantable central venous access device (Port-a-Cath)
2013, 3Q, 18 Placement of peripherally inserted central catheter (PICC)

AHA Coding Clinic for table Ø2J

2015, 3Q, 9 Failed attempt to treat coronary artery occlusion

AHA Coding Clinic for table Ø2K

2020, 1Q, 32 Ablation convergent procedure (catheter-based and thoracoscopic ablations)

AHA Coding Clinic for table Ø2L

2018, 4Q, 94 Insertion and removal of failed Watchman™ device
2017, 4Q, 31 Resuscitative endovascular balloon occlusion of the aorta
2017, 4Q, 33-34 Occlusion/ligation of pulmonary trunk & right pulmonary artery
2016, 4Q, 102-109 Correction of congenital heart defects
2016, 2Q, 26 Embolization of pulmonary arteriovenous fistula
2015, 4Q, 23 Congenital heart corrective procedures
2014, 3Q, 20 MAZE procedure performed with coronary artery bypass graft

AHA Coding Clinic for table Ø2N

2019, 2Q, 13 Unroofing of anomalous coronary artery
2019, 2Q, 20 Pericardiectomy for constrictive pericarditis
2017, 4Q, 35 Release of myocardial bridge
2016, 4Q, 80-81 Thoracic aorta, ascending/arch and descending
2014, 3Q, 16 Repair of Tetralogy of Fallot

AHA Coding Clinic for table Ø2P

2019, 1Q, 24 Replacement of left ventricular assist device with retention of outflow graft
2018, 4Q, 52-54 Percutaneous extracorporeal membrane oxygenation
2018, 4Q, 85 Externalization of lumboatrial shunt
2018, 4Q, 94 Insertion and removal of failed Watchman™ device
2018, 2Q, 3-5 Intra-aortic balloon pump
2017, 4Q, 42-45 Insertion of external heart assist devices
2017, 4Q, 104 Placement of Watchman™ left atrial appendage device
2017, 3Q, 18 Intra-aortic balloon pump removal
2017, 2Q, 24 Tunneled catheter versus totally implantable catheter
2017, 2Q, 26 Exchange of tunneled catheter
2017, 1Q, 11 External heart assist device
2017, 1Q, 13 SynCardia total artificial heart
2016, 4Q, 95-96 Intracardiac pacemaker
2016, 4Q, 137-139 Heart assist device systems
2016, 3Q, 19 Nonoperative removal of peripherally inserted central catheter
2016, 2Q, 15 Removal and replacement of tunneled internal jugular catheter
2015, 4Q, 31 Vascular access devices
2015, 3Q, 33 Approach values for repositioning and removal of cardiac lead

AHA Coding Clinic for table Ø2Q

2018, 1Q, 12 Percutaneous balloon valvuloplasty & cardiac catheterization with ventriculogram
2017, 1Q, 18 Sutureless repair of pulmonary vein stenosis
2016, 4Q, 80-81 Thoracic aorta, ascending/arch and descending
2016, 4Q, 82-83 Coronary artery, number of arteries
2016, 4Q, 101 Root operation Creation
2016, 4Q, 102-109 Correction of congenital heart defects
2015, 4Q, 23 Congenital heart corrective procedures
2015, 3Q, 16 Vascular ring surgery and double aortic arch
2015, 2Q, 23 Annuloplasty ring
2013, 3Q, 26 Transcatheter replacement of heart valve (TAVR) with measurements

AHA Coding Clinic for table Ø2R

2020, 1Q, 25 Elephant trunk repair of aortic dissection
2019, 4Q, 24 Coronary artery Body Part to root operation Insertion
2019, 4Q, 46 Cerebral embolic filtration
2019, 3Q, 23 Replacement of atrioventricular valve
2019, 3Q, 24 Valve sparing aortic root replacement with modified Gleason Vascutek® graft to ascending aorta
2019, 1Q, 31 Transcatheter aortic valve in valve replacement
2018, 3Q, 11 Transcatheter aortic valve replacement via transaortic approach
2018, 1Q, 12 Percutaneous balloon valvuloplasty & cardiac catheterization with ventriculogram
2017, 4Q, 55-56 Added approach values - Percutaneous heart valve procedures
2017, 1Q, 13 SynCardia total artificial heart
2016, 4Q, 80-81 Thoracic aorta, ascending/arch and descending
2016, 3Q, 32 Transcatheter tricuspid valve replacement
2014, 1Q, 10 Repair of thoracic aortic aneurysm & coronary artery bypass graft

AHA Coding Clinic for table Ø2S

2016, 4Q, 80-81 Thoracic aorta, ascending/arch and descending
2016, 4Q, 82-83 Coronary artery, number of arteries
2016, 4Q, 102-109 Correction of congenital heart defects
2015, 4Q, 23 Congenital heart corrective procedures

AHA Coding Clinic for table Ø2U

2020, 1Q, 24 Pulmonary artery unifocalization
2019, 4Q, 25 Coronary artery to root operation Supplement
2018, 1Q, 12 Percutaneous balloon valvuloplasty & cardiac catheterization with ventriculogram
2017, 4Q, 36 Alfieri stitch procedure
2017, 3Q, 7 Senning procedure (arterial switch)
2017, 1Q, 19 Norwood Sano procedure
2016, 4Q, 80-81 Thoracic aorta, ascending/arch and descending
2016, 4Q, 101 Root operation Creation
2016, 4Q, 102-109 Correction of congenital heart defects
2016, 2Q, 23 Repair of tetralogy of Fallot with autologous pericardial patch graft
2016, 2Q, 26 Aortic valve replacement with aortic root enlargement
2015, 4Q, 22-24 Congenital heart corrective procedures
2015, 3Q, 16 Revision of previous truncus arteriosus surgery with ventricle to pulmonary artery conduit
2015, 2Q, 23 Annuloplasty ring
2014, 3Q, 16 Repair of Tetralogy of Fallot

AHA Coding Clinic for table Ø2V

2020, 1Q, 25 Elephant trunk repair of aortic dissection
2017, 4Q, 35-36 Alfieri stitch procedure
2016, 4Q, 80-81 Thoracic aorta, ascending/arch and descending
2016, 4Q, 89-92 Branched and fenestrated endograft repair of aneurysms

AHA Coding Clinic for table Ø2W

2019, 1Q, 24 Replacement of left ventricular assist device with retention of outflow graft
2018, 3Q, 8 Coronary artery bypass graft surgery (revision versus total redo)
2018, 3Q, 9 Fibrin sheath stripping of malfunctioning port-a-cath
2018, 1Q, 17 Repositioning of Impella short-term external heart assist device
2017, 4Q, 42-45 Insertion of external heart assist devices
2017, 4Q, 55-56 Added approach values - Percutaneous heart valve procedures
2016, 4Q, 85 Coronary Artery, number of stents
2016, 4Q, 95-96 Intracardiac pacemaker
2015, 3Q, 32 Approach values for repositioning and removal of cardiac lead
2014, 3Q, 31 Closure of paravalvular leak using Amplatzer® vascular plug

AHA Coding Clinic for table Ø2Y

2013, 3Q, 18 Heart transplant surgery

Coronary Arteries

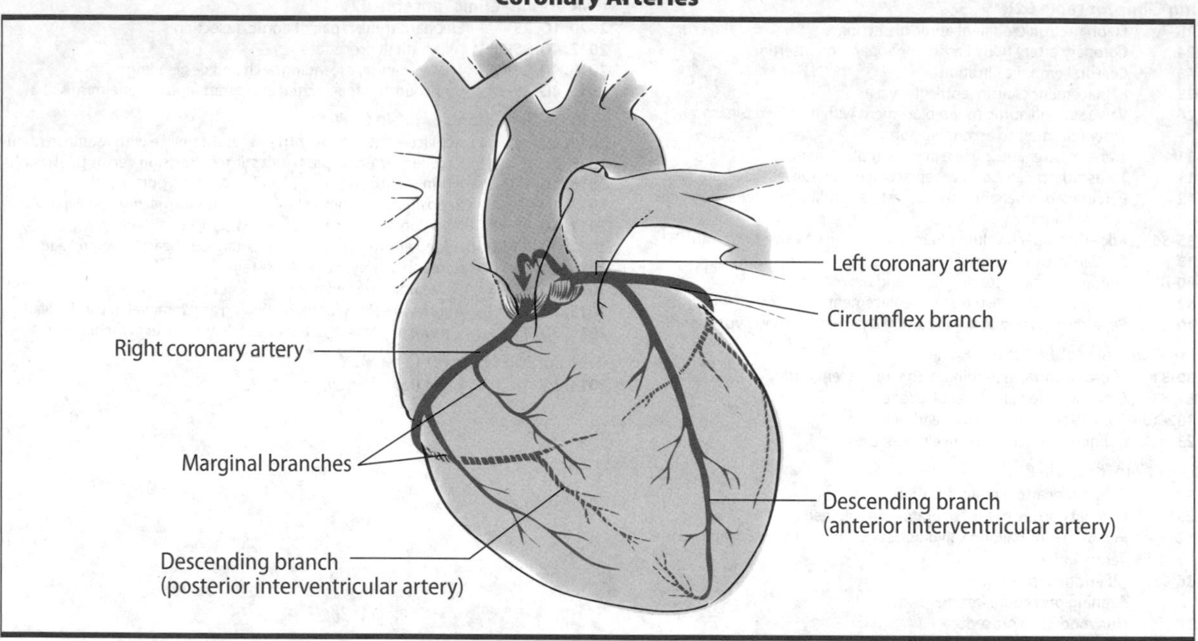

Heart Anatomy

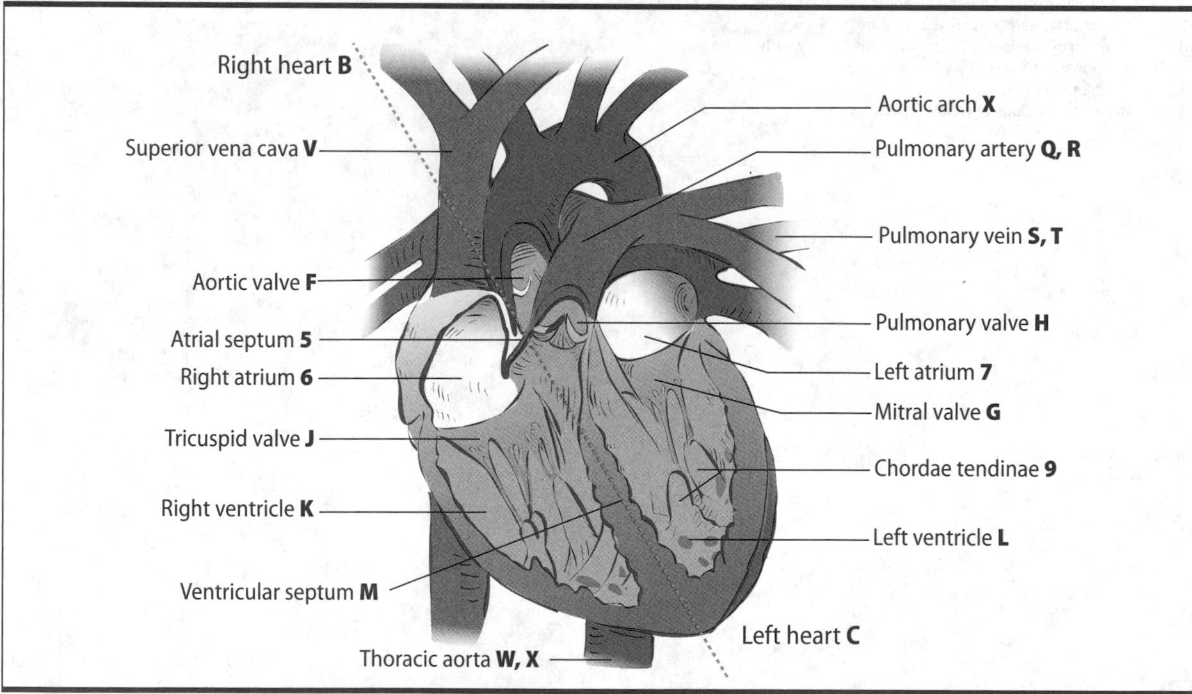

Ø Medical and Surgical
2 Heart and Great Vessels
1 Bypass Definition: Altering the route of passage of the contents of a tubular body part

Explanation: Rerouting contents of a body part to a downstream area of the normal route, to a similar route and body part, or to an abnormal route and dissimilar body part. Includes one or more anastomoses, with or without the use of a device.

Body Part Character 4	Approach Character 5	Device Character 6	Qualifier Character 7
Ø Coronary Artery, One Artery 1 Coronary Artery, Two Arteries 2 Coronary Artery, Three Arteries 3 Coronary Artery, Four or More Arteries	Ø Open	8 Zooplastic Tissue 9 Autologous Venous Tissue A Autologous Arterial Tissue J Synthetic Substitute K Nonautologous Tissue Substitute	3 Coronary Artery 8 Internal Mammary, Right 9 Internal Mammary, Left C Thoracic Artery F Abdominal Artery W Aorta
Ø Coronary Artery, One Artery 1 Coronary Artery, Two Arteries 2 Coronary Artery, Three Arteries 3 Coronary Artery, Four or More Arteries	Ø Open	Z No Device	3 Coronary Artery 8 Internal Mammary, Right 9 Internal Mammary, Left C Thoracic Artery F Abdominal Artery
Ø Coronary Artery, One Artery 1 Coronary Artery, Two Arteries 2 Coronary Artery, Three Arteries 3 Coronary Artery, Four or More Arteries	3 Percutaneous	4 Intraluminal Device, Drug-eluting D Intraluminal Device	4 Coronary Vein
Ø Coronary Artery, One Artery 1 Coronary Artery, Two Arteries 2 Coronary Artery, Three Arteries 3 Coronary Artery, Four or More Arteries	4 Percutaneous Endoscopic	4 Intraluminal Device, Drug-eluting D Intraluminal Device	4 Coronary Vein
Ø Coronary Artery, One Artery 1 Coronary Artery, Two Arteries 2 Coronary Artery, Three Arteries 3 Coronary Artery, Four or More Arteries	4 Percutaneous Endoscopic	8 Zooplastic Tissue 9 Autologous Venous Tissue A Autologous Arterial Tissue J Synthetic Substitute K Nonautologous Tissue Substitute	3 Coronary Artery 8 Internal Mammary, Right 9 Internal Mammary, Left C Thoracic Artery F Abdominal Artery W Aorta
Ø Coronary Artery, One Artery 1 Coronary Artery, Two Arteries 2 Coronary Artery, Three Arteries 3 Coronary Artery, Four or More Arteries	4 Percutaneous Endoscopic	Z No Device	3 Coronary Artery 8 Internal Mammary, Right 9 Internal Mammary, Left C Thoracic Artery F Abdominal Artery
6 Atrium, Right Atrium dextrum cordis Right auricular appendix Sinus venosus	Ø Open 4 Percutaneous Endoscopic	8 Zooplastic Tissue 9 Autologous Venous Tissue A Autologous Arterial Tissue J Synthetic Substitute K Nonautologous Tissue Substitute	P Pulmonary Trunk Q Pulmonary Artery, Right R Pulmonary Artery, Left
6 Atrium, Right Atrium dextrum cordis Right auricular appendix Sinus venosus	Ø Open 4 Percutaneous Endoscopic	Z No Device	7 Atrium, Left P Pulmonary Trunk Q Pulmonary Artery, Right R Pulmonary Artery, Left
6 Atrium, Right Atrium dextrum cordis Right auricular appendix Sinus venosus	3 Percutaneous	Z No Device	7 Atrium, Left
7 Atrium, Left Atrium pulmonale Left auricular appendix	Ø Open 4 Percutaneous Endoscopic	8 Zooplastic Tissue 9 Autologous Venous Tissue A Autologous Arterial Tissue J Synthetic Substitute K Nonautologous Tissue Substitute Z No Device	P Pulmonary Trunk Q Pulmonary Artery, Right R Pulmonary Artery, Left S Pulmonary Vein, Right T Pulmonary Vein, Left U Pulmonary Vein, Confluence
7 Atrium, Left Atrium pulmonale Left auricular appendix	3 Percutaneous	J Synthetic Substitute	6 Atrium, Right
K Ventricle, Right Conus arteriosus L Ventricle, Left	Ø Open 4 Percutaneous Endoscopic	8 Zooplastic Tissue 9 Autologous Venous Tissue A Autologous Arterial Tissue J Synthetic Substitute K Nonautologous Tissue Substitute	P Pulmonary Trunk Q Pulmonary Artery, Right R Pulmonary Artery, Left

HAC Ø21[Ø,1,2,3]Ø[8,9,A,J,K][3,8,9,C,F,W] when reported with SDx J98.51 or J98.59
HAC Ø21[Ø,1,2,3]ØZ[3,8,9,C,F] when reported with SDx J98.51 or J98.59
HAC Ø21[Ø,1,2,3]4[8,9,A,J,K][3,8,9,C,F,W] when reported with SDx J98.51 or J98.59
HAC Ø21[Ø,1,2,3]4Z[3,8,9,C,F] when reported with SDx J98.51 or J98.59

Ø21 Continued on next page

Ø Medical and Surgical
2 Heart and Great Vessels
1 Bypass Definition: Altering the route of passage of the contents of a tubular body part

Explanation: Rerouting contents of a body part to a downstream area of the normal route, to a similar route and body part, or to an abnormal route and dissimilar body part. Includes one or more anastomoses, with or without the use of a device.

Ø21 Continued

Body Part Character 4	Approach Character 5	Device Character 6	Qualifier Character 7
K Ventricle, Right Conus arteriosus **L** Ventricle, Left	**Ø** Open **4** Percutaneous Endoscopic	**Z** No Device	**5** Coronary Circulation **8** Internal Mammary, Right **9** Internal Mammary, Left **C** Thoracic Artery **F** Abdominal Artery **P** Pulmonary Trunk **Q** Pulmonary Artery, Right **R** Pulmonary Artery, Left **W** Aorta
P Pulmonary Trunk **Q** Pulmonary Artery, Right **R** Pulmonary Artery, Left Arterial canal (duct) Botallo's duct Pulmoaortic canal	**Ø** Open **4** Percutaneous Endoscopic	**8** Zooplastic Tissue **9** Autologous Venous Tissue **A** Autologous Arterial Tissue **J** Synthetic Substitute **K** Nonautologous Tissue Substitute **Z** No Device	**A** Innominate Artery **B** Subclavian **D** Carotid
V Superior Vena Cava Precava	**Ø** Open **4** Percutaneous Endoscopic	**8** Zooplastic Tissue **9** Autologous Venous Tissue **A** Autologous Arterial Tissue **J** Synthetic Substitute **K** Nonautologous Tissue Substitute **Z** No Device	**P** Pulmonary Trunk **Q** Pulmonary Artery, Right **R** Pulmonary Artery, Left **S** Pulmonary Vein, Right **T** Pulmonary Vein, Left **U** Pulmonary Vein, Confluence
W Thoracic Aorta, Descending	**Ø** Open	**8** Zooplastic Tissue **9** Autologous Venous Tissue **A** Autologous Arterial Tissue **J** Synthetic Substitute **K** Nonautologous Tissue Substitute	**A** Innominate Artery **B** Subclavian **D** Carotid **F** Abdominal Artery **G** Axillary Artery **H** Brachial Artery **P** Pulmonary Trunk **Q** Pulmonary Artery, Right **R** Pulmonary Artery, Left **V** Lower Extremity Artery
W Thoracic Aorta, Descending	**Ø** Open	**Z** No Device	**A** Innominate Artery **B** Subclavian **D** Carotid **P** Pulmonary Trunk **Q** Pulmonary Artery, Right **R** Pulmonary Artery, Left
W Thoracic Aorta, Descending	**4** Percutaneous Endoscopic	**8** Zooplastic Tissue **9** Autologous Venous Tissue **A** Autologous Arterial Tissue **J** Synthetic Substitute **K** Nonautologous Tissue Substitute **Z** No Device	**A** Innominate Artery **B** Subclavian **D** Carotid **P** Pulmonary Trunk **Q** Pulmonary Artery, Right **R** Pulmonary Artery, Left
X Thoracic Aorta, Ascending/Arch Aortic arch Ascending aorta	**Ø** Open **4** Percutaneous Endoscopic	**8** Zooplastic Tissue **9** Autologous Venous Tissue **A** Autologous Arterial Tissue **J** Synthetic Substitute **K** Nonautologous Tissue Substitute **Z** No Device	**A** Innominate Artery **B** Subclavian **D** Carotid **P** Pulmonary Trunk **Q** Pulmonary Artery, Right **R** Pulmonary Artery, Left

Ø Medical and Surgical
2 Heart and Great Vessels
4 Creation Definition: Putting in or on biological or synthetic material to form a new body part that to the extent possible replicates the anatomic structure or function of an absent body part

Explanation: Used for gender reassignment surgery and corrective procedures in individuals with congenital anomalies

Body Part Character 4	Approach Character 5	Device Character 6	Qualifier Character 7
F Aortic Valve Aortic annulus	**Ø** Open	**7** Autologous Tissue **8** Zooplastic Tissue **J** Synthetic Substitute **K** Nonautologous Tissue Substitute	**J** Truncal Valve
G Mitral Valve Bicuspid valve Left atrioventricular valve Mitral annulus **J** Tricuspid Valve Right atrioventricular valve Tricuspid annulus	**Ø** Open	**7** Autologous Tissue **8** Zooplastic Tissue **J** Synthetic Substitute **K** Nonautologous Tissue Substitute	**2** Common Atrioventricular Valve

Ø Medical and Surgical
2 Heart and Great Vessels
5 Destruction Definition: Physical eradication of all or a portion of a body part by the direct use of energy, force, or a destructive agent
Explanation: None of the body part is physically taken out

Body Part Character 4	Approach Character 5	Device Character 6	Qualifier Character 7
4 Coronary Vein **5 Atrial Septum** Interatrial septum **6 Atrium, Right** Atrium dextrum cordis Right auricular appendix Sinus venosus **8 Conduction Mechanism** Atrioventricular node Bundle of His Bundle of Kent Sinoatrial node **9 Chordae Tendineae** **D Papillary Muscle** **F Aortic Valve** Aortic annulus **G Mitral Valve** Bicuspid valve Left atrioventricular valve Mitral annulus **H Pulmonary Valve** Pulmonary annulus Pulmonic valve **J Tricuspid Valve** Right atrioventricular valve Tricuspid annulus **K Ventricle, Right** Conus arteriosus **L Ventricle, Left** **M Ventricular Septum** Interventricular septum **N Pericardium** **P Pulmonary Trunk** **Q Pulmonary Artery, Right** **R Pulmonary Artery, Left** Arterial canal (duct) Botallo's duct Pulmoaortic canal **S Pulmonary Vein, Right** Right inferior pulmonary vein Right superior pulmonary vein **T Pulmonary Vein, Left** Left inferior pulmonary vein Left superior pulmonary vein **V Superior Vena Cava** Precava **W Thoracic Aorta, Descending** **X Thoracic Aorta, Ascending/Arch** Aortic arch Ascending aorta	**Ø Open** **3 Percutaneous** **4 Percutaneous Endoscopic**	**Z No Device**	**Z No Qualifier**
7 Atrium, Left Atrium pulmonale Left auricular appendix	**Ø Open** **3 Percutaneous** **4 Percutaneous Endoscopic**	**Z No Device**	**K Left Atrial Appendage** **Z No Qualifier**

DRG Non-OR Ø257[Ø,3,4]ZK

0 Medical and Surgical
2 Heart and Great Vessels
7 Dilation Definition: Expanding an orifice or the lumen of a tubular body part

Explanation: The orifice can be a natural orifice or an artificially created orifice. Accomplished by stretching a tubular body part using intraluminal pressure or by cutting part of the orifice or wall of the tubular body part.

Body Part Character 4	Approach Character 5	Device Character 6	Qualifier Character 7
0 Coronary Artery, One Artery **1** Coronary Artery, Two Arteries **2** Coronary Artery, Three Arteries **3** Coronary Artery, Four or More Arteries	**0** Open **3** Percutaneous **4** Percutaneous Endoscopic	**4** Intraluminal Device, Drug-eluting **5** Intraluminal Device, Drug-eluting, Two **6** Intraluminal Device, Drug-eluting, Three **7** Intraluminal Device, Drug-eluting, Four or More **D** Intraluminal Device **E** Intraluminal Device, Two **F** Intraluminal Device, Three **G** Intraluminal Device, Four or More **T** Intraluminal Device, Radioactive **Z** No Device	**6** Bifurcation **Z** No Qualifier
F Aortic Valve Aortic annulus **G** Mitral Valve Bicuspid valve Left atrioventricular valve Mitral annulus **H** Pulmonary Valve Pulmonary annulus Pulmonic valve **J** Tricuspid Valve Right atrioventricular valve Tricuspid annulus **K** Ventricle, Right Conus arteriosus **L** Ventricle, Left **P** Pulmonary Trunk **Q** Pulmonary Artery, Right **S** Pulmonary Vein, Right Right inferior pulmonary vein Right superior pulmonary vein **T** Pulmonary Vein, Left Left inferior pulmonary vein Left superior pulmonary vein **V** Superior Vena Cava Precava **W** Thoracic Aorta, Descending **X** Thoracic Aorta, Ascending/Arch Aortic arch Ascending aorta	**0** Open **3** Percutaneous **4** Percutaneous Endoscopic	**4** Intraluminal Device, Drug-eluting **D** Intraluminal Device **Z** No Device	**Z** No Qualifier
R Pulmonary Artery, Left Arterial canal (duct) Botallo's duct Pulmoaortic canal	**0** Open **3** Percutaneous **4** Percutaneous Endoscopic	**4** Intraluminal Device, Drug-eluting **D** Intraluminal Device **Z** No Device	**T** Ductus Arteriosus **Z** No Qualifier

0 Medical and Surgical
2 Heart and Great Vessels
8 Division Definition: Cutting into a body part, without draining fluids and/or gases from the body part, in order to separate or transect a body part

Explanation: All or a portion of the body part is separated into two or more portions

Body Part Character 4	Approach Character 5	Device Character 6	Qualifier Character 7
8 Conduction Mechanism Atrioventricular node Bundle of His Bundle of Kent Sinoatrial node **9** Chordae Tendineae **D** Papillary Muscle	**0** Open **3** Percutaneous **4** Percutaneous Endoscopic	**Z** No Device	**Z** No Qualifier

Ø Medical and Surgical
2 Heart and Great Vessels
B Excision Definition: Cutting out or off, without replacement, a portion of a body part
Explanation: The qualifier DIAGNOSTIC is used to identify excision procedures that are biopsies

Body Part Character 4	Approach Character 5	Device Character 6	Qualifier Character 7
4 Coronary Vein **5** Atrial Septum Interatrial septum **6** Atrium, Right Atrium dextrum cordis Right auricular appendix Sinus venosus **8** Conduction Mechanism Atrioventricular node Bundle of His Bundle of Kent Sinoatrial node **9** Chordae Tendineae **D** Papillary Muscle **F** Aortic Valve Aortic annulus **G** Mitral Valve Bicuspid valve Left atrioventricular valve Mitral annulus **H** Pulmonary Valve Pulmonary annulus Pulmonic valve **J** Tricuspid Valve Right atrioventricular valve Tricuspld annulus **K** Ventricle, Right NC Conus arteriosus **L** Ventricle, Left NC **M** Ventricular Septum Interventricular septum **N** Pericardium **P** Pulmonary Trunk **Q** Pulmonary Artery, Right **R** Pulmonary Artery, Left Arterial canal (duct) Botallo's duct Pulmoaortic canal **S** Pulmonary Vein, Right Right inferior pulmonary vein Right superior pulmonary vein **T** Pulmonary Veln, Left Left inferior pulmonary vein Left superior pulmonary vein **V** Superior Vena Cava Precava **W** Thoracic Aorta, Descending **X** Thoracic Aorta, Ascending/Arch Aortic arch Ascending aorta	**Ø** Open **3** Percutaneous **4** Percutaneous Endoscopic	**Z** No Device	**X** Diagnostic **Z** No Qualifier
7 Atrium, Left Atrium pulmonale Left auricular appendix	**Ø** Open **3** Percutaneous **4** Percutaneous Endoscopic	**Z** No Device	**K** Left Atrial Appendage **X** Diagnostic **Z** No Qualifier

DRG Non-OR Ø2B7[Ø,3,4]ZK
Non-OR Ø2B[4,5,6,8,9,D,F,G,H,J,K,L,M][Ø,3,4]ZX
NC Ø2B[K,L][Ø,3,4]ZZ

Ø Medical and Surgical
2 Heart and Great Vessels
C Extirpation Definition: Taking or cutting out solid matter from a body part

Explanation: The solid matter may be an abnormal byproduct of a biological function or a foreign body; it may be imbedded in a body part or in the lumen of a tubular body part. The solid matter may or may not have been previously broken into pieces.

Body Part Character 4	Approach Character 5	Device Character 6	Qualifier Character 7
Ø Coronary Artery, One Artery 1 Coronary Artery, Two Arteries 2 Coronary Artery, Three Arteries 3 Coronary Artery, Four or More Arteries	Ø Open 3 Percutaneous 4 Percutaneous Endoscopic	Z No Device	6 Bifurcation Z No Qualifier
4 **Coronary Vein** 5 **Atrial Septum** Interatrial septum 6 **Atrium, Right** Atrium dextrum cordis Right auricular appendix Sinus venosus 7 **Atrium, Left** Atrium pulmonale Left auricular appendix 8 **Conduction Mechanism** Atrioventricular node Bundle of His Bundle of Kent Sinoatrial node 9 **Chordae Tendineae** D **Papillary Muscle** F **Aortic Valve** Aortic annulus G **Mitral Valve** Bicuspid valve Left atrioventricular valve Mitral annulus H **Pulmonary Valve** Pulmonary annulus Pulmonic valve J **Tricuspid Valve** Right atrioventricular valve Tricuspid annulus K **Ventricle, Right** Conus arteriosus L **Ventricle, Left** M **Ventricular Septum** Interventricular septum N **Pericardium** P **Pulmonary Trunk** Q **Pulmonary Artery, Right** R **Pulmonary Artery, Left** Arterial canal (duct) Botallo's duct Pulmoaortic canal S **Pulmonary Vein, Right** Right inferior pulmonary vein Right superior pulmonary vein T **Pulmonary Vein, Left** Left inferior pulmonary vein Left superior pulmonary vein V **Superior Vena Cava** Precava W **Thoracic Aorta, Descending** X **Thoracic Aorta, Ascending/Arch** Aortic arch Ascending aorta	Ø Open 3 Percutaneous 4 Percutaneous Endoscopic	Z No Device	Z No Qualifier

Ø Medical and Surgical
2 Heart and Great Vessels
F Fragmentation Definition: Breaking solid matter in a body part into pieces

Explanation: Physical force (e.g., manual, ultrasonic) applied directly or indirectly is used to break the solid matter into pieces. The solid matter may be an abnormal byproduct of a biological function or a foreign body. The pieces of solid matter are not taken out.

Body Part Character 4	Approach Character 5	Device Character 6	Qualifier Character 7
N Pericardium NC	**Ø Open** **3 Percutaneous** **4 Percutaneous Endoscopic** **X External**	**Z No Device**	**Z No Qualifier**
P Pulmonary Trunk **Q Pulmonary Artery, Right** **R Pulmonary Artery, Left** Arterial canal (duct) Botallo's duct Pulmoaortic canal **S Pulmonary Vein, Right** Right inferior pulmonary vein Right superior pulmonary vein **T Pulmonary Vein, Left** Left inferior pulmonary vein Left superior pulmonary vein	**3 Percutaneous**	**Z No Device**	**Ø Ultrasonic** **Z No Qualifier**

Non-OR Ø2FNXZZ
NC Ø2FNXZZ

Ø Medical and Surgical
2 Heart and Great Vessels
H Insertion Definition: Putting in a nonbiological appliance that monitors, assists, performs, or prevents a physiological function but does not physically take the place of a body part
Explanation: None

Body Part Character 4	Approach Character 5	Device Character 6	Qualifier Character 7
Ø Coronary Artery, One Artery 1 Coronary Artery, Two Arteries 2 Coronary Artery, Three Arteries 3 Coronary Artery, Four or More Arteries	Ø Open 3 Percutaneous 4 Percutaneous Endoscopic	D Intraluminal Device Y Other Device	Z No Qualifier
4 Coronary Vein ⊞ 6 Atrium, Right ⊞ Atrium dextrum cordis Right auricular appendix Sinus venosus 7 Atrium, Left ⊞ Atrium pulmonale Left auricular appendix K Ventricle, Right ⊞ Conus arteriosus L Ventricle, Left ⊞	Ø Open 3 Percutaneous 4 Percutaneous Endoscopic	Ø Monitoring Device, Pressure Sensor 2 Monitoring Device 3 Infusion Device D Intraluminal Device J Cardiac Lead, Pacemaker K Cardiac Lead, Defibrillator M Cardiac Lead N Intracardiac Pacemaker Y Other Device	Z No Qualifier
A Heart LC NC	Ø Open 3 Percutaneous 4 Percutaneous Endoscopic	Q Implantable Heart Assist System Y Other Device	Z No Qualifier
A Heart ⊞	Ø Open 3 Percutaneous 4 Percutaneous Endoscopic	R Short-term External Heart Assist System	J Intraoperative S Biventricular Z No Qualifier
N Pericardium ⊞	Ø Open 3 Percutaneous 4 Percutaneous Endoscopic	Ø Monitoring Device, Pressure Sensor 2 Monitoring Device J Cardiac Lead, Pacemaker K Cardiac Lead, Defibrillator M Cardiac Lead Y Other Device	Z No Qualifier
P Pulmonary Trunk Q Pulmonary Artery, Right R Pulmonary Artery, Left Arterial canal (duct) Botallo's duct Pulmoaortic canal S Pulmonary Vein, Right Right inferior pulmonary vein Right superior pulmonary vein T Pulmonary Vein, Left Left inferior pulmonary vein Left superior pulmonary vein V Superior Vena Cava Precava W Thoracic Aorta, Descending	Ø Open 3 Percutaneous 4 Percutaneous Endoscopic	Ø Monitoring Device, Pressure Sensor 2 Monitoring Device 3 Infusion Device D Intraluminal Device Y Other Device	Z No Qualifier
X Thoracic Aorta, Ascending/Arch Aortic arch Ascending aorta	Ø Open 3 Percutaneous 4 Percutaneous Endoscopic	Ø Monitoring Device, Pressure Sensor 2 Monitoring Device 3 Infusion Device D Intraluminal Device	Z No Qualifier

DRG Non-OR Ø2H[4,6,7,K,L][Ø,3,4][J,M]Z
DRG Non-OR Ø2HK32Z
DRG Non-OR Ø2HN[Ø,3,4][J,M]Z
Non-OR Ø2H[4,6,7,L]3[2,3]Z
Non-OR Ø2H[6,7]3MZ
Non-OR Ø2HK3[Ø,3]Z
Non-OR Ø2HN32Z
Non-OR Ø2HP[Ø,3,4][Ø,2,3]Z
Non-OR Ø2H[Q,R][Ø,3,4][2,3]Z
Non-OR Ø2H[S,T,V,W][Ø,3,4]3Z
Non-OR Ø2H[S,T,V,W]32Z
Non-OR Ø2HW[Ø,3]ØZ
Non-OR Ø2HX[Ø,3,4][Ø,3]Z

HAC Ø2H43[J,K,M]Z when reported with SDx K68.11 or T81.4Ø-T81.49, T82.6-T82.7 with 7th character A
HAC Ø2H[6,K]33Z when reported with SDx J95.811
HAC Ø2H[6,7]3[J,M]Z when reported with SDx K68.11 or T81.4Ø-T81.49, T82.6-T82.7 with 7th character A
HAC Ø2H[K,L]3JZ when reported with SDx K68.11 or T81.4Ø-T81.49, T82.6-T82.7 with 7th character A
HAC Ø2HN[Ø,3,4][J,M]Z when reported with SDx K68.11 or T81.4Ø-T81.49, T82.6-T82.7 with 7th character A
HAC Ø2H[S,T,V][3,4]3Z when reported with SDx J95.811
LC Ø2HAØQZ
NC Ø2HA[3,4]QZ

See Appendix L for Procedure Combinations
⊞ Ø2H[4,6,7,K,L][Ø,3,4][J,K,M]Z
⊞ Ø2HA[Ø,4]R[S,Z]
⊞ Ø2HA3RS
⊞ Ø2HN[Ø,3,4][J,K,M]Z

Ø Medical and Surgical
2 Heart and Great Vessels
J Inspection Definition: Visually and/or manually exploring a body part

Explanation: Visual exploration may be performed with or without optical instrumentation. Manual exploration may be performed directly or through intervening body layers.

Body Part Character 4	Approach Character 5	Device Character 6	Qualifier Character 7
A Heart Y Great Vessel	Ø Open 3 Percutaneous 4 Percutaneous Endoscopic	Z No Device	Z No Qualifier

Non-OR Ø2J[A,Y]3ZZ

Ø Medical and Surgical
2 Heart and Great Vessels
K Map Definition: Locating the route of passage of electrical impulses and/or locating functional areas in a body part

Explanation: Applicable only to the cardiac conduction mechanism and the central nervous system

Body Part Character 4	Approach Character 5	Device Character 6	Qualifier Character 7
8 Conduction Mechanism Atrioventricular node Bundle of His Bundle of Kent Sinoatrial node	Ø Open 3 Percutaneous 4 Percutaneous Endoscopic	Z No Device	Z No Qualifier

DRG Non-OR Ø2K8[Ø,3,4]ZZ

Ø Medical and Surgical
2 Heart and Great Vessels
L Occlusion Definition: Completely closing an orifice or the lumen of a tubular body part

Explanation: The orifice can be a natural orifice or an artificially created orifice

Body Part Character 4	Approach Character 5	Device Character 6	Qualifier Character 7
7 Atrium, Left Atrium pulmonale Left auricular appendix	Ø Open 3 Percutaneous 4 Percutaneous Endoscopic	C Extraluminal Device D Intraluminal Device Z No Device	K Left Atrial Appendage
H Pulmonary Valve Pulmonary annulus Pulmonic valve P Pulmonary Trunk Q Pulmonary Artery, Right S Pulmonary Vein, Right Right inferior pulmonary vein Right superior pulmonary vein T Pulmonary Vein, Left Left inferior pulmonary vein Left superior pulmonary vein V Superior Vena Cava Precava	Ø Open 3 Percutaneous 4 Percutaneous Endoscopic	C Extraluminal Device D Intraluminal Device Z No Device	Z No Qualifier
R Pulmonary Artery, Left Arterial canal (duct) Botallo's duct Pulmoaortic canal	Ø Open 3 Percutaneous 4 Percutaneous Endoscopic	C Extraluminal Device D Intraluminal Device Z No Device	T Ductus Arteriosus Z No Qualifier
W Thoracic Aorta, Descending	3 Percutaneous	D Intraluminal Device	J Temporary

DRG Non-OR Ø2L7[Ø,3,4][C,D,Z]K

Ø Medical and Surgical
2 Heart and Great Vessels
N Release Definition: Freeing a body part from an abnormal physical constraint by cutting or by the use of force
Explanation: Some of the restraining tissue may be taken out but none of the body part is taken out

Body Part Character 4	Approach Character 5	Device Character 6	Qualifier Character 7
Ø Coronary Artery, One Artery **1** Coronary Artery, Two Arteries **2** Coronary Artery, Three Arteries **3** Coronary Artery, Four or More Arteries **4** Coronary Vein **5** Atrial Septum Interatrial septum **6** Atrium, Right Atrium dextrum cordis Right auricular appendix Sinus venosus **7** Atrium, Left Atrium pulmonale Left auricular appendix **8** Conduction Mechanism Atrioventricular node Bundle of His Bundle of Kent Sinoatrial node **9** Chordae Tendineae **D** Papillary Muscle **F** Aortic Valve Aortic annulus **G** Mitral Valve Bicuspid valve Left atrioventricular valve Mitral annulus **H** Pulmonary Valve Pulmonary annulus Pulmonic valve **J** Tricuspid Valve Right atrioventricular valve Tricuspid annulus **K** Ventricle, Right Conus arteriosus **L** Ventricle, Left **M** Ventricular Septum Interventricular septum **N** Pericardium **P** Pulmonary Trunk **Q** Pulmonary Artery, Right **R** Pulmonary Artery, Left Arterial canal (duct) Botallo's duct Pulmoaortic canal **S** Pulmonary Vein, Right Right inferior pulmonary vein Right superior pulmonary vein **T** Pulmonary Vein, Left Left inferior pulmonary vein Left superior pulmonary vein **V** Superior Vena Cava Precava **W** Thoracic Aorta, Descending **X** Thoracic Aorta, Ascending/Arch Aortic arch Ascending aorta	**Ø** Open **3** Percutaneous **4** Percutaneous Endoscopic	**Z** No Device	**Z** No Qualifier

Ø Medical and Surgical
2 Heart and Great Vessels
P Removal Definition: Taking out or off a device from a body part

Explanation: If a device is taken out and a similar device put in without cutting or puncturing the skin or mucous membrane, the procedure is coded to the root operation CHANGE. Otherwise, the procedure for taking out a device is coded to the root operation REMOVAL.

Body Part Character 4	Approach Character 5	Device Character 6	Qualifier Character 7
A Heart	Ø Open 3 Percutaneous 4 Percutaneous Endoscopic	2 Monitoring Device 3 Infusion Device 7 Autologous Tissue Substitute 8 Zooplastic Tissue C Extraluminal Device D Intraluminal Device J Synthetic Substitute K Nonautologous Tissue Substitute M Cardiac Lead N Intracardiac Pacemaker Q Implantable Heart Assist System Y Other Device	Z No Qualifier
A Heart ⊞	Ø Open 3 Percutaneous 4 Percutaneous Endoscopic	R Short-term External Heart Assist System	S Biventricular Z No Qualifier
A Heart	X External	2 Monitoring Device 3 Infusion Device D Intraluminal Device M Cardiac Lead	Z No Qualifier
Y Great Vessel	Ø Open 3 Percutaneous 4 Percutaneous Endoscopic	2 Monitoring Device 3 Infusion Device 7 Autologous Tissue Substitute 8 Zooplastic Tissue C Extraluminal Device D Intraluminal Device J Synthetic Substitute K Nonautologous Tissue Substitute Y Other Device	Z No Qualifier
Y Great Vessel	X External	2 Monitoring Device 3 Infusion Device D Intraluminal Device	Z No Qualifier

Non-OR Ø2PA3[2,3,D]Z
Non-OR Ø2PA[3,4]YZ
Non-OR Ø2PAX[2,3,D,M]Z
Non-OR Ø2PY3[2,3,D]Z
Non-OR Ø2PY[3,4]YZ
Non-OR Ø2PYX[2,3,D]Z
HAC Ø2PA[Ø,3,4]MZ when reported with SDx K68.11 or T81.4Ø-T81.49, T82.6-T82.7 with 7th character A
HAC Ø2PAXMZ when reported with SDx K68.11 or T81.4Ø-T81.49, T82.6-T82.7 with 7th character A

See Appendix L for Procedure Combinations
⊞ Ø2PA[Ø,3,4]RZ

Ø Medical and Surgical
2 Heart and Great Vessels
Q Repair Definition: Restoring, to the extent possible, a body part to its normal anatomic structure and function
Explanation: Used only when the method to accomplish the repair is not one of the other root operations

Body Part Character 4	Approach Character 5	Device Character 6	Qualifier Character 7
Ø Coronary Artery, One Artery **1 Coronary Artery, Two Arteries** **2 Coronary Artery, Three Arteries** **3 Coronary Artery, Four or More Arteries** **4 Coronary Vein** **5 Atrial Septum** Interatrial septum **6 Atrium, Right** Atrium dextrum cordis Right auricular appendix Sinus venosus **7 Atrium, Left** Atrium pulmonale Left auricular appendix **8 Conduction Mechanism** Atrioventricular node Bundle of His Bundle of Kent Sinoatrial node **9 Chordae Tendineae** **A Heart** **B Heart, Right** Right coronary sulcus **C Heart, Left** Left coronary sulcus Obtuse margin **D Papillary Muscle** **H Pulmonary Valve** Pulmonary annulus Pulmonic valve **K Ventricle, Right** Conus arteriosus **L Ventricle, Left** **M Ventricular Septum** Interventricular septum **N Pericardium** **P Pulmonary Trunk** **Q Pulmonary Artery, Right** **R Pulmonary Artery, Left** Arterial canal (duct) Botallo's duct Pulmoaortic canal **S Pulmonary Vein, Right** Right inferior pulmonary vein Right superior pulmonary vein **T Pulmonary Vein, Left** Left inferior pulmonary vein Left superior pulmonary vein **V Superior Vena Cava** Precava **W Thoracic Aorta, Descending** **X Thoracic Aorta, Ascending/Arch** Aortic arch Ascending aorta	**Ø Open** **3 Percutaneous** **4 Percutaneous Endoscopic**	**Z No Device**	**Z No Qualifier**
F Aortic Valve Aortic annulus	**Ø Open** **3 Percutaneous** **4 Percutaneous Endoscopic**	**Z No Device**	**J Truncal Valve** **Z No Qualifier**
G Mitral Valve Bicuspid valve Left atrioventricular valve Mitral annulus	**Ø Open** **3 Percutaneous** **4 Percutaneous Endoscopic**	**Z No Device**	**E Atrioventricular Valve, Left** **Z No Qualifier**
J Tricuspid Valve Right atrioventricular valve Tricuspid annulus	**Ø Open** **3 Percutaneous** **4 Percutaneous Endoscopic**	**Z No Device**	**G Atrioventricular Valve, Right** **Z No Qualifier**

Ø Medical and Surgical
2 Heart and Great Vessels
R Replacement Definition: Putting in or on biological or synthetic material that physically takes the place and/or function of all or a portion of a body part

Explanation: The body part may have been taken out or replaced, or may be taken out, physically eradicated, or rendered nonfunctional during the REPLACEMENT procedure. A REMOVAL procedure is coded for taking out the device used in a previous replacement procedure.

Body Part Character 4	Approach Character 5	Device Character 6	Qualifier Character 7
5 Atrial Septum Interatrial septum **6 Atrium, Right** Atrium dextrum cordis Right auricular appendix Sinus venosus **7 Atrium, Left** Atrium pulmonale Left auricular appendix **9 Chordae Tendineae** **D Papillary Muscle** **K Ventricle, Right** LC NC ⊞ Conus arteriosus **L Ventricle, Left** LC NC ⊞ **M Ventricular Septum** Interventricular septum **N Pericardium** **P Pulmonary Trunk** **Q Pulmonary Artery, Right** **R Pulmonary Artery, Left** Arterial canal (duct) Botallo's duct Pulmoaortic canal **S Pulmonary Vein, Right** Right inferior pulmonary vein Right superior pulmonary vein **T Pulmonary Vein, Left** Left inferior pulmonary vein Left superior pulmonary vein **V Superior Vena Cava** Precava **W Thoracic Aorta, Descending** **X Thoracic Aorta, Ascending/Arch** Aortic arch Ascending aorta	**Ø Open** **4 Percutaneous Endoscopic**	**7 Autologous Tissue Substitute** **8 Zooplastic Tissue** **J Synthetic Substitute** **K Nonautologous Tissue Substitute**	**Z No Qualifier**
F Aortic Valve Aortic annulus **G Mitral Valve** Bicuspid valve Left atrioventricular valve Mitral annulus **H Pulmonary Valve** Pulmonary annulus Pulmonic valve **J Tricuspid Valve** Right atrioventricular valve Tricuspid annulus	**Ø Open** **4 Percutaneous Endoscopic**	**7 Autologous Tissue Substitute** **8 Zooplastic Tissue** **J Synthetic Substitute** **K Nonautologous Tissue Substitute**	**Z No Qualifier**
F Aortic Valve Aortic annulus **G Mitral Valve** Bicuspid valve Left atrioventricular valve Mitral annulus **H Pulmonary Valve** Pulmonary annulus Pulmonic valve **J Tricuspid Valve** Right atrioventricular valve Tricuspid annulus	**3 Percutaneous**	**7 Autologous Tissue Substitute** **8 Zooplastic Tissue** **J Synthetic Substitute** **K Nonautologous Tissue Substitute**	**H Transapical** **Z No Qualifier**

LC Ø2RKØJZ with Ø2RLØJZ with diagnosis code ZØØ.6
NC Ø2RKØJZ with Ø2RLØJZ without diagnosis code ZØØ.6

See Appendix L for Procedure Combinations
⊞ Ø2R[K,L]ØJZ

Ø Medical and Surgical
2 Heart and Great Vessels
S Reposition Definition: Moving to its normal location, or other suitable location, all or a portion of a body part

Explanation: The body part is moved to a new location from an abnormal location, or from a normal location where it is not functioning correctly. The body part may or may not be cut out or off to be moved to the new location.

Body Part Character 4	Approach Character 5	Device Character 6	Qualifier Character 7
Ø Coronary Artery, One Artery **1 Coronary Artery, Two Arteries** **P Pulmonary Trunk** **Q Pulmonary Artery, Right** **R Pulmonary Artery, Left** Arterial canal (duct) Botallo's duct Pulmoaortic canal **S Pulmonary Vein, Right** Right inferior pulmonary vein Right superior pulmonary vein **T Pulmonary Vein, Left** Left inferior pulmonary vein Left superior pulmonary vein **V Superior Vena Cava** Precava **W Thoracic Aorta, Descending** **X Thoracic Aorta, Ascending/Arch** Aortic arch Ascending aorta	**Ø Open**	**Z No Device**	**Z No Qualifier**

Ø Medical and Surgical
2 Heart and Great Vessels
T Resection Definition: Cutting out or off, without replacement, all of a body part

Explanation: None

Body Part Character 4	Approach Character 5	Device Character 6	Qualifier Character 7
5 Atrial Septum Interatrial septum **8 Conduction Mechanism** Atrioventricular node Bundle of His Bundle of Kent Sinoatrial node **9 Chordae Tendineae** **D Papillary Muscle** **H Pulmonary Valve** Pulmonary annulus Pulmonic valve **M Ventricular Septum** Interventricular septum **N Pericardium**	**Ø Open** **3 Percutaneous** **4 Percutaneous Endoscopic**	**Z No Device**	**Z No Qualifier**

Ø Medical and Surgical
2 Heart and Great Vessels
U Supplement Definition: Putting in or on biological or synthetic material that physically reinforces and/or augments the function of a portion of a body part

Explanation: The biological material is non-living, or is living and from the same individual. The body part may have been previously replaced, and the SUPPLEMENT procedure is performed to physically reinforce and/or augment the function of the replaced body part.

Body Part Character 4	Approach Character 5	Device Character 6	Qualifier Character 7
Ø Coronary Artery, One Artery **1 Coronary Artery, Two Arteries** **2 Coronary Artery, Three Arteries** **3 Coronary Artery, Four or More Arteries** **5 Atrial Septum** Interatrial septum **6 Atrium, Right** Atrium dextrum cordis Right auricular appendix Sinus venosus **7 Atrium, Left** Atrium pulmonale Left auricular appendix **9 Chordae Tendineae** **A Heart** **D Papillary Muscle** **H Pulmonary Valve** Pulmonary annulus Pulmonic valve **K Ventricle, Right** Conus arteriosus **L Ventricle, Left** **M Ventricular Septum** Interventricular septum **N Pericardium** **P Pulmonary Trunk** **Q Pulmonary Artery, Right** **R Pulmonary Artery, Left** Arterial canal (duct) Botallo's duct Pulmoaortic canal **S Pulmonary Vein, Right** Right inferior pulmonary vein Right superior pulmonary vein **T Pulmonary Vein, Left** Left inferior pulmonary vein Left superior pulmonary vein **V Superior Vena Cava** Precava **W Thoracic Aorta, Descending** **X Thoracic Aorta, Ascending/Arch** Aortic arch Ascending aorta	**Ø Open** **3 Percutaneous** **4 Percutaneous Endoscopic**	**7 Autologous Tissue Substitute** **8 Zooplastic Tissue** **J Synthetic Substitute** **K Nonautologous Tissue Substitute**	**Z No Qualifier**
F Aortic Valve Aortic annulus	**Ø Open** **3 Percutaneous** **4 Percutaneous Endoscopic**	**7 Autologous Tissue Substitute** **8 Zooplastic Tissue** **J Synthetic Substitute** **K Nonautologous Tissue Substitute**	**J Truncal Valve** **Z No Qualifier**
G Mitral Valve Bicuspid valve Left atrioventricular valve Mitral annulus	**Ø Open** **4 Percutaneous Endoscopic**	**7 Autologous Tissue Substitute** **8 Zooplastic Tissue** **J Synthetic Substitute** **K Nonautologous Tissue Substitute**	**E Atrioventricular Valve, Left** **Z No Qualifier**
G Mitral Valve Bicuspid valve Left atrioventricular valve Mitral annulus	**3 Percutaneous**	**7 Autologous Tissue Substitute** **8 Zooplastic Tissue** **K Nonautologous Tissue Substitute**	**E Atrioventricular Valve, Left** **Z No Qualifier**
G Mitral Valve Bicuspid valve Left atrioventricular valve Mitral annulus	**3 Percutaneous**	**J Synthetic Substitute**	**E Atrioventricular Valve, Left** **H Transapical** **Z No Qualifier**
J Tricuspid Valve Right atrioventricular valve Tricuspid annulus	**Ø Open** **3 Percutaneous** **4 Percutaneous Endoscopic**	**7 Autologous Tissue Substitute** **8 Zooplastic Tissue** **J Synthetic Substitute** **K Nonautologous Tissue Substitute**	**G Atrioventricular Valve, Right** **Z No Qualifier**

DRG Non-OR Ø2U7[3,4]JZ

Ø Medical and Surgical
2 Heart and Great Vessels
V Restriction Definition: Partially closing an orifice or the lumen of a tubular body part
Explanation: The orifice can be a natural orifice or an artificially created orifice

Body Part Character 4	Approach Character 5	Device Character 6	Qualifier Character 7
A Heart	**Ø Open** **3 Percutaneous** **4 Percutaneous Endoscopic**	**C Extraluminal Device** **Z No Device**	**Z No Qualifier**
G Mitral Valve Bicuspid valve Left atrioventricular valve Mitral annulus	**Ø Open** **3 Percutaneous** **4 Percutaneous Endoscopic**	**Z No Device**	**Z No Qualifier**
P Pulmonary Trunk **Q Pulmonary Artery, Right** **S Pulmonary Vein, Right** Right inferior pulmonary vein Right superior pulmonary vein **T Pulmonary Vein, Left** Left inferior pulmonary vein Left superior pulmonary vein **V Superior Vena Cava** Precava	**Ø Open** **3 Percutaneous** **4 Percutaneous Endoscopic**	**C Extraluminal Device** **D Intraluminal Device** **Z No Device**	**Z No Qualifier**
R Pulmonary Artery, Left Arterial canal (duct) Botallo's duct Pulmoaortic canal	**Ø Open** **3 Percutaneous** **4 Percutaneous Endoscopic**	**C Extraluminal Device** **D Intraluminal Device** **Z No Device**	**T Ductus Arteriosus** **Z No Qualifier**
W Thoracic Aorta, Descending **X Thoracic Aorta, Ascending/Arch** Aortic arch Ascending aorta	**Ø Open** **3 Percutaneous** **4 Percutaneous Endoscopic**	**C Extraluminal Device** **D Intraluminal Device** **E Intraluminal Device, Branched or Fenestrated, One or Two Arteries** **F Intraluminal Device, Branched or Fenestrated, Three or More Arteries** **Z No Device**	**Z No Qualifier**

Ø Medical and Surgical
2 Heart and Great Vessels
W Revision Definition: Correcting, to the extent possible, a portion of a malfunctioning device or the position of a displaced device

Explanation: Revision can include correcting a malfunctioning or displaced device by taking out or putting in components of the device such as a screw or pin

Body Part Character 4	Approach Character 5	Device Character 6	Qualifier Character 7
5 Atrial Septum Interatrial septum **M Ventricular Septum** Interventricular septum	**Ø Open** **4 Percutaneous Endoscopic**	**J Synthetic Substitute**	**Z No Qualifier**
A Heart LC NC ⊞	**Ø Open** **3 Percutaneous** **4 Percutaneous Endoscopic**	**2 Monitoring Device** **3 Infusion Device** **7 Autologous Tissue Substitute** **8 Zooplastic Tissue** **C Extraluminal Device** **D Intraluminal Device** **J Synthetic Substitute** **K Nonautologous Tissue Substitute** **M Cardiac Lead** **N Intracardiac Pacemaker** **Q Implantable Heart Assist System** **Y Other Device**	**Z No Qualifier**
A Heart ⊞	**Ø Open** **3 Percutaneous** **4 Percutaneous Endoscopic**	**R Short-term External Heart Assist System**	**S Biventricular** **Z No Qualifier**
A Heart	**X External**	**2 Monitoring Device** **3 Infusion Device** **7 Autologous Tissue Substitute** **8 Zooplastic Tissue** **C Extraluminal Device** **D Intraluminal Device** **J Synthetic Substitute** **K Nonautologous Tissue Substitute** **M Cardiac Lead** **N Intracardiac Pacemaker** **Q Implantable Heart Assist System**	**Z No Qualifier**
A Heart	**X External**	**R Short-term External Heart Assist System**	**S Biventricular** **Z No Qualifier**
F Aortic Valve Aortic annulus **G Mitral Valve** Bicuspid valve Left atrioventricular valve Mitral annulus **H Pulmonary Valve** Pulmonary annulus Pulmonic valve **J Tricuspid Valve** Right atrioventricular valve Tricuspid annulus	**Ø Open** **3 Percutaneous** **4 Percutaneous Endoscopic**	**7 Autologous Tissue Substitute** **8 Zooplastic Tissue** **J Synthetic Substitute** **K Nonautologous Tissue Substitute**	**Z No Qualifier**
Y Great Vessel	**Ø Open** **3 Percutaneous** **4 Percutaneous Endoscopic**	**2 Monitoring Device** **3 Infusion Device** **7 Autologous Tissue Substitute** **8 Zooplastic Tissue** **C Extraluminal Device** **D Intraluminal Device** **J Synthetic Substitute** **K Nonautologous Tissue Substitute** **Y Other Device**	**Z No Qualifier**
Y Great Vessel	**X External**	**2 Monitoring Device** **3 Infusion Device** **7 Autologous Tissue Substitute** **8 Zooplastic Tissue** **C Extraluminal Device** **D Intraluminal Device** **J Synthetic Substitute** **K Nonautologous Tissue Substitute**	**Z No Qualifier**

Non-OR Ø2WA3[2,3,D]Z
Non-OR Ø2WA[3,4]YZ
Non-OR Ø2WAX[2,3,7,8,C,D,J,K,M,N,Q]Z
Non-OR Ø2WAXRZ
Non-OR Ø2WY3[2,3,D]Z
Non-OR Ø2WY[3,4]YZ
Non-OR Ø2WYX[2,3,7,8,C,D,J,K]Z

HAC Ø2WA[Ø,3,4]MZ when reported with T81.4Ø–T81.49, T82.6–T82.7 with 7th character A
LC Ø2WAØ[J,Q]Z
NC Ø2WA[3,4]QZ

See Appendix L for Procedure Combinations
⊞ Ø2WA[Ø,3,4]QZ
⊞ Ø2WA[Ø,3,4]RZ

Ø Medical and Surgical
2 Heart and Great Vessels
Y Transplantation Definition: Putting in or on all or a portion of a living body part taken from another individual or animal to physically take the place and/or function of all or a portion of a similar body part
Explanation: The native body part may or may not be taken out, and the transplanted body part may take over all or a portion of its function

Body Part Character 4	Approach Character 5	Device Character 6	Qualifier Character 7
A Heart LC	Ø Open	Z No Device	Ø Allogeneic 1 Syngeneic 2 Zooplastic

LC Ø2YAØZ[Ø,1,2]

Upper Arteries Ø31–Ø3W

Character Meanings

This Character Meaning table is provided as a guide to assist the user in the identification of character members that may be found in this section of code tables. It **SHOULD NOT** be used to build a PCS code.

Operation–Character 3	Body Part–Character 4	Approach–Character 5	Device–Character 6	Qualifier–Character 7
1 Bypass	Ø Internal Mammary Artery, Right	Ø Open	Ø Drainage Device	Ø Upper Arm Artery, Right OR Ultrasonic
5 Destruction	1 Internal Mammary Artery, Left	3 Percutaneous	2 Monitoring Device	1 Upper Arm Artery, Left OR Drug-Coated Balloon
7 Dilation	2 Innominate Artery	4 Percutaneous Endoscopic	3 Infusion Device	2 Upper Arm Artery, Bilateral
9 Drainage	3 Subclavian Artery, Right	X External	4 Intraluminal Device, Drug-eluting	3 Lower Arm Artery, Right
B Excision	4 Subclavian Artery, Left		5 Intraluminal Device, Drug-eluting, Two	4 Lower Arm Artery, Left
C Extirpation	5 Axillary Artery, Right		6 Intraluminal Device, Drug-eluting, Three	5 Lower Arm Artery, Bilateral
F Fragmentation	6 Axillary Artery, Left		7 Intraluminal Device, Drug-eluting, Four or More OR Autologous Tissue Substitute	6 Upper Leg Artery, Right
H Insertion	7 Brachial Artery, Right		9 Autologous Venous Tissue	7 Upper Leg Artery, Left OR Stent Retriever
J Inspection	8 Brachial Artery, Left		A Autologous Arterial Tissue	8 Upper Leg Artery, Bilateral
L Occlusion	9 Ulnar Artery, Right		B Intraluminal Device, Bioactive	9 Lower Leg Artery, Right
N Release	A Ulnar Artery, Left		C Extraluminal Device	B Lower Leg Artery, Left
P Removal	B Radial Artery, Right		D Intraluminal Device	C Lower Leg Artery, Bilateral
Q Repair	C Radial Artery, Left		E Intraluminal Device, Two	D Upper Arm Vein
R Replacement	D Hand Artery, Right		F Intraluminal Device, Three	F Lower Arm Vein
S Reposition	F Hand Artery, Left		G Intraluminal Device, Four or More	G Intracranial Artery
U Supplement	G Intracranial Artery		H Intraluminal Device, Flow Diverter	J Extracranial Artery, Right
V Restriction	H Common Carotid Artery, Right		J Synthetic Substitute	K Extracranial Artery, Left
W Revision	J Common Carotid Artery, Left		K Nonautologous Tissue Substitute	M Pulmonary Artery, Right
	K Internal Carotid Artery, Right		M Stimulator Lead	N Pulmonary Artery, Left
	L Internal Carotid Artery, Left		Y Other Device	T Abdominal Artery
	M External Carotid Artery, Right		Z No Device	V Superior Vena Cava
	N External Carotid Artery, Left			W Lower Extremity Vein
	P Vertebral Artery, Right			X Diagnostic
	Q Vertebral Artery, Left			Y Upper Artery
	R Face Artery			Z No Qualifier
	S Temporal Artery, Right			
	T Temporal Artery, Left			
	U Thyroid Artery, Right			
	V Thyroid Artery, Left			
	Y Upper Artery			

AHA Coding Clinic for table Ø31

2019, 4Q, 26 Upper artery bypass Qualifier
2019, 4Q, 26 Percutaneous approach upper artery bypass
2017, 4Q, 64-65 New qualifier values - Left to right carotid bypass
2017, 2Q, 22 Carotid artery to subclavian artery transposition
2017, 1Q, 31 Left to right common carotid artery bypass
2016, 3Q, 37 Insertion of arteriovenous graft using HeRO device
2016, 3Q, 39 Revision of arteriovenous graft
2013, 4Q, 125 Stage II cephalic vein transposition (superficialization) of arteriovenous fistula
2013, 1Q, 27 Creation of radial artery fistula

AHA Coding Clinic for table Ø37

2019, 4Q, 27 Bifurcation Qualifier
2019, 3Q, 29 Transcarotid arterial catheterization
2018, 2Q, 24 Coronary artery bifurcation
2016, 4Q, 86 Peripheral artery, number of stents
2016, 4Q, 86-87 Coronary and peripheral artery bifurcation
2015, 1Q, 32 Deployment of stent for herniated/migrated coil in basilar artery

AHA Coding Clinic for table Ø3B

2016, 2Q, 12 Resection of malignant neoplasm of infratemporal fossa

AHA Coding Clinic for table Ø3C

2019, 4Q, 27 Bifurcation Qualifier
2018, 4Q, 47-48 Endovascular thrombectomy with stent retriever
2018, 2Q, 24 Coronary artery bifurcation
2017, 4Q, 64-65 New qualifier values - Left to right carotid bypass
2017, 2Q, 23 Thrombectomy via Fogarty catheter
2016, 4Q, 86-87 Coronary and peripheral artery bifurcation
2016, 2Q, 11 Carotid endarterectomy with patch angioplasty
2015, 1Q, 29 Discontinued carotid endarterectomy

AHA Coding Clinic for table Ø3H

2020, 1Q, 25 Elephant trunk repair of aortic dissection
2016, 2Q, 32 Arterial catheter placement

AHA Coding Clinic for table Ø3J

2015, 1Q, 29 Discontinued carotid endarterectomy

AHA Coding Clinic for table Ø3L

2016, 2Q, 30 Clipping (occlusion) of cerebral artery, decompressive craniectomy and storage of bone flap in abdominal wall
2014, 4Q, 20 Control of epistaxis
2014, 4Q, 37 Endovascular embolization of arteriovenous malformation using Onyx-18 liquid

AHA Coding Clinic for table Ø3Q

2017, 1Q, 31 Left to right common carotid artery bypass

AHA Coding Clinic for table Ø3S

2017, 2Q, 22 Carotid artery to subclavian artery transposition
2015, 3Q, 27 Moyamoya disease and hemispheric pial synagiosis with craniotomy

AHA Coding Clinic for table Ø3U

2019, 1Q, 22 Cerebral artery fusiform aneurysm repair via wrapping
2016, 2Q, 11 Carotid endarterectomy with patch angioplasty

AHA Coding Clinic for table Ø3V

2019, 4Q, 27-28 Aneurysm treatment using flow diverter stent
2019, 1Q, 22 Cerebral artery fusiform aneurysm repair via wrapping
2016, 1Q, 19 Embolization of superior hypophyseal aneurysm using stent-assisted coil

AHA Coding Clinic for table Ø3W

2016, 3Q, 39 Revision of arteriovenous graft
2015, 1Q, 32 Deployment of stent for herniated/migrated coil in basilar artery

Upper Arteries

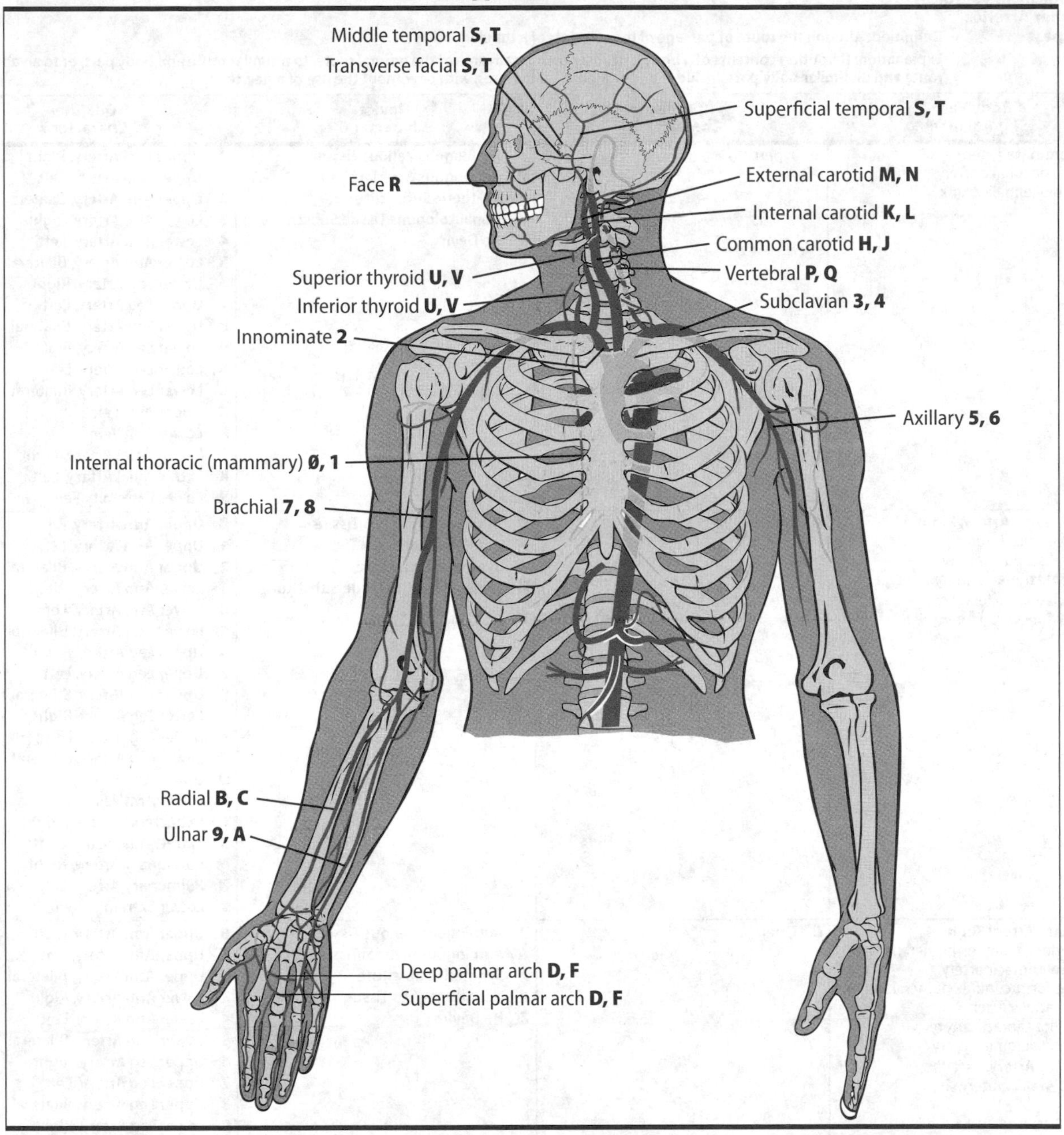

Middle temporal **S, T**
Transverse facial **S, T**
Superficial temporal **S, T**
Face **R**
External carotid **M, N**
Internal carotid **K, L**
Common carotid **H, J**
Superior thyroid **U, V**
Vertebral **P, Q**
Inferior thyroid **U, V**
Subclavian **3, 4**
Innominate **2**
Axillary **5, 6**
Internal thoracic (mammary) **Ø, 1**
Brachial **7, 8**
Radial **B, C**
Ulnar **9, A**
Deep palmar arch **D, F**
Superficial palmar arch **D, F**

Head and Neck Arteries

Middle cerebral **G**
Anterior cerebral **G**
Posterior communicating **G**
Anterior communicating **G**
Posterior cerebral **G**
Ophthalmic **G**
Basilar **G**
Internal carotid **K,L**
External carotid **M,N**
Vertebral **P,Q**
Common carotid **H,J**

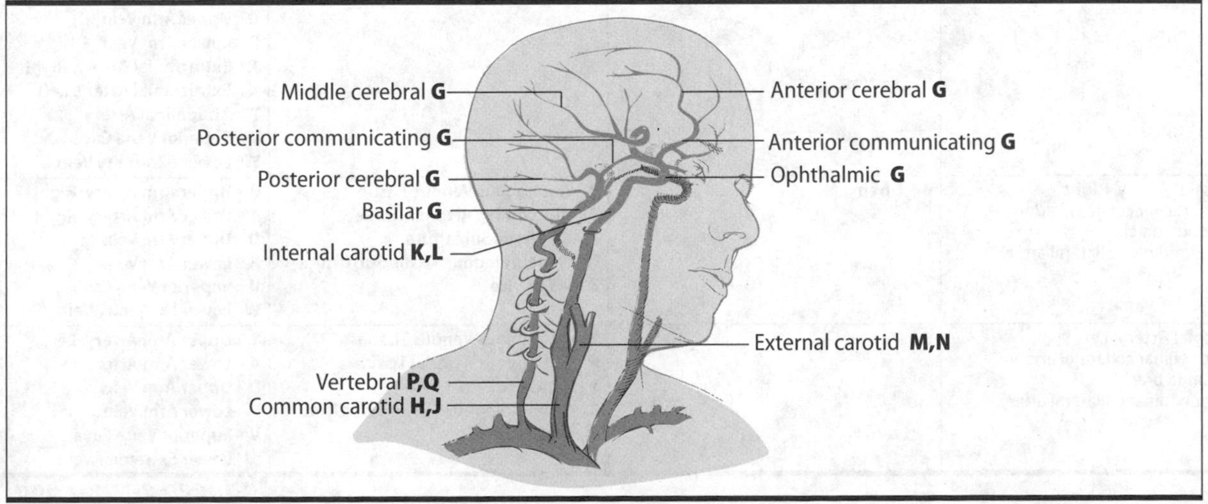

Ø Medical and Surgical
3 Upper Arteries
1 Bypass Definition: Altering the route of passage of the contents of a tubular body part

Explanation: Rerouting contents of a body part to a downstream area of the normal route, to a similar route and body part, or to an abnormal route and dissimilar body part. Includes one or more anastomoses, with or without the use of a device.

Body Part Character 4	Approach Character 5	Device Character 6	Qualifier Character 7
2 Innominate Artery Brachiocephalic artery Brachiocephalic trunk	**Ø Open**	**9 Autologous Venous Tissue** **A Autologous Arterial Tissue** **J Synthetic Substitute** **K Nonautologous Tissue Substitute** **Z No Device**	**Ø Upper Arm Artery, Right** **1 Upper Arm Artery, Left** **2 Upper Arm Artery, Bilateral** **3 Lower Arm Artery, Right** **4 Lower Arm Artery, Left** **5 Lower Arm Artery, Bilateral** **6 Upper Leg Artery, Right** **7 Upper Leg Artery, Left** **8 Upper Leg Artery, Bilateral** **9 Lower Leg Artery, Right** **B Lower Leg Artery, Left** **C Lower Leg Artery, Bilateral** **D Upper Arm Vein** **F Lower Arm Vein** **J Extracranial Artery, Right** **K Extracranial Artery, Left** **W Lower Extremity Vein**
3 Subclavian Artery, Right Costocervical trunk Dorsal scapular artery Internal thoracic artery **4 Subclavian Artery, Left** *See 3 Subclavian Artery, Right*	**Ø Open**	**9 Autologous Venous Tissue** **A Autologous Arterial Tissue** **J Synthetic Substitute** **K Nonautologous Tissue Substitute** **Z No Device**	**Ø Upper Arm Artery, Right** **1 Upper Arm Artery, Left** **2 Upper Arm Artery, Bilateral** **3 Lower Arm Artery, Right** **4 Lower Arm Artery, Left** **5 Lower Arm Artery, Bilateral** **6 Upper Leg Artery, Right** **7 Upper Leg Artery, Left** **8 Upper Leg Artery, Bilateral** **9 Lower Leg Artery, Right** **B Lower Leg Artery, Left** **C Lower Leg Artery, Bilateral** **D Upper Arm Vein** **F Lower Arm Vein** **J Extracranial Artery, Right** **K Extracranial Artery, Left** **M Pulmonary Artery, Right** **N Pulmonary Artery, Left** **W Lower Extremity Vein**
5 Axillary Artery, Right Anterior circumflex humeral artery Lateral thoracic artery Posterior circumflex humeral artery Subscapular artery Superior thoracic artery Thoracoacromial artery **6 Axillary Artery, Left** *See 5 Axillary Artery, Right*	**Ø Open**	**9 Autologous Venous Tissue** **A Autologous Arterial Tissue** **J Synthetic Substitute** **K Nonautologous Tissue Substitute** **Z No Device**	**Ø Upper Arm Artery, Right** **1 Upper Arm Artery, Left** **2 Upper Arm Artery, Bilateral** **3 Lower Arm Artery, Right** **4 Lower Arm Artery, Left** **5 Lower Arm Artery, Bilateral** **6 Upper Leg Artery, Right** **7 Upper Leg Artery, Left** **8 Upper Leg Artery, Bilateral** **9 Lower Leg Artery, Right** **B Lower Leg Artery, Left** **C Lower Leg Artery, Bilateral** **D Upper Arm Vein** **F Lower Arm Vein** **J Extracranial Artery, Right** **K Extracranial Artery, Left** **T Abdominal Artery** **V Superior Vena Cava** **W Lower Extremity Vein**
7 Brachial Artery, Right Inferior ulnar collateral artery Profunda brachii Superior ulnar collateral artery	**Ø Open**	**9 Autologous Venous Tissue** **A Autologous Arterial Tissue** **J Synthetic Substitute** **K Nonautologous Tissue Substitute** **Z No Device**	**Ø Upper Arm Artery, Right** **3 Lower Arm Artery, Right** **D Upper Arm Vein** **F Lower Arm Vein** **V Superior Vena Cava** **W Lower Extremity Vein**
8 Brachial Artery, Left Inferior ulnar collateral artery Profunda brachii Superior ulnar collateral artery	**Ø Open**	**9 Autologous Venous Tissue** **A Autologous Arterial Tissue** **J Synthetic Substitute** **K Nonautologous Tissue Substitute** **Z No Device**	**1 Upper Arm Artery, Left** **4 Lower Arm Artery, Left** **D Upper Arm Vein** **F Lower Arm Vein** **V Superior Vena Cava** **W Lower Extremity Vein**

Ø31 Continued on next page

Ø Medical and Surgical
3 Upper Arteries
1 Bypass Definition: Altering the route of passage of the contents of a tubular body part

Explanation: Rerouting contents of a body part to a downstream area of the normal route, to a similar route and body part, or to an abnormal route and dissimilar body part. Includes one or more anastomoses, with or without the use of a device.

Ø31 Continued

Body Part Character 4	Approach Character 5	Device Character 6	Qualifier Character 7
9 Ulnar Artery, Right Anterior ulnar recurrent artery Common interosseous artery Posterior ulnar recurrent artery **B Radial Artery, Right** Radial recurrent artery	**Ø Open**	**9 Autologous Venous Tissue** **A Autologous Arterial Tissue** **J Synthetic Substitute** **K Nonautologous Tissue Substitute** **Z No Device**	**3 Lower Arm Artery, Right** **F Lower Arm Vein**
9 Ulnar Artery, Right Anterior ulnar recurrent artery Common interosseous artery Posterior ulnar recurrent artery **B Radial Artery, Right** Radial recurrent artery	**3 Percutaneous**	**Z No Device**	**F Lower Arm Vein**
A Ulnar Artery, Left Anterior ulnar recurrent artery Common interosseous artery Posterior ulnar recurrent artery **C Radial Artery, Left** Radial recurrent artery	**Ø Open**	**9 Autologous Venous Tissue** **A Autologous Arterial Tissue** **J Synthetic Substitute** **K Nonautologous Tissue Substitute** **Z No Device**	**4 Lower Arm Artery, Left** **F Lower Arm Vein**
A Ulnar Artery, Left Anterior ulnar recurrent artery Common interosseous artery Posterior ulnar recurrent artery **C Radial Artery, Left** Radial recurrent artery	**3 Percutaneous**	**Z No Device**	**F Lower Arm Vein**
G Intracranial Artery Anterior cerebral artery Anterior choroidal artery Anterior communicating artery Basilar artery Circle of Willis Internal carotid artery, intracranial portion Middle cerebral artery Ophthalmic artery Posterior cerebral artery Posterior communicating artery Posterior inferior cerebellar artery (PICA) **S Temporal Artery, Right** Middle temporal artery Superficial temporal artery Transverse facial artery **T Temporal Artery, Left** ***See*** *S Temporal Artery, Right*	**Ø Open**	**9 Autologous Venous Tissue** **A Autologous Arterial Tissue** **J Synthetic Substitute** **K Nonautologous Tissue Substitute** **Z No Device**	**G Intracranial Artery**
H Common Carotid Artery, Right **J Common Carotid Artery, Left**	**Ø Open**	**9 Autologous Venous Tissue** **A Autologous Arterial Tissue** **J Synthetic Substitute** **K Nonautologous Tissue Substitute** **Z No Device**	**G Intracranial Artery** **J Extracranial Artery, Right** **K Extracranial Artery, Left** **Y Upper Artery**
K Internal Carotid Artery, Right Caroticotympanic artery Carotid sinus **L Internal Carotid Artery, Left** Caroticotympanic artery Carotid sinus **M External Carotid Artery, Right** Ascending pharyngeal artery Internal maxillary artery Lingual artery Maxillary artery Occipital artery Posterior auricular artery Superior thyroid artery **N External Carotid Artery, Left** Ascending pharyngeal artery Internal maxillary artery Lingual artery Maxillary artery Occipital artery Posterior auricular artery Superior thyroid artery	**Ø Open**	**9 Autologous Venous Tissue** **A Autologous Arterial Tissue** **J Synthetic Substitute** **K Nonautologous Tissue Substitute** **Z No Device**	**J Extracranial Artery, Right** **K Extracranial Artery, Left**

Ø Medical and Surgical
3 Upper Arteries
5 Destruction Definition: Physical eradication of all or a portion of a body part by the direct use of energy, force, or a destructive agent
Explanation: None of the body part is physically taken out

Body Part Character 4		Approach Character 5	Device Character 6	Qualifier Character 7
Ø Internal Mammary Artery, Right Anterior intercostal artery Internal thoracic artery Musculophrenic artery Pericardiophrenic artery Superior epigastric artery **1 Internal Mammary Artery, Left** *See Ø Internal Mammary Artery, Right* **2 Innominate Artery** Brachiocephalic artery Brachiocephalic trunk **3 Subclavian Artery, Right** Costocervical trunk Dorsal scapular artery Internal thoracic artery **4 Subclavian Artery, Left** *See 3 Subclavian Artery, Right* **5 Axillary Artery, Right** Anterior circumflex humeral artery Lateral thoracic artery Posterior circumflex humeral artery Subscapular artery Superior thoracic artery Thoracoacromial artery **6 Axillary Artery, Left** *See 5 Axillary Artery, Right* **7 Brachial Artery, Right** Inferior ulnar collateral artery Profunda brachii Superior ulnar collateral artery **8 Brachial Artery, Left** *See 7 Brachial Artery, Right* **9 Ulnar Artery, Right** Anterior ulnar recurrent artery Common interosseous artery Posterior ulnar recurrent artery **A Ulnar Artery, Left** *See 9 Ulnar Artery, Right* **B Radial Artery, Right** Radial recurrent artery **C Radial Artery, Left** *See B Radial Artery, Right* **D Hand Artery, Right** Deep palmar arch Princeps pollicis artery Radialis indicis Superficial palmar arch **F Hand Artery, Left** *See D Hand Artery, Right* **G Intracranial Artery** Anterior cerebral artery Anterior choroidal artery Anterior communicating artery Basilar artery Circle of Willis Internal carotid artery, intracranial portion Middle cerebral artery Ophthalmic artery Posterior cerebral artery Posterior communicating artery Posterior inferior cerebellar artery (PICA)	**H Common Carotid Artery, Right** **J Common Carotid Artery, Left** **K Internal Carotid Artery, Right** Caroticotympanic artery Carotid sinus **L Internal Carotid Artery, Left** *See K Internal Carotid Artery, Right* **M External Carotid Artery, Right** Ascending pharyngeal artery Internal maxillary artery Lingual artery Maxillary artery Occipital artery Posterior auricular artery Superior thyroid artery **N External Carotid Artery, Left** *See M External Carotid Artery, Right* **P Vertebral Artery, Right** Anterior spinal artery Posterior spinal artery **Q Vertebral Artery, Left** *See P Vertebral Artery, Right* **R Face Artery** Angular artery Ascending palatine artery External maxillary artery Facial artery Inferior labial artery Submental artery Superior labial artery **S Temporal Artery, Right** Middle temporal artery Superficial temporal artery Transverse facial artery **T Temporal Artery, Left** *See S Temporal Artery, Right* **U Thyroid Artery, Right** Cricothyroid artery Hyoid artery Sternocleidomastoid artery Superior laryngeal artery Superior thyroid artery Thyrocervical trunk **V Thyroid Artery, Left** *See U Thyroid Artery, Right* **Y Upper Artery** Aortic intercostal artery Bronchial artery Esophageal artery Subcostal artery	**Ø Open** **3 Percutaneous** **4 Percutaneous Endoscopic**	**Z No Device**	**Z No Qualifier**

Ø Medical and Surgical
3 Upper Arteries
7 Dilation Definition: Expanding an orifice or the lumen of a tubular body part

Explanation: The orifice can be a natural orifice or an artificially created orifice. Accomplished by stretching a tubular body part using intraluminal pressure or by cutting part of the orifice or wall of the tubular body part.

Body Part Character 4		Approach Character 5	Device Character 6	Qualifier Character 7
Ø Internal Mammary Artery, Right Anterior intercostal artery Internal thoracic artery Musculophrenic artery Pericardiophrenic artery Superior epigastric artery **1 Internal Mammary Artery, Left** *See Ø Internal Mammary Artery, Right* **2 Innominate Artery** Brachiocephalic artery Brachiocephalic trunk **3 Subclavian Artery, Right** Costocervical trunk Dorsal scapular artery Internal thoracic artery **4 Subclavian Artery, Left** *See 3 Subclavian Artery, Right* **5 Axillary Artery, Right** Anterior circumflex humeral artery Lateral thoracic artery Posterior circumflex humeral artery Subscapular artery Superior thoracic artery Thoracoacromial artery	**6 Axillary Artery, Left** *See 5 Axillary Artery, Right* **7 Brachial Artery, Right** Inferior ulnar collateral artery Profunda brachii Superior ulnar collateral artery **8 Brachial Artery, Left** *See 7 Brachial Artery, Right* **9 Ulnar Artery, Right** Anterior ulnar recurrent artery Common interosseous artery Posterior ulnar recurrent artery **A Ulnar Artery, Left** *See 9 Ulnar Artery, Right* **B Radial Artery, Right** Radial recurrent artery **C Radial Artery, Left** *See B Radial Artery, Right*	**Ø Open** **3 Percutaneous** **4 Percutaneous Endoscopic**	**4 Intraluminal Device, Drug-eluting** **5 Intraluminal Device, Drug-eluting, Two** **6 Intraluminal Device, Drug-eluting, Three** **7 Intraluminal Device, Drug-eluting, Four or More** **E Intraluminal Device, Two** **F Intraluminal Device, Three** **G Intraluminal Device, Four or More**	**Z No Qualifier**
Ø Internal Mammary Artery, Right Anterior intercostal artery Internal thoracic artery Musculophrenic artery Pericardiophrenic artery Superior epigastric artery **1 Internal Mammary Artery, Left** *See Ø Internal Mammary Artery, Right* **2 Innominate Artery** Brachiocephalic artery Brachiocephalic trunk **3 Subclavian Artery, Right** Costocervical trunk Dorsal scapular artery Internal thoracic artery **4 Subclavian Artery, Left** *See 3 Subclavian Artery, Right* **5 Axillary Artery, Right** Anterior circumflex humeral artery Lateral thoracic artery Posterior circumflex humeral artery Subscapular artery Superior thoracic artery Thoracoacromial artery	**6 Axillary Artery, Left** *See 5 Axillary Artery, Right* **7 Brachial Artery, Right** Inferior ulnar collateral artery Profunda brachii Superior ulnar collateral artery **8 Brachial Artery, Left** *See 7 Brachial Artery, Right* **9 Ulnar Artery, Right** Anterior ulnar recurrent artery Common interosseous artery Posterior ulnar recurrent artery **A Ulnar Artery, Left** *See 9 Ulnar Artery, Right* **B Radial Artery, Right** Radial recurrent artery **C Radial Artery, Left** *See B Radial Artery, Right*	**Ø Open** **3 Percutaneous** **4 Percutaneous Endoscopic**	**D Intraluminal Device** **Z No Device**	**1 Drug-Coated Balloon** **Z No Qualifier**

Ø37 Continued on next page

Ø Medical and Surgical
3 Upper Arteries
7 Dilation

Ø37 Continued

Definition: Expanding an orifice or the lumen of a tubular body part

Explanation: The orifice can be a natural orifice or an artificially created orifice. Accomplished by stretching a tubular body part using intraluminal pressure or by cutting part of the orifice or wall of the tubular body part.

Body Part Character 4	Approach Character 5	Device Character 6	Qualifier Character 7
D Hand Artery, Right Deep palmar arch Princeps pollicis artery Radialis indicis Superficial palmar arch **F Hand Artery, Left** *See D Hand Artery, Right* **G Intracranial Artery** NC Anterior cerebral artery Anterior choroidal artery Anterior communicating artery Basilar artery Circle of Willis Internal carotid artery, intracranial portion Middle cerebral artery Ophthalmic artery Posterior cerebral artery Posterior communicating artery Posterior inferior cerebellar artery (PICA) **H Common Carotid Artery, Right** **J Common Carotid Artery, Left** **K Internal Carotid Artery, Right** Caroticotympanic artery Carotid sinus **L Internal Carotid Artery, Left** *See K Internal Carotid Artery, Right* **M External Carotid Artery, Right** Ascending pharyngeal artery Internal maxillary artery Lingual artery Maxillary artery Occipital artery Posterior auricular artery Superior thyroid artery **N External Carotid Artery, Left** *See M External Carotid Artery, Right* **P Vertebral Artery, Right** Anterior spinal artery Posterior spinal artery **Q Vertebral Artery, Left** *See P Vertebral Artery, Right* **R Face Artery** Angular artery Ascending palatine artery External maxillary artery Facial artery Inferior labial artery Submental artery Superior labial artery **S Temporal Artery, Right** Middle temporal artery Superficial temporal artery Transverse facial artery **T Temporal Artery, Left** *See S Temporal Artery, Right* **U Thyroid Artery, Right** Cricothyroid artery Hyoid artery Sternocleidomastoid artery Superior laryngeal artery Superior thyroid artery Thyrocervical trunk **V Thyroid Artery, Left** *See U Thyroid Artery, Right* **Y Upper Artery** Aortic intercostal artery Bronchial artery Esophageal artery Subcostal artery	**Ø** Open **3** Percutaneous **4** Percutaneous Endoscopic	**4** Intraluminal Device, Drug-eluting **5** Intraluminal Device, Drug-eluting, Two **6** Intraluminal Device, Drug-eluting, Three **7** Intraluminal Device, Drug-eluting, Four or More **D** Intraluminal Device **E** Intraluminal Device, Two **F** Intraluminal Device, Three **G** Intraluminal Device, Four or More **Z** No Device	**Z** No Qualifier

NC Ø37G[3,4]ZZ

Ø Medical and Surgical
3 Upper Arteries
9 Drainage Definition: Taking or letting out fluids and/or gases from a body part
Explanation: The qualifier DIAGNOSTIC is used to identify drainage procedures that are biopsies

Body Part Character 4	Body Part Character 4	Approach Character 5	Device Character 6	Qualifier Character 7
Ø **Internal Mammary Artery, Right** Anterior intercostal artery Internal thoracic artery Musculophrenic artery Pericardiophrenic artery Superior epigastric artery 1 **Internal Mammary Artery, Left** *See Ø Internal Mammary Artery, Right above* 2 **Innominate Artery** Brachiocephalic artery Brachiocephalic trunk 3 **Subclavian Artery, Right** Costocervical trunk Dorsal scapular artery Internal thoracic artery 4 **Subclavian Artery, Left** *See 3 Subclavian Artery, Right* 5 **Axillary Artery, Right** Anterior circumflex humeral artery Lateral thoracic artery Posterior circumflex humeral artery Subscapular artery Superior thoracic artery Thoracoacromial artery 6 **Axillary Artery, Left** *See 5 Axillary Artery, Right* 7 **Brachial Artery, Right** Inferior ulnar collateral artery Profunda brachii Superior ulnar collateral artery 8 **Brachial Artery, Left** *See 7 Brachial Artery, Right* 9 **Ulnar Artery, Right** Anterior ulnar recurrent artery Common interosseous artery Posterior ulnar recurrent artery A **Ulnar Artery, Left** *See 9 Ulnar Artery, Right* B **Radial Artery, Right** Radial recurrent artery C **Radial Artery, Left** *See B Radial Artery, Right* D **Hand Artery, Right** Deep palmar arch Princeps pollicis artery Radialis indicis Superficial palmar arch F **Hand Artery, Left** *See D Hand Artery, Right* G **Intracranial Artery** Anterior cerebral artery Anterior choroidal artery Anterior communicating artery Basilar artery Circle of Willis Internal carotid artery, intracranial portion Middle cerebral artery Ophthalmic artery Posterior cerebral artery Posterior communicating artery Posterior inferior cerebellar artery (PICA)	H **Common Carotid Artery, Right** J **Common Carotid Artery, Left** K **Internal Carotid Artery, Right** Caroticotympanic artery Carotid sinus L **Internal Carotid Artery, Left** *See K Internal Carotid Artery, Right* M **External Carotid Artery, Right** Ascending pharyngeal artery Internal maxillary artery Lingual artery Maxillary artery Occipital artery Posterior auricular artery Superior thyroid artery N **External Carotid Artery, Left** *See M External Carotid Artery, Right* P **Vertebral Artery, Right** Anterior spinal artery Posterior spinal artery Q **Vertebral Artery, Left** *See P Vertebral Artery, Right* R **Face Artery** Angular artery Ascending palatine artery External maxillary artery Facial artery Inferior labial artery Submental artery Superior labial artery S **Temporal Artery, Right** Middle temporal artery Superficial temporal artery Transverse facial artery T **Temporal Artery, Left** *See S Temporal Artery, Right* U **Thyroid Artery, Right** Cricothyroid artery Hyoid artery Sternocleidomastoid artery Superior laryngeal artery Superior thyroid artery Thyrocervical trunk V **Thyroid Artery, Left** *See U Thyroid Artery, Right* Y **Upper Artery** Aortic intercostal artery Bronchial artery Esophageal artery Subcostal artery	Ø Open 3 Percutaneous 4 Percutaneous Endoscopic	Ø Drainage Device	Z No Qualifier

Non-OR Ø39[Ø,1,2,3,4,5,6,7,8,9,A,B,C,D,F,G,H,J,K,L,M,N,P,Q,R,S,T,U,V,Y][Ø,3,4]ØZ

Ø39 Continued on next page

Ø Medical and Surgical
3 Upper Arteries
9 Drainage Definition: Taking or letting out fluids and/or gases from a body part
Explanation: The qualifier DIAGNOSTIC is used to identify drainage procedures that are biopsies

Ø39 Continued

Body Part Character 4		Approach Character 5	Device Character 6	Qualifier Character 7
Ø Internal Mammary Artery, Right Anterior intercostal artery Internal thoracic artery Musculophrenic artery Pericardiophrenic artery Superior epigastric artery **1 Internal Mammary Artery, Left** **See** *Ø Internal Mammary Artery, Right* **2 Innominate Artery** Brachiocephalic artery Brachiocephalic trunk **3 Subclavian Artery, Right** Costocervical trunk Dorsal scapular artery Internal thoracic artery **4 Subclavian Artery, Left** **See** *3 Subclavian Artery, Right* **5 Axillary Artery, Right** Anterior circumflex humeral artery Lateral thoracic artery Posterior circumflex humeral artery Subscapular artery Superior thoracic artery Thoracoacromial artery **6 Axillary Artery, Left** **See** *5 Axillary Artery, Right* **7 Brachial Artery, Right** Inferior ulnar collateral artery Profunda brachii Superior ulnar collateral artery **8 Brachial Artery, Left** **See** *7 Brachial Artery, Right* **9 Ulnar Artery, Right** Anterior ulnar recurrent artery Common interosseous artery Posterior ulnar recurrent artery **A Ulnar Artery, Left** **See** *9 Ulnar Artery, Right* **B Radial Artery, Right** Radial recurrent artery **C Radial Artery, Left** **See** *B Radial Artery, Right* **D Hand Artery, Right** Deep palmar arch Princeps pollicis artery Radialis indicis Superficial palmar arch **F Hand Artery, Left** **See** *D Hand Artery, Right* **G Intracranial Artery** Anterior cerebral artery Anterior choroidal artery Anterior communicating artery Basilar artery Circle of Willis Internal carotid artery, intracranial portion Middle cerebral artery Ophthalmic artery Posterior cerebral artery Posterior communicating artery Posterior inferior cerebellar artery (PICA)	**H Common Carotid Artery, Right** **J Common Carotid Artery, Left** **K Internal Carotid Artery, Right** Caroticotympanic artery Carotid sinus **L Internal Carotid Artery, Left** **See** *K Internal Carotid Artery, Right* **M External Carotid Artery, Right** Ascending pharyngeal artery Internal maxillary artery LIngual artery Maxillary artery Occipital artery Posterior auricular artery Superior thyroid artery **N External Carotid Artery, Left** **See** *M External Carotid Artery, Right* **P Vertebral Artery, Right** Anterior spinal artery Posterior spinal artery **Q Vertebral Artery, Left** **See** *P Vertebral Artery, Right* **R Face Artery** Angular artery Ascending palatine artery External maxillary artery Facial artery Inferior labial artery Submental artery Superior labial artery **S Temporal Artery, Right** Middle temporal artery Superficial temporal artery Transverse facial artery **T Temporal Artery, Left** **See** *S Temporal Artery, Right* **U Thyroid Artery, Right** Cricothyroid artery Hyoid artery Sternocleidomastoid artery Superior laryngeal artery Superior thyroid artery Thyrocervical trunk **V Thyroid Artery, Left** **See** *U Thyroid Artery, Right* **Y Upper Artery** Aortic intercostal artery Bronchial artery Esophageal artery Subcostal artery	**Ø Open** **3 Percutaneous** **4 Percutaneous Endoscopic**	**Z No Device**	**X Diagnostic** **Z No Qualifier**

Non-OR Ø39[Ø,1,2,3,4,5,6,7,8,9,A,B,C,D,F,G,H,J,K,L,M,N,P,Q,R,S,T,U,V,Y]3ZX
Non-OR Ø39[Ø,1,2,3,4,5,6,7,8,9,A,B,C,D,F,G,H,J,K,L,M,N,P,Q,R,S,T,U,V,Y][Ø,3,4]ZZ

Ø Medical and Surgical
3 Upper Arteries
B Excision Definition: Cutting out or off, without replacement, a portion of a body part
Explanation: The qualifier DIAGNOSTIC is used to identify excision procedures that are biopsies

Body Part Character 4		Approach Character 5	Device Character 6	Qualifier Character 7
Ø Internal Mammary Artery, Right Anterior intercostal artery Internal thoracic artery Musculophrenic artery Pericardiophrenic artery Superior epigastric artery **1 Internal Mammary Artery, Left** *See Ø Internal Mammary Artery, Right* **2 Innominate Artery** Brachiocephalic artery Brachiocephalic trunk **3 Subclavian Artery, Right** Costocervical trunk Dorsal scapular artery Internal thoracic artery **4 Subclavian Artery, Left** *See 3 Subclavian Artery, Right* **5 Axillary Artery, Right** Anterior circumflex humeral artery Lateral thoracic artery Posterior circumflex humeral artery Subscapular artery Superior thoracic artery Thoracoacromial artery **6 Axillary Artery, Left** *See 5 Axillary Artery, Right* **7 Brachial Artery, Right** Inferior ulnar collateral artery Profunda brachii Superior ulnar collateral artery **8 Brachial Artery, Left** *See 7 Brachial Artery, Right* **9 Ulnar Artery, Right** Anterior ulnar recurrent artery Common interosseous artery Posterior ulnar recurrent artery **A Ulnar Artery, Left** *See 9 Ulnar Artery, Right* **B Radial Artery, Right** Radial recurrent artery **C Radial Artery, Left** *See B Radial Artery, Right* **D Hand Artery, Right** Deep palmar arch Princeps pollicis artery Radialis indicis Superficial palmar arch **F Hand Artery, Left** *See D Hand Artery, Right* **G Intracranial Artery** Anterior cerebral artery Anterior choroidal artery Anterior communicating artery Basilar artery Circle of Willis Internal carotid artery, intracranial portion Middle cerebral artery Ophthalmic artery Posterior cerebral artery Posterior communicating artery Posterior inferior cerebellar artery (PICA)	**H Common Carotid Artery, Right** **J Common Carotid Artery, Left** **K Internal Carotid Artery, Right** Caroticotympanic artery Carotid sinus **L Internal Carotid Artery, Left** *See K Internal Carotid Artery, Right* **M External Carotid Artery, Right** Ascending pharyngeal artery Internal maxillary artery Lingual artery Maxillary artery Occipital artery Posterior auricular artery Superior thyroid artery **N External Carotid Artery, Left** *See M External Carotid Artery, Right* **P Vertebral Artery, Right** Anterior spinal artery Posterior spinal artery **Q Vertebral Artery, Left** *See P Vertebral Artery, Right* **R Face Artery** Angular artery Ascending palatine artery External maxillary artery Facial artery Inferior labial artery Submental artery Superior labial artery **S Temporal Artery, Right** Middle temporal artery Superficial temporal artery Transverse facial artery **T Temporal Artery, Left** *See S Temporal Artery, Right* **U Thyroid Artery, Right** Cricothyroid artery Hyoid artery Sternocleidomastoid artery Superior laryngeal artery Superior thyroid artery Thyrocervical trunk **V Thyroid Artery, Left** *See U Thyroid Artery, Right* **Y Upper Artery** Aortic intercostal artery Bronchial artery Esophageal artery Subcostal artery	**Ø Open** **3 Percutaneous** **4 Percutaneous Endoscopic**	**Z No Device**	**X Diagnostic** **Z No Qualifier**

Ø Medical and Surgical
3 Upper Arteries
C Extirpation Definition: Taking or cutting out solid matter from a body part

Explanation: The solid matter may be an abnormal byproduct of a biological function or a foreign body; it may be imbedded in a body part or in the lumen of a tubular body part. The solid matter may or may not have been previously broken into pieces.

Body Part Character 4		Approach Character 5	Device Character 6	Qualifier Character 7
Ø Internal Mammary Artery, Right Anterior intercostal artery Internal thoracic artery Musculophrenic artery Pericardiophrenic artery Superior epigastric artery **1 Internal Mammary Artery, Left** *See Ø Internal Mammary Artery, Right* **2 Innominate Artery** Brachiocephalic artery Brachiocephalic trunk **3 Subclavian Artery, Right** Costocervical trunk Dorsal scapular artery Internal thoracic artery **4 Subclavian Artery, Left** *See 3 Subclavian Artery, Right* **5 Axillary Artery, Right** Anterior circumflex humeral artery Lateral thoracic artery Posterior circumflex humeral artery Subscapular artery Superior thoracic artery Thoracoacromial artery **6 Axillary Artery, Left** *See 5 Axillary Artery, Right* **7 Brachial Artery, Right** Inferior ulnar collateral artery Profunda brachii Superior ulnar collateral artery **8 Brachial Artery, Left** *See 7 Brachial Artery, Right* **9 Ulnar Artery, Right** Anterior ulnar recurrent artery Common interosseous artery Posterior ulnar recurrent artery	**A Ulnar Artery, Left** *See 9 Ulnar Artery, Right* **B Radial Artery, Right** Radial recurrent artery **C Radial Artery, Left** *See B Radial Artery, Right* **D Hand Artery, Right** Deep palmar arch Princeps pollicis artery Radialis indicis Superficial palmar arch **F Hand Artery, Left** *See D Hand Artery, Right* **R Face Artery** Angular artery Ascending palatine artery External maxillary artery Facial artery Inferior labial artery Submental artery Superior labial artery **S Temporal Artery, Right** Middle temporal artery Superficial temporal artery Transverse facial artery **T Temporal Artery, Left** *See S Temporal Artery, Right* **U Thyroid Artery, Right** Cricothyroid artery Hyoid artery Sternocleidomastoid artery Superior laryngeal artery Superior thyroid artery Thyrocervical trunk **V Thyroid Artery, Left** *See U Thyroid Artery, Right* **Y Upper Artery** Aortic intercostal artery Bronchial artery Esophageal artery Subcostal artery	**Ø Open** **3 Percutaneous** **4 Percutaneous Endoscopic**	**Z No Device**	**Z No Qualifier**
G Intracranial Artery Anterior cerebral artery Anterior choroidal artery Anterior communicating artery Basilar artery Circle of Willis Internal carotid artery, intracranial portion Middle cerebral artery Ophthalmic artery Posterior cerebral artery Posterior communicating artery Posterior inferior cerebellar artery (PICA) **H Common Carotid Artery, Right** **J Common Carotid Artery, Left** **K Internal Carotid Artery, Right** Caroticotympanic artery Carotid sinus	**L Internal Carotid Artery, Left** *See K Internal Carotid Artery, Right* **M External Carotid Artery, Right** Ascending pharyngeal artery Internal maxillary artery Lingual artery Maxillary artery Occipital artery Posterior auricular artery Superior thyroid artery **N External Carotid Artery, Left** *See M External Carotid Artery, Right* **P Vertebral Artery, Right** Anterior spinal artery Posterior spinal artery **Q Vertebral Artery, Left** *See P Vertebral Artery, Right*	**Ø Open** **4 Percutaneous Endoscopic**	**Z No Device**	**Z No Qualifier**

Ø3C Continued on next page

Ø3C Continued

Ø Medical and Surgical
3 Upper Arteries
C Extirpation Definition: Taking or cutting out solid matter from a body part

Explanation: The solid matter may be an abnormal byproduct of a biological function or a foreign body; it may be imbedded in a body part or in the lumen of a tubular body part. The solid matter may or may not have been previously broken into pieces.

Body Part Character 4		Approach Character 5	Device Character 6	Qualifier Character 7
G Intracranial Artery Anterior cerebral artery Anterior choroidal artery Anterior communicating artery Basilar artery Circle of Willis Internal carotid artery, intracranial portion Middle cerebral artery Ophthalmic artery Posterior cerebral artery Posterior communicating artery Posterior inferior cerebellar artery (PICA) **H Common Carotid Artery, Right** **J Common Carotid Artery, Left** **K Internal Carotid Artery, Right** Caroticotympanic artery Carotid sinus	**L Internal Carotid Artery, Left** *See K Internal Carotid Artery, Right* **M External Carotid Artery, Right** Ascending pharyngeal artery Internal maxillary artery Lingual artery Maxillary artery Occipital artery Posterior auricular artery Superior thyroid artery **N External Carotid Artery, Left** *See M External Carotid Artery, Right* **P Vertebral Artery, Right** Anterior spinal artery Posterior spinal artery **Q Vertebral Artery, Left** *See P Vertebral Artery, Right*	**3 Percutaneous**	**Z No Device**	**7 Stent Retriever** **Z No Qualifier**

Ø Medical and Surgical
3 Upper Arteries
F Fragmentation Definition: Breaking solid matter in a body part into pieces

Explanation: Physical force (e.g., manual, ultrasonic) applied directly or indirectly is used to break the solid matter into pieces. The solid matter may be an abnormal byproduct of a biological function or a foreign body. The pieces of solid matter are not taken out.

Body Part Character 4		Approach Character 5	Device Character 6	Qualifier Character 7
2 Innominate Artery Brachiocephalic artery Brachiocephalic trunk **3 Subclavian Artery, Right** Costocervical trunk Dorsal scapular artery Internal thoracic artery **4 Subclavian Artery, Left** *See 3 Subclavian Artery, Right* **5 Axillary Artery, Right** Anterior circumflex humeral artery Lateral thoracic artery Posterior circumflex humeral artery Subscapular artery Superior thoracic artery Thoracoacromial artery **6 Axillary Artery, Left** *See 5 Axillary Artery, Right* **7 Brachial Artery, Right** Inferior ulnar collateral artery Profunda brachii Superior ulnar collateral artery **8 Brachial Artery, Left** *See 7 Brachial Artery, Right*	**9 Ulnar Artery, Right** Anterior ulnar recurrent artery Common interosseous artery Posterior ulnar recurrent artery **A Ulnar Artery, Left** *See 9 Ulnar Artery, Right* **B Radial Artery, Right** Radial recurrent artery **C Radial Artery, Left** *See B Radial Artery, Right* **Y Upper Artery** Aortic intercostal artery Bronchial artery Esophageal artery Subcostal artery	**3 Percutaneous**	**Z No Device**	**Ø Ultrasonic** **Z No Qualifier**

Ø Medical and Surgical
3 Upper Arteries
H Insertion **Definition: Putting in a nonbiological appliance that monitors, assists, performs, or prevents a physiological function but does not physically take the place of a body part**
Explanation: None

Body Part Character 4	Approach Character 5	Device Character 6	Qualifier Character 7
Ø Internal Mammary Artery, Right Anterior intercostal artery Internal thoracic artery Musculophrenic artery Pericardiophrenic artery Superior epigastric artery **1 Internal Mammary Artery, Left** *See Ø Internal Mammary Artery, Right* **2 Innominate Artery** Brachiocephalic artery Brachiocephalic trunk **3 Subclavian Artery, Right** Costocervical trunk Dorsal scapular artery Internal thoracic artery **4 Subclavian Artery, Left** *See 3 Subclavian Artery, Right* **5 Axillary Artery, Right** Anterior circumflex humeral artery Lateral thoracic artery Posterior circumflex humeral artery Subscapular artery Superior thoracic artery Thoracoacromial artery **6 Axillary Artery, Left** *See 5 Axillary Artery, Right* **7 Brachial Artery, Right** Inferior ulnar collateral artery Profunda brachii Superior ulnar collateral artery **8 Brachial Artery, Left** *See 7 Brachial Artery, Right* **9 Ulnar Artery, Right** Anterior ulnar recurrent artery Common interosseous artery Posterior ulnar recurrent artery **A Ulnar Artery, Left** *See 9 Ulnar Artery, Right* **B Radial Artery, Right** Radial recurrent artery **C Radial Artery, Left** *See B Radial Artery, Right* **D Hand Artery, Right** Deep palmar arch Princeps pollicis artery Radialis indicis Superficial palmar arch **F Hand Artery, Left** *See D Hand Artery, Right* **G Intracranial Artery** Anterior cerebral artery Anterior choroidal artery Anterior communicating artery Basilar artery Circle of Willis Internal carotid artery, intracranial portion Middle cerebral artery Ophthalmic artery Posterior cerebral artery Posterior communicating artery Posterior inferior cerebellar artery (PICA) **H Common Carotid Artery, Right** **J Common Carotid Artery, Left** **M External Carotid Artery, Right** Ascending pharyngeal artery Internal maxillary artery Lingual artery Maxillary artery Occipital artery Posterior auricular artery Superior thyroid artery **N External Carotid Artery, Left** *See M External Carotid Artery, Right* **P Vertebral Artery, Right** Anterior spinal artery Posterior spinal artery **Q Vertebral Artery, Left** *See P Vertebral Artery, Right* **R Face Artery** Angular artery Ascending palatine artery External maxillary artery Facial artery Inferior labial artery Submental artery Superior labial artery **S Temporal Artery, Right** Middle temporal artery Superficial temporal artery Transverse facial artery **T Temporal Artery, Left** *See S Temporal Artery, Right* **U Thyroid Artery, Right** Cricothyroid artery Hyoid artery Sternocleidomastoid artery Superior laryngeal artery Superior thyroid artery Thyrocervical trunk **V Thyroid Artery, Left** *See U Thyroid Artery, Right*	**Ø Open** **3 Percutaneous** **4 Percutaneous Endoscopic**	**3 Infusion Device** **D Intraluminal Device**	**Z No Qualifier**
K Internal Carotid Artery, Right Caroticotympanic artery Carotid sinus **L Internal Carotid Artery, Left** *See K Internal Carotid Artery, Right*	**Ø Open** **3 Percutaneous** **4 Percutaneous Endoscope**	**3 Infusion Device** **D Intraluminal Device** **M Stimulator Lead**	**Z No Qualifier**
Y Upper Artery Aortic intercostal artery Bronchial artery Esophageal artery Subcostal artery	**Ø Open** **3 Percutaneous** **4 Percutaneous Endoscopic**	**2 Monitoring Device** **3 Infusion Device** **D Intraluminal Device** **Y Other Device**	**Z No Qualifier**

Non-OR Ø3H[Ø,1,2,3,4,5,6,7,8,9,A,B,C,D,F,G,H,J,M,N,P,Q,R,S,T,U,V][Ø,3,4]3Z
Non-OR Ø3H[K,L][Ø,3,4]3Z
Non-OR Ø3HY[Ø,3,4]3Z
Non-OR Ø3HY32Z
Non-OR Ø3HY[3,4]YZ

Ø Medical and Surgical
3 Upper Arteries
J Inspection Definition: Visually and/or manually exploring a body part

Explanation: Visual exploration may be performed with or without optical instrumentation. Manual exploration may be performed directly or through intervening body layers.

Body Part Character 4	Approach Character 5	Device Character 6	Qualifier Character 7
Y Upper Artery Aortic intercostal artery Bronchial artery Esophageal artery Subcostal artery	**Ø Open** **3 Percutaneous** **4 Percutaneous Endoscopic** **X External**	**Z No Device**	**Z No Qualifier**

Non-OR Ø3JY[3,4,X]ZZ

Ø Medical and Surgical
3 Upper Arteries
L Occlusion Definition: Completely closing an orifice or the lumen of a tubular body part
Explanation: The orifice can be a natural orifice or an artificially created orifice

Body Part Character 4		Approach Character 5	Device Character 6	Qualifier Character 7
Ø Internal Mammary Artery, Right Anterior intercostal artery Internal thoracic artery Musculophrenic artery Pericardiophrenic artery Superior epigastric artery **1 Internal Mammary Artery, Left** *See Ø Internal Mammary Artery, Left* **2 Innominate Artery** Brachiocephalic artery Brachiocephalic trunk **3 Subclavian Artery, Right** Costocervical trunk Dorsal scapular artery Internal thoracic artery **4 Subclavian Artery, Left** *See 3 Subclavian Artery, Right* **5 Axillary Artery, Right** Anterior circumflex humeral artery Lateral thoracic artery Posterior circumflex humeral artery Subscapular artery Superior thoracic artery Thoracoacromial artery **6 Axillary Artery, Left** *See 5 Axillary Artery, Right* **7 Brachial Artery, Right** Inferior ulnar collateral artery Profunda brachii Superior ulnar collateral artery **8 Brachial Artery, Left** *See 7 Brachial Artery, Right* **9 Ulnar Artery, Right** Anterior ulnar recurrent artery Common interosseous artery Posterior ulnar recurrent artery	**A Ulnar Artery, Left** *See 9 Ulnar Artery, Right* **B Radial Artery, Right** Radial recurrent artery **C Radial Artery, Left** *See B Radial Artery, Right* **D Hand Artery, Right** Deep palmar arch Princeps pollicis artery Radialis indicis Superficial palmar arch **F Hand Artery, Left** *See D Hand Artery, Right* **R Face Artery** Angular artery Ascending palatine artery External maxillary artery Facial artery Inferior labial artery Submental artery Superior labial artery **S Temporal Artery, Right** Middle temporal artery Superficial temporal artery Transverse facial artery **T Temporal Artery, Left** *See S Temporal Artery, Right* **U Thyroid Artery, Right** Cricothyroid artery Hyoid artery Sternocleidomastoid artery Superior laryngeal artery Superior thyroid artery Thyrocervical trunk **V Thyroid Artery, Left** *See U Thyroid Artery, Right* **Y Upper Artery** Aortic intercostal artery Bronchial artery Esophageal artery Subcostal artery	**Ø** Open **3** Percutaneous **4** Percutaneous Endoscopic	**C** Extraluminal Device **D** Intraluminal Device **Z** No Device	**Z** No Qualifier
G Intracranial Artery Anterior cerebral artery Anterior choroidal artery Anterior communicating artery Basilar artery Circle of Willis Internal carotid artery, intracranial portion Middle cerebral artery Ophthalmic artery Posterior cerebral artery Posterior communicating artery Posterior inferior cerebellar artery (PICA) **H Common Carotid Artery, Right** **J Common Carotid Artery, Left** **K Internal Carotid Artery, Right** Caroticotympanic artery Carotid sinus	**L Internal Carotid Artery, Left** *See K Internal Carotid Artery, Right* **M External Carotid Artery, Right** Ascending pharyngeal artery Internal maxillary artery Lingual artery Maxillary artery Occipital artery Posterior auricular artery Superior thyroid artery **N External Carotid Artery, Left** *See M External Carotid Artery, Right* **P Vertebral Artery, Right** Anterior spinal artery Posterior spinal artery **Q Vertebral Artery, Left** *See P Vertebral Artery, Right*	**Ø** Open **3** Percutaneous **4** Percutaneous Endoscopic	**B** Intraluminal Device, Bioactive **C** Extraluminal Device **D** Intraluminal Device **Z** No Device	**Z** No Qualifier

Ø Medical and Surgical
3 Upper Arteries
N Release Definition: Freeing a body part from an abnormal physical constraint by cutting or by the use of force
Explanation: Some of the restraining tissue may be taken out but none of the body part is taken out

Body Part Character 4	Approach Character 5	Device Character 6	Qualifier Character 7
Ø Internal Mammary Artery, Right Anterior intercostal artery Internal thoracic artery Musculophrenic artery Pericardiophrenic artery Superior epigastric artery **1 Internal Mammary Artery, Left** *See Ø Internal Mammary Artery, Right* **2 Innominate Artery** Brachiocephalic artery Brachiocephalic trunk **3 Subclavian Artery, Right** Costocervical trunk Dorsal scapular artery Internal thoracic artery **4 Subclavian Artery, Left** *See 3 Subclavian Artery, Right* **5 Axillary Artery, Right** Anterior circumflex humeral artery Lateral thoracic artery Posterior circumflex humeral artery Subscapular artery Superior thoracic artery Thoracoacromial artery **6 Axillary Artery, Left** *See 5 Axillary Artery, Right* **7 Brachial Artery, Right** Inferior ulnar collateral artery Profunda brachii Superior ulnar collateral artery **8 Brachial Artery, Left** *See 7 Brachial Artery, Right* **9 Ulnar Artery, Right** Anterior ulnar recurrent artery Common interosseous artery Posterior ulnar recurrent artery **A Ulnar Artery, Left** *See 9 Ulnar Artery, Right* **B Radial Artery, Right** Radial recurrent artery **C Radial Artery, Left** *See B Radial Artery, Right* **D Hand Artery, Right** Deep palmar arch Princeps pollicis artery Radialis indicis Superficial palmar arch **F Hand Artery, Left** *See D Hand Artery, Right* **G Intracranial Artery** Anterior cerebral artery Anterior choroidal artery Anterior communicating artery Basilar artery Circle of Willis Internal carotid artery, intracranial portion Middle cerebral artery Ophthalmic artery Posterior cerebral artery Posterior communicating artery Posterior inferior cerebellar artery (PICA) **H Common Carotid Artery, Right** **J Common Carotid Artery, Left** **K Internal Carotid Artery, Right** Caroticotympanic artery Carotid sinus **L Internal Carotid Artery, Left** *See K Internal Carotid Artery, Right* **M External Carotid Artery, Right** Ascending pharyngeal artery Internal maxillary artery Lingual artery Maxillary artery Occipital artery Posterior auricular artery Superior thyroid artery **N External Carotid Artery, Left** *See M External Carotid Artery, Right* **P Vertebral Artery, Right** Anterior spinal artery Posterior spinal artery **Q Vertebral Artery, Left** *See P Vertebral Artery, Right* **R Face Artery** Angular artery Ascending palatine artery External maxillary artery Facial artery Inferior labial artery Submental artery Superior labial artery **S Temporal Artery, Right** Middle temporal artery Superficial temporal artery Transverse facial artery **T Temporal Artery, Left** *See S Temporal Artery, Right* **U Thyroid Artery, Right** Cricothyroid artery Hyoid artery Sternocleidomastoid artery Superior laryngeal artery Superior thyroid artery Thyrocervical trunk **V Thyroid Artery, Left** *See U Thyroid Artery, Right* **Y Upper Artery** Aortic intercostal artery Bronchial artery Esophageal artery Subcostal artery	**Ø Open** **3 Percutaneous** **4 Percutaneous Endoscopic**	**Z No Device**	**Z No Qualifier**

Ø Medical and Surgical
3 Upper Arteries
P Removal Definition: Taking out or off a device from a body part

Explanation: If a device is taken out and a similar device put in without cutting or puncturing the skin or mucous membrane, the procedure is coded to the root operation CHANGE. Otherwise, the procedure for taking out a device is coded to the root operation REMOVAL.

Body Part Character 4	Approach Character 5	Device Character 6	Qualifier Character 7
Y Upper Artery Aortic intercostal artery Bronchial artery Esophageal artery Subcostal artery	**Ø Open** **3 Percutaneous** **4 Percutaneous Endoscopic**	**Ø Drainage Device** **2 Monitoring Device** **3 Infusion Device** **7 Autologous Tissue Substitute** **C Extraluminal Device** **D Intraluminal Device** **J Synthetic Substitute** **K Nonautologous Tissue Substitute** **M Stimulator Lead** **Y Other Device**	**Z No Qualifier**
Y Upper Artery Aortic intercostal artery Bronchial artery Esophageal artery Subcostal artery	**X External**	**Ø Drainage Device** **2 Monitoring Device** **3 Infusion Device** **D Intraluminal Device** **M Stimulator Lead**	**Z No Qualifier**

Non-OR Ø3PY3[Ø,2,3,D]Z
Non-OR Ø3PY[3,4]YZ
Non-OR Ø3PYX[Ø,2,3,D,M]Z

Ø Medical and Surgical
3 Upper Arteries
Q Repair Definition: Restoring, to the extent possible, a body part to its normal anatomic structure and function
Explanation: Used only when the method to accomplish the repair is not one of the other root operations

Body Part Character 4		Approach Character 5	Device Character 6	Qualifier Character 7
Ø Internal Mammary Artery, Right Anterior intercostal artery Internal thoracic artery Musculophrenic artery Pericardiophrenic artery Superior epigastric artery **1 Internal Mammary Artery, Left** *See Ø Internal Mammary Artery, Right* **2 Innominate Artery** Brachiocephalic artery Brachiocephalic trunk **3 Subclavian Artery, Right** Costocervical trunk Dorsal scapular artery Internal thoracic artery **4 Subclavian Artery, Left** *See 3 Subclavian Artery, Right* **5 Axillary Artery, Right** Anterior circumflex humeral artery Lateral thoracic artery Posterior circumflex humeral artery Subscapular artery Superior thoracic artery Thoracoacromial artery **6 Axillary Artery, Left** *See 5 Axillary Artery, Right* **7 Brachial Artery, Right** Inferior ulnar collateral artery Profunda brachii Superior ulnar collateral artery **8 Brachial Artery, Left** *See 7 Brachial Artery, Right* **9 Ulnar Artery, Right** Anterior ulnar recurrent artery Common interosseous artery Posterior ulnar recurrent artery **A Ulnar Artery, Left** *See 9 Ulnar Artery, Right* **B Radial Artery, Right** Radial recurrent artery **C Radial Artery, Left** *See B Radial Artery, Right* **D Hand Artery, Right** Deep palmar arch Princeps pollicis artery Radialis indicis Superficial palmar arch **F Hand Artery, Left** *See D Hand Artery, Right* **G Intracranial Artery** Anterior cerebral artery Anterior choroidal artery Anterior communicating artery Basilar artery Circle of Willis Internal carotid artery, intracranial portion Middle cerebral artery Ophthalmic artery Posterior cerebral artery Posterior communicating artery Posterior inferior cerebellar artery (PICA)	**H Common Carotid Artery, Right** **J Common Carotid Artery, Left** **K Internal Carotid Artery, Right** Caroticotympanic artery Carotid sinus **L Internal Carotid Artery, Left** *See K Internal Carotid Artery, Right* **M External Carotid Artery, Right** Ascending pharyngeal artery Internal maxillary artery Lingual artery Maxillary artery Occipital artery Posterior auricular artery Superior thyroid artery **N External Carotid Artery, Left** *See M External Carotid Artery, Right* **P Vertebral Artery, Right** Anterior spinal artery Posterior spinal artery **Q Vertebral Artery, Left** *See P Vertebral Artery, Right* **R Face Artery** Angular artery Ascending palatine artery External maxillary artery Facial artery Inferior labial artery Submental artery Superior labial artery **S Temporal Artery, Right** Middle temporal artery Superficial temporal artery Transverse facial artery **T Temporal Artery, Left** *See S Temporal Artery, Right* **U Thyroid Artery, Right** Cricothyroid artery Hyoid artery Sternocleidomastoid artery Superior laryngeal artery Superior thyroid artery Thyrocervical trunk **V Thyroid Artery, Left** *See U Thyroid Artery, Right* **Y Upper Artery** Aortic intercostal artery Bronchial artery Esophageal artery Subcostal artery	**Ø Open** **3 Percutaneous** **4 Percutaneous Endoscopic**	**Z No Device**	**Z No Qualifier**

Ø Medical and Surgical
3 Upper Arteries
R Replacement Definition: Putting in or on biological or synthetic material that physically takes the place and/or function of all or a portion of a body part

Explanation: The body part may have been taken out or replaced, or may be taken out, physically eradicated, or rendered nonfunctional during the REPLACEMENT procedure. A REMOVAL procedure is coded for taking out the device used in a previous replacement procedure.

Body Part Character 4	Approach Character 5	Device Character 6	Qualifier Character 7
Ø Internal Mammary Artery, Right Anterior intercostal artery Internal thoracic artery Musculophrenic artery Pericardiophrenic artery Superior epigastric artery **1 Internal Mammary Artery, Left** *See Ø Internal Mammary Artery, Right* **2 Innominate Artery** Brachiocephalic artery Brachiocephalic trunk **3 Subclavian Artery, Right** Costocervical trunk Dorsal scapular artery Internal thoracic artery **4 Subclavian Artery, Left** *See 3 Subclavian Artery, Right* **5 Axillary Artery, Right** Anterior circumflex humeral artery Lateral thoracic artery Posterior circumflex humeral artery Subscapular artery Superior thoracic artery Thoracoacromial artery **6 Axillary Artery, Left** *See 5 Axillary Artery, Right* **7 Brachial Artery, Right** Inferior ulnar collateral artery Profunda brachii Superior ulnar collateral artery **8 Brachial Artery, Left** *See 7 Brachial Artery, Right* **9 Ulnar Artery, Right** Anterior ulnar recurrent artery Common interosseous artery Posterior ulnar recurrent artery **A Ulnar Artery, Left** *See 9 Ulnar Artery, Right* **B Radial Artery, Right** Radial recurrent artery **C Radial Artery, Left** *See B Radial Artery, Right* **D Hand Artery, Right** Deep palmar arch Princeps pollicis artery Radialis indicis Superficial palmar arch **F Hand Artery, Left** *See D Hand Artery, Right* **G Intracranial Artery** Anterior cerebral artery Anterior choroidal artery Anterior communicating artery Basilar artery Circle of Willis Internal carotid artery, intracranial portion Middle cerebral artery Ophthalmic artery Posterior cerebral artery Posterior communicating artery Posterior inferior cerebellar artery (PICA) **H Common Carotid Artery, Right** **J Common Carotid Artery, Left** **K Internal Carotid Artery, Right** Caroticotympanic artery Carotid sinus **L Internal Carotid Artery, Left** *See K Internal Carotid Artery, Right* **M External Carotid Artery, Right** Ascending pharyngeal artery Internal maxillary artery Lingual artery Maxillary artery Occipital artery Posterior auricular artery Superior thyroid artery **N External Carotid Artery, Left** *See M External Carotid Artery, Right* **P Vertebral Artery, Right** Anterior spinal artery Posterior spinal artery **Q Vertebral Artery, Left** *See P Vertebral Artery, Right* **R Face Artery** Angular artery Ascending palatine artery External maxillary artery Facial artery Inferior labial artery Submental artery Superior labial artery **S Temporal Artery, Right** Middle temporal artery Superficial temporal artery Transverse facial artery **T Temporal Artery, Left** *See S Temporal Artery, Right* **U Thyroid Artery, Right** Cricothyroid artery Hyoid artery Sternocleidomastoid artery Superior laryngeal artery Superior thyroid artery Thyrocervical trunk **V Thyroid Artery, Left** *See U Thyroid Artery, Right* **Y Upper Artery** Aortic intercostal artery Bronchial artery Esophageal artery Subcostal artery	**Ø Open** **4 Percutaneous Endoscopic**	**7 Autologous Tissue Substitute** **J Synthetic Substitute** **K Nonautologous Tissue Substitute**	**Z No Qualifier**

Ø Medical and Surgical
3 Upper Arteries
S Reposition Definition: Moving to its normal location, or other suitable location, all or a portion of a body part

Explanation: The body part is moved to a new location from an abnormal location, or from a normal location where it is not functioning correctly. The body part may or may not be cut out or off to be moved to the new location.

Body Part Character 4	Approach Character 5	Device Character 6	Qualifier Character 7
Ø Internal Mammary Artery, Right Anterior intercostal artery Internal thoracic artery Musculophrenic artery Pericardiophrenic artery Superior epigastric artery **1 Internal Mammary Artery, Left** **See** *Ø Internal Mammary Artery, Right* **2 Innominate Artery** Brachiocephalic artery Brachiocephalic trunk **3 Subclavian Artery, Right** Costocervical trunk Dorsal scapular artery Internal thoracic artery **4 Subclavian Artery, Left** **See** *3 Subclavian Artery, Right* **5 Axillary Artery, Right** Anterior circumflex humeral artery Lateral thoracic artery Posterior circumflex humeral artery Subscapular artery Superior thoracic artery Thoracoacromial artery **6 Axillary Artery, Left** **See** *5 Axillary Artery, Right* **7 Brachial Artery, Right** Inferior ulnar collateral artery Profunda brachii Superior ulnar collateral artery **8 Brachial Artery, Left** **See** *7 Brachial Artery, Right* **9 Ulnar Artery, Right** Anterior ulnar recurrent artery Common interosseous artery Posterior ulnar recurrent artery **A Ulnar Artery, Left** **See** *9 Ulnar Artery, Right* **B Radial Artery, Right** Radial recurrent artery **C Radial Artery, Left** **See** *B Radial Artery, Right* **D Hand Artery, Right** Deep palmar arch Princeps pollicis artery Radialis indicis Superficial palmar arch **F Hand Artery, Left** **See** *D Hand Artery, Right* **G Intracranial Artery** Anterior cerebral artery Anterior choroidal artery Anterior communicating artery Basilar artery Circle of Willis Internal carotid artery, intracranial portion Middle cerebral artery Ophthalmic artery Posterior cerebral artery Posterior communicating artery Posterior inferior cerebellar artery (PICA) **H Common Carotid Artery, Right** **J Common Carotid Artery, Left** **K Internal Carotid Artery, Right** Caroticotympanic artery Carotid sinus **L Internal Carotid Artery, Left** **See** *K Internal Carotid Artery, Right* **M External Carotid Artery, Right** Ascending pharyngeal artery Internal maxillary artery Lingual artery Maxillary artery Occipital artery Posterior auricular artery Superior thyroid artery **N External Carotid Artery, Left** **See** *M External Carotid Artery, Right* **P Vertebral Artery, Right** Anterior spinal artery Posterior spinal artery **Q Vertebral Artery, Left** **See** *P Vertebral Artery, Right* **R Face Artery** Angular artery Ascending palatine artery External maxillary artery Facial artery Inferior labial artery Submental artery Superior labial artery **S Temporal Artery, Right** Middle temporal artery Superficial temporal artery Transverse facial artery **T Temporal Artery, Left** **See** *S Temporal Artery, Right* **U Thyroid Artery, Right** Cricothyroid artery Hyoid artery Sternocleidomastoid artery Superior laryngeal artery Superior thyroid artery Thyrocervical trunk **V Thyroid Artery, Left** **See** *U Thyroid Artery, Right* **Y Upper Artery** Aortic intercostal artery Bronchial artery Esophageal artery Subcostal artery	**Ø Open** **3 Percutaneous** **4 Percutaneous Endoscopic**	**Z No Device**	**Z No Qualifier**

Ø Medical and Surgical
3 Upper Arteries
U Supplement Definition: Putting in or on biological or synthetic material that physically reinforces and/or augments the function of a portion of a body part

Explanation: The biological material is non-living, or is living and from the same individual. The body part may have been previously replaced, and the SUPPLEMENT procedure is performed to physically reinforce and/or augment the function of the replaced body part.

Body Part Character 4	Approach Character 5	Device Character 6	Qualifier Character 7
Ø Internal Mammary Artery, Right Anterior intercostal artery Internal thoracic artery Musculophrenic artery Pericardiophrenic artery Superior epigastric artery **1 Internal Mammary Artery, Left** *See Ø Internal Mammary Artery, Right* **2 Innominate Artery** Brachiocephalic artery Brachiocephalic trunk **3 Subclavian Artery, Right** Costocervical trunk Dorsal scapular artery Internal thoracic artery **4 Subclavian Artery, Left** *See 3 Subclavian Artery, Right* **5 Axillary Artery, Right** Anterior circumflex humeral artery Lateral thoracic artery Posterior circumflex humeral artery Subscapular artery Superior thoracic artery Thoracoacromial artery **6 Axillary Artery, Left** *See 5 Axillary Artery, Right* **7 Brachial Artery, Right** Inferior ulnar collateral artery Profunda brachii Superior ulnar collateral artery **8 Brachial Artery, Left** *See 7 Brachial Artery, Right* **9 Ulnar Artery, Right** Anterior ulnar recurrent artery Common interosseous artery Posterior ulnar recurrent artery **A Ulnar Artery, Left** *See 9 Ulnar Artery, Right* **B Radial Artery, Right** Radial recurrent artery **C Radial Artery, Left** *See B Radial Artery, Right* **D Hand Artery, Right** Deep palmar arch Princeps pollicis artery Radialis indicis Superficial palmar arch **F Hand Artery, Left** *See D Hand Artery, Right* **G Intracranial Artery** Anterior cerebral artery Anterior choroidal artery Anterior communicating artery Basilar artery Circle of Willis Internal carotid artery, intracranial portion Middle cerebral artery Ophthalmic artery Posterior cerebral artery Posterior communicating artery Posterior inferior cerebellar artery (PICA) **H Common Carotid Artery, Right** **J Common Carotid Artery, Left** **K Internal Carotid Artery, Right** Caroticotympanic artery Carotid sinus **L Internal Carotid Artery, Left** *See K Internal Carotid Artery, Right* **M External Carotid Artery, Right** Ascending pharyngeal artery Internal maxillary artery Lingual artery Maxillary artery Occipital artery Posterior auricular artery Superior thyroid artery **N External Carotid Artery, Left** *See M External Carotid Artery, Right* **P Vertebral Artery, Right** Anterior spinal artery Posterior spinal artery **Q Vertebral Artery, Left** *See P Vertebral Artery, Right* **R Face Artery** Angular artery Ascending palatine artery External maxillary artery Facial artery Inferior labial artery Submental artery Superior labial artery **S Temporal Artery, Right** Middle temporal artery Superficial temporal artery Transverse facial artery **T Temporal Artery, Left** *See S Temporal Artery, Right* **U Thyroid Artery, Right** Cricothyroid artery Hyoid artery Sternocleidomastoid artery Superior laryngeal artery Superior thyroid artery Thyrocervical trunk **V Thyroid Artery, Left** *See U Thyroid Artery, Right* **Y Upper Artery** Aortic intercostal artery Bronchial artery Esophageal artery Subcostal artery	**Ø Open** **3 Percutaneous** **4 Percutaneous Endoscopic**	**7 Autologous Tissue Substitute** **J Synthetic Substitute** **K Nonautologous Tissue Substitute**	**Z No Qualifier**

Ø Medical and Surgical
3 Upper Arteries
V Restriction Definition: Partially closing an orifice or the lumen of a tubular body part

Explanation: The orifice can be a natural orifice or an artificially created orifice

Body Part Character 4		Approach Character 5	Device Character 6	Qualifier Character 7
Ø Internal Mammary Artery, Right Anterior intercostal artery Internal thoracic artery Musculophrenic artery Pericardiophrenic artery Superior epigastric artery **1 Internal Mammary Artery, Left** ***See*** *Ø Internal Mammary Artery, Right* **2 Innominate Artery** Brachiocephalic artery Brachiocephalic trunk **3 Subclavian Artery, Right** Costocervical trunk Dorsal scapular artery Internal thoracic artery **4 Subclavian Artery, Left** ***See*** *3 Subclavian Artery, Right* **5 Axillary Artery, Right** Anterior circumflex humeral artery Lateral thoracic artery Posterior circumflex humeral artery Subscapular artery Superior thoracic artery Thoracoacromial artery **6 Axillary Artery, Left** ***See*** *5 Axillary Artery, Right* **7 Brachial Artery, Right** Inferior ulnar collateral artery Profunda brachii Superior ulnar collateral artery **8 Brachial Artery, Left** ***See*** *7 Brachial Artery, Right* **9 Ulnar Artery, Right** Anterior ulnar recurrent artery Common interosseous artery Posterior ulnar recurrent artery **A Ulnar Artery, Left** ***See*** *9 Ulnar Artery, Right*	**B Radial Artery, Right** Radial recurrent artery **C Radial Artery, Left** ***See*** *B Radial Artery, Right* **D Hand Artery, Right** Deep palmar arch Princeps pollicis artery Radialis indicis Superficial palmar arch **F Hand Artery, Left** ***See*** *D Hand Artery, Right* **R Face Artery** Angular artery Ascending palatine artery External maxillary artery Facial artery Inferior labial artery Submental artery Superior labial artery **S Temporal Artery, Right** Middle temporal artery Superficial temporal artery Transverse facial artery **T Temporal Artery, Left** ***See*** *S Temporal Artery, Right* **U Thyroid Artery, Right** Cricothyroid artery Hyoid artery Sternocleidomastoid artery Superior laryngeal artery Superior thyroid artery Thyrocervical trunk **V Thyroid Artery, Left** ***See*** *U Thyroid Artery, Right* **Y Upper Artery** Aortic intercostal artery Bronchial artery Esophageal artery Subcostal artery	**Ø Open** **3 Percutaneous** **4 Percutaneous Endoscopic**	**C Extraluminal Device** **D Intraluminal Device** **Z No Device**	**Z No Qualifier**
G Intracranial Artery Anterior cerebral artery Anterior choroidal artery Anterior communicating artery Basilar artery Circle of Willis Internal carotid artery, intracranial portion Middle cerebral artery Ophthalmic artery Posterior cerebral artery Posterior communicating artery Posterior inferior cerebellar artery (PICA) **H Common Carotid Artery, Right** **J Common Carotid Artery, Left** **K Internal Carotid Artery, Right** Caroticotympanic artery Carotid sinus	**L Internal Carotid Artery, Left** ***See*** *K Internal Carotid Artery, Right* **M External Carotid Artery, Right** Ascending pharyngeal artery Internal maxillary artery Lingual artery Maxillary artery Occipital artery Posterior auricular artery Superior thyroid artery **N External Carotid Artery, Left** ***See*** *M External Carotid Artery, Right* **P Vertebral Artery, Right** Anterior spinal artery Posterior spinal artery **Q Vertebral Artery, Left** ***See*** *P Vertebral Artery, Right*	**Ø Open** **3 Percutaneous** **4 Percutaneous Endoscopic**	**B Intraluminal Device, Bioactive** **C Extraluminal Device** **D Intraluminal Device** **H Intraluminal Device, Flow Diverter** **Z No Device**	**Z No Qualifier**

Ø Medical and Surgical
3 Upper Arteries
W Revision Definition: Correcting, to the extent possible, a portion of a malfunctioning device or the position of a displaced device

Explanation: Revision can include correcting a malfunctioning or displaced device by taking out or putting in components of the device such as a screw or pin

Body Part Character 4	Approach Character 5	Device Character 6	Qualifier Character 7
Y Upper Artery Aortic intercostal artery Bronchial artery Esophageal artery Subcostal artery	**Ø** Open **3** Percutaneous **4** Percutaneous Endoscopic	**Ø** Drainage Device **2** Monitoring Device **3** Infusion Device **7** Autologous Tissue Substitute **C** Extraluminal Device **D** Intraluminal Device **J** Synthetic Substitute **K** Nonautologous Tissue Substitute **M** Stimulator Lead **Y** Other Device	**Z** No Qualifier
Y Upper Artery Aortic intercostal artery Bronchial artery Esophageal artery Subcostal artery	**X** External	**Ø** Drainage Device **2** Monitoring Device **3** Infusion Device **7** Autologous Tissue Substitute **C** Extraluminal Device **D** Intraluminal Device **J** Synthetic Substitute **K** Nonautologous Tissue Substitute **M** Stimulator Lead	**Z** No Qualifier

Non-OR Ø3WY3[Ø,2,3,D]Z
Non-OR Ø3WY[3,4]YZ
Non-OR Ø3WYX[Ø,2,3,7,C,D,J,K,M]Z

Lower Arteries Ø41–Ø4W

Character Meanings

This Character Meaning table is provided as a guide to assist the user in the identification of character members that may be found in this section of code tables. It **SHOULD NOT** be used to build a PCS code.

Operation–Character 3	Body Part–Character 4	Approach–Character 5	Device–Character 6	Qualifier–Character 7
1 Bypass	Ø Abdominal Aorta	Ø Open	Ø Drainage Device	Ø Abdominal Aorta OR Ultrasonic
5 Destruction	1 Celiac Artery	3 Percutaneous	1 Radioactive Element	1 Celiac Artery OR Drug-Coated Balloon
7 Dilation	2 Gastric Artery	4 Percutaneous Endoscopic	2 Monitoring Device	2 Mesenteric Artery
9 Drainage	3 Hepatic Artery	X External	3 Infusion Device	3 Renal Artery, Right
B Excision	4 Splenic Artery		4 Intraluminal Device, Drug-eluting	4 Renal Artery, Left
C Extirpation	5 Superior Mesenteric Artery		5 Intraluminal Device, Drug-eluting, Two	5 Renal Artery, Bilateral
F Fragmentation	6 Colic Artery, Right		6 Intraluminal Device, Drug-eluting, Three	6 Common Iliac Artery, Right
H Insertion	7 Colic Artery, Left		7 Intraluminal Device, Drug-eluting, Four or More OR Autologous Tissue Substitute	7 Common Iliac Artery, Left
J Inspection	8 Colic Artery, Middle		9 Autologous Venous Tissue	8 Common Iliac Arteries, Bilateral
L Occlusion	9 Renal Artery, Right		A Autologous Arterial Tissue	9 Internal Iliac Artery, Right
N Release	A Renal Artery, Left		C Extraluminal Device	B Internal Iliac Artery, Left
P Removal	B Inferior Mesenteric Artery		D Intraluminal Device	C Internal Iliac Arteries, Bilateral
Q Repair	C Common Iliac Artery, Right		E Intraluminal Device, Two OR Intraluminal Device, Branched or Fenestrated, One or Two Arteries	D External Iliac Artery, Right
R Replacement	D Common Iliac Artery, Left		F Intraluminal Device, Three OR Intraluminal Device, Branched or Fenestrated, Three or More Arteries	F External Iliac Artery, Left
S Reposition	E Internal Iliac Artery, Right		G Intraluminal Device, Four or More	G External Iliac Arteries, Bilateral
U Supplement	F Internal Iliac Artery, Left		J Synthetic Substitute	H Femoral Artery, Right
V Restriction	H External Iliac Artery, Right		K Nonautologous Tissue Substitute	J Femoral Artery, Left OR Temporary
W Revision	J External Iliac Artery, Left		Y Other Device	K Femoral Arteries, Bilateral
	K Femoral Artery, Right		Z No Device	L Popliteal Artery
	L Femoral Artery, Left			M Peroneal Artery
	M Popliteal Artery, Right			N Posterior Tibial Artery
	N Popliteal Artery, Left			P Foot Artery
	P Anterior Tibial Artery, Right			Q Lower Extremity Artery
	Q Anterior Tibial Artery, Left			R Lower Artery
	R Posterior Tibial Artery, Right			S Lower Extremity Vein
	S Posterior Tibial Artery, Left			T Uterine Artery, Right
	T Peroneal Artery, Right			U Uterine Artery, Left
	U Peroneal Artery, Left			X Diagnostic
	V Foot Artery, Right			Z No Qualifier
	W Foot Artery, Left			
	Y Lower Artery			

AHA Coding Clinic for table Ø41
2019, 1Q, 23 Endovascular repair of shaggy aorta and deployment of chimney stent grafts
2018, 3Q, 25 Femoral artery to tibioperoneal trunk bypass
2017, 4Q, 46-47 New and revised body part values - Bypass hepatic artery to renal artery
2017, 3Q, 5 Femoral artery to posterior tibial artery bypass using autologous and synthetic grafts
2017, 3Q, 16 Abdominal aortic debranching with bypass of external iliac artery to bilateral renal arteries and superior mesenteric artery
2017, 1Q, 32 Peroneal artery to dorsalis pedis artery bypass using saphenous vein graft
2016, 2Q, 18 Femoral-tibial artery bypass and saphenous vein graft
2015, 3Q, 28 Bilateral renal artery bypass

AHA Coding Clinic for table Ø47
2019, 4Q, 27 Bifurcation Qualifier
2019, 2Q, 14 Revision of occluded femoral-popliteal bypass graft
2018, 2Q, 24 Coronary artery bifurcation
2016, 4Q, 86 Peripheral artery, number of stents
2016, 4Q, 86-88 Coronary and peripheral artery bifurcation
2016, 3Q, 39 Infrarenal abdominal aortic aneurysm repair with iliac graft extension
2015, 4Q, 4-7, 15 Drug-coated balloon angioplasty in peripheral vessels
2015, 3Q, 9 Aborted endovascular stenting of superficial femoral artery

AHA Coding Clinic for table Ø4C
2019, 4Q, 27 Bifurcation Qualifier
2019, 1Q, 23 Endovascular repair of shaggy aorta and deployment of chimney stent grafts
2018, 2Q, 24 Coronary artery bifurcation
2017, 2Q, 23 Thrombectomy via Fogarty catheter
2016, 4Q, 86-88 Coronary and peripheral artery bifurcation
2016, 1Q, 31 Iliofemoral endarterectomy with patch repair
2015, 1Q, 29 Discontinued carotid endarterectomy
2015, 1Q, 36 Percutaneous mechanical thrombectomy of femoropopliteal bypass graft

AHA Coding Clinic for table Ø4H
2019, 3Q, 20 Removal and revision of ECMO component
2019, 1Q, 23 Endovascular repair of shaggy aorta and deployment of chimney stent grafts
2017, 1Q, 30 Insertion of umbilical artery catheter

AHA Coding Clinic for table Ø4L
2018, 2Q, 18 Transverse rectus abdominis myocutaneous (TRAM) delay
2017, 4Q, 31 Resuscitative endovascular balloon occlusion of the aorta
2015, 2Q, 27 Uterine artery embolization using Gelfoam
2014, 3Q, 26 Coil embolization of gastroduodenal artery with chemoembolization of hepatic artery
2014, 1Q, 24 Endovascular embolization for gastrointestinal bleeding

AHA Coding Clinic for table Ø4N
2015, 2Q, 28 Release and replacement of celiac artery

AHA Coding Clinic for table Ø4P
2019, 3Q, 20 Removal and revision of ECMO component

AHA Coding Clinic for table Ø4Q
2014, 1Q, 21 Repair of femoral artery pseudoaneurysm

AHA Coding Clinic for table Ø4R
2019, 1Q, 22 Abdominal aortic aneurysm repair using tube graft
2015, 2Q, 28 Release and replacement of celiac artery

AHA Coding Clinic for table Ø4U
2019, 1Q, 22 Abdominal aortic aneurysm repair using tube graft
2016, 2Q, 18 Femoral-tibial artery bypass and saphenous vein graft
2016, 1Q, 31 Iliofemoral endarterectomy with patch repair
2014, 4Q, 37 Bovine patch arterioplasty
2014, 1Q, 22 Repair of pseudoaneurysm of femoral-popliteal bypass graft

AHA Coding Clinic for table Ø4V
2019, 4Q, 27 Bifurcation Qualifier
2019, 1Q, 22 Abdominal aortic aneurysm repair using tube graft
2018, 2Q, 24 Coronary artery bifurcation
2016, 4Q, 86-87 Coronary and peripheral artery bifurcation
2016, 4Q, 89-93 Branched and fenestrated endograft repair of aneurysms
2016, 3Q, 39 Infrarenal abdominal aortic aneurysm repair with iliac graft extension
2014, 1Q, 9 Endovascular repair of abdominal aortic aneurysm

AHA Coding Clinic for table Ø4W
2019, 2Q, 14 Revision of occluded femoral-popliteal bypass graft
2015, 1Q, 36 Revision of femoropopliteal bypass graft
2014, 1Q, 9 Endovascular repair of endoleak
2014, 1Q, 22 Repair of pseudoaneurysm of femoral-popliteal bypass graft

Lower Arteries

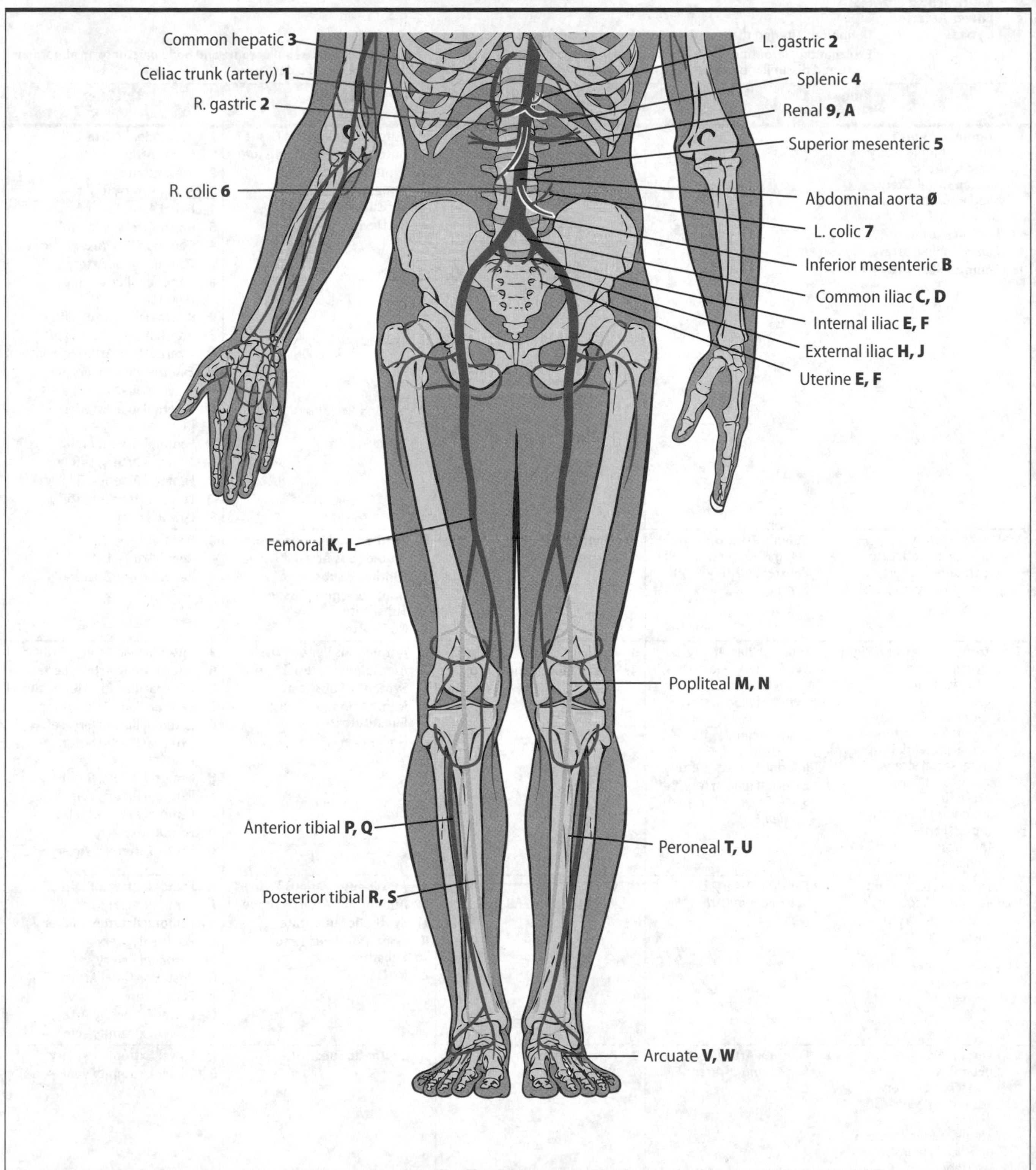

Ø Medical and Surgical
4 Lower Arteries
1 Bypass Definition: Altering the route of passage of the contents of a tubular body part

Explanation: Rerouting contents of a body part to a downstream area of the normal route, to a similar route and body part, or to an abnormal route and dissimilar body part. Includes one or more anastomoses, with or without the use of a device.

Body Part Character 4	Approach Character 5	Device Character 6	Qualifier Character 7
Ø Abdominal Aorta Inferior phrenic artery Lumbar artery Median sacral artery Middle suprarenal artery Ovarian artery Testicular artery **C Common Iliac Artery, Right** **D Common Iliac Artery, Left**	**Ø Open** **4 Percutaneous Endoscopic**	**9 Autologous Venous Tissue** **A Autologous Arterial Tissue** **J Synthetic Substitute** **K Nonautologous Tissue Substitute** **Z No Device**	**Ø Abdominal Aorta** **1 Celiac Artery** **2 Mesenteric Artery** **3 Renal Artery, Right** **4 Renal Artery, Left** **5 Renal Artery, Bilateral** **6 Common Iliac Artery, Right** **7 Common Iliac Artery, Left** **8 Common Iliac Arteries, Bilateral** **9 Internal Iliac Artery, Right** **B Internal Iliac Artery, Left** **C Internal Iliac Arteries, Bilateral** **D External Iliac Artery, Right** **F External Iliac Artery, Left** **G External Iliac Arteries, Bilateral** **H Femoral Artery, Right** **J Femoral Artery, Left** **K Femoral Arteries, Bilateral** **Q Lower Extremity Artery** **R Lower Artery**
3 Hepatic Artery Common hepatic artery Gastroduodenal artery Hepatic artery proper **4 Splenic Artery** Left gastroepiploic artery Pancreatic artery Short gastric artery	**Ø Open** **4 Percutaneous Endoscopic**	**9 Autologous Venous Tissue** **A Autologous Arterial Tissue** **J Synthetic Substitute** **K Nonautologous Tissue Substitute** **Z No Device**	**3 Renal Artery, Right** **4 Renal Artery, Left** **5 Renal Artery, Bilateral**
E Internal Iliac Artery, Right Deferential artery Hypogastric artery Iliolumbar artery Inferior gluteal artery Inferior vesical artery Internal pudendal artery Lateral sacral artery Middle rectal artery Obturator artery Superior gluteal artery Umbilical artery Uterine artery Vaginal artery **F Internal Iliac Artery, Left** *See E Internal Iliac Artery, Right* **H External Iliac Artery, Right** Deep circumflex iliac artery Inferior epigastric artery **J External Iliac Artery, Left** *See H External Iliac Artery, Right*	**Ø Open** **4 Percutaneous Endoscopic**	**9 Autologous Venous Tissue** **A Autologous Arterial Tissue** **J Synthetic Substitute** **K Nonautologous Tissue Substitute** **Z No Device**	**9 Internal Iliac Artery, Right** **B Internal Iliac Artery, Left** **C Internal Iliac Arteries, Bilateral** **D External Iliac Artery, Right** **F External Iliac Artery, Left** **G External Iliac Arteries, Bilateral** **H Femoral Artery, Right** **J Femoral Artery, Left** **K Femoral Arteries, Bilateral** **P Foot Artery** **Q Lower Extremity Artery**
K Femoral Artery, Right Circumflex iliac artery Deep femoral artery Descending genicular artery External pudendal artery Superficial epigastric artery **L Femoral Artery, Left** *See K Femoral Artery, Right*	**Ø Open** **4 Percutaneous Endoscopic**	**9 Autologous Venous Tissue** **A Autologous Arterial Tissue** **J Synthetic Substitute** **K Nonautologous Tissue Substitute** **Z No Device**	**H Femoral Artery, Right** **J Femoral Artery, Left** **K Femoral Arteries, Bilateral** **L Popliteal Artery** **M Peroneal Artery** **N Posterior Tibial Artery** **P Foot Artery** **Q Lower Extremity Artery** **S Lower Extremity Vein**
K Femoral Artery, Right Circumflex iliac artery Deep femoral artery Descending genicular artery External pudendal artery Superficial epigastric artery **L Femoral Artery, Left** *See K Femoral Artery, Right*	**3 Percutaneous**	**J Synthetic Substitute**	**Q Lower Extremity Artery** **S Lower Extremity Vein**
M Popliteal Artery, Right Inferior genicular artery Middle genicular artery Superior genicular artery Sural artery Tibioperoneal trunk **N Popliteal Artery, Left** *See M Popliteal Artery, Right*	**Ø Open** **4 Percutaneous Endoscopic**	**9 Autologous Venous Tissue** **A Autologous Arterial Tissue** **J Synthetic Substitute** **K Nonautologous Tissue Substitute** **Z No Device**	**L Popliteal Artery** **M Peroneal Artery** **P Foot Artery** **Q Lower Extremity Artery** **S Lower Extremity Vein**

Ø41 Continued on next page

Ø Medical and Surgical
4 Lower Arteries
1 Bypass Definition: Altering the route of passage of the contents of a tubular body part

Explanation: Rerouting contents of a body part to a downstream area of the normal route, to a similar route and body part, or to an abnormal route and dissimilar body part. Includes one or more anastomoses, with or without the use of a device.

Ø41 Continued

Body Part Character 4	Approach Character 5	Device Character 6	Qualifier Character 7
M Popliteal Artery, Right Inferior genicular artery Middle genicular artery Superior genicular artery Sural artery Tibioperoneal trunk **N Popliteal Artery, Left** *See M Popliteal Artery, Right*	**3 Percutaneous**	**J Synthetic Substitute**	**Q Lower Extremity Artery** **S Lower Extremity Vein**
P Anterior Tibial Artery, Right Anterior lateral malleolar artery Anterior medial malleolar artery Anterior tibial recurrent artery Dorsalis pedis artery Posterior tibial recurrent artery **Q Anterior Tibial Artery, Left** *See P Anterior Tibial Artery, Right* **R Posterior Tibial Artery, Right** **S Posterior Tibial Artery, Left**	**Ø Open** **3 Percutaneous** **4 Percutaneous Endoscopic**	**J Synthetic Substitute**	**Q Lower Extremity Artery** **S Lower Extremity Vein**
T Peroneal Artery, Right Fibular artery **U Peroneal Artery, Left** *See T Peroneal Artery, Right* **V Foot Artery, Right** Arcuate artery Dorsal metatarsal artery Lateral plantar artery Lateral tarsal artery Medial plantar artery **W Foot Artery, Left** *See V Foot Artery, Right*	**Ø Open** **4 Percutaneous Endoscopic**	**9 Autologous Venous Tissue** **A Autologous Arterial Tissue** **J Synthetic Substitute** **K Nonautologous Tissue Substitute** **Z No Device**	**P Foot Artery** **Q Lower Extremity Artery** **S Lower Extremity Vein**
T Peroneal Artery, Right Fibular artery **U Peroneal Artery, Left** *See T Peroneal Artery, Right* **V Foot Artery, Right** Arcuate artery Dorsal metatarsal artery Lateral plantar artery Lateral tarsal artery Medial plantar artery **W Foot Artery, Left** *See V Foot Artery, Right*	**3 Percutaneous**	**J Synthetic Substitute**	**Q Lower Extremity Artery** **S Lower Extremity Vein**

Ø Medical and Surgical
4 Lower Arteries
5 Destruction Definition: Physical eradication of all or a portion of a body part by the direct use of energy, force, or a destructive agent
Explanation: None of the body part is physically taken out

Body Part Character 4	Approach Character 5	Device Character 6	Qualifier Character 7
Ø Abdominal Aorta Inferior phrenic artery Lumbar artery Median sacral artery Middle suprarenal artery Ovarian artery Testicular artery **1 Celiac Artery** Celiac trunk **2 Gastric Artery** Left gastric artery Right gastric artery **3 Hepatic Artery** Common hepatic artery Gastroduodenal artery Hepatic artery proper **4 Splenic Artery** Left gastroepiploic artery Pancreatic artery Short gastric artery **5 Superior Mesenteric Artery** Ileal artery Ileocolic artery Inferior pancreaticoduodenal artery Jejunal artery **6 Colic Artery, Right** **7 Colic Artery, Left** **8 Colic Artery, Middle** **9 Renal Artery, Right** Inferior suprarenal artery Renal segmental artery **A Renal Artery, Left** ***See*** *9 Renal Artery, Right* **B Inferior Mesenteric Artery** Sigmoid artery Superior rectal artery **C Common Iliac Artery, Right** **D Common Iliac Artery, Left** **E Internal Iliac Artery, Right** Deferential artery Hypogastric artery Iliolumbar artery Inferior gluteal artery Inferior vesical artery Internal pudendal artery Lateral sacral artery Middle rectal artery Obturator artery Superior gluteal artery Umbilical artery Uterine artery Vaginal artery **F Internal Iliac Artery, Left** ***See*** *E Internal Iliac Artery, Right* **H External Iliac Artery, Right** Deep circumflex iliac artery Inferior epigastric artery **J External Iliac Artery, Left** ***See*** *H External Iliac Artery, Right* **K Femoral Artery, Right** Circumflex iliac artery Deep femoral artery Descending genicular artery External pudendal artery Superficial epigastric artery **L Femoral Artery, Left** ***See*** *K Femoral Artery, Right* **M Popliteal Artery, Right** Inferior genicular artery Middle genicular artery Superior genicular artery Sural artery Tibioperoneal trunk **N Popliteal Artery, Left** ***See*** *M Popliteal Artery, Right* **P Anterior Tibial Artery, Right** Anterior lateral malleolar artery Anterior medial malleolar artery Anterior tibial recurrent artery Dorsalis pedis artery Posterior tibial recurrent artery **Q Anterior Tibial Artery, Left** ***See*** *P Anterior Tibial Artery, Right* **R Posterior Tibial Artery, Right** **S Posterior Tibial Artery, Left** **T Peroneal Artery, Right** Fibular artery **U Peroneal Artery, Left** ***See*** *T Peroneal Artery, Right* **V Foot Artery, Right** Arcuate artery Dorsal metatarsal artery Lateral plantar artery Lateral tarsal artery Medial plantar artery **W Foot Artery, Left** ***See*** *V Foot Artery, Right* **Y Lower Artery** Umbilical artery	**Ø Open** **3 Percutaneous** **4 Percutaneous Endoscopic**	**Z No Device**	**Z No Qualifier**

Ø Medical and Surgical
4 Lower Arteries
7 Dilation Definition: Expanding an orifice or the lumen of a tubular body part

Explanation: The orifice can be a natural orifice or an artificially created orifice. Accomplished by stretching a tubular body part using intraluminal pressure or by cutting part of the orifice or wall of the tubular body part.

Body Part Character 4		Approach Character 5	Device Character 6	Qualifier Character 7
Ø Abdominal Aorta Inferior phrenic artery Lumbar artery Median sacral artery Middle suprarenal artery Ovarian artery Testicular artery **1 Celiac Artery** Celiac trunk **2 Gastric Artery** Left gastric artery Right gastric artery **3 Hepatic Artery** Common hepatic artery Gastroduodenal artery Hepatic artery proper **4 Splenic Artery** Left gastroepiploic artery Pancreatic artery Short gastric artery **5 Superior Mesenteric Artery** Ileal artery Ileocolic artery Inferior pancreaticoduodenal artery Jejunal artery **6 Colic Artery, Right** **7 Colic Artery, Left** **8 Colic Artery, Middle** **9 Renal Artery, Right** Inferior suprarenal artery Renal segmental artery **A Renal Artery, Left** *See 9 Renal Artery, Right* **B Inferior Mesenteric Artery** Sigmoid artery Superior rectal artery **C Common Iliac Artery, Right** **D Common Iliac Artery, Left** **E Internal Iliac Artery, Right** Deferential artery Hypogastric artery Iliolumbar artery Inferior gluteal artery Inferior vesical artery Internal pudendal artery Lateral sacral artery Middle rectal artery Obturator artery Superior gluteal artery Umbilical artery Uterine artery Vaginal artery	**F Internal Iliac Artery, Left** *See E Internal Iliac Artery, Right* **H External Iliac Artery, Right** Deep circumflex iliac artery Inferior epigastric artery **J External Iliac Artery, Left** *See H External Iliac Artery, Right* **K Femoral Artery, Right** Circumflex iliac artery Deep femoral artery Descending genicular artery External pudendal artery Superficial epigastric artery **L Femoral Artery, Left** *See K Femoral Artery, Right* **M Popliteal Artery, Right** Inferior genicular artery Middle genicular artery Superior genicular artery Sural artery Tibioperoneal trunk **N Popliteal Artery, Left** *See M Popliteal Artery, Right* **P Anterior Tibial Artery, Right** Anterior lateral malleolar artery Anterior medial malleolar artery Anterior tibial recurrent artery Dorsalis pedis artery Posterior tibial recurrent artery **Q Anterior Tibial Artery, Left** *See P Anterior Tibial Artery, Right* **R Posterior Tibial Artery, Right** **S Posterior Tibial Artery, Left** **T Peroneal Artery, Right** Fibular artery **U Peroneal Artery, Left** *See T Peroneal Artery, Right* **V Foot Artery, Right** Arcuate artery Dorsal metatarsal artery Lateral plantar artery Lateral tarsal artery Medial plantar artery **W Foot Artery, Left** *See V Foot Artery, Right* **Y Lower Artery** Umbilical artery	**Ø Open** **3 Percutaneous** **4 Percutaneous Endoscopic**	**4 Intraluminal Device, Drug-eluting** **D Intraluminal Device** **Z No Device**	**1 Drug-Coated Balloon** **Z No Qualifier**

Ø47 Continued on next page

Ø Medical and Surgical
4 Lower Arteries
7 Dilation Definition: Expanding an orifice or the lumen of a tubular body part

Explanation: The orifice can be a natural orifice or an artificially created orifice. Accomplished by stretching a tubular body part using intraluminal pressure or by cutting part of the orifice or wall of the tubular body part.

Ø47 Continued

Body Part Character 4		Approach Character 5	Device Character 6	Qualifier Character 7
Ø Abdominal Aorta Inferior phrenic artery Lumbar artery Median sacral artery Middle suprarenal artery Ovarian artery Testicular artery **1 Celiac Artery** Celiac trunk **2 Gastric Artery** Left gastric artery Right gastric artery **3 Hepatic Artery** Common hepatic artery Gastroduodenal artery Hepatic artery proper **4 Splenic Artery** Left gastroepiploic artery Pancreatic artery Short gastric artery **5 Superior Mesenteric Artery** Ileal artery Ileocolic artery Inferior pancreaticoduodenal artery Jejunal artery **6 Colic Artery, Right** **7 Colic Artery, Left** **8 Colic Artery, Middle** **9 Renal Artery, Right** Inferior suprarenal artery Renal segmental artery **A Renal Artery, Left** *See 9 Renal Artery, Right* **B Inferior Mesenteric Artery** Sigmoid artery Superior rectal artery **C Common Iliac Artery, Right** **D Common Iliac Artery, Left** **E Internal Iliac Artery, Right** Deferential artery Hypogastric artery Iliolumbar artery Inferior gluteal artery Inferior vesical artery Internal pudendal artery Lateral sacral artery Middle rectal artery Obturator artery Superior gluteal artery Umbilical artery Uterine artery Vaginal artery	**F Internal Iliac Artery, Left** *See E Internal Iliac Artery, Right* **H External Iliac Artery, Right** Deep circumflex iliac artery Inferior epigastric artery **J External Iliac Artery, Left** *See H External Iliac Artery, Right* **K Femoral Artery, Right** Circumflex iliac artery Deep femoral artery Descending genicular artery External pudendal artery Superficial epigastric artery **L Femoral Artery, Left** *See K Femoral Artery, Right* **M Popliteal Artery, Right** Inferior genicular artery Middle genicular artery Superior genicular artery Sural artery Tibioperoneal trunk **N Popliteal Artery, Left** *See M Popliteal Artery, Right* **P Anterior Tibial Artery, Right** Anterior lateral malleolar artery Anterior medial malleolar artery Anterior tibial recurrent artery Dorsalis pedis artery Posterior tibial recurrent artery **Q Anterior Tibial Artery, Left** *See P Anterior Tibial Artery, Right* **R Posterior Tibial Artery, Right** **S Posterior Tibial Artery, Left** **T Peroneal Artery, Right** Fibular artery **U Peroneal Artery, Left** *See T Peroneal Artery, Right* **V Foot Artery, Right** Arcuate artery Dorsal metatarsal artery Lateral plantar artery Lateral tarsal artery Medial plantar artery **W Foot Artery, Left** *See V Foot Artery, Right* **Y Lower Artery** Umbilical artery	**Ø Open** **3 Percutaneous** **4 Percutaneous Endoscopic**	**5 Intraluminal Device, Drug-eluting, Two** **6 Intraluminal Device, Drug-eluting, Three** **7 Intraluminal Device, Drug-eluting, Four or More** **E Intraluminal Device, Two** **F Intraluminal Device, Three** **G Intraluminal Device, Four or More**	**Z No Qualifier**

Ø Medical and Surgical
4 Lower Arteries
9 Drainage Definition: Taking or letting out fluids and/or gases from a body part
Explanation: The qualifier DIAGNOSTIC is used to identify drainage procedures that are biopsies

Body Part Character 4	Approach Character 5	Device Character 6	Qualifier Character 7
Ø Abdominal Aorta Inferior phrenic artery Lumbar artery Median sacral artery Middle suprarenal artery Ovarian artery Testicular artery **1 Celiac Artery** Celiac trunk **2 Gastric Artery** Left gastric artery Right gastric artery **3 Hepatic Artery** Common hepatic artery Gastroduodenal artery Hepatic artery proper **4 Splenic Artery** Left gastroepiploic artery Pancreatic artery Short gastric artery **5 Superior Mesenteric Artery** Ileal artery Ileocolic artery Inferior pancreaticoduodenal artery Jejunal artery **6 Colic Artery, Right** **7 Colic Artery, Left** **8 Colic Artery, Middle** **9 Renal Artery, Right** Inferior suprarenal artery Renal segmental artery **A Renal Artery, Left** *See 9 Renal Artery, Right* **B Inferior Mesenteric Artery** Sigmoid artery Superior rectal artery **C Common Iliac Artery, Right** **D Common Iliac Artery, Left** **E Internal Iliac Artery, Right** Deferential artery Hypogastric artery Iliolumbar artery Inferior gluteal artery Inferior vesical artery Internal pudendal artery Lateral sacral artery Middle rectal artery Obturator artery Superior gluteal artery Umbilical artery Uterine artery Vaginal artery **F Internal Iliac Artery, Left** *See E Internal Iliac Artery, Right* **H External Iliac Artery, Right** Deep circumflex iliac artery Inferior epigastric artery **J External Iliac Artery, Left** *See H External Iliac Artery, Right* **K Femoral Artery, Right** Circumflex iliac artery Deep femoral artery Descending genicular artery External pudendal artery Superficial epigastric artery **L Femoral Artery, Left** *See K Femoral Artery, Right* **M Popliteal Artery, Right** Inferior genicular artery Middle genicular artery Superior genicular artery Sural artery Tibioperoneal trunk **N Popliteal Artery, Left** *See M Popliteal Artery, Right* **P Anterior Tibial Artery, Right** Anterior lateral malleolar artery Anterior medial malleolar artery Anterior tibial recurrent artery Dorsalis pedis artery Posterior tibial recurrent artery **Q Anterior Tibial Artery, Left** *See P Anterior Tibial Artery, Right* **R Posterior Tibial Artery, Right** **S Posterior Tibial Artery, Left** **T Peroneal Artery, Right** Fibular artery **U Peroneal Artery, Left** *See T Peroneal Artery, Right* **V Foot Artery, Right** Arcuate artery Dorsal metatarsal artery Lateral plantar artery Lateral tarsal artery Medial plantar artery **W Foot Artery, Left** *See V Foot Artery, Right* **Y Lower Artery** Umbilical artery	**Ø Open** **3 Percutaneous** **4 Percutaneous Endoscopic**	**Ø Drainage Device**	**Z No Qualifier**

Non-OR Ø49[Ø,1,2,3,4,5,6,7,8,9,A,B,C,D,E,F,H,J,K,L,M,N,P,Q,R,S,T,U,V,W,Y][Ø,3,4]ØZ

Ø49 Continued on next page

Ø Medical and Surgical
4 Lower Arteries
9 Drainage Definition: Taking or letting out fluids and/or gases from a body part
Explanation: The qualifier DIAGNOSTIC is used to identify drainage procedures that are biopsies

Ø49 Continued

Body Part Character 4	Approach Character 5	Device Character 6	Qualifier Character 7
Ø Abdominal Aorta Inferior phrenic artery Lumbar artery Median sacral artery Middle suprarenal artery Ovarian artery Testicular artery **1 Celiac Artery** Celiac trunk **2 Gastric Artery** Left gastric artery Right gastric artery **3 Hepatic Artery** Common hepatic artery Gastroduodenal artery Hepatic artery proper **4 Splenic Artery** Left gastroepiploic artery Pancreatic artery Short gastric artery **5 Superior Mesenteric Artery** Ileal artery Ileocolic artery Inferior pancreaticoduodenal artery Jejunal artery **6 Colic Artery, Right** **7 Colic Artery, Left** **8 Colic Artery, Middle** **9 Renal Artery, Right** Inferior suprarenal artery Renal segmental artery **A Renal Artery, Left** ***See*** *9 Renal Artery, Right* **B Inferior Mesenteric Artery** Sigmoid artery Superior rectal artery **C Common Iliac Artery, Right** **D Common Iliac Artery, Left** **E Internal Iliac Artery, Right** Deferential artery Hypogastric artery Iliolumbar artery Inferior gluteal artery Inferior vesical artery Internal pudendal artery Lateral sacral artery Middle rectal artery Obturator artery Superior gluteal artery Umbilical artery Uterine artery Vaginal artery **F Internal Iliac Artery, Left** ***See*** *E Internal Iliac Artery, Right* **H External Iliac Artery, Right** Deep circumflex iliac artery Inferior epigastric artery **J External Iliac Artery, Left** ***See*** *H External Iliac Artery, Right* **K Femoral Artery, Right** Circumflex iliac artery Deep femoral artery Descending genicular artery External pudendal artery Superficial epigastric artery **L Femoral Artery, Left** ***See*** *K Femoral Artery, Right* **M Popliteal Artery, Right** Inferior genicular artery Middle genicular artery Superior genicular artery Sural artery Tibioperoneal trunk **N Popliteal Artery, Left** ***See*** *M Popliteal Artery, Right* **P Anterior Tibial Artery, Right** Anterior lateral malleolar artery Anterior medial malleolar artery Anterior tibial recurrent artery Dorsalis pedis artery Posterior tibial recurrent artery **Q Anterior Tibial Artery, Left** ***See*** *P Anterior Tibial Artery, Right* **R Posterior Tibial Artery, Right** **S Posterior Tibial Artery, Left** **T Peroneal Artery, Right** Fibular artery **U Peroneal Artery, Left** ***See*** *T Peroneal Artery, Right* **V Foot Artery, Right** Arcuate artery Dorsal metatarsal artery Lateral plantar artery Lateral tarsal artery Medial plantar artery **W Foot Artery, Left** ***See*** *V Foot Artery, Right* **Y Lower Artery** Umbilical artery	Ø Open 3 Percutaneous 4 Percutaneous Endoscopic	Z No Device	X Diagnostic Z No Qualifier

Non-OR Ø49[Ø,1,2,3,4,5,6,7,8,9,A,B,C,D,E,F,H,J,K,L,M,N,P,Q,R,S,T,U,V,W,Y]3ZX
Non-OR Ø49[Ø,1,2,3,4,5,6,7,8,9,A,B,C,D,E,F,H,J,K,L,M,N,P,Q,R,S,T,U,V,W,Y][Ø,3,4]ZZ

Ø Medical and Surgical
4 Lower Arteries
B Excision Definition: Cutting out or off, without replacement, a portion of a body part
Explanation: The qualifier DIAGNOSTIC is used to identify excision procedures that are biopsies

Body Part Character 4	Body Part Character 4	Approach Character 5	Device Character 6	Qualifier Character 7
Ø Abdominal Aorta Inferior phrenic artery Lumbar artery Median sacral artery Middle suprarenal artery Ovarian artery Testicular artery **1 Celiac Artery** Celiac trunk **2 Gastric Artery** Left gastric artery Right gastric artery **3 Hepatic Artery** Common hepatic artery Gastroduodenal artery Hepatic artery proper **4 Splenic Artery** Left gastroepiploic artery Pancreatic artery Short gastric artery **5 Superior Mesenteric Artery** Ileal artery Ileocolic artery Inferior pancreaticoduodenal artery Jejunal artery **6 Colic Artery, Right** **7 Colic Artery, Left** **8 Colic Artery, Middle** **9 Renal Artery, Right** Inferior suprarenal artery Renal segmental artery **A Renal Artery, Left** ***See*** *9 Renal Artery, Right* **B Inferior Mesenteric Artery** Sigmoid artery Superior rectal artery **C Common Iliac Artery, Right** **D Common Iliac Artery, Left** **E Internal Iliac Artery, Right** Deferential artery Hypogastric artery Iliolumbar artery Inferior gluteal artery Inferior vesical artery Internal pudendal artery Lateral sacral artery Middle rectal artery Obturator artery Superior gluteal artery Umbilical artery Uterine artery Vaginal artery	**F Internal Iliac Artery, Left** ***See*** *E Internal Iliac Artery, Right* **H External Iliac Artery, Right** Deep circumflex iliac artery Inferior epigastric artery **J External Iliac Artery, Left** ***See*** *H External Iliac Artery, Right* **K Femoral Artery, Right** Circumflex iliac artery Deep femoral artery Descending genicular artery External pudendal artery Superficial epigastric artery **L Femoral Artery, Left** ***See*** *K Femoral Artery, Right* **M Popliteal Artery, Right** Inferior genicular artery Middle genicular artery Superior genicular artery Sural artery Tibioperoneal trunk **N Popliteal Artery, Left** ***See*** *M Popliteal Artery, Right* **P Anterior Tibial Artery, Right** Anterior lateral malleolar artery Anterior medial malleolar artery Anterior tibial recurrent artery Dorsalis pedis artery Posterior tibial recurrent artery **Q Anterior Tibial Artery, Left** ***See*** *P Anterior Tibial Artery, Right* **R Posterior Tibial Artery, Right** **S Posterior Tibial Artery, Left** **T Peroneal Artery, Right** Fibular artery **U Peroneal Artery, Left** ***See*** *T Peroneal Artery, Right* **V Foot Artery, Right** Arcuate artery Dorsal metatarsal artery Lateral plantar artery Lateral tarsal artery Medial plantar artery **W Foot Artery, Left** ***See*** *V Foot Artery, Right* **Y Lower Artery** Umbilical artery	**Ø Open** **3 Percutaneous** **4 Percutaneous Endoscopic**	**Z No Device**	**X Diagnostic** **Z No Qualifier**

Ø Medical and Surgical
4 Lower Arteries
C Extirpation Definition: Taking or cutting out solid matter from a body part

Explanation: The solid matter may be an abnormal byproduct of a biological function or a foreign body; it may be imbedded in a body part or in the lumen of a tubular body part. The solid matter may or may not have been previously broken into pieces.

Body Part Character 4		Approach Character 5	Device Character 6	Qualifier Character 7
Ø Abdominal Aorta Inferior phrenic artery Lumbar artery Median sacral artery Middle suprarenal artery Ovarian artery Testicular artery **1 Celiac Artery** Celiac trunk **2 Gastric Artery** Left gastric artery Right gastric artery **3 Hepatic Artery** Common hepatic artery Gastroduodenal artery Hepatic artery proper **4 Splenic Artery** Left gastroepiploic artery Pancreatic artery Short gastric artery **5 Superior Mesenteric Artery** Ileal artery Ileocolic artery Inferior pancreaticoduodenal artery Jejunal artery **6 Colic Artery, Right** **7 Colic Artery, Left** **8 Colic Artery, Middle** **9 Renal Artery, Right** Inferior suprarenal artery Renal segmental artery **A Renal Artery, Left** ***See*** *9 Renal Artery, Right* **B Inferior Mesenteric Artery** Sigmoid artery Superior rectal artery **C Common Iliac Artery, Right** **D Common Iliac Artery, Left** **E Internal Iliac Artery, Right** Deferential artery Hypogastric artery Iliolumbar artery Inferior gluteal artery Inferior vesical artery Internal pudendal artery Lateral sacral artery Middle rectal artery Obturator artery Superior gluteal artery Umbilical artery Uterine artery Vaginal artery	**F Internal Iliac Artery, Left** ***See*** *E Internal Iliac Artery, Right* **H External Iliac Artery, Right** Deep circumflex iliac artery Inferior epigastric artery **J External Iliac Artery, Left** ***See*** *H External Iliac Artery, Right* **K Femoral Artery, Right** Circumflex iliac artery Deep femoral artery Descending genicular artery External pudendal artery Superficial epigastric artery **L Femoral Artery, Left** ***See*** *K Femoral Artery, Right* **M Popliteal Artery, Right** Inferior genicular artery Middle genicular artery Superior genicular artery Sural artery Tibioperoneal trunk **N Popliteal Artery, Left** ***See*** *M Popliteal Artery, Right* **P Anterior Tibial Artery, Right** Anterior lateral malleolar artery Anterior medial malleolar artery Anterior tibial recurrent artery Dorsalis pedis artery Posterior tibial recurrent artery **Q Anterior Tibial Artery, Left** ***See*** *P Anterior Tibial Artery, Right* **R Posterior Tibial Artery, Right** **S Posterior Tibial Artery, Left** **T Peroneal Artery, Right** Fibular artery **U Peroneal Artery, Left** ***See*** *T Peroneal Artery, Right* **V Foot Artery, Right** Arcuate artery Dorsal metatarsal artery Lateral plantar artery Lateral tarsal artery Medial plantar artery **W Foot Artery, Left** ***See*** *V Foot Artery, Right* **Y Lower Artery** Umbilical artery	**Ø Open** **3 Percutaneous** **4 Percutaneous Endoscopic**	**Z No Device**	**Z No Qualifier**

Ø Medical and Surgical
4 Lower Arteries
F Fragmentation Definition: Breaking solid matter in a body part into pieces

Explanation: Physical force (e.g., manual, ultrasonic) applied directly or indirectly is used to break the solid matter into pieces. The solid matter may be an abnormal byproduct of a biological function or a foreign body. The pieces of solid matter are not taken out.

Body Part Character 4		Approach Character 5	Device Character 6	Qualifier Character 7
C Common Iliac Artery, Right **D Common Iliac Artery, Left** **E Internal Iliac Artery, Right** Deferential artery Hypogastric artery Iliolumbar artery Inferior gluteal artery Inferior vesical artery Internal pudendal artery Lateral sacral artery Middle rectal artery Obturator artery Superior gluteal artery Umbilical artery Uterine artery Vaginal artery **F Internal Iliac Artery, Left** *See E Internal Iliac Artery, Right* **H External Iliac Artery, Right** Deep circumflex iliac artery Inferior epigastric artery **J External Iliac Artery, Left** *See H External Iliac Artery, Right* **K Femoral Artery, Right** Circumflex Iliac artery Deep femoral artery Descending genicular artery External pudendal artery Superficial epigastric artery	**L Femoral Artery, Left** *See K Femoral Artery, Right* **M Popliteal Artery, Right** Inferior genicular artery Middle genicular artery Superior genicular artery Sural artery Tibioperoneal trunk **N Popliteal Artery, Left** *See M Popliteal Artery, Right* **P Anterior Tibial Artery, Right** Anterior lateral malleolar artery Anterior medial malleolar artery Anterior tibial recurrent artery Dorsalis pedis artery Posterior tibial recurrent artery **Q Anterior Tibial Artery, Left** *See P Anterior Tibial Artery, Right* **R Posterior Tibial Artery, Right** **S Posterior Tibial Artery, Left** **T Peroneal Artery, Right** Fibular artery **U Peroneal Artery, Left** *See T Peroneal Artery, Right* **Y Lower Artery** Umbilical artery	**3** Percutaneous	**Z** No Device	**Ø** Ultrasonic **Z** No Qualifier

Ø Medical and Surgical
4 Lower Arteries
H Insertion Definition: Putting in a nonbiological appliance that monitors, assists, performs, or prevents a physiological function but does not physically take the place of a body part

Explanation: None

Body Part Character 4	Approach Character 5	Device Character 6	Qualifier Character 7
Ø Abdominal Aorta Inferior phrenic artery Lumbar artery Median sacral artery Middle suprarenal artery Ovarian artery Testicular artery	**Ø Open** **3 Percutaneous** **4 Percutaneous Endoscopic**	**2 Monitoring Device** **3 Infusion Device** **D Intraluminal Device**	**Z No Qualifier**
1 Celiac Artery Celiac trunk **2 Gastric Artery** Left gastric artery Right gastric artery **3 Hepatic Artery** Common hepatic artery Gastroduodenal artery Hepatic artery proper **4 Splenic Artery** Left gastroepiploic artery Pancreatic artery Short gastric artery **5 Superior Mesenteric Artery** Ileal artery Ileocolic artery Inferior pancreaticoduodenal artery Jejunal artery **6 Colic Artery, Right** **7 Colic Artery, Left** **8 Colic Artery, Middle** **9 Renal Artery, Right** Inferior suprarenal artery Renal segmental artery **A Renal Artery, Left** *See 9 Renal Artery, Right* **B Inferior Mesenteric Artery** Sigmoid artery Superior rectal artery **C Common Iliac Artery, Right** **D Common Iliac Artery, Left** **E Internal Iliac Artery, Right** Deferential artery Hypogastric artery Iliolumbar artery Inferior gluteal artery Inferior vesical artery Internal pudendal artery Lateral sacral artery Middle rectal artery Obturator artery Superior gluteal artery Umbilical artery Uterine artery Vaginal artery **F Internal Iliac Artery, Left** *See E Internal Iliac Artery, Right* **H External Iliac Artery, Right** Deep circumflex iliac artery Inferior epigastric artery **J External Iliac Artery, Left** *See H External Iliac Artery, Right* **K Femoral Artery, Right** Circumflex iliac artery Deep femoral artery Descending genicular artery External pudendal artery Superficial epigastric artery **L Femoral Artery, Left** *See K Femoral Artery, Right* **M Popliteal Artery, Right** Inferior genicular artery Middle genicular artery Superior genicular artery Sural artery Tibioperoneal trunk **N Popliteal Artery, Left** *See M Popliteal Artery, Right* **P Anterior Tibial Artery, Right** Anterior lateral malleolar artery Anterior medial malleolar artery Anterior tibial recurrent artery Dorsalis pedis artery Posterior tibial recurrent artery **Q Anterior Tibial Artery, Left** *See P Anterior Tibial Artery, Right* **R Posterior Tibial Artery, Right** **S Posterior Tibial Artery, Left** **T Peroneal Artery, Right** Fibular artery **U Peroneal Artery, Left** *See T Peroneal Artery, Right* **V Foot Artery, Right** Arcuate artery Dorsal metatarsal artery Lateral plantar artery Lateral tarsal artery Medial plantar artery **W Foot Artery, Left** *See V Foot Artery, Right*	**Ø Open** **3 Percutaneous** **4 Percutaneous Endoscopic**	**3 Infusion Device** **D Intraluminal Device**	**Z No Qualifier**
Y Lower Artery Umbilical artery	**Ø Open** **3 Percutaneous** **4 Percutaneous Endoscopic**	**2 Monitoring Device** **3 Infusion Device** **D Intraluminal Device** **Y Other Device**	**Z No Qualifier**

Non-OR Ø4HØ[Ø,3,4][2,3]Z
Non-OR Ø4H[1,2,3,4,5,6,7,8,9,A,B,C,D,E,F,H,J,K,L,M,N,P,Q,R,S,T,U,V,W][Ø,3,4]3Z
Non-OR Ø4HY32Z
Non-OR Ø4HY[Ø,3,4]3Z
Non-OR Ø4HY[3,4]YZ

Ø Medical and Surgical
4 Lower Arteries
J Inspection Definition: Visually and/or manually exploring a body part

Explanation: Visual exploration may be performed with or without optical instrumentation. Manual exploration may be performed directly or through intervening body layers.

Body Part Character 4	Approach Character 5	Device Character 6	Qualifier Character 7
Y Lower Artery Umbilical artery	Ø Open 3 Percutaneous 4 Percutaneous Endoscopic X External	Z No Device	Z No Qualifier

Non-OR Ø4JY[3,4,X]ZZ

Ø Medical and Surgical
4 Lower Arteries
L Occlusion Definition: Completely closing an orifice or the lumen of a tubular body part

Explanation: The orifice can be a natural orifice or an artificially created orifice

Body Part Character 4	Approach Character 5	Device Character 6	Qualifier Character 7
Ø Abdominal Aorta Inferior phrenic artery Lumbar artery Median sacral artery Middle suprarenal artery Ovarian artery Testicular artery	Ø Open 4 Percutaneous Endoscopic	C Extraluminal Device D Intraluminal Device Z No Device	Z No Qualifier
Ø Abdominal Aorta Inferior phrenic artery Lumbar artery Median sacral artery Middle suprarenal artery Ovarian artery Testicular artery	3 Percutaneous	C Extraluminal Device Z No Device	Z No Qualifier
Ø Abdominal Aorta Inferior phrenic artery Lumbar artery Median sacral artery Middle suprarenal artery Ovarian artery Testicular artery	3 Percutaneous	D Intraluminal Device	J Temporary Z No Qualifier

Ø4L Continued on next page

Ø Medical and Surgical
4 Lower Arteries
L Occlusion Definition: Completely closing an orifice or the lumen of a tubular body part

Explanation: The orifice can be a natural orifice or an artificially created orifice

Ø4L Continued

Body Part Character 4	Approach Character 5	Device Character 6	Qualifier Character 7
1 Celiac Artery Celiac trunk **2 Gastric Artery** Left gastric artery, Right gastric artery **3 Hepatic Artery** Common hepatic artery, Gastroduodenal artery, Hepatic artery proper **4 Splenic Artery** Left gastroepiploic artery, Pancreatic artery, Short gastric artery **5 Superior Mesenteric Artery** Ileal artery, Ileocolic artery, Inferior pancreaticoduodenal artery, Jejunal artery **6 Colic Artery, Right** **7 Colic Artery, Left** **8 Colic Artery, Middle** **9 Renal Artery, Right** Inferior suprarenal artery, Renal segmental artery **A Renal Artery, Left** *See 9 Renal Artery, Right* **B Inferior Mesenteric Artery** Sigmoid artery, Superior rectal artery **C Common Iliac Artery, Right** **D Common Iliac Artery, Left** **H External Iliac Artery, Right** Deep circumflex iliac artery, Inferior epigastric artery **J External Iliac Artery, Left** *See H External Iliac Artery, Right* **K Femoral Artery, Right** Circumflex iliac artery, Deep femoral artery, Descending genicular artery, External pudendal artery, Superficial epigastric artery **L Femoral Artery, Left** *See K Femoral Artery, Right* **M Popliteal Artery, Right** Inferior genicular artery, Middle genicular artery, Superior genicular artery, Sural artery, Tibioperoneal trunk **N Popliteal Artery, Left** *See M Popliteal Artery, Right* **P Anterior Tibial Artery, Right** Anterior lateral malleolar artery, Anterior medial malleolar artery, Anterior tibial recurrent artery, Dorsalis pedis artery, Posterior tibial recurrent artery **Q Anterior Tibial Artery, Left** *See P Anterior Tibial Artery, Right* **R Posterior Tibial Artery, Right** **S Posterior Tibial Artery, Left** **T Peroneal Artery, Right** Fibular artery **U Peroneal Artery, Left** *See T Peroneal Artery, Right* **V Foot Artery, Right** Arcuate artery, Dorsal metatarsal artery, Lateral plantar artery, Lateral tarsal artery, Medial plantar artery **W Foot Artery, Left** *See V Foot Artery, Right* **Y Lower Artery** Umbilical artery	**Ø Open** **3 Percutaneous** **4 Percutaneous Endoscopic**	**C Extraluminal Device** **D Intraluminal Device** **Z No Device**	**Z No Qualifier**
E Internal Iliac Artery, Right Deferential artery, Hypogastric artery, Iliolumbar artery, Inferior gluteal artery, Inferior vesical artery, Internal pudendal artery, Lateral sacral artery, Middle rectal artery, Obturator artery, Superior gluteal artery, Umbilical artery, Uterine artery, Vaginal artery	**Ø Open** **3 Percutaneous** **4 Percutaneous Endoscopic**	**C Extraluminal Device** **D Intraluminal Device** **Z No Device**	**T Uterine Artery, Right** ♀ **Z No Qualifier**
F Internal Iliac Artery, Left Deferential artery, Hypogastric artery, Iliolumbar artery, Inferior gluteal artery, Inferior vesical artery, Internal pudendal artery, Lateral sacral artery, Middle rectal artery, Obturator artery, Superior gluteal artery, Umbilical artery, Uterine Artery, Vaginal artery	**Ø Open** **3 Percutaneous** **4 Percutaneous Endoscopic**	**C Extraluminal Device** **D Intraluminal Device** **Z No Device**	**U Uterine Artery, Left** ♀ **Z No Qualifier**

♀ Ø4LE[Ø,3,4][C,D,Z]T
♀ Ø4LF[Ø,3,4][C,D,Z]U

Ø Medical and Surgical
4 Lower Arteries
N Release Definition: Freeing a body part from an abnormal physical constraint by cutting or by the use of force
Explanation: Some of the restraining tissue may be taken out but none of the body part is taken out

Body Part Character 4		Approach Character 5	Device Character 6	Qualifier Character 7
Ø Abdominal Aorta Inferior phrenic artery Lumbar artery Median sacral artery Middle suprarenal artery Ovarian artery Testicular artery **1 Celiac Artery** Celiac trunk **2 Gastric Artery** Left gastric artery Right gastric artery **3 Hepatic Artery** Common hepatic artery Gastroduodenal artery Hepatic artery proper **4 Splenic Artery** Left gastroepiploic artery Pancreatic artery Short gastric artery **5 Superior Mesenteric Artery** Ileal artery Ileocolic artery Inferior pancreaticoduodenal artery Jejunal artery **6 Colic Artery, Right** **7 Colic Artery, Left** **8 Colic Artery, Middle** **9 Renal Artery, Right** Inferior suprarenal artery Renal segmental artery **A Renal Artery, Left** *See 9 Renal Artery, Right* **B Inferior Mesenteric Artery** Sigmoid artery Superior rectal artery **C Common Iliac Artery, Right** **D Common Iliac Artery, Left** **E Internal Iliac Artery, Right** Deferential artery Hypogastric artery Iliolumbar artery Inferior gluteal artery Inferior vesical artery Internal pudendal artery Lateral sacral artery Middle rectal artery Obturator artery Superior gluteal artery Umbilical artery Uterine artery Vaginal artery	**F Internal Iliac Artery, Left** *See E Internal Iliac Artery, Right* **H External Iliac Artery, Right** Deep circumflex iliac artery Inferior epigastric artery **J External Iliac Artery, Left** *See H External Iliac Artery, Right* **K Femoral Artery, Right** Circumflex iliac artery Deep femoral artery Descending genicular artery External pudendal artery Superficial epigastric artery **L Femoral Artery, Left** *See K Femoral Artery, Right* **M Popliteal Artery, Right** Inferior genicular artery Middle genicular artery Superior genicular artery Sural artery Tibioperoneal trunk **N Popliteal Artery, Left** *See M Popliteal Artery, Right* **P Anterior Tibial Artery, Right** Anterior lateral malleolar artery Anterior medial malleolar artery Anterior tibial recurrent artery Dorsalis pedis artery Posterior tibial recurrent artery **Q Anterior Tibial Artery, Left** *See P Anterior Tibial Artery, Right* **R Posterior Tibial Artery, Right** **S Posterior Tibial Artery, Left** **T Peroneal Artery, Right** Fibular artery **U Peroneal Artery, Left** *See T Peroneal Artery, Right* **V Foot Artery, Right** Arcuate artery Dorsal metatarsal artery Lateral plantar artery Lateral tarsal artery Medial plantar artery **W Foot Artery, Left** *See V Foot Artery, Right* **Y Lower Artery** Umbilical artery	**Ø Open** **3 Percutaneous** **4 Percutaneous Endoscopic**	**Z No Device**	**Z No Qualifier**

Ø Medical and Surgical
4 Lower Arteries
P Removal Definition: Taking out or off a device from a body part

Explanation: If a device is taken out and a similar device put in without cutting or puncturing the skin or mucous membrane, the procedure is coded to the root operation CHANGE. Otherwise, the procedure for taking out a device is coded to the root operation REMOVAL.

Body Part Character 4	Approach Character 5	Device Character 6	Qualifier Character 7
Y Lower Artery Umbilical artery	Ø Open 3 Percutaneous 4 Percutaneous Endoscopic	Ø Drainage Device 2 Monitoring Device 3 Infusion Device 7 Autologous Tissue Substitute C Extraluminal Device D Intraluminal Device J Synthetic Substitute K Nonautologous Tissue Substitute Y Other Device	Z No Qualifier
Y Lower Artery Umbilical artery	X External	Ø Drainage Device 1 Radioactive Element 2 Monitoring Device 3 Infusion Device D Intraluminal Device	Z No Qualifier

Non-OR Ø4PY3[Ø,2,3,D]Z
Non-OR Ø4PY[3,4]YZ
Non-OR Ø4PYX[Ø,1,2,3,D]Z

Ø Medical and Surgical
4 Lower Arteries
Q Repair Definition: Restoring, to the extent possible, a body part to its normal anatomic structure and function

Explanation: Used only when the method to accomplish the repair is not one of the other root operations

Body Part Character 4	Approach Character 5	Device Character 6	Qualifier Character 7
Ø Abdominal Aorta Inferior phrenic artery Lumbar artery Median sacral artery Middle suprarenal artery Ovarian artery Testicular artery **1 Celiac Artery** Celiac trunk **2 Gastric Artery** Left gastric artery Right gastric artery **3 Hepatic Artery** Common hepatic artery Gastroduodenal artery Hepatic artery proper **4 Splenic Artery** Left gastroepiploic artery Pancreatic artery Short gastric artery **5 Superior Mesenteric Artery** Ileal artery Ileocolic artery Inferior pancreaticoduodenal artery Jejunal artery **6 Colic Artery, Right** **7 Colic Artery, Left** **8 Colic Artery, Middle** **9 Renal Artery, Right** Inferior suprarenal artery Renal segmental artery **A Renal Artery, Left** ***See*** *9 Renal Artery, Right* **B Inferior Mesenteric Artery** Sigmoid artery Superior rectal artery **C Common Iliac Artery, Right** **D Common Iliac Artery, Left** **E Internal Iliac Artery, Right** Deferential artery Hypogastric artery Iliolumbar artery Inferior gluteal artery Inferior vesical artery Internal pudendal artery Lateral sacral artery Middle rectal artery Obturator artery Superior gluteal artery Umbilical artery Uterine artery Vaginal artery **F Internal Iliac Artery, Left** ***See*** *E Internal Iliac Artery, Right* **H External Iliac Artery, Right** Deep circumflex iliac artery Inferior epigastric artery **J External Iliac Artery, Left** ***See*** *H External Iliac Artery, Right* **K Femoral Artery, Right** Circumflex iliac artery Deep femoral artery Descending genicular artery External pudendal artery Superficial epigastric artery **L Femoral Artery, Left** ***See*** *K Femoral Artery, Right* **M Popliteal Artery, Right** Inferior genicular artery Middle genicular artery Superior genicular artery Sural artery Tibioperoneal trunk **N Popliteal Artery, Left** ***See*** *M Popliteal Artery, Right* **P Anterior Tibial Artery, Right** Anterior lateral malleolar artery Anterior medial malleolar artery Anterior tibial recurrent artery Dorsalis pedis artery Posterior tibial recurrent artery **Q Anterior Tibial Artery, Left** ***See*** *P Anterior Tibial Artery, Right* **R Posterior Tibial Artery, Right** **S Posterior Tibial Artery, Left** **T Peroneal Artery, Right** Fibular artery **U Peroneal Artery, Left** ***See*** *T Peroneal Artery, Right* **V Foot Artery, Right** Arcuate artery Dorsal metatarsal artery Lateral plantar artery Lateral tarsal artery Medial plantar artery **W Foot Artery, Left** ***See*** *V Foot Artery, Right* **Y Lower Artery** Umbilical artery	**Ø Open** **3 Percutaneous** **4 Percutaneous Endoscopic**	**Z No Device**	**Z No Qualifier**

Ø Medical and Surgical
4 Lower Arteries
R Replacement Definition: Putting in or on biological or synthetic material that physically takes the place and/or function of all or a portion of a body part

Explanation: The body part may have been taken out or replaced, or may be taken out, physically eradicated, or rendered nonfunctional during the REPLACEMENT procedure. A REMOVAL procedure is coded for taking out the device used in a previous replacement procedure.

Body Part Character 4	Approach Character 5	Device Character 6	Qualifier Character 7
Ø Abdominal Aorta Inferior phrenic artery Lumbar artery Median sacral artery Middle suprarenal artery Ovarian artery Testicular artery **1 Celiac Artery** Celiac trunk **2 Gastric Artery** Left gastric artery Right gastric artery **3 Hepatic Artery** Common hepatic artery Gastroduodenal artery Hepatic artery proper **4 Splenic Artery** Left gastroepiploic artery Pancreatic artery Short gastric artery **5 Superior Mesenteric Artery** Ileal artery Ileocolic artery Inferior pancreaticoduodenal artery Jejunal artery **6 Colic Artery, Right** **7 Colic Artery, Left** **8 Colic Artery, Middle** **9 Renal Artery, Right** Inferior suprarenal artery Renal segmental artery **A Renal Artery, Left** *See 9 Renal Artery, Right* **B Inferior Mesenteric Artery** Sigmoid artery Superior rectal artery **C Common Iliac Artery, Right** **D Common Iliac Artery, Left** **E Internal Iliac Artery, Right** Deferential artery Hypogastric artery Iliolumbar artery Inferior gluteal artery Inferior vesical artery Internal pudendal artery Lateral sacral artery Middle rectal artery Obturator artery Superior gluteal artery Umbilical artery Uterine artery Vaginal artery **F Internal Iliac Artery, Left** *See E Internal Iliac Artery, Right* **H External Iliac Artery, Right** Deep circumflex iliac artery Inferior epigastric artery **J External Iliac Artery, Left** *See H External Iliac Artery, Right* **K Femoral Artery, Right** Circumflex iliac artery Deep femoral artery Descending genicular artery External pudendal artery Superficial epigastric artery **L Femoral Artery, Left** *See K Femoral Artery, Right* **M Popliteal Artery, Right** Inferior genicular artery Middle genicular artery Superior genicular artery Sural artery Tibioperoneal trunk **N Popliteal Artery, Left** *See M Popliteal Artery, Right* **P Anterior Tibial Artery, Right** Anterior lateral malleolar artery Anterior medial malleolar artery Anterior tibial recurrent artery Dorsalis pedis artery Posterior tibial recurrent artery **Q Anterior Tibial Artery, Left** *See P Anterior Tibial Artery, Right* **R Posterior Tibial Artery, Right** **S Posterior Tibial Artery, Left** **T Peroneal Artery, Right** Fibular artery **U Peroneal Artery, Left** *See T Peroneal Artery, Right* **V Foot Artery, Right** Arcuate artery Dorsal metatarsal artery Lateral plantar artery Lateral tarsal artery Medial plantar artery **W Foot Artery, Left** *See V Foot Artery, Right* **Y Lower Artery** Umbilical artery	**Ø Open** **4 Percutaneous Endoscopic**	**7 Autologous Tissue Substitute** **J Synthetic Substitute** **K Nonautologous Tissue Substitute**	**Z No Qualifier**

Ø Medical and Surgical
4 Lower Arteries
S Reposition Definition: Moving to its normal location, or other suitable location, all or a portion of a body part

Explanation: The body part is moved to a new location from an abnormal location, or from a normal location where it is not functioning correctly. The body part may or may not be cut out or off to be moved to the new location.

Body Part Character 4	Approach Character 5	Device Character 6	Qualifier Character 7
Ø Abdominal Aorta Inferior phrenic artery Lumbar artery Median sacral artery Middle suprarenal artery Ovarian artery Testicular artery **1 Celiac Artery** Celiac trunk **2 Gastric Artery** Left gastric artery Right gastric artery **3 Hepatic Artery** Common hepatic artery Gastroduodenal artery Hepatic artery proper **4 Splenic Artery** Left gastroepiploic artery Pancreatic artery Short gastric artery **5 Superior Mesenteric Artery** Ileal artery Ileocolic artery Inferior pancreaticoduodenal artery Jejunal artery **6 Colic Artery, Right** **7 Colic Artery, Left** **8 Colic Artery, Middle** **9 Renal Artery, Right** Inferior suprarenal artery Renal segmental artery **A Renal Artery, Left** ***See*** *9 Renal Artery, Right* **B Inferior Mesenteric Artery** Sigmoid artery Superior rectal artery **C Common Iliac Artery, Right** **D Common Iliac Artery, Left** **E Internal Iliac Artery, Right** Deferential artery Hypogastric artery Iliolumbar artery Inferior gluteal artery Inferior vesical artery Internal pudendal artery Lateral sacral artery Middle rectal artery Obturator artery Superior gluteal artery Umbilical artery Uterine artery Vaginal artery **F Internal Iliac Artery, Left** ***See*** *E Internal Iliac Artery, Right* **H External Iliac Artery, Right** Deep circumflex iliac artery Inferior epigastric artery **J External Iliac Artery, Left** ***See*** *H External Iliac Artery, Right* **K Femoral Artery, Right** Circumflex iliac artery Deep femoral artery Descending genicular artery External pudendal artery Superficial epigastric artery **L Femoral Artery, Left** ***See*** *K Femoral Artery, Right* **M Popliteal Artery, Right** Inferior genicular artery Middle genicular artery Superior genicular artery Sural artery Tibioperoneal trunk **N Popliteal Artery, Left** ***See*** *M Popliteal Artery, Right* **P Anterior Tibial Artery, Right** Anterior lateral malleolar artery Anterior medial malleolar artery Anterior tibial recurrent artery Dorsalis pedis artery Posterior tibial recurrent artery **Q Anterior Tibial Artery, Left** ***See*** *P Anterior Tibial Artery, Right* **R Posterior Tibial Artery, Right** **S Posterior Tibial Artery, Left** **T Peroneal Artery, Right** Fibular artery **U Peroneal Artery, Left** ***See*** *T Peroneal Artery, Right* **V Foot Artery, Right** Arcuate artery Dorsal metatarsal artery Lateral plantar artery Lateral tarsal artery Medial plantar artery **W Foot Artery, Left** ***See*** *V Foot Artery, Right* **Y Lower Artery** Umbilical artery	**Ø Open** **3 Percutaneous** **4 Percutaneous Endoscopic**	**Z No Device**	**Z No Qualifier**

Ø Medical and Surgical
4 Lower Arteries
U Supplement

Definition: Putting in or on biological or synthetic material that physically reinforces and/or augments the function of a portion of a body part

Explanation: The biological material is non-living, or is living and from the same individual. The body part may have been previously replaced, and the SUPPLEMENT procedure is performed to physically reinforce and/or augment the function of the replaced body part.

Body Part Character 4	Approach Character 5	Device Character 6	Qualifier Character 7
Ø Abdominal Aorta Inferior phrenic artery Lumbar artery Median sacral artery Middle suprarenal artery Ovarian artery Testicular artery **1 Celiac Artery** Celiac trunk **2 Gastric Artery** Left gastric artery Right gastric artery **3 Hepatic Artery** Common hepatic artery Gastroduodenal artery Hepatic artery proper **4 Splenic Artery** Left gastroepiploic artery Pancreatic artery Short gastric artery **5 Superior Mesenteric Artery** Ileal artery Ileocolic artery Inferior pancreaticoduodenal artery Jejunal artery **6 Colic Artery, Right** **7 Colic Artery, Left** **8 Colic Artery, Middle** **9 Renal Artery, Right** Inferior suprarenal artery Renal segmental artery **A Renal Artery, Left** *See 9 Renal Artery, Right* **B Inferior Mesenteric Artery** Sigmoid artery Superior rectal artery **C Common Iliac Artery, Right** **D Common Iliac Artery, Left** **E Internal Iliac Artery, Right** Deferential artery Hypogastric artery Iliolumbar artery Inferior gluteal artery Inferior vesical artery Internal pudendal artery Lateral sacral artery Middle rectal artery Obturator artery Superior gluteal artery Umbilical artery Uterine artery Vaginal artery **F Internal Iliac Artery, Left** *See E Internal Iliac Artery, Right* **H External Iliac Artery, Right** Deep circumflex iliac artery Inferior epigastric artery **J External Iliac Artery, Left** *See H External Iliac Artery, Right* **K Femoral Artery, Right** Circumflex iliac artery Deep femoral artery Descending genicular artery External pudendal artery Superficial epigastric artery **L Femoral Artery, Left** *See K Femoral Artery, Right* **M Popliteal Artery, Right** Inferior genicular artery Middle genicular artery Superior genicular artery Sural artery Tibioperoneal trunk **N Popliteal Artery, Left** *See M Popliteal Artery, Right* **P Anterior Tibial Artery, Right** Anterior lateral malleolar artery Anterior medial malleolar artery Anterior tibial recurrent artery Dorsalis pedis artery Posterior tibial recurrent artery **Q Anterior Tibial Artery, Left** *See P Anterior Tibial Artery, Right* **R Posterior Tibial Artery, Right** **S Posterior Tibial Artery, Left** **T Peroneal Artery, Right** Fibular artery **U Peroneal Artery, Left** *See T Peroneal Artery, Right* **V Foot Artery, Right** Arcuate artery Dorsal metatarsal artery Lateral plantar artery Lateral tarsal artery Medial plantar artery **W Foot Artery, Left** *See V Foot Artery, Right* **Y Lower Artery** Umbilical artery	**Ø Open** **3 Percutaneous** **4 Percutaneous Endoscopic**	**7 Autologous Tissue Substitute** **J Synthetic Substitute** **K Nonautologous Tissue Substitute**	**Z No Qualifier**

Ø Medical and Surgical
4 Lower Arteries
V Restriction Definition: Partially closing an orifice or the lumen of a tubular body part
Explanation: The orifice can be a natural orifice or an artificially created orifice

Body Part Character 4	Approach Character 5	Device Character 6	Qualifier Character 7
Ø Abdominal Aorta Inferior phrenic artery Lumbar artery Median sacral artery Middle suprarenal artery Ovarian artery Testicular artery	**Ø Open** **3 Percutaneous** **4 Percutaneous Endoscopic**	**C Extraluminal Device** **E Intraluminal Device, Branched or Fenestrated, One or Two Arteries** **F Intraluminal Device, Branched or Fenestrated, Three or More Arteries** **Z No Device**	**Z No Qualifier**
Ø Abdominal Aorta Inferior phrenic artery Lumbar artery Median sacral artery Middle suprarenal artery Ovarian artery Testicular artery	**Ø Open** **3 Percutaneous** **4 Percutaneous Endoscopic**	**D Intraluminal Device**	**J Temporary** **Z No Qualifier**
1 Celiac Artery Celiac trunk **2 Gastric Artery** Left gastric artery Right gastric artery **3 Hepatic Artery** Common hepatic artery Gastroduodenal artery Hepatic artery proper **4 Splenic Artery** Left gastroepiploic artery Pancreatic artery Short gastric artery **5 Superior Mesenteric Artery** Ileal artery Ileocolic artery Inferior pancreaticoduodenal artery Jejunal artery **6 Colic Artery, Right** **7 Colic Artery, Left** **8 Colic Artery, Middle** **9 Renal Artery, Right** Inferior suprarenal artery Renal segmental artery **A Renal Artery, Left** *See 9 Renal Artery, Right* **B Inferior Mesenteric Artery** Sigmoid artery Superior rectal artery **E Internal Iliac Artery, Right** Deferential artery Hypogastric artery Iliolumbar artery Inferior gluteal artery Inferior vesical artery Internal pudendal artery Lateral sacral artery Middle rectal artery Obturator artery Superior gluteal artery Umbilical artery Uterine artery Vaginal artery **F Internal Iliac Artery, Left** *See E Internal Iliac Artery, Right* **H External Iliac Artery, Right** Deep circumflex iliac artery Inferior epigastric artery **J External Iliac Artery, Left** *See H External Iliac Artery, Right* **K Femoral Artery, Right** Circumflex iliac artery Deep femoral artery Descending genicular artery External pudendal artery Superficial epigastric artery **L Femoral Artery, Left** *See K Femoral Artery, Right* **M Popliteal Artery, Right** Inferior genicular artery Middle genicular artery Superior genicular artery Sural artery Tibioperoneal trunk **N Popliteal Artery, Left** *See M Popliteal Artery, Right* **P Anterior Tibial Artery, Right** Anterior lateral malleolar artery Anterior medial malleolar artery Anterior tibial recurrent artery Dorsalis pedis artery Posterior tibial recurrent artery **Q Anterior Tibial Artery, Left** *See P Anterior Tibial Artery, Right* **R Posterior Tibial Artery, Right** **S Posterior Tibial Artery, Left** **T Peroneal Artery, Right** Fibular artery **U Peroneal Artery, Left** *See T Peroneal Artery, Right* **V Foot Artery, Right** Arcuate artery Dorsal metatarsal artery Lateral plantar artery Lateral tarsal artery Medial plantar artery **W Foot Artery, Left** *See V Foot Artery, Right* **Y Lower Artery** Umbilical artery	**Ø Open** **3 Percutaneous** **4 Percutaneous Endoscopic**	**C Extraluminal Device** **D Intraluminal Device** **Z No Device**	**Z No Qualifier**
C Common Iliac Artery, Right **D Common Iliac Artery, Left**	**Ø Open** **3 Percutaneous** **4 Percutaneous Endoscopic**	**C Extraluminal Device** **D Intraluminal Device** **E Intraluminal Device, Branched or Fenestrated, One or Two Arteries** **Z No Device**	**Z No Qualifier**

Ø Medical and Surgical
4 Lower Arteries
W Revision

Definition: Correcting, to the extent possible, a portion of a malfunctioning device or the position of a displaced device

Explanation: Revision can include correcting a malfunctioning or displaced device by taking out or putting in components of the device such as a screw or pin

Body Part Character 4	Approach Character 5	Device Character 6	Qualifier Character 7
Y Lower Artery Umbilical artery	**Ø Open** **3 Percutaneous** **4 Percutaneous Endoscopic**	**Ø Drainage Device** **2 Monitoring Device** **3 Infusion Device** **7 Autologous Tissue Substitute** **C Extraluminal Device** **D Intraluminal Device** **J Synthetic Substitute** **K Nonautologous Tissue Substitute** **Y Other Device**	**Z No Qualifier**
Y Lower Artery Umbilical artery	**X External**	**Ø Drainage Device** **2 Monitoring Device** **3 Infusion Device** **7 Autologous Tissue Substitute** **C Extraluminal Device** **D Intraluminal Device** **J Synthetic Substitute** **K Nonautologous Tissue Substitute**	**Z No Qualifier**

Non-OR Ø4WY3[Ø,2,3,D]Z
Non-OR Ø4WY[3,4]YZ
Non-OR Ø4WYX[Ø,2,3,7,C,D,J,K]Z

Upper Veins Ø51–Ø5W

Character Meanings

This Character Meaning table is provided as a guide to assist the user in the identification of character members that may be found in this section of code tables. It **SHOULD NOT** be used to build a PCS code.

Operation–Character 3		Body Part–Character 4		Approach–Character 5		Device–Character 6		Qualifier–Character 7	
1	Bypass	Ø	Azygos Vein	Ø	Open	Ø	Drainage Device	Ø	Ultrasonic
5	Destruction	1	Hemiazygos Vein	3	Percutaneous	2	Monitoring Device	1	Drug-Coated Balloon
7	Dilation	3	Innominate Vein, Right	4	Percutaneous Endoscopic	3	Infusion Device	X	Diagnostic
9	Drainage	4	Innominate Vein, Left	X	External	7	Autologous Tissue Substitute	Y	Upper Vein
B	Excision	5	Subclavian Vein, Right			9	Autologous Venous Tissue	Z	No Qualifier
C	Extirpation	6	Subclavian Vein, Left			A	Autologous Arterial Tissue		
D	Extraction	7	Axillary Vein, Right			C	Extraluminal Device		
F	Fragmentation	8	Axillary Vein, Left			D	Intraluminal Device		
H	Insertion	9	Brachial Vein, Right			J	Synthetic Substitute		
J	Inspection	A	Brachial Vein, Left			K	Nonautologous Tissue Substitute		
L	Occlusion	B	Basilic Vein, Right			M	Neurostimulator Lead		
N	Release	C	Basilic Vein, Left			Y	Other Device		
P	Removal	D	Cephalic Vein, Right			Z	No Device		
Q	Repair	F	Cephalic Vein, Left						
R	Replacement	G	Hand Vein, Right						
S	Reposition	H	Hand Vein, Left						
U	Supplement	L	Intracranial Vein						
V	Restriction	M	Internal Jugular Vein, Right						
W	Revision	N	Internal Jugular Vein, Left						
		P	External Jugular Vein, Right						
		Q	External Jugular Vein, Left						
		R	Vertebral Vein, Right						
		S	Vertebral Vein, Left						
		T	Face Vein, Right						
		V	Face Vein, Left						
		Y	Upper Vein						

AHA Coding Clinic for table Ø51
2020, 1Q, 28 Free flap microvascular breast reconstruction
2017, 3Q, 15 Bypass of innominate vein to atrial appendage

AHA Coding Clinic for table Ø59
2018, 3Q, 7 Catheter placement for treatment of congestive heart failure

AHA Coding Clinic for table Ø5B
2020, 1Q, 24 Resection of vascular malformation, likely cavernoma
2016, 2Q, 12 Resection of malignant neoplasm of infratemporal fossa

AHA Coding Clinic for table Ø5H
2016, 4Q, 97-98 Phrenic neurostimulator

AHA Coding Clinic for table Ø5P
2016, 4Q, 97-98 Phrenic neurostimulator

AHA Coding Clinic for table Ø5Q
2017, 3Q, 15 Bypass of innominate vein to atrial appendage

AHA Coding Clinic for table Ø5S
2013, 4Q, 125 Stage II cephalic vein transposition (superficialization) of arteriovenous fistula

AHA Coding Clinic for table Ø5W
2016, 4Q, 97-98 Phrenic neurostimulator

Head and Neck Veins

Superficial temporal **L**
Superior ophthalmic **L**
Retromandibular **T, V**
Facial **T, V**
Lingual **T, V**
Thyroid **P, Q**
Anterior jugular **P, Q**
External jugular **P, Q**
Bracheocephalic **3, 4**
Superior sagittal sinus **L**
Inferior sagittal sinus **L**
Straight sinus **L**
Transverse sinus **L**
Occipital sinus **L**
Posterior auricular **P, Q**
Deep cervical **R, S**
External jugular **P, Q**
Vertebral **R, S**
Subclavian **5, 6**

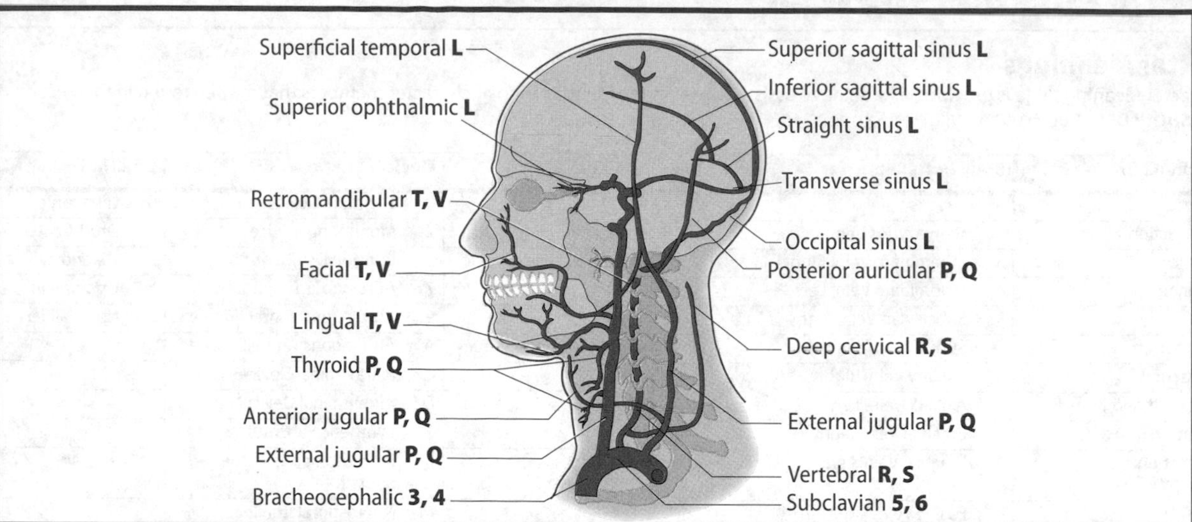

Upper Veins

Superficial temporal **L**
Vertebral **R, S**
Internal jugular **M, N**
External jugular **P, Q**
Subclavian **5, 6**
Innominate **3, 4**
Azygos **Ø**
Brachial **9, A**
Axillary **7,8**
Hemiazygos **1**
Cephalic **D, F**
Basilic **B, C**
Radial **9, A**
Ulnar **9, A**
Digital **G, H**

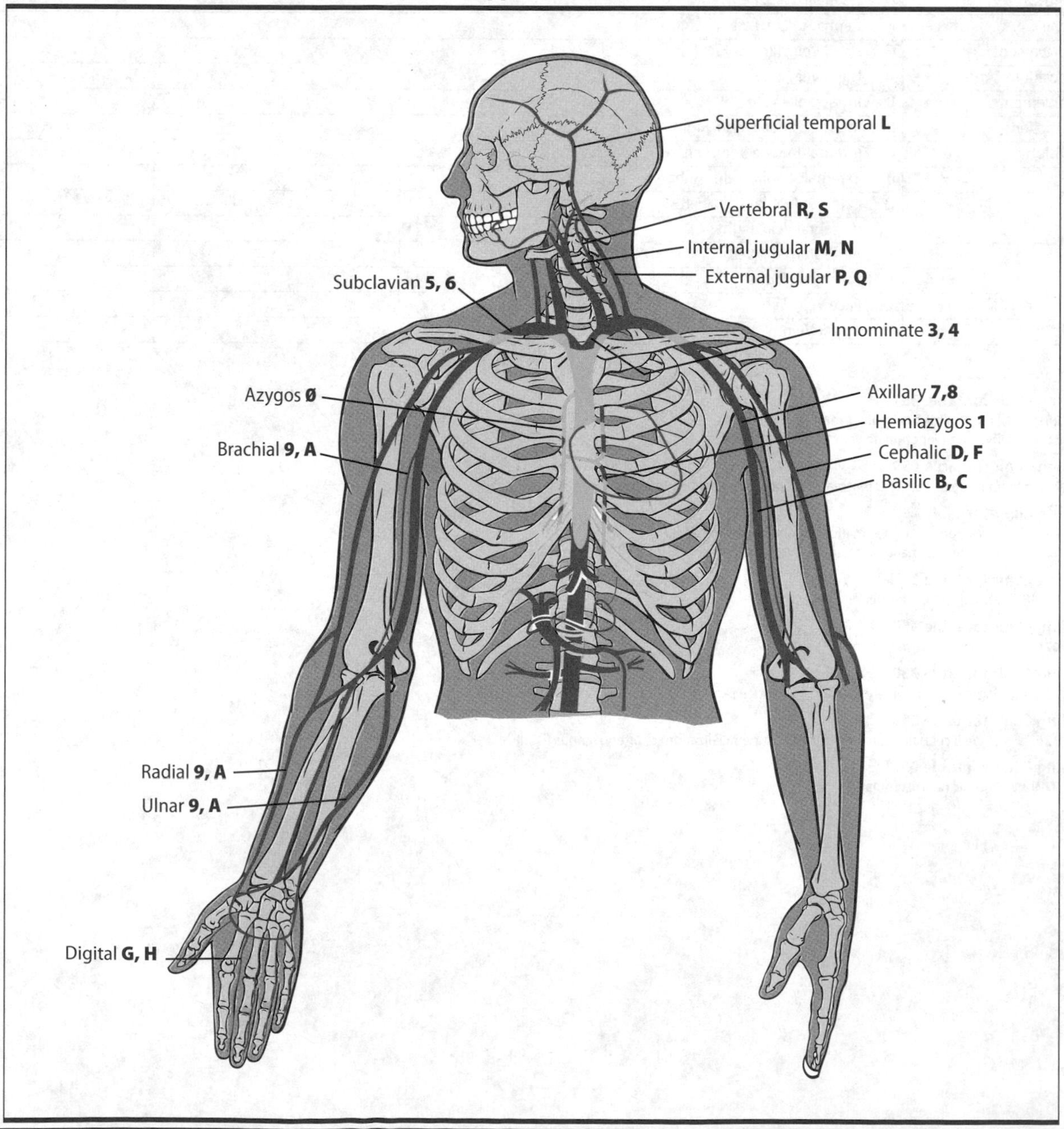

Ø Medical and Surgical
5 Upper Veins
1 Bypass

Definition: Altering the route of passage of the contents of a tubular body part

Explanation: Rerouting contents of a body part to a downstream area of the normal route, to a similar route and body part, or to an abnormal route and dissimilar body part. Includes one or more anastomoses, with or without the use of a device.

Body Part Character 4	Body Part Character 4	Approach Character 5	Device Character 6	Qualifier Character 7
Ø Azygos Vein Right ascending lumbar vein Right subcostal vein **1 Hemiazygos Vein** Left ascending lumbar vein Left subcostal vein **3 Innominate Vein, Right** Brachiocephalic vein Inferior thyroid vein **4 Innominate Vein, Left** *See 3 Innominate Vein, Right* **5 Subclavian Vein, Right** **6 Subclavian Vein, Left** **7 Axillary Vein, Right** **8 Axillary Vein, Left** **9 Brachial Vein, Right** Radial vein Ulnar vein **A Brachial Vein, Left** *See 9 Brachial Vein, Right* **B Basilic Vein, Right** Median antebrachial vein Median cubital vein **C Basilic Vein, Left** *See B Basilic Vein, Right* **D Cephalic Vein, Right** Accessory cephalic vein **F Cephalic Vein, Left** *See D Cephalic Vein, Right* **G Hand Vein, Right** Dorsal metacarpal vein Palmar (volar) digital vein Palmar (volar) metacarpal vein Superficial palmar venous arch Volar (palmar) digital vein Volar (palmar) metacarpal vein	**H Hand Vein, Left** *See G Hand Vein, Right* **L Intracranial Vein** Anterior cerebral vein Basal (internal) cerebral vein Dural venous sinus Great cerebral vein Inferior cerebellar vein Inferior cerebral vein Internal (basal) cerebral vein Middle cerebral vein Ophthalmic vein Superior cerebellar vein Superior cerebral vein **M Internal Jugular Vein, Right** **N Internal Jugular Vein, Left** **P External Jugular Vein, Right** Posterior auricular vein **Q External Jugular Vein, Left** *See P External Jugular Vein, Right* **R Vertebral Vein, Right** Deep cervical vein Suboccipital venous plexus **S Vertebral Vein, Left** *See R Vertebral Vein, Right* **T Face Vein, Right** Angular vein Anterior facial vein Common facial vein Deep facial vein Frontal vein Posterior facial (retromandibular) vein Supraorbital vein **V Face Vein, Left** *See T Face Vein, Right*	**Ø Open** **4 Percutaneous Endoscopic**	**7 Autologous Tissue Substitute** **9 Autologous Venous Tissue** **A Autologous Arterial Tissue** **J Synthetic Substitute** **K Nonautologous Tissue Substitute** **Z No Device**	**Y Upper Vein**

Upper Veins
Ø51–Ø51

Ø Medical and Surgical
5 Upper Veins
5 Destruction Definition: Physical eradication of all or a portion of a body part by the direct use of energy, force, or a destructive agent

Explanation: None of the body part is physically taken out

Body Part Character 4	Approach Character 5	Device Character 6	Qualifier Character 7
Ø Azygos Vein Right ascending lumbar vein Right subcostal vein **1 Hemiazygos Vein** Left ascending lumbar vein Left subcostal vein **3 Innominate Vein, Right** Brachlocephalic vein Inferior thyroid vein **4 Innominate Vein, Left** *See 3 Innominate Vein, Right* **5 Subclavian Vein, Right** **6 Subclavian Vein, Left** **7 Axillary Vein, Right** **8 Axillary Vein, Left** **9 Brachial Vein, Right** Radial vein Ulnar vein **A Brachial Vein, Left** *See 9 Brachial Vein, Right* **B Basilic Vein, Right** Median antebrachial vein Median cubital vein **C Basilic Vein, Left** *See B Basilic Vein, Right* **D Cephalic Vein, Right** Accessory cephalic vein **F Cephalic Vein, Left** *See D Cephalic Vein, Right* **G Hand Vein, Right** Dorsal metacarpal vein Palmar (volar) digital vein Palmar (volar) metacarpal vein Superficial palmar venous arch Volar (palmar) digital vein Volar (palmar) metacarpal vein **H Hand Vein, Left** *See G Hand Vein, Right* **L Intracranial Vein** Anterior cerebral vein Basal (internal) cerebral vein Dural venous sinus Great cerebral vein Inferior cerebellar vein Inferior cerebral vein Internal (basal) cerebral vein Middle cerebral vein Ophthalmic vein Superior cerebellar vein Superior cerebral vein **M Internal Jugular Vein, Right** **N Internal Jugular Vein, Left** **P External Jugular Vein, Right** Posterior auricular vein **Q External Jugular Vein, Left** *See P External Jugular Vein, Right* **R Vertebral Vein, Right** Deep cervical vein Suboccipital venous plexus **S Vertebral Vein, Left** *See R Vertebral Vein, Right* **T Face Vein, Right** Angular vein Anterior facial vein Common facial vein Deep facial vein Frontal vein Posterior facial (retromandibular) vein Supraorbital vein **V Face Vein, Left** *See T Face Vein, Right* **Y Upper Vein**	**Ø Open** **3 Percutaneous** **4 Percutaneous Endoscopic**	**Z No Device**	**Z No Qualifier**

Ø Medical and Surgical
5 Upper Veins
7 Dilation

Definition: Expanding an orifice or the lumen of a tubular body part

Explanation: The orifice can be a natural orifice or an artificially created orifice. Accomplished by stretching a tubular body part using intraluminal pressure or by cutting part of the orifice or wall of the tubular body part.

Body Part Character 4		Approach Character 5	Device Character 6	Qualifier Character 7
Ø Azygos Vein Right ascending lumbar vein Right subcostal vein **1 Hemiazygos Vein** Left ascending lumbar vein Left subcostal vein **G Hand Vein, Right** Dorsal metacarpal vein Palmar (volar) digital vein Palmar (volar) metacarpal vein Superficial palmar venous arch Volar (palmar) digital vein Volar (palmar) metacarpal vein **H Hand Vein, Left** *See G Hand Vein, Right* **L Intracranial Vein** NC Anterior cerebral vein Basal (internal) cerebral vein Dural venous sinus Great cerebral vein Inferior cerebellar vein Inferior cerebral vein Internal (basal) cerebral vein Middle cerebral vein Ophthalmic vein Superior cerebellar vein Superior cerebral vein	**M Internal Jugular Vein, Right** **N Internal Jugular Vein, Left** **P External Jugular Vein, Right** Posterior auricular vein **Q External Jugular Vein, Left** *See P External Jugular Vein, Right* **R Vertebral Vein, Right** Deep cervical vein Suboccipital venous plexus **S Vertebral Vein, Left** *See R Vertebral Vein, Right* **T Face Vein, Right** Angular vein Anterior facial vein Common facial vein Deep facial vein Frontal vein Posterior facial (retromandibular) vein Supraorbital vein **V Face Vein, Left** *See T Face Vein, Right* **Y Upper Vein**	Ø Open 3 Percutaneous 4 Percutaneous Endoscopic	D Intraluminal Device Z No Device	Z No Qualifier
3 Innominate Vein, Right Brachiocephalic vein Inferior thyroid vein **4 Innominate Vein, Left** *See 3 Innominate Vein, Right* **5 Subclavian Vein, Right** **6 Subclavian Vein, Left** **7 Axillary Vein, Right** **8 Axillary Vein, Left** **9 Brachial Vein, Right** Radial vein Ulnar vein	**A Brachial Vein, Left** *See 9 Brachial Vein, Right* **B Basilic Vein, Right** Median antebrachial vein Median cubital vein **C Basilic Vein, Left** *See B Basilic Vein, Right* **D Cephalic Vein, Right** Accessory cephalic vein **F Cephalic Vein, Left** *See D Cephalic Vein, Right*	Ø Open 3 Percutaneous 4 Percutaneous Endoscopic	D Intraluminal Device Z No Device	1 Drug-Coated Balloon Z No Qualifier

NC Ø57L[3,4]ZZ

Ø Medical and Surgical
5 Upper Veins
9 Drainage Definition: Taking or letting out fluids and/or gases from a body part
Explanation: The qualifier DIAGNOSTIC is used to identify drainage procedures that are biopsies

Body Part Character 4		Approach Character 5	Device Character 6	Qualifier Character 7
Ø Azygos Vein Right ascending lumbar vein Right subcostal vein **1 Hemiazygos Vein** Left ascending lumbar vein Left subcostal vein **3 Innominate Vein, Right** Brachiocephalic vein Inferior thyroid vein **4 Innominate Vein, Left** *See 3 Innominate Vein, Right* **5 Subclavian Vein, Right** **6 Subclavian Vein, Left** **7 Axillary Vein, Right** **8 Axillary Vein, Left** **9 Brachial Vein, Right** Radial vein Ulnar vein **A Brachial Vein, Left** *See 9 Brachial Vein, Right* **B Basilic Vein, Right** Median antebrachial vein Median cubital vein **C Basilic Vein, Left** *See B Basilic Vein, Right* **D Cephalic Vein, Right** Accessory cephalic vein **F Cephalic Vein, Left** *See D Cephalic Vein, Right* **G Hand Vein, Right** Dorsal metacarpal vein Palmar (volar) digital vein Palmar (volar) metacarpal vein Superficial palmar venous arch Volar (palmar) digital vein Volar (palmar) metacarpal vein	**H Hand Vein, Left** *See G Hand Vein, Right* **L Intracranial Vein** Anterior cerebral vein Basal (internal) cerebral vein Dural venous sinus Great cerebral vein Inferior cerebellar vein Inferior cerebral vein Internal (basal) cerebral vein Middle cerebral vein Ophthalmic vein Superior cerebellar vein Superior cerebral vein **M Internal Jugular Vein, Right** **N Internal Jugular Vein, Left** **P External Jugular Vein, Right** Posterior auricular vein **Q External Jugular Vein, Left** *See P External Jugular Vein, Right* **R Vertebral Vein, Right** Deep cervical vein Suboccipital venous plexus **S Vertebral Vein, Left** *See R Vertebral Vein, Right* **T Face Vein, Right** Angular vein Anterior facial vein Common facial vein Deep facial vein Frontal vein Posterior facial (retromandibular) vein Supraorbital vein **V Face Vein, Left** *See T Face Vein, Right* **Y Upper Vein**	**Ø Open** **3 Percutaneous** **4 Percutaneous Endoscopic**	**Ø Drainage Device**	**Z No Qualifier**
Ø Azygos Vein Right ascending lumbar vein Right subcostal vein **1 Hemiazygos Vein** Left ascending lumbar vein Left subcostal vein **3 Innominate Vein, Right** Brachiocephalic vein Inferior thyroid vein **4 Innominate Vein, Left** *See 3 Innominate Vein, Right* **5 Subclavian Vein, Right** **6 Subclavian Vein, Left** **7 Axillary Vein, Right** **8 Axillary Vein, Left** **9 Brachial Vein, Right** Radial vein Ulnar vein **A Brachial Vein, Left** *See 9 Brachial Vein, Right* **B Basilic Vein, Right** Median antebrachial vein Median cubital vein **C Basilic Vein, Left** *See B Basilic Vein, Right* **D Cephalic Vein, Right** Accessory cephalic vein **F Cephalic Vein, Left** *See D Cephalic Vein, Right* **G Hand Vein, Right** Dorsal metacarpal vein Palmar (volar) digital vein Palmar (volar) metacarpal vein Superficial palmar venous arch Volar (palmar) digital vein Volar (palmar) metacarpal vein	**H Hand Vein, Left** *See G Hand Vein, Right* **L Intracranial Vein** Anterior cerebral vein Basal (internal) cerebral vein Dural venous sinus Great cerebral vein Inferior cerebellar vein Inferior cerebral vein Internal (basal) cerebral vein Middle cerebral vein Ophthalmic vein Superior cerebellar vein Superior cerebral vein **M Internal Jugular Vein, Right** **N Internal Jugular Vein, Left** **P External Jugular Vein, Right** Posterior auricular vein **Q External Jugular Vein, Left** *See P External Jugular Vein, Right* **R Vertebral Vein, Right** Deep cervical vein Suboccipital venous plexus **S Vertebral Vein, Left** *See R Vertebral Vein, Right* **T Face Vein, Right** Angular vein Anterior facial vein Common facial vein Deep facial vein Frontal vein Posterior facial (retromandibular) vein Supraorbital vein **V Face Vein, Left** *See T Face Vein, Right* **Y Upper Vein**	**Ø Open** **3 Percutaneous** **4 Percutaneous Endoscopic**	**Z No Device**	**X Diagnostic** **Z No Qualifier**

Non-OR Ø59[Ø,1,3,4,5,6,7,8,9,A,B,C,D,F,G,H,L,M,N,P,Q,R,S,T,V,Y][Ø,3,4]ØZ
Non-OR Ø59[Ø,1,3,4,5,6,7,8,9,A,B,C,D,F,G,H,L,M,N,P,Q,R,S,T,V,Y]3ZX
Non-OR Ø59[Ø,1,3,4,5,6,7,8,9,A,B,C,D,F,G,H,L,M,N,P,Q,R,S,T,V,Y][Ø,3,4]ZZ

Ø Medical and Surgical
5 Upper Veins
B Excision Definition: Cutting out or off, without replacement, a portion of a body part
Explanation: The qualifier DIAGNOSTIC is used to identify excision procedures that are biopsies

Body Part Character 4		Approach Character 5	Device Character 6	Qualifier Character 7
Ø Azygos Vein Right ascending lumbar vein Right subcostal vein **1 Hemiazygos Vein** Left ascending lumbar vein Left subcostal vein **3 Innominate Vein, Right** Brachiocephalic vein Inferior thyroid vein **4 Innominate Vein, Left** ***See*** *3 Innominate Vein, Right* **5 Subclavian Vein, Right** **6 Subclavian Vein, Left** **7 Axillary Vein, Right** **8 Axillary Vein, Left** **9 Brachial Vein, Right** Radial vein Ulnar vein **A Brachial Vein, Left** ***See*** *9 Brachial Vein, Right* **B Basilic Vein, Right** Median antebrachial vein Median cubital vein **C Basilic Vein, Left** ***See*** *B Basilic Vein, Right* **D Cephalic Vein, Right** Accessory cephalic vein **F Cephalic Vein, Left** ***See*** *D Cephalic Vein, Right* **G Hand Vein, Right** Dorsal metacarpal vein Palmar (volar) digital vein Palmar (volar) metacarpal vein Superficial palmar venous arch Volar (palmar) digital vein Volar (palmar) metacarpal vein	**H Hand Vein, Left** ***See*** *G Hand Vein, Right* **L Intracranial Vein** Anterior cerebral vein Basal (internal) cerebral vein Dural venous sinus Great cerebral vein Inferior cerebellar vein Inferior cerebral vein Internal (basal) cerebral vein Middle cerebral vein Ophthalmic vein Superior cerebellar vein Superior cerebral vein **M Internal Jugular Vein, Right** **N Internal Jugular Vein, Left** **P External Jugular Vein, Right** Posterior auricular vein **Q External Jugular Vein, Left** ***See*** *P External Jugular Vein, Right* **R Vertebral Vein, Right** Deep cervical vein Suboccipital venous plexus **S Vertebral Vein, Left** ***See*** *R Vertebral Vein, Right* **T Face Vein, Right** Angular vein Anterior facial vein Common facial vein Deep facial vein Frontal vein Posterior facial (retromandibular) vein Supraorbital vein **V Face Vein, Left** ***See*** *T Face Vein, Right* **Y Upper Vein**	**Ø Open** **3 Percutaneous** **4 Percutaneous Endoscopic**	**Z No Device**	**X Diagnostic** **Z No Qualifier**

Ø Medical and Surgical
5 Upper Veins
C Extirpation Definition: Taking or cutting out solid matter from a body part

Explanation: The solid matter may be an abnormal byproduct of a biological function or a foreign body; it may be imbedded in a body part or in the lumen of a tubular body part. The solid matter may or may not have been previously broken into pieces.

Body Part Character 4		Approach Character 5	Device Character 6	Qualifier Character 7
Ø Azygos Vein Right ascending lumbar vein Right subcostal vein **1 Hemiazygos Vein** Left ascending lumbar vein Left subcostal vein **3 Innominate Vein, Right** Brachiocephalic vein Inferior thyroid vein **4 Innominate Vein, Left** *See 3 Innominate Vein, Right* **5 Subclavian Vein, Right** **6 Subclavian Vein, Left** **7 Axillary Vein, Right** **8 Axillary Vein, Left** **9 Brachial Vein, Right** Radial vein Ulnar vein **A Brachial Vein, Left** *See 9 Brachial Vein, Right* **B Basilic Vein, Right** Median antebrachial vein Median cubital vein **C Basilic Vein, Left** *See B Basilic Vein, Right* **D Cephalic Vein, Right** Accessory cephalic vein **F Cephalic Vein, Left** *See D Cephalic Vein, Right* **G Hand Vein, Right** Dorsal metacarpal vein Palmar (volar) digital vein Palmar (volar) metacarpal vein Superficial palmar venous arch Volar (palmar) digital vein Volar (palmar) metacarpal vein	**H Hand Vein, Left** *See G Hand Vein, Right* **L Intracranial Vein** Anterior cerebral vein Basal (internal) cerebral vein Dural venous sinus Great cerebral vein Inferior cerebellar vein Inferior cerebral vein Internal (basal) cerebral vein Middle cerebral vein Ophthalmic vein Superior cerebellar vein Superior cerebral vein **M Internal Jugular Vein, Right** **N Internal Jugular Vein, Left** **P External Jugular Vein, Right** Posterior auricular vein **Q External Jugular Vein, Left** *See P External Jugular Vein, Right* **R Vertebral Vein, Right** Deep cervical vein Suboccipital venous plexus **S Vertebral Vein, Left** *See R Vertebral Vein, Right* **T Face Vein, Right** Angular vein Anterior facial vein Common facial vein Deep facial vein Frontal vein Posterior facial (retromandibular) vein Supraorbital vein **V Face Vein, Left** *See T Face Vein, Right* **Y Upper Vein**	**Ø Open** **3 Percutaneous** **4 Percutaneous Endoscopic**	**Z No Device**	**Z No Qualifier**

Ø Medical and Surgical
5 Upper Veins
D Extraction Definition: Pulling or stripping out or off all or a portion of a body part by the use of force

Explanation: The qualifier DIAGNOSTIC is used to identify extraction procedures that are biopsies

Body Part Character 4		Approach Character 5	Device Character 6	Qualifier Character 7
9 Brachial Vein, Right Radial vein Ulnar vein **A Brachial Vein, Left** *See 9 Brachial Vein, Right* **B Basilic Vein, Right** Median antebrachial vein Median cubital vein **C Basilic Vein, Left** *See B Basilic Vein, Right* **D Cephalic Vein, Right** Accessory cephalic vein	**F Cephalic Vein, Left** *See D Cephalic Vein, Right* **G Hand Vein, Right** Dorsal metacarpal vein Palmar (volar) digital vein Palmar (volar) metacarpal vein Superficial palmar venous arch Volar (palmar) digital vein Volar (palmar) metacarpal vein **H Hand Vein, Left** *See G Hand Vein, Right* **Y Upper Vein**	**Ø Open** **3 Percutaneous**	**Z No Device**	**Z No Qualifier**

Ø Medical and Surgical
5 Upper Veins
F Fragmentation Definition: Breaking solid matter in a body part into pieces

Explanation: Physical force (e.g., manual, ultrasonic) applied directly or indirectly is used to break the solid matter into pieces. The solid matter may be an abnormal byproduct of a biological function or a foreign body. The pieces of solid matter are not taken out.

Body Part Character 4		Approach Character 5	Device Character 6	Qualifier Character 7
3 Innominate Vein, Right Brachiocephalic vein Inferior thyroid vein **4 Innominate Vein, Left** *See 3 Innominate Vein, Right* **5 Subclavian Vein, Right** **6 Subclavian Vein, Left** **7 Axillary Vein, Right** **8 Axillary Vein, Left** **9 Brachial Vein, Right** Radial vein Ulnar vein	**A Brachial Vein, Left** *See 9 Brachial Vein, Right* **B Basilic Vein, Right** Median antebrachial vein Median cubital vein **C Basilic Vein, Left** *See B Basilic Vein, Right* **D Cephalic Vein, Right** Accessory cephalic vein **F Cephalic Vein, Left** *See D Cephalic Vein, Right* **Y Upper Vein**	**3 Percutaneous**	**Z No Device**	**Ø Ultrasonic** **Z No Qualifier**

Ø Medical and Surgical
5 Upper Veins
H Insertion Definition: Putting in a nonbiological appliance that monitors, assists, performs, or prevents a physiological function but does not physically take the place of a body part
Explanation: None

Body Part Character 4		Approach Character 5	Device Character 6	Qualifier Character 7
Ø Azygos Vein ⊞ Right ascending lumbar vein Right subcostal vein		**Ø Open** **3 Percutaneous** **4 Percutaneous Endoscopic**	**2 Monitoring Device** **3 Infusion Device** **D Intraluminal Device** **M Neurostimulator Lead**	**Z No Qualifier**
1 Hemiazygos Vein Left ascending lumbar vein Left subcostal vein **5 Subclavian Vein, Right** **6 Subclavian Vein, Left** **7 Axillary Vein, Right** **8 Axillary Vein, Left** **9 Brachial Vein, Right** Radial vein Ulnar vein **A Brachial Vein, Left** *See 9 Brachial Vein, Right* **B Basilic Vein, Right** Median antebrachial vein Median cubital vein **C Basilic Vein, Left** *See B Basilic Vein, Right* **D Cephalic Vein, Right** Accessory cephalic vein **F Cephalic Vein, Left** *See D Cephalic Vein, Right* **G Hand Vein, Right** Dorsal metacarpal vein Palmar (volar) digital vein Palmar (volar) metacarpal vein Superficial palmar venous arch Volar (palmar) digital vein Volar (palmar) metacarpal vein **H Hand Vein, Left** *See G Hand Vein, Right*	**L Intracranial Vein** Anterior cerebral vein Basal (internal) cerebral vein Dural venous sinus Great cerebral vein Inferior cerebellar vein Inferior cerebral vein Internal (basal) cerebral vein Middle cerebral vein Ophthalmic vein Superior cerebellar vein Superior cerebral vein **M Internal Jugular Vein, Right** **N Internal Jugular Vein, Left** **P External Jugular Vein, Right** Posterior auricular vein **Q External Jugular Vein, Left** *See P External Jugular Vein, Right* **R Vertebral Vein, Right** Deep cervical vein Suboccipital venous plexus **S Vertebral Vein, Left** *See R Vertebral Vein, Right* **T Face Vein, Right** Angular vein Anterior facial vein Common facial vein Deep facial vein Frontal vein Posterior facial (retromandibular) vein Supraorbital vein **V Face Vein, Left** *See T Face Vein, Right*	**Ø Open** **3 Percutaneous** **4 Percutaneous Endoscopic**	**3 Infusion Device** **D Intraluminal Device**	**Z No Qualifier**
3 Innominate Vein, Right ⊞ Brachiocephalic vein Inferior thyroid vein **4 Innominate Vein, Left** ⊞ *See 3 Innominate Vein, Right*		**Ø Open** **3 Percutaneous** **4 Percutaneous Endoscopic**	**3 Infusion Device** **D Intraluminal Device** **M Neurostimulator Lead**	**Z No Qualifier**
Y Upper Vein		**Ø Open** **3 Percutaneous** **4 Percutaneous Endoscopic**	**2 Monitoring Device** **3 Infusion Device** **D Intraluminal Device** **Y Other Device**	**Z No Qualifier**

Non-OR Ø5HØ[Ø,3,4]3Z
Non-OR Ø5H[1,5,6,7,8,9,A,B,C,D,F,G,H,L,M,N,P,Q,R,S,T,V][Ø,3,4]3Z
Non-OR Ø5H[3,4][Ø,3,4]3Z
Non-OR Ø5HY[Ø,3,4]3Z
Non-OR Ø5HY32Z
Non-OR Ø5HY[3,4]YZ
HAC Ø5HØ[3,4]3Z when reported with SDx J95.811
HAC Ø5H[1,5,6][3,4]3Z when reported with SDx J95.811
HAC Ø5H[M,N,P,Q]33Z when reported with SDx J95.811
HAC Ø5H[3,4][3,4]3Z when reported with SDx J95.811

See Appendix L for Procedure Combinations
⊞ Ø5HØ[Ø,3,4]MZ
⊞ Ø5H[3,4][Ø,3,4]MZ

Ø Medical and Surgical
5 Upper Veins
J Inspection Definition: Visually and/or manually exploring a body part

Explanation: Visual exploration may be performed with or without optical instrumentation. Manual exploration may be performed directly or through intervening body layers.

Body Part Character 4	Approach Character 5	Device Character 6	Qualifier Character 7
Y Upper Vein	Ø Open 3 Percutaneous 4 Percutaneous Endoscopic X External	Z No Device	Z No Qualifier

Non-OR Ø5JY[3,X]ZZ

Ø Medical and Surgical
5 Upper Veins
L Occlusion Definition: Completely closing an orifice or the lumen of a tubular body part

Explanation: The orifice can be a natural orifice or an artificially created orifice

Body Part Character 4	Body Part Character 4	Approach Character 5	Device Character 6	Qualifier Character 7
Ø Azygos Vein Right ascending lumbar vein Right subcostal vein **1 Hemiazygos Vein** Left ascending lumbar vein Left subcostal vein **3 Innominate Vein, Right** Brachiocephalic vein Inferior thyroid vein **4 Innominate Vein, Left** *See 3 Innominate Vein, Right* **5 Subclavian Vein, Right** **6 Subclavian Vein, Left** **7 Axillary Vein, Right** **8 Axillary Vein, Left** **9 Brachial Vein, Right** Radial vein Ulnar vein **A Brachial Vein, Left** *See 9 Brachial Vein, Right* **B Basilic Vein, Right** Median antebrachial vein Median cubital vein **C Basilic Vein, Left** *See B Basilic Vein, Right* **D Cephalic Vein, Right** Accessory cephalic vein **F Cephalic Vein, Left** *See D Cephalic Vein, Right* **G Hand Vein, Right** Dorsal metacarpal vein Palmar (volar) digital vein Palmar (volar) metacarpal vein Superficial palmar venous arch Volar (palmar) digital vein Volar (palmar) metacarpal vein	**H Hand Vein, Left** *See G Hand Vein, Right* **L Intracranial Vein** Anterior cerebral vein Basal (internal) cerebral vein Dural venous sinus Great cerebral vein Inferior cerebellar vein Inferior cerebral vein Internal (basal) cerebral vein Middle cerebral vein Ophthalmic vein Superior cerebellar vein Superior cerebral vein **M Internal Jugular Vein, Right** **N Internal Jugular Vein, Left** **P External Jugular Vein, Right** Posterior auricular vein **Q External Jugular Vein, Left** *See P External Jugular Vein, Right* **R Vertebral Vein, Right** Deep cervical vein Suboccipital venous plexus **S Vertebral Vein, Left** *See R Vertebral Vein, Right* **T Face Vein, Right** Angular vein Anterior facial vein Common facial vein Deep facial vein Frontal vein Posterior facial (retromandibular) vein Supraorbital vein **V Face Vein, Left** *See T Face Vein, Right* **Y Upper Vein**	Ø Open 3 Percutaneous 4 Percutaneous Endoscopic	C Extraluminal Device D Intraluminal Device Z No Device	Z No Qualifier

Ø Medical and Surgical
5 Upper Veins
N Release Definition: Freeing a body part from an abnormal physical constraint by cutting or by the use of force
Explanation: Some of the restraining tissue may be taken out but none of the body part is taken out

Body Part Character 4		Approach Character 5	Device Character 6	Qualifier Character 7
Ø Azygos Vein Right ascending lumbar vein Right subcostal vein **1 Hemiazygos Vein** Left ascending lumbar vein Left subcostal vein **3 Innominate Vein, Right** Brachlocephalic vein Inferior thyroid vein **4 Innominate Vein, Left** ***See*** *3 Innominate Vein, Right* **5 Subclavian Vein, Right** **6 Subclavian Vein, Left** **7 Axillary Vein, Right** **8 Axillary Vein, Left** **9 Brachial Vein, Right** Radial vein Ulnar vein **A Brachial Vein, Left** ***See*** *9 Brachial Vein, Right* **B Basilic Vein, Right** Median antebrachial vein Median cubital vein **C Basilic Vein, Left** ***See*** *B Basilic Vein, Right* **D Cephalic Vein, Right** Accessory cephalic vein **F Cephalic Vein, Left** ***See*** *D Cephalic Vein, Right* **G Hand Vein, Right** Dorsal metacarpal vein Palmar (volar) digital vein Palmar (volar) metacarpal vein Superficial palmar venous arch Volar (palmar) digital vein Volar (palmar) metacarpal vein	**H Hand Vein, Left** ***See*** *G Hand Vein, Right* **L Intracranial Vein** Anterior cerebral vein Basal (internal) cerebral vein Dural venous sinus Great cerebral vein Inferior cerebellar vein Inferior cerebral vein Internal (basal) cerebral vein Middle cerebral vein Ophthalmic vein Superior cerebellar vein Superior cerebral vein **M Internal Jugular Vein, Right** **N Internal Jugular Vein, Left** **P External Jugular Vein, Right** Posterior auricular vein **Q External Jugular Vein, Left** ***See*** *P External Jugular Vein, Right* **R Vertebral Vein, Right** Deep cervical vein Suboccipital venous plexus **S Vertebral Vein, Left** ***See*** *R Vertebral Vein, Right* **T Face Vein, Right** Angular vein Anterior facial vein Common facial vein Deep facial vein Frontal vein Posterior facial (retromandibular) vein Supraorbital vein **V Face Vein, Left** ***See*** *T Face Vein, Right* **Y Upper Vein**	**Ø Open** **3 Percutaneous** **4 Percutaneous Endoscopic**	**Z No Device**	**Z No Qualifier**

Ø Medical and Surgical
5 Upper Veins
P Removal Definition: Taking out or off a device from a body part

Explanation: If a device is taken out and a similar device put in without cutting or puncturing the skin or mucous membrane, the procedure is coded to the root operation CHANGE. Otherwise, the procedure for taking out a device is coded to the root operation REMOVAL.

Body Part Character 4	Approach Character 5	Device Character 6	Qualifier Character 7
Ø Azygos Vein Right ascending lumbar vein Right subcostal vein	**Ø Open** **3 Percutaneous** **4 Percutaneous Endoscopic** **X External**	**2 Monitoring Device** **M Neurostimulator Lead**	**Z No Qualifier**
3 Innominate Vein, Right Brachiocephalic vein Inferior thyroid vein **4 Innominate Vein, Left** *See 3 Innominate Vein, Right*	**Ø Open** **3 Percutaneous** **4 Percutaneous Endoscopic** **X External**	**M Neurostimulator Lead**	**Z No Qualifier**
Y Upper Vein	**Ø Open** **3 Percutaneous** **4 Percutaneous Endoscopic**	**Ø Drainage Device** **2 Monitoring Device** **3 Infusion Device** **7 Autologous Tissue Substitute** **C Extraluminal Device** **D Intraluminal Device** **J Synthetic Substitute** **K Nonautologous Tissue Substitute** **Y Other Device**	**Z No Qualifier**
Y Upper Vein	**X External**	**Ø Drainage Device** **2 Monitoring Device** **3 Infusion Device** **D Intraluminal Device**	**Z No Qualifier**

Non-OR Ø5PØ[Ø,3,4,X]2Z
Non-OR Ø5PY3[Ø,2,3]Z
Non-OR Ø5PY[3,4]YZ
Non-OR Ø5PYX[Ø,2,3,D]Z

Ø Medical and Surgical
5 Upper Veins
Q Repair Definition: Restoring, to the extent possible, a body part to its normal anatomic structure and function
Explanation: Used only when the method to accomplish the repair is not one of the other root operations

Body Part Character 4		Approach Character 5	Device Character 6	Qualifier Character 7
Ø Azygos Vein Right ascending lumbar vein Right subcostal vein **1 Hemiazygos Vein** Left ascending lumbar vein Left subcostal vein **3 Innominate Vein, Right** Brachiocephalic vein Inferior thyroid vein **4 Innominate Vein, Left** *See 3 Innominate Vein, Right* **5 Subclavian Vein, Right** **6 Subclavian Vein, Left** **7 Axillary Vein, Right** **8 Axillary Vein, Left** **9 Brachial Vein, Right** Radial vein Ulnar vein **A Brachial Vein, Left** *See 9 Brachial Vein, Right* **B Basilic Vein, Right** Median antebrachial vein Median cubital vein **C Basilic Vein, Left** *See B Basilic Vein, Right* **D Cephalic Vein, Right** Accessory cephalic vein **F Cephalic Vein, Left** *See D Cephalic Vein, Right* **G Hand Vein, Right** Dorsal metacarpal vein Palmar (volar) digital vein Palmar (volar) metacarpal vein Superficial palmar venous arch Volar (palmar) digital vein Volar (palmar) metacarpal vein	**H Hand Vein, Left** *See G Hand Vein, Right* **L Intracranial Vein** Anterior cerebral vein Basal (internal) cerebral vein Dural venous sinus Great cerebral vein Inferior cerebellar vein Inferior cerebral vein Internal (basal) cerebral vein Middle cerebral vein Ophthalmic vein Superior cerebellar vein Superior cerebral vein **M Internal Jugular Vein, Right** **N Internal Jugular Vein, Left** **P External Jugular Vein, Right** Posterior auricular vein **Q External Jugular Vein, Left** *See P External Jugular Vein, Right* **R Vertebral Vein, Right** Deep cervical vein Suboccipital venous plexus **S Vertebral Vein, Left** *See R Vertebral Vein, Right* **T Face Vein, Right** Angular vein Anterior facial vein Common facial vein Deep facial vein Frontal vein Posterior facial (retromandibular) vein Supraorbital vein **V Face Vein, Left** *See T Face Vein, Right* **Y Upper Vein**	**Ø Open** **3 Percutaneous** **4 Percutaneous Endoscopic**	**Z No Device**	**Z No Qualifier**

Ø Medical and Surgical
5 Upper Veins
R Replacement Definition: Putting in or on biological or synthetic material that physically takes the place and/or function of all or a portion of a body part

Explanation: The body part may have been taken out or replaced, or may be taken out, physically eradicated, or rendered nonfunctional during the REPLACEMENT procedure. A REMOVAL procedure is coded for taking out the device used in a previous replacement procedure.

Body Part Character 4		Approach Character 5	Device Character 6	Qualifier Character 7
Ø Azygos Vein Right ascending lumbar vein Right subcostal vein **1 Hemiazygos Vein** Left ascending lumbar vein Left subcostal vein **3 Innominate Vein, Right** Brachiocephalic vein Inferior thyroid vein **4 Innominate Vein, Left** *See 3 Innominate Vein, Right* **5 Subclavian Vein, Right** **6 Subclavian Vein, Left** **7 Axillary Vein, Right** **8 Axillary Vein, Left** **9 Brachial Vein, Right** Radial vein Ulnar vein **A Brachial Vein, Left** *See 9 Brachial Vein, Right* **B Basilic Vein, Right** Median antebrachial vein Median cubital vein **C Basilic Vein, Left** *See B Basilic Vein, Right* **D Cephalic Vein, Right** Accessory cephalic vein **F Cephalic Vein, Left** *See D Cephalic Vein, Right* **G Hand Vein, Right** Dorsal metacarpal vein Palmar (volar) digital vein Palmar (volar) metacarpal vein Superficial palmar venous arch Volar (palmar) digital vein Volar (palmar) metacarpal vein	**H Hand Vein, Left** *See G Hand Vein, Right* **L Intracranial Vein** Anterior cerebral vein Basal (internal) cerebral vein Dural venous sinus Great cerebral vein Inferior cerebellar vein Inferior cerebral vein Internal (basal) cerebral vein Middle cerebral vein Ophthalmic vein Superior cerebellar vein Superior cerebral vein **M Internal Jugular Vein, Right** **N Internal Jugular Vein, Left** **P External Jugular Vein, Right** Posterior auricular vein **Q External Jugular Vein, Left** *See P External Jugular Vein, Right* **R Vertebral Vein, Right** Deep cervical vein Suboccipital venous plexus **S Vertebral Vein, Left** *See R Vertebral Vein, Right* **T Face Vein, Right** Angular vein Anterior facial vein Common facial vein Deep facial vein Frontal vein Posterior facial (retromandibular) vein Supraorbital vein **V Face Vein, Left** *See T Face Vein, Right* **Y Upper Vein**	**Ø Open** **4 Percutaneous Endoscopic**	**7 Autologous Tissue Substitute** **J Synthetic Substitute** **K Nonautologous Tissue Substitute**	**Z No Qualifier**

Ø Medical and Surgical
5 Upper Veins
S Reposition Definition: Moving to its normal location, or other suitable location, all or a portion of a body part

Explanation: The body part is moved to a new location from an abnormal location, or from a normal location where it is not functioning correctly. The body part may or may not be cut out or off to be moved to the new location.

Body Part Character 4		Approach Character 5	Device Character 6	Qualifier Character 7
Ø Azygos Vein Right ascending lumbar vein Right subcostal vein **1 Hemiazygos Vein** Left ascending lumbar vein Left subcostal vein **3 Innominate Vein, Right** Brachiocephalic vein Inferior thyroid vein **4 Innominate Vein, Left** *See 3 Innominate Vein, Right* **5 Subclavian Vein, Right** **6 Subclavian Vein, Left** **7 Axillary Vein, Right** **8 Axillary Vein, Left** **9 Brachial Vein, Right** Radial vein Ulnar vein **A Brachial Vein, Left** *See 9 Brachial Vein, Right* **B Basilic Vein, Right** Median antebrachial vein Median cubital vein **C Basilic Vein, Left** *See B Basilic Vein, Right* **D Cephalic Vein, Right** Accessory cephalic vein **F Cephalic Vein, Left** *See D Cephalic Vein, Right* **G Hand Vein, Right** Dorsal metacarpal vein Palmar (volar) digital vein Palmar (volar) metacarpal vein Superficial palmar venous arch Volar (palmar) digital vein Volar (palmar) metacarpal vein	**H Hand Vein, Left** *See G Hand Vein, Right* **L Intracranial Vein** Anterior cerebral vein Basal (internal) cerebral vein Dural venous sinus Great cerebral vein Inferior cerebellar vein Inferior cerebral vein Internal (basal) cerebral vein Middle cerebral vein Ophthalmic vein Superior cerebellar vein Superior cerebral vein **M Internal Jugular Vein, Right** **N Internal Jugular Vein, Left** **P External Jugular Vein, Right** Posterior auricular vein **Q External Jugular Vein, Left** *See P External Jugular Vein, Right* **R Vertebral Vein, Right** Deep cervical vein Suboccipital venous plexus **S Vertebral Vein, Left** *See R Vertebral Vein, Right* **T Face Vein, Right** Angular vein Anterior facial vein Common facial vein Deep facial vein Frontal vein Posterior facial (retromandibular) vein Supraorbital vein **V Face Vein, Left** *See T Face Vein, Right* **Y Upper Vein**	**Ø Open** **3 Percutaneous** **4 Percutaneous Endoscopic**	**Z No Device**	**Z No Qualifier**

Ø Medical and Surgical
5 Upper Veins
U Supplement

Definition: Putting in or on biological or synthetic material that physically reinforces and/or augments the function of a portion of a body part

Explanation: The biological material is non-living, or is living and from the same individual. The body part may have been previously replaced, and the SUPPLEMENT procedure is performed to physically reinforce and/or augment the function of the replaced body part.

Body Part Character 4		Approach Character 5	Device Character 6	Qualifier Character 7
Ø Azygos Vein Right ascending lumbar vein Right subcostal vein **1 Hemiazygos Vein** Left ascending lumbar vein Left subcostal vein **3 Innominate Vein, Right** Brachiocephalic vein Inferior thyroid vein **4 Innominate Vein, Left** *See 3 Innominate Vein, Right* **5 Subclavian Vein, Right** **6 Subclavian Vein, Left** **7 Axillary Vein, Right** **8 Axillary Vein, Left** **9 Brachial Vein, Right** Radial vein Ulnar vein **A Brachial Vein, Left** *See 9 Brachial Vein, Right* **B Basilic Vein, Right** Median antebrachial vein Median cubital vein **C Basilic Vein, Left** *See B Basilic Vein, Right* **D Cephalic Vein, Right** Accessory cephalic vein **F Cephalic Vein, Left** *See D Cephalic Vein, Right* **G Hand Vein, Right** Dorsal metacarpal vein Palmar (volar) digital vein Palmar (volar) metacarpal vein Superficial palmar venous arch Volar (palmar) digital vein Volar (palmar) metacarpal vein	**H Hand Vein, Left** *See G Hand Vein, Right* **L Intracranial Vein** Anterior cerebral vein Basal (internal) cerebral vein Dural venous sinus Great cerebral vein Inferior cerebellar vein Inferior cerebral vein Internal (basal) cerebral vein Middle cerebral vein Ophthalmic vein Superior cerebellar vein Superior cerebral vein **M Internal Jugular Vein, Right** **N Internal Jugular Vein, Left** **P External Jugular Vein, Right** Posterior auricular vein **Q External Jugular Vein, Left** *See P External Jugular Vein, Right* **R Vertebral Vein, Right** Deep cervical vein Suboccipital venous plexus **S Vertebral Vein, Left** *See R Vertebral Vein, Right* **T Face Vein, Right** Angular vein Anterior facial vein Common facial vein Deep facial vein Frontal vein Posterior facial (retromandibular) vein Supraorbital vein **V Face Vein, Left** *See T Face Vein, Right* **Y Upper Vein**	**Ø Open** **3 Percutaneous** **4 Percutaneous Endoscopic**	**7 Autologous Tissue Substitute** **J Synthetic Substitute** **K Nonautologous Tissue Substitute**	**Z No Qualifier**

Ø Medical and Surgical
5 Upper Veins
V Restriction Definition: Partially closing an orifice or the lumen of a tubular body part
Explanation: The orifice can be a natural orifice or an artificially created orifice

Body Part Character 4	Approach Character 5	Device Character 6	Qualifier Character 7
Ø Azygos Vein Right ascending lumbar vein Right subcostal vein **1 Hemiazygos Vein** Left ascending lumbar vein Left subcostal vein **3 Innominate Vein, Right** Brachiocephalic vein Inferior thyroid vein **4 Innominate Vein, Left** *See 3 Innominate Vein, Right* **5 Subclavian Vein, Right** **6 Subclavian Vein, Left** **7 Axillary Vein, Right** **8 Axillary Vein, Left** **9 Brachial Vein, Right** Radial vein Ulnar vein **A Brachial Vein, Left** *See 9 Brachial Vein, Right* **B Basilic Vein, Right** Median antebrachial vein Median cubital vein **C Basilic Vein, Left** *See B Basilic Vein, Right* **D Cephalic Vein, Right** Accessory cephalic vein **F Cephalic Vein, Left** *See D Cephalic Vein, Right* **G Hand Vein, Right** Dorsal metacarpal vein Palmar (volar) digital vein Palmar (volar) metacarpal vein Superficial palmar venous arch Volar (palmar) digital vein Volar (palmar) metacarpal vein **H Hand Vein, Left** *See G Hand Vein, Right* **L Intracranial Vein** Anterior cerebral vein Basal (internal) cerebral vein Dural venous sinus Great cerebral vein Inferior cerebellar vein Inferior cerebral vein Internal (basal) cerebral vein Middle cerebral vein Ophthalmic vein Superior cerebellar vein Superior cerebral vein **M Internal Jugular Vein, Right** **N Internal Jugular Vein, Left** **P External Jugular Vein, Right** Posterior auricular vein **Q External Jugular Vein, Left** *See P External Jugular Vein, Right* **R Vertebral Vein, Right** Deep cervical vein Suboccipital venous plexus **S Vertebral Vein, Left** *See R Vertebral Vein, Right* **T Face Vein, Right** Angular vein Anterior facial vein Common facial vein Deep facial vein Frontal vein Posterior facial (retromandibular) vein Supraorbital vein **V Face Vein, Left** *See T Face Vein, Right* **Y Upper Vein**	**Ø Open** **3 Percutaneous** **4 Percutaneous Endoscopic**	**C Extraluminal Device** **D Intraluminal Device** **Z No Device**	**Z No Qualifier**

Ø Medical and Surgical
5 Upper Veins
W Revision

Definition: Correcting, to the extent possible, a portion of a malfunctioning device or the position of a displaced device

Explanation: Revision can include correcting a malfunctioning or displaced device by taking out or putting in components of the device such as a screw or pin

Body Part Character 4	Approach Character 5	Device Character 6	Qualifier Character 7
Ø Azygos Vein Right ascending lumbar vein Right subcostal vein	**Ø Open** **3 Percutaneous** **4 Percutaneous Endoscopic** **X External**	**2 Monitoring Device** **M Neurostimulator Lead**	**Z No Qualifier**
3 Innominate Vein, Right Brachiocephalic vein Inferior thyroid vein **4 Innominate Vein, Left** *See 3 Innominate Vein, Right*	**Ø Open** **3 Percutaneous** **4 Percutaneous Endoscopic** **X External**	**M Neurostimulator Lead**	**Z No Qualifier**
Y Upper Vein	**Ø Open** **3 Percutaneous** **4 Percutaneous Endoscopic**	**Ø Drainage Device** **2 Monitoring Device** **3 Infusion Device** **7 Autologous Tissue Substitute** **C Extraluminal Device** **D Intraluminal Device** **J Synthetic Substitute** **K Nonautologous Tissue Substitute** **Y Other Device**	**Z No Qualifier**
Y Upper Vein	**X External**	**Ø Drainage Device** **2 Monitoring Device** **3 Infusion Device** **7 Autologous Tissue Substitute** **C Extraluminal Device** **D Intraluminal Device** **J Synthetic Substitute** **K Nonautologous Tissue Substitute**	**Z No Qualifier**

Non-OR Ø5WØXMZ
Non-OR Ø5W[3,4]XMZ
Non-OR Ø5WY3[Ø,2,3,D]Z
Non-OR Ø5WY[3,4]YZ
Non-OR Ø5WYX[Ø,2,3,7,C,D,J,K]Z

Lower Veins Ø61–Ø6W

Character Meanings

This Character Meaning table is provided as a guide to assist the user in the identification of character members that may be found in this section of code tables. It **SHOULD NOT** be used to build a PCS code.

Operation–Character 3	Body Part–Character 4	Approach–Character 5	Device–Character 6	Qualifier–Character 7
1 Bypass	Ø Inferior Vena Cava	Ø Open	Ø Drainage Device	Ø Ultrasonic
5 Destruction	1 Splenic Vein	3 Percutaneous	2 Monitoring Device	4 Hepatic Vein
7 Dilation	2 Gastric Vein	4 Percutaneous Endoscopic	3 Infusion Device	5 Superior Mesenteric Vein
9 Drainage	3 Esophageal Vein	7 Via Natural or Artificial Opening	7 Autologous Tissue Substitute	6 Inferior Mesenteric Vein
B Excision	4 Hepatic Vein	8 Via Natural or Artificial Opening Endoscopic	9 Autologous Venous Tissue	9 Renal Vein, Right
C Extirpation	5 Superior Mesenteric Vein	X External	A Autologous Arterial Tissue	B Renal Vein, Left
D Extraction	6 Inferior Mesenteric Vein		C Extraluminal Device	C Hemorrhoidal Plexus
F Fragmentation	7 Colic Vein		D Intraluminal Device	P Pulmonary Trunk
H Insertion	8 Portal Vein		J Synthetic Substitute	Q Pulmonary Artery, Right
J Inspection	9 Renal Vein, Right		K Nonautologous Tissue Substitute	R Pulmonary Artery, Left
L Occlusion	B Renal Vein, Left		Y Other Device	T Via Umbilical Vein
N Release	C Common Iliac Vein, Right		Z No Device	X Diagnostic
P Removal	D Common Iliac Vein, Left			Y Lower Vein
Q Repair	F External Iliac Vein, Right			Z No Qualifier
R Replacement	G External Iliac Vein, Left			
S Reposition	H Hypogastric Vein, Right			
U Supplement	J Hypogastric Vein, Left			
V Restriction	M Femoral Vein, Right			
W Revision	N Femoral Vein, Left			
	P Saphenous Vein, Right			
	Q Saphenous Vein, Left			
	T Foot Vein, Right			
	V Foot Vein, Left			
	Y Lower Vein			

AHA Coding Clinic for table Ø61
2017, 4Q, 36-38 Fontan completion procedure
2017, 4Q, 66-67 New qualifier values - Portal to hepatic shunt

AHA Coding Clinic for table Ø6B
2020, 1Q, 28 Free flap microvascular breast reconstruction
2017, 3Q, 5 Femoral artery to posterior tibial artery bypass using autologous and synthetic grafts
2017, 1Q, 31 Left to right common carotid artery bypass
2017, 1Q, 32 Peroneal artery to dorsalis pedis artery bypass using saphenous vein graft
2016, 3Q, 31 Femoral to peroneal artery bypass with in-situ saphenous vein graft and lysis of valves
2016, 2Q, 18 Femoral-tibial artery bypass and saphenous vein graft
2016, 1Q, 27 Aortocoronary bypass graft utilizing Y-graft
2014, 3Q, 8 Excision of saphenous vein for coronary artery bypass graft
2014, 3Q, 20 MAZE procedure performed with coronary artery bypass graft
2014, 1Q, 10 Repair of thoracic aortic aneurysm & coronary artery bypass graft

AHA Coding Clinic for table Ø6H
2017, 3Q, 11 Placement of peripherally inserted central catheter using 3CG ECG technology
2017, 1Q, 31 Umbilical vein catheterization
2017, 1Q, 31 Central catheter placement in femoral vein
2013, 3Q, 18 Heart transplant surgery

AHA Coding Clinic for table Ø6L
2019, 4Q, 28 Transorifice occlusion of gastric varices
2018, 2Q, 18 Transverse rectus abdominis myocutaneous (TRAM) delay
2017, 4Q, 57-58 Added approach values - Transorifice esophageal vein banding
2013, 4Q, 112 Endoscopic banding of esophageal varices

AHA Coding Clinic for table Ø6V
2018, 3Q, 11 Transvenous transcatheter placement of valve in inferior vena cava
2018, 1Q, 10 Revision of transjugular intrahepatic portosystemic shunt

AHA Coding Clinic for table Ø6W
2019, 2Q, 39 Transjugular intrahepatic portosystemic shunt revision
2018, 1Q, 10 Revision of transjugular intrahepatic portosystemic shunt
2014, 3Q, 25 Revision of transjugular intrahepatic portosystemic shunt (TIPS)

Lower Veins

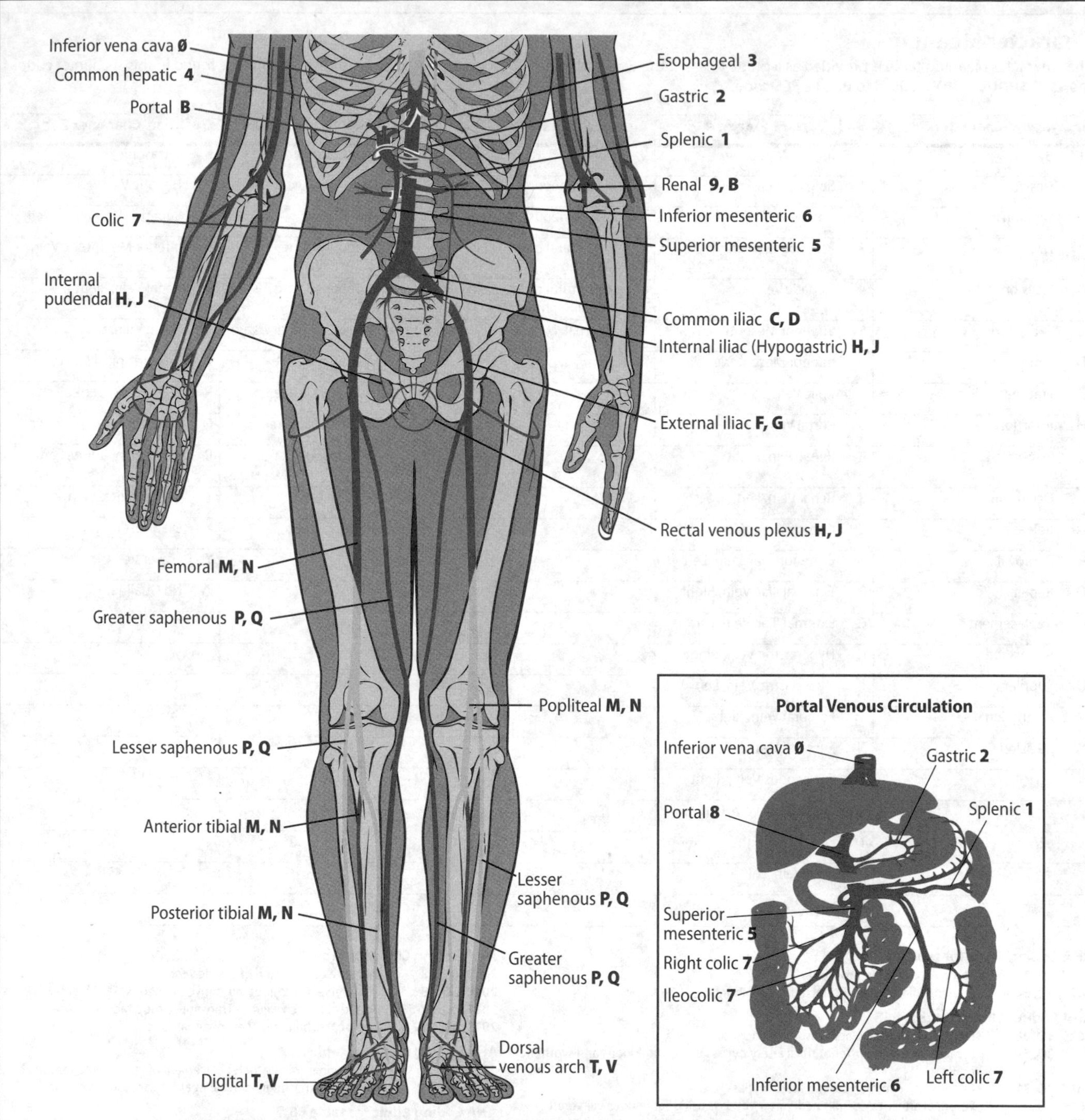
Inferior vena cava Ø
Common hepatic 4
Portal B
Colic 7
Internal pudendal H, J
Esophageal 3
Gastric 2
Splenic 1
Renal 9, B
Inferior mesenteric 6
Superior mesenteric 5
Common iliac C, D
Internal iliac (Hypogastric) H, J
External iliac F, G
Rectal venous plexus H, J
Femoral M, N
Greater saphenous P, Q
Popliteal M, N
Lesser saphenous P, Q
Anterior tibial M, N
Lesser saphenous P, Q
Posterior tibial M, N
Greater saphenous P, Q
Dorsal venous arch T, V
Digital T, V
Portal Venous Circulation
Inferior vena cava Ø
Gastric 2
Splenic 1
Portal 8
Superior mesenteric 5
Right colic 7
Ileocolic 7
Inferior mesenteric 6
Left colic 7

Ø Medical and Surgical
6 Lower Veins
1 Bypass

Definition: Altering the route of passage of the contents of a tubular body part

Explanation: Rerouting contents of a body part to a downstream area of the normal route, to a similar route and body part, or to an abnormal route and dissimilar body part. Includes one or more anastomoses, with or without the use of a device.

Body Part Character 4	Approach Character 5	Device Character 6	Qualifier Character 7
Ø Inferior Vena Cava Postcava Right inferior phrenic vein Right ovarian vein Right second lumbar vein Right suprarenal vein Right testicular vein	**Ø Open** **4 Percutaneous Endoscopic**	**7 Autologous Tissue Substitute** **9 Autologous Venous Tissue** **A Autologous Arterial Tissue** **J Synthetic Substitute** **K Nonautologous Tissue Substitute** **Z No Device**	**5 Superior Mesenteric Vein** **6 Inferior Mesenteric Vein** **P Pulmonary Trunk** **Q Pulmonary Artery, Right** **R Pulmonary Artery, Left** **Y Lower Vein**
1 Splenic Vein Left gastroepiploic vein Pancreatic vein	**Ø Open** **4 Percutaneous Endoscopic**	**7 Autologous Tissue Substitute** **9 Autologous Venous Tissue** **A Autologous Arterial Tissue** **J Synthetic Substitute** **K Nonautologous Tissue Substitute** **Z No Device**	**9 Renal Vein, Right** **B Renal Vein, Left** **Y Lower Vein**
2 Gastric Vein **3 Esophageal Vein** **4 Hepatic Vein** **5 Superior Mesenteric Vein** Right gastroepiploic vein **6 Inferior Mesenteric Vein** Sigmoid vein Superior rectal vein **7 Colic Vein** Ileocolic vein Left colic vein Middle colic vein Right colic vein **9 Renal Vein, Right** **B Renal Vein, Left** Left inferior phrenic vein Left ovarian vein Left second lumbar vein Left suprarenal vein Left testicular vein **C Common Iliac Vein, Right** **D Common Iliac Vein, Left** **F External Iliac Vein, Right** **G External Iliac Vein, Left** **H Hypogastric Vein, Right** Gluteal vein Internal iliac vein Internal pudendal vein Lateral sacral vein Middle hemorrhoidal vein Obturator vein Uterine vein Vaginal vein Vesical vein **J Hypogastric Vein, Left** *See H Hypogastric Vein, Right* **M Femoral Vein, Right** Deep femoral (profunda femoris) vein Popliteal vein Profunda femoris (deep femoral) vein **N Femoral Vein, Left** *See M Femoral Vein, Right* **P Saphenous Vein, Right** External pudendal vein Great(er) saphenous vein Lesser saphenous vein Small saphenous vein Superficial circumflex iliac vein Superficial epigastric vein **Q Saphenous Vein, Left** *See P Saphenous Vein, Right* **T Foot Vein, Right** Common digital vein Dorsal metatarsal vein Dorsal venous arch Plantar digital vein Plantar metatarsal vein Plantar venous arch **V Foot Vein, Left** *See T Foot Vein, Right*	**Ø Open** **4 Percutaneous Endoscopic**	**7 Autologous Tissue Substitute** **9 Autologous Venous Tissue** **A Autologous Arterial Tissue** **J Synthetic Substitute** **K Nonautologous Tissue Substitute** **Z No Device**	**Y Lower Vein**
8 Portal Vein Hepatic portal vein	**Ø Open**	**7 Autologous Tissue Substitute** **9 Autologous Venous Tissue** **A Autologous Arterial Tissue** **J Synthetic Substitute** **K Nonautologous Tissue Substitute** **Z No Device**	**9 Renal Vein, Right** **B Renal Vein, Left** **Y Lower Vein**
8 Portal Vein Hepatic portal vein	**3 Percutaneous**	**J Synthetic Substitute**	**4 Hepatic Vein** **Y Lower Vein**
8 Portal Vein Hepatic portal vein	**4 Percutaneous Endoscopic**	**7 Autologous Tissue Substitute** **9 Autologous Venous Tissue** **A Autologous Arterial Tissue** **K Nonautologous Tissue Substitute** **Z No Device**	**9 Renal Vein, Right** **B Renal Vein, Left** **Y Lower Vein**
8 Portal Vein Hepatic portal vein	**4 Percutaneous Endoscopic**	**J Synthetic Substitute**	**4 Hepatic Vein** **9 Renal Vein, Right** **B Renal Vein, Left** **Y Lower Vein**

Ø Medical and Surgical
6 Lower Veins
5 Destruction Definition: Physical eradication of all or a portion of a body part by the direct use of energy, force, or a destructive agent
Explanation: None of the body part is physically taken out

Body Part Character 4	Approach Character 5	Device Character 6	Qualifier Character 7
Ø Inferior Vena Cava Postcava Right inferior phrenic vein Right ovarian vein Right second lumbar vein Right suprarenal vein Right testicular vein **1 Splenic Vein** Left gastroepiploic vein Pancreatic vein **2 Gastric Vein** **3 Esophageal Vein** **4 Hepatic Vein** **5 Superior Mesenteric Vein** Right gastroepiploic vein **6 Inferior Mesenteric Vein** Sigmoid vein Superior rectal vein **7 Colic Vein** Ileocolic vein Left colic vein Middle colic vein Right colic vein **8 Portal Vein** Hepatic portal vein **9 Renal Vein, Right** **B Renal Vein, Left** Left inferior phrenic vein Left ovarian vein Left second lumbar vein Left suprarenal vein Left testicular vein **C Common Iliac Vein, Right** **D Common Iliac Vein, Left** **F External Iliac Vein, Right** **G External Iliac Vein, Left** **H Hypogastric Vein, Right** Gluteal vein Internal iliac vein Internal pudendal vein Lateral sacral vein Middle hemorrhoidal vein Obturator vein Uterine vein Vaginal vein Vesical vein **J Hypogastric Vein, Left** **See** *H Hypogastric Vein, Right* **M Femoral Vein, Right** Deep femoral (profunda femoris) vein Popliteal vein Profunda femoris (deep femoral) vein **N Femoral Vein, Left** **See** *M Femoral Vein, Right* **P Saphenous Vein, Right** External pudendal vein Great(er) saphenous vein Lesser saphenous vein Small saphenous vein Superficial circumflex iliac vein Superficial epigastric vein **Q Saphenous Vein, Left** **See** *P Saphenous Vein, Right* **T Foot Vein, Right** Common digital vein Dorsal metatarsal vein Dorsal venous arch Plantar digital vein Plantar metatarsal vein Plantar venous arch **V Foot Vein, Left** **See** *T Foot Vein, Right*	**Ø Open** **3 Percutaneous** **4 Percutaneous Endoscopic**	**Z No Device**	**Z No Qualifier**
Y Lower Vein	**Ø Open** **3 Percutaneous** **4 Percutaneous Endoscopic**	**Z No Device**	**C Hemorrhoidal Plexus** **Z No Qualifier**

Ø Medical and Surgical
6 Lower Veins
7 Dilation Definition: Expanding an orifice or the lumen of a tubular body part

Explanation: The orifice can be a natural orifice or an artificially created orifice. Accomplished by stretching a tubular body part using intraluminal pressure or by cutting part of the orifice or wall of the tubular body part.

Body Part Character 4	Approach Character 5	Device Character 6	Qualifier Character 7
Ø Inferior Vena Cava Postcava Right inferior phrenic vein Right ovarian vein Right second lumbar vein Right suprarenal vein Right testicular vein **1 Splenic Vein** Left gastroepiploic vein Pancreatic vein **2 Gastric Vein** **3 Esophageal Vein** **4 Hepatic Vein** **5 Superior Mesenteric Vein** Right gastroepiploic vein **6 Inferior Mesenteric Vein** Sigmoid vein Superior rectal vein **7 Colic Vein** Ileocolic vein Left colic vein Middle colic vein Right colic vein **8 Portal Vein** Hepatic portal vein **9 Renal Vein, Right** **B Renal Vein, Left** Left inferior phrenic vein Left ovarian vein Left second lumbar vein Left suprarenal vein Left testicular vein **C Common Iliac Vein, Right** **D Common Iliac Vein, Left** **F External Iliac Vein, Right** **G External Iliac Vein, Left** **H Hypogastric Vein, Right** Gluteal vein Internal iliac vein Internal pudendal vein Lateral sacral vein Middle hemorrhoidal vein Obturator vein Uterine vein Vaginal vein Vesical vein **J Hypogastric Vein, Left** ***See*** *H Hypogastric Vein, Right* **M Femoral Vein, Right** Deep femoral (profunda femoris) vein Popliteal vein Profunda femoris (deep femoral) vein **N Femoral Vein, Left** ***See*** *M Femoral Vein, Right* **P Saphenous Vein, Right** External pudendal vein Great(er) saphenous vein Lesser saphenous vein Small saphenous vein Superficial circumflex iliac vein Superficial epigastric vein **Q Saphenous Vein, Left** ***See*** *P Saphenous Vein, Right* **T Foot Vein, Right** Common digital vein Dorsal metatarsal vein Dorsal venous arch Plantar digital vein Plantar metatarsal vein Plantar venous arch **V Foot Vein, Left** ***See*** *T Foot Vein, Right* **Y Lower Vein**	**Ø Open** **3 Percutaneous** **4 Percutaneous Endoscopic**	**D Intraluminal Device** **Z No Device**	**Z No Qualifier**

Ø Medical and Surgical
6 Lower Veins
9 Drainage Definition: Taking or letting out fluids and/or gases from a body part
Explanation: The qualifier DIAGNOSTIC is used to identify drainage procedures that are biopsies

Body Part Character 4	Approach Character 5	Device Character 6	Qualifier Character 7
Ø Inferior Vena Cava Postcava Right inferior phrenic vein Right ovarian vein Right second lumbar vein Right suprarenal vein Right testicular vein **1 Splenic Vein** Left gastroepiploic vein Pancreatic vein **2 Gastric Vein** **3 Esophageal Vein** **4 Hepatic Vein** **5 Superior Mesenteric Vein** Right gastroepiploic vein **6 Inferior Mesenteric Vein** Sigmoid vein Superior rectal vein **7 Colic Vein** Ileocolic vein Left colic vein Middle colic vein Right colic vein **8 Portal Vein** Hepatic portal vein **9 Renal Vein, Right** **B Renal Vein, Left** Left inferior phrenic vein Left ovarian vein Left second lumbar vein Left suprarenal vein Left testicular vein **C Common Iliac Vein, Right** **D Common Iliac Vein, Left** **F External Iliac Vein, Right** **G External Iliac Vein, Left** **H Hypogastric Vein, Right** Gluteal vein Internal iliac vein Internal pudendal vein Lateral sacral vein Middle hemorrhoidal vein Obturator vein Uterine vein Vaginal vein Vesical vein **J Hypogastric Vein, Left** ***See** H Hypogastric Vein, Right* **M Femoral Vein, Right** Deep femoral (profunda femoris) vein Popliteal vein Profunda femoris (deep femoral) vein **N Femoral Vein, Left** ***See** M Femoral Vein, Right* **P Saphenous Vein, Right** External pudendal vein Great(er) saphenous vein Lesser saphenous vein Small saphenous vein Superficial circumflex iliac vein Superficial epigastric vein **Q Saphenous Vein, Left** ***See** P Saphenous Vein, Right* **T Foot Vein, Right** Common digital vein Dorsal metatarsal vein Dorsal venous arch Plantar digital vein Plantar metatarsal vein Plantar venous arch **V Foot Vein, Left** ***See** T Foot Vein, Right* **Y Lower Vein**	**Ø Open** **3 Percutaneous** **4 Percutaneous Endoscopic**	**Ø Drainage Device**	**Z No Qualifier**

Non-OR Ø69[Ø,1,2,4,5,6,7,8,9,B,C,D,F,G,H,J,M,N,P,Q,T,V,Y][Ø,3,4]ØZ
Non-OR Ø6933ØZ

Ø69 Continued on next page

Ø Medical and Surgical
6 Lower Veins
9 Drainage Definition: Taking or letting out fluids and/or gases from a body part
Explanation: The qualifier DIAGNOSTIC is used to identify drainage procedures that are biopsies

Ø69 Continued

Body Part Character 4	Approach Character 5	Device Character 6	Qualifier Character 7
Ø Inferior Vena Cava Postcava Right inferior phrenic vein Right ovarian vein Right second lumbar vein Right suprarenal vein Right testicular vein **1 Splenic Vein** Left gastroepiploic vein Pancreatic vein **2 Gastric Vein** **3 Esophageal Vein** **4 Hepatic Vein** **5 Superior Mesenteric Vein** Right gastroepiploic vein **6 Inferior Mesenteric Vein** Sigmoid vein Superior rectal vein **7 Colic Vein** Ileocolic vein Left colic vein Middle colic vein Right colic vein **8 Portal Vein** Hepatic portal vein **9 Renal Vein, Right** **B Renal Vein, Left** Left inferior phrenic vein Left ovarian vein Left second lumbar vein Left suprarenal vein Left testicular vein **C Common Iliac Vein, Right** **D Common Iliac Vein, Left** **F External Iliac Vein, Right** **G External Iliac Vein, Left** **H Hypogastric Vein, Right** Gluteal vein Internal iliac vein Internal pudendal vein Lateral sacral vein Middle hemorrhoidal vein Obturator vein Uterine vein Vaginal vein Vesical vein **J Hypogastric Vein, Left** ***See** H Hypogastric Vein, Right* **M Femoral Vein, Right** Deep femoral (profunda femoris) vein Popliteal vein Profunda femoris (deep femoral) vein **N Femoral Vein, Left** ***See** M Femoral Vein, Right* **P Saphenous Vein, Right** External pudendal vein Great(er) saphenous vein Lesser saphenous vein Small saphenous vein Superficial circumflex iliac vein Superficial epigastric vein **Q Saphenous Vein, Left** ***See** P Saphenous Vein, Right* **T Foot Vein, Right** Common digital vein Dorsal metatarsal vein Dorsal venous arch Plantar digital vein Plantar metatarsal vein Plantar venous arch **V Foot Vein, Left** ***See** T Foot Vein, Right* **Y Lower Vein**	**Ø Open** **3 Percutaneous** **4 Percutaneous Endoscopic**	**Z No Device**	**X Diagnostic** **Z No Qualifier**

Non-OR Ø69[Ø,1,2,3,4,5,6,7,8,9,B,C,D,F,G,H,J,M,N,P,Q,T,V,Y]3ZX
Non-OR Ø69[Ø,1,2,4,5,6,7,8,9,B,C,D,F,G,H,J,M,N,P,Q,T,V,Y][Ø,3,4]ZZ
Non-OR Ø6933ZZ

Ø Medical and Surgical
6 Lower Veins
B Excision Definition: Cutting out or off, without replacement, a portion of a body part
Explanation: The qualifier DIAGNOSTIC is used to identify excision procedures that are biopsies

Body Part Character 4		Approach Character 5	Device Character 6	Qualifier Character 7
Ø Inferior Vena Cava Postcava Right inferior phrenic vein Right ovarian vein Right second lumbar vein Right suprarenal vein Right testicular vein **1 Splenic Vein** Left gastroepiploic vein Pancreatic vein **2 Gastric Vein** **3 Esophageal Vein** **4 Hepatic Vein** **5 Superior Mesenteric Vein** Right gastroepiploic vein **6 Inferior Mesenteric Vein** Sigmoid vein Superior rectal vein **7 Colic Vein** Ileocolic vein Left colic vein Middle colic vein Right colic vein **8 Portal Vein** Hepatic portal vein **9 Renal Vein, Right** **B Renal Vein, Left** Left inferior phrenic vein Left ovarian vein Left second lumbar vein Left suprarenal vein Left testicular vein **C Common Iliac Vein, Right** **D Common Iliac Vein, Left** **F External Iliac Vein, Right** **G External Iliac Vein, Left**	**H Hypogastric Vein, Right** Gluteal vein Internal iliac vein Internal pudendal vein Lateral sacral vein Middle hemorrhoidal vein Obturator vein Uterine vein Vaginal vein Vesical vein **J Hypogastric Vein, Left** *See H Hypogastric Vein, Right* **M Femoral Vein, Right** Deep femoral (profunda femoris) vein Popliteal vein Profunda femoris (deep femoral) vein **N Femoral Vein, Left** *See M Femoral Vein, Right* **P Saphenous Vein, Right** External pudendal vein Great(er) saphenous vein Lesser saphenous vein Small saphenous vein Superficial circumflex iliac vein Superficial epigastric vein **Q Saphenous Vein, Left** *See P Saphenous Vein, Right* **T Foot Vein, Right** Common digital vein Dorsal metatarsal vein Dorsal venous arch Plantar digital vein Plantar metatarsal vein Plantar venous arch **V Foot Vein, Left** *See T Foot Vein, Right*	**Ø Open** **3 Percutaneous** **4 Percutaneous Endoscopic**	**Z No Device**	**X Diagnostic** **Z No Qualifier**
Y Lower Vein		**Ø Open** **3 Percutaneous** **4 Percutaneous Endoscopic**	**Z No Device**	**C Hemorrhoidal Plexus** **X Diagnostic** **Z No Qualifier**

Ø Medical and Surgical
6 Lower Veins
C Extirpation Definition: Taking or cutting out solid matter from a body part

Explanation: The solid matter may be an abnormal byproduct of a biological function or a foreign body; it may be imbedded in a body part or in the lumen of a tubular body part. The solid matter may or may not have been previously broken into pieces.

Body Part Character 4		Approach Character 5	Device Character 6	Qualifier Character 7
Ø Inferior Vena Cava Postcava Right inferior phrenic vein Right ovarian vein Right second lumbar vein Right suprarenal vein Right testicular vein **1 Splenic Vein** Left gastroepiploic vein Pancreatic vein **2 Gastric Vein** **3 Esophageal Vein** **4 Hepatic Vein** **5 Superior Mesenteric Vein** Right gastroepiploic vein **6 Inferior Mesenteric Vein** Sigmoid vein Superior rectal vein **7 Colic Vein** Ileocolic vein Left colic vein Middle colic vein Right colic vein **8 Portal Vein** Hepatic portal vein **9 Renal Vein, Right** **B Renal Vein, Left** Left inferior phrenic vein Left ovarian vein Left second lumbar vein Left suprarenal vein Left testicular vein **C Common Iliac Vein, Right** **D Common Iliac Vein, Left** **F External Iliac Vein, Right** **G External Iliac Vein, Left**	**H Hypogastric Vein, Right** Gluteal vein Internal iliac vein Internal pudendal vein Lateral sacral vein Middle hemorrhoidal vein Obturator vein Uterine vein Vaginal vein Vesical vein **J Hypogastric Vein, Left** *See H Hypogastric Vein, Right* **M Femoral Vein, Right** Deep femoral (profunda femoris) vein Popliteal vein Profunda femoris (deep femoral) vein **N Femoral Vein, Left** *See M Femoral Vein, Right* **P Saphenous Vein, Right** External pudendal vein Great(er) saphenous vein Lesser saphenous vein Small saphenous vein Superficial circumflex iliac vein Superficial epigastric vein **Q Saphenous Vein, Left** *See P Saphenous Vein, Right* **T Foot Vein, Right** Common digital vein Dorsal metatarsal vein Dorsal venous arch Plantar digital vein Plantar metatarsal vein Plantar venous arch **V Foot Vein, Left** *See T Foot Vein, Right* **Y Lower Vein**	**Ø Open** **3 Percutaneous** **4 Percutaneous Endoscopic**	**Z No Device**	**Z No Qualifier**

Ø Medical and Surgical
6 Lower Veins
D Extraction Definition: Pulling or stripping out or off all or a portion of a body part by the use of force

Explanation: The qualifier DIAGNOSTIC is used to identify extraction procedures that are biopsies

Body Part Character 4		Approach Character 5	Device Character 6	Qualifier Character 7
M Femoral Vein, Right Deep femoral (profunda femoris) vein Popliteal vein Profunda femoris (deep femoral) vein **N Femoral Vein, Left** *See M Femoral Vein, Right* **P Saphenous Vein, Right** External pudendal vein Great(er) saphenous vein Lesser saphenous vein Small saphenous vein Superficial circumflex iliac vein Superficial epigastric vein **Q Saphenous Vein, Left** *See P Saphenous Vein, Right*	**T Foot Vein, Right** Common digital vein Dorsal metatarsal vein Dorsal venous arch Plantar digital vein Plantar metatarsal vein Plantar venous arch **V Foot Vein, Left** *See T Foot Vein, Right* **Y Lower Vein**	**Ø Open** **3 Percutaneous** **4 Percutaneous Endoscopic**	**Z No Device**	**Z No Qualifier**

Ø Medical and Surgical
6 Lower Veins
F Fragmentation Definition: Breaking solid matter in a body part into pieces

Explanation: Physical force (e.g., manual, ultrasonic) applied directly or indirectly is used to break the solid matter into pieces. The solid matter may be an abnormal byproduct of a biological function or a foreign body. The pieces of solid matter are not taken out.

Body Part Character 4		Approach Character 5	Device Character 6	Qualifier Character 7
C Common Iliac Vein, Right **D Common Iliac Vein, Left** **F External Iliac Vein, Right** **G External Iliac Vein, Left** **H Hypogastric Vein, Right** Gluteal vein Internal iliac vein Internal pudendal vein Lateral sacral vein Middle hemorrhoidal vein Obturator vein Uterine vein Vaginal vein Vesical vein **J Hypogastric Vein, Left** *See H Hypogastric Vein, Right*	**M Femoral Vein, Right** Deep femoral (profunda femoris) vein Popliteal vein Profunda femoris (deep femoral) vein **N Femoral Vein, Left** *See M Femoral Vein, Right* **P Saphenous Vein, Right** External pudendal vein Great(er) saphenous vein Lesser saphenous vein Small saphenous vein Superficial circumflex iliac vein Superficial epigastric vein **Q Saphenous Vein, Left** *See P Saphenous Vein, Right* **Y Lower Vein**	**3 Percutaneous**	**Z No Device**	**Ø Ultrasonic** **Z No Qualifier**

Ø Medical and Surgical
6 Lower Veins
H Insertion Definition: Putting in a nonbiological appliance that monitors, assists, performs, or prevents a physiological function but does not physically take the place of a body part

Explanation: None

Body Part Character 4		Approach Character 5	Device Character 6	Qualifier Character 7
Ø Inferior Vena Cava Postcava Right inferior phrenic vein Right ovarian vein Right second lumbar vein Right suprarenal vein Right testicular vein		**Ø Open** **3 Percutaneous**	**3 Infusion Device**	**T Via Umbilical Vein** **Z No Qualifier**
Ø Inferior Vena Cava Postcava Right inferior phrenic vein Right ovarian vein Right second lumbar vein Right suprarenal vein Right testicular vein		**Ø Open** **3 Percutaneous**	**D Intraluminal Device**	**Z No Qualifier**
Ø Inferior Vena Cava Postcava Right inferior phrenic vein Right ovarian vein Right second lumbar vein Right suprarenal vein Right testicular vein		**4 Percutaneous Endoscopic**	**3 Infusion Device** **D Intraluminal Device**	**Z No Qualifier**
1 Splenic Vein Left gastroepiploic vein Pancreatic vein **2 Gastric Vein** **3 Esophageal Vein** **4 Hepatic Vein** **5 Superior Mesenteric Vein** Right gastroepiploic vein **6 Inferior Mesenteric Vein** Sigmoid vein Superior rectal vein **7 Colic Vein** Ileocolic vein Left colic vein Middle colic vein Right colic vein **8 Portal Vein** Hepatic portal vein **9 Renal Vein, Right** **B Renal Vein, Left** Left inferior phrenic vein Left ovarian vein Left second lumbar vein Left suprarenal vein Left testicular vein **C Common Iliac Vein, Right** **D Common Iliac Vein, Left** **F External Iliac Vein, Right** **G External Iliac Vein, Left**	**H Hypogastric Vein, Right** Gluteal vein Internal iliac vein Internal pudendal vein Lateral sacral vein Middle hemorrhoidal vein Obturator vein Uterine vein Vaginal vein Vesical vein **J Hypogastric Vein, Left** ***See*** *H Hypogastric Vein, Right* **M Femoral Vein, Right** Deep femoral (profunda femoris) vein Popliteal vein Profunda femoris (deep femoral) vein **N Femoral Vein, Left** ***See*** *M Femoral Vein, Right* **P Saphenous Vein, Right** External pudendal vein Great(er) saphenous vein Lesser saphenous vein Small saphenous vein Superficial circumflex iliac vein Superficial epigastric vein **Q Saphenous Vein, Left** ***See*** *P Saphenous Vein, Right* **T Foot Vein, Right** Common digital vein Dorsal metatarsal vein Dorsal venous arch Plantar digital vein Plantar metatarsal vein Plantar venous arch **V Foot Vein, Left** ***See*** *T Foot Vein, Right*	**Ø Open** **3 Percutaneous** **4 Percutaneous Endoscopic**	**3 Infusion Device** **D Intraluminal Device**	**Z No Qualifier**
Y Lower Vein		**Ø Open** **3 Percutaneous** **4 Percutaneous Endoscopic**	**2 Monitoring Device** **3 Infusion Device** **D Intraluminal Device** **Y Other Device**	**Z No Qualifier**

Non-OR Ø6HØ[Ø,3]3[T,Z]
Non-OR Ø6HØ[Ø,3]DZ
Non-OR Ø6HØ4[3,D]Z
Non-OR Ø6H[1,2,3,4,5,6,7,8,9,B,C,D,F,G,H,J,M,N,P,Q,T,V][Ø,3,4]3Z
Non-OR Ø6HY[Ø,3,4]3Z
Non-OR Ø6HY32Z
Non-OR Ø6HY[3,4]YZ

Ø Medical and Surgical
6 Lower Veins
J Inspection Definition: Visually and/or manually exploring a body part

Explanation: Visual exploration may be performed with or without optical instrumentation. Manual exploration may be performed directly or through intervening body layers.

Body Part Character 4	Approach Character 5	Device Character 6	Qualifier Character 7
Y Lower Vein	Ø Open 3 Percutaneous 4 Percutaneous Endoscopic X External	Z No Device	Z No Qualifier

Non-OR Ø6JY[3,X]ZZ

Ø Medical and Surgical
6 Lower Veins
L Occlusion Definition: Completely closing an orifice or the lumen of a tubular body part

Explanation: The orifice can be a natural orifice or an artificially created orifice

Body Part Character 4	Approach Character 5	Device Character 6	Qualifier Character 7
Ø **Inferior Vena Cava** Postcava Right inferior phrenic vein Right ovarian vein Right second lumbar vein Right suprarenal vein Right testicular vein 1 **Splenic Vein** Left gastroepiploic vein Pancreatic vein 4 **Hepatic Vein** 5 **Superior Mesenteric Vein** Right gastroepiploic vein 6 **Inferior Mesenteric Vein** Sigmoid vein Superior rectal vein 7 **Colic Vein** Ileocolic vein Left colic vein Middle colic vein Right colic vein 8 **Portal Vein** Hepatic portal vein 9 **Renal Vein, Right** B **Renal Vein, Left** Left inferior phrenic vein Left ovarian vein Left second lumbar vein Left suprarenal vein Left testicular vein C **Common Iliac Vein, Right** D **Common Iliac Vein, Left** F **External Iliac Vein, Right** G **External Iliac Vein, Left** H **Hypogastric Vein, Right** Gluteal vein Internal iliac vein Internal pudendal vein Lateral sacral vein Middle hemorrhoidal vein Obturator vein Uterine vein Vaginal vein Vesical vein J **Hypogastric Vein, Left** *See H Hypogastric Vein, Right* M **Femoral Vein, Right** Deep femoral (profunda femoris) vein Popliteal vein Profunda femoris (deep femoral) vein N **Femoral Vein, Left** *See M Femoral Vein, Right* P **Saphenous Vein, Right** External pudendal vein Great(er) saphenous vein Lesser saphenous vein Small saphenous vein Superficial circumflex iliac vein Superficial epigastric vein Q **Saphenous Vein, Left** *See P Saphenous Vein, Right* T **Foot Vein, Right** Common digital vein Dorsal metatarsal vein Dorsal venous arch Plantar digital vein Plantar metatarsal vein Plantar venous arch V **Foot Vein, Left** *See T Foot Vein, Right*	Ø Open 3 Percutaneous 4 Percutaneous Endoscopic	C Extraluminal Device D Intraluminal Device Z No Device	Z No Qualifier
2 Gastric Vein 3 Esophageal Vein	Ø Open 3 Percutaneous 4 Percutaneous Endoscopic 7 Via Natural or Artificial Opening 8 Via Natural or Artificial Opening Endoscopic	C Extraluminal Device D Intraluminal Device Z No Device	Z No Qualifier
Y Lower Vein	Ø Open 3 Percutaneous 4 Percutaneous Endoscopic	C Extraluminal Device D Intraluminal Device Z No Device	C Hemorrhoidal Plexus Z No Qualifier

Non-OR Ø6L2[7,8][C,D,Z]Z
Non-OR Ø6L3[3,4,7,8][C,D,Z]Z

Ø Medical and Surgical
6 Lower Veins
N Release Definition: Freeing a body part from an abnormal physical constraint by cutting or by the use of force
Explanation: Some of the restraining tissue may be taken out but none of the body part is taken out

Body Part Character 4		Approach Character 5	Device Character 6	Qualifier Character 7
Ø Inferior Vena Cava Postcava Right inferior phrenic vein Right ovarian vein Right second lumbar vein Right suprarenal vein Right testicular vein **1 Splenic Vein** Left gastroepiploic vein Pancreatic vein **2 Gastric Vein** **3 Esophageal Vein** **4 Hepatic Vein** **5 Superior Mesenteric Vein** Right gastroepiploic vein **6 Inferior Mesenteric Vein** Sigmoid vein Superior rectal vein **7 Colic Vein** Ileocolic vein Left colic vein Middle colic vein Right colic vein **8 Portal Vein** Hepatic portal vein **9 Renal Vein, Right** **B Renal Vein, Left** Left inferior phrenic vein Left ovarian vein Left second lumbar vein Left suprarenal vein Left testicular vein **C Common Iliac Vein, Right** **D Common Iliac Vein, Left** **F External Iliac Vein, Right** **G External Iliac Vein, Left**	**H Hypogastric Vein, Right** Gluteal vein Internal iliac vein Internal pudendal vein Lateral sacral vein Middle hemorrhoidal vein Obturator vein Uterine vein Vaginal vein Vesical vein **J Hypogastric Vein, Left** *See H Hypogastric Vein, Right* **M Femoral Vein, Right** Deep femoral (profunda femoris) vein Popliteal vein Profunda femoris (deep femoral) vein **N Femoral Vein, Left** *See M Femoral Vein, Right* **P Saphenous Vein, Right** External pudendal vein Great(er) saphenous vein Lesser saphenous vein Small saphenous vein Superficial circumflex iliac vein Superficial epigastric vein **Q Saphenous Vein, Left** *See P Saphenous Vein, Right* **T Foot Vein, Right** Common digital vein Dorsal metatarsal vein Dorsal venous arch Plantar digital vein Plantar metatarsal vein Plantar venous arch **V Foot Vein, Left** *See T Foot Vein, Right* **Y Lower Vein**	**Ø Open** **3 Percutaneous** **4 Percutaneous Endoscopic**	**Z No Device**	**Z No Qualifier**

Ø Medical and Surgical
6 Lower Veins
P Removal Definition: Taking out or off a device from a body part
Explanation: If a device is taken out and a similar device put in without cutting or puncturing the skin or mucous membrane, the procedure is coded to the root operation CHANGE. Otherwise, the procedure for taking out a device is coded to the root operation REMOVAL.

Body Part Character 4	Approach Character 5	Device Character 6	Qualifier Character 7
Y Lower Vein	**Ø Open** **3 Percutaneous** **4 Percutaneous Endoscopic**	**Ø Drainage Device** **2 Monitoring Device** **3 Infusion Device** **7 Autologous Tissue Substitute** **C Extraluminal Device** **D Intraluminal Device** **J Synthetic Substitute** **K Nonautologous Tissue Substitute** **Y Other Device**	**Z No Qualifier**
Y Lower Vein	**X External**	**Ø Drainage Device** **2 Monitoring Device** **3 Infusion Device** **D Intraluminal Device**	**Z No Qualifier**

Non-OR Ø6PY3[Ø,2,3]Z
Non-OR Ø6PY[3,4]YZ
Non-OR Ø6PYX[Ø,2,3,D]Z

Ø Medical and Surgical
6 Lower Veins
Q Repair **Definition: Restoring, to the extent possible, a body part to its normal anatomic structure and function**
Explanation: Used only when the method to accomplish the repair is not one of the other root operations

Body Part Character 4	Approach Character 5	Device Character 6	Qualifier Character 7
Ø Inferior Vena Cava Postcava Right inferior phrenic vein Right ovarian vein Right second lumbar vein Right suprarenal vein Right testicular vein	**Ø Open** **3 Percutaneous** **4 Percutaneous Endoscopic**	**Z No Device**	**Z No Qualifier**
1 Splenic Vein Left gastroepiploic vein Pancreatic vein			
2 Gastric Vein			
3 Esophageal Vein			
4 Hepatic Vein			
5 Superior Mesenteric Vein Right gastroepiploic vein			
6 Inferior Mesenteric Vein Sigmoid vein Superior rectal vein			
7 Colic Vein Ileocolic vein Left colic vein Middle colic vein Right colic vein			
8 Portal Vein Hepatic portal vein			
9 Renal Vein, Right			
B Renal Vein, Left Left inferior phrenic vein Left ovarian vein Left second lumbar vein Left suprarenal vein Left testicular vein			
C Common Iliac Vein, Right			
D Common Iliac Vein, Left			
F External Iliac Vein, Right			
G External Iliac Vein, Left			
H Hypogastric Vein, Right Gluteal vein Internal iliac vein Internal pudendal vein Lateral sacral vein Middle hemorrhoidal vein Obturator vein Uterine vein Vaginal vein Vesical vein			
J Hypogastric Vein, Left ***See** H Hypogastric Vein, Right*			
M Femoral Vein, Right Deep femoral (profunda femoris) vein Popliteal vein Profunda femoris (deep femoral) vein			
N Femoral Vein, Left ***See** M Femoral Vein, Right*			
P Saphenous Vein, Right External pudendal vein Great(er) saphenous vein Lesser saphenous vein Small saphenous vein Superficial circumflex iliac vein Superficial epigastric vein			
Q Saphenous Vein, Left ***See** P Saphenous Vein, Right*			
T Foot Vein, Right Common digital vein Dorsal metatarsal vein Dorsal venous arch Plantar digital vein Plantar metatarsal vein Plantar venous arch			
V Foot Vein, Left ***See** T Foot Vein, Right*			
Y Lower Vein			

Ø Medical and Surgical
6 Lower Veins
R Replacement Definition: Putting in or on biological or synthetic material that physically takes the place and/or function of all or a portion of a body part

Explanation: The body part may have been taken out or replaced, or may be taken out, physically eradicated, or rendered nonfunctional during the REPLACEMENT procedure. A REMOVAL procedure is coded for taking out the device used in a previous replacement procedure.

Body Part Character 4	Approach Character 5	Device Character 6	Qualifier Character 7
Ø Inferior Vena Cava Postcava Right inferior phrenic vein Right ovarian vein Right second lumbar vein Right suprarenal vein Right testicular vein **1 Splenic Vein** Left gastroepiploic vein Pancreatic vein **2 Gastric Vein** **3 Esophageal Vein** **4 Hepatic Vein** **5 Superior Mesenteric Vein** Right gastroepiploic vein **6 Inferior Mesenteric Vein** Sigmoid vein Superior rectal vein **7 Colic Vein** Ileocolic vein Left colic vein Middle colic vein Right colic vein **8 Portal Vein** Hepatic portal vein **9 Renal Vein, Right** **B Renal Vein, Left** Left inferior phrenic vein Left ovarian vein Left second lumbar vein Left suprarenal vein Left testicular vein **C Common Iliac Vein, Right** **D Common Iliac Vein, Left** **F External Iliac Vein, Right** **G External Iliac Vein, Left** **H Hypogastric Vein, Right** Gluteal vein Internal iliac vein Internal pudendal vein Lateral sacral vein Middle hemorrhoidal vein Obturator vein Uterine vein Vaginal vein Vesical vein **J Hypogastric Vein, Left** ***See*** *H Hypogastric Vein, Right* **M Femoral Vein, Right** Deep femoral (profunda femoris) vein Popliteal vein Profunda femoris (deep femoral) vein **N Femoral Vein, Left** ***See*** *M Femoral Vein, Right* **P Saphenous Vein, Right** External pudendal vein Great(er) saphenous vein Lesser saphenous vein Small saphenous vein Superficial circumflex iliac vein Superficial epigastric vein **Q Saphenous Vein, Left** ***See*** *P Saphenous Vein, Right* **T Foot Vein, Right** Common digital vein Dorsal metatarsal vein Dorsal venous arch Plantar digital vein Plantar metatarsal vein Plantar venous arch **V Foot Vein, Left** ***See*** *T Foot Vein, Right* **Y Lower Vein**	**Ø Open** **4 Percutaneous Endoscopic**	**7 Autologous Tissue Substitute** **J Synthetic Substitute** **K Nonautologous Tissue Substitute**	**Z No Qualifier**

Ø Medical and Surgical
6 Lower Veins
S Reposition Definition: Moving to its normal location, or other suitable location, all or a portion of a body part

Explanation: The body part is moved to a new location from an abnormal location, or from a normal location where it is not functioning correctly. The body part may or may not be cut out or off to be moved to the new location.

Body Part Character 4	Approach Character 5	Device Character 6	Qualifier Character 7
Ø Inferior Vena Cava Postcava Right inferior phrenic vein Right ovarian vein Right second lumbar vein Right suprarenal vein Right testicular vein **1 Splenic Vein** Left gastroepiploic vein Pancreatic vein **2 Gastric Vein** **3 Esophageal Vein** **4 Hepatic Vein** **5 Superior Mesenteric Vein** Right gastroepiploic vein **6 Inferior Mesenteric Vein** Sigmoid vein Superior rectal vein **7 Colic Vein** Ileocolic vein Left colic vein Middle colic vein Right colic vein **8 Portal Vein** Hepatic portal vein **9 Renal Vein, Right** **B Renal Vein, Left** Left inferior phrenic vein Left ovarian vein Left second lumbar vein Left suprarenal vein Left testicular vein **C Common Iliac Vein, Right** **D Common Iliac Vein, Left** **F External Iliac Vein, Right** **G External Iliac Vein, Left** **H Hypogastric Vein, Right** Gluteal vein Internal iliac vein Internal pudendal vein Lateral sacral vein Middle hemorrhoidal vein Obturator vein Uterine vein Vaginal vein Vesical vein **J Hypogastric Vein, Left** *See H Hypogastric Vein, Right* **M Femoral Vein, Right** Deep femoral (profunda femoris) vein Popliteal vein Profunda femoris (deep femoral) vein **N Femoral Vein, Left** *See M Femoral Vein, Right* **P Saphenous Vein, Right** External pudendal vein Great(er) saphenous vein Lesser saphenous vein Small saphenous vein Superficial circumflex iliac vein Superficial epigastric vein **Q Saphenous Vein, Left** *See P Saphenous Vein, Right* **T Foot Vein, Right** Common digital vein Dorsal metatarsal vein Dorsal venous arch Plantar digital vein Plantar metatarsal vein Plantar venous arch **V Foot Vein, Left** *See T Foot Vein, Right* **Y Lower Vein**	**Ø Open** **3 Percutaneous** **4 Percutaneous Endoscopic**	**Z No Device**	**Z No Qualifier**

Ø Medical and Surgical
6 Lower Veins
U Supplement Definition: Putting in or on biological or synthetic material that physically reinforces and/or augments the function of a portion of a body part

Explanation: The biological material is non-living, or is living and from the same individual. The body part may have been previously replaced, and the SUPPLEMENT procedure is performed to physically reinforce and/or augment the function of the replaced body part.

Body Part Character 4	Approach Character 5	Device Character 6	Qualifier Character 7
Ø Inferior Vena Cava Postcava Right inferior phrenic vein Right ovarian vein Right second lumbar vein Right suprarenal vein Right testicular vein **1 Splenic Vein** Left gastroepiploic vein Pancreatic vein **2 Gastric Vein** **3 Esophageal Vein** **4 Hepatic Vein** **5 Superior Mesenteric Vein** Right gastroepiploic vein **6 Inferior Mesenteric Vein** Sigmoid vein Superior rectal vein **7 Colic Vein** Ileocolic vein Left colic vein Middle colic vein Right colic vein **8 Portal Vein** Hepatic portal vein **9 Renal Vein, Right** **B Renal Vein, Left** Left inferior phrenic vein Left ovarian vein Left second lumbar vein Left suprarenal vein Left testicular vein **C Common Iliac Vein, Right** **D Common Iliac Vein, Left** **F External Iliac Vein, Right** **G External Iliac Vein, Left** **H Hypogastric Vein, Right** Gluteal vein Internal iliac vein Internal pudendal vein Lateral sacral vein Middle hemorrhoidal vein Obturator vein Uterine vein Vaginal vein Vesical vein **J Hypogastric Vein, Left** ***See** H Hypogastric Vein, Right* **M Femoral Vein, Right** Deep femoral (profunda femoris) vein Popliteal vein Profunda femoris (deep femoral) vein **N Femoral Vein, Left** ***See** M Femoral Vein, Right* **P Saphenous Vein, Right** External pudendal vein Great(er) saphenous vein Lesser saphenous vein Small saphenous vein Superficial circumflex iliac vein Superficial epigastric vein **Q Saphenous Vein, Left** ***See** P Saphenous Vein, Right* **T Foot Vein, Right** Common digital vein Dorsal metatarsal vein Dorsal venous arch Plantar digital vein Plantar metatarsal vein Plantar venous arch **V Foot Vein, Left** ***See** T Foot Vein, Right* **Y Lower Vein**	**Ø Open** **3 Percutaneous** **4 Percutaneous Endoscopic**	**7 Autologous Tissue Substitute** **J Synthetic Substitute** **K Nonautologous Tissue Substitute**	**Z No Qualifier**

Ø Medical and Surgical
6 Lower Veins
V Restriction Definition: Partially closing an orifice or the lumen of a tubular body part
Explanation: The orifice can be a natural orifice or an artificially created orifice

Body Part Character 4	Approach Character 5	Device Character 6	Qualifier Character 7
Ø Inferior Vena Cava Postcava Right inferior phrenic vein Right ovarian vein Right second lumbar vein Right suprarenal vein Right testicular vein **1 Splenic Vein** Left gastroepiploic vein Pancreatic vein **2 Gastric Vein** **3 Esophageal Vein** **4 Hepatic Vein** **5 Superior Mesenteric Vein** Right gastroepiploic vein **6 Inferior Mesenteric Vein** Sigmoid vein Superior rectal vein **7 Colic Vein** Ileocolic vein Left colic vein Middle colic vein Right colic vein **8 Portal Vein** Hepatic portal vein **9 Renal Vein, Right** **B Renal Vein, Left** Left inferior phrenic vein Left ovarian vein Left second lumbar vein Left suprarenal vein Left testicular vein **C Common Iliac Vein, Right** **D Common Iliac Vein, Left** **F External Iliac Vein, Right** **G External Iliac Vein, Left** **H Hypogastric Vein, Right** Gluteal vein Internal iliac vein Internal pudendal vein Lateral sacral vein Middle hemorrhoidal vein Obturator vein Uterine vein Vaginal vein Vesical vein **J Hypogastric Vein, Left** *See H Hypogastric Vein, Right* **M Femoral Vein, Right** Deep femoral (profunda femoris) vein Popliteal vein Profunda femoris (deep femoral) vein **N Femoral Vein, Left** *See M Femoral Vein, Right* **P Saphenous Vein, Right** External pudendal vein Great(er) saphenous vein Lesser saphenous vein Small saphenous vein Superficial circumflex iliac vein Superficial epigastric vein **Q Saphenous Vein, Left** *See P Saphenous Vein, Right* **T Foot Vein, Right** Common digital vein Dorsal metatarsal vein Dorsal venous arch Plantar digital vein Plantar metatarsal vein Plantar venous arch **V Foot Vein, Left** *See T Foot Vein, Right* **Y Lower Vein**	**Ø Open** **3 Percutaneous** **4 Percutaneous Endoscopic**	**C Extraluminal Device** **D Intraluminal Device** **Z No Device**	**Z No Qualifier**

Ø Medical and Surgical
6 Lower Veins
W Revision

Definition: Correcting, to the extent possible, a portion of a malfunctioning device or the position of a displaced device

Explanation: Revision can include correcting a malfunctioning or displaced device by taking out or putting in components of the device such as a screw or pin

Body Part Character 4	Approach Character 5	Device Character 6	Qualifier Character 7
Y Lower Vein	Ø Open 3 Percutaneous 4 Percutaneous Endoscopic	Ø Drainage Device 2 Monitoring Device 3 Infusion Device 7 Autologous Tissue Substitute C Extraluminal Device D Intraluminal Device J Synthetic Substitute K Nonautologous Tissue Substitute Y Other Device	Z No Qualifier
Y Lower Vein	X External	Ø Drainage Device 2 Monitoring Device 3 Infusion Device 7 Autologous Tissue Substitute C Extraluminal Device D Intraluminal Device J Synthetic Substitute K Nonautologous Tissue Substitute	Z No Qualifier

Non-OR Ø6WY3[Ø,2,3,D]Z
Non-OR Ø6WY[3,4]YZ
Non-OR Ø6WYX[Ø,2,3,7,C,D,J,K]Z

Lymphatic and Hemic Systems Ø72–Ø7Y

Character Meanings*

This Character Meaning table is provided as a guide to assist the user in the identification of character members that may be found in this section of code tables. It **SHOULD NOT** be used to build a PCS code.

Operation–Character 3		Body Part–Character 4		Approach–Character 5		Device–Character 6		Qualifier–Character 7	
2	Change	Ø	Lymphatic, Head	Ø	Open	Ø	Drainage Device	Ø	Allogeneic
5	Destruction	1	Lymphatic, Right Neck	3	Percutaneous	1	Radioactive Element	1	Syngeneic
9	Drainage	2	Lymphatic, Left Neck	4	Percutaneous Endoscopic	3	Infusion Device	2	Zooplastic
B	Excision	3	Lymphatic, Right Upper Extremity	8	Via Natural or Artificial Opening Endoscopic	7	Autologous Tissue Substitute	X	Diagnostic
C	Extirpation	4	Lymphatic, Left Upper Extremity	X	External	C	Extraluminal Device	Z	No Qualifier
D	Extraction	5	Lymphatic, Right Axillary			D	Intraluminal Device		
H	Insertion	6	Lymphatic, Left Axillary			J	Synthetic Substitute		
J	Inspection	7	Lymphatic, Thorax			K	Nonautologous Tissue Substitute		
L	Occlusion	8	Lymphatic, Internal Mammary, Right			Y	Other Device		
N	Release	9	Lymphatic, Internal Mammary, Left			Z	No Device		
P	Removal	B	Lymphatic, Mesenteric						
Q	Repair	C	Lymphatic, Pelvis						
S	Reposition	D	Lymphatic, Aortic						
T	Resection	F	Lymphatic, Right Lower Extremity						
U	Supplement	G	Lymphatic, Left Lower Extremity						
V	Restriction	H	Lymphatic, Right Inguinal						
W	Revision	J	Lymphatic, Left Inguinal						
Y	Transplantation	K	Thoracic Duct						
		L	Cisterna Chyli						
		M	Thymus						
		N	Lymphatic						
		P	Spleen						
		Q	Bone Marrow, Sternum						
		R	Bone Marrow, Iliac						
		S	Bone Marrow, Vertebral						
		T	Bone Marrow						

* Includes lymph vessels and lymph nodes.

AHA Coding Clinic for table Ø79
2018, 4Q, 84 Fine needle aspiration biopsy of lymphatic tissue
2017, 1Q, 34 Lymphovenous bypass following mastectomy
2014, 1Q, 26 Transbronchial needle aspiration lymph node biopsy
2013, 4Q, 111 Transbronchial needle aspiration lymph node biopsy

AHA Coding Clinic for table Ø7B
2019, 1Q, 3-8 Whipple procedure
2018, 4Q, 84 Fine needle aspiration biopsy of lymphatic tissue
2018, 1Q, 22 Resection of lymph node chains
2016, 1Q, 30 Axillary lymph node resection with modified radical mastectomy
2014, 3Q, 10 Selective excision of paratracheal lymph nodes
2014, 1Q, 20 Fiducial marker placement
2014, 1Q, 26 Transbronchial endoscopic lymph node aspiration biopsy

AHA Coding Clinic for table Ø7D
2018, 4Q, 84 Fine needle aspiration biopsy of lymphatic tissue
2013, 4Q, 111 Root operation for bone marrow biopsy

AHA Coding Clinic for table Ø7Q
2017, 1Q, 34 Lymphovenous bypass following mastectomy

AHA Coding Clinic for table Ø7S
2019, 3Q, 29 Thymus transplant for T-Cell production

AHA Coding Clinic for table Ø7T
2018, 1Q, 22 Resection of lymph node chains
2016, 2Q, 12 Resection of malignant neoplasm of infratemporal fossa
2016, 1Q, 30 Axillary lymph node resection with modified radical mastectomy
2015, 4Q, 13 New Section X codes—New Technology procedures
2014, 3Q, 9 Radical resection of level I lymph nodes
2014, 3Q, 16 Repair of Tetralogy of Fallot

AHA Coding Clinic for table Ø7Y
2019, 3Q, 29 Thymus transplant for T-Cell production

Lymphatic and Hemic Systems

Lymphatic System

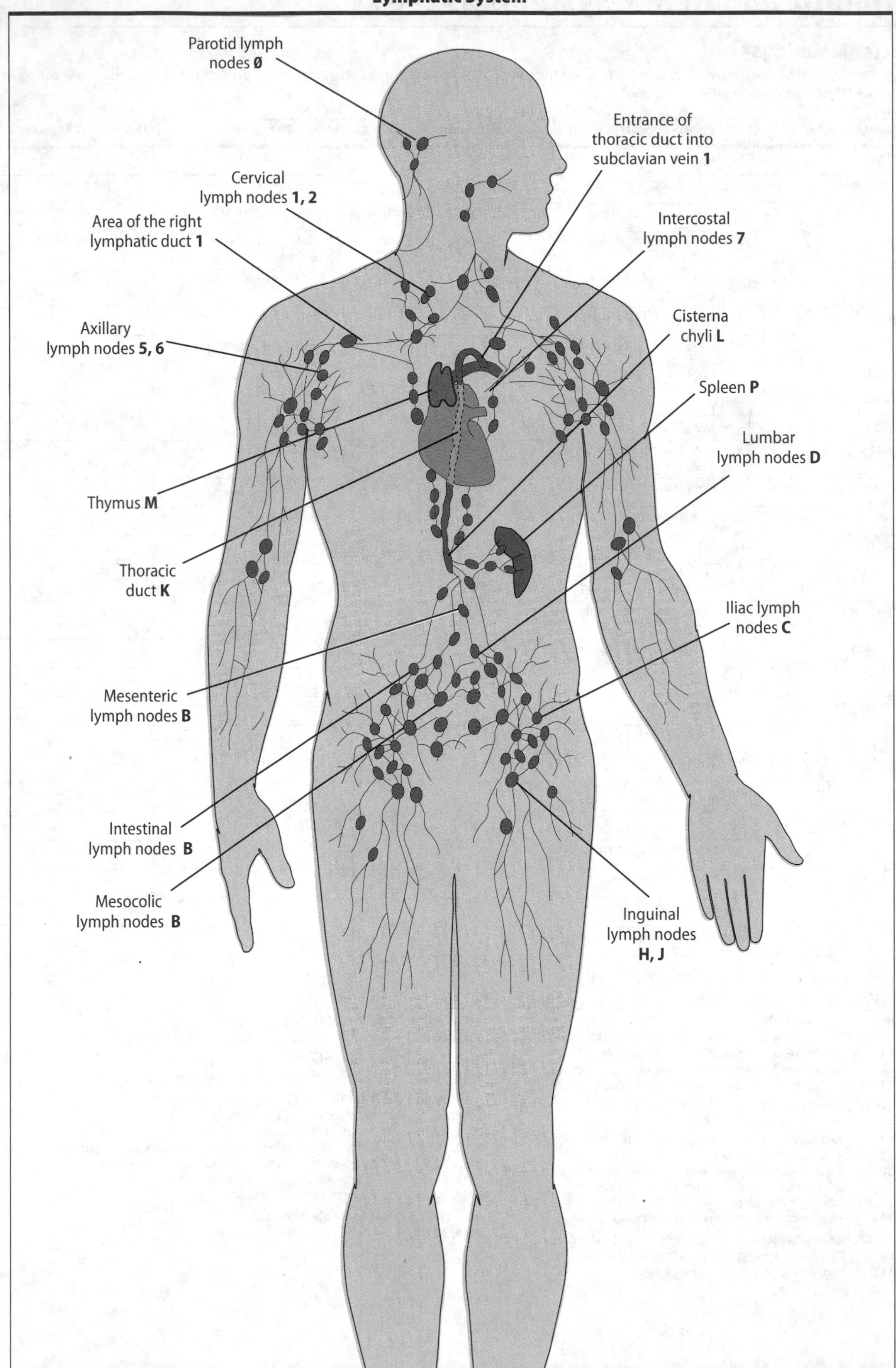

Ø Medical and Surgical
7 Lymphatic and Hemic Systems
2 Change Definition: Taking out or off a device from a body part and putting back an identical or similar device in or on the same body part without cutting or puncturing the skin or a mucous membrane

Explanation: All CHANGE procedures are coded using the approach EXTERNAL

Body Part Character 4		Approach Character 5	Device Character 6	Qualifier Character 7
K Thoracic Duct Left jugular trunk Left subclavian trunk L Cisterna Chyli Intestinal lymphatic trunk Lumbar lymphatic trunk	M Thymus Thymus gland N Lymphatic P Spleen Accessory spleen T Bone Marrow	X External	Ø Drainage Device Y Other Device	Z No Qualifier

Non-OR All body part, approach, device, and qualifier values

Ø Medical and Surgical
7 Lymphatic and Hemic Systems
5 Destruction Definition: Physical eradication of all or a portion of a body part by the direct use of energy, force, or a destructive agent

Explanation: None of the body part is physically taken out

Body Part Character 4		Approach Character 5	Device Character 6	Qualifier Character 7
Ø Lymphatic, Head Buccinator lymph node Infraauricular lymph node Infraparotid lymph node Parotid lymph node Preauricular lymph node Submandibular lymph node Submaxillary lymph node Submental lymph node Subparotid lymph node Suprahyoid lymph node 1 Lymphatic, Right Neck Cervical lymph node Jugular lymph node Mastoid (postauricular) lymph node Occipital lymph node Postauricular (mastoid) lymph node Retropharyngeal lymph node Right jugular trunk Right lymphatic duct Right subclavian trunk Supraclavicular (Virchow's) lymph node Virchow's (supraclavicular) lymph node 2 Lymphatic, Left Neck Cervical lymph node Jugular lymph node Mastoid (postauricular) lymph node Occipital lymph node Postauricular (mastoid) lymph node Retropharyngeal lymph node Supraclavicular (Virchow's) lymph node Virchow's (supraclavicular) lymph node 3 Lymphatic, Right Upper Extremity Cubital lymph node Deltopectoral (infraclavicular) lymph node Epitrochlear lymph node Infraclavicular (deltopectoral) lymph node Supratrochlear lymph node 4 Lymphatic, Left Upper Extremity *See 3 Lymphatic, Right Upper Extremity* 5 Lymphatic, Right Axillary Anterior (pectoral) lymph node Apical (subclavicular) lymph node Brachial (lateral) lymph node Central axillary lymph node Lateral (brachial) lymph node Pectoral (anterior) lymph node Posterior (subscapular) lymph node Subclavicular (apical) lymph node Subscapular (posterior) lymph node	6 Lymphatic, Left Axillary *See 5 Lymphatic, Right Axillary* 7 Lymphatic, Thorax Intercostal lymph node Mediastinal lymph node Parasternal lymph node Paratracheal lymph node Tracheobronchial lymph node 8 Lymphatic, Internal Mammary, Right 9 Lymphatic, Internal Mammary, Left B Lymphatic, Mesenteric Inferior mesenteric lymph node Pararectal lymph node Superior mesenteric lymph node C Lymphatic, Pelvis Common iliac (subaortic) lymph node Gluteal lymph node Iliac lymph node Inferior epigastric lymph node Obturator lymph node Sacral lymph node Subaortic (common iliac) lymph node Suprainguinal lymph node D Lymphatic, Aortic Celiac lymph node Gastric lymph node Hepatic lymph node Lumbar lymph node Pancreaticosplenic lymph node Paraaortic lymph node Retroperitoneal lymph node F Lymphatic, Right Lower Extremity Femoral lymph node Popliteal lymph node G Lymphatic, Left Lower Extremity *See F Lymphatic, Right Lower Extremity* H Lymphatic, Right Inguinal J Lymphatic, Left Inguinal K Thoracic Duct Left jugular trunk Left subclavian trunk L Cisterna Chyli Intestinal lymphatic trunk Lumbar lymphatic trunk M Thymus Thymus gland P Spleen Accessory spleen	Ø Open 3 Percutaneous 4 Percutaneous Endoscopic	Z No Device	Z No Qualifier

Ø Medical and Surgical
7 Lymphatic and Hemic Systems
9 Drainage Definition: Taking or letting out fluids and/or gases from a body part
Explanation: The qualifier DIAGNOSTIC is used to identify drainage procedures that are biopsies

Body Part Character 4		Approach Character 5	Device Character 6	Qualifier Character 7
Ø Lymphatic, Head Buccinator lymph node Infraauricular lymph node Infraparotid lymph node Parotid lymph node Preauricular lymph node Submandibular lymph node Submaxillary lymph node Submental lymph node Subparotid lymph node Suprahyoid lymph node **1 Lymphatic, Right Neck** Cervical lymph node Jugular lymph node Mastoid (postauricular) lymph node Occipital lymph node Postauricular (mastoid) lymph node Retropharyngeal lymph node Right jugular trunk Right lymphatic duct Right subclavian trunk Supraclavicular (Virchow's) lymph node Virchow's (supraclavicular) lymph node **2 Lymphatic, Left Neck** Cervical lymph node Jugular lymph node Mastoid (postauricular) lymph node Occipital lymph node Postauricular (mastoid) lymph node Retropharyngeal lymph node Supraclavicular (Virchow's) lymph node Virchow's (supraclavicular) lymph node **3 Lymphatic, Right Upper Extremity** Cubital lymph node Deltopectoral (infraclavicular) lymph node Epitrochlear lymph node Infraclavicular (deltopectoral) lymph node Supratrochlear lymph node **4 Lymphatic, Left Upper Extremity** *See 3 Lymphatic, Right Upper Extremity* **5 Lymphatic, Right Axillary** Anterior (pectoral) lymph node Apical (subclavicular) lymph node Brachial (lateral) lymph node Central axillary lymph node Lateral (brachial) lymph node Pectoral (anterior) lymph node Posterior (subscapular) lymph node Subclavicular (apical) lymph node Subscapular (posterior) lymph node	**6 Lymphatic, Left Axillary** *See 5 Lymphatic, Right Axillary* **7 Lymphatic, Thorax** Intercostal lymph node Mediastinal lymph node Parasternal lymph node Paratracheal lymph node Tracheobronchial lymph node **8 Lymphatic, Internal Mammary, Right** **9 Lymphatic, Internal Mammary, Left** **B Lymphatic, Mesenteric** Inferior mesenteric lymph node Pararectal lymph node Superior mesenteric lymph node **C Lymphatic, Pelvis** Common iliac (subaortic) lymph node Gluteal lymph node Iliac lymph node Inferior epigastric lymph node Obturator lymph node Sacral lymph node Subaortic (common iliac) lymph node Suprainguinal lymph node **D Lymphatic, Aortic** Celiac lymph node Gastric lymph node Hepatic lymph node Lumbar lymph node Pancreaticosplenic lymph node Paraaortic lymph node Retroperitoneal lymph node **F Lymphatic, Right Lower Extremity** Femoral lymph node Popliteal lymph node **G Lymphatic, Left Lower Extremity** *See F Lymphatic, Right Lower Extremity* **H Lymphatic, Right Inguinal** **J Lymphatic, Left Inguinal** **K Thoracic Duct** Left jugular trunk Left subclavian trunk **L Cisterna Chyli** Intestinal lymphatic trunk Lumbar lymphatic trunk	**Ø Open** **3 Percutaneous** **4 Percutaneous Endoscopic** **8 Via Natural or Artificial Opening Endoscopic**	**Ø Drainage Device**	**Z No Qualifier**

Non-OR Ø79[Ø,1,2,3,4,5,6,7,8,9,B,C,D,F,G,H,J,K,L][3,8]ØZ

Ø79 Continued on next page

Ø Medical and Surgical
7 Lymphatic and Hemic Systems
9 Drainage Definition: Taking or letting out fluids and/or gases from a body part
Explanation: The qualifier DIAGNOSTIC is used to identify drainage procedures that are biopsies

Ø79 Continued

Body Part Character 4		Approach Character 5	Device Character 6	Qualifier Character 7
Ø Lymphatic, Head Buccinator lymph node Infraauricular lymph node Infraparotid lymph node Parotid lymph node Preauricular lymph node Submandibular lymph node Submaxillary lymph node Submental lymph node Subparotid lymph node Suprahyoid lymph node **1 Lymphatic, Right Neck** Cervical lymph node Jugular lymph node Mastoid (postauricular) lymph node Occipital lymph node Postauricular (mastoid) lymph node Retropharyngeal lymph node Right jugular trunk Right lymphatic duct Right subclavian trunk Supraclavicular (Virchow's) lymph node Virchow's (supraclavicular) lymph node **2 Lymphatic, Left Neck** Cervical lymph node Jugular lymph node Mastoid (postauricular) lymph node Occipital lymph node Postauricular (mastoid) lymph node Retropharyngeal lymph node Supraclavicular (Virchow's) lymph node Virchow's (supraclavicular) lymph node **3 Lymphatic, Right Upper Extremity** Cubital lymph node Deltopectoral (infraclavicular) lymph node Epitrochlear lymph node Infraclavicular (deltopectoral) lymph node Supratrochlear lymph node **4 Lymphatic, Left Upper Extremity** *See 3 Lymphatic, Right Upper Extremity* **5 Lymphatic, Right Axillary** Anterior (pectoral) lymph node Apical (subclavicular) lymph node Brachial (lateral) lymph node Central axillary lymph node Lateral (brachial) lymph node Pectoral (anterior) lymph node Posterior (subscapular) lymph node Subclavicular (apical) lymph node Subscapular (posterior) lymph node	**6 Lymphatic, Left Axillary** *See 5 Lymphatic, Right Axillary* **7 Lymphatic, Thorax** Intercostal lymph node Mediastinal lymph node Parasternal lymph node Paratracheal lymph node Tracheobronchial lymph node **8 Lymphatic, Internal Mammary, Right** **9 Lymphatic, Internal Mammary, Left** **B Lymphatic, Mesenteric** Inferior mesenteric lymph node Pararectal lymph node Superior mesenteric lymph node **C Lymphatic, Pelvis** Common iliac (subaortic) lymph node Gluteal lymph node Iliac lymph node Inferior epigastric lymph node Obturator lymph node Sacral lymph node Subaortic (common iliac) lymph node Suprainguinal lymph node **D Lymphatic, Aortic** Celiac lymph node Gastric lymph node Hepatic lymph node Lumbar lymph node Pancreaticosplenic lymph node Paraaortic lymph node Retroperitoneal lymph node **F Lymphatic, Right Lower Extremity** Femoral lymph node Popliteal lymph node **G Lymphatic, Left Lower Extremity** *See F Lymphatic, Right Lower Extremity* **H Lymphatic, Right Inguinal** **J Lymphatic, Left Inguinal** **K Thoracic Duct** Left jugular trunk Left subclavian trunk **L Cisterna Chyli** Intestinal lymphatic trunk Lumbar lymphatic trunk	**Ø Open** **3 Percutaneous** **4 Percutaneous Endoscopic** **8 Via Natural or Artificial Opening Endoscopic**	**Z No Device**	**X Diagnostic** **Z No Qualifier**
M Thymus Thymus gland **P Spleen** Accessory spleen **T Bone Marrow**		**Ø Open** **3 Percutaneous** **4 Percutaneous Endoscopic**	**Ø Drainage Device**	**Z No Qualifier**
M Thymus Thymus gland **P Spleen** Accessory spleen **T Bone Marrow**		**Ø Open** **3 Percutaneous** **4 Percutaneous Endoscopic**	**Z No Device**	**X Diagnostic** **Z No Qualifier**

Non-OR Ø79[Ø,1,2,3,4,5,6,7,8,9,B,C,D,F,G,H,J,K,L]8ZX
Non-OR Ø79[Ø,1,2,3,4,5,6,7,8,9,B,C,D,F,G,H,J,K,L][3,8]ZZ
Non-OR Ø79M3ØZ
Non-OR Ø79P[3,4]ØZ
Non-OR Ø79T[Ø,3,4]ØZ
Non-OR Ø79M3ZZ
Non-OR Ø79P[3,4]Z[X,Z]
Non-OR Ø79T[Ø,3,4]Z[X,Z]

0 Medical and Surgical
7 Lymphatic and Hemic Systems
B Excision Definition: Cutting out or off, without replacement, a portion of a body part
Explanation: The qualifier DIAGNOSTIC is used to identify excision procedures that are biopsies

Body Part Character 4	Approach Character 5	Device Character 6	Qualifier Character 7
0 Lymphatic, Head Buccinator lymph node Infraauricular lymph node Infraparotid lymph node Parotid lymph node Preauricular lymph node Submandibular lymph node Submaxillary lymph node Submental lymph node Subparotid lymph node Suprahyoid lymph node **1 Lymphatic, Right Neck** Cervical lymph node Jugular lymph node Mastoid (postauricular) lymph node Occipital lymph node Postauricular (mastoid) lymph node Retropharyngeal lymph node Right jugular trunk Right lymphatic duct Right subclavian trunk Supraclavicular (Virchow's) lymph node Virchow's (supraclavicular) lymph node **2 Lymphatic, Left Neck** Cervical lymph node Jugular lymph node Mastoid (postauricular) lymph node Occipital lymph node Postauricular (mastoid) lymph node Retropharyngeal lymph node Supraclavicular (Virchow's) lymph node Virchow's (supraclavicular) lymph node **3 Lymphatic, Right Upper Extremity** Cubital lymph node Deltopectoral (infraclavicular) lymph node Epitrochlear lymph node Infraclavicular (deltopectoral) lymph node Supratrochlear lymph node **4 Lymphatic, Left Upper Extremity** *See 3 Lymphatic, Right Upper Extremity* **5 Lymphatic, Right Axillary** Anterior (pectoral) lymph node Apical (subclavicular) lymph node Brachial (lateral) lymph node Central axillary lymph node Lateral (brachial) lymph node Pectoral (anterior) lymph node Posterior (subscapular) lymph node Subclavicular (apical) lymph node Subscapular (posterior) lymph node **6 Lymphatic, Left Axillary** *See 5 Lymphatic, Right Axillary* **7 Lymphatic, Thorax** Intercostal lymph node Mediastinal lymph node Parasternal lymph node Paratracheal lymph node Tracheobronchial lymph node **8 Lymphatic, Internal Mammary, Right** **9 Lymphatic, Internal Mammary, Left** **B Lymphatic, Mesenteric** Inferior mesenteric lymph node Pararectal lymph node Superior mesenteric lymph node **C Lymphatic, Pelvis** Common iliac (subaortic) lymph node Gluteal lymph node Iliac lymph node Inferior epigastric lymph node Obturator lymph node Sacral lymph node Subaortic (common iliac) lymph node Suprainguinal lymph node **D Lymphatic, Aortic** Celiac lymph node Gastric lymph node Hepatic lymph node Lumbar lymph node Pancreaticosplenic lymph node Paraaortic lymph node Retroperitoneal lymph node **F Lymphatic, Right Lower Extremity** Femoral lymph node Popliteal lymph node **G Lymphatic, Left Lower Extremity** *See F Lymphatic, Right Lower Extremity* **H Lymphatic, Right Inguinal** ⊞ **J Lymphatic, Left Inguinal** ⊞ **K Thoracic Duct** Left jugular trunk Left subclavian trunk **L Cisterna Chyli** Intestinal lymphatic trunk Lumbar lymphatic trunk **M Thymus** Thymus gland **P Spleen** Accessory spleen	**0 Open** **3 Percutaneous** **4 Percutaneous Endoscopic**	**Z No Device**	**X Diagnostic** **Z No Qualifier**

Non-OR 07BP[3,4]ZX

See Appendix L for Procedure Combinations
⊞ 07B[H,J][0,4]ZZ

Ø Medical and Surgical
7 Lymphatic and Hemic Systems
C Extirpation Definition: Taking or cutting out solid matter from a body part

Explanation: The solid matter may be an abnormal byproduct of a biological function or a foreign body; it may be imbedded in a body part or in the lumen of a tubular body part. The solid matter may or may not have been previously broken into pieces.

Body Part Character 4	Approach Character 5	Device Character 6	Qualifier Character 7
Ø Lymphatic, Head Buccinator lymph node Infraauricular lymph node Infraparotid lymph node Parotid lymph node Preauricular lymph node Submandibular lymph node Submaxillary lymph node Submental lymph node Subparotid lymph node Suprahyoid lymph node **1 Lymphatic, Right Neck** Cervical lymph node Jugular lymph node Mastoid (postauricular) lymph node Occipital lymph node Postauricular (mastoid) lymph node Retropharyngeal lymph node Right jugular trunk Right lymphatic duct Right subclavian trunk Supraclavicular (Virchow's) lymph node Virchow's (supraclavicular) lymph node **2 Lymphatic, Left Neck** Cervical lymph node Jugular lymph node Mastoid (postauricular) lymph node Occipital lymph node Postauricular (mastoid) lymph node Retropharyngeal lymph node Supraclavicular (Virchow's) lymph node Virchow's (supraclavicular) lymph node **3 Lymphatic, Right Upper Extremity** Cubital lymph node Deltopectoral (infraclavicular) lymph node Epitrochlear lymph node Infraclavicular (deltopectoral) lymph node Supratrochlear lymph node **4 Lymphatic, Left Upper Extremity** *See 3 Lymphatic, Right Upper Extremity* **5 Lymphatic, Right Axillary** Anterior (pectoral) lymph node Apical (subclavicular) lymph node Brachial (lateral) lymph node Central axillary lymph node Lateral (brachial) lymph node Pectoral (anterior) lymph node Posterior (subscapular) lymph node Subclavicular (apical) lymph node Subscapular (posterior) lymph node **6 Lymphatic, Left Axillary** *See 5 Lymphatic, Right Axillary* **7 Lymphatic, Thorax** Intercostal lymph node Mediastinal lymph node Parasternal lymph node Paratracheal lymph node Tracheobronchial lymph node **8 Lymphatic, Internal Mammary, Right** **9 Lymphatic, Internal Mammary, Left** **B Lymphatic, Mesenteric** Inferior mesenteric lymph node Pararectal lymph node Superior mesenteric lymph node **C Lymphatic, Pelvis** Common iliac (subaortic) lymph node Gluteal lymph node Iliac lymph node Inferior epigastric lymph node Obturator lymph node Sacral lymph node Subaortic (common iliac) lymph node Suprainguinal lymph node **D Lymphatic, Aortic** Celiac lymph node Gastric lymph node Hepatic lymph node Lumbar lymph node Pancreaticosplenic lymph node Paraaortic lymph node Retroperitoneal lymph node **F Lymphatic, Right Lower Extremity** Femoral lymph node Popliteal lymph node **G Lymphatic, Left Lower Extremity** *See F Lymphatic, Right Lower Extremity* **H Lymphatic, Right Inguinal** **J Lymphatic, Left Inguinal** **K Thoracic Duct** Left jugular trunk Left subclavian trunk **L Cisterna Chyli** Intestinal lymphatic trunk Lumbar lymphatic trunk **M Thymus** Thymus gland **P Spleen** Accessory spleen	**Ø Open** **3 Percutaneous** **4 Percutaneous Endoscopic**	**Z No Device**	**Z No Qualifier**

Non-OR Ø7CP[3,4]ZZ

Ø Medical and Surgical
7 Lymphatic and Hemic Systems
D Extraction Definition: Pulling or stripping out or off all or a portion of a body part by the use of force
Explanation: The qualifier DIAGNOSTIC is used to identify extraction procedures that are biopsies

Body Part Character 4	Approach Character 5	Device Character 6	Qualifier Character 7
Ø Lymphatic, Head Buccinator lymph node Infraauricular lymph node Infraparotid lymph node Parotid lymph node Preauricular lymph node Submandibular lymph node Submaxillary lymph node Submental lymph node Subparotid lymph node Suprahyoid lymph node **1 Lymphatic, Right Neck** Cervical lymph node Jugular lymph node Mastoid (postauricular) lymph node Occipital lymph node Postauricular (mastoid) lymph node Retropharyngeal lymph node Right jugular trunk Right lymphatic duct Right subclavian trunk Supraclavicular (Virchow's) lymph node Virchow's (supraclavicular) lymph node **2 Lymphatic, Left Neck** Cervical lymph node Jugular lymph node Mastoid (postauricular) lymph node Occipital lymph node Postauricular (mastoid) lymph node Retropharyngeal lymph node Supraclavicular (Virchow's) lymph node Virchow's (supraclavicular) lymph node **3 Lymphatic, Right Upper Extremity** Cubital lymph node Deltopectoral (infraclavicular) lymph node Epitrochlear lymph node Infraclavicular (deltopectoral) lymph node Supratrochlear lymph node **4 Lymphatic, Left Upper Extremity** ***See*** *3 Lymphatic, Right Upper Extremity* **5 Lymphatic, Right Axillary** Anterior (pectoral) lymph node Apical (subclavicular) lymph node Brachial (lateral) lymph node Central axillary lymph node Lateral (brachial) lymph node Pectoral (anterior) lymph node Posterior (subscapular) lymph node Subclavicular (apical) lymph node Subscapular (posterior) lymph node **6 Lymphatic, Left Axillary** ***See*** *5 Lymphatic, Right Axillary* **7 Lymphatic, Thorax** Intercostal lymph node Mediastinal lymph node Parasternal lymph node Paratracheal lymph node Tracheobronchial lymph node **8 Lymphatic, Internal Mammary, Right** **9 Lymphatic, Internal Mammary, Left** **B Lymphatic, Mesenteric** Inferior mesenteric lymph node Pararectal lymph node Superior mesenteric lymph node **C Lymphatic, Pelvis** Common iliac (subaortic) lymph node Gluteal lymph node Iliac lymph node Inferior epigastric lymph node Obturator lymph node Sacral lymph node Subaortic (common iliac) lymph node Suprainguinal lymph node **D Lymphatic, Aortic** Celiac lymph node Gastric lymph node Hepatic lymph node Lumbar lymph node Pancreaticosplenic lymph node Paraaortic lymph node Retroperitoneal lymph node **F Lymphatic, Right Lower Extremity** Femoral lymph node Popliteal lymph node **G Lymphatic, Left Lower Extremity** ***See*** *F Lymphatic, Right Lower Extremity* **H Lymphatic, Right Inguinal** **J Lymphatic, Left Inguinal** **K Thoracic Duct** Left jugular trunk Left subclavian trunk **L Cisterna Chyli** Intestinal lymphatic trunk Lumbar lymphatic trunk	**3 Percutaneous** **4 Percutaneous Endoscopic** **8 Via Natural or Artificial Opening Endoscopic**	**Z No Device**	**X Diagnostic**
M Thymus Thymus gland **P Spleen** Accessory spleen	**3 Percutaneous** **4 Percutaneous Endoscopic**	**Z No Device**	**X Diagnostic**
Q Bone Marrow, Sternum **R Bone Marrow, Iliac** **S Bone Marrow, Vertebral**	**Ø Open** **3 Percutaneous**	**Z No Device**	**X Diagnostic** **Z No Qualifier**

Non-OR All body part, approach, device, and qualifier values

Ø Medical and Surgical
7 Lymphatic and Hemic Systems
H Insertion Definition: Putting in a nonbiological appliance that monitors, assists, performs, or prevents a physiological function but does not physically take the place of a body part

Explanation: None

Body Part Character 4	Approach Character 5	Device Character 6	Qualifier Character 7
K Thoracic Duct Left jugular trunk Left subclavian trunk L Cisterna Chyli Intestinal lymphatic trunk Lumbar lymphatic trunk M Thymus Thymus gland N Lymphatic P Spleen Accessory spleen T Bone Marrow	Ø Open 3 Percutaneous 4 Percutaneous Endoscopic	1 Radioactive Element 3 Infusion Device Y Other Device	Z No Qualifier

Non-OR Ø7H[K,L,M,N,P][Ø,3,4]3Z
Non-OR Ø7H[K,L,M]3YZ
Non-OR Ø7H[N,P][3,4]YZ

Ø Medical and Surgical
7 Lymphatic and Hemic Systems
J Inspection Definition: Visually and/or manually exploring a body part

Explanation: Visual exploration may be performed with or without optical instrumentation. Manual exploration may be performed directly or through intervening body layers.

Body Part Character 4	Approach Character 5	Device Character 6	Qualifier Character 7
K Thoracic Duct Left jugular trunk Left subclavian trunk L Cisterna Chyli Intestinal lymphatic trunk Lumbar lymphatic trunk M Thymus Thymus gland T Bone Marrow	Ø Open 3 Percutaneous 4 Percutaneous Endoscopic	Z No Device	Z No Qualifier
N Lymphatic	Ø Open 3 Percutaneous 4 Percutaneous Endoscopic 8 Via Natural or Artificial Opening Endoscopic X External	Z No Device	Z No Qualifier
P Spleen Accessory spleen	Ø Open 3 Percutaneous 4 Percutaneous Endoscopic X External	Z No Device	Z No Qualifier

Non-OR Ø7J[K,L,M]3ZZ
Non-OR Ø7JT[Ø,3,4]ZZ
Non-OR Ø7JN[3,8,X]ZZ
Non-OR Ø7JP[3,4,X]ZZ

Ø Medical and Surgical
7 Lymphatic and Hemic Systems
L Occlusion Definition: Completely closing an orifice or the lumen of a tubular body part
Explanation: The orifice can be a natural orifice or an artificially created orifice

Body Part Character 4	Approach Character 5	Device Character 6	Qualifier Character 7
Ø Lymphatic, Head Buccinator lymph node Infraauricular lymph node Infraparotid lymph node Parotid lymph node Preauricular lymph node Submandibular lymph node Submaxillary lymph node Submental lymph node Subparotid lymph node Suprahyoid lymph node **1 Lymphatic, Right Neck** Cervical lymph node Jugular lymph node Mastoid (postauricular) lymph node Occipital lymph node Postauricular (mastoid) lymph node Retropharyngeal lymph node Right jugular trunk Right lymphatic duct Right subclavian trunk Supraclavicular (Virchow's) lymph node Virchow's (supraclavicular) lymph node **2 Lymphatic, Left Neck** Cervical lymph node Jugular lymph node Mastoid (postauricular) lymph node Occipital lymph node Postauricular (mastoid) lymph node Retropharyngeal lymph node Supraclavicular (Virchow's) lymph node Virchow's (supraclavicular) lymph node **3 Lymphatic, Right Upper Extremity** Cubital lymph node Deltopectoral (infraclavicular) lymph node Epitrochlear lymph node Infraclavicular (deltopectoral) lymph node Supratrochlear lymph node **4 Lymphatic, Left Upper Extremity** *See 3 Lymphatic, Right Upper Extremity* **5 Lymphatic, Right Axillary** Anterior (pectoral) lymph node Apical (subclavicular) lymph node Brachial (lateral) lymph node Central axillary lymph node Lateral (brachial) lymph node Pectoral (anterior) lymph node Posterior (subscapular) lymph node Subclavicular (apical) lymph node Subscapular (posterior) lymph node **6 Lymphatic, Left Axillary** *See 5 Lymphatic, Right Axillary* **7 Lymphatic, Thorax** Intercostal lymph node Mediastinal lymph node Parasternal lymph node Paratracheal lymph node Tracheobronchial lymph node **8 Lymphatic, Internal Mammary, Right** **9 Lymphatic, Internal Mammary, Left** **B Lymphatic, Mesenteric** Inferior mesenteric lymph node Pararectal lymph node Superior mesenteric lymph node **C Lymphatic, Pelvis** Common iliac (subaortic) lymph node Gluteal lymph node Iliac lymph node Inferior epigastric lymph node Obturator lymph node Sacral lymph node Subaortic (common iliac) lymph node Suprainguinal lymph node **D Lymphatic, Aortic** Celiac lymph node Gastric lymph node Hepatic lymph node Lumbar lymph node Pancreaticosplenic lymph node Paraaortic lymph node Retroperitoneal lymph node **F Lymphatic, Right Lower Extremity** Femoral lymph node Popliteal lymph node **G Lymphatic, Left Lower Extremity** *See F Lymphatic, Right Lower Extremity* **H Lymphatic, Right Inguinal** **J Lymphatic, Left Inguinal** **K Thoracic Duct** Left jugular trunk Left subclavian trunk **L Cisterna Chyli** Intestinal lymphatic trunk Lumbar lymphatic trunk	**Ø Open** **3 Percutaneous** **4 Percutaneous Endoscopic**	**C Extraluminal Device** **D Intraluminal Device** **Z No Device**	**Z No Qualifier**

Ø Medical and Surgical
7 Lymphatic and Hemic Systems
N Release Definition: Freeing a body part from an abnormal physical constraint by cutting or by the use of force
Explanation: Some of the restraining tissue may be taken out but none of the body part is taken out

Body Part Character 4	Approach Character 5	Device Character 6	Qualifier Character 7
Ø Lymphatic, Head Buccinator lymph node Infraauricular lymph node Infraparotid lymph node Parotid lymph node Preauricular lymph node Submandibular lymph node Submaxillary lymph node Submental lymph node Subparotid lymph node Suprahyoid lymph node **1 Lymphatic, Right Neck** Cervical lymph node Jugular lymph node Mastoid (postauricular) lymph node Occipital lymph node Postauricular (mastoid) lymph node Retropharyngeal lymph node Right jugular trunk Right lymphatic duct Right subclavian trunk Supraclavicular (Virchow's) lymph node Virchow's (supraclavicular) lymph node **2 Lymphatic, Left Neck** Cervical lymph node Jugular lymph node Mastoid (postauricular) lymph node Occipital lymph node Postauricular (mastoid) lymph node Retropharyngeal lymph node Supraclavicular (Virchow's) lymph node Virchow's (supraclavicular) lymph node **3 Lymphatic, Right Upper Extremity** Cubital lymph node Deltopectoral (infraclavicular) lymph node Epitrochlear lymph node Infraclavicular (deltopectoral) lymph node Supratrochlear lymph node **4 Lymphatic, Left Upper Extremity** ***See** 3 Lymphatic, Right Upper Extremity* **5 Lymphatic, Right Axillary** Anterior (pectoral) lymph node Apical (subclavicular) lymph node Brachial (lateral) lymph node Central axillary lymph node Lateral (brachial) lymph node Pectoral (anterior) lymph node Posterior (subscapular) lymph node Subclavicular (apical) lymph node Subscapular (posterior) lymph node **6 Lymphatic, Left Axillary** ***See** 5 Lymphatic, Right Axillary* **7 Lymphatic, Thorax** Intercostal lymph node Mediastinal lymph node Parasternal lymph node Paratracheal lymph node Tracheobronchial lymph node **8 Lymphatic, Internal Mammary, Right** **9 Lymphatic, Internal Mammary, Left** **B Lymphatic, Mesenteric** Inferior mesenteric lymph node Pararectal lymph node Superior mesenteric lymph node **C Lymphatic, Pelvis** Common iliac (subaortic) lymph node Gluteal lymph node Iliac lymph node Inferior epigastric lymph node Obturator lymph node Sacral lymph node Subaortic (common iliac) lymph node Suprainguinal lymph node **D Lymphatic, Aortic** Celiac lymph node Gastric lymph node Hepatic lymph node Lumbar lymph node Pancreaticosplenic lymph node Paraaortic lymph node Retroperitoneal lymph node **F Lymphatic, Right Lower Extremity** Femoral lymph node Popliteal lymph node **G Lymphatic, Left Lower Extremity** ***See** F Lymphatic, Right Lower Extremity* **H Lymphatic, Right Inguinal** **J Lymphatic, Left Inguinal** **K Thoracic Duct** Left jugular trunk Left subclavian trunk **L Cisterna Chyli** Intestinal lymphatic trunk Lumbar lymphatic trunk **M Thymus** Thymus gland **P Spleen** Accessory spleen	**Ø Open** **3 Percutaneous** **4 Percutaneous Endoscopic**	**Z No Device**	**Z No Qualifier**

Lymphatic and Hemic Systems

Ø7N–Ø7N

Ø Medical and Surgical
7 Lymphatic and Hemic Systems
P Removal Definition: Taking out or off a device from a body part

Explanation: If a device is taken out and a similar device put in without cutting or puncturing the skin or mucous membrane, the procedure is coded to the root operation CHANGE. Otherwise, the procedure for taking out a device is coded to the root operation REMOVAL.

Body Part Character 4	Approach Character 5	Device Character 6	Qualifier Character 7
K Thoracic Duct Left jugular trunk Left subclavian trunk **L Cisterna Chyli** Intestinal lymphatic trunk Lumbar lymphatic trunk **N Lymphatic**	**Ø Open** **3 Percutaneous** **4 Percutaneous Endoscopic**	**Ø Drainage Device** **3 Infusion Device** **7 Autologous Tissue Substitute** **C Extraluminal Device** **D Intraluminal Device** **J Synthetic Substitute** **K Nonautologous Tissue Substitute** **Y Other Device**	**Z No Qualifier**
K Thoracic Duct Left jugular trunk Left subclavian trunk **L Cisterna Chyli** Intestinal lymphatic trunk Lumbar lymphatic trunk **N Lymphatic**	**X External**	**Ø Drainage Device** **3 Infusion Device** **D Intraluminal Device**	**Z No Qualifier**
M Thymus Thymus gland **P Spleen** Accessory spleen	**Ø Open** **3 Percutaneous** **4 Percutaneous Endoscopic**	**Ø Drainage Device** **3 Infusion Device** **Y Other Device**	**Z No Qualifier**
M Thymus Thymus gland **P Spleen** Accessory spleen	**X External**	**Ø Drainage Device** **3 Infusion Device**	**Z No Qualifier**
T Bone Marrow	**Ø Open** **3 Percutaneous** **4 Percutaneous Endoscopic** **X External**	**Ø Drainage Device**	**Z No Qualifier**

Non-OR Ø7P[K,L,N][3,4]YZ
Non-OR Ø7P[K,L,N]X[Ø,3,D]Z
Non-OR Ø7P[M,P][3,4]YZ
Non-OR Ø7P[M,P]X[Ø,3]Z
Non-OR Ø7PT[Ø,3,4,X]ØZ

Ø **Medical and Surgical**
7 **Lymphatic and Hemic Systems**
Q **Repair** Definition: Restoring, to the extent possible, a body part to its normal anatomic structure and function
Explanation: Used only when the method to accomplish the repair is not one of the other root operations

Body Part Character 4	Approach Character 5	Device Character 6	Qualifier Character 7
Ø **Lymphatic, Head** Buccinator lymph node Infraauricular lymph node Infraparotid lymph node Parotid lymph node Preauricular lymph node Submandibular lymph node Submaxillary lymph node Submental lymph node Subparotid lymph node Suprahyoid lymph node 1 **Lymphatic, Right Neck** Cervical lymph node Jugular lymph node Mastoid (postauricular) lymph node Occipital lymph node Postauricular (mastoid) lymph node Retropharyngeal lymph node Right jugular trunk Right lymphatic duct Right subclavian trunk Supraclavicular (Virchow's) lymph node Virchow's (supraclavicular) lymph node 2 **Lymphatic, Left Neck** Cervical lymph node Jugular lymph node Mastoid (postauricular) lymph node Occipital lymph node Postauricular (mastoid) lymph node Retropharyngeal lymph node Supraclavicular (Virchow's) lymph node Virchow's (supraclavicular) lymph node 3 **Lymphatic, Right Upper Extremity** Cubital lymph node Deltopectoral (infraclavicular) lymph node Epitrochlear lymph node Infraclavicular (deltopectoral) lymph node Supratrochlear lymph node 4 **Lymphatic, Left Upper Extremity** *See 3 Lymphatic, Right Upper Extremity* 5 **Lymphatic, Right Axillary** Anterior (pectoral) lymph node Apical (subclavicular) lymph node Brachial (lateral) lymph node Central axillary lymph node Lateral (brachial) lymph node Pectoral (anterior) lymph node Posterior (subscapular) lymph node Subclavicular (apical) lymph node Subscapular (posterior) lymph node 6 **Lymphatic, Left Axillary** *See 5 Lymphatic, Right Axillary* 7 **Lymphatic, Thorax** Intercostal lymph node Mediastinal lymph node Parasternal lymph node Paratracheal lymph node Tracheobronchial lymph node 8 **Lymphatic, Internal Mammary, Right** 9 **Lymphatic, Internal Mammary, Left** B **Lymphatic, Mesenteric** Inferior mesenteric lymph node Pararectal lymph node Superior mesenteric lymph node C **Lymphatic, Pelvis** Common iliac (subaortic) lymph node Gluteal lymph node Iliac lymph node Inferior epigastric lymph node Obturator lymph node Sacral lymph node Subaortic (common iliac) lymph node Suprainguinal lymph node D **Lymphatic, Aortic** Celiac lymph node Gastric lymph node Hepatic lymph node Lumbar lymph node Pancreaticosplenic lymph node Paraaortic lymph node Retroperitoneal lymph node F **Lymphatic, Right Lower Extremity** Femoral lymph node Popliteal lymph node G **Lymphatic, Left Lower Extremity** *See F Lymphatic, Right Lower Extremity* H **Lymphatic, Right Inguinal** J **Lymphatic, Left Inguinal** K **Thoracic Duct** Left jugular trunk Left subclavian trunk L **Cisterna Chyli** Intestinal lymphatic trunk Lumbar lymphatic trunk	Ø **Open** 3 **Percutaneous** 4 **Percutaneous Endoscopic** 8 **Via Natural or Artificial Opening Endoscopic**	Z **No Device**	Z **No Qualifier**
M **Thymus** Thymus gland P **Spleen** Accessory spleen	Ø **Open** 3 **Percutaneous** 4 **Percutaneous Endoscopic**	Z **No Device**	Z **No Qualifier**

Ø Medical and Surgical
7 Lymphatic and Hemic Systems
S Reposition Definition: Moving to its normal location, or other suitable location, all or a portion of a body part

Explanation: The body part is moved to a new location from an abnormal location, or from a normal location where it is not functioning correctly. The body part may or may not be cut out or off to be moved to the new location.

Body Part Character 4	Approach Character 5	Device Character 6	Qualifier Character 7
M Thymus Thymus gland **P Spleen** Accessory spleen	**Ø Open**	**Z No Device**	**Z No Qualifier**

Ø Medical and Surgical
7 Lymphatic and Hemic Systems
T Resection Definition: Cutting out or off, without replacement, all of a body part

Explanation: None

Body Part Character 4	Approach Character 5	Device Character 6	Qualifier Character 7
Ø Lymphatic, Head Buccinator lymph node Infraauricular lymph node Infraparotid lymph node Parotid lymph node Preauricular lymph node Submandibular lymph node Submaxillary lymph node Submental lymph node Subparotid lymph node Suprahyoid lymph node **1 Lymphatic, Right Neck** Cervical lymph node Jugular lymph node Mastoid (postauricular) lymph node Occipital lymph node Postauricular (mastoid) lymph node Retropharyngeal lymph node Right jugular trunk Right lymphatic duct Right subclavian trunk Supraclavicular (Virchow's) lymph node Virchow's (supraclavicular) lymph node **2 Lymphatic, Left Neck** Cervical lymph node Jugular lymph node Mastoid (postauricular) lymph node Occipital lymph node Postauricular (mastoid) lymph node Retropharyngeal lymph node Supraclavicular (Virchow's) lymph node Virchow's (supraclavicular) lymph node **3 Lymphatic, Right Upper Extremity** Cubital lymph node Deltopectoral (infraclavicular) lymph node Epitrochlear lymph node Infraclavicular (deltopectoral) lymph node Supratrochlear lymph node **4 Lymphatic, Left Upper Extremity** *See 3 Lymphatic, Right Upper Extremity* **5 Lymphatic, Right Axillary** ⊞ Anterior (pectoral) lymph node Apical (subclavicular) lymph node Brachial (lateral) lymph node Central axillary lymph node Lateral (brachial) lymph node Pectoral (anterior) lymph node Posterior (subscapular) lymph node Subclavicular (apical) lymph node Subscapular (posterior) lymph node **6 Lymphatic, Left Axillary** ⊞ *See 5 Lymphatic, Right Axillary* **7 Lymphatic, Thorax** ⊞ Intercostal lymph node Mediastinal lymph node Parasternal lymph node Paratracheal lymph node Tracheobronchial lymph node **8 Lymphatic, Internal Mammary, Right** ⊞ **9 Lymphatic, Internal Mammary, Left** ⊞ **B Lymphatic, Mesenteric** Inferior mesenteric lymph node Pararectal lymph node Superior mesenteric lymph node **C Lymphatic, Pelvis** Common iliac (subaortic) lymph node Gluteal lymph node Iliac lymph node Inferior epigastric lymph node Obturator lymph node Sacral lymph node Subaortic (common iliac) lymph node Suprainguinal lymph node **D Lymphatic, Aortic** Celiac lymph node Gastric lymph node Hepatic lymph node Lumbar lymph node Pancreaticosplenic lymph node Paraaortic lymph node Retroperitoneal lymph node **F Lymphatic, Right Lower Extremity** Femoral lymph node Popliteal lymph node **G Lymphatic, Left Lower Extremity** *See F Lymphatic, Right Lower Extremity* **H Lymphatic, Right Inguinal** **J Lymphatic, Left Inguinal** **K Thoracic Duct** Left jugular trunk Left subclavian trunk **L Cisterna Chyli** Intestinal lymphatic trunk Lumbar lymphatic trunk **M Thymus** Thymus gland **P Spleen** Accessory spleen	**Ø Open** **4 Percutaneous Endoscopic**	**Z No Device**	**Z No Qualifier**

See Appendix L for Procedure Combinations

⊞ Ø7T[5,6,7,8,9]ØZZ

Ø Medical and Surgical
7 Lymphatic and Hemic Systems
U Supplement Definition: Putting in or on biological or synthetic material that physically reinforces and/or augments the function of a portion of a body part

Explanation: The biological material is non-living, or is living and from the same individual. The body part may have been previously replaced, and the SUPPLEMENT procedure is performed to physically reinforce and/or augment the function of the replaced body part.

Body Part Character 4		Approach Character 5	Device Character 6	Qualifier Character 7
Ø Lymphatic, Head Buccinator lymph node Infraauricular lymph node Infraparotid lymph node Parotid lymph node Preauricular lymph node Submandibular lymph node Submaxillary lymph node Submental lymph node Subparotid lymph node Suprahyoid lymph node **1 Lymphatic, Right Neck** Cervical lymph node Jugular lymph node Mastoid (postauricular) lymph node Occipital lymph node Postauricular (mastoid) lymph node Retropharyngeal lymph node Right jugular trunk Right lymphatic duct Right subclavian trunk Supraclavicular (Virchow's) lymph node Virchow's (supraclavicular) lymph node **2 Lymphatic, Left Neck** Cervical lymph node Jugular lymph node Mastoid (postauricular) lymph node Occipital lymph node Postauricular (mastoid) lymph node Retropharyngeal lymph node Supraclavicular (Virchow's) lymph node Virchow's (supraclavicular) lymph node **3 Lymphatic, Right Upper Extremity** Cubital lymph node Deltopectoral (infraclavicular) lymph node Epitrochlear lymph node Infraclavicular (deltopectoral) lymph node Supratrochlear lymph node **4 Lymphatic, Left Upper Extremity** *See 3 Lymphatic, Right Upper Extremity* **5 Lymphatic, Right Axillary** Anterior (pectoral) lymph node Apical (subclavicular) lymph node Brachial (lateral) lymph node Central axillary lymph node Lateral (brachial) lymph node Pectoral (anterior) lymph node Posterior (subscapular) lymph node Subclavicular (apical) lymph node Subscapular (posterior) lymph node	**6 Lymphatic, Left Axillary** *See 5 Lymphatic, Right Axillary* **7 Lymphatic, Thorax** Intercostal lymph node Mediastinal lymph node Parasternal lymph node Paratracheal lymph node Tracheobronchial lymph node **8 Lymphatic, Internal Mammary, Right** **9 Lymphatic, Internal Mammary, Left** **B Lymphatic, Mesenteric** Inferior mesenteric lymph node Pararectal lymph node Superior mesenteric lymph node **C Lymphatic, Pelvis** Common iliac (subaortic) lymph node Gluteal lymph node Iliac lymph node Inferior epigastric lymph node Obturator lymph node Sacral lymph node Subaortic (common iliac) lymph node Suprainguinal lymph node **D Lymphatic, Aortic** Celiac lymph node Gastric lymph node Hepatic lymph node Lumbar lymph node Pancreaticosplenic lymph node Paraaortic lymph node Retroperitoneal lymph node **F Lymphatic, Right Lower Extremity** Femoral lymph node Popliteal lymph node **G Lymphatic, Left Lower Extremity** *See F Lymphatic, Right Lower Extremity* **H Lymphatic, Right Inguinal** **J Lymphatic, Left Inguinal** **K Thoracic Duct** Left jugular trunk Left subclavian trunk **L Cisterna Chyli** Intestinal lymphatic trunk Lumbar lymphatic trunk	**Ø Open** **4 Percutaneous Endoscopic**	**7 Autologous Tissue Substitute** **J Synthetic Substitute** **K Nonautologous Tissue Substitute**	**Z No Qualifier**

Ø Medical and Surgical
7 Lymphatic and Hemic Systems
V Restriction Definition: Partially closing an orifice or the lumen of a tubular body part
Explanation: The orifice can be a natural orifice or an artificially created orifice

Body Part Character 4		Approach Character 5	Device Character 6	Qualifier Character 7
Ø Lymphatic, Head Buccinator lymph node Infraauricular lymph node Infraparotid lymph node Parotid lymph node Preauricular lymph node Submandibular lymph node Submaxillary lymph node Submental lymph node Subparotid lymph node Suprahyoid lymph node **1 Lymphatic, Right Neck** Cervical lymph node Jugular lymph node Mastoid (postauricular) lymph node Occipital lymph node Postauricular (mastoid) lymph node Retropharyngeal lymph node Right jugular trunk Right lymphatic duct Right subclavian trunk Supraclavicular (Virchow's) lymph node Virchow's (supraclavicular) lymph node **2 Lymphatic, Left Neck** Cervical lymph node Jugular lymph node Mastoid (postauricular) lymph node Occipital lymph node Postauricular (mastoid) lymph node Retropharyngeal lymph node Supraclavicular (Virchow's) lymph node Virchow's (supraclavicular) lymph node **3 Lymphatic, Right Upper Extremity** Cubital lymph node Deltopectoral (infraclavicular) lymph node Epitrochlear lymph node Infraclavicular (deltopectoral) lymph node Supratrochlear lymph node **4 Lymphatic, Left Upper Extremity** *See 3 Lymphatic, Right Upper Extremity* **5 Lymphatic, Right Axillary** Anterior (pectoral) lymph node Apical (subclavicular) lymph node Brachial (lateral) lymph node Central axillary lymph node Lateral (brachial) lymph node Pectoral (anterior) lymph node Posterior (subscapular) lymph node Subclavicular (apical) lymph node Subscapular (posterior) lymph node	**6 Lymphatic, Left Axillary** *See 5 Lymphatic, Right Axillary* **7 Lymphatic, Thorax** Intercostal lymph node Mediastinal lymph node Parasternal lymph node Paratracheal lymph node Tracheobronchial lymph node **8 Lymphatic, Internal Mammary, Right** **9 Lymphatic, Internal Mammary, Left** **B Lymphatic, Mesenteric** Inferior mesenteric lymph node Pararectal lymph node Superior mesenteric lymph node **C Lymphatic, Pelvis** Common iliac (subaortic) lymph node Gluteal lymph node Iliac lymph node Inferior epigastric lymph node Obturator lymph node Sacral lymph node Subaortic (common iliac) lymph node Suprainguinal lymph node **D Lymphatic, Aortic** Celiac lymph node Gastric lymph node Hepatic lymph node Lumbar lymph node Pancreaticosplenic lymph node Paraaortic lymph node Retroperitoneal lymph node **F Lymphatic, Right Lower Extremity** Femoral lymph node Popliteal lymph node **G Lymphatic, Left Lower Extremity** *See F Lymphatic, Right Lower Extremity* **H Lymphatic, Right Inguinal** **J Lymphatic, Left Inguinal** **K Thoracic Duct** Left jugular trunk Left subclavian trunk **L Cisterna Chyli** Intestinal lymphatic trunk Lumbar lymphatic trunk	**Ø Open** **3 Percutaneous** **4 Percutaneous Endoscopic**	**C Extraluminal Device** **D Intraluminal Device** **Z No Device**	**Z No Qualifier**

Ø Medical and Surgical
7 Lymphatic and Hemic Systems
W Revision Definition: Correcting, to the extent possible, a portion of a malfunctioning device or the position of a displaced device

Explanation: Revision can include correcting a malfunctioning or displaced device by taking out or putting in components of the device such as a screw or pin

Body Part Character 4	Approach Character 5	Device Character 6	Qualifier Character 7
K Thoracic Duct Left jugular trunk Left subclavian trunk **L** Cisterna Chyli Intestinal lymphatic trunk Lumbar lymphatic trunk **N** Lymphatic	**Ø** Open **3** Percutaneous **4** Percutaneous Endoscopic	**Ø** Drainage Device **3** Infusion Device **7** Autologous Tissue Substitute **C** Extraluminal Device **D** Intraluminal Device **J** Synthetic Substitute **K** Nonautologous Tissue Substitute **Y** Other Device	**Z** No Qualifier
K Thoracic Duct Left jugular trunk Left subclavian trunk **L** Cisterna Chyli Intestinal lymphatic trunk Lumbar lymphatic trunk **N** Lymphatic	**X** External	**Ø** Drainage Device **3** Infusion Device **7** Autologous Tissue Substitute **C** Extraluminal Device **D** Intraluminal Device **J** Synthetic Substitute **K** Nonautologous Tissue Substitute	**Z** No Qualifier
M Thymus Thymus gland **P** Spleen Accessory spleen	**Ø** Open **3** Percutaneous **4** Percutaneous Endoscopic	**Ø** Drainage Device **3** Infusion Device **Y** Other Device	**Z** No Qualifier
M Thymus Thymus gland **P** Spleen Accessory spleen	**X** External	**Ø** Drainage Device **3** Infusion Device	**Z** No Qualifier
T Bone Marrow	**Ø** Open **3** Percutaneous **4** Percutaneous Endoscopic **X** External	**Ø** Drainage Device	**Z** No Qualifier

Non-OR Ø7W[K,L,N][3,4]YZ
Non-OR Ø7W[K,L,N]X[Ø,3,7,C,D,J,K]Z
Non-OR Ø7W[M,P][3,4]YZ
Non-OR Ø7W[M,P]X[Ø,3]Z
Non-OR Ø7WT[Ø,3,4,X]ØZ

Ø Medical and Surgical
7 Lymphatic and Hemic Systems
Y Transplantation Definition: Putting in or on all or a portion of a living body part taken from another individual or animal to physically take the place and/or function of all or a portion of a similar body part

Explanation: The native body part may or may not be taken out, and the transplanted body part may take over all or a portion of its function

Body Part Character 4	Approach Character 5	Device Character 6	Qualifier Character 7
M Thymus Thymus gland **P** Spleen Accessory spleen	**Ø** Open	**Z** No Device	**Ø** Allogeneic **1** Syngeneic **2** Zooplastic

Eye Ø8Ø–Ø8X

Character Meanings

This Character Meaning table is provided as a guide to assist the user in the identification of character members that may be found in this section of code tables. It **SHOULD NOT** be used to build a PCS code.

Operation–Character 3	Body Part–Character 4	Approach–Character 5	Device–Character 6	Qualifier–Character 7
Ø Alteration	Ø Eye, Right	Ø Open	Ø Drainage Device OR Synthetic Substitute, Intraocular Telescope	3 Nasal Cavity
1 Bypass	1 Eye, Left	3 Percutaneous	1 Radioactive Element	4 Sclera
2 Change	2 Anterior Chamber, Right	7 Via Natural or Artificial Opening	3 Infusion Device	X Diagnostic
5 Destruction	3 Anterior Chamber, Left	8 Via Natural or Artificial Opening Endoscopic	5 Epiretinal Visual Prosthesis	Z No Qualifier
7 Dilation	4 Vitreous, Right	X External	7 Autologous Tissue Substitute	
9 Drainage	5 Vitreous, Left		C Extraluminal Device	
B Excision	6 Sclera, Right		D Intraluminal Device	
C Extirpation	7 Sclera, Left		J Synthetic Substitute	
D Extraction	8 Cornea, Right		K Nonautologous Tissue Substitute	
F Fragmentation	9 Cornea, Left		Y Other Device	
H Insertion	A Choroid, Right		Z No Device	
J Inspection	B Choroid, Left			
L Occlusion	C Iris, Right			
M Reattachment	D Iris, Left			
N Release	E Retina, Right			
P Removal	F Retina, Left			
Q Repair	G Retinal Vessel, Right			
R Replacement	H Retinal Vessel, Left			
S Reposition	J Lens, Right			
T Resection	K Lens, Left			
U Supplement	L Extraocular Muscle, Right			
V Restriction	M Extraocular Muscle, Left			
W Revision	N Upper Eyelid, Right			
X Transfer	P Upper Eyelid, Left			
	Q Lower Eyelid, Right			
	R Lower Eyelid, Left			
	S Conjunctiva, Right			
	T Conjunctiva, Left			
	V Lacrimal Gland, Right			
	W Lacrimal Gland, Left			
	X Lacrimal Duct, Right			
	Y Lacrimal Duct, Left			

AHA Coding Clinic for table Ø81
2019, 1Q, 27 Glaucoma tube shunt

AHA Coding Clinic for table Ø89
2016, 2Q, 21 Laser trabeculoplasty

AHA Coding Clinic for table Ø8B
2014, 4Q, 35 Vitrectomy with air/fluid exchange
2014, 4Q, 36 Pars plans vitrectomy without mention of instillation of oil, air or fluid

AHA Coding Clinic for table Ø8J
2015, 1Q, 35 Attempted removal of foreign body from cornea

AHA Coding Clinic for table Ø8N
2015, 2Q, 24 Penetrating keratoplasty and anterior segment reconstruction

AHA Coding Clinic for table Ø8Q
2018, 3Q, 13 Repair of ruptured globe

AHA Coding Clinic for table Ø8R
2015, 2Q, 24 Penetrating keratoplasty and anterior segment reconstruction
2015, 2Q, 25 Penetrating keratoplasty and placement of viscoelastic eye with paracentesis

AHA Coding Clinic for table Ø8T
2015, 2Q, 12 Orbital exenteration

AHA Coding Clinic for table Ø8U
2014, 3Q, 31 Corneal amniotic membrane transplantation

Eye

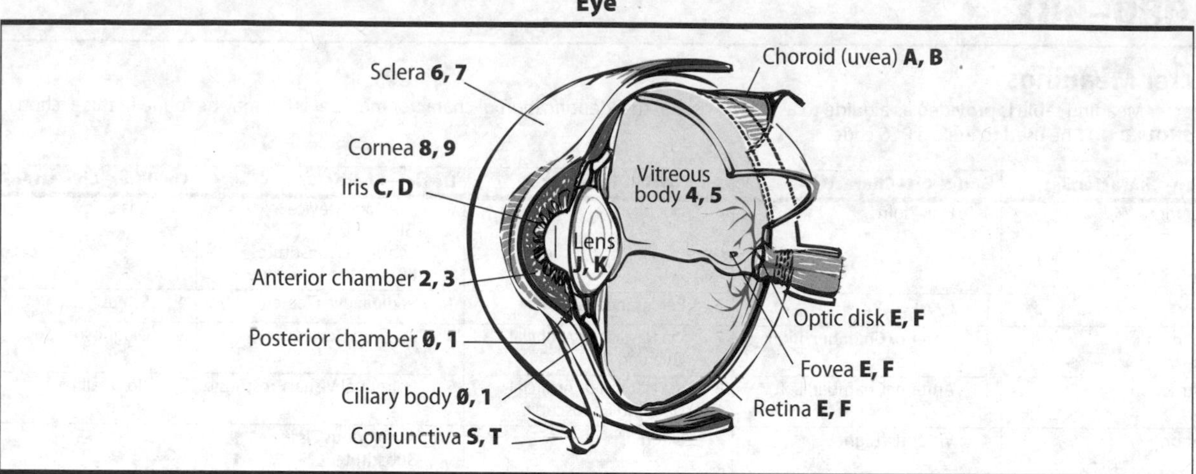

Eye Musculature

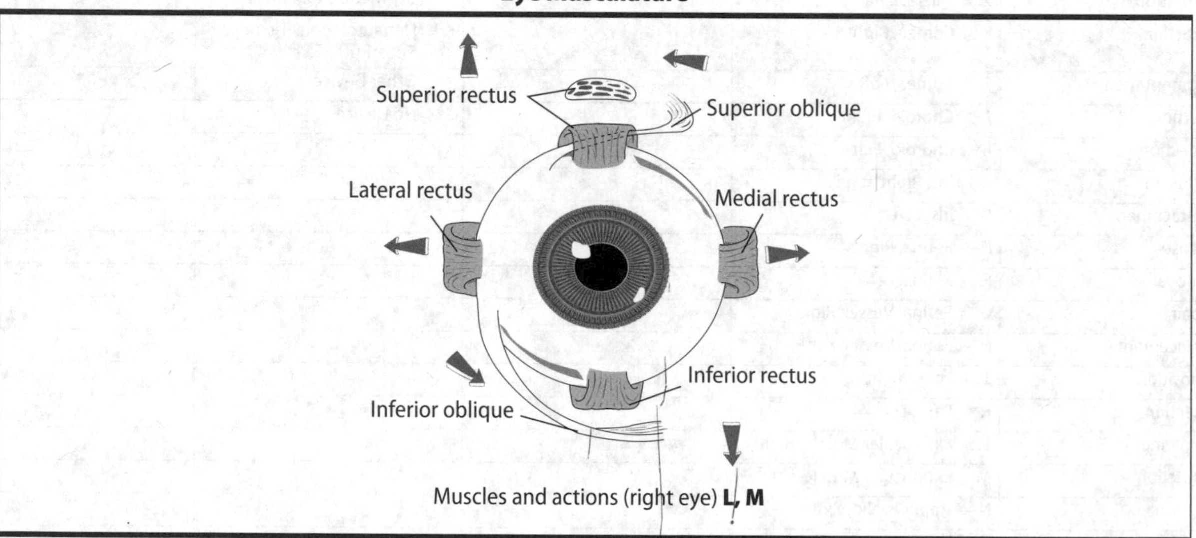

Lacrimal System

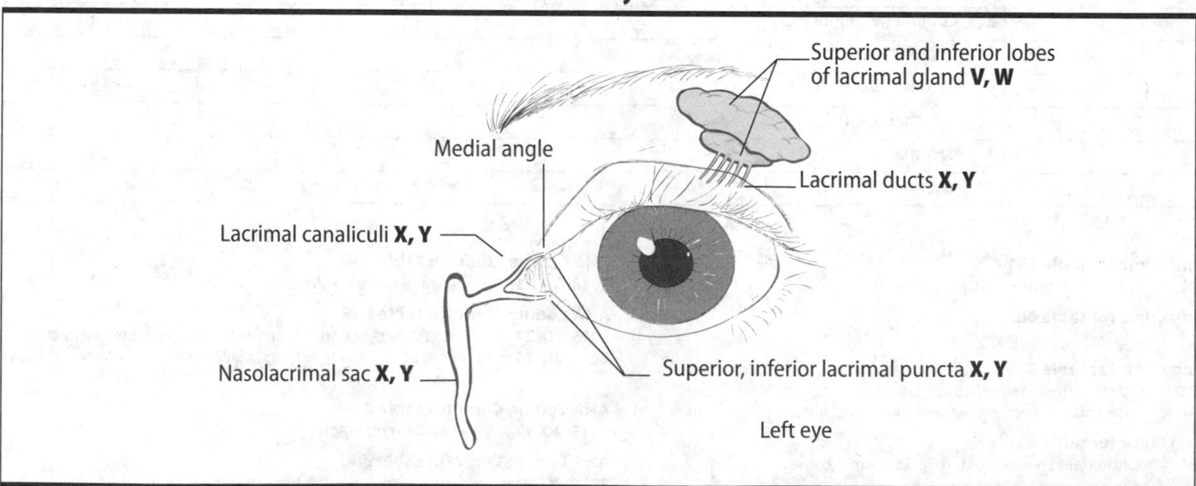

Ø Medical and Surgical
8 Eye
Ø Alteration Definition: Modifying the anatomic structure of a body part without affecting the function of the body part

Explanation: Principal purpose is to improve appearance

Body Part Character 4	Approach Character 5	Device Character 6	Qualifier Character 7
N Upper Eyelid, Right Lateral canthus Levator palpebrae superioris muscle Orbicularis oculi muscle Superior tarsal plate **P Upper Eyelid, Left** *See N Upper Eyelid, Right* **Q Lower Eyelid, Right** Inferior tarsal plate Medial canthus **R Lower Eyelid, Left** *See Q Lower Eyelid, Right*	**Ø Open** **3 Percutaneous** **X External**	**7 Autologous Tissue Substitute** **J Synthetic Substitute** **K Nonautologous Tissue Substitute** **Z No Device**	**Z No Qualifier**

Non-OR All body part, approach, device, and qualifier values

Ø Medical and Surgical
8 Eye
1 Bypass Definition: Altering the route of passage of the contents of a tubular body part

Explanation: Rerouting contents of a body part to a downstream area of the normal route, to a similar route and body part, or to an abnormal route and dissimilar body part. Includes one or more anastomoses, with or without the use of a device.

Body Part Character 4	Approach Character 5	Device Character 6	Qualifier Character 7
2 Anterior Chamber, Right Aqueous humour **3 Anterior Chamber, Left** *See 2 Anterior Chamber, Right*	**3 Percutaneous**	**J Synthetic Substitute** **K Nonautologous Tissue Substitute** **Z No Device**	**4 Sclera**
X Lacrimal Duct, Right Lacrimal canaliculus Lacrimal punctum Lacrimal sac Nasolacrimal duct **Y Lacrimal Duct, Left** *See X Lacrimal Duct, Right*	**Ø Open** **3 Percutaneous**	**J Synthetic Substitute** **K Nonautologous Tissue Substitute** **Z No Device**	**3 Nasal Cavity**

Ø Medical and Surgical
8 Eye
2 Change Definition: Taking out or off a device from a body part and putting back an identical or similar device in or on the same body part without cutting or puncturing the skin or a mucous membrane

Explanation: All CHANGE procedures are coded using the approach EXTERNAL

Body Part Character 4	Approach Character 5	Device Character 6	Qualifier Character 7
Ø Eye, Right Ciliary body Posterior chamber **1 Eye, Left** *See Ø Eye, Right*	**X External**	**Ø Drainage Device** **Y Other Device**	**Z No Qualifier**

Non-OR All body part, approach, device, and qualifier values

Ø Medical and Surgical
8 Eye
5 Destruction

Definition: Physical eradication of all or a portion of a body part by the direct use of energy, force, or a destructive agent
Explanation: None of the body part is physically taken out

Body Part Character 4		Approach Character 5	Device Character 6	Qualifier Character 7
Ø Eye, Right Ciliary body Posterior chamber **1 Eye, Left** *See Ø Eye, Right* **6 Sclera, Right** **7 Sclera, Left**	**8 Cornea, Right** **9 Cornea, Left** **S Conjunctiva, Right** Plica semilunaris **T Conjunctiva, Left** *See S Conjunctiva, Right*	**X External**	**Z No Device**	**Z No Qualifier**
2 Anterior Chamber, Right Aqueous humour **3 Anterior Chamber, Left** *See 2 Anterior Chamber, Right* **4 Vitreous, Right** Vitreous body **5 Vitreous, Left** *See 4 Vitreous, Right* **C Iris, Right** **D Iris, Left**	**E Retina, Right** Fovea Macula Optic disc **F Retina, Left** *See E Retina, Right* **G Retinal Vessel, Right** **H Retinal Vessel, Left** **J Lens, Right** Zonule of Zinn **K Lens, Left** *See J Lens, Right*	**3 Percutaneous**	**Z No Device**	**Z No Qualifier**
A Choroid, Right **B Choroid, Left** **L Extraocular Muscle, Right** Inferior oblique muscle Inferior rectus muscle Lateral rectus muscle Medial rectus muscle Superior oblique muscle Superior rectus muscle	**M Extraocular Muscle, Left** *See L Extraocular Muscle, Right* **V Lacrimal Gland, Right** **W Lacrimal Gland, Left**	**Ø Open** **3 Percutaneous**	**Z No Device**	**Z No Qualifier**
N Upper Eyelid, Right Lateral canthus Levator palpebrae superioris muscle Orbicularis oculi muscle Superior tarsal plate **P Upper Eyelid, Left** *See N Upper Eyelid, Right*	**Q Lower Eyelid, Right** Inferior tarsal plate Medial canthus **R Lower Eyelid, Left** *See Q Lower Eyelid, Right*	**Ø Open** **3 Percutaneous** **X External**	**Z No Device**	**Z No Qualifier**
X Lacrimal Duct, Right Lacrimal canaliculus Lacrimal punctum Lacrimal sac Nasolacrimal duct	**Y Lacrimal Duct, Left** *See X Lacrimal Duct, Right*	**Ø Open** **3 Percutaneous** **7 Via Natural or Artificial Opening** **8 Via Natural or Artificial Opening Endoscopic**	**Z No Device**	**Z No Qualifier**

Non-OR Ø85[E,F]3ZZ

Ø Medical and Surgical
8 Eye
7 Dilation

Definition: Expanding an orifice or the lumen of a tubular body part
Explanation: The orifice can be a natural orifice or an artificially created orifice. Accomplished by stretching a tubular body part using intraluminal pressure or by cutting part of the orifice or wall of the tubular body part.

Body Part Character 4	Approach Character 5	Device Character 6	Qualifier Character 7
X Lacrimal Duct, Right Lacrimal canaliculus Lacrimal punctum Lacrimal sac Nasolacrimal duct **Y Lacrimal Duct, Left** *See X Lacrimal Duct, Right*	**Ø Open** **3 Percutaneous** **7 Via Natural or Artificial Opening** **8 Via Natural or Artificial Opening Endoscopic**	**D Intraluminal Device** **Z No Device**	**Z No Qualifier**

Ø Medical and Surgical
8 Eye
9 Drainage Definition: Taking or letting out fluids and/or gases from a body part
Explanation: The qualifier DIAGNOSTIC is used to identify drainage procedures that are biopsies

Body Part Character 4		Approach Character 5	Device Character 6	Qualifier Character 7
Ø Eye, Right Ciliary body Posterior chamber **1 Eye, Left** *See Ø Eye, Right* **6 Sclera, Right** **7 Sclera, Left**	**8 Cornea, Right** **9 Cornea, Left** **S Conjunctiva, Right** Plica semilunaris **T Conjunctiva, Left** *See S Conjunctiva, Right*	**X External**	**Ø Drainage Device**	**Z No Qualifier**
Ø Eye, Right Ciliary body Posterior chamber **1 Eye, Left** *See Ø Eye, Right* **6 Sclera, Right** **7 Sclera, Left**	**8 Cornea, Right** **9 Cornea, Left** **S Conjunctiva, Right** Plica semilunaris **T Conjunctiva, Left** *See S Conjunctiva, Right*	**X External**	**Z No Device**	**X Diagnostic** **Z No Qualifier**
2 Anterior Chamber, Right Aqueous humour **3 Anterior Chamber, Left** *See 2 Anterior Chamber, Right* **4 Vitreous, Right** Vitreous body **5 Vitreous, Left** *See 4 Vitreous, Right* **C Iris, Right** **D Iris, Left**	**E Retina, Right** Fovea Macula Optic disc **F Retina, Left** *See E Retina, Right* **G Retinal Vessel, Right** **H Retinal Vessel, Left** **J Lens, Right** Zonule of Zinn **K Lens, Left** *See J Lens, Right*	**3 Percutaneous**	**Ø Drainage Device**	**Z No Qualifier**
2 Anterior Chamber, Right Aqueous humour **3 Anterior Chamber, Left** *See 2 Anterior Chamber, Right* **4 Vitreous, Right** Vitreous body **5 Vitreous, Left** *See 4 Vitreous, Right* **C Iris, Right** **D Iris, Left**	**E Retina, Right** Fovea Macula Optic disc **F Retina, Left** *See E Retina, Right* **G Retinal Vessel, Right** **H Retinal Vessel, Left** **J Lens, Right** Zonule of Zinn **K Lens, Left** *See J Lens, Right*	**3 Percutaneous**	**Z No Device**	**X Diagnostic** **Z No Qualifier**
A Choroid, Right **B Choroid, Left** **L Extraocular Muscle, Right** Inferior oblique muscle Inferior rectus muscle Lateral rectus muscle Medial rectus muscle Superior oblique muscle Superior rectus muscle	**M Extraocular Muscle, Left** *See L Extraocular Muscle, Right* **V Lacrimal Gland, Right** **W Lacrimal Gland, Left**	**Ø Open** **3 Percutaneous**	**Ø Drainage Device**	**Z No Qualifier**
A Choroid, Right **B Choroid, Left** **L Extraocular Muscle, Right** Inferior oblique muscle Inferior rectus muscle Lateral rectus muscle Medial rectus muscle Superior oblique muscle Superior rectus muscle	**M Extraocular Muscle, Left** *See L Extraocular Muscle, Right* **V Lacrimal Gland, Right** **W Lacrimal Gland, Left**	**Ø Open** **3 Percutaneous**	**Z No Device**	**X Diagnostic** **Z No Qualifier**
N Upper Eyelid, Right Lateral canthus Levator palpebrae superioris muscle Orbicularis oculi muscle Superior tarsal plate **P Upper Eyelid, Left** *See N Upper Eyelid, Right*	**Q Lower Eyelid, Right** Inferior tarsal plate Medial canthus **R Lower Eyelid, Left** *See Q Lower Eyelid, Right*	**Ø Open** **3 Percutaneous** **X External**	**Ø Drainage Device**	**Z No Qualifier**

Non-OR Ø89[Ø,1,6,7,8,9,S,T]XZ[X,Z]
Non-OR Ø89[N,P,Q,R][Ø,3,X]ØZ

Ø89 Continued on next page

Ø Medical and Surgical
8 Eye
9 Drainage

Ø89 Continued

Definition: Taking or letting out fluids and/or gases from a body part
Explanation: The qualifier DIAGNOSTIC is used to identify drainage procedures that are biopsies

Body Part Character 4		Approach Character 5	Device Character 6	Qualifier Character 7
N Upper Eyelid, Right Lateral canthus Levator palpebrae superioris muscle Orbicularis oculi muscle Superior tarsal plate **P Upper Eyelid, Left** *See N Upper Eyelid, Right*	**Q Lower Eyelid, Right** Inferior tarsal plate Medial canthus **R Lower Eyelid, Left** *See Q Lower Eyelid, Right*	**Ø Open** **3 Percutaneous** **X External**	**Z No Device**	**X Diagnostic** **Z No Qualifier**
X Lacrimal Duct, Right Lacrimal canaliculus Lacrimal punctum Lacrimal sac Nasolacrimal duct	**Y Lacrimal Duct, Left** *See X Lacrimal Duct, Right*	**Ø Open** **3 Percutaneous** **7 Via Natural or Artificial Opening** **8 Via Natural or Artificial Opening Endoscopic**	**Ø Drainage Device**	**Z No Qualifier**
X Lacrimal Duct, Right Lacrimal canaliculus Lacrimal punctum Lacrimal sac Nasolacrimal duct	**Y Lacrimal Duct, Left** *See X Lacrimal Duct, Right*	**Ø Open** **3 Percutaneous** **7 Via Natural or Artificial Opening** **8 Via Natural or Artificial Opening Endoscopic**	**Z No Device**	**X Diagnostic** **Z No Qualifier**

Non-OR Ø89[N,P,Q,R]ØZZ
Non-OR Ø89[N,P,Q,R][3,X]Z[X,Z]

Ø Medical and Surgical
8 Eye
B Excision

Definition: Cutting out or off, without replacement, a portion of a body part
Explanation: The qualifier DIAGNOSTIC is used to identify excision procedures that are biopsies

Body Part Character 4		Approach Character 5	Device Character 6	Qualifier Character 7
Ø Eye, Right Ciliary body Posterior chamber **1 Eye, Left** *See Ø Eye, Right* **N Upper Eyelid, Right** Lateral canthus Levator palpebrae superioris muscle Orbicularis oculi muscle Superior tarsal plate	**P Upper Eyelid, Left** *See N Upper Eyelid, Right* **Q Lower Eyelid, Right** Inferior tarsal plate Medial canthus **R Lower Eyelid, Left** *See Q Lower Eyelid, Right*	**Ø Open** **3 Percutaneous** **X External**	**Z No Device**	**X Diagnostic** **Z No Qualifier**
4 Vitreous, Right Vitreous body **5 Vitreous, Left** *See 4 Vitreous, Right* **C Iris, Right** **D Iris, Left** **E Retina, Right** Fovea Macula Optic disc	**F Retina, Left** *See E Retina, Right* **J Lens, Right** Zonule of Zinn **K Lens, Left** *See J Lens, Right*	**3 Percutaneous**	**Z No Device**	**X Diagnostic** **Z No Qualifier**
6 Sclera, Right **7 Sclera, Left** **8 Cornea, Right** **9 Cornea, Left**	**S Conjunctiva, Right** Plica semilunaris **T Conjunctiva, Left** *See S Conjunctiva, Right*	**X External**	**Z No Device**	**X Diagnostic** **Z No Qualifier**
A Choroid, Right **B Choroid, Left** **L Extraocular Muscle, Right** Inferior oblique muscle Inferior rectus muscle Lateral rectus muscle Medial rectus muscle Superior oblique muscle Superior rectus muscle	**M Extraocular Muscle, Left** *See L Extraocular Muscle, Right* **V Lacrimal Gland, Right** **W Lacrimal Gland, Left**	**Ø Open** **3 Percutaneous**	**Z No Device**	**X Diagnostic** **Z No Qualifier**
X Lacrimal Duct, Right Lacrimal canaliculus Lacrimal punctum Lacrimal sac Nasolacrimal duct	**Y Lacrimal Duct, Left** *See X Lacrimal Duct, Right*	**Ø Open** **3 Percutaneous** **7 Via Natural or Artificial Opening** **8 Via Natural or Artificial Opening Endoscopic**	**Z No Device**	**X Diagnostic** **Z No Qualifier**

Ø Medical and Surgical
8 Eye
C Extirpation Definition: Taking or cutting out solid matter from a body part

Explanation: The solid matter may be an abnormal byproduct of a biological function or a foreign body; it may be imbedded in a body part or in the lumen of a tubular body part. The solid matter may or may not have been previously broken into pieces.

Body Part Character 4	Approach Character 5	Device Character 6	Qualifier Character 7
Ø Eye, Right Ciliary body Posterior chamber **1 Eye, Left** *See Ø Eye, Right* **6 Sclera, Right** **7 Sclera, Left** **8 Cornea, Right** **9 Cornea, Left** **S Conjunctiva, Right** Plica semilunaris **T Conjunctiva, Left** *See S Conjunctiva, Right*	**X External**	**Z No Device**	**Z No Qualifier**
2 Anterior Chamber, Right Aqueous humour **3 Anterior Chamber, Left** *See 2 Anterior Chamber, Right* **4 Vitreous, Right** Vitreous body **5 Vitreous, Left** *See 4 Vitreous, Right* **C Iris, Right** **D Iris, Left** **E Retina, Right** Fovea Macula Optic disc **F Retina, Left** *See* E Retina, Right **G Retinal Vessel, Right** **H Retinal Vessel, Left** **J Lens, Right** Zonule of Zinn **K Lens, Left** *See J Lens, Right*	**3 Percutaneous** **X External**	**Z No Device**	**Z No Qualifier**
A Choroid, Right **B Choroid, Left** **L Extraocular Muscle, Right** Inferior oblique muscle Inferior rectus muscle Lateral rectus muscle Medial rectus muscle Superior oblique muscle Superior rectus muscle **M Extraocular Muscle, Left** *See L Extraocular Muscle, Right* **N Upper Eyelid, Right** Lateral canthus Levator palpebrae superioris muscle Orbicularis oculi muscle Superior tarsal plate **P Upper Eyelid, Left** *See N Upper Eyelid, Right* **Q Lower Eyelid, Right** Inferior tarsal plate Medial canthus **R Lower Eyelid, Left** *See Q Lower Eyelid, Right* **V Lacrimal Gland, Right** **W Lacrimal Gland, Left**	**Ø Open** **3 Percutaneous** **X External**	**Z No Device**	**Z No Qualifier**
X Lacrimal Duct, Right Lacrimal canaliculus Lacrimal punctum Lacrimal sac Nasolacrimal duct **Y Lacrimal Duct, Left** *See X Lacrimal Duct, Right*	**Ø Open** **3 Percutaneous** **7 Via Natural or Artificial Opening** **8 Via Natural or Artificial Opening Endoscopic**	**Z No Device**	**Z No Qualifier**

Non-OR Ø8C[Ø,1,6,7,S,T]XZZ
Non-OR Ø8C[2,3]XZZ
Non-OR Ø8C[N,P,Q,R][Ø,3,X]ZZ

Ø Medical and Surgical
8 Eye
D Extraction Definition: Pulling or stripping out or off all or a portion of a body part by the use of force
Explanation: The qualifier DIAGNOSTIC is used to identify extraction procedures that are biopsies

Body Part Character 4	Approach Character 5	Device Character 6	Qualifier Character 7
8 Cornea, Right **9** Cornea, Left	**X** External	**Z** No Device	**X** Diagnostic **Z** No Qualifier
J Lens, Right Zonule of Zinn **K** Lens, Left *See J Lens, Right*	**3** Percutaneous	**Z** No Device	**Z** No Qualifier

Ø Medical and Surgical
8 Eye
F Fragmentation Definition: Breaking solid matter in a body part into pieces
Explanation: Physical force (e.g., manual, ultrasonic) applied directly or indirectly is used to break the solid matter into pieces. The solid matter may be an abnormal byproduct of a biological function or a foreign body. The pieces of solid matter are not taken out.

Body Part Character 4	Approach Character 5	Device Character 6	Qualifier Character 7
4 Vitreous, Right NC Vitreous body **5** Vitreous, Left NC *See 4 Vitreous, Right*	**3** Percutaneous **X** External	**Z** No Device	**Z** No Qualifier

Non-OR Ø8F[4,5]XZZ
NC Ø8F[4,5]XZZ

Ø Medical and Surgical
8 Eye
H Insertion Definition: Putting in a nonbiological appliance that monitors, assists, performs, or prevents a physiological function but does not physically take the place of a body part
Explanation: None

Body Part Character 4	Approach Character 5	Device Character 6	Qualifier Character 7
Ø Eye, Right Ciliary body Posterior chamber **1** Eye, Left *See Ø Eye, Right*	**Ø** Open	**5** Epiretinal Visual Prosthesis **Y** Other Device	**Z** No Qualifier
Ø Eye, Right Ciliary body Posterior chamber **1** Eye, Left *See Ø Eye, Right*	**3** Percutaneous	**1** Radioactive Element **3** Infusion Device **Y** Other Device	**Z** No Qualifier
Ø Eye, Right Ciliary body Posterior chamber **1** Eye, Left *See Ø Eye, Right*	**7** Via Natural or Artificial Opening **8** Via Natural or Artificial Opening Endoscopic	**Y** Other Device	**Z** No Qualifier
Ø Eye, Right Ciliary body Posterior chamber **1** Eye, Left *See Ø Eye, Right*	**X** External	**1** Radioactive Element **3** Infusion Device	**Z** No Qualifier

Non-OR Ø8H[Ø,1]3YZ
Non-OR Ø8H[Ø,1][7,8]YZ

Ø Medical and Surgical
8 Eye
J Inspection Definition: Visually and/or manually exploring a body part

Explanation: Visual exploration may be performed with or without optical instrumentation. Manual exploration may be performed directly or through intervening body layers.

Body Part Character 4	Approach Character 5	Device Character 6	Qualifier Character 7
Ø Eye, Right Ciliary body Posterior chamber **1** Eye, Left *See Ø Eye, Right* **J** Lens, Right Zonule of Zinn **K** Lens, Left *See J Lens, Right*	**X** External	**Z** No Device	**Z** No Qualifier
L Extraocular Muscle, Right Inferior oblique muscle Inferior rectus muscle Lateral rectus muscle Medial rectus muscle Superior oblique muscle Superior rectus muscle **M** Extraocular Muscle, Left *See L Extraocular Muscle, Right*	**Ø** Open **X** External	**Z** No Device	**Z** No Qualifier

Non-OR Ø8J[Ø,1,J,K]XZZ
Non-OR Ø8J[L,M]XZZ

Ø Medical and Surgical
8 Eye
L Occlusion Definition: Completely closing an orifice or the lumen of a tubular body part

Explanation: The orifice can be a natural orifice or an artificially created orifice

Body Part Character 4	Approach Character 5	Device Character 6	Qualifier Character 7
X Lacrimal Duct, Right Lacrimal canaliculus Lacrimal punctum Lacrimal sac Nasolacrimal duct **Y** Lacrimal Duct, Left *See X Lacrimal Duct, Right*	**Ø** Open **3** Percutaneous	**C** Extraluminal Device **D** Intraluminal Device **Z** No Device	**Z** No Qualifier
X Lacrimal Duct, Right Lacrimal canaliculus Lacrimal punctum Lacrimal sac Nasolacrimal duct **Y** Lacrimal Duct, Left *See X Lacrimal Duct, Right*	**7** Via Natural or Artificial Opening **8** Via Natural or Artificial Opening Endoscopic	**D** Intraluminal Device **Z** No Device	**Z** No Qualifier

Ø Medical and Surgical
8 Eye
M Reattachment Definition: Putting back in or on all or a portion of a separated body part to its normal location or other suitable location

Explanation: Vascular circulation and nervous pathways may or may not be reestablished

Body Part Character 4	Approach Character 5	Device Character 6	Qualifier Character 7
N Upper Eyelid, Right Lateral canthus Levator palpebrae superioris muscle Orbicularis oculi muscle Superior tarsal plate **P** Upper Eyelid, Left *See N Upper Eyelid, Right* **Q** Lower Eyelid, Right Inferior tarsal plate Medial canthus **R** Lower Eyelid, Left *See Q Lower Eyelid, Right*	**X** External	**Z** No Device	**Z** No Qualifier

Ø Medical and Surgical
8 Eye
N Release Definition: Freeing a body part from an abnormal physical constraint by cutting or by the use of force
Explanation: Some of the restraining tissue may be taken out but none of the body part is taken out

Body Part Character 4	Approach Character 5	Device Character 6	Qualifier Character 7
Ø Eye, Right Ciliary body Posterior chamber **1 Eye, Left** *See Ø Eye, Right* **6 Sclera, Right** **7 Sclera, Left** **8 Cornea, Right** **9 Cornea, Left** **S Conjunctiva, Right** Plica semilunaris **T Conjunctiva, Left** *See S Conjunctiva, Right*	**X External**	**Z No Device**	**Z No Qualifier**
2 Anterior Chamber, Right Aqueous humour **3 Anterior Chamber, Left** *See 2 Anterior Chamber, Right* **4 Vitreous, Right** Vitreous body **5 Vitreous, Left** *See 4 Vitreous, Right* **C Iris, Right** **D Iris, Left** **E Retina, Right** Fovea Macula Optic disc **F Retina, Left** *See E Retina, Right* **G Retinal Vessel, Right** **H Retinal Vessel, Left** **J Lens, Right** Zonule of Zinn **K Lens, Left** *See J Lens, Right*	**3 Percutaneous**	**Z No Device**	**Z No Qualifier**
A Choroid, Right **B Choroid, Left** **L Extraocular Muscle, Right** Inferior oblique muscle Inferior rectus muscle Lateral rectus muscle Medial rectus muscle Superior oblique muscle Superior rectus muscle **M Extraocular Muscle, Left** *See L Extraocular Muscle, Right* **V Lacrimal Gland, Right** **W Lacrimal Gland, Left**	**Ø Open** **3 Percutaneous**	**Z No Device**	**Z No Qualifier**
N Upper Eyelid, Right Lateral canthus Levator palpebrae superioris muscle Orbicularis oculi muscle Superior tarsal plate **P Upper Eyelid, Left** *See N Upper Eyelid, Right* **Q Lower Eyelid, Right** Inferior tarsal plate Medial canthus **R Lower Eyelid, Left** *See Q Lower Eyelid, Right*	**Ø Open** **3 Percutaneous** **X External**	**Z No Device**	**Z No Qualifier**
X Lacrimal Duct, Right Lacrimal canaliculus Lacrimal punctum Lacrimal sac Nasolacrimal duct **Y Lacrimal Duct, Left** *See X Lacrimal Duct, Right*	**Ø Open** **3 Percutaneous** **7 Via Natural or Artificial Opening** **8 Via Natural or Artificial Opening Endoscopic**	**Z No Device**	**Z No Qualifier**

Ø Medical and Surgical
8 Eye
P Removal Definition: Taking out or off a device from a body part

Explanation: If a device is taken out and a similar device put in without cutting or puncturing the skin or mucous membrane, the procedure is coded to the root operation CHANGE. Otherwise, the procedure for taking out a device is coded to the root operation REMOVAL.

Body Part Character 4	Approach Character 5	Device Character 6	Qualifier Character 7
Ø Eye, Right Ciliary body Posterior chamber **1 Eye, Left** *See Ø Eye, Right*	**Ø Open** **3 Percutaneous** **7 Via Natural or Artificial Opening** **8 Via Natural or Artificial Opening Endoscopic**	**Ø Drainage Device** **1 Radioactive Element** **3 Infusion Device** **7 Autologous Tissue Substitute** **C Extraluminal Device** **D Intraluminal Device** **J Synthetic Substitute** **K Nonautologous Tissue Substitute** **Y Other Device**	**Z No Qualifier**
Ø Eye, Right Ciliary body Posterior chamber **1 Eye, Left** *See Ø Eye, Right*	**X External**	**Ø Drainage Device** **1 Radioactive Element** **3 Infusion Device** **7 Autologous Tissue Substitute** **C Extraluminal Device** **D Intraluminal Device** **J Synthetic Substitute** **K Nonautologous Tissue Substitute**	**Z No Qualifier**
J Lens, Right Zonule of Zinn **K Lens, Left** *See J Lens, Right*	**3 Percutaneous**	**J Synthetic Substitute** **Y Other Device**	**Z No Qualifier**
L Extraocular Muscle, Right Inferior oblique muscle Inferior rectus muscle Lateral rectus muscle Medial rectus muscle Superior oblique muscle Superior rectus muscle **M Extraocular Muscle, Left** *See L Extraocular Muscle, Right*	**Ø Open** **3 Percutaneous**	**Ø Drainage Device** **7 Autologous Tissue Substitute** **J Synthetic Substitute** **K Nonautologous Tissue Substitute** **Y Other Device**	**Z No Qualifier**

Non-OR Ø8P[Ø,1]3YZ
Non-OR Ø8P[Ø,1][7,8][Ø,3,D,Y]Z
Non-OR Ø8P[Ø,1]X[Ø,1,3,C,D,J]Z
Non-OR Ø8P[J,K]3YZ
Non-OR Ø8P[L,M]3YZ

Ø Medical and Surgical
8 Eye
Q Repair Definition: Restoring, to the extent possible, a body part to its normal anatomic structure and function
Explanation: Used only when the method to accomplish the repair is not one of the other root operations

Body Part Character 4	Approach Character 5	Device Character 6	Qualifier Character 7
Ø Eye, Right Ciliary body Posterior chamber **1 Eye, Left** *See Ø Eye, Right* **6 Sclera, Right** **7 Sclera, Left** **8 Cornea, Right** NC **9 Cornea, Left** NC **S Conjunctiva, Right** Plica semilunaris **T Conjunctiva, Left** *See S Conjunctiva, Right*	**X External**	**Z No Device**	**Z No Qualifier**
2 Anterior Chamber, Right Aqueous humour **3 Anterior Chamber, Left** *See 2 Anterior Chamber, Right* **4 Vitreous, Right** Vitreous body **5 Vitreous, Left** *See 4 Vitreous, Right* **C Iris, Right** **D Iris, Left** **E Retina, Right** Fovea Macula Optic disc **F Retina, Left** *See E Retina, Right* **G Retinal Vessel, Right** **H Retinal Vessel, Left** **J Lens, Right** Zonule of Zinn **K Lens, Left** *See J Lens, Right*	**3 Percutaneous**	**Z No Device**	**Z No Qualifier**
A Choroid, Right **B Choroid, Left** **L Extraocular Muscle, Right** Inferior oblique muscle Inferior rectus muscle Lateral rectus muscle Medial rectus muscle Superior oblique muscle Superior rectus muscle **M Extraocular Muscle, Left** *See L Extraocular Muscle, Right* **V Lacrimal Gland, Right** **W Lacrimal Gland, Left**	**Ø Open** **3 Percutaneous**	**Z No Device**	**Z No Qualifier**
N Upper Eyelid, Right Lateral canthus Levator palpebrae superioris muscle Orbicularis oculi muscle Superior tarsal plate **P Upper Eyelid, Left** *See N Upper Eyelid, Right* **Q Lower Eyelid, Right** Inferior tarsal plate Medial canthus **R Lower Eyelid, Left** *See Q Lower Eyelid, Right*	**Ø Open** **3 Percutaneous** **X External**	**Z No Device**	**Z No Qualifier**
X Lacrimal Duct, Right Lacrimal canaliculus Lacrimal punctum Lacrimal sac Nasolacrimal duct **Y Lacrimal Duct, Left** *See X Lacrimal Duct, Right*	**Ø Open** **3 Percutaneous** **7 Via Natural or Artificial Opening** **8 Via Natural or Artificial Opening Endoscopic**	**Z No Device**	**Z No Qualifier**

Non-OR Ø8Q[N,P,Q,R][Ø,3,X]ZZ
NC Ø8Q[8,9]XZZ

Ø Medical and Surgical
8 Eye
R Replacement Definition: Putting in or on biological or synthetic material that physically takes the place and/or function of all or a portion of a body part

Explanation: The body part may have been taken out or replaced, or may be taken out, physically eradicated, or rendered nonfunctional during the REPLACEMENT procedure. A REMOVAL procedure is coded for taking out the device used in a previous replacement procedure.

Body Part Character 4	Approach Character 5	Device Character 6	Qualifier Character 7
Ø Eye, Right Ciliary body Posterior chamber **1 Eye, Left** *See Ø Eye, Right* **A Choroid, Right** **B Choroid, Left**	**Ø Open** **3 Percutaneous**	**7 Autologous Tissue Substitute** **J Synthetic Substitute** **K Nonautologous Tissue Substitute**	**Z No Qualifier**
4 Vitreous, Right Vitreous body **5 Vitreous, Left** *See 4 Vitreous, Right* **C Iris, Right** **D Iris, Left** **G Retinal Vessel, Right** **H Retinal Vessel, Left**	**3 Percutaneous**	**7 Autologous Tissue Substitute** **J Synthetic Substitute** **K Nonautologous Tissue Substitute**	**Z No Qualifier**
6 Sclera, Right **7 Sclera, Left** **S Conjunctiva, Right** Plica semilunaris **T Conjunctiva, Left** *See S Conjunctiva, Right*	**X External**	**7 Autologous Tissue Substitute** **J Synthetic Substitute** **K Nonautologous Tissue Substitute**	**Z No Qualifier**
8 Cornea, Right **9 Cornea, Left**	**3 Percutaneous** **X External**	**7 Autologous Tissue Substitute** **J Synthetic Substitute** **K Nonautologous Tissue Substitute**	**Z No Qualifier**
J Lens, Right Zonule of Zinn **K Lens, Left** *See J Lens, Right*	**3 Percutaneous**	**Ø Synthetic Substitute, Intraocular Telescope** **7 Autologous Tissue Substitute** **J Synthetic Substitute** **K Nonautologous Tissue Substitute**	**Z No Qualifier**
N Upper Eyelid, Right Lateral canthus Levator palpebrae superioris muscle Orbicularis oculi muscle Superior tarsal plate **P Upper Eyelid, Left** *See N Upper Eyelid, Right* **Q Lower Eyelid, Right** Inferior tarsal plate Medial canthus **R Lower Eyelid, Left** *See Q Lower Eyelid, Right*	**Ø Open** **3 Percutaneous** **X External**	**7 Autologous Tissue Substitute** **J Synthetic Substitute** **K Nonautologous Tissue Substitute**	**Z No Qualifier**
X Lacrimal Duct, Right Lacrimal canaliculus Lacrimal punctum Lacrimal sac Nasolacrimal duct **Y Lacrimal Duct, Left** *See X Lacrimal Duct, Right*	**Ø Open** **3 Percutaneous** **7 Via Natural or Artificial Opening** **8 Via Natural or Artificial Opening Endoscopic**	**7 Autologous Tissue Substitute** **J Synthetic Substitute** **K Nonautologous Tissue Substitute**	**Z No Qualifier**

Ø Medical and Surgical
8 Eye
S Reposition Definition: Moving to its normal location, or other suitable location, all or a portion of a body part

Explanation: The body part is moved to a new location from an abnormal location, or from a normal location where it is not functioning correctly. The body part may or may not be cut out or off to be moved to the new location.

Body Part Character 4	Approach Character 5	Device Character 6	Qualifier Character 7
C Iris, Right **D Iris, Left** **G Retinal Vessel, Right** **H Retinal Vessel, Left** **J Lens, Right** Zonule of Zinn **K Lens, Left** *See J Lens, Right*	**3 Percutaneous**	**Z No Device**	**Z No Qualifier**
L Extraocular Muscle, Right Inferior oblique muscle Inferior rectus muscle Lateral rectus muscle Medial rectus muscle Superior oblique muscle Superior rectus muscle **M Extraocular Muscle, Left** *See L Extraocular Muscle, Right* **V Lacrimal Gland, Right** **W Lacrimal Gland, Left**	**Ø Open** **3 Percutaneous**	**Z No Device**	**Z No Qualifier**
N Upper Eyelid, Right Lateral canthus Levator palpebrae superioris muscle Orbicularis oculi muscle Superior tarsal plate **P Upper Eyelid, Left** *See N Upper Eyelid, Right* **Q Lower Eyelid, Right** Inferior tarsal plate Medial canthus **R Lower Eyelid, Left** *See Q Lower Eyelid, Right*	**Ø Open** **3 Percutaneous** **X External**	**Z No Device**	**Z No Qualifier**
X Lacrimal Duct, Right Lacrimal canaliculus Lacrimal punctum Lacrimal sac Nasolacrimal duct **Y Lacrimal Duct, Left** *See X Lacrimal Duct, Right*	**Ø Open** **3 Percutaneous** **7 Via Natural or Artificial Opening** **8 Via Natural or Artificial Opening Endoscopic**	**Z No Device**	**Z No Qualifier**

Ø Medical and Surgical
8 Eye
T Resection Definition: Cutting out or off, without replacement, all of a body part
Explanation: None

Body Part Character 4	Approach Character 5	Device Character 6	Qualifier Character 7
Ø Eye, Right Ciliary body Posterior chamber **1 Eye, Left** *See Ø Eye, Right* **8 Cornea, Right** **9 Cornea, Left**	**X External**	**Z No Device**	**Z No Qualifier**
4 Vitreous, Right Vitreous body **5 Vitreous, Left** *See 4 Vitreous, Right* **C Iris, Right** **D Iris, Left** **J Lens, Right** Zonule of Zinn **K Lens, Left** *See J Lens, Right*	**3 Percutaneous**	**Z No Device**	**Z No Qualifier**
L Extraocular Muscle, Right Inferior oblique muscle Inferior rectus muscle Lateral rectus muscle Medial rectus muscle Superior oblique muscle Superior rectus muscle **M Extraocular Muscle, Left** *See L Extraocular Muscle, Right* **V Lacrimal Gland, Right** **W Lacrimal Gland, Left**	**Ø Open** **3 Percutaneous**	**Z No Device**	**Z No Qualifier**
N Upper Eyelid, Right Lateral canthus Levator palpebrae superioris muscle Orbicularis oculi muscle Superior tarsal plate **P Upper Eyelid, Left** *See N Upper Eyelid, Right* **Q Lower Eyelid, Right** Inferior tarsal plate Medial canthus **R Lower Eyelid, Left** *See Q Lower Eyelid, Right*	**Ø Open** **X External**	**Z No Device**	**Z No Qualifier**
X Lacrimal Duct, Right Lacrimal canaliculus Lacrimal punctum Lacrimal sac Nasolacrimal duct **Y Lacrimal Duct, Left** *See X Lacrimal Duct, Right*	**Ø Open** **3 Percutaneous** **7 Via Natural or Artificial Opening** **8 Via Natural or Artificial Opening Endoscopic**	**Z No Device**	**Z No Qualifier**

Ø Medical and Surgical
8 Eye
U Supplement Definition: Putting in or on biological or synthetic material that physically reinforces and/or augments the function of a portion of a body part

Explanation: The biological material is non-living, or is living and from the same individual. The body part may have been previously replaced, and the SUPPLEMENT procedure is performed to physically reinforce and/or augment the function of the replaced body part.

Body Part Character 4	Approach Character 5	Device Character 6	Qualifier Character 7
Ø Eye, Right Ciliary body Posterior chamber **1 Eye, Left** *See Ø Eye, Right* **C Iris, Right** **D Iris, Left** **E Retina, Right** Fovea Macula Optic disc **F Retina, Left** *See E Retina, Right* **G Retinal Vessel, Right** **H Retinal Vessel, Left** **L Extraocular Muscle, Right** Inferior oblique muscle Inferior rectus muscle Lateral rectus muscle Medial rectus muscle Superior oblique muscle Superior rectus muscle **M Extraocular Muscle, Left** *See L Extraocular Muscle, Right*	**Ø Open** **3 Percutaneous**	**7 Autologous Tissue Substitute** **J Synthetic Substitute** **K Nonautologous Tissue Substitute**	**Z No Qualifier**
8 Cornea, Right NC **9 Cornea, Left** NC **N Upper Eyelid, Right** Lateral canthus Levator palpebrae superioris muscle Orbicularis oculi muscle Superior tarsal plate **P Upper Eyelid, Left** *See N Upper Eyelid, Right* **Q Lower Eyelid, Right** Inferior tarsal plate Medial canthus **R Lower Eyelid, Left** *See Q Lower Eyelid, Right*	**Ø Open** **3 Percutaneous** **X External**	**7 Autologous Tissue Substitute** **J Synthetic Substitute** **K Nonautologous Tissue Substitute**	**Z No Qualifier**
X Lacrimal Duct, Right Lacrimal canaliculus Lacrimal punctum Lacrimal sac Nasolacrimal duct **Y Lacrimal Duct, Left** *See X Lacrimal Duct, Right*	**Ø Open** **3 Percutaneous** **7 Via Natural or Artificial Opening** **8 Via Natural or Artificial Opening Endoscopic**	**7 Autologous Tissue Substitute** **J Synthetic Substitute** **K Nonautologous Tissue Substitute**	**Z No Qualifier**

NC Ø8U[8,9][Ø,3,X]KZ

Ø Medical and Surgical
8 Eye
V Restriction Definition: Partially closing an orifice or the lumen of a tubular body part

Explanation: The orifice can be a natural orifice or an artificially created orifice

Body Part Character 4	Approach Character 5	Device Character 6	Qualifier Character 7
X Lacrimal Duct, Right Lacrimal canaliculus Lacrimal punctum Lacrimal sac Nasolacrimal duct **Y Lacrimal Duct, Left** *See X Lacrimal Duct, Right*	**Ø Open** **3 Percutaneous**	**C Extraluminal Device** **D Intraluminal Device** **Z No Device**	**Z No Qualifier**
X Lacrimal Duct, Right Lacrimal canaliculus Lacrimal punctum Lacrimal sac Nasolacrimal duct **Y Lacrimal Duct, Left** *See X Lacrimal Duct, Right*	**7 Via Natural or Artificial Opening** **8 Via Natural or Artificial Opening Endoscopic**	**D Intraluminal Device** **Z No Device**	**Z No Qualifier**

Ø Medical and Surgical
8 Eye
W Revision Definition: Correcting, to the extent possible, a portion of a malfunctioning device or the position of a displaced device

Explanation: Revision can include correcting a malfunctioning or displaced device by taking out or putting in components of the device such as a screw or pin

Body Part Character 4	Approach Character 5	Device Character 6	Qualifier Character 7
Ø Eye, Right Ciliary body Posterior chamber **1 Eye, Left** *See Ø Eye, Right*	**Ø Open** **3 Percutaneous** **7 Via Natural or Artificial Opening** **8 Via Natural or Artificial Opening Endoscopic**	**Ø Drainage Device** **3 Infusion Device** **7 Autologous Tissue Substitute** **C Extraluminal Device** **D Intraluminal Device** **J Synthetic Substitute** **K Nonautologous Tissue Substitute** **Y Other Device**	**Z No Qualifier**
Ø Eye, Right Ciliary body Posterior chamber **1 Eye, Left** *See Ø Eye, Right*	**X External**	**Ø Drainage Device** **3 Infusion Device** **7 Autologous Tissue Substitute** **C Extraluminal Device** **D Intraluminal Device** **J Synthetic Substitute** **K Nonautologous Tissue Substitute**	**Z No Qualifier**
J Lens, Right Zonule of Zinn **K Lens, Left** *See J Lens, Right*	**3 Percutaneous**	**J Synthetic Substitute** **Y Other Device**	**Z No Qualifier**
J Lens, Right Zonule of Zinn **K Lens, Left** *See J Lens, Right*	**X External**	**J Synthetic Substitute**	**Z No Qualifier**
L Extraocular Muscle, Right Inferior oblique muscle Inferior rectus muscle Lateral rectus muscle Medial rectus muscle Superior oblique muscle Superior rectus muscle **M Extraocular Muscle, Left** *See L Extraocular Muscle, Right*	**Ø Open** **3 Percutaneous**	**Ø Drainage Device** **7 Autologous Tissue Substitute** **J Synthetic Substitute** **K Nonautologous Tissue Substitute** **Y Other Device**	**Z No Qualifier**

Non-OR Ø8W[Ø,1][3,7,8]YZ
Non-OR Ø8W[Ø,1]X[Ø,3,7,C,D,J,K]Z
Non-OR Ø8W[J,K]3YZ
Non-OR Ø8W[J,K]XJZ
Non-OR Ø8W[L,M]3YZ

Ø Medical and Surgical
8 Eye
X Transfer Definition: Moving, without taking out, all or a portion of a body part to another location to take over the function of all or a portion of a body part

Explanation: The body part transferred remains connected to its vascular and nervous supply

Body Part Character 4	Approach Character 5	Device Character 6	Qualifier Character 7
L Extraocular Muscle, Right Inferior oblique muscle Inferior rectus muscle Lateral rectus muscle Medial rectus muscle Superior oblique muscle Superior rectus muscle **M Extraocular Muscle, Left** *See L Extraocular Muscle, Right*	**Ø Open** **3 Percutaneous**	**Z No Device**	**Z No Qualifier**

Ear, Nose, Sinus Ø9Ø–Ø9W

Character Meanings*

This Character Meaning table is provided as a guide to assist the user in the identification of character members that may be found in this section of code tables. It **SHOULD NOT** be used to build a PCS code.

Operation–Character 3		Body Part–Character 4		Approach–Character 5		Device–Character 6		Qualifier–Character 7	
Ø	Alteration	Ø	External Ear, Right	Ø	Open	Ø	Drainage Device	Ø	Endolymphatic
1	Bypass	1	External Ear, Left	3	Percutaneous	1	Radioactive Element	X	Diagnostic
2	Change	2	External Ear, Bilateral	4	Percutaneous Endoscopic	4	Hearing Device, Bone Conduction	Z	No Qualifier
3	Control	3	External Auditory Canal, Right	7	Via Natural or Artificial Opening	5	Hearing Device, Single Channel Cochlear Prosthesis		
5	Destruction	4	External Auditory Canal, Left	8	Via Natural or Artificial Opening Endoscopic	6	Hearing Device, Multiple Channel Cochlear Prosthesis		
7	Dilation	5	Middle Ear, Right	X	External	7	Autologous Tissue Substitute		
8	Division	6	Middle Ear, Left			B	Intraluminal Device, Airway		
9	Drainage	7	Tympanic Membrane, Right			D	Intraluminal Device		
B	Excision	8	Tympanic Membrane, Left			J	Synthetic Substitute		
C	Extirpation	9	Auditory Ossicle, Right			K	Nonautologous Tissue Substitute		
D	Extraction	A	Auditory Ossicle, Left			S	Hearing Device		
H	Insertion	B	Mastoid Sinus, Right			Y	Other Device		
J	Inspection	C	Mastoid Sinus, Left			Z	No Device		
M	Reattachment	D	Inner Ear, Right						
N	Release	E	Inner Ear, Left						
P	Removal	F	Eustachian Tube, Right						
Q	Repair	G	Eustachian Tube, Left						
R	Replacement	H	Ear, Right						
S	Reposition	J	Ear, Left						
T	Resection	K	Nasal Mucosa and Soft Tissue						
U	Supplement	L	Nasal Turbinate						
W	Revision	M	Nasal Septum						
		N	Nasopharynx						
		P	Accessory Sinus						
		Q	Maxillary Sinus, Right						
		R	Maxillary Sinus, Left						
		S	Frontal Sinus, Right						
		T	Frontal Sinus, Left						
		U	Ethmoid Sinus, Right						
		V	Ethmoid Sinus, Left						
		W	Sphenoid Sinus, Right						
		X	Sphenoid Sinus, Left						
		Y	Sinus						

* Includes sinus ducts.

AHA Coding Clinic for table Ø93
2018, 4Q, 38 Control of epistaxis

AHA Coding Clinic for table Ø95
2018, 1Q, 19 Control of epistaxis via silver nitrate cauterization

AHA Coding Clinic for table Ø9Q
2018, 1Q, 19 Control of epistaxis via silver nitrate cauterization
2017, 4Q, 106 Control of bleeding of external naris using suture
2014, 4Q, 20 Control of epistaxis
2014, 3Q, 22 Transsphenoidal removal of pituitary tumor and fat graft placement
2013, 4Q, 114 Balloon sinuplasty

AHA Coding Clinic for table Ø9U
2019, 4Q, 28-29 Sinus supplement

Ear Anatomy

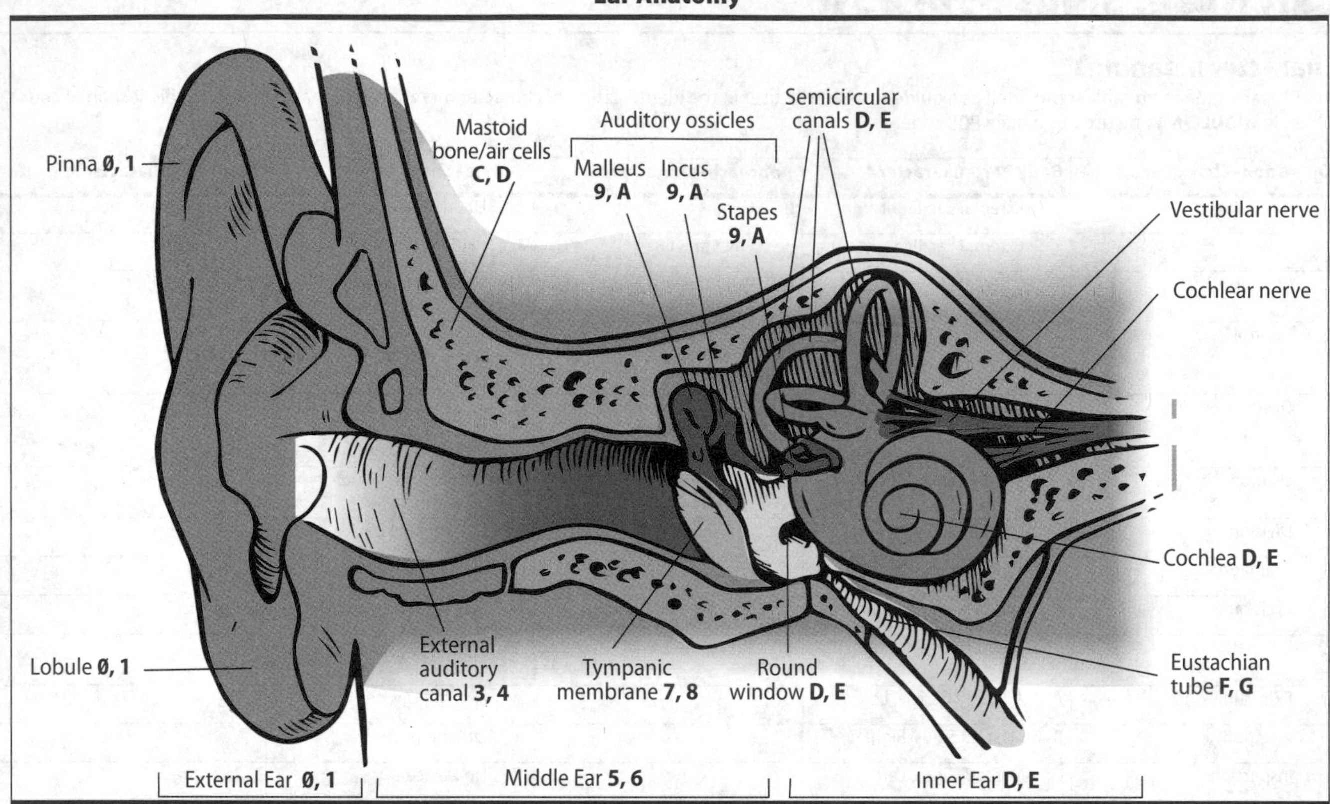

Nasal Turbinates

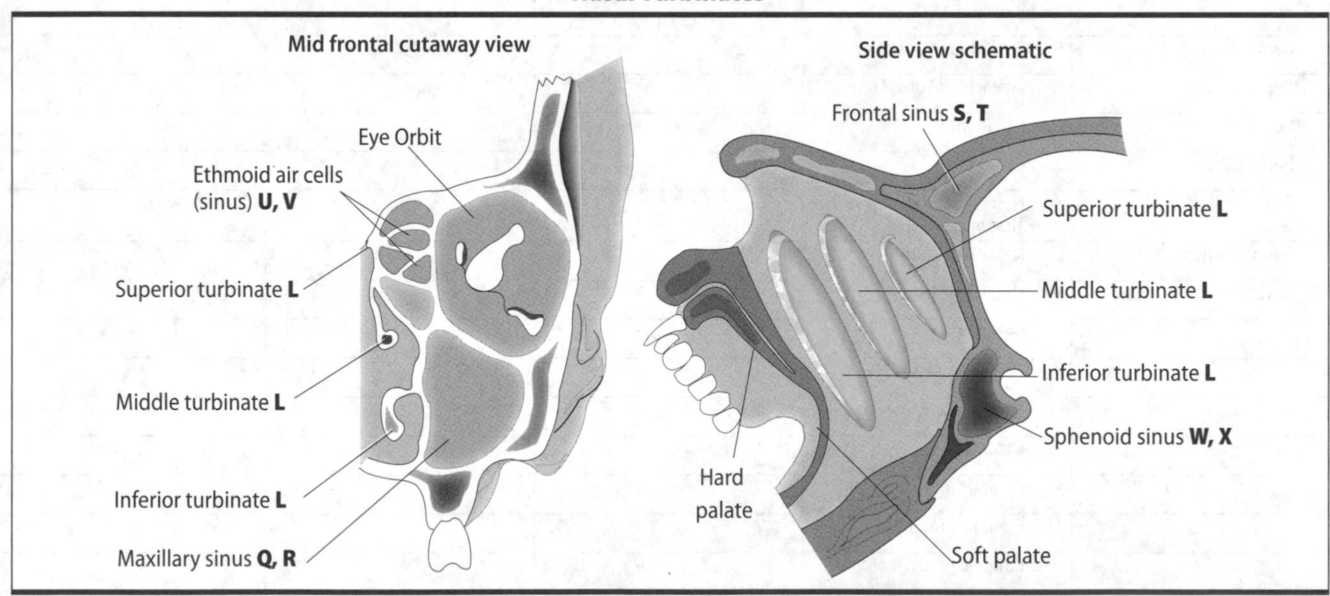

Paranasal Sinuses

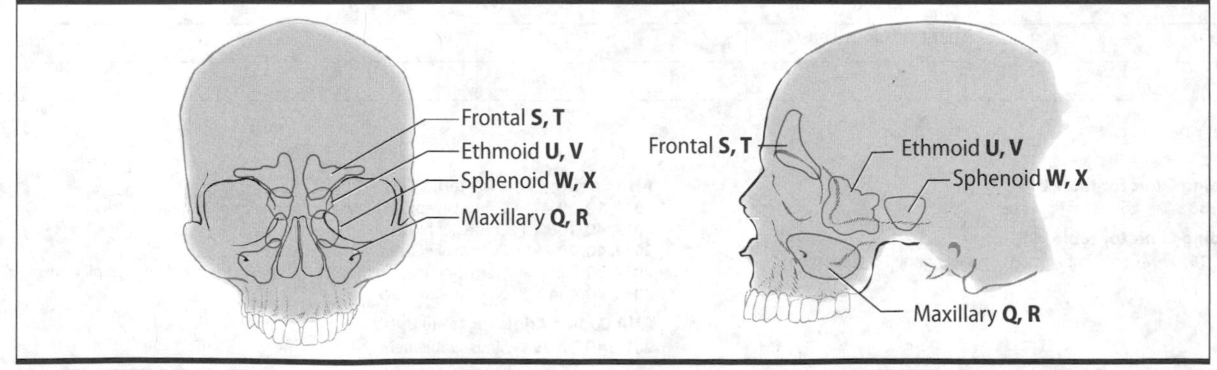

Ø Medical and Surgical
9 Ear, Nose, Sinus
Ø Alteration Definition: Modifying the anatomic structure of a body part without affecting the function of the body part
Explanation: Principal purpose is to improve appearance

Body Part Character 4		Approach Character 5	Device Character 6	Qualifier Character 7
Ø External Ear, Right Antihelix Antitragus Auricle Earlobe Helix Pinna Tragus **1 External Ear, Left** *See Ø External Ear, Right*	**2 External Ear, Bilateral** *See Ø External Ear, Right* **K Nasal Mucosa and Soft Tissue** Columella External naris Greater alar cartilage Internal naris Lateral nasal cartilage Lesser alar cartilage Nasal cavity Nostril	**Ø Open** **3 Percutaneous** **4 Percutaneous Endoscopic** **X External**	**7 Autologous Tissue Substitute** **J Synthetic Substitute** **K Nonautologous Tissue Substitute** **Z No Device**	**Z No Qualifier**

Ø Medical and Surgical
9 Ear, Nose, Sinus
1 Bypass Definition: Altering the route of passage of the contents of a tubular body part
Explanation: Rerouting contents of a body part to a downstream area of the normal route, to a similar route and body part, or to an abnormal route and dissimilar body part. Includes one or more anastomoses, with or without the use of a device.

Body Part Character 4	Approach Character 5	Device Character 6	Qualifier Character 7
D Inner Ear, Right Bony labyrinth Bony vestibule Cochlea Round window Semicircular canal **E Inner Ear, Left** *See D Inner Ear, Right*	**Ø Open**	**7 Autologous Tissue Substitute** **J Synthetic Substitute** **K Nonautologous Tissue Substitute** **Z No Device**	**Ø Endolymphatic**

Ø Medical and Surgical
9 Ear, Nose, Sinus
2 Change Definition: Taking out or off a device from a body part and putting back an identical or similar device in or on the same body part without cutting or puncturing the skin or a mucous membrane
Explanation: All CHANGE procedures are coded using the approach EXTERNAL

Body Part Character 4	Approach Character 5	Device Character 6	Qualifier Character 7
H Ear, Right **J Ear, Left** **K Nasal Mucosa and Soft Tissue** Columella External naris Greater alar cartilage Internal naris Lateral nasal cartilage Lesser alar cartilage Nasal cavity Nostril **Y Sinus**	**X External**	**Ø Drainage Device** **Y Other Device**	**Z No Qualifier**

Non-OR All body part, approach, device, and qualifier values

Ø Medical and Surgical
9 Ear, Nose, Sinus
3 Control Definition: Stopping, or attempting to stop, postprocedural or other acute bleeding
Explanation: None

Body Part Character 4	Approach Character 5	Device Character 6	Qualifier Character 7
K Nasal Mucosa and Soft Tissue Columella External naris Greater alar cartilage Internal naris Lateral nasal cartilage Lesser alar cartilage Nasal cavity Nostril	**7 Via Natural or Artificial Opening** **8 Via Natural or Artificial Opening Endoscopic**	**Z No Device**	**Z No Qualifier**

Non-OR Ø93K[7,8]ZZ

Ø Medical and Surgical
9 Ear, Nose, Sinus
5 Destruction Definition: Physical eradication of all or a portion of a body part by the direct use of energy, force, or a destructive agent
Explanation: None of the body part is physically taken out

Body Part Character 4		Approach Character 5	Device Character 6	Qualifier Character 7
Ø External Ear, Right Antihelix Antitragus Auricle Earlobe Helix Pinna Tragus	**1 External Ear, Left** *See Ø External Ear, Right*	**Ø Open** **3 Percutaneous** **4 Percutaneous Endoscopic** **X External**	**Z No Device**	**Z No Qualifier**
3 External Auditory Canal, Right External auditory meatus	**4 External Auditory Canal, Left** *See 3 External Auditory Canal, Right*	**Ø Open** **3 Percutaneous** **4 Percutaneous Endoscopic** **7 Via Natural or Artificial Opening** **8 Via Natural or Artificial Opening Endoscopic** **X External**	**Z No Device**	**Z No Qualifier**
5 Middle Ear, Right Oval window Tympanic cavity **6 Middle Ear, Left** *See 5 Middle Ear, Right* **9 Auditory Ossicle, Right** Incus Malleus Stapes **A Auditory Ossicle, Left** *See 9 Auditory Ossicle, Right*	**D Inner Ear, Right** Bony labyrinth Bony vestibule Cochlea Round window Semicircular canal **E Inner Ear, Left** *See D Inner Ear, Right*	**Ø Open** **8 Via Natural or Artificial Opening Endoscopic**	**Z No Device**	**Z No Qualifier**
7 Tympanic Membrane, Right Pars flaccida **8 Tympanic Membrane, Left** *See 7 Tympanic Membrane, Right* **F Eustachian Tube, Right** Auditory tube Pharyngotympanic tube **G Eustachian Tube, Left** *See F Eustachian Tube, Right*	**L Nasal Turbinate** Inferior turbinate Middle turbinate Nasal concha Superior turbinate **N Nasopharynx** Choana Fossa of Rosenmuller Pharyngeal recess Rhinopharynx	**Ø Open** **3 Percutaneous** **4 Percutaneous Endoscopic** **7 Via Natural or Artificial Opening** **8 Via Natural or Artificial Opening Endoscopic**	**Z No Device**	**Z No Qualifier**
B Mastoid Sinus, Right Mastoid air cells **C Mastoid Sinus, Left** *See B Mastoid Sinus, Right* **M Nasal Septum** Quadrangular cartilage Septal cartilage Vomer bone **P Accessory Sinus** **Q Maxillary Sinus, Right** Antrum of Highmore	**R Maxillary Sinus, Left** *See Q Maxillary Sinus, Right* **S Frontal Sinus, Right** **T Frontal Sinus, Left** **U Ethmoid Sinus, Right** Ethmoidal air cell **V Ethmoid Sinus, Left** *See U Ethmoid Sinus, Right* **W Sphenoid Sinus, Right** **X Sphenoid Sinus, Left**	**Ø Open** **3 Percutaneous** **4 Percutaneous Endoscopic** **8 Via Natural or Artificial Opening Endoscopic**	**Z No Device**	**Z No Qualifier**
K Nasal Mucosa and Soft Tissue Columella External naris Greater alar cartilage Internal naris Lateral nasal cartilage Lesser alar cartilage Nasal cavity Nostril		**Ø Open** **3 Percutaneous** **4 Percutaneous Endoscopic** **8 Via Natural or Artificial Opening Endoscopic** **X External**	**Z No Device**	**Z No Qualifier**

Non-OR Ø95[Ø,1][Ø,3,4,X]ZZ
Non-OR Ø95[3,4][Ø,3,4,7,8,X]ZZ
Non-OR Ø95[F,G][Ø,3,4,7,8]ZZ
Non-OR Ø95M[Ø,3,4,8]ZZ
Non-OR Ø95K[Ø,3,4,8,X]ZZ

Ø Medical and Surgical
9 Ear, Nose, Sinus
7 Dilation Definition: Expanding an orifice or the lumen of a tubular body part

Explanation: The orifice can be a natural orifice or an artificially created orifice. Accomplished by stretching a tubular body part using intraluminal pressure or by cutting part of the orifice or wall of the tubular body part.

Body Part Character 4	Approach Character 5	Device Character 6	Qualifier Character 7
F Eustachian Tube, Right Auditory tube Pharyngotympanic tube **G Eustachian Tube, Left** *See F Eustachian Tube, Right*	**Ø Open** **7 Via Natural or Artificial Opening** **8 Via Natural or Artificial Opening Endoscopic**	**D Intraluminal Device** **Z No Device**	**Z No Qualifier**
F Eustachian Tube, Right Auditory tube Pharyngotympanic tube **G Eustachian Tube, Left** *See F Eustachian Tube, Right*	**3 Percutaneous** **4 Percutaneous Endoscopic**	**Z No Device**	**Z No Qualifier**

Non-OR All body part, approach, device, and qualifier values

Ø Medical and Surgical
9 Ear, Nose, Sinus
8 Division Definition: Cutting into a body part, without draining fluids and/or gases from the body part, in order to separate or transect a body part

Explanation: All or a portion of the body part is separated into two or more portions

Body Part Character 4	Approach Character 5	Device Character 6	Qualifier Character 7
L Nasal Turbinate Inferior turbinate Middle turbinate Nasal concha Superior turbinate	**Ø Open** **3 Percutaneous** **4 Percutaneous Endoscopic** **7 Via Natural or Artificial Opening** **8 Via Natural or Artificial Opening Endoscopic**	**Z No Device**	**Z No Qualifier**

Ear, Nose, Sinus

Ø97–Ø98

Ø Medical and Surgical
9 Ear, Nose, Sinus
9 Drainage Definition: Taking or letting out fluids and/or gases from a body part
Explanation: The qualifier DIAGNOSTIC is used to identify drainage procedures that are biopsies

Body Part Character 4		Approach Character 5	Device Character 6	Qualifier Character 7
Ø External Ear, Right Antihelix Antitragus Auricle Earlobe Helix Pinna Tragus	**1 External Ear, Left** *See Ø External Ear, Right*	**Ø Open** **3 Percutaneous** **4 Percutaneous Endoscopic** **X External**	**Ø Drainage Device**	**Z No Qualifier**
Ø External Ear, Right Antihelix Antitragus Auricle Earlobe Helix Pinna Tragus	**1 External Ear, Left** *See Ø External Ear, Right*	**Ø Open** **3 Percutaneous** **4 Percutaneous Endoscopic** **X External**	**Z No Device**	**X Diagnostic** **Z No Qualifier**
3 External Auditory Canal, Right External auditory meatus **4 External Auditory Canal, Left** *See 3 External Auditory Canal, Right*	**K Nasal Mucosa and Soft Tissue** Columella External naris Greater alar cartilage Internal naris Lateral nasal cartilage Lesser alar cartilage Nasal cavity Nostril	**Ø Open** **3 Percutaneous** **4 Percutaneous Endoscopic** **7 Via Natural or Artificial Opening** **8 Via Natural or Artificial Opening Endoscopic** **X External**	**Ø Drainage Device**	**Z No Qualifier**
3 External Auditory Canal, Right External auditory meatus **4 External Auditory Canal, Left** *See 3 External Auditory Canal, Right*	**K Nasal Mucosa and Soft Tissue** Columella External naris Greater alar cartilage Internal naris Lateral nasal cartilage Lesser alar cartilage Nasal cavity Nostril	**Ø Open** **3 Percutaneous** **4 Percutaneous Endoscopic** **7 Via Natural or Artificial Opening** **8 Via Natural or Artificial Opening Endoscopic** **X External**	**Z No Device**	**X Diagnostic** **Z No Qualifier**
5 Middle Ear, Right Oval window Tympanic cavity **6 Middle Ear, Left** *See 5 Middle Ear, Right* **9 Auditory Ossicle, Right** Incus Malleus Stapes	**A Auditory Ossicle, Left** *See 9 Auditory Ossicle, Right* **D Inner Ear, Right** Bony labyrinth Bony vestibule Cochlea Round window Semicircular canal **E Inner Ear, Left** *See D Inner Ear, Right*	**Ø Open** **7 Via Natural or Artificial Opening** **8 Via Natural or Artificial Opening Endoscopic**	**Ø Drainage Device**	**Z No Qualifier**
5 Middle Ear, Right Oval window Tympanic cavity **6 Middle Ear, Left** *See 5 Middle Ear, Right* **9 Auditory Ossicle, Right** Incus Malleus Stapes	**A Auditory Ossicle, Left** *See 9 Auditory Ossicle, Right* **D Inner Ear, Right** Bony labyrinth Bony vestibule Cochlea Round window Semicircular canal **E Inner Ear, Left** *See D Inner Ear, Right*	**Ø Open** **7 Via Natural or Artificial Opening** **8 Via Natural or Artificial Opening Endoscopic**	**Z No Device**	**X Diagnostic** **Z No Qualifier**

Non-OR Ø99[Ø,1][Ø,3,4,X]ØZ
Non-OR Ø99[Ø,1][Ø,3,4,X]Z[X,Z]
Non-OR Ø99[3,4,K][Ø,3,4,7,8,X]ØZ
Non-OR Ø99[3,4,K][Ø,3,4,7,8,X]Z[X,Z]
Non-OR Ø99[5,6]8ØZ
Non-OR Ø99[9,A,D,E][7,8]ØZ
Non-OR Ø99[5,6]ØZZ
Non-OR Ø99[5,6,9,A,D,E][7,8]Z[X,Z]

Ø99 Continued on next page

Ø99 Continued

Ø Medical and Surgical
9 Ear, Nose, Sinus
9 Drainage Definition: Taking or letting out fluids and/or gases from a body part
Explanation: The qualifier DIAGNOSTIC is used to identify drainage procedures that are biopsies

Body Part Character 4	Approach Character 5	Device Character 6	Qualifier Character 7
7 Tympanic Membrane, Right Pars flaccida **8 Tympanic Membrane, Left** *See 7 Tympanic Membrane, Right* **B Mastoid Sinus, Right** Mastoid air cells **C Mastoid Sinus, Left** *See B Mastoid Sinus, Right* **F Eustachian Tube, Right** Auditory tube, Pharyngotympanic tube **G Eustachian Tube, Left** *See F Eustachian Tube, Right* **L Nasal Turbinate** Inferior turbinate, Middle turbinate, Nasal concha, Superior turbinate **M Nasal Septum** Quadrangular cartilage, Septal cartilage, Vomer bone **N Nasopharynx** Choana, Fossa of Rosenmuller, Pharyngeal recess, Rhinopharynx **P Accessory Sinus** **Q Maxillary Sinus, Right** Antrum of Highmore **R Maxillary Sinus, Left** *See Q Maxillary Sinus, Right* **S Frontal Sinus, Right** **T Frontal Sinus, Left** **U Ethmoid Sinus, Right** Ethmoidal air cell **V Ethmoid Sinus, Left** *See U Ethmoid Sinus, Right* **W Sphenoid Sinus, Right** **X Sphenoid Sinus, Left**	**Ø Open** **3 Percutaneous** **4 Percutaneous Endoscopic** **7 Via Natural or Artificial Opening** **8 Via Natural or Artificial Opening Endoscopic**	**Ø Drainage Device**	**Z No Qualifier**
7 Tympanic Membrane, Right Pars flaccida **8 Tympanic Membrane, Left** *See 7 Tympanic Membrane, Right* **B Mastoid Sinus, Right** Mastoid air cells **C Mastoid Sinus, Left** *See B Mastoid Sinus, Right* **F Eustachian Tube, Right** Auditory tube, Pharyngotympanic tube **G Eustachian Tube, Left** *See F Eustachian Tube, Right* **L Nasal Turbinate** Inferior turbinate, Middle turbinate, Nasal concha, Superior turbinate **M Nasal Septum** Quadrangular cartilage, Septal cartilage, Vomer bone **N Nasopharynx** Choana, Fossa of Rosenmuller, Pharyngeal recess, Rhinopharynx **P Accessory Sinus** **Q Maxillary Sinus, Right** Antrum of Highmore **R Maxillary Sinus, Left** *See Q Maxillary Sinus, Right* **S Frontal Sinus, Right** **T Frontal Sinus, Left** **U Ethmoid Sinus, Right** Ethmoidal air cell **V Ethmoid Sinus, Left** *See U Ethmoid Sinus, Right* **W Sphenoid Sinus, Right** **X Sphenoid Sinus, Left**	**Ø Open** **3 Percutaneous** **4 Percutaneous Endoscopic** **7 Via Natural or Artificial Opening** **8 Via Natural or Artificial Opening Endoscopic**	**Z No Device**	**X Diagnostic** **Z No Qualifier**

Non-OR Ø99[B,C][3,7,8]ØZ
Non-OR Ø99[F,G,L,M][Ø,3,4,7,8]ØZ
Non-OR Ø99N3ØZ
Non-OR Ø99[P,Q,R,S,T,U,V,W,X][3,4,7,8]ØZ
Non-OR Ø99[7,8][Ø,3,4,7,8]ZZ
Non-OR Ø99[7,8][7,8]ZX
Non-OR Ø99[B,C]3ZZ
Non-OR Ø99[B,C][7,8]Z[X,Z]
Non-OR Ø99[F,G][Ø,3,4,7,8]ZZ
Non-OR Ø99[F,G][7,8]ZX
Non-OR Ø99[L,M][Ø,3,4,7,8]Z[X,Z]
Non-OR Ø99N[Ø,3,4,7,8]ZX
Non-OR Ø99N3ZZ
Non-OR Ø99[P,Q,R,S,T,U,V,W,X][3,4,7,8]Z[X,Z]

Ø Medical and Surgical
9 Ear, Nose, Sinus
B Excision Definition: Cutting out or off, without replacement, a portion of a body part
Explanation: The qualifier DIAGNOSTIC is used to identify excision procedures that are biopsies

Body Part Character 4		Approach Character 5	Device Character 6	Qualifier Character 7
Ø External Ear, Right Antihelix Antitragus Auricle Earlobe Helix Pinna Tragus	**1 External Ear, Left** *See Ø External Ear, Right*	**Ø Open** **3 Percutaneous** **4 Percutaneous Endoscopic** **X External**	**Z No Device**	**X Diagnostic** **Z No Qualifier**
3 External Auditory Canal, Right External auditory meatus	**4 External Auditory Canal, Left** *See 3 External Auditory Canal, Right*	**Ø Open** **3 Percutaneous** **4 Percutaneous Endoscopic** **7 Via Natural or Artificial Opening** **8 Via Natural or Artificial Opening Endoscopic** **X External**	**Z No Device**	**X Diagnostic** **Z No Qualifier**
5 Middle Ear, Right Oval window Tympanic cavity **6 Middle Ear, Left** *See 5 Middle Ear, Right* **9 Auditory Ossicle, Right** Incus Malleus Stapes	**A Auditory Ossicle, Left** *See 9 Auditory Ossicle, Right* **D Inner Ear, Right** Bony labyrinth Bony vestibule Cochlea Round window Semicircular canal **E Inner Ear, Left** *See D Inner Ear, Right*	**Ø Open** **8 Via Natural or Artificial Opening Endoscopic**	**Z No Device**	**X Diagnostic** **Z No Qualifier**
7 Tympanic Membrane, Right Pars flaccida **8 Tympanic Membrane, Left** *See 7 Tympanic Membrane, Right* **F Eustachian Tube, Right** Auditory tube Pharyngotympanic tube **G Eustachian Tube, Left** *See F Eustachian Tube, Right*	**L Nasal Turbinate** Inferior turbinate Middle turbinate Nasal concha Superior turbinate **N Nasopharynx** Choana Fossa of Rosenmuller Pharyngeal recess Rhinopharynx	**Ø Open** **3 Percutaneous** **4 Percutaneous Endoscopic** **7 Via Natural or Artificial Opening** **8 Via Natural or Artificial Opening Endoscopic**	**Z No Device**	**X Diagnostic** **Z No Qualifier**
B Mastoid Sinus, Right Mastoid air cells **C Mastoid Sinus, Left** *See B Mastoid Sinus, Right* **M Nasal Septum** Quadrangular cartilage Septal cartilage Vomer bone **P Accessory Sinus** **Q Maxillary Sinus, Right** Antrum of Highmore	**R Maxillary Sinus, Left** *See Q Maxillary Sinus, Right* **S Frontal Sinus, Right** **T Frontal Sinus, Left** **U Ethmoid Sinus, Right** Ethmoidal air cell **V Ethmoid Sinus, Left** *See U Ethmoid Sinus, Right* **W Sphenoid Sinus, Right** **X Sphenoid Sinus, Left**	**Ø Open** **3 Percutaneous** **4 Percutaneous Endoscopic** **8 Via Natural or Artificial Opening Endoscopic**	**Z No Device**	**X Diagnostic** **Z No Qualifier**
K Nasal Mucosa and Soft Tissue Columella External naris Greater alar cartilage Internal naris Lateral nasal cartilage Lesser alar cartilage Nasal cavity Nostril		**Ø Open** **3 Percutaneous** **4 Percutaneous Endoscopic** **8 Via Natural or Artificial Opening Endoscopic** **X External**	**Z No Device**	**X Diagnostic** **Z No Qualifier**

Non-OR Ø9B[Ø,1][Ø,3,4,X]Z[X,Z]
Non-OR Ø9B[3,4][Ø,3,4,7,8,X]Z[X,Z]
Non-OR Ø9B[F,G,L,N][Ø,3,4,7,8]Z[X,Z]
Non-OR Ø9BM[Ø,3,4,8]ZX
Non-OR Ø9B[P,Q,R,S,T,U,V,W,X][3,4,8]ZX
Non-OR Ø9BK8Z[X,Z]

Ø Medical and Surgical
9 Ear, Nose, Sinus
C Extirpation Definition: Taking or cutting out solid matter from a body part

Explanation: The solid matter may be an abnormal byproduct of a biological function or a foreign body; it may be imbedded in a body part or in the lumen of a tubular body part. The solid matter may or may not have been previously broken into pieces.

Body Part Character 4		Approach Character 5	Device Character 6	Qualifier Character 7
Ø External Ear, Right Antihelix Antitragus Auricle Earlobe Helix Pinna Tragus	1 External Ear, Left *See Ø External Ear, Right*	Ø Open 3 Percutaneous 4 Percutaneous Endoscopic X External	Z No Device	Z No Qualifier
3 External Auditory Canal, Right External auditory meatus	4 External Auditory Canal, Left *See 3 External Auditory Canal, Right*	Ø Open 3 Percutaneous 4 Percutaneous Endoscopic 7 Via Natural or Artificial Opening 8 Via Natural or Artificial Opening Endoscopic X External	Z No Device	Z No Qualifier
5 Middle Ear, Right Oval window Tympanic cavity 6 Middle Ear, Left *See 5 Middle Ear, Right* 9 Auditory Ossicle, Right Incus Malleus Stapes	A Auditory Ossicle, Left *See 9 Auditory Ossicle, Right* D Inner Ear, Right Bony labyrinth Bony vestibule Cochlea Round window Semicircular canal E Inner Ear, Left *See D Inner Ear, Right*	Ø Open 8 Via Natural or Artificial Opening Endoscopic	Z No Device	Z No Qualifier
7 Tympanic Membrane, Right Pars flaccida 8 Tympanic Membrane, Left *See 7 Tympanic Membrane, Right* F Eustachian Tube, Right Auditory tube Pharyngotympanic tube G Eustachian Tube, Left *See F Eustachian Tube, Right*	L Nasal Turbinate Inferior turbinate Middle turbinate Nasal concha Superior turbinate N Nasopharynx Choana Fossa of Rosenmuller Pharyngeal recess Rhinopharynx	Ø Open 3 Percutaneous 4 Percutaneous Endoscopic 7 Via Natural or Artificial Opening 8 Via Natural or Artificial Opening Endoscopic	Z No Device	Z No Qualifier
B Mastoid Sinus, Right Mastoid air cells C Mastoid Sinus, Left *See B Mastoid Sinus, Right* M Nasal Septum Quadrangular cartilage Septal cartilage Vomer bone P Accessory Sinus Q Maxillary Sinus, Right Antrum of Highmore	R Maxillary Sinus, Left *See Q Maxillary Sinus, Right* S Frontal Sinus, Right T Frontal Sinus, Left U Ethmoid Sinus, Right Ethmoidal air cell V Ethmoid Sinus, Left *See U Ethmoid Sinus, Right* W Sphenoid Sinus, Right X Sphenoid Sinus, Left	Ø Open 3 Percutaneous 4 Percutaneous Endoscopic 8 Via Natural or Artificial Opening Endoscopic	Z No Device	Z No Qualifier
K Nasal Mucosa and Soft Tissue Columella External naris Greater alar cartilage Internal naris Lateral nasal cartilage Lesser alar cartilage Nasal cavity Nostril		Ø Open 3 Percutaneous 4 Percutaneous Endoscopic 8 Via Natural or Artificial Opening Endoscopic X External	Z No Device	Z No Qualifier

Non-OR Ø9C[Ø,1][Ø,3,4,X]ZZ
Non-OR Ø9C[3,4][Ø,3,4,7,8,X]ZZ
Non-OR Ø9C[7,8,F,G,L][Ø,3,4,7,8]ZZ
Non-OR Ø9CM[Ø,3,4,8]ZZ
Non-OR Ø9CK8ZZ

Ø Medical and Surgical
9 Ear, Nose, Sinus
D Extraction Definition: Pulling or stripping out or off all or a portion of a body part by the use of force
Explanation: The qualifier DIAGNOSTIC is used to identify extraction procedures that are biopsies

Body Part Character 4	Approach Character 5	Device Character 6	Qualifier Character 7
7 Tympanic Membrane, Right Pars flaccida **8 Tympanic Membrane, Left** *See 7 Tympanic Membrane, Right* **L Nasal Turbinate** Inferior turbinate Middle turbinate Nasal concha Superior turbinate	**Ø Open** **3 Percutaneous** **4 Percutaneous Endoscopic** **7 Via Natural or Artificial Opening** **8 Via Natural or Artificial Opening Endoscopic**	**Z No Device**	**Z No Qualifier**
9 Auditory Ossicle, Right Incus Malleus Stapes **A Auditory Ossicle, Left** *See 9 Auditory Ossicle, Right*	**Ø Open**	**Z No Device**	**Z No Qualifier**
B Mastoid Sinus, Right Mastoid air cells **C Mastoid Sinus, Left** *See B Mastoid Sinus, Right* **M Nasal Septum** Quadrangular cartilage Septal cartilage Vomer bone **P Accessory Sinus** **Q Maxillary Sinus, Right** Antrum of Highmore **R Maxillary Sinus, Left** *See Q Maxillary Sinus, Right* **S Frontal Sinus, Right** **T Frontal Sinus, Left** **U Ethmoid Sinus, Right** Ethmoidal air cell **V Ethmoid Sinus, Left** *See U Ethmoid Sinus, Right* **W Sphenoid Sinus, Right** **X Sphenoid Sinus, Left**	**Ø Open** **3 Percutaneous** **4 Percutaneous Endoscopic**	**Z No Device**	**Z No Qualifier**

Ø Medical and Surgical
9 Ear, Nose, Sinus
H Insertion Definition: Putting in a nonbiological appliance that monitors, assists, performs, or prevents a physiological function but does not physically take the place of a body part
Explanation: None

Body Part Character 4	Approach Character 5	Device Character 6	Qualifier Character 7
D Inner Ear, Right Bony labyrinth Bony vestibule Cochlea Round window Semicircular canal **E Inner Ear, Left** *See D Inner Ear, Right*	**Ø Open** **3 Percutaneous** **4 Percutaneous Endoscopic**	**1 Radioactive Element** **4 Hearing Device, Bone Conduction** **5 Hearing Device, Single Channel Cochlear Prosthesis** **6 Hearing Device, Multiple Channel Cochlear Prosthesis** **S Hearing Device**	**Z No Qualifier**
H Ear, Right **J Ear, Left** **K Nasal Mucosa and Soft Tissue** Columella External naris Greater alar cartilage Internal naris Lateral nasal cartilage Lesser alar cartilage Nasal cavity Nostril **Y Sinus**	**Ø Open** **3 Percutaneous** **4 Percutaneous Endoscopic** **7 Via Natural or Artificial Opening** **8 Via Natural or Artificial Opening Endoscopic**	**1 Radioactive Element** **Y Other Device**	**Z No Qualifier**
N Nasopharynx Choana Fossa of Rosenmuller Pharyngeal recess Rhinopharynx	**7 Via Natural or Artificial Opening** **8 Via Natural or Artificial Opening Endoscopic**	**1 Radioactive Element** **B Intraluminal Device, Airway**	**Z No Qualifier**

Non-OR Ø9H[H,J][3,4,7,8]YZ
Non-OR Ø9H[K,Y][Ø,3,4,7,8]YZ
Non-OR Ø9HN[7,8]BZ

Ø Medical and Surgical
9 Ear, Nose, Sinus
J Inspection Definition: Visually and/or manually exploring a body part
Explanation: Visual exploration may be performed with or without optical instrumentation. Manual exploration may be performed directly or through intervening body layers.

Body Part Character 4	Approach Character 5	Device Character 6	Qualifier Character 7
7 Tympanic Membrane, Right Pars flaccida **8 Tympanic Membrane, Left** *See 7 Tympanic Membrane, Right* **H Ear, Right** **J Ear, Left**	**Ø Open** **3 Percutaneous** **4 Percutaneous Endoscopic** **7 Via Natural or Artificial Opening** **8 Via Natural or Artificial Opening Endoscopic** **X External**	**Z No Device**	**Z No Qualifier**
D Inner Ear, Right Bony labyrinth Bony vestibule Cochlea Round window Semicircular canal **E Inner Ear, Left** *See D Inner Ear, Right* **K Nasal Mucosa and Soft Tissue** Columella External naris Greater alar cartilage Internal naris Lateral nasal cartilage Lesser alar cartilage Nasal cavity Nostril **Y Sinus**	**Ø Open** **3 Percutaneous** **4 Percutaneous Endoscopic** **8 Via Natural or Artificial Opening Endoscopic** **X External**	**Z No Device**	**Z No Qualifier**

Non-OR Ø9J[7,8][3,7,8,X]ZZ
Non-OR Ø9J[H,J][Ø,3,4,7,8,X]ZZ
Non-OR Ø9J[D,E][3,8,X]ZZ
Non-OR Ø9J[K,Y][Ø,3,4,8,X]ZZ

Ø Medical and Surgical
9 Ear, Nose, Sinus
M Reattachment Definition: Putting back in or on all or a portion of a separated body part to its normal location or other suitable location
Explanation: Vascular circulation and nervous pathways may or may not be reestablished

Body Part Character 4	Approach Character 5	Device Character 6	Qualifier Character 7
Ø External Ear, Right Antihelix Antitragus Auricle Earlobe Helix Pinna Tragus **1 External Ear, Left** *See Ø External Ear, Right* **K Nasal Mucosa and Soft Tissue** Columella External naris Greater alar cartilage Internal naris Lateral nasal cartilage Lesser alar cartilage Nasal cavity Nostril	**X External**	**Z No Device**	**Z No Qualifier**

Ø Medical and Surgical
9 Ear, Nose, Sinus
N Release Definition: Freeing a body part from an abnormal physical constraint by cutting or by the use of force
Explanation: Some of the restraining tissue may be taken out but none of the body part is taken out

Body Part Character 4		Approach Character 5	Device Character 6	Qualifier Character 7
Ø External Ear, Right Antihelix Antitragus Auricle Earlobe Helix Pinna Tragus	**1 External Ear, Left** *See Ø External Ear, Right*	**Ø Open** **3 Percutaneous** **4 Percutaneous Endoscopic** **X External**	**Z No Device**	**Z No Qualifier**
3 External Auditory Canal, Right External auditory meatus	**4 External Auditory Canal, Left** *See 3 External Auditory Canal, Right*	**Ø Open** **3 Percutaneous** **4 Percutaneous Endoscopic** **7 Via Natural or Artificial Opening** **8 Via Natural or Artificial Opening Endoscopic** **X External**	**Z No Device**	**Z No Qualifier**
5 Middle Ear, Right Oval window Tympanic cavity **6 Middle Ear, Left** *See 5 Middle Ear, Right* **9 Auditory Ossicle, Right** Incus Malleus Stapes	**A Auditory Ossicle, Left** *See 9 Auditory Ossicle, Right* **D Inner Ear, Right** Bony labyrinth Bony vestibule Cochlea Round window Semicircular canal **E Inner Ear, Left** *See D Inner Ear, Right*	**Ø Open** **8 Via Natural or Artificial Opening Endoscopic**	**Z No Device**	**Z No Qualifier**
7 Tympanic Membrane, Right Pars flaccida **8 Tympanic Membrane, Left** *See 7 Tympanic Membrane, Right* **F Eustachian Tube, Right** Auditory tube Pharyngotympanic tube **G Eustachian Tube, Left** *See F Eustachian Tube, Right*	**L Nasal Turbinate** Inferior turbinate Middle turbinate Nasal concha Superior turbinate **N Nasopharynx** Choana Fossa of Rosenmuller Pharyngeal recess Rhinopharynx	**Ø Open** **3 Percutaneous** **4 Percutaneous Endoscopic** **7 Via Natural or Artificial Opening** **8 Via Natural or Artificial Opening Endoscopic**	**Z No Device**	**Z No Qualifier**
B Mastoid Sinus, Right Mastoid air cells **C Mastoid Sinus, Left** *See B Mastoid Sinus, Right* **M Nasal Septum** Quadrangular cartilage Septal cartilage Vomer bone **P Accessory Sinus** **Q Maxillary Sinus, Right** Antrum of Highmore	**R Maxillary Sinus, Left** *See Q Maxillary Sinus, Right* **S Frontal Sinus, Right** **T Frontal Sinus, Left** **U Ethmoid Sinus, Right** Ethmoidal air cell **V Ethmoid Sinus, Left** *See U Ethmoid Sinus, Right* **W Sphenoid Sinus, Right** **X Sphenoid Sinus, Left**	**Ø Open** **3 Percutaneous** **4 Percutaneous Endoscopic** **8 Via Natural or Artificial Opening Endoscopic**	**Z No Device**	**Z No Qualifier**
K Nasal Mucosa and Soft Tissue Columella External naris Greater alar cartilage Internal naris Lateral nasal cartilage Lesser alar cartilage Nasal cavity Nostril		**Ø Open** **3 Percutaneous** **4 Percutaneous Endoscopic** **8 Via Natural or Artificial Opening Endoscopic** **X External**	**Z No Device**	**Z No Qualifier**

Non-OR Ø9N[Ø,1]XZZ
Non-OR Ø9N[3,4]XZZ
Non-OR Ø9N[F,G,L][Ø,3,4,7,8]ZZ
Non-OR Ø9NM[Ø,3,4,8]ZZ
Non-OR Ø9NK[Ø,3,4,8,X]ZZ

Ø Medical and Surgical
9 Ear, Nose, Sinus
P Removal Definition: Taking out or off a device from a body part

Explanation: If a device is taken out and a similar device put in without cutting or puncturing the skin or mucous membrane, the procedure is coded to the root operation CHANGE. Otherwise, the procedure for taking out a device is coded to the root operation REMOVAL.

Body Part Character 4	Approach Character 5	Device Character 6	Qualifier Character 7
7 Tympanic Membrane, Right Pars flaccida **8 Tympanic Membrane, Left** *See 7 Tympanic Membrane, Right*	**Ø Open** **7 Via Natural or Artificial Opening** **8 Via Natural or Artificial Opening Endoscopic** **X External**	**Ø Drainage Device**	**Z No Qualifier**
D Inner Ear, Right Bony labyrinth Bony vestibule Cochlea Round window Semicircular canal **E Inner Ear, Left** *See D Inner Ear, Right*	**Ø Open** **7 Via Natural or Artificial Opening** **8 Via Natural or Artificial Opening Endoscopic**	**S Hearing Device**	**Z No Qualifier**
H Ear, Right **J Ear, Left** **K Nasal Mucosa and Soft Tissue** Columella External naris Greater alar cartilage Internal naris Lateral nasal cartilage Lesser alar cartilage Nasal cavity Nostril	**Ø Open** **3 Percutaneous** **4 Percutaneous Endoscopic** **7 Via Natural or Artificial Opening** **8 Via Natural or Artificial Opening Endoscopic**	**Ø Drainage Device** **7 Autologous Tissue Substitute** **D Intraluminal Device** **J Synthetic Substitute** **K Nonautologous Tissue Substitute** **Y Other Device**	**Z No Qualifier**
H Ear, Right **J Ear, Left** **K Nasal Mucosa and Soft Tissue** Columella External naris Greater alar cartilage Internal naris Lateral nasal cartilage Lesser alar cartilage Nasal cavity Nostril	**X External**	**Ø Drainage Device** **7 Autologous Tissue Substitute** **D Intraluminal Device** **J Synthetic Substitute** **K Nonautologous Tissue Substitute**	**Z No Qualifier**
Y Sinus	**Ø Open** **3 Percutaneous** **4 Percutaneous Endoscopic**	**Ø Drainage Device** **Y Other Device**	**Z No Qualifier**
Y Sinus	**7 Via Natural or Artificial Opening** **8 Via Natural or Artificial Opening Endoscopic**	**Y Other Device**	**Z No Qualifier**
Y Sinus	**X External**	**Ø Drainage Device**	**Z No Qualifier**

Non-OR Ø9P[7,8][Ø,7,8,X]ØZ
Non-OR Ø9P[H,J][3,4][Ø,J,K,Y]Z
Non-OR Ø9P[H,J][7,8][Ø,D,Y]Z
Non-OR Ø9PK[Ø,3,4,7,8][Ø,7,D,J,K,Y]Z
Non-OR Ø9P[H,J]X[Ø,7,D,J,K]Z
Non-OR Ø9PKX[Ø,7,D,J,K]Z
Non-OR Ø9PY[3,4]YZ
Non-OR Ø9PY[7,8]YZ
Non-OR Ø9PYXØZ

Ø Medical and Surgical
9 Ear, Nose, Sinus
Q Repair Definition: Restoring, to the extent possible, a body part to its normal anatomic structure and function
Explanation: Used only when the method to accomplish the repair is not one of the other root operations

Body Part Character 4		Approach Character 5	Device Character 6	Qualifier Character 7
Ø External Ear, Right Antihelix Antitragus Auricle Earlobe Helix Pinna Tragus	**1 External Ear, Left** *See Ø External Ear, Right* **2 External Ear, Bilateral** *See Ø External Ear, Right*	**Ø Open** **3 Percutaneous** **4 Percutaneous Endoscopic** **X External**	**Z No Device**	**Z No Qualifier**
3 External Auditory Canal, Right External auditory meatus **4 External Auditory Canal, Left** *See 3 External Auditory Canal, Right*	**F Eustachian Tube, Right** Auditory tube Pharyngotympanic tube **G Eustachian Tube, Left** *See F Eustachian Tube, Right*	**Ø Open** **3 Percutaneous** **4 Percutaneous Endoscopic** **7 Via Natural or Artificial Opening** **8 Via Natural or Artificial Opening Endoscopic** **X External**	**Z No Device**	**Z No Qualifier**
5 Middle Ear, Right Oval window Tympanic cavity **6 Middle Ear, Left** *See 5 Middle Ear, Right* **9 Auditory Ossicle, Right** Incus Malleus Stapes	**A Auditory Ossicle, Left** *See 9 Auditory Ossicle, Right* **D Inner Ear, Right** Bony labyrinth Bony vestibule Cochlea Round window Semicircular canal **E Inner Ear, Left** *See D Inner Ear, Right*	**Ø Open** **8 Via Natural or Artificial Opening Endoscopic**	**Z No Device**	**Z No Qualifier**
7 Tympanic Membrane, Right Pars flaccida **8 Tympanic Membrane, Left** *See 7 Tympanic Membrane, Right* **L Nasal Turbinate** Inferior turbinate Middle turbinate Nasal concha Superior turbinate	**N Nasopharynx** Choana Fossa of Rosenmuller Pharyngeal recess Rhinopharynx	**Ø Open** **3 Percutaneous** **4 Percutaneous Endoscopic** **7 Via Natural or Artificial Opening** **8 Via Natural or Artificial Opening Endoscopic**	**Z No Device**	**Z No Qualifier**
B Mastoid Sinus, Right Mastoid air cells **C Mastoid Sinus, Left** *See B Mastoid Sinus, Right* **M Nasal Septum** Quadrangular cartilage Septal cartilage Vomer bone **P Accessory Sinus** **Q Maxillary Sinus, Right** Antrum of Highmore	**R Maxillary Sinus, Left** *See Q Maxillary Sinus, Right* **S Frontal Sinus, Right** **T Frontal Sinus, Left** **U Ethmoid Sinus, Right** Ethmoidal air cell **V Ethmoid Sinus, Left** *See U Ethmoid Sinus, Right* **W Sphenoid Sinus, Right** **X Sphenoid Sinus, Left**	**Ø Open** **3 Percutaneous** **4 Percutaneous Endoscopic** **8 Via Natural or Artificial Opening Endoscopic**	**Z No Device**	**Z No Qualifier**
K Nasal Mucosa and Soft Tissue Columella External naris Greater alar cartilage Internal naris Lateral nasal cartilage Lesser alar cartilage Nasal cavity Nostril		**Ø Open** **3 Percutaneous** **4 Percutaneous Endoscopic** **8 Via Natural or Artificial Opening Endoscopic** **X External**	**Z No Device**	**Z No Qualifier**

Non-OR Ø9Q[Ø,1,2]XZZ
Non-OR Ø9Q[3,4]XZZ
Non-OR Ø9Q[F,G][Ø,3,4,7,8,X]ZZ
Non-OR Ø9QKXZZ

Ø Medical and Surgical
9 Ear, Nose, Sinus
R Replacement Definition: Putting in or on biological or synthetic material that physically takes the place and/or function of all or a portion of a body part

Explanation: The body part may have been taken out or replaced, or may be taken out, physically eradicated, or rendered nonfunctional during the REPLACEMENT procedure. A REMOVAL procedure is coded for taking out the device used in a previous replacement procedure.

Body Part Character 4	Approach Character 5	Device Character 6	Qualifier Character 7
Ø External Ear, Right Antihelix Antitragus Auricle Earlobe Helix Pinna Tragus **1 External Ear, Left** *See Ø External Ear, Right* **2 External Ear, Bilateral** *See Ø External Ear, Right* **K Nasal Mucosa and Soft Tissue** Columella External naris Greater alar cartilage Internal naris Lateral nasal cartilage Lesser alar cartilage Nasal cavity Nostril	**Ø Open** **X External**	**7 Autologous Tissue Substitute** **J Synthetic Substitute** **K Nonautologous Tissue Substitute**	**Z No Qualifier**
5 Middle Ear, Right Oval window Tympanic cavity **6 Middle Ear, Left** *See 5 Middle Ear, Right* **9 Auditory Ossicle, Right** Incus Malleus Stapes **A Auditory Ossicle, Left** *See 9 Auditory Ossicle, Right* **D Inner Ear, Right** Bony labyrinth Bony vestibule Cochlea Round window Semicircular canal **E Inner Ear, Left** *See D Inner Ear, Right*	**Ø Open**	**7 Autologous Tissue Substitute** **J Synthetic Substitute** **K Nonautologous Tissue Substitute**	**Z No Qualifier**
7 Tympanic Membrane, Right Pars flaccida **8 Tympanic Membrane, Left** *See 7 Tympanic Membrane, Right* **N Nasopharynx** Choana Fossa of Rosenmuller Pharyngeal recess Rhinopharynx	**Ø Open** **7 Via Natural or Artificial Opening** **8 Via Natural or Artificial Opening Endoscopic**	**7 Autologous Tissue Substitute** **J Synthetic Substitute** **K Nonautologous Tissue Substitute**	**Z No Qualifier**
L Nasal Turbinate Inferior turbinate Middle turbinate Nasal concha Superior turbinate	**Ø Open** **3 Percutaneous** **4 Percutaneous Endoscopic** **7 Via Natural or Artificial Opening** **8 Via Natural or Artificial Opening Endoscopic**	**7 Autologous Tissue Substitute** **J Synthetic Substitute** **K Nonautologous Tissue Substitute**	**Z No Qualifier**
M Nasal Septum Quadrangular cartilage Septal cartilage Vomer bone	**Ø Open** **3 Percutaneous** **4 Percutaneous Endoscopic**	**7 Autologous Tissue Substitute** **J Synthetic Substitute** **K Nonautologous Tissue Substitute**	**Z No Qualifier**

Ø Medical and Surgical
9 Ear, Nose, Sinus
S Reposition Definition: Moving to its normal location, or other suitable location, all or a portion of a body part

Explanation: The body part is moved to a new location from an abnormal location, or from a normal location where it is not functioning correctly. The body part may or may not be cut out or off to be moved to the new location.

Body Part Character 4	Approach Character 5	Device Character 6	Qualifier Character 7
Ø External Ear, Right Antihelix Antitragus Auricle Earlobe Helix Pinna Tragus **1 External Ear, Left** *See Ø External Ear, Right* **2 External Ear, Bilateral** *See Ø External Ear, Right* **K Nasal Mucosa and Soft Tissue** Columella External naris Greater alar cartilage Internal naris Lateral nasal cartilage Lesser alar cartilage Nasal cavity Nostril	**Ø Open** **4 Percutaneous Endoscopic** **X External**	**Z No Device**	**Z No Qualifier**
7 Tympanic Membrane, Right Pars flaccida **8 Tympanic Membrane, Left** *See 7 Tympanic Membrane, Right* **F Eustachian Tube, Right** Auditory tube Pharyngotympanic tube **G Eustachian Tube, Left** *See F Eustachian Tube, Right* **L Nasal Turbinate** Inferior turbinate Middle turbinate Nasal concha Superior turbinate	**Ø Open** **4 Percutaneous Endoscopic** **7 Via Natural or Artificial Opening** **8 Via Natural or Artificial Opening Endoscopic**	**Z No Device**	**Z No Qualifier**
9 Auditory Ossicle, Right Incus Malleus Stapes **A Auditory Ossicle, Left** *See 9 Auditory Ossicle, Right* **M Nasal Septum** Quadrangular cartilage Septal cartilage Vomer bone	**Ø Open** **4 Percutaneous Endoscopic**	**Z No Device**	**Z No Qualifier**

Non-OR Ø9S[F,G][Ø,4,7,8]ZZ

Ø Medical and Surgical
9 Ear, Nose, Sinus
T Resection Definition: Cutting out or off, without replacement, all of a body part

Explanation: None

Body Part Character 4		Approach Character 5	Device Character 6	Qualifier Character 7
Ø External Ear, Right Antihelix Antitragus Auricle Earlobe Helix Pinna Tragus	**1 External Ear, Left** *See Ø External Ear, Right*	**Ø Open** **4 Percutaneous Endoscopic** **X External**	**Z No Device**	**Z No Qualifier**
5 Middle Ear, Right Oval window Tympanic cavity **6 Middle Ear, Left** *See 5 Middle Ear, Right* **9 Auditory Ossicle, Right** Incus Malleus Stapes	**A Auditory Ossicle, Left** *See 9 Auditory Ossicle, Right* **D Inner Ear, Right** Bony labyrinth Bony vestibule Cochlea Round window Semicircular canal **E Inner Ear, Left** *See D Inner Ear, Right*	**Ø Open** **8 Via Natural or Artificial Opening Endoscopic**	**Z No Device**	**Z No Qualifier**
7 Tympanic Membrane, Right Pars flaccida **8 Tympanic Membrane, Left** *See 7 Tympanic Membrane, Right* **F Eustachian Tube, Right** Auditory tube Pharyngotympanic tube **G Eustachian Tube, Left** *See F Eustachian Tube, Right*	**L Nasal Turbinate** Inferior turbinate Middle turbinate Nasal concha Superior turbinate **N Nasopharynx** Choana Fossa of Rosenmuller Pharyngeal recess Rhinopharynx	**Ø Open** **4 Percutaneous Endoscopic** **7 Via Natural or Artificial Opening** **8 Via Natural or Artificial Opening Endoscopic**	**Z No Device**	**Z No Qualifier**
B Mastoid Sinus, Right Mastoid air cells **C Mastoid Sinus, Left** *See B Mastoid Sinus, Right* **M Nasal Septum** Quadrangular cartilage Septal cartilage Vomer bone **P Accessory Sinus** **Q Maxillary Sinus, Right** Antrum of Highmore	**R Maxillary Sinus, Left** *See Q Maxillary Sinus, Right* **S Frontal Sinus, Right** **T Frontal Sinus, Left** **U Ethmoid Sinus, Right** Ethmoidal air cell **V Ethmoid Sinus, Left** *See U Ethmoid Sinus, Right* **W Sphenoid Sinus, Right** **X Sphenoid Sinus, Left**	**Ø Open** **4 Percutaneous Endoscopic** **8 Via Natural or Artificial Opening Endoscopic**	**Z No Device**	**Z No Qualifier**
K Nasal Mucosa and Soft Tissue Columella External naris Greater alar cartilage Internal naris Lateral nasal cartilage Lesser alar cartilage Nasal cavity Nostril		**Ø Open** **4 Percutaneous Endoscopic** **8 Via Natural or Artificial Opening Endoscopic** **X External**	**Z No Device**	**Z No Qualifier**

Non-OR Ø9T[F,G][Ø,4,7,8]ZZ

Ø Medical and Surgical
9 Ear, Nose, Sinus
U Supplement Definition: Putting in or on biological or synthetic material that physically reinforces and/or augments the function of a portion of a body part

Explanation: The biological material is non-living, or is living and from the same individual. The body part may have been previously replaced, and the SUPPLEMENT procedure is performed to physically reinforce and/or augment the function of the replaced body part.

Body Part Character 4		Approach Character 5	Device Character 6	Qualifier Character 7
Ø External Ear, Right Antihelix Antitragus Auricle Earlobe Helix Pinna Tragus	**1 External Ear, Left** *See Ø External Ear, Right* **2 External Ear, Bilateral** *See Ø External Ear, Right*	**Ø Open** **X External**	**7 Autologous Tissue Substitute** **J Synthetic Substitute** **K Nonautologous Tissue Substitute**	**Z No Qualifier**
5 Middle Ear, Right Oval window Tympanic cavity **6 Middle Ear, Left** *See 5 Middle Ear, Right* **9 Auditory Ossicle, Right** Incus Malleus Stapes **A Auditory Ossicle, Left** *See 9 Auditory Ossicle, Right*	**D Inner Ear, Right** Bony labyrinth Bony vestibule Cochlea Round window Semicircular canal **E Inner Ear, Left** *See D Inner Ear, Right*	**Ø Open** **8 Via Natural or Artificial Opening Endoscopic**	**7 Autologous Tissue Substitute** **J Synthetic Substitute** **K Nonautologous Tissue Substitute**	**Z No Qualifier**
7 Tympanic Membrane, Right Pars flaccida **8 Tympanic Membrane, Left** *See 7 Tympanic Membrane, Right*	**N Nasopharynx** Choana Fossa of Rosenmuller Pharyngeal recess Rhinopharynx	**Ø Open** **7 Via Natural or Artificial Opening** **8 Via Natural or Artificial Opening Endoscopic**	**7 Autologous Tissue Substitute** **J Synthetic Substitute** **K Nonautologous Tissue Substitute**	**Z No Qualifier**
B Mastoid Sinus, Right Mastoid air cells **C Mastoid Sinus, Left** *See B Mastoid Sinus, Right* **L Nasal Turbinate** Inferior turbinate Middle turbinate Nasal concha Superior turbinate **P Accessory Sinus** **Q Maxillary Sinus, Right** Antrum of Highmore	**R Maxillary Sinus, Left** *See Q Maxillary Sinus, Right* **S Frontal Sinus, Right** **T Frontal Sinus, Left** **U Ethmoid Sinus, Right** Ethmoidal air cell **V Ethmoid Sinus, Left** *See U Ethmoid Sinus, Right* **W Sphenoid Sinus, Right** **X Sphenoid Sinus, Left**	**Ø Open** **3 Percutaneous** **4 Percutaneous Endoscopic** **7 Via Natural or Artificial Opening** **8 Via Natural or Artificial Opening Endoscopic**	**7 Autologous Tissue Substitute** **J Synthetic Substitute** **K Nonautologous Tissue Substitute**	**Z No Qualifier**
K Nasal Mucosa and Soft Tissue Columella External naris Greater alar cartilage Internal naris Lateral nasal cartilage Lesser alar cartilage Nasal cavity Nostril		**Ø Open** **8 Via Natural or Artificial Opening Endoscopic** **X External**	**7 Autologous Tissue Substitute** **J Synthetic Substitute** **K Nonautologous Tissue Substitute**	**Z No Qualifier**
M Nasal Septum Quadrangular cartilage Septal cartilage Vomer bone		**Ø Open** **3 Percutaneous** **4 Percutaneous Endoscopic** **8 Via Natural or Artificial Opening Endoscopic**	**7 Autologous Tissue Substitute** **J Synthetic Substitute** **K Nonautologous Tissue Substitute**	**Z No Qualifier**

Ø Medical and Surgical
9 Ear, Nose, Sinus
W Revision Definition: Correcting, to the extent possible, a portion of a malfunctioning device or the position of a displaced device

Explanation: Revision can include correcting a malfunctioning or displaced device by taking out or putting in components of the device such as a screw or pin

Body Part Character 4	Approach Character 5	Device Character 6	Qualifier Character 7
7 Tympanic Membrane, Right Pars flaccida **8 Tympanic Membrane, Left** *See 7 Tympanic Membrane, Right* **9 Auditory Ossicle, Right** Incus Malleus Stapes **A Auditory Ossicle, Left** *See 9 Auditory Ossicle, Right*	**Ø Open** **7 Via Natural or Artificial Opening** **8 Via Natural or Artificial Opening Endoscopic**	**7 Autologous Tissue Substitute** **J Synthetic Substitute** **K Nonautologous Tissue Substitute**	**Z No Qualifier**
D Inner Ear, Right Bony labyrinth Bony vestibule Cochlea Round window Semicircular canal **E Inner Ear, Left** *See D Inner Ear, Right*	**Ø Open** **7 Via Natural or Artificial Opening** **8 Via Natural or Artificial Opening Endoscopic**	**S Hearing Device**	**Z No Qualifier**
H Ear, Right **J Ear, Left** **K Nasal Mucosa and Soft Tissue** Columella External naris Greater alar cartilage Internal naris Lateral nasal cartilage Lesser alar cartilage Nasal cavity Nostril	**Ø Open** **3 Percutaneous** **4 Percutaneous Endoscopic** **7 Via Natural or Artificial Opening** **8 Via Natural or Artificial Opening Endoscopic**	**Ø Drainage Device** **7 Autologous Tissue Substitute** **D Intraluminal Device** **J Synthetic Substitute** **K Nonautologous Tissue Substitute** **Y Other Device**	**Z No Qualifier**
H Ear, Right **J Ear, Left** **K Nasal Mucosa and Soft Tissue** Columella External naris Greater alar cartilage Internal naris Lateral nasal cartilage Lesser alar cartilage Nasal cavity Nostril	**X External**	**Ø Drainage Device** **7 Autologous Tissue Substitute** **D Intraluminal Device** **J Synthetic Substitute** **K Nonautologous Tissue Substitute**	**Z No Qualifier**
Y Sinus	**Ø Open** **3 Percutaneous** **4 Percutaneous Endoscopic**	**Ø Drainage Device** **Y Other Device**	**Z No Qualifier**
Y Sinus	**7 Via Natural or Artificial Opening** **8 Via Natural or Artificial Opening Endoscopic**	**Y Other Device**	**Z No Qualifier**
Y Sinus	**X External**	**Ø Drainage Device**	**Z No Qualifier**

Non-OR Ø9W[H,J][3,4][J,K,Y]Z
Non-OR Ø9W[H,J][7,8][D,Y]Z
Non-OR Ø9WK[Ø,3,4,7,8][Ø,7,D,J,K,Y]Z
Non-OR Ø9W[H,J,K]X[Ø,7,D,J,K]Z
Non-OR Ø9WY[3,4]YZ
Non-OR Ø9WY[7,8]YZ
Non-OR Ø9WYXØZ

Respiratory System ØB1–ØBY

Character Meanings

This Character Meaning table is provided as a guide to assist the user in the identification of character members that may be found in this section of code tables. It **SHOULD NOT** be used to build a PCS code.

Operation–Character 3	Body Part–Character 4	Approach–Character 5	Device–Character 6	Qualifier–Character 7
1 Bypass	Ø Tracheobronchial Tree	Ø Open	Ø Drainage Device	Ø Allogeneic
2 Change	1 Trachea	3 Percutaneous	1 Radioactive Element	1 Syngeneic
5 Destruction	2 Carina	4 Percutaneous Endoscopic	2 Monitoring Device	2 Zooplastic
7 Dilation	3 Main Bronchus, Right	7 Via Natural or Artificial Opening	3 Infusion Device	4 Cutaneous
9 Drainage	4 Upper Lobe Bronchus, Right	8 Via Natural or Artificial Opening Endoscopic	7 Autologous Tissue Substitute	6 Esophagus
B Excision	5 Middle Lobe Bronchus, Right	X External	C Extraluminal Device	X Diagnostic
C Extirpation	6 Lower Lobe Bronchus, Right		D Intraluminal Device	Z No Qualifier
D Extraction	7 Main Bronchus, Left		E Intraluminal Device, Endotracheal Airway	
F Fragmentation	8 Upper Lobe Bronchus, Left		F Tracheostomy Device	
H Insertion	9 Lingula Bronchus		G Intraluminal Device, Endobronchial Valve	
J Inspection	B Lower Lobe Bronchus, Left		J Synthetic Substitute	
L Occlusion	C Upper Lung Lobe, Right		K Nonautologous Tissue Substitute	
M Reattachment	D Middle Lung Lobe, Right		M Diaphragmatic Pacemaker Lead	
N Release	F Lower Lung Lobe, Right		Y Other Device	
P Removal	G Upper Lung Lobe, Left		Z No Device	
Q Repair	H Lung Lingula			
R Replacement	J Lower Lung Lobe, Left			
S Reposition	K Lung, Right			
T Resection	L Lung, Left			
U Supplement	M Lungs, Bilateral			
V Restriction	N Pleura, Right			
W Revision	P Pleura, Left			
Y Transplantation	Q Pleura			
	T Diaphragm			

AHA Coding Clinic for table ØB5
2016, 2Q, 17 Photodynamic therapy for treatment of malignant mesothelioma
2015, 2Q, 31 Thoracoscopic talc pleurodesis

AHA Coding Clinic for table ØB9
2017, 3Q, 15 Bronchoscopy with suctioning for removal of retained secretions
2017, 1Q, 51 Bronchoalveolar lavage
2016, 1Q, 26 Bronchoalveolar lavage, endobronchial biopsy and transbronchial biopsy
2016, 1Q, 27 Fiberoptic bronchoscopy with brushings and bronchoalveolar lavage

AHA Coding Clinic for table ØBB
2016, 1Q, 26 Bronchoalveolar lavage, endobronchial biopsy and transbronchial biopsy
2016, 1Q, 27 Fiberoptic bronchoscopy with brushings and bronchoalveolar lavage
2014, 1Q, 20 Fiducial marker placement

AHA Coding Clinic for table ØBC
2017, 3Q, 14 Bronchoscopy with suctioning and washings for removal of mucus plug

AHA Coding Clinic for table ØBD
2018, 3Q, 28 Lung decortication for empyema

AHA Coding Clinic for table ØBH
2019, 3Q, 33 Insertion of endobronchial valve
2014, 4Q, 3-10 Mechanical ventilation

AHA Coding Clinic for table ØBJ
2015, 2Q, 31 Thoracoscopic talc pleurodesis
2014, 1Q, 20 Fiducial marker placement

AHA Coding Clinic for table ØBL
2019, 3Q, 33 Insertion of endobronchial valve

AHA Coding Clinic for table ØBN
2019, 2Q, 20 Pericardiectomy for constrictive pericarditis
2018, 3Q, 28 Lung decortication
2018, 3Q, 28 Lung decortication for empyema
2015, 3Q, 15 Vascular ring surgery with release of esophagus and trachea

AHA Coding Clinic for table ØBQ
2016, 2Q, 22 Esophageal lengthening Collis gastroplasty with Nissen fundoplication and hiatal hernia
2014, 3Q, 28 Laparoscopic Nissen fundoplication and diaphragmatic hernia repair

AHA Coding Clinic for table ØBU
2015, 1Q, 28 Repair of bronchopleural fistula using omental pedicle graft

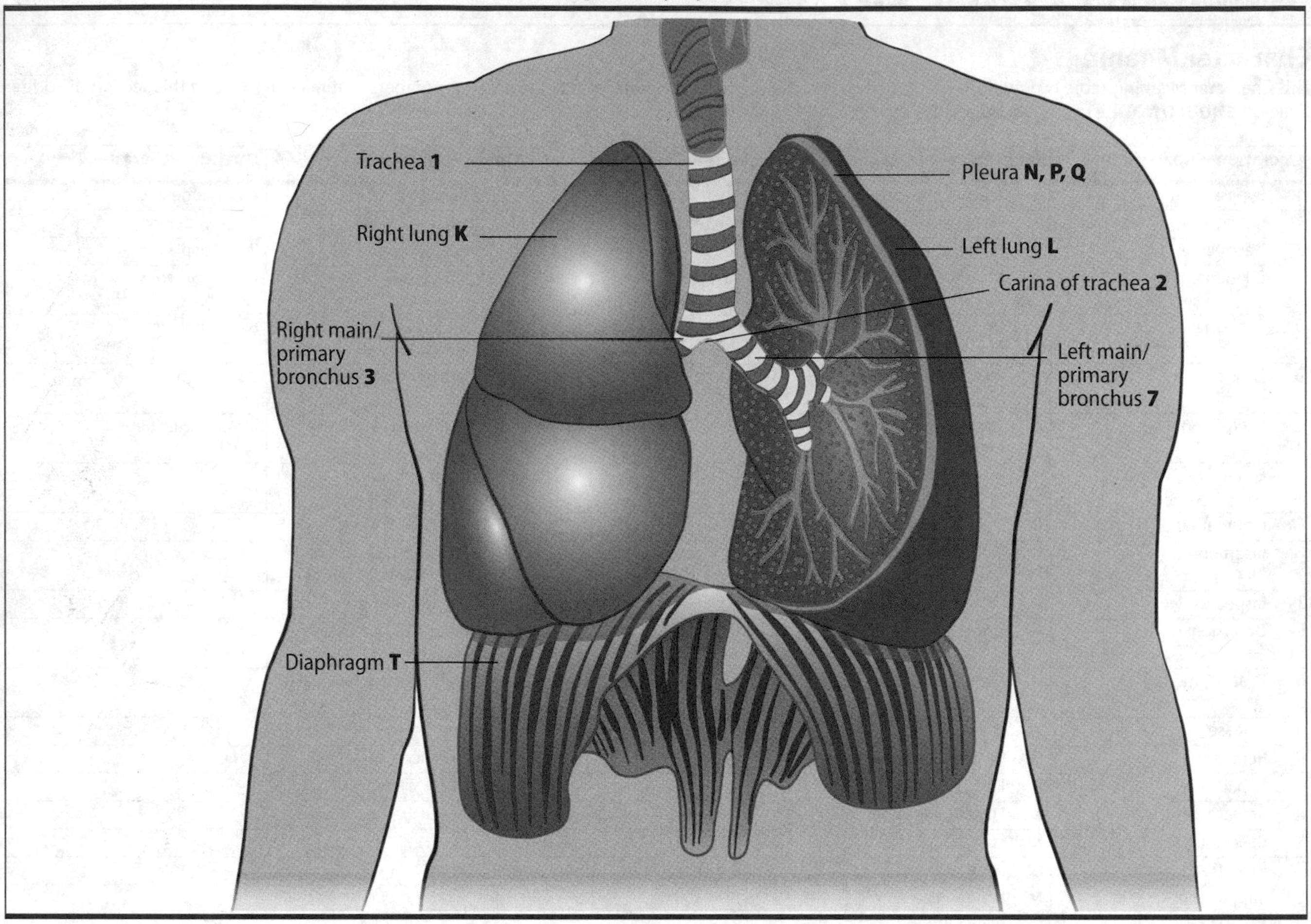

Respiratory System

Trachea **1**
Pleura **N, P, Q**
Right lung **K**
Left lung **L**
Carina of trachea **2**
Right main/
primary
bronchus **3**
Left main/
primary
bronchus **7**
Diaphragm **T**

Right Lung Bronchi

Right lung **K**
R. main
bronchus **3**
Trachea **1**
R. upper lobe
bronchus **4**
Tracheobronchial tree **Ø**
R. middle lobe
bronchus **5**
Carini **2**
R. lower lobe
bronchus **6**

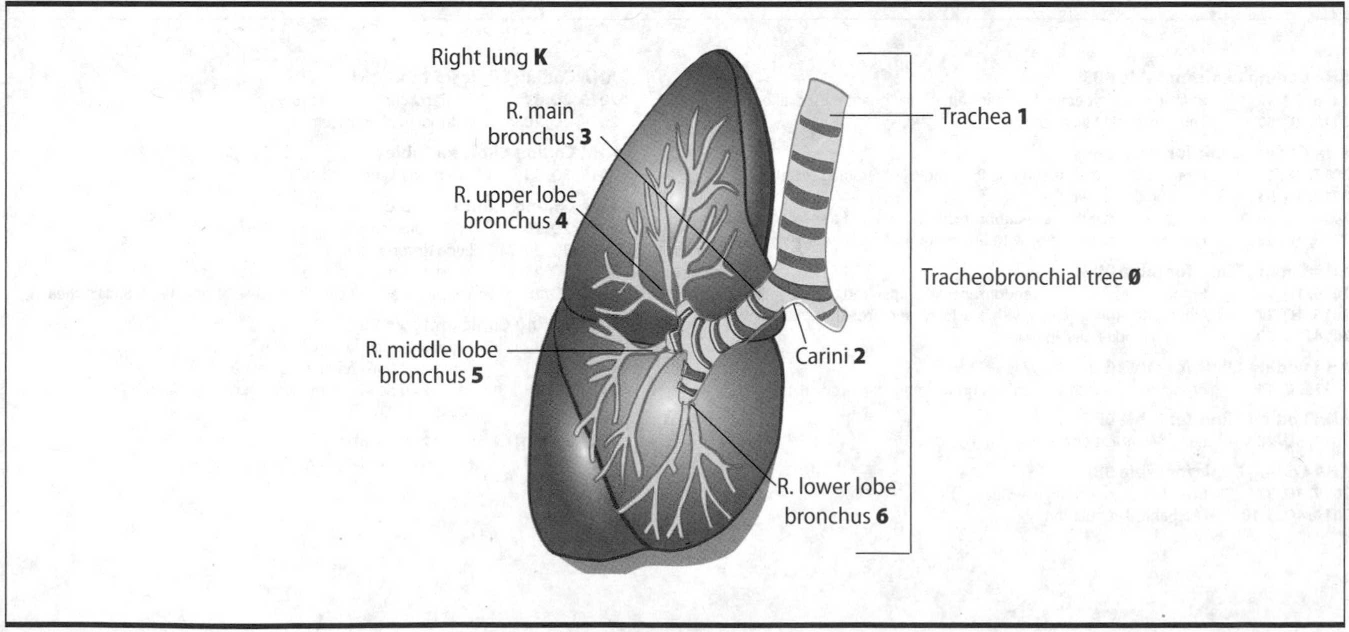

Ø Medical and Surgical
B Respiratory System
1 Bypass Definition: Altering the route of passage of the contents of a tubular body part

Explanation: Rerouting contents of a body part to a downstream area of the normal route, to a similar route and body part, or to an abnormal route and dissimilar body part. Includes one or more anastomoses, with or without the use of a device.

Body Part Character 4	Approach Character 5	Device Character 6	Qualifier Character 7
1 Trachea Cricoid cartilage	Ø Open	D Intraluminal Device	6 Esophagus
1 Trachea Cricoid cartilage	Ø Open	F Tracheostomy Device Z No Device	4 Cutaneous
1 Trachea Cricoid cartilage	3 Percutaneous 4 Percutaneous Endoscopic	F Tracheostomy Device Z No Device	4 Cutaneous

DRG Non-OR ØB113[F,Z]4
Non-OR ØB11ØD6

Ø Medical and Surgical
B Respiratory System
2 Change Definition: Taking out or off a device from a body part and putting back an identical or similar device in or on the same body part without cutting or puncturing the skin or a mucous membrane

Explanation: All CHANGE procedures are coded using the approach EXTERNAL

Body Part Character 4	Approach Character 5	Device Character 6	Qualifier Character 7
Ø Tracheobronchial Tree K Lung, Right L Lung, Left Q Pleura T Diaphragm	X External	Ø Drainage Device Y Other Device	Z No Qualifier
1 Trachea Cricoid cartilage	X External	Ø Drainage Device E Intraluminal Device, Endotracheal Airway F Tracheostomy Device Y Other Device	Z No Qualifier

Non-OR All body part, approach, device, and qualifier values

Ø Medical and Surgical
B Respiratory System
5 Destruction Definition: Physical eradication of all or a portion of a body part by the direct use of energy, force, or a destructive agent

Explanation: None of the body part is physically taken out

Body Part Character 4	Approach Character 5	Device Character 6	Qualifier Character 7
1 Trachea Cricoid cartilage 2 Carina 3 Main Bronchus, Right Bronchus intermedius Intermediate bronchus 4 Upper Lobe Bronchus, Right 5 Middle Lobe Bronchus, Right 6 Lower Lobe Bronchus, Right 7 Main Bronchus, Left 8 Upper Lobe Bronchus, Left 9 Lingula Bronchus B Lower Lobe Bronchus, Left C Upper Lung Lobe, Right D Middle Lung Lobe, Right F Lower Lung Lobe, Right G Upper Lung Lobe, Left H Lung Lingula J Lower Lung Lobe, Left K Lung, Right L Lung, Left M Lungs, Bilateral	Ø Open 3 Percutaneous 4 Percutaneous Endoscopic 7 Via Natural or Artificial Opening 8 Via Natural or Artificial Opening Endoscopic	Z No Device	Z No Qualifier
N Pleura, Right P Pleura, Left T Diaphragm	Ø Open 3 Percutaneous 4 Percutaneous Endoscopic	Z No Device	Z No Qualifier

Non-OR ØB5[3,4,5,6,7,8,9,B][4,8]ZZ
Non-OR ØB5[C,D,F,G,H,J,K,L,M]8ZZ

Ø Medical and Surgical
B Respiratory System
7 Dilation Definition: Expanding an orifice or the lumen of a tubular body part

Explanation: The orifice can be a natural orifice or an artificially created orifice. Accomplished by stretching a tubular body part using intraluminal pressure or by cutting part of the orifice or wall of the tubular body part.

Body Part Character 4	Approach Character 5	Device Character 6	Qualifier Character 7
1 Trachea Cricoid cartilage 2 Carina 3 Main Bronchus, Right Bronchus intermedius Intermediate bronchus 4 Upper Lobe Bronchus, Right 5 Middle Lobe Bronchus, Right 6 Lower Lobe Bronchus, Right 7 Main Bronchus, Left 8 Upper Lobe Bronchus, Left 9 Lingula Bronchus B Lower Lobe Bronchus, Left	Ø Open 3 Percutaneous 4 Percutaneous Endoscopic 7 Via Natural or Artificial Opening 8 Via Natural or Artificial Opening Endoscopic	D Intraluminal Device Z No Device	Z No Qualifier

Non-OR ØB7[3,4,5,6,7,8,9,B][Ø,3,4,7,8][D,Z]Z

Ø Medical and Surgical
B Respiratory System
9 Drainage Definition: Taking or letting out fluids and/or gases from a body part

Explanation: The qualifier DIAGNOSTIC is used to identify drainage procedures that are biopsies

Body Part Character 4	Approach Character 5	Device Character 6	Qualifier Character 7
1 Trachea Cricoid cartilage 2 Carina 3 Main Bronchus, Right Bronchus intermedius Intermediate bronchus 4 Upper Lobe Bronchus, Right 5 Middle Lobe Bronchus, Right 6 Lower Lobe Bronchus, Right 7 Main Bronchus, Left 8 Upper Lobe Bronchus, Left 9 Lingula Bronchus B Lower Lobe Bronchus, Left C Upper Lung Lobe, Right D Middle Lung Lobe, Right F Lower Lung Lobe, Right G Upper Lung Lobe, Left H Lung Lingula J Lower Lung Lobe, Left K Lung, Right L Lung, Left M Lungs, Bilateral	Ø Open 3 Percutaneous 4 Percutaneous Endoscopic 7 Via Natural or Artificial Opening 8 Via Natural or Artificial Opening Endoscopic	Ø Drainage Device	Z No Qualifier
1 Trachea Cricoid cartilage 2 Carina 3 Main Bronchus, Right Bronchus intermedius Intermediate bronchus 4 Upper Lobe Bronchus, Right 5 Middle Lobe Bronchus, Right 6 Lower Lobe Bronchus, Right 7 Main Bronchus, Left 8 Upper Lobe Bronchus, Left 9 Lingula Bronchus B Lower Lobe Bronchus, Left C Upper Lung Lobe, Right D Middle Lung Lobe, Right F Lower Lung Lobe, Right G Upper Lung Lobe, Left H Lung Lingula J Lower Lung Lobe, Left K Lung, Right L Lung, Left M Lungs, Bilateral	Ø Open 3 Percutaneous 4 Percutaneous Endoscopic 7 Via Natural or Artificial Opening 8 Via Natural or Artificial Opening Endoscopic	Z No Device	X Diagnostic Z No Qualifier
N Pleura, Right P Pleura, Left	Ø Open 3 Percutaneous 4 Percutaneous Endoscopic 8 Via Natural or Artificial Opening Endoscopic	Ø Drainage Device	Z No Qualifier
N Pleura, Right P Pleura, Left	Ø Open 3 Percutaneous 4 Percutaneous Endoscopic 8 Via Natural or Artificial Opening Endoscopic	Z No Device	X Diagnostic Z No Qualifier
T Diaphragm	Ø Open 3 Percutaneous 4 Percutaneous Endoscopic	Ø Drainage Device	Z No Qualifier
T Diaphragm	Ø Open 3 Percutaneous 4 Percutaneous Endoscopic	Z No Device	X Diagnostic Z No Qualifier

Non-OR ØB9[1,2,3,4,5,6,7,8,9,B][7,8]ØZ
Non-OR ØB9[1,2,3,4,5,6,7,8,9,B][3,4]ZX
Non-OR ØB9[1,2,3,4,5,6,7,8,9,B][7,8]Z[X,Z]
Non-OR ØB9[C,D,F,G,H,J,K,L,M][3,4,7]ZX
Non-OR ØB9[C,D,F,G,H,J,K,L,M]8Z[X,Z]
Non-OR ØB9[N,P][Ø,3,8]ØZ
Non-OR ØB9[N,P][Ø,3,8]Z[X,Z]
Non-OR ØB9[N,P]4ZX
Non-OR ØB9T[3,4]ØZ
Non-OR ØB9T[3,4]Z[X,Z]

Ø Medical and Surgical
B Respiratory System
B Excision Definition: Cutting out or off, without replacement, a portion of a body part

Explanation: The qualifier DIAGNOSTIC is used to identify excision procedures that are biopsies

Body Part Character 4	Approach Character 5	Device Character 6	Qualifier Character 7
1 Trachea Cricoid cartilage **2 Carina** **3 Main Bronchus, Right** Bronchus intermedius Intermediate bronchus **4 Upper Lobe Bronchus, Right** **5 Middle Lobe Bronchus, Right** **6 Lower Lobe Bronchus, Right** **7 Main Bronchus, Left** **8 Upper Lobe Bronchus, Left** **9 Lingula Bronchus** **B Lower Lobe Bronchus, Left** **C Upper Lung Lobe, Right** **D Middle Lung Lobe, Right** **F Lower Lung Lobe, Right** **G Upper Lung Lobe, Left** **H Lung Lingula** **J Lower Lung Lobe, Left** **K Lung, Right** **L Lung, Left** **M Lungs, Bilateral**	**Ø Open** **3 Percutaneous** **4 Percutaneous Endoscopic** **7 Via Natural or Artificial Opening** **8 Via Natural or Artificial Opening Endoscopic**	**Z No Device**	**X Diagnostic** **Z No Qualifier**
N Pleura, Right **P Pleura, Left**	**Ø Open** **3 Percutaneous** **4 Percutaneous Endoscopic** **8 Via Natural or Artificial Opening Endoscopic**	**Z No Device**	**X Diagnostic** **Z No Qualifier**
T Diaphragm	**Ø Open** **3 Percutaneous** **4 Percutaneous Endoscopic**	**Z No Device**	**X Diagnostic** **Z No Qualifier**

Non-OR ØBB[1,2,3,4,5,6,7,8,9,B][3,4,7,8]ZX
Non-OR ØBB[3,4,5,6,7,8,9,B,M][4,8]ZZ
Non-OR ØBB[C,D,F,G,H,J,K,L,M]3ZX
Non-OR ØBB[C,D,F,G,H,J,K,L]8ZZ
Non-OR ØBB[N,P][Ø,3]ZX

Ø Medical and Surgical
B Respiratory System
C Extirpation Definition: Taking or cutting out solid matter from a body part

Explanation: The solid matter may be an abnormal byproduct of a biological function or a foreign body; it may be imbedded in a body part or in the lumen of a tubular body part. The solid matter may or may not have been previously broken into pieces.

Body Part Character 4	Approach Character 5	Device Character 6	Qualifier Character 7
1 Trachea Cricoid cartilage **2 Carina** **3 Main Bronchus, Right** Bronchus intermedius Intermediate bronchus **4 Upper Lobe Bronchus, Right** **5 Middle Lobe Bronchus, Right** **6 Lower Lobe Bronchus, Right** **7 Main Bronchus, Left** **8 Upper Lobe Bronchus, Left** **9 Lingula Bronchus** **B Lower Lobe Bronchus, Left** **C Upper Lung Lobe, Right** **D Middle Lung Lobe, Right** **F Lower Lung Lobe, Right** **G Upper Lung Lobe, Left** **H Lung Lingula** **J Lower Lung Lobe, Left** **K Lung, Right** **L Lung, Left** **M Lungs, Bilateral**	**Ø Open** **3 Percutaneous** **4 Percutaneous Endoscopic** **7 Via Natural or Artificial Opening** **8 Via Natural or Artificial Opening Endoscopic**	**Z No Device**	**Z No Qualifier**
N Pleura, Right **P Pleura, Left** **T Diaphragm**	**Ø Open** **3 Percutaneous** **4 Percutaneous Endoscopic**	**Z No Device**	**Z No Qualifier**

Non-OR ØBC[1,2,3,4,5,6,7,8,9,B][7,8]ZZ
Non-OR ØBC[N,P]3ZZ

Ø Medical and Surgical
B Respiratory System
D Extraction Definition: Pulling or stripping out or off all or a portion of a body part by the use of force

Explanation: The qualifier DIAGNOSTIC is used to identify extraction procedures that are biopsies

Body Part Character 4	Approach Character 5	Device Character 6	Qualifier Character 7
1 Trachea Cricoid cartilage 2 Carina 3 Main Bronchus, Right Bronchus intermedius Intermediate bronchus 4 Upper Lobe Bronchus, Right 5 Middle Lobe Bronchus, Right 6 Lower Lobe Bronchus, Right 7 Main Bronchus, Left 8 Upper Lobe Bronchus, Left 9 Lingula Bronchus B Lower Lobe Bronchus, Left C Upper Lung Lobe, Right D Middle Lung Lobe, Right F Lower Lung Lobe, Right G Upper Lung Lobe, Left H Lung Lingula J Lower Lung Lobe, Left K Lung, Right L Lung, Left M Lungs, Bilateral	4 Percutaneous Endoscopic 8 Via Natural or Artificial Opening Endoscopic	Z No Device	X Diagnostic
N Pleura, Right P Pleura, Left	Ø Open 3 Percutaneous 4 Percutaneous Endoscopic	Z No Device	X Diagnostic Z No Qualifier

Non-OR ØBD[1,2,3,4,5,6,7,8,9,B,C,D,F,G,H,J,K,L,M][4,8]ZX

Ø Medical and Surgical
B Respiratory System
F Fragmentation Definition: Breaking solid matter in a body part into pieces

Explanation: Physical force (e.g., manual, ultrasonic) applied directly or indirectly is used to break the solid matter into pieces. The solid matter may be an abnormal byproduct of a biological function or a foreign body. The pieces of solid matter are not taken out.

Body Part Character 4	Approach Character 5	Device Character 6	Qualifier Character 7
1 Trachea NC Cricoid cartilage 2 Carina NC 3 Main Bronchus, Right NC Bronchus intermedius Intermediate bronchus 4 Upper Lobe Bronchus, Right NC 5 Middle Lobe Bronchus, Right NC 6 Lower Lobe Bronchus, Right NC 7 Main Bronchus, Left NC 8 Upper Lobe Bronchus, Left NC 9 Lingula Bronchus NC B Lower Lobe Bronchus, Left NC	Ø Open 3 Percutaneous 4 Percutaneous Endoscopic 7 Via Natural or Artificial Opening 8 Via Natural or Artificial Opening Endoscopic X External	Z No Device	Z No Qualifier

Non-OR ØBF[1,2,3,4,5,6,7,8,9,B]XZZ
Non-OR ØBF[3,4,5,6,7,8,9,B][7,8]ZZ
NC ØBF[1,2,3,4,5,6,7,8,9,B]XZZ

Ø Medical and Surgical
B Respiratory System
H Insertion Definition: Putting in a nonbiological appliance that monitors, assists, performs, or prevents a physiological function but does not physically take the place of a body part

Explanation: None

Body Part Character 4	Approach Character 5	Device Character 6	Qualifier Character 7
Ø Tracheobronchial Tree	**Ø** Open **3** Percutaneous **4** Percutaneous Endoscopic **7** Via Natural or Artificial Opening **8** Via Natural or Artificial Opening Endoscopic	**1** Radioactive Element **2** Monitoring Device **3** Infusion Device **D** Intraluminal Device **Y** Other Device	**Z** No Qualifier
1 Trachea Cricoid cartilage	**Ø** Open	**2** Monitoring Device **D** Intraluminal Device **Y** Other Device	**Z** No Qualifier
1 Trachea Cricoid cartilage	**3** Percutaneous	**D** Intraluminal Device **E** Intraluminal Device, Endotracheal Airway **Y** Other Device	**Z** No Qualifier
1 Trachea Cricoid cartilage	**4** Percutaneous Endoscopic	**D** Intraluminal Device **Y** Other Device	**Z** No Qualifier
1 Trachea Cricoid cartilage	**7** Via Natural or Artificial Opening **8** Via Natural or Artificial Opening Endoscopic	**2** Monitoring Device **D** Intraluminal Device **E** Intraluminal Device, Endotracheal Airway **Y** Other Device	**Z** No Qualifier
3 Main Bronchus, Right Bronchus intermedius Intermediate bronchus **4** Upper Lobe Bronchus, Right **5** Middle Lobe Bronchus, Right **6** Lower Lobe Bronchus, Right **7** Main Bronchus, Left **8** Upper Lobe Bronchus, Left **9** Lingula Bronchus **B** Lower Lobe Bronchus, Left	**Ø** Open **3** Percutaneous **4** Percutaneous Endoscopic **7** Via Natural or Artificial Opening **8** Via Natural or Artificial Opening Endoscopic	**G** Intraluminal Device, Endobronchial Valve	**Z** No Qualifier
K Lung, Right **L** Lung, Left	**Ø** Open **3** Percutaneous **4** Percutaneous Endoscopic **7** Via Natural or Artificial Opening **8** Via Natural or Artificial Opening Endoscopic	**1** Radioactive Element **2** Monitoring Device **3** Infusion Device **Y** Other Device	**Z** No Qualifier
Q Pleura	**Ø** Open **3** Percutaneous **4** Percutaneous Endoscopic **7** Via Natural or Artificial Opening **8** Via Natural or Artificial Opening Endoscopic	**Y** Other Device	**Z** No Qualifier
T Diaphragm	**Ø** Open **3** Percutaneous **4** Percutaneous Endoscopic	**2** Monitoring Device **M** Diaphragmatic Pacemaker Lead **Y** Other Device	**Z** No Qualifier
T Diaphragm	**7** Via Natural or Artificial Opening **8** Via Natural or Artificial Opening Endoscopic	**Y** Other Device	**Z** No Qualifier

DRG Non-OR ØBH[3,4,5,6,7,8,9,B]8GZ
Non-OR ØBHØ3YZ
Non-OR ØBHØ[7,8][2,3,D,Y]Z
Non-OR ØBH13[E,Y]Z
Non-OR ØBH1[7,8][2,D,E,Y]Z
Non-OR ØBH[K,L]3YZ
Non-OR ØBH[K,L]7[2,3,Y]Z
Non-OR ØBH[K,L]8[2,3]Z
Non-OR ØBHQ[3,7]YZ
Non-OR ØBHT3YZ
Non-OR ØBHT[7,8]YZ

Ø Medical and Surgical
B Respiratory System
J Inspection Definition: Visually and/or manually exploring a body part

Explanation: Visual exploration may be performed with or without optical instrumentation. Manual exploration may be performed directly or through intervening body layers.

Body Part Character 4	Approach Character 5	Device Character 6	Qualifier Character 7
Ø Tracheobronchial Tree 1 Trachea Cricoid cartilage K Lung, Right L Lung, Left Q Pleura T Diaphragm	Ø Open 3 Percutaneous 4 Percutaneous Endoscopic 7 Via Natural or Artificial Opening 8 Via Natural or Artificial Opening Endoscopic X External	Z No Device	Z No Qualifier

Non-OR ØBJ[Ø,K,L,Q,T][3,7,8,X]ZZ
Non-OR ØBJ1[3,4,7,8,X]ZZ

Ø Medical and Surgical
B Respiratory System
L Occlusion Definition: Completely closing an orifice or the lumen of a tubular body part

Explanation: The orifice can be a natural orifice or an artificially created orifice

Body Part Character 4	Approach Character 5	Device Character 6	Qualifier Character 7
1 Trachea Cricoid cartilage 2 Carina 3 Main Bronchus, Right Bronchus intermedius Intermediate bronchus 4 Upper Lobe Bronchus, Right 5 Middle Lobe Bronchus, Right 6 Lower Lobe Bronchus, Right 7 Main Bronchus, Left 8 Upper Lobe Bronchus, Left 9 Lingula Bronchus B Lower Lobe Bronchus, Left	Ø Open 3 Percutaneous 4 Percutaneous Endoscopic	C Extraluminal Device D Intraluminal Device Z No Device	Z No Qualifier
1 Trachea Cricoid cartilage 2 Carina 3 Main Bronchus, Right Bronchus intermedius Intermediate bronchus 4 Upper Lobe Bronchus, Right 5 Middle Lobe Bronchus, Right 6 Lower Lobe Bronchus, Right 7 Main Bronchus, Left 8 Upper Lobe Bronchus, Left 9 Lingula Bronchus B Lower Lobe Bronchus, Left	7 Via Natural or Artificial Opening 8 Via Natural or Artificial Opening Endoscopic	D Intraluminal Device Z No Device	Z No Qualifier

Ø Medical and Surgical
B Respiratory System
M Reattachment Definition: Putting back in or on all or a portion of a separated body part to its normal location or other suitable location
Explanation: Vascular circulation and nervous pathways may or may not be reestablished

Body Part Character 4	Approach Character 5	Device Character 6	Qualifier Character 7
1 Trachea Cricoid cartilage **2 Carina** **3 Main Bronchus, Right** Bronchus intermedius Intermediate bronchus **4 Upper Lobe Bronchus, Right** **5 Middle Lobe Bronchus, Right** **6 Lower Lobe Bronchus, Right** **7 Main Bronchus, Left** **8 Upper Lobe Bronchus, Left** **9 Lingula Bronchus** **B Lower Lobe Bronchus, Left** **C Upper Lung Lobe, Right** **D Middle Lung Lobe, Right** **F Lower Lung Lobe, Right** **G Upper Lung Lobe, Left** **H Lung Lingula** **J Lower Lung Lobe, Left** **K Lung, Right** **L Lung, Left** **T Diaphragm**	**Ø Open**	**Z No Device**	**Z No Qualifier**

Ø Medical and Surgical
B Respiratory System
N Release Definition: Freeing a body part from an abnormal physical constraint by cutting or by the use of force
Explanation: Some of the restraining tissue may be taken out but none of the body part is taken out

Body Part Character 4	Approach Character 5	Device Character 6	Qualifier Character 7
1 Trachea Cricoid cartilage **2 Carina** **3 Main Bronchus, Right** Bronchus intermedius Intermediate bronchus **4 Upper Lobe Bronchus, Right** **5 Middle Lobe Bronchus, Right** **6 Lower Lobe Bronchus, Right** **7 Main Bronchus, Left** **8 Upper Lobe Bronchus, Left** **9 Lingula Bronchus** **B Lower Lobe Bronchus, Left** **C Upper Lung Lobe, Right** **D Middle Lung Lobe, Right** **F Lower Lung Lobe, Right** **G Upper Lung Lobe, Left** **H Lung Lingula** **J Lower Lung Lobe, Left** **K Lung, Right** **L Lung, Left** **M Lungs, Bilateral**	**Ø Open** **3 Percutaneous** **4 Percutaneous Endoscopic** **7 Via Natural or Artificial Opening** **8 Via Natural or Artificial Opening Endoscopic**	**Z No Device**	**Z No Qualifier**
N Pleura, Right **P Pleura, Left** **T Diaphragm**	**Ø Open** **3 Percutaneous** **4 Percutaneous Endoscopic**	**Z No Device**	**Z No Qualifier**

Ø Medical and Surgical
B Respiratory System
P Removal Definition: Taking out or off a device from a body part

Explanation: If a device is taken out and a similar device put in without cutting or puncturing the skin or mucous membrane, the procedure is coded to the root operation CHANGE. Otherwise, the procedure for taking out a device is coded to the root operation REMOVAL.

Body Part Character 4	Approach Character 5	Device Character 6	Qualifier Character 7
Ø Tracheobronchial Tree	Ø Open 3 Percutaneous 4 Percutaneous Endoscopic 7 Via Natural or Artificial Opening 8 Via Natural or Artificial Opening Endoscopic	Ø Drainage Device 1 Radioactive Element 2 Monitoring Device 3 Infusion Device 7 Autologous Tissue Substitute C Extraluminal Device D Intraluminal Device J Synthetic Substitute K Nonautologous Tissue Substitute Y Other Device	Z No Qualifier
Ø Tracheobronchial Tree	X External	Ø Drainage Device 1 Radioactive Element 2 Monitoring Device 3 Infusion Device D Intraluminal Device	Z No Qualifier
1 Trachea Cricoid cartilage	Ø Open 3 Percutaneous 4 Percutaneous Endoscopic 7 Via Natural or Artificial Opening 8 Via Natural or Artificial Opening Endoscopic	Ø Drainage Device 2 Monitoring Device 7 Autologous Tissue Substitute C Extraluminal Device D Intraluminal Device F Tracheostomy Device J Synthetic Substitute K Nonautologous Tissue Substitute	Z No Qualifier
1 Trachea Cricoid cartilage	X External	Ø Drainage Device 2 Monitoring Device D Intraluminal Device F Tracheostomy Device	Z No Qualifier
K Lung, Right L Lung, Left	Ø Open 3 Percutaneous 4 Percutaneous Endoscopic 7 Via Natural or Artificial Opening 8 Via Natural or Artificial Opening Endoscopic	Ø Drainage Device 1 Radioactive Element 2 Monitoring Device 3 Infusion Device Y Other Device	Z No Qualifier
K Lung, Right L Lung, Left	X External	Ø Drainage Device 1 Radioactive Element 2 Monitoring Device 3 Infusion Device	Z No Qualifier
Q Pleura	Ø Open 3 Percutaneous 4 Percutaneous Endoscopic 7 Via Natural or Artificial Opening 8 Via Natural or Artificial Opening Endoscopic	Ø Drainage Device 1 Radioactive Element 2 Monitoring Device Y Other Device	Z No Qualifier
Q Pleura	X External	Ø Drainage Device 1 Radioactive Element 2 Monitoring Device	Z No Qualifier
T Diaphragm	Ø Open 3 Percutaneous 4 Percutaneous Endoscopic 7 Via Natural or Artificial Opening 8 Via Natural or Artificial Opening Endoscopic	Ø Drainage Device 2 Monitoring Device 7 Autologous Tissue Substitute J Synthetic Substitute K Nonautologous Tissue Substitute M Diaphragmatic Pacemaker Lead Y Other Device	Z No Qualifier
T Diaphragm	X External	Ø Drainage Device 2 Monitoring Device M Diaphragmatic Pacemaker Lead	Z No Qualifier

Non-OR ØBPØ[3,4]YZ
Non-OR ØBPØ[7,8][Ø,2,3,D,Y]Z
Non-OR ØBPØX[Ø,1,2,3,D]Z
Non-OR ØBP1[Ø,3,4]FZ
Non-OR ØBP1[7,8][Ø,2,D,F]Z
Non-OR ØBP1X[Ø,2,D,F]Z
Non-OR ØBP[K,L]3YZ
Non-OR ØBPK7[Ø,1,2,3,Y]Z
Non-OR ØBPK8[Ø,1,2,3]Z
Non-OR ØBPL7[Ø,2,3,Y]Z
Non-OR ØBPL8[Ø,2,3]Z
Non-OR ØBP[K,L]X[Ø,1,2,3]Z
Non-OR ØBPQ[Ø,3,4,7,8][Ø,1,2,]Z
Non-OR ØBPQ[3,7]YZ
Non-OR ØBPQX[Ø,1,2]Z
Non-OR ØBPT3YZ
Non-OR ØBPT[7,8][Ø,2,Y]Z
Non-OR ØBPTX[Ø,2,M]Z

Ø Medical and Surgical
B Respiratory System
Q Repair Definition: Restoring, to the extent possible, a body part to its normal anatomic structure and function
Explanation: Used only when the method to accomplish the repair is not one of the other root operations

Body Part Character 4	Approach Character 5	Device Character 6	Qualifier Character 7
1 Trachea Cricoid cartilage **2 Carina** **3 Main Bronchus, Right** Bronchus intermedius Intermediate bronchus **4 Upper Lobe Bronchus, Right** **5 Middle Lobe Bronchus, Right** **6 Lower Lobe Bronchus, Right** **7 Main Bronchus, Left** **8 Upper Lobe Bronchus, Left** **9 Lingula Bronchus** **B Lower Lobe Bronchus, Left** **C Upper Lung Lobe, Right** **D Middle Lung Lobe, Right** **F Lower Lung Lobe, Right** **G Upper Lung Lobe, Left** **H Lung Lingula** **J Lower Lung Lobe, Left** **K Lung, Right** **L Lung, Left** **M Lungs, Bilateral**	**Ø Open** **3 Percutaneous** **4 Percutaneous Endoscopic** **7 Via Natural or Artificial Opening** **8 Via Natural or Artificial Opening Endoscopic**	**Z No Device**	**Z No Qualifier**
N Pleura, Right **P Pleura, Left** **T Diaphragm**	**Ø Open** **3 Percutaneous** **4 Percutaneous Endoscopic**	**Z No Device**	**Z No Qualifier**

Ø Medical and Surgical
B Respiratory System
R Replacement Definition: Putting in or on biological or synthetic material that physically takes the place and/or function of all or a portion of a body part

Explanation: The body part may have been taken out or replaced, or may be taken out, physically eradicated, or rendered nonfunctional during the REPLACEMENT procedure. A REMOVAL procedure is coded for taking out the device used in a previous replacement procedure.

Body Part Character 4	Approach Character 5	Device Character 6	Qualifier Character 7
1 Trachea Cricoid cartilage **2 Carina** **3 Main Bronchus, Right** Bronchus intermedius Intermediate bronchus **4 Upper Lobe Bronchus, Right** **5 Middle Lobe Bronchus, Right** **6 Lower Lobe Bronchus, Right** **7 Main Bronchus, Left** **8 Upper Lobe Bronchus, Left** **9 Lingula Bronchus** **B Lower Lobe Bronchus, Left** **T Diaphragm**	**Ø Open** **4 Percutaneous Endoscopic**	**7 Autologous Tissue Substitute** **J Synthetic Substitute** **K Nonautologous Tissue Substitute**	**Z No Qualifier**

Ø Medical and Surgical
B Respiratory System
S Reposition Definition: Moving to its normal location, or other suitable location, all or a portion of a body part

Explanation: The body part is moved to a new location from an abnormal location, or from a normal location where it is not functioning correctly. The body part may or may not be cut out or off to be moved to the new location.

Body Part Character 4	Approach Character 5	Device Character 6	Qualifier Character 7
1 Trachea Cricoid cartilage **2 Carina** **3 Main Bronchus, Right** Bronchus intermedius Intermediate bronchus **4 Upper Lobe Bronchus, Right** **5 Middle Lobe Bronchus, Right** **6 Lower Lobe Bronchus, Right** **7 Main Bronchus, Left** **8 Upper Lobe Bronchus, Left** **9 Lingula Bronchus** **B Lower Lobe Bronchus, Left** **C Upper Lung Lobe, Right** **D Middle Lung Lobe, Right** **F Lower Lung Lobe, Right** **G Upper Lung Lobe, Left** **H Lung Lingula** **J Lower Lung Lobe, Left** **K Lung, Right** **L Lung, Left** **T Diaphragm**	**Ø Open**	**Z No Device**	**Z No Qualifier**

Ø Medical and Surgical
B Respiratory System
T Resection Definition: Cutting out or off, without replacement, all of a body part

Explanation: None

Body Part Character 4	Approach Character 5	Device Character 6	Qualifier Character 7
1 Trachea Cricoid cartilage **2** Carina **3** Main Bronchus, Right Bronchus intermedius Intermediate bronchus **4** Upper Lobe Bronchus, Right **5** Middle Lobe Bronchus, Right **6** Lower Lobe Bronchus, Right **7** Main Bronchus, Left **8** Upper Lobe Bronchus, Left **9** Lingula Bronchus **B** Lower Lobe Bronchus, Left **C** Upper Lung Lobe, Right **D** Middle Lung Lobe, Right **F** Lower Lung Lobe, Right **G** Upper Lung Lobe, Left **H** Lung Lingula **J** Lower Lung Lobe, Left **K** Lung, Right **L** Lung, Left **M** Lungs, Bilateral **T** Diaphragm	**Ø** Open **4** Percutaneous Endoscopic	**Z** No Device	**Z** No Qualifier

Ø Medical and Surgical
B Respiratory System
U Supplement Definition: Putting in or on biological or synthetic material that physically reinforces and/or augments the function of a portion of a body part

Explanation: The biological material is non-living, or is living and from the same individual. The body part may have been previously replaced, and the SUPPLEMENT procedure is performed to physically reinforce and/or augment the function of the replaced body part.

Body Part Character 4	Approach Character 5	Device Character 6	Qualifier Character 7
1 Trachea Cricoid cartilage **2** Carina **3** Main Bronchus, Right Bronchus intermedius Intermediate bronchus **4** Upper Lobe Bronchus, Right **5** Middle Lobe Bronchus, Right **6** Lower Lobe Bronchus, Right **7** Main Bronchus, Left **8** Upper Lobe Bronchus, Left **9** Lingula Bronchus **B** Lower Lobe Bronchus, Left	**Ø** Open **4** Percutaneous Endoscopic **8** Via Natural or Artificial Opening Endoscopic	**7** Autologous Tissue Substitute **J** Synthetic Substitute **K** Nonautologous Tissue Substitute	**Z** No Qualifier
T Diaphragm	**Ø** Open **4** Percutaneous Endoscopic	**7** Autologous Tissue Substitute **J** Synthetic Substitute **K** Nonautologous Tissue Substitute	**Z** No Qualifier

Ø Medical and Surgical
B Respiratory System
V Restriction Definition: Partially closing an orifice or the lumen of a tubular body part

Explanation: The orifice can be a natural orifice or an artificially created orifice

Body Part Character 4	Approach Character 5	Device Character 6	Qualifier Character 7
1 Trachea Cricoid cartilage **2 Carina** **3 Main Bronchus, Right** Bronchus intermedius Intermediate bronchus **4 Upper Lobe Bronchus, Right** **5 Middle Lobe Bronchus, Right** **6 Lower Lobe Bronchus, Right** **7 Main Bronchus, Left** **8 Upper Lobe Bronchus, Left** **9 Lingula Bronchus** **B Lower Lobe Bronchus, Left**	**Ø Open** **3 Percutaneous** **4 Percutaneous Endoscopic**	**C Extraluminal Device** **D Intraluminal Device** **Z No Device**	**Z No Qualifier**
1 Trachea Cricoid cartilage **2 Carina** **3 Main Bronchus, Right** Bronchus intermedius Intermediate bronchus **4 Upper Lobe Bronchus, Right** **5 Middle Lobe Bronchus, Right** **6 Lower Lobe Bronchus, Right** **7 Main Bronchus, Left** **8 Upper Lobe Bronchus, Left** **9 Lingula Bronchus** **B Lower Lobe Bronchus, Left**	**7 Via Natural or Artificial Opening** **8 Via Natural or Artificial Opening Endoscopic**	**D Intraluminal Device** **Z No Device**	**Z No Qualifier**

Ø Medical and Surgical
B Respiratory System
W Revision Definition: Correcting, to the extent possible, a portion of a malfunctioning device or the position of a displaced device

Explanation: Revision can include correcting a malfunctioning or displaced device by taking out or putting in components of the device such as a screw or pin

Body Part Character 4	Approach Character 5	Device Character 6	Qualifier Character 7
Ø Tracheobronchial Tree	Ø Open 3 Percutaneous 4 Percutaneous Endoscopic 7 Via Natural or Artificial Opening 8 Via Natural or Artificial Opening Endoscopic	Ø Drainage Device 2 Monitoring Device 3 Infusion Device 7 Autologous Tissue Substitute C Extraluminal Device D Intraluminal Device J Synthetic Substitute K Nonautologous Tissue Substitute Y Other Device	Z No Qualifier
Ø Tracheobronchial Tree	X External	Ø Drainage Device 2 Monitoring Device 3 Infusion Device 7 Autologous Tissue Substitute C Extraluminal Device D Intraluminal Device J Synthetic Substitute K Nonautologous Tissue Substitute	Z No Qualifier
1 Trachea Cricoid cartilage	Ø Open 3 Percutaneous 4 Percutaneous Endoscopic 7 Via Natural or Artificial Opening 8 Via Natural or Artificial Opening Endoscopic X External	Ø Drainage Device 2 Monitoring Device 7 Autologous Tissue Substitute C Extraluminal Device D Intraluminal Device F Tracheostomy Device J Synthetic Substitute K Nonautologous Tissue Substitute	Z No Qualifier
K Lung, Right L Lung, Left	Ø Open 3 Percutaneous 4 Percutaneous Endoscopic 7 Via Natural or Artificial Opening 8 Via Natural or Artificial Opening Endoscopic	Ø Drainage Device 2 Monitoring Device 3 Infusion Device Y Other Device	Z No Qualifier
K Lung, Right L Lung, Left	X External	Ø Drainage Device 2 Monitoring Device 3 Infusion Device	Z No Qualifier
Q Pleura	Ø Open 3 Percutaneous 4 Percutaneous Endoscopic 7 Via Natural or Artificial Opening 8 Via Natural or Artificial Opening Endoscopic	Ø Drainage Device 2 Monitoring Device Y Other Device	Z No Qualifier
Q Pleura	X External	Ø Drainage Device 2 Monitoring Device	Z No Qualifier
T Diaphragm	Ø Open 3 Percutaneous 4 Percutaneous Endoscopic 7 Via Natural or Artificial Opening 8 Via Natural or Artificial Opening Endoscopic	Ø Drainage Device 2 Monitoring Device 7 Autologous Tissue Substitute J Synthetic Substitute K Nonautologous Tissue Substitute M Diaphragmatic Pacemaker Lead Y Other Device	Z No Qualifier
T Diaphragm	X External	Ø Drainage Device 2 Monitoring Device 7 Autologous Tissue Substitute J Synthetic Substitute K Nonautologous Tissue Substitute M Diaphragmatic Pacemaker Lead	Z No Qualifier

Non-OR ØBWØ[3,4]YZ
Non-OR ØBWØ[7,8][2,3,D,Y]Z
Non-OR ØBWØX[Ø,2,3,7,C,D,J,K]Z
Non-OR ØBW1X[Ø,2,7,C,D,F,J,K]Z
Non-OR ØBW[K,L]3YZ
Non-OR ØBW[K,L]7[Ø,2,3,Y]Z
Non-OR ØBW[K,L]8[Ø,2,3]Z
Non-OR ØBW[K,L]X[Ø,2,3]Z
Non-OR ØBWQ[Ø,3,4,7,8][Ø,2]Z
Non-OR ØBWQ[Ø,3,7]YZ
Non-OR ØBWQX[Ø,2]Z
Non-OR ØBWT[3,7,8]YZ
Non-OR ØBWTX[Ø,2,7,J,K,M]Z

Ø Medical and Surgical
B Respiratory System
Y Transplantation Definition: Putting in or on all or a portion of a living body part taken from another individual or animal to physically take the place and/or function of all or a portion of a similar body part

Explanation: The native body part may or may not be taken out, and the transplanted body part may take over all or a portion of its function

Body Part Character 4	Approach Character 5	Device Character 6	Qualifier Character 7
C Upper Lung Lobe, Right LC D Middle Lung Lobe, Right LC F Lower Lung Lobe, Right LC G Upper Lung Lobe, Left LC H Lung Lingula LC J Lower Lung Lobe, Left LC K Lung, Right LC L Lung, Left LC M Lungs, Bilateral LC	Ø Open	Z No Device	Ø Allogeneic 1 Syngeneic 2 Zooplastic

LC ØBY[C,D,F,G,H,J,K,L,M]ØZ[Ø,1,2]

Mouth and Throat ØCØ–ØCX

Character Meanings

This Character Meaning table is provided as a guide to assist the user in the identification of character members that may be found in this section of code tables. It **SHOULD NOT** be used to build a PCS code.

Operation–Character 3		Body Part–Character 4		Approach–Character 5		Device–Character 6		Qualifier–Character 7	
Ø	Alteration	Ø	Upper Lip	Ø	Open	Ø	Drainage Device	Ø	Single
2	Change	1	Lower Lip	3	Percutaneous	1	Radioactive Element	1	Multiple
5	Destruction	2	Hard Palate	4	Percutaneous Endoscopic	5	External Fixation Device	2	All
7	Dilation	3	Soft Palate	7	Via Natural or Artificial Opening	7	Autologous Tissue Substitute	X	Diagnostic
9	Drainage	4	Buccal Mucosa	8	Via Natural or Artificial Opening Endoscopic	B	Intraluminal Device, Airway	Z	No Qualifier
B	Excision	5	Upper Gingiva	X	External	C	Extraluminal Device		
C	Extirpation	6	Lower Gingiva			D	Intraluminal Device		
D	Extraction	7	Tongue			J	Synthetic Substitute		
F	Fragmentation	8	Parotid Gland, Right			K	Nonautologous Tissue Substitute		
H	Insertion	9	Parotid Gland, Left			Y	Other Device		
J	Inspection	A	Salivary Gland			Z	No Device		
L	Occlusion	B	Parotid Duct, Right						
M	Reattachment	C	Parotid Duct, Left						
N	Release	D	Sublingual Gland, Right						
P	Removal	F	Sublingual Gland, Left						
Q	Repair	G	Submaxillary Gland, Right						
R	Replacement	H	Submaxillary Gland, Left						
S	Reposition	J	Minor Salivary Gland						
T	Resection	M	Pharynx						
U	Supplement	N	Uvula						
V	Restriction	P	Tonsils						
W	Revision	Q	Adenoids						
X	Transfer	R	Epiglottis						
		S	Larynx						
		T	Vocal Cord, Right						
		V	Vocal Cord, Left						
		W	Upper Tooth						
		X	Lower Tooth						
		Y	Mouth and Throat						

AHA Coding Clinic for table ØC9
2017, 2Q, 16 Incision and drainage of floor of mouth

AHA Coding Clinic for table ØCB
2017, 2Q, 16 Excision of floor of mouth
2016, 3Q, 28 Lingual tonsillectomy, tongue base excision and epiglottopexy
2016, 2Q, 19 Biopsy of the base of tongue
2014, 3Q, 21 Superficial parotidectomy

AHA Coding Clinic for table ØCC
2016, 2Q, 20 Sialendoscopy with stone removal

AHA Coding Clinic for table ØCQ
2017, 1Q, 20 Preparatory nasal adhesion repair before definitive cleft palate repair

AHA Coding Clinic for table ØCR
2014, 3Q, 25 Excision of soft palate with placement of surgical obturator
2014, 2Q, 5 Oasis acellular matrix graft
2014, 2Q, 6 Composite grafting (synthetic versus nonautologous tissue substitute)

AHA Coding Clinic for table ØCS
2016, 3Q, 28 Lingual tonsillectomy, tongue base excision and epiglottopexy

AHA Coding Clinic for table ØCT
2016, 2Q, 12 Resection of malignant neoplasm of infratemporal fossa
2014, 3Q, 21 Superficial parotidectomy
2014, 3Q, 23 Le Fort I osteotomy

Salivary Glands

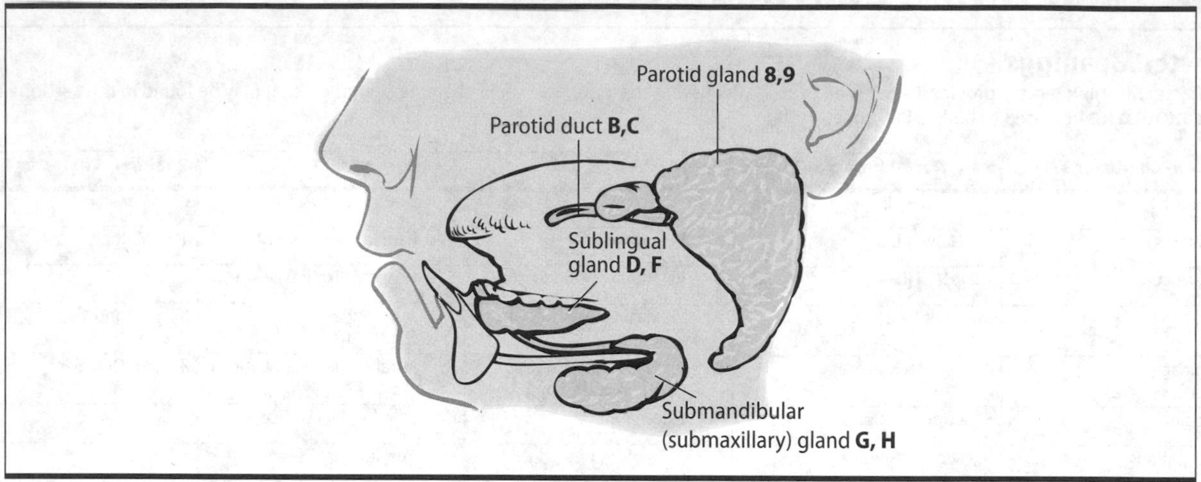

Oral Anatomy

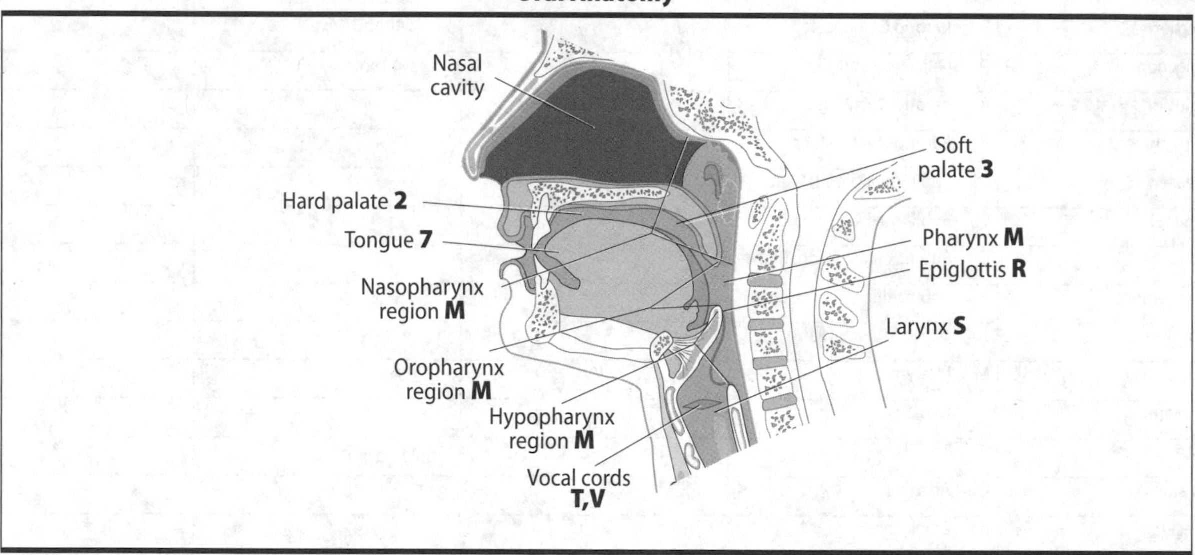

Mouth Frontal View (Upper)

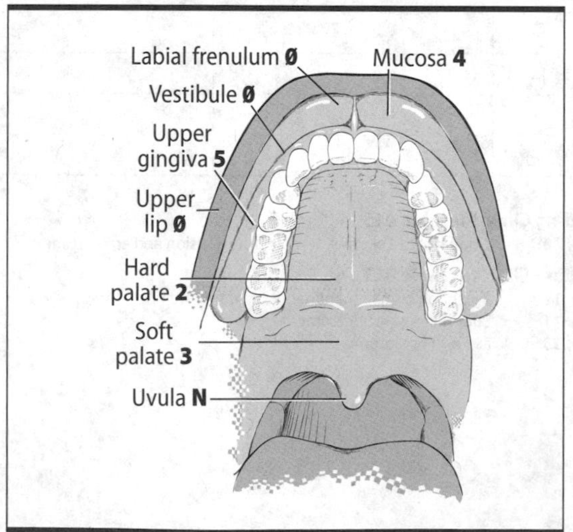

Mouth Frontal View (Lower)

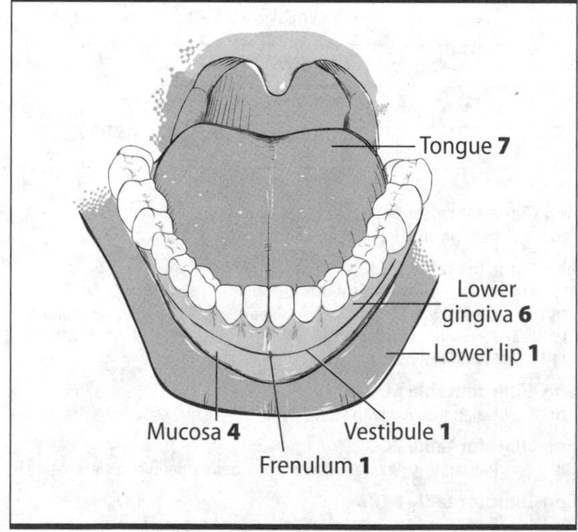

Ø Medical and Surgical
C Mouth and Throat
Ø Alteration Definition: Modifying the anatomic structure of a body part without affecting the function of the body part
Explanation: Principal purpose is to improve appearance

Body Part Character 4	Approach Character 5	Device Character 6	Qualifier Character 7
Ø Upper Lip Frenulum labii superioris Labial gland Vermilion border **1** Lower Lip Frenulum labii inferioris Labial gland Vermilion border	**X** External	**7** Autologous Tissue Substitute **J** Synthetic Substitute **K** Nonautologous Tissue Substitute **Z** No Device	**Z** No Qualifier

Ø Medical and Surgical
C Mouth and Throat
2 Change Definition: Taking out or off a device from a body part and putting back an identical or similar device in or on the same body part without cutting or puncturing the skin or a mucous membrane
Explanation: All CHANGE procedures are coded using the approach EXTERNAL

Body Part Character 4	Approach Character 5	Device Character 6	Qualifier Character 7
A Salivary Gland **S** Larynx Aryepiglottic fold Arytenoid cartilage Corniculate cartilage Cuneiform cartilage False vocal cord Glottis Rima glottidis Thyroid cartilage Ventricular fold **Y** Mouth and Throat	**X** External	**Ø** Drainage Device **Y** Other Device	**Z** No Qualifier

Non-OR All body part, approach, device, and qualifier values

Ø Medical and Surgical
C Mouth and Throat
5 Destruction Definition: Physical eradication of all or a portion of a body part by the direct use of energy, force, or a destructive agent
Explanation: None of the body part is physically taken out

Body Part Character 4	Approach Character 5	Device Character 6	Qualifier Character 7
Ø Upper Lip Frenulum labii superioris; Labial gland; Vermilion border **1 Lower Lip** Frenulum labii inferioris; Labial gland; Vermilion border **2 Hard Palate** **3 Soft Palate** **4 Buccal Mucosa** Buccal gland; Molar gland; Palatine gland **5 Upper Gingiva** **6 Lower Gingiva** **7 Tongue** Frenulum linguae **N Uvula** Palatine uvula **P Tonsils** Palatine tonsil **Q Adenoids** Pharyngeal tonsil	**Ø Open** **3 Percutaneous** **X External**	**Z No Device**	**Z No Qualifier**
8 Parotid Gland, Right **9 Parotid Gland, Left** **B Parotid Duct, Right** Stensen's duct **C Parotid Duct, Left** *See B Parotid Duct, Right* **D Sublingual Gland, Right** **F Sublingual Gland, Left** **G Submaxillary Gland, Right** Submandibular gland **H Submaxillary Gland, Left** *See G Submaxillary Gland, Right* **J Minor Salivary Gland** Anterior lingual gland	**Ø Open** **3 Percutaneous**	**Z No Device**	**Z No Qualifier**
M Pharynx Base of tongue; Hypopharynx; Laryngopharynx; Lingual tonsil; Oropharynx; Piriform recess (sinus); Tongue, base of **R Epiglottis** Glossoepiglottic fold **S Larynx** Aryepiglottic fold; Arytenoid cartilage; Corniculate cartilage; Cuneiform cartilage; False vocal cord; Glottis; Rima glottidis; Thyroid cartilage; Ventricular fold **T Vocal Cord, Right** Vocal fold **V Vocal Cord, Left** *See T Vocal Cord, Right*	**Ø Open** **3 Percutaneous** **4 Percutaneous Endoscopic** **7 Via Natural or Artificial Opening** **8 Via Natural or Artificial Opening Endoscopic**	**Z No Device**	**Z No Qualifier**
W Upper Tooth **X Lower Tooth**	**Ø Open** **X External**	**Z No Device**	**Ø Single** **1 Multiple** **2 All**

Non-OR ØC5[5,6][Ø,3,X]ZZ
Non-OR ØC5[W,X][Ø,X]Z[Ø,1,2]

Ø Medical and Surgical
C Mouth and Throat
7 Dilation Definition: Expanding an orifice or the lumen of a tubular body part
Explanation: The orifice can be a natural orifice or an artificially created orifice. Accomplished by stretching a tubular body part using intraluminal pressure or by cutting part of the orifice or wall of the tubular body part.

Body Part Character 4	Approach Character 5	Device Character 6	Qualifier Character 7
B Parotid Duct, Right Stensen's duct **C Parotid Duct, Left** *See B Parotid Duct, Right*	**Ø Open** **3 Percutaneous** **7 Via Natural or Artificial Opening**	**D Intraluminal Device** **Z No Device**	**Z No Qualifier**
M Pharynx Base of tongue; Hypopharynx; Laryngopharynx; Lingual tonsil; Oropharynx; Piriform recess (sinus); Tongue, base of	**7 Via Natural or Artificial Opening** **8 Via Natural or Artificial Opening Endoscopic**	**D Intraluminal Device** **Z No Device**	**Z No Qualifier**
S Larynx Aryepiglottic fold; Arytenoid cartilage; Corniculate cartilage; Cuneiform cartilage; False vocal cord; Glottis; Rima glottidis; Thyroid cartilage; Ventricular fold	**Ø Open** **3 Percutaneous** **4 Percutaneous Endoscopic** **7 Via Natural or Artificial Opening** **8 Via Natural or Artificial Opening Endoscopic**	**D Intraluminal Device** **Z No Device**	**Z No Qualifier**

Non-OR ØC7[B,C][Ø,3,7][D,Z]Z
Non-OR ØC7M[7,8][D,Z]Z

Ø Medical and Surgical
C Mouth and Throat
9 Drainage Definition: Taking or letting out fluids and/or gases from a body part
Explanation: The qualifier DIAGNOSTIC is used to identify drainage procedures that are biopsies

Body Part Character 4		Approach Character 5	Device Character 6	Qualifier Character 7
Ø Upper Lip Frenulum labii superioris Labial gland Vermilion border **1 Lower Lip** Frenulum labii inferioris Labial gland Vermilion border **2 Hard Palate** **3 Soft Palate** **4 Buccal Mucosa** Buccal gland Molar gland Palatine gland	**5 Upper Gingiva** **6 Lower Gingiva** **7 Tongue** Frenulum linguae **N Uvula** Palatine uvula **P Tonsils** Palatine tonsil **Q Adenoids** Pharyngeal tonsil	Ø Open 3 Percutaneous X External	Ø Drainage Device	Z No Qualifier
Ø Upper Lip Frenulum labii superioris Labial gland Vermilion border **1 Lower Lip** Frenulum labii inferioris Labial gland Vermilion border **2 Hard Palate** **3 Soft Palate** **4 Buccal Mucosa** Buccal gland Molar gland Palatine gland	**5 Upper Gingiva** **6 Lower Gingiva** **7 Tongue** Frenulum linguae **N Uvula** Palatine uvula **P Tonsils** Palatine tonsil **Q Adenoids** Pharyngeal tonsil	Ø Open 3 Percutaneous X External	Z No Device	X Diagnostic Z No Qualifier
8 Parotid Gland, Right **9 Parotid Gland, Left** **B Parotid Duct, Right** Stensen's duct **C Parotid Duct, Left** *See B Parotid Duct, Right* **D Sublingual Gland, Right**	**F Sublingual Gland, Left** **G Submaxillary Gland, Right** Submandibular gland **H Submaxillary Gland, Left** *See G Submaxillary Gland, Right* **J Minor Salivary Gland** Anterior lingual gland	Ø Open 3 Percutaneous	Ø Drainage Device	Z No Qualifier
8 Parotid Gland, Right **9 Parotid Gland, Left** **B Parotid Duct, Right** Stensen's duct **C Parotid Duct, Left** *See B Parotid Duct, Right*	**D Sublingual Gland, Right** **F Sublingual Gland, Left** **G Submaxillary Gland, Right** Submandibular gland **H Submaxillary Gland, Left** *See G Submaxillary Gland, Right* **J Minor Salivary Gland** Anterior lingual gland	Ø Open 3 Percutaneous	Z No Device	X Diagnostic Z No Qualifier
M Pharynx Base of tongue Hypopharynx Laryngopharynx Lingual tonsil Oropharynx Piriform recess (sinus) Tongue, base of **R Epiglottis** Glossoepiglottic fold	**S Larynx** Aryepiglottic fold Arytenoid cartilage Corniculate cartilage Cuneiform cartilage False vocal cord Glottis Rima glottidis Thyroid cartilage Ventricular fold **T Vocal Cord, Right** Vocal fold **V Vocal Cord, Left** *See T Vocal Cord, Right*	Ø Open 3 Percutaneous 4 Percutaneous Endoscopic 7 Via Natural or Artificial Opening 8 Via Natural or Artificial Opening Endoscopic	Ø Drainage Device	Z No Qualifier

Non-OR ØC9[Ø,1,2,3,4,7,N,P,Q]3ØZ
Non-OR ØC9[5,6][Ø,3,X]ØZ
Non-OR ØC9[Ø,1,4][Ø,3,X]ZX
Non-OR ØC9[Ø,1,2,3,4,7,N,P,Q]3ZZ
Non-OR ØC9[5,6][Ø,3,X]Z[X,Z]
Non-OR ØC97[3,X]ZX
Non-OR ØC9[8,9,B,C,D,F,G,H,J][Ø,3]ØZ
Non-OR ØC9[8,9,B,C,D,F,G,H,J]3ZX
Non-OR ØC9[8,9,G,H]3ZZ
Non-OR ØC9[B,C,D, F,J][Ø,3]ZZ
Non-OR ØC9[M,R,S,T,V]3ØZ

ØC9 Continued on next page

ØC9 Continued

Ø Medical and Surgical
C Mouth and Throat
9 Drainage Definition: Taking or letting out fluids and/or gases from a body part
Explanation: The qualifier DIAGNOSTIC is used to identify drainage procedures that are biopsies

Body Part Character 4		Approach Character 5	Device Character 6	Qualifier Character 7
M Pharynx Base of tongue Hypopharynx Laryngopharynx Lingual tonsil Oropharynx Piriform recess (sinus) Tongue, base of **R Epiglottis** Glossoepiglottic fold	**S Larynx** Aryepiglottic fold Arytenoid cartilage Corniculate cartilage Cuneiform cartilage False vocal cord Glottis Rima glottidis Thyroid cartilage Ventricular fold **T Vocal Cord, Right** Vocal fold **V Vocal Cord, Left** *See T Vocal Cord, Right*	**Ø Open** **3 Percutaneous** **4 Percutaneous Endoscopic** **7 Via Natural or Artificial Opening** **8 Via Natural or Artificial Opening Endoscopic**	**Z No Device**	**X Diagnostic** **Z No Qualifier**
W Upper Tooth **X Lower Tooth**		**Ø Open** **X External**	**Ø Drainage Device** **Z No Device**	**Ø Single** **1 Multiple** **2 All**

Non-OR ØC9M[Ø,3,4,7,8]ZX
Non-OR ØC9[M,R,S,T,V]3ZZ
Non-OR ØC9[R,S,T,V][3,4,7,8]ZX
Non-OR ØC9[W,X][Ø,X][Ø,Z][Ø,1,2]

Ø Medical and Surgical
C Mouth and Throat
B Excision Definition: Cutting out or off, without replacement, a portion of a body part
Explanation: The qualifier DIAGNOSTIC is used to identify excision procedures that are biopsies

Body Part Character 4		Approach Character 5	Device Character 6	Qualifier Character 7
Ø Upper Lip Frenulum labii superioris Labial gland Vermilion border **1 Lower Lip** Frenulum labii inferioris Labial gland Vermilion border **2 Hard Palate** **3 Soft Palate** **4 Buccal Mucosa** Buccal gland Molar gland Palatine gland	**5 Upper Gingiva** **6 Lower Gingiva** **7 Tongue** Frenulum linguae **N Uvula** Palatine uvula **P Tonsils** Palatine tonsil **Q Adenoids** Pharyngeal tonsil	**Ø Open** **3 Percutaneous** **X External**	**Z No Device**	**X Diagnostic** **Z No Qualifier**
8 Parotid Gland, Right **9 Parotid Gland, Left** **B Parotid Duct, Right** Stensen's duct **C Parotid Duct, Left** *See B Parotid Duct, Right* **D Sublingual Gland, Right**	**F Sublingual Gland, Left** **G Submaxillary Gland, Right** Submandibular gland **H Submaxillary Gland, Left** *See G Submaxillary Gland, Right* **J Minor Salivary Gland** Anterior lingual gland	**Ø Open** **3 Percutaneous**	**Z No Device**	**X Diagnostic** **Z No Qualifier**
M Pharynx Base of tongue Hypopharynx Laryngopharynx Lingual tonsil Oropharynx Piriform recess (sinus) Tongue, base of **R Epiglottis** Glossoepiglottic fold	**S Larynx** Aryepiglottic fold Arytenoid cartilage Corniculate cartilage Cuneiform cartilage False vocal cord Glottis Rima glottidis Thyroid cartilage Ventricular fold **T Vocal Cord, Right** Vocal fold **V Vocal Cord, Left** *See T Vocal Cord, Right*	**Ø Open** **3 Percutaneous** **4 Percutaneous Endoscopic** **7 Via Natural or Artificial Opening** **8 Via Natural or Artificial Opening Endoscopic**	**Z No Device**	**X Diagnostic** **Z No Qualifier**
W Upper Tooth **X Lower Tooth**		**Ø Open** **X External**	**Z No Device**	**Ø Single** **1 Multiple** **2 All**

Non-OR ØCB[Ø,1,4][Ø,3,X]ZX
Non-OR ØCB[5,6][Ø,3,X]Z[X,Z]
Non-OR ØCB7[3,X]ZX
Non-OR ØCB[8,9,B,C,D,F,G,H,J]3ZX
Non-OR ØCBM[Ø,3,4,7,8]ZX
Non-OR ØCB[R,S,T,V][3,4,7,8]ZX
Non-OR ØCB[W,X][Ø,X]Z[Ø,1,2]

Ø Medical and Surgical
C Mouth and Throat
C Extirpation Definition: Taking or cutting out solid matter from a body part

Explanation: The solid matter may be an abnormal byproduct of a biological function or a foreign body; it may be imbedded in a body part or in the lumen of a tubular body part. The solid matter may or may not have been previously broken into pieces.

Body Part Character 4		Approach Character 5	Device Character 6	Qualifier Character 7
Ø Upper Lip Frenulum labii superioris Labial gland Vermilion border 1 Lower Lip Frenulum labii inferioris Labial gland Vermilion border 2 Hard Palate 3 Soft Palate 4 Buccal Mucosa Buccal gland Molar gland Palatine gland	5 Upper Gingiva 6 Lower Gingiva 7 Tongue Frenulum linguae N Uvula Palatine uvula P Tonsils Palatine tonsil Q Adenoids Pharyngeal tonsil	Ø Open 3 Percutaneous X External	Z No Device	Z No Qualifier
8 Parotid Gland, Right 9 Parotid Gland, Left B Parotid Duct, Right Stensen's duct C Parotid Duct, Left *See B Parotid Duct, Right* D Sublingual Gland, Right	F Sublingual Gland, Left G Submaxillary Gland, Right Submandibular gland H Submaxillary Gland, Left *See G Submaxillary Gland, Right* J Minor Salivary Gland Anterior lingual gland	Ø Open 3 Percutaneous	Z No Device	Z No Qualifier
M Pharynx Base of tongue Hypopharynx Laryngopharynx Lingual tonsil Oropharynx Piriform recess (sinus) Tongue, base of R Epiglottis Glossoepiglottic fold	S Larynx Aryepiglottic fold Arytenoid cartilage Corniculate cartilage Cuneiform cartilage False vocal cord Glottis Rima glottidis Thyroid cartilage Ventricular fold T Vocal Cord, Right Vocal fold V Vocal Cord, Left *See T Vocal Cord, Right*	Ø Open 3 Percutaneous 4 Percutaneous Endoscopic 7 Via Natural or Artificial Opening 8 Via Natural or Artificial Opening Endoscopic	Z No Device	Z No Qualifier
W Upper Tooth X Lower Tooth		Ø Open X External	Z No Device	Ø Single 1 Multiple 2 All

Non-OR ØCC[Ø,1,2,3,4,7,N,P,Q]XZZ
Non-OR ØCC[5,6][Ø,3,X]ZZ
Non-OR ØCC[8,9,G,H]3ZZ
Non-OR ØCC[B,C,D, F,J][Ø,3]ZZ
Non-OR ØCC[M,S][7,8]ZZ
Non-OR ØCC[W,X][Ø,X]Z[Ø,1,2]

Ø Medical and Surgical
C Mouth and Throat
D Extraction Definition: Pulling or stripping out or off all or a portion of a body part by the use of force

Explanation: The qualifier DIAGNOSTIC is used to identify extraction procedures that are biopsies

Body Part Character 4	Approach Character 5	Device Character 6	Qualifier Character 7
T Vocal Cord, Right Vocal fold V Vocal Cord, Left *See T Vocal Cord, Right*	Ø Open 3 Percutaneous 4 Percutaneous Endoscopic 7 Via Natural or Artificial Opening 8 Via Natural or Artificial Opening Endoscopic	Z No Device	Z No Qualifier
W Upper Tooth X Lower Tooth	X External	Z No Device	Ø Single 1 Multiple 2 All

Non-OR ØCD[W,X]XZ[Ø,1,2]

Ø Medical and Surgical
C Mouth and Throat
F Fragmentation Definition: Breaking solid matter in a body part into pieces

Explanation: Physical force (e.g., manual, ultrasonic) applied directly or indirectly is used to break the solid matter into pieces. The solid matter may be an abnormal byproduct of a biological function or a foreign body. The pieces of solid matter are not taken out.

Body Part Character 4	Approach Character 5	Device Character 6	Qualifier Character 7
B Parotid Duct, Right NC Stensen's duct **C** Parotid Duct, Left NC *See B Parotid Duct, Right*	**Ø** Open **3** Percutaneous **7** Via Natural or Artificial Opening **X** External	**Z** No Device	**Z** No Qualifier

Non-OR All body part, approach, device, and qualifier values
NC ØCF[B,C]XZZ

Ø Medical and Surgical
C Mouth and Throat
H Insertion Definition: Putting in a nonbiological appliance that monitors, assists, performs, or prevents a physiological function but does not physically take the place of a body part

Explanation: None

Body Part Character 4	Approach Character 5	Device Character 6	Qualifier Character 7
7 Tongue Frenulum linguae	**Ø** Open **3** Percutaneous **X** External	**1** Radioactive Element	**Z** No Qualifier
A Salivary Gland **S** Larynx Aryepiglottic fold Arytenoid cartilage Corniculate cartilage Cuneiform cartilage False vocal cord Glottis Rima glottidis Thyroid cartilage Ventricular fold	**Ø** Open **3** Percutaneous **7** Via Natural or Artificial Opening **8** Via Natural or Artificial Opening Endoscopic	**1** Radioactive Element **Y** Other Device	**Z** No Qualifier
Y Mouth and Throat	**Ø** Open **3** Percutaneous	**1** Radioactive Element **Y** Other Device	**Z** No Qualifier
Y Mouth and Throat	**7** Via Natural or Artificial Opening **8** Via Natural or Artificial Opening Endoscopic	**1** Radioactive Element **B** Intraluminal Device, Airway **Y** Other Device	**Z** No Qualifier

Non-OR ØCH[A,S][3,7,8]YZ
Non-OR ØCHSØYZ
Non-OR ØCHY[Ø,3]YZ
Non-OR ØCHY[7,8][B,Y]Z

Ø Medical and Surgical
C Mouth and Throat
J Inspection Definition: Visually and/or manually exploring a body part

Explanation: Visual exploration may be performed with or without optical instrumentation. Manual exploration may be performed directly or through intervening body layers.

Body Part Character 4	Approach Character 5	Device Character 6	Qualifier Character 7
A Salivary Gland	**Ø** Open **3** Percutaneous **X** External	**Z** No Device	**Z** No Qualifier
S Larynx Aryepiglottic fold Arytenoid cartilage Corniculate cartilage Cuneiform cartilage False vocal cord Glottis Rima glottidis Thyroid cartilage Ventricular fold **Y** Mouth and Throat	**Ø** Open **3** Percutaneous **4** Percutaneous Endoscopic **7** Via Natural or Artificial Opening **8** Via Natural or Artificial Opening Endoscopic **X** External	**Z** No Device	**Z** No Qualifier

Non-OR All body part, approach, device, and qualifier values

Ø Medical and Surgical
C Mouth and Throat
L Occlusion Definition: Completely closing an orifice or the lumen of a tubular body part
Explanation: The orifice can be a natural orifice or an artificially created orifice

Body Part Character 4	Approach Character 5	Device Character 6	Qualifier Character 7
B Parotid Duct, Right Stensen's duct **C** Parotid Duct, Left *See B Parotid Duct, Right*	**Ø** Open **3** Percutaneous **4** Percutaneous Endoscopic	**C** Extraluminal Device **D** Intraluminal Device **Z** No Device	**Z** No Qualifier
B Parotid Duct, Right Stensen's duct **C** Parotid Duct, Left *See B Parotid Duct, Right*	**7** Via Natural or Artificial Opening **8** Via Natural or Artificial Opening Endoscopic	**D** Intraluminal Device **Z** No Device	**Z** No Qualifier

Ø Medical and Surgical
C Mouth and Throat
M Reattachment Definition: Putting back in or on all or a portion of a separated body part to its normal location or other suitable location
Explanation: Vascular circulation and nervous pathways may or may not be reestablished

Body Part Character 4	Approach Character 5	Device Character 6	Qualifier Character 7
Ø Upper Lip Frenulum labii superioris Labial gland Vermilion border **1** Lower Lip Frenulum labii inferioris Labial gland Vermilion border **3** Soft Palate **7** Tongue Frenulum linguae **N** Uvula Palatine uvula	**Ø** Open	**Z** No Device	**Z** No Qualifier
W Upper Tooth **X** Lower Tooth	**Ø** Open **X** External	**Z** No Device	**Ø** Single **1** Multiple **2** All

Non-OR ØCM[W,X][Ø,X]Z[Ø,1,2]

Ø Medical and Surgical
C Mouth and Throat
N Release Definition: Freeing a body part from an abnormal physical constraint by cutting or by the use of force
Explanation: Some of the restraining tissue may be taken out but none of the body part is taken out

Body Part Character 4	Approach Character 5	Device Character 6	Qualifier Character 7
Ø Upper Lip Frenulum labii superioris Labial gland Vermilion border **1 Lower Lip** Frenulum labii inferioris Labial gland Vermilion border **2 Hard Palate** **3 Soft Palate** **4 Buccal Mucosa** Buccal gland Molar gland Palatine gland **5 Upper Gingiva** **6 Lower Gingiva** **7 Tongue** Frenulum linguae **N Uvula** Palatine uvula **P Tonsils** Palatine tonsil **Q Adenoids** Pharyngeal tonsil	**Ø Open** **3 Percutaneous** **X External**	**Z No Device**	**Z No Qualifier**
8 Parotid Gland, Right **9 Parotid Gland, Left** **B Parotid Duct, Right** Stensen's duct **C Parotid Duct, Left** *See B Parotid Duct, Right* **D Sublingual Gland, Right** **F Sublingual Gland, Left** **G Submaxillary Gland, Right** Submandibular gland **H Submaxillary Gland, Left** *See G Submaxillary Gland, Right* **J Minor Salivary Gland** Anterior lingual gland	**Ø Open** **3 Percutaneous**	**Z No Device**	**Z No Qualifier**
M Pharynx Base of tongue Hypopharynx Laryngopharynx Lingual tonsil Oropharynx Piriform recess (sinus) Tongue, base of **R Epiglottis** Glossoepiglottic fold **S Larynx** Aryepiglottic fold Arytenoid cartilage Corniculate cartilage Cuneiform cartilage False vocal cord Glottis Rima glottidis Thyroid cartilage Ventricular fold **T Vocal Cord, Right** Vocal fold **V Vocal Cord, Left** *See T Vocal Cord, Right*	**Ø Open** **3 Percutaneous** **4 Percutaneous Endoscopic** **7 Via Natural or Artificial Opening** **8 Via Natural or Artificial Opening Endoscopic**	**Z No Device**	**Z No Qualifier**
W Upper Tooth **X Lower Tooth**	**Ø Open** **X External**	**Z No Device**	**Ø Single** **1 Multiple** **2 All**

Non-OR ØCN[Ø,1,5,6,7][Ø,3,X]ZZ
Non-OR ØCN[W,X][Ø,X]Z[Ø,1,2]

Ø Medical and Surgical
C Mouth and Throat
P Removal Definition: Taking out or off a device from a body part

Explanation: If a device is taken out and a similar device put in without cutting or puncturing the skin or mucous membrane, the procedure is coded to the root operation CHANGE. Otherwise, the procedure for taking out a device is coded to the root operation REMOVAL.

Body Part Character 4	Approach Character 5	Device Character 6	Qualifier Character 7
A Salivary Gland	**Ø Open** **3 Percutaneous**	**Ø Drainage Device** **C Extraluminal Device** **Y Other Device**	**Z No Qualifier**
A Salivary Gland	**7 Via Natural or Artificial Opening** **8 Via Natural or Artificial Opening Endoscopic**	**Y Other Device**	**Z No Qualifier**
S Larynx Aryepiglottic fold Arytenoid cartilage Corniculate cartilage Cuneiform cartilage False vocal cord Glottis Rima glottidis Thyroid cartilage Ventricular fold	**Ø Open** **3 Percutaneous** **7 Via Natural or Artificial Opening** **8 Via Natural or Artificial Opening Endoscopic**	**Ø Drainage Device** **7 Autologous Tissue Substitute** **D Intraluminal Device** **J Synthetic Substitute** **K Nonautologous Tissue Substitute** **Y Other Device**	**Z No Qualifier**
S Larynx Aryepiglottic fold Arytenoid cartilage Corniculate cartilage Cuneiform cartilage False vocal cord Glottis Rima glottidis Thyroid cartilage Ventricular fold	**X External**	**Ø Drainage Device** **7 Autologous Tissue Substitute** **D Intraluminal Device** **J Synthetic Substitute** **K Nonautologous Tissue Substitute**	**Z No Qualifier**
Y Mouth and Throat	**Ø Open** **3 Percutaneous** **7 Via Natural or Artificial Opening** **8 Via Natural or Artificial Opening Endoscopic**	**Ø Drainage Device** **1 Radioactive Element** **7 Autologous Tissue Substitute** **D Intraluminal Device** **J Synthetic Substitute** **K Nonautologous Tissue Substitute** **Y Other Device**	**Z No Qualifier**
Y Mouth and Throat	**X External**	**Ø Drainage Device** **1 Radioactive Element** **7 Autologous Tissue Substitute** **D Intraluminal Device** **J Synthetic Substitute** **K Nonautologous Tissue Substitute**	**Z No Qualifier**

Non-OR ØCPA[Ø,3][Ø,C,Y]Z
Non-OR ØCPA[7,8]YZ
Non-OR ØCPS3YZ
Non-OR ØCPS[7,8][Ø,D,Y]Z
Non-OR ØCPSX[Ø,7,D,J,K]Z
Non-OR ØCPY3YZ
Non-OR ØCPY[7,8][Ø,D,Y]Z
Non-OR ØCPYX[Ø,1,7,D,J,K]Z

Ø Medical and Surgical
C Mouth and Throat
Q Repair Definition: Restoring, to the extent possible, a body part to its normal anatomic structure and function
Explanation: Used only when the method to accomplish the repair is not one of the other root operations

Body Part Character 4	Approach Character 5	Device Character 6	Qualifier Character 7
Ø Upper Lip Frenulum labii superioris Labial gland Vermilion border **1 Lower Lip** Frenulum labii inferioris Labial gland Vermilion border **2 Hard Palate** **3 Soft Palate** **4 Buccal Mucosa** Buccal gland Molar gland Palatine gland **5 Upper Gingiva** **6 Lower Gingiva** **7 Tongue** Frenulum linguae **N Uvula** Palatine uvula **P Tonsils** Palatine tonsil **Q Adenoids** Pharyngeal tonsil	**Ø Open** **3 Percutaneous** **X External**	**Z No Device**	**Z No Qualifier**
8 Parotid Gland, Right **9 Parotid Gland, Left** **B Parotid Duct, Right** Stensen's duct **C Parotid Duct, Left** *See B Parotid Duct, Right* **D Sublingual Gland, Right** **F Sublingual Gland, Left** **G Submaxillary Gland, Right** Submandibular gland **H Submaxillary Gland, Left** *See G Submaxillary Gland, Right* **J Minor Salivary Gland** Anterior lingual gland	**Ø Open** **3 Percutaneous**	**Z No Device**	**Z No Qualifier**
M Pharynx Base of tongue Hypopharynx Laryngopharynx Lingual tonsil Oropharynx Piriform recess (sinus) Tongue, base of **R Epiglottis** Glossoepiglottic fold **S Larynx** Aryepiglottic fold Arytenoid cartilage Corniculate cartilage Cuneiform cartilage False vocal cord Glottis Rima glottidis Thyroid cartilage Ventricular fold **T Vocal Cord, Right** Vocal fold **V Vocal Cord, Left** *See T Vocal Cord, Right*	**Ø Open** **3 Percutaneous** **4 Percutaneous Endoscopic** **7 Via Natural or Artificial Opening** **8 Via Natural or Artificial Opening Endoscopic**	**Z No Device**	**Z No Qualifier**
W Upper Tooth **X Lower Tooth**	**Ø Open** **X External**	**Z No Device**	**Ø Single** **1 Multiple** **2 All**

Non-OR ØCQ[Ø,1,4,7]XZZ
Non-OR ØCQ[5,6][Ø,3,X]ZZ
Non-OR ØCQ[W,X][Ø,X]Z[Ø,1,2]

Ø Medical and Surgical
C Mouth and Throat
R Replacement Definition: Putting in or on biological or synthetic material that physically takes the place and/or function of all or a portion of a body part

Explanation: The body part may have been taken out or replaced, or may be taken out, physically eradicated, or rendered nonfunctional during the REPLACEMENT procedure. A REMOVAL procedure is coded for taking out the device used in a previous replacement procedure.

Body Part Character 4	Approach Character 5	Device Character 6	Qualifier Character 7
Ø Upper Lip Frenulum labii superioris Labial gland Vermilion border **1 Lower Lip** Frenulum labii inferioris Labial gland Vermilion border **2 Hard Palate** **3 Soft Palate** **4 Buccal Mucosa** Buccal gland Molar gland Palatine gland **5 Upper Gingiva** **6 Lower Gingiva** **7 Tongue** Frenulum linguae **N Uvula** Palatine uvula	**Ø Open** **3 Percutaneous** **X External**	**7 Autologous Tissue Substitute** **J Synthetic Substitute** **K Nonautologous Tissue Substitute**	**Z No Qualifier**
B Parotid Duct, Right Stensen's duct **C Parotid Duct, Left** *See B Parotid Duct, Right*	**Ø Open** **3 Percutaneous**	**7 Autologous Tissue Substitute** **J Synthetic Substitute** **K Nonautologous Tissue Substitute**	**Z No Qualifier**
M Pharynx Base of tongue Hypopharynx Laryngopharynx Lingual tonsil Oropharynx Piriform recess (sinus) Tongue, base of **R Epiglottis** Glossoepiglottic fold **S Larynx** Aryepiglottic fold Arytenoid cartilage Corniculate cartilage Cuneiform cartilage False vocal cord Glottis Rima glottidis Thyroid cartilage Ventricular fold **T Vocal Cord, Right** Vocal fold **V Vocal Cord, Left** *See T Vocal Cord, Right*	**Ø Open** **7 Via Natural or Artificial Opening** **8 Via Natural or Artificial Opening Endoscopic**	**7 Autologous Tissue Substitute** **J Synthetic Substitute** **K Nonautologous Tissue Substitute**	**Z No Qualifier**
W Upper Tooth **X Lower Tooth**	**Ø Open** **X External**	**7 Autologous Tissue Substitute** **J Synthetic Substitute** **K Nonautologous Tissue Substitute**	**Ø Single** **1 Multiple** **2 All**

Non-OR ØCR[W,X][Ø,X][7,J,K][Ø,1,2]

Ø Medical and Surgical
C Mouth and Throat
S Reposition Definition: Moving to its normal location, or other suitable location, all or a portion of a body part

Explanation: The body part is moved to a new location from an abnormal location, or from a normal location where it is not functioning correctly. The body part may or may not be cut out or off to be moved to the new location.

Body Part Character 4	Approach Character 5	Device Character 6	Qualifier Character 7
Ø Upper Lip Frenulum labii superioris Labial gland Vermilion border **1 Lower Lip** Frenulum labii inferioris Labial gland Vermilion border **2 Hard Palate** **3 Soft Palate** **7 Tongue** Frenulum linguae **N Uvula** Palatine uvula	**Ø Open** **X External**	**Z No Device**	**Z No Qualifier**
B Parotid Duct, Right Stensen's duct **C Parotid Duct, Left** *See B Parotid Duct, Right*	**Ø Open** **3 Percutaneous**	**Z No Device**	**Z No Qualifier**
R Epiglottis Glossoepiglottic fold **T Vocal Cord, Right** Vocal fold **V Vocal Cord, Left** *See T Vocal Cord, Right*	**Ø Open** **7 Via Natural or Artificial Opening** **8 Via Natural or Artificial Opening Endoscopic**	**Z No Device**	**Z No Qualifier**
W Upper Tooth **X Lower Tooth**	**Ø Open** **X External**	**5 External Fixation Device** **Z No Device**	**Ø Single** **1 Multiple** **2 All**

Non-OR ØCS[W,X][Ø,X][5,Z][Ø,1,2]

Ø Medical and Surgical
C Mouth and Throat
T Resection Definition: Cutting out or off, without replacement, all of a body part
Explanation: None

Body Part Character 4	Approach Character 5	Device Character 6	Qualifier Character 7
Ø Upper Lip Frenulum labii superioris Labial gland Vermilion border **1 Lower Lip** Frenulum labii inferioris Labial gland Vermilion border **2 Hard Palate** **3 Soft Palate** **7 Tongue** Frenulum linguae **N Uvula** Palatine uvula **P Tonsils** Palatine tonsil **Q Adenoids** Pharyngeal tonsil	**Ø Open** **X External**	**Z No Device**	**Z No Qualifier**
8 Parotid Gland, Right **9 Parotid Gland, Left** **B Parotid Duct, Right** Stensen's duct **C Parotid Duct, Left** *See B Parotid Duct, Right* **D Sublingual Gland, Right** **F Sublingual Gland, Left** **G Submaxillary Gland, Right** Submandibular gland **H Submaxillary Gland, Left** *See G Submaxillary Gland, Right* **J Minor Salivary Gland** Anterior lingual gland	**Ø Open**	**Z No Device**	**Z No Qualifier**
M Pharynx Base of tongue Hypopharynx Laryngopharynx Lingual tonsil Oropharynx Piriform recess (sinus) Tongue, base of **R Epiglottis** Glossoepiglottic fold **S Larynx** Aryepiglottic fold Arytenoid cartilage Corniculate cartilage Cuneiform cartilage False vocal cord Glottis Rima glottidis Thyroid cartilage Ventricular fold **T Vocal Cord, Right** Vocal fold **V Vocal Cord, Left** *See T Vocal Cord, Right*	**Ø Open** **4 Percutaneous Endoscopic** **7 Via Natural or Artificial Opening** **8 Via Natural or Artificial Opening Endoscopic**	**Z No Device**	**Z No Qualifier**
W Upper Tooth **X Lower Tooth**	**Ø Open**	**Z No Device**	**Ø Single** **1 Multiple** **2 All**

Non-OR ØCT[W,X]ØZ[Ø,1,2]

Ø Medical and Surgical
C Mouth and Throat
U Supplement Definition: Putting in or on biological or synthetic material that physically reinforces and/or augments the function of a portion of a body part

Explanation: The biological material is non-living, or is living and from the same individual. The body part may have been previously replaced, and the SUPPLEMENT procedure is performed to physically reinforce and/or augment the function of the replaced body part.

Body Part Character 4	Approach Character 5	Device Character 6	Qualifier Character 7
Ø Upper Lip Frenulum labii superioris Labial gland Vermilion border **1 Lower Lip** Frenulum labii inferioris Labial gland Vermilion border **2 Hard Palate** **3 Soft Palate** **4 Buccal Mucosa** Buccal gland Molar gland Palatine gland **5 Upper Gingiva** **6 Lower Gingiva** **7 Tongue** Frenulum linguae **N Uvula** Palatine uvula	**Ø Open** **3 Percutaneous** **X External**	**7 Autologous Tissue Substitute** **J Synthetic Substitute** **K Nonautologous Tissue Substitute**	**Z No Qualifier**
M Pharynx Base of tongue Hypopharynx Laryngopharynx Lingual tonsil Oropharynx Piriform recess (sinus) Tongue, base of **R Epiglottis** Glossoepiglottic fold **S Larynx** Aryepiglottic fold Arytenoid cartilage Corniculate cartilage Cuneiform cartilage False vocal cord Glottis Rima glottidis Thyroid cartilage Ventricular fold **T Vocal Cord, Right** Vocal fold **V Vocal Cord, Left** *See T Vocal Cord, Right*	**Ø Open** **7 Via Natural or Artificial Opening** **8 Via Natural or Artificial Opening Endoscopic**	**7 Autologous Tissue Substitute** **J Synthetic Substitute** **K Nonautologous Tissue Substitute**	**Z No Qualifier**

Non-OR ØCU2[Ø,3]JZ

Ø Medical and Surgical
C Mouth and Throat
V Restriction Definition: Partially closing an orifice or the lumen of a tubular body part

Explanation: The orifice can be a natural orifice or an artificially created orifice

Body Part Character 4	Approach Character 5	Device Character 6	Qualifier Character 7
B Parotid Duct, Right Stensen's duct **C Parotid Duct, Left** *See B Parotid Duct, Right*	**Ø Open** **3 Percutaneous**	**C Extraluminal Device** **D Intraluminal Device** **Z No Device**	**Z No Qualifier**
B Parotid Duct, Right Stensen's duct **C Parotid Duct, Left** *See B Parotid Duct, Right*	**7 Via Natural or Artificial Opening** **8 Via Natural or Artificial Opening Endoscopic**	**D Intraluminal Device** **Z No Device**	**Z No Qualifier**

Ø Medical and Surgical
C Mouth and Throat
W Revision Definition: Correcting, to the extent possible, a portion of a malfunctioning device or the position of a displaced device

Explanation: Revision can include correcting a malfunctioning or displaced device by taking out or putting in components of the device such as a screw or pin

Body Part Character 4	Approach Character 5	Device Character 6	Qualifier Character 7
A Salivary Gland	Ø Open 3 Percutaneous	Ø Drainage Device C Extraluminal Device Y Other Device	Z No Qualifier
A Salivary Gland	7 Via Natural or Artificial Opening 8 Via Natural or Artificial Opening Endoscopic	Y Other Device	Z No Qualifier
A Salivary Gland	X External	Ø Drainage Device C Extraluminal Device	Z No Qualifier
S Larynx Aryepiglottic fold Arytenoid cartilage Corniculate cartilage Cuneiform cartilage False vocal cord Glottis Rima glottidis Thyroid cartilage Ventricular fold	Ø Open 3 Percutaneous 7 Via Natural or Artificial Opening 8 Via Natural or Artificial Opening Endoscopic	Ø Drainage Device 7 Autologous Tissue Substitute D Intraluminal Device J Synthetic Substitute K Nonautologous Tissue Substitute Y Other Device	Z No Qualifier
S Larynx Aryepiglottic fold Arytenoid cartilage Corniculate cartilage Cuneiform cartilage False vocal cord Glottis Rima glottidis Thyroid cartilage Ventricular fold	X External	Ø Drainage Device 7 Autologous Tissue Substitute D Intraluminal Device J Synthetic Substitute K Nonautologous Tissue Substitute	Z No Qualifier
Y Mouth and Throat	Ø Open 3 Percutaneous 7 Via Natural or Artificial Opening 8 Via Natural or Artificial Opening Endoscopic	Ø Drainage Device 1 Radioactive Element 7 Autologous Tissue Substitute D Intraluminal Device J Synthetic Substitute K Nonautologous Tissue Substitute Y Other Device	Z No Qualifier
Y Mouth and Throat	X External	Ø Drainage Device 1 Radioactive Element 7 Autologous Tissue Substitute D Intraluminal Device J Synthetic Substitute K Nonautologous Tissue Substitute	Z No Qualifier

Non-OR ØCWA[Ø,3][Ø,C,Y]Z
Non-OR ØCWA[7,8]YZ
Non-OR ØCWAX[Ø,C]Z
Non-OR ØCWS[3,7,8]YZ
Non-OR ØCWSX[Ø,7,D,J,K]Z
Non-OR ØCWYØ7Z
Non-OR ØCWY[3,7,8]YZ
Non-OR ØCWYX[Ø,1,7,D,J,K]Z

Ø Medical and Surgical
C Mouth and Throat
X Transfer

Definition: Moving, without taking out, all or a portion of a body part to another location to take over the function of all or a portion of a body part
Explanation: The body part transferred remains connected to its vascular and nervous supply

Body Part Character 4	Approach Character 5	Device Character 6	Qualifier Character 7
Ø Upper Lip Frenulum labii superioris Labial gland Vermilion border **1 Lower Lip** Frenulum labii inferioris Labial gland Vermilion border **3 Soft Palate** **4 Buccal Mucosa** Buccal gland Molar gland Palatine gland **5 Upper Gingiva** **6 Lower Gingiva** **7 Tongue** Frenulum linguae	**Ø Open** **X External**	**Z No Device**	**Z No Qualifier**

Gastrointestinal System ØD1–ØDY

Character Meanings

This Character Meaning table is provided as a guide to assist the user in the identification of character members that may be found in this section of code tables. It **SHOULD NOT** be used to build a PCS code.

Operation–Character 3		Body Part–Character 4		Approach–Character 5		Device–Character 6		Qualifier–Character 7	
1	Bypass	Ø	Upper Intestinal Tract	Ø	Open	Ø	Drainage Device	Ø	Allogeneic
2	Change	1	Esophagus, Upper	3	Percutaneous	1	Radioactive Element	1	Syngeneic
5	Destruction	2	Esophagus, Middle	4	Percutaneous Endoscopic	2	Monitoring Device	2	Zooplastic
7	Dilation	3	Esophagus, Lower	7	Via Natural or Artificial Opening	3	Infusion Device	3	Vertical
8	Division	4	Esophagogastric Junction	8	Via Natural or Artificial Opening Endoscopic	7	Autologous Tissue Substitute	4	Cutaneous
9	Drainage	5	Esophagus	F	Via Natural or Artificial Opening with Percutaneous Endoscopic Assistance	B	Intraluminal Device, Airway	5	Esophagus
B	Excision	6	Stomach	X	External	C	Extraluminal Device	6	Stomach
C	Extirpation	7	Stomach, Pylorus			D	Intraluminal Device	7	Vagina
D	Extraction	8	Small Intestine			J	Synthetic Substitute	8	Small Intestine
F	Fragmentation	9	Duodenum			K	Nonautologous Tissue Substitute	9	Duodenum
H	Insertion	A	Jejunum			L	Artificial Sphincter	A	Jejunum
J	Inspection	B	Ileum			M	Stimulator Lead	B	Ileum
L	Occlusion	C	Ileocecal Valve			U	Feeding Device	E	Large Intestine
M	Reattachment	D	Lower Intestinal Tract			Y	Other Device	H	Cecum
N	Release	E	Large Intestine			Z	No Device	K	Ascending Colon
P	Removal	F	Large Intestine, Right					L	Transverse Colon
Q	Repair	G	Large Intestine, Left					M	Descending Colon
R	Replacement	H	Cecum					N	Sigmoid Colon
S	Reposition	J	Appendix					P	Rectum
T	Resection	K	Ascending Colon					Q	Anus
U	Supplement	L	Transverse Colon					X	Diagnostic
V	Restriction	M	Descending Colon					Z	No Qualifier
W	Revision	N	Sigmoid Colon						
X	Transfer	P	Rectum						
Y	Transplantation	Q	Anus						
		R	Anal Sphincter						
		U	Omentum						
		V	Mesentery						
		W	Peritoneum						

AHA Coding Clinic for table ØD1
2019, 4Q, 29 Intestinal bypass
2017, 2Q, 17 Billroth II (distal gastrectomy and gastrojejunostomy)
2016, 2Q, 31 Laparoscopic biliopancreatic diversion with duodenal switch
2014, 4Q, 41 Abdominoperineal resection (APR) with flap closure of perineum and colostomy

AHA Coding Clinic for table ØD2
2019, 1Q, 26 Exchange of clogged gastrojejunostomy tube

AHA Coding Clinic for table ØD5
2017, 1Q, 34 Debulking of tumor and peritoneum ablation

AHA Coding Clinic for table ØD7
2017, 3Q, 23 Laparoscopic pyloromyotomy
2014, 4Q, 40 Dilation of gastrojejunostomy anastomosis stricture

AHA Coding Clinic for table ØD8
2019, 2Q, 15 Reversal of Roux-en-Y bypass
2017, 3Q, 22 Laparoscopic esophagomyotomy (Heller type) and Toupet fundoplication
2017, 3Q, 23 Laparoscopic pyloromyotomy

AHA Coding Clinic for table ØD9
2015, 2Q, 29 Insertion of nasogastric tube for drainage and feeding

AHA Coding Clinic for table ØDB
2019, 2Q, 15 Reversal of Roux-en-Y bypass
2019, 1Q, 3-8 Whipple procedure
2019, 1Q, 27 Excision of pelvic sidewall mass
2017, 2Q, 17 Billroth II (distal gastrectomy and gastrojejunostomy)
2017, 1Q, 16 Hepatic flexure versus transverse colon
2016, 3Q, 3-7 Stoma creation & takedown procedures
2016, 2Q, 31 Laparoscopic biliopancreatic diversion with duodenal switch
2016, 1Q, 22 Perineal proctectomy
2016, 1Q, 24 Endoscopic brush biopsy of esophagus
2014, 4Q, 40 Abdominoperineal resection (APR) with flap closure of perineum and colostomy
2014, 3Q, 28 Ileostomy takedown and parastomal hernia repair
2014, 3Q, 32 Pyloric-sparing Whipple procedure

AHA Coding Clinic for table ØDD
2017, 4Q, 41-42 Extraction procedures

AHA Coding Clinic for table ØDH
2019, 2Q, 18 Endoscopic wound VAC placement
2016, 3Q, 26 Insertion of gastrostomy tube
2013, 4Q, 117 Percutaneous endoscopic placement of gastrostomy tube

AHA Coding Clinic for table ØDJ
2019, 1Q, 25 Laparoscopic appendectomy converted to open procedure
2019, 1Q, 25 Milking of inspissated material from ileum to colon
2017, 2Q, 15 Low anterior resection with sigmoidoscopy
2016, 2Q, 20 Capsule endoscopy of small intestine
2015, 3Q, 24 Esophagogastroduodenoscopy with epinephrine injection for control of bleeding

AHA Coding Clinic for table ØDL
2013, 4Q, 112 Endoscopic banding of esophageal varices

AHA Coding Clinic for table ØDN
2017, 4Q, 49-50 New and revised body part values - Repositioning of the intestine
2017, 1Q, 35 Lysis of omental and peritoneal adhesions
2015, 3Q, 15 Vascular ring surgery with release of esophagus and trachea
2015, 3Q, 16 Vascular ring surgery and double aortic arch

AHA Coding Clinic for table ØDP
2019, 2Q, 18 Removal of wound VAC

AHA Coding Clinic for table ØDQ
2019, 2Q, 15 Reversal of Roux-en-Y bypass
2018, 2Q, 25 Third and fourth degree obstetric lacerations
2018, 1Q, 11 Repair of internal hernia at Petersen space
2017, 3Q, 17 Posterior sagittal anorectoplasty
2016, 3Q, 3-7 Stoma creation & takedown procedures
2016, 3Q, 26 Insertion of gastrostomy tube
2016, 1Q, 7 Obstetrical perineal laceration repair
2016, 1Q, 8 Obstetrical perineal laceration repair
2014, 4Q, 20 Control of bleeding duodenal ulcer

AHA Coding Clinic for table ØDS
2019, 1Q, 30 Laparoscopic-assisted rectopexy with manual reduction of prolapse
2017, 4Q, 49-50 New and revised body part values - Repositioning of the intestine
2017, 3Q, 9 Ileocolic intussusception reduction via air enema
2017, 3Q, 17 Posterior sagittal anorectoplasty
2016, 3Q, 3-5 Stoma creation & takedown procedures

AHA Coding Clinic for table ØDT
2019, 1Q, 3-8 Whipple procedure
2019, 1Q, 14 Esophagectomy with colon interposition
2017, 4Q, 49-50 New and revised body part values - Repositioning of the intestine
2014, 4Q, 40 Abdominoperineal resection (APR) with flap closure of perineum and colostomy
2014, 4Q, 42 Right colectomy with side-to-side functional end-to-end anastomosis
2014, 3Q, 6 Ileocecectomy including cecum, terminal ileum and appendix
2014, 3Q, 6 Right colectomy

AHA Coding Clinic for table ØDU
2019, 1Q, 30 Laparoscopic-assisted rectopexy with manual reduction of prolapse

AHA Coding Clinic for table ØDV
2017, 3Q, 22 Laparoscopic esophagomyotomy (Heller type) and Toupet fundoplication
2016, 2Q, 22 Esophageal lengthening Collis gastroplasty with Nissen fundoplication and hiatal hernia
2014, 3Q, 28 Laparoscopic Nissen fundoplication and diaphragmatic hernia repair

AHA Coding Clinic for table ØDW
2018, 1Q, 20 Adjustment of gastric band

AHA Coding Clinic for table ØDX
2019, 4Q, 29-30 Transfer large intestine to vagina
2019, 1Q, 14 Esophagectomy with colon interposition
2017, 2Q, 18 Esophagectomy and esophagogastrectomy with cervical esophagogastrostomy
2016, 2Q, 22 Esophageal lengthening Collis gastroplasty with Nissen fundoplication and hiatal hernia
2015, 1Q, 28 Repair of bronchopleural fistula using omental pedicle graft

Upper Intestinal Tract (Ø) and Lower Intestinal Tract (D)

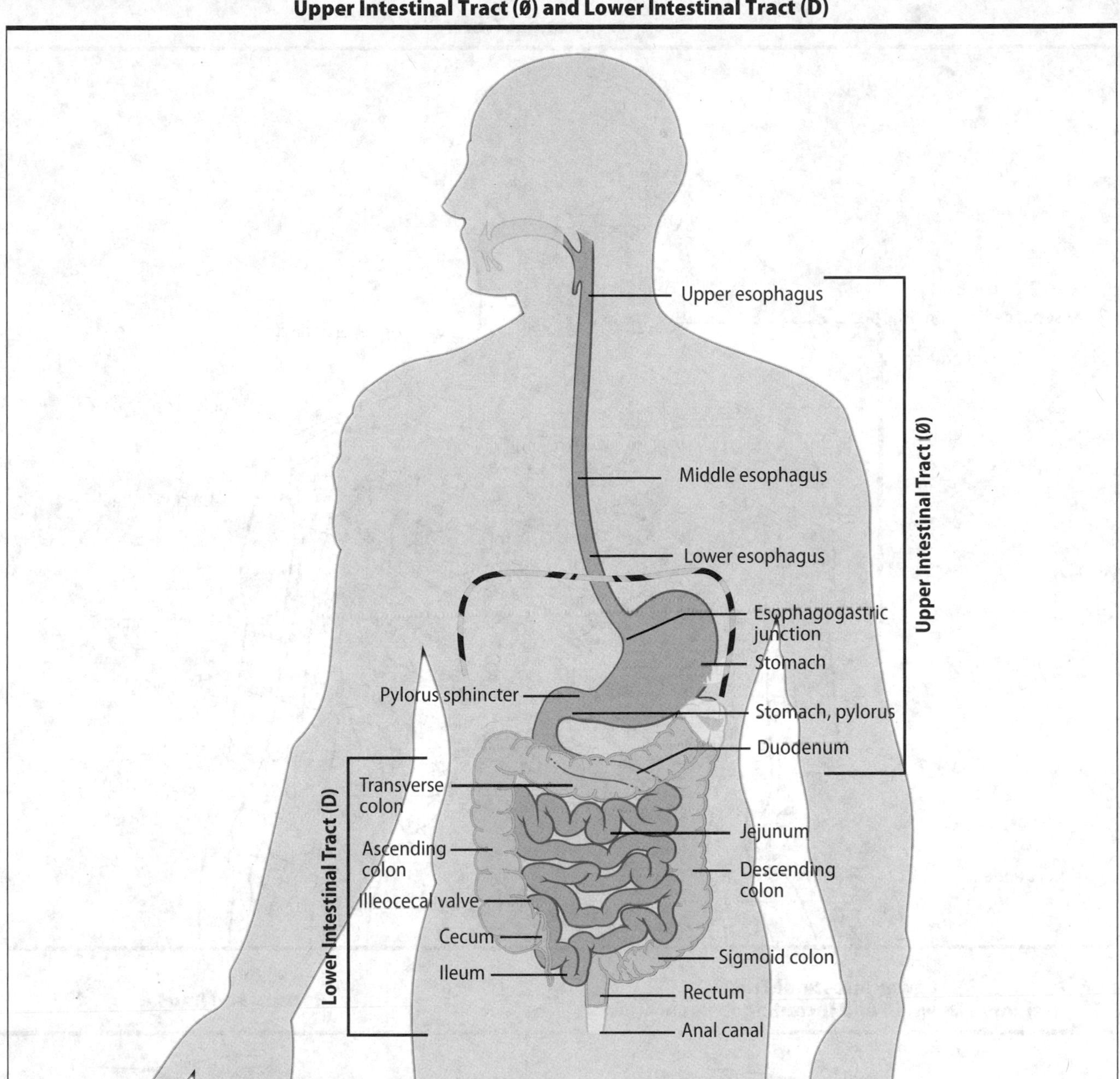

Upper Intestinal Tract

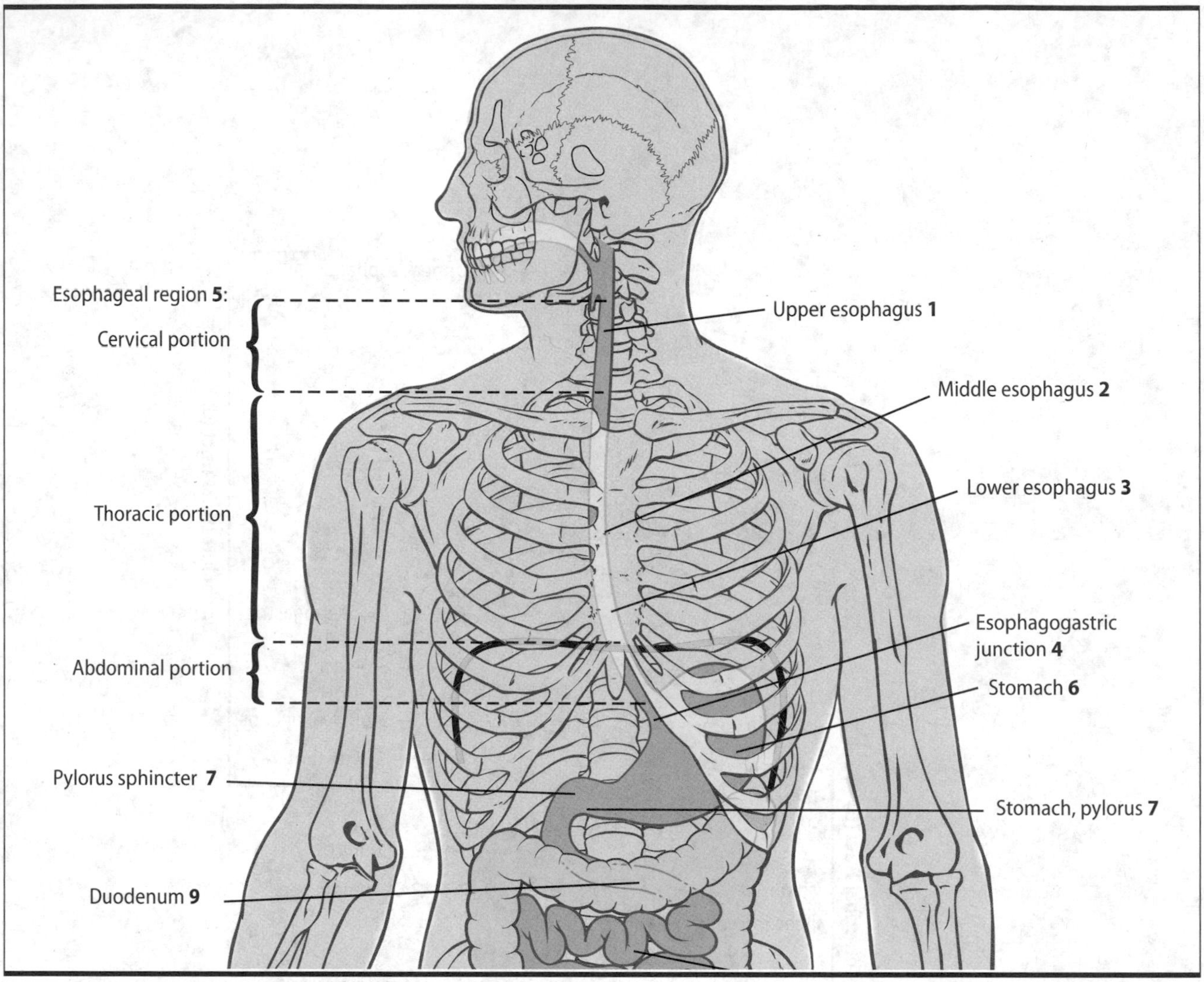

Esophageal region **5**:

Cervical portion

Thoracic portion

Abdominal portion

Upper esophagus **1**

Middle esophagus **2**

Lower esophagus **3**

Esophagogastric junction **4**

Stomach **6**

Pylorus sphincter **7**

Stomach, pylorus **7**

Duodenum **9**

Lower Intestinal Tract (Jejunum Down to and Including Rectum/Anus)

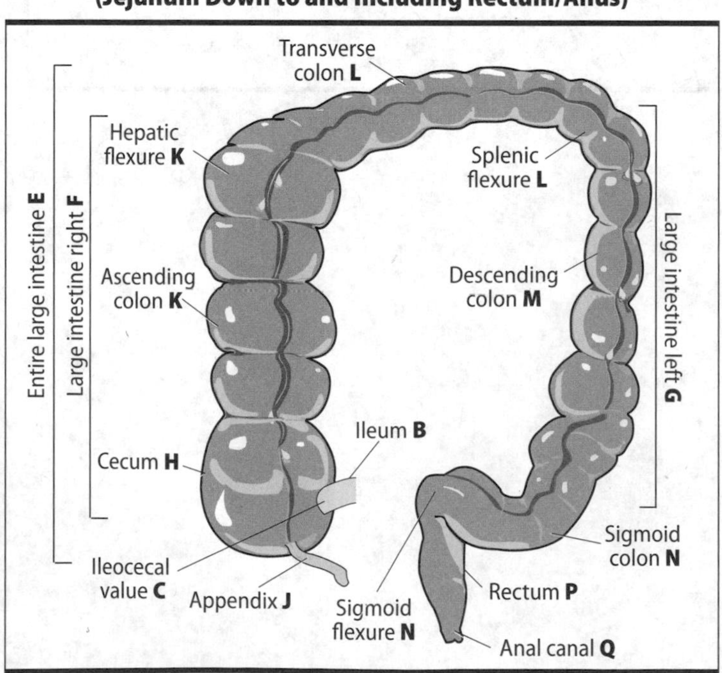

Rectum and Anus

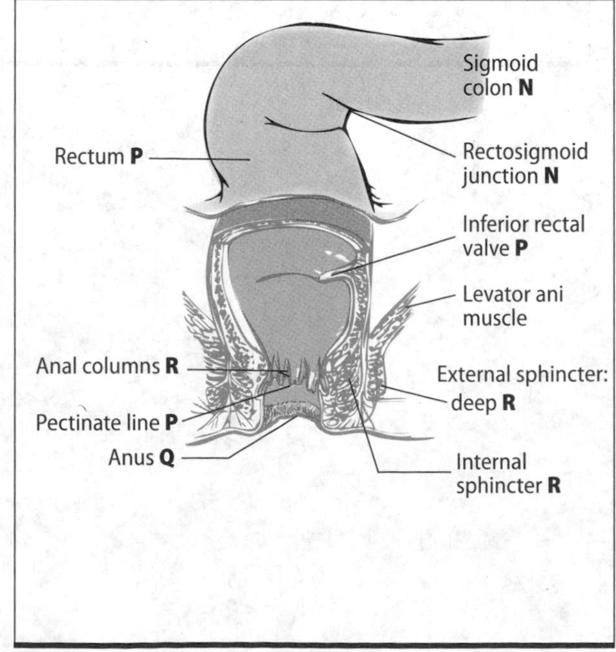

Ø **Medical and Surgical**
D **Gastrointestinal System**
1 **Bypass** Definition: Altering the route of passage of the contents of a tubular body part

Explanation: Rerouting contents of a body part to a downstream area of the normal route, to a similar route and body part, or to an abnormal route and dissimilar body part. Includes one or more anastomoses, with or without the use of a device.

Body Part Character 4	Approach Character 5	Device Character 6	Qualifier Character 7
1 Esophagus, Upper Cervical esophagus 2 Esophagus, Middle Thoracic esophagus 3 Esophagus, Lower Abdominal esophagus 5 Esophagus	Ø Open 4 Percutaneous Endoscopic 8 Via Natural or Artificial Opening Endoscopic	7 Autologous Tissue Substitute J Synthetic Substitute K Nonautologous Tissue Substitute Z No Device	4 Cutaneous 6 Stomach 9 Duodenum A Jejunum B Ileum
1 Esophagus, Upper Cervical esophagus 2 Esophagus, Middle Thoracic esophagus 3 Esophagus, Lower Abdominal esophagus 5 Esophagus	3 Percutaneous	J Synthetic Substitute	4 Cutaneous
6 Stomach 9 Duodenum	Ø Open 4 Percutaneous Endoscopic 8 Via Natural or Artificial Opening Endoscopic	7 Autologous Tissue Substitute J Synthetic Substitute K Nonautologous Tissue Substitute Z No Device	4 Cutaneous 9 Duodenum A Jejunum B Ileum L Transverse Colon
6 Stomach 9 Duodenum	3 Percutaneous	J Synthetic Substitute	4 Cutaneous
8 Small Intestine	Ø Open 4 Percutaneous Endoscopic 8 Via Natural or Artificial Opening Endoscopic	7 Autologous Tissue Substitute J Synthetic Substitute K Nonautologous Tissue Substitute Z No Device	4 Cutaneous 8 Small Intestine H Cecum K Ascending Colon L Transverse Colon M Descending Colon N Sigmoid Colon P Rectum Q Anus
A Jejunum Duodenojejunal flexure	Ø Open 4 Percutaneous Endoscopic 8 Via Natural or Artificial Opening Endoscopic	7 Autologous Tissue Substitute J Synthetic Substitute K Nonautologous Tissue Substitute Z No Device	4 Cutaneous A Jejunum B Ileum H Cecum K Ascending Colon L Transverse Colon M Descending Colon N Sigmoid Colon P Rectum Q Anus
A Jejunum Duodenojejunal flexure	3 Percutaneous	J Synthetic Substitute	4 Cutaneous
B Ileum	Ø Open 4 Percutaneous Endoscopic 8 Via Natural or Artificial Opening Endoscopic	7 Autologous Tissue Substitute J Synthetic Substitute K Nonautologous Tissue Substitute Z No Device	4 Cutaneous B Ileum H Cecum K Ascending Colon L Transverse Colon M Descending Colon N Sigmoid Colon P Rectum Q Anus
B Ileum	3 Percutaneous	J Synthetic Substitute	4 Cutaneous
E Large Intestine	Ø Open 4 Percutaneous Endoscopic 8 Via Natural or Artificial Opening Endoscopic	7 Autologous Tissue Substitute J Synthetic Substitute K Nonautologous Tissue Substitute Z No Device	4 Cutaneous E Large Intestine P Rectum
H Cecum	Ø Open 4 Percutaneous Endoscopic 8 Via Natural or Artificial Opening Endoscopic	7 Autologous Tissue Substitute J Synthetic Substitute K Nonautologous Tissue Substitute Z No Device	4 Cutaneous H Cecum K Ascending Colon L Transverse Colon M Descending Colon N Sigmoid Colon P Rectum
H Cecum	3 Percutaneous	J Synthetic Substitute	4 Cutaneous

Non-OR ØD16[Ø,4,8][7,J,K,Z]4
Non-OR ØD163J4
HAC ØD16[Ø,4,8][7,J,K,Z][9,A,B,L] when reported with PDx E66.Ø1 and SDx K68.11, K95.Ø1, K95.81 or T81.4Ø–T81.49 with7th character A

ØD1 Continued on next page

Ø Medical and Surgical
D Gastrointestinal System
1 Bypass Definition: Altering the route of passage of the contents of a tubular body part

Explanation: Rerouting contents of a body part to a downstream area of the normal route, to a similar route and body part, or to an abnormal route and dissimilar body part. Includes one or more anastomoses, with or without the use of a device.

ØD1 Continued

Body Part Character 4	Approach Character 5	Device Character 6	Qualifier Character 7
K Ascending Colon	**Ø** Open **4** Percutaneous Endoscopic **8** Via Natural or Artificial Opening Endoscopic	**7** Autologous Tissue Substitute **J** Synthetic Substitute **K** Nonautologous Tissue Substitute **Z** No Device	**4** Cutaneous **K** Ascending Colon **L** Transverse Colon **M** Descending Colon **N** Sigmoid Colon **P** Rectum
K Ascending Colon	**3** Percutaneous	**J** Synthetic Substitute	**4** Cutaneous
L Transverse Colon Hepatic flexure Splenic flexure	**Ø** Open **4** Percutaneous Endoscopic **8** Via Natural or Artificial Opening Endoscopic	**7** Autologous Tissue Substitute **J** Synthetic Substitute **K** Nonautologous Tissue Substitute **Z** No Device	**4** Cutaneous **L** Transverse Colon **M** Descending Colon **N** Sigmoid Colon **P** Rectum
L Transverse Colon Hepatic flexure Splenic flexure	**3** Percutaneous	**J** Synthetic Substitute	**4** Cutaneous
M Descending Colon	**Ø** Open **4** Percutaneous Endoscopic **8** Via Natural or Artificial Opening Endoscopic	**7** Autologous Tissue Substitute **J** Synthetic Substitute **K** Nonautologous Tissue Substitute **Z** No Device	**4** Cutaneous **M** Descending Colon **N** Sigmoid Colon **P** Rectum
M Descending Colon	**3** Percutaneous	**J** Synthetic Substitute	**4** Cutaneous
N Sigmoid Colon Rectosigmoid junction Sigmoid flexure	**Ø** Open **4** Percutaneous Endoscopic **8** Via Natural or Artificial Opening Endoscopic	**7** Autologous Tissue Substitute **J** Synthetic Substitute **K** Nonautologous Tissue Substitute **Z** No Device	**4** Cutaneous **N** Sigmoid Colon **P** Rectum
N Sigmoid Colon Rectosigmoid junction Sigmoid flexure	**3** Percutaneous	**J** Synthetic Substitute	**4** Cutaneous

Ø Medical and Surgical
D Gastrointestinal System
2 Change Definition: Taking out or off a device from a body part and putting back an identical or similar device in or on the same body part without cutting or puncturing the skin or a mucous membrane

Explanation: All CHANGE procedures are coded using the approach EXTERNAL

Body Part Character 4	Approach Character 5	Device Character 6	Qualifier Character 7
Ø Upper Intestinal Tract **D** Lower Intestinal Tract	**X** External	**Ø** Drainage Device **U** Feeding Device **Y** Other Device	**Z** No Qualifier
U Omentum Gastrocolic ligament Gastrocolic omentum Gastrohepatic omentum Gastrophrenic ligament Gastrosplenic ligament Greater Omentum Hepatogastric ligament Lesser Omentum **V** Mesentery Mesoappendix Mesocolon **W** Peritoneum Epiploic foramen	**X** External	**Ø** Drainage Device **Y** Other Device	**Z** No Qualifier

Non-OR All body part, approach, device, and qualifier values

Ø Medical and Surgical
D Gastrointestinal System
5 Destruction Definition: Physical eradication of all or a portion of a body part by the direct use of energy, force, or a destructive agent
Explanation: None of the body part is physically taken out

Body Part Character 4	Approach Character 5	Device Character 6	Qualifier Character 7
1 Esophagus, Upper Cervical esophagus **2 Esophagus, Middle** Thoracic esophagus **3 Esophagus, Lower** Abdominal esophagus **4 Esophagogastric Junction** Cardia Cardioesophageal junction Gastroesophageal (GE) junction **5 Esophagus** **6 Stomach** **7 Stomach, Pylorus** Pyloric antrum Pyloric canal Pyloric sphincter **8 Small Intestine** **9 Duodenum** **A Jejunum** Duodenojejunal flexure **B Ileum** **C Ileocecal Valve** **E Large Intestine** **F Large Intestine, Right** **G Large Intestine, Left** **H Cecum** **J Appendix** Vermiform appendix **K Ascending Colon** **L Transverse Colon** Hepatic flexure Splenic flexure **M Descending Colon** **N Sigmoid Colon** Rectosigmoid junction Sigmoid flexure **P Rectum** Anorectal junction	**Ø Open** **3 Percutaneous** **4 Percutaneous Endoscopic** **7 Via Natural or Artificial Opening** **8 Via Natural or Artificial Opening Endoscopic**	**Z No Device**	**Z No Qualifier**
Q Anus Anal orifice	**Ø Open** **3 Percutaneous** **4 Percutaneous Endoscopic** **7 Via Natural or Artificial Opening** **8 Via Natural or Artificial Opening Endoscopic** **X External**	**Z No Device**	**Z No Qualifier**
R Anal Sphincter External anal sphincter Internal anal sphincter **U Omentum** Gastrocolic ligament Gastrocolic omentum Gastrohepatic omentum Gastrophrenic ligament Gastrosplenic ligament Greater Omentum Hepatogastric ligament Lesser Omentum **V Mesentery** Mesoappendix Mesocolon **W Peritoneum** Epiploic foramen	**Ø Open** **3 Percutaneous** **4 Percutaneous Endoscopic**	**Z No Device**	**Z No Qualifier**

Non-OR ØD5[1,2,3,4,5,6,7,9,E,F,G,H,K,L,M,N][4,8]ZZ
Non-OR ØD5[8,A,B,C]8ZZ
Non-OR ØD5P[Ø,3,4,7,8]ZZ
Non-OR ØD5Q[4,8]ZZ
Non-OR ØD5R4ZZ

Ø Medical and Surgical
D Gastrointestinal System
7 Dilation Definition: Expanding an orifice or the lumen of a tubular body part

Explanation: The orifice can be a natural orifice or an artificially created orifice. Accomplished by stretching a tubular body part using intraluminal pressure or by cutting part of the orifice or wall of the tubular body part.

Body Part Character 4	Approach Character 5	Device Character 6	Qualifier Character 7
1 Esophagus, Upper Cervical esophagus 2 Esophagus, Middle Thoracic esophagus 3 Esophagus, Lower Abdominal esophagus 4 Esophagogastric Junction Cardia Cardioesophageal junction Gastroesophageal (GE) junction 5 Esophagus 6 Stomach 7 Stomach, Pylorus Pyloric antrum Pyloric canal Pyloric sphincter 8 Small Intestine 9 Duodenum A Jejunum Duodenojejunal flexure B Ileum C Ileocecal Valve E Large Intestine F Large Intestine, Right G Large Intestine, Left H Cecum K Ascending Colon L Transverse Colon Hepatic flexure Splenic flexure M Descending Colon N Sigmoid Colon Rectosigmoid junction Sigmoid flexure P Rectum Anorectal junction Q Anus Anal orifice	Ø Open 3 Percutaneous 4 Percutaneous Endoscopic 7 Via Natural or Artificial Opening 8 Via Natural or Artificial Opening Endoscopic	D Intraluminal Device Z No Device	Z No Qualifier

Non-OR ØD7[1,2,3,4,5,6,8,9,A,B,C,E,F,G,H,K,L,M,N,P,Q][7,8][D,Z]Z
Non-OR ØD77[4,8]DZ
Non-OR ØD777[D,Z]Z
Non-OR ØD7[8,9,A,B,C,E,F,G,H,K,L,M,N][Ø,3,4]DZ

Ø Medical and Surgical
D Gastrointestinal System
8 Division Definition: Cutting into a body part, without draining fluids and/or gases from the body part, in order to separate or transect a body part

Explanation: All or a portion of the body part is separated into two or more portions

Body Part Character 4	Approach Character 5	Device Character 6	Qualifier Character 7
4 Esophagogastric Junction Cardia Cardioesophageal junction Gastroesophageal (GE) junction 7 Stomach, Pylorus Pyloric antrum Pyloric canal Pyloric sphincter	Ø Open 3 Percutaneous 4 Percutaneous Endoscopic 7 Via Natural or Artificial Opening 8 Via Natural or Artificial Opening Endoscopic	Z No Device	Z No Qualifier
R Anal Sphincter External anal sphincter Internal anal sphincter	Ø Open 3 Percutaneous	Z No Device	Z No Qualifier

Ø Medical and Surgical
D Gastrointestinal System
9 Drainage Definition: Taking or letting out fluids and/or gases from a body part
Explanation: The qualifier DIAGNOSTIC is used to identify drainage procedures that are biopsies

Body Part Character 4	Approach Character 5	Device Character 6	Qualifier Character 7
1 Esophagus, Upper Cervical esophagus **2 Esophagus, Middle** Thoracic esophagus **3 Esophagus, Lower** Abdominal esophagus **4 Esophagogastric Junction** Cardia Cardioesophageal junction Gastroesophageal (GE) junction **5 Esophagus** **6 Stomach** **7 Stomach, Pylorus** Pyloric antrum Pyloric canal Pyloric sphincter **8 Small Intestine** **9 Duodenum** **A Jejunum** Duodenojejunal flexure **B Ileum** **C Ileocecal Valve** **E Large Intestine** **F Large Intestine, Right** **G Large Intestine, Left** **H Cecum** **J Appendix** Vermiform appendix **K Ascending Colon** **L Transverse Colon** Hepatic flexure Splenic flexure **M Descending Colon** **N Sigmoid Colon** Rectosigmoid junction Sigmoid flexure **P Rectum** Anorectal junction	**Ø Open** **3 Percutaneous** **4 Percutaneous Endoscopic** **7 Via Natural or Artificial Opening** **8 Via Natural or Artificial Opening Endoscopic**	**Ø Drainage Device**	**Z No Qualifier**
1 Esophagus, Upper Cervical esophagus **2 Esophagus, Middle** Thoracic esophagus **3 Esophagus, Lower** Abdominal esophagus **4 Esophagogastric Junction** Cardia Cardioesophageal junction Gastroesophageal (GE) junction **5 Esophagus** **6 Stomach** **7 Stomach, Pylorus** Pyloric antrum Pyloric canal Pyloric sphincter **8 Small Intestine** **9 Duodenum** **A Jejunum** Duodenojejunal flexure **B Ileum** **C Ileocecal Valve** **E Large Intestine** **F Large Intestine, Right** **G Large Intestine, Left** **H Cecum** **J Appendix** Vermiform appendix **K Ascending Colon** **L Transverse Colon** Hepatic flexure Splenic flexure **M Descending Colon** **N Sigmoid Colon** Rectosigmoid junction Sigmoid flexure **P Rectum** Anorectal junction	**Ø Open** **3 Percutaneous** **4 Percutaneous Endoscopic** **7 Via Natural or Artificial Opening** **8 Via Natural or Artificial Opening Endoscopic**	**Z No Device**	**X Diagnostic** **Z No Qualifier**
Q Anus Anal orifice	**Ø Open** **3 Percutaneous** **4 Percutaneous Endoscopic** **7 Via Natural or Artificial Opening** **8 Via Natural or Artificial Opening Endoscopic** **X External**	**Ø Drainage Device**	**Z No Qualifier**
Q Anus Anal orifice	**Ø Open** **3 Percutaneous** **4 Percutaneous Endoscopic** **7 Via Natural or Artificial Opening** **8 Via Natural or Artificial Opening Endoscopic** **X External**	**Z No Device**	**X Diagnostic** **Z No Qualifier**

Non-OR ØD9[1,2,3,4,5,C,J]3ØZ
Non-OR ØD9[6,7,8,9,A,B,E,F,G,H,K,L,M,N,P][3,7,8]ØZ
Non-OR ØD9[1,2,3,4,5,6,7,8,9,A,B,C,E,F,G,H,K,L,M,N,P][3,4,7,8]ZX
Non-OR ØD9[1,2,3,4,5,6,7,8,9,A,B,C,E,F,G,H,J,K,L,M,N,P]3ZZ
Non-OR ØD9Q3ØZ
Non-OR ØD9Q[Ø,4,7,8,X]ZX
Non-OR ØD9Q3Z[X,Z]

ØD9 Continued on next page

Ø Medical and Surgical
D Gastrointestinal System
9 Drainage Definition: Taking or letting out fluids and/or gases from a body part
Explanation: The qualifier DIAGNOSTIC is used to identify drainage procedures that are biopsies

ØD9 Continued

Body Part Character 4	Approach Character 5	Device Character 6	Qualifier Character 7
R Anal Sphincter External anal sphincter Internal anal sphincter **U Omentum** Gastrocolic ligament Gastrocolic omentum Gastrohepatic omentum Gastrophrenic ligament Gastrosplenic ligament Greater Omentum Hepatogastric ligament Lesser Omentum **V Mesentery** Mesoappendix Mesocolon **W Peritoneum** Epiploic foramen	**Ø Open** **3 Percutaneous** **4 Percutaneous Endoscopic**	**Ø Drainage Device**	**Z No Qualifier**
R Anal Sphincter External anal sphincter Internal anal sphincter **U Omentum** Gastrocolic ligament Gastrocolic omentum Gastrohepatic omentum Gastrophrenic ligament Gastrosplenic ligament Greater Omentum Hepatogastric ligament Lesser Omentum **V Mesentery** Mesoappendix Mesocolon **W Peritoneum** Epiploic foramen	**Ø Open** **3 Percutaneous** **4 Percutaneous Endoscopic**	**Z No Device**	**X Diagnostic** **Z No Qualifier**

Non-OR ØD9R3ØZ
Non-OR ØD9[U,V,W][3,4]ØZ
Non-OR ØD9R[Ø,4]ZX
Non-OR ØD9[R,U,V,W]3Z[X,Z]
Non-OR ØD9[U,V,W]4ZZ

Ø Medical and Surgical
D Gastrointestinal System
B Excision Definition: Cutting out or off, without replacement, a portion of a body part
Explanation: The qualifier DIAGNOSTIC is used to identify excision procedures that are biopsies

Body Part Character 4	Approach Character 5	Device Character 6	Qualifier Character 7
1 Esophagus, Upper Cervical esophagus 2 Esophagus, Middle Thoracic esophagus 3 Esophagus, Lower Abdominal esophagus 4 Esophagogastric Junction Cardia Cardioesophageal junction Gastroesophageal (GE) junction 5 Esophagus 7 Stomach, Pylorus Pyloric antrum Pyloric canal Pyloric sphincter 8 Small Intestine 9 Duodenum A Jejunum Duodenojejunal flexure B Ileum C Ileocecal Valve E Large Intestine F Large Intestine, Right H Cecum J Appendix Vermiform appendix K Ascending Colon P Rectum Anorectal junction	Ø Open 3 Percutaneous 4 Percutaneous Endoscopic 7 Via Natural or Artificial Opening 8 Via Natural or Artificial Opening Endoscopic	Z No Device	X Diagnostic Z No Qualifier
6 Stomach	Ø Open 3 Percutaneous 4 Percutaneous Endoscopic 7 Via Natural or Artificial Opening 8 Via Natural or Artificial Opening Endoscopic	Z No Device	3 Vertical X Diagnostic Z No Qualifier
G Large Intestine, Left L Transverse Colon Hepatic flexure Splenic flexure M Descending Colon N Sigmoid Colon Rectosigmoid junction Sigmoid flexure	Ø Open 3 Percutaneous 4 Percutaneous Endoscopic 7 Via Natural or Artificial Opening 8 Via Natural or Artificial Opening Endoscopic	Z No Device	X Diagnostic Z No Qualifier
G Large Intestine, Left L Transverse Colon Hepatic flexure Splenic flexure M Descending Colon N Sigmoid Colon Rectosigmoid junction Sigmoid flexure	F Via Natural or Artificial Opening with Percutaneous Endoscopic Assistance	Z No Device	Z No Qualifier
Q Anus Anal orifi	Ø Open 3 Percutaneous 4 Percutaneous Endoscopic 7 Via Natural or Artificial Opening 8 Via Natural or Artificial Opening Endoscopic X External	Z No Device	X Diagnostic Z No Qualifier
R Anal Sphincter External anal sphincter Internal anal sphincter U Omentum Gastrocolic ligament Gastrocolic omentum Gastrohepatic omentum Gastrophrenic ligament Gastrosplenic ligament Greater Omentum Hepatogastric ligament Lesser Omentum V Mesentery Mesoappendix Mesocolon W Peritoneum Epiploic foramen	Ø Open 3 Percutaneous 4 Percutaneous Endoscopic	Z No Device	X Diagnostic Z No Qualifier

Non-OR ØDB[1,2,3,4,5,7,8,9,A,B,C,E,F,H,K,P][3,4,7,8]ZX
Non-OR ØDB[1,2,3,5,7,9][4,8]ZZ
Non-OR ØDB[4,E,F,H,K,P]8ZZ
Non-OR ØDB6[3,7,8]Z[3,X,Z]
Non-OR ØDB[G,L,M,N][3,4,7,8]ZX
Non-OR ØDB[G,L,M,N]8ZZ
Non-OR ØDBQ[Ø,3,4,7,8,X]ZX
Non-OR ØDBQ8ZZ
Non-OR ØDBR[Ø,3,4]ZX
Non-OR ØDB[U,V,W][3,4]ZX

Ø Medical and Surgical
D Gastrointestinal System
C Extirpation Definition: Taking or cutting out solid matter from a body part

Explanation: The solid matter may be an abnormal byproduct of a biological function or a foreign body; it may be imbedded in a body part or in the lumen of a tubular body part. The solid matter may or may not have been previously broken into pieces.

Body Part Character 4	Approach Character 5	Device Character 6	Qualifier Character 7
1 Esophagus, Upper Cervical esophagus **2 Esophagus, Middle** Thoracic esophagus **3 Esophagus, Lower** Abdominal esophagus **4 Esophagogastric Junction** Cardia Cardioesophageal junction Gastroesophageal (GE) junction **5 Esophagus** **6 Stomach** **7 Stomach, Pylorus** Pyloric antrum Pyloric canal Pyloric sphincter **8 Small Intestine** **9 Duodenum** **A Jejunum** Duodenojejunal flexure **B Ileum** **C Ileocecal Valve** **E Large Intestine** **F Large Intestine, Right** **G Large Intestine, Left** **H Cecum** **J Appendix** Vermiform appendix **K Ascending Colon** **L Transverse Colon** Hepatic flexure Splenic flexure **M Descending Colon** **N Sigmoid Colon** Rectosigmoid junction Sigmoid flexure **P Rectum** Anorectal junction	**Ø Open** **3 Percutaneous** **4 Percutaneous Endoscopic** **7 Via Natural or Artificial Opening** **8 Via Natural or Artificial Opening Endoscopic**	**Z No Device**	**Z No Qualifier**
Q Anus Anal orifice	**Ø Open** **3 Percutaneous** **4 Percutaneous Endoscopic** **7 Via Natural or Artificial Opening** **8 Via Natural or Artificial Opening Endoscopic** **X External**	**Z No Device**	**Z No Qualifier**
R Anal Sphincter External anal sphincter Internal anal sphincter **U Omentum** Gastrocolic ligament Gastrocolic omentum Gastrohepatic omentum Gastrophrenic ligament Gastrosplenic ligament Greater Omentum Hepatogastric ligament Lesser Omentum **V Mesentery** Mesoappendix Mesocolon **W Peritoneum** Epiploic foramen	**Ø Open** **3 Percutaneous** **4 Percutaneous Endoscopic**	**Z No Device**	**Z No Qualifier**

Non-OR ØDC[1,2,3,4,5,6,7,8,9,A,B,C,E,F,G,H,K,L,M,N,P][7,8]ZZ
Non-OR ØDCQ[7,8,X]ZZ

Ø Medical and Surgical
D Gastrointestinal System
D Extraction Definition: Pulling or stripping out or off all or a portion of a body part by the use of force
Explanation: The qualifier DIAGNOSTIC is used to identify extraction procedures that are biopsies

Body Part Character 4	Approach Character 5	Device Character 6	Qualifier Character 7
1 Esophagus, Upper Cervical esophagus **2 Esophagus, Middle** Thoracic esophagus **3 Esophagus, Lower** Abdominal esophagus **4 Esophagogastric Junction** Cardia Cardioesophageal junction Gastroesophageal (GE) junction **5 Esophagus** **6 Stomach** **7 Stomach, Pylorus** Pyloric antrum Pyloric canal Pyloric sphincter **8 Small Intestine** **9 Duodenum** **A Jejunum** Duodenojejunal flexure **B Ileum** **C Ileocecal Valve** **E Large Intestine** **F Large Intestine, Right** **G Large Intestine, Left** **H Cecum** **J Appendix** Vermiform appendix **K Ascending Colon** **L Transverse Colon** Hepatic flexure Splenic flexure **M Descending Colon** **N Sigmoid Colon** Rectosigmoid junction Sigmoid flexure **P Rectum** Anorectal junction	**3 Percutaneous** **4 Percutaneous Endoscopic** **8 Via Natural or Artificial Opening Endoscopic**	**Z No Device**	**X Diagnostic**
Q Anus Anal orifice	**3 Percutaneous** **4 Percutaneous Endoscopic** **8 Via Natural or Artificial Opening Endoscopic** **X External**	**Z No Device**	**X Diagnostic**

Non-OR ØDD[1,2,3,4,5,6,7,8,9,A,B,C,E,F,G,H,K,L,M,N,P][3,4,8]ZX
Non-OR ØDDQ[3,4,8,X]ZX

Ø Medical and Surgical
D Gastrointestinal System
F Fragmentation Definition: Breaking solid matter in a body part into pieces

Explanation: Physical force (e.g., manual, ultrasonic) applied directly or indirectly is used to break the solid matter into pieces. The solid matter may be an abnormal byproduct of a biological function or a foreign body. The pieces of solid matter are not taken out.

Body Part Character 4	Approach Character 5	Device Character 6	Qualifier Character 7
5 Esophagus NC **6 Stomach** NC **8 Small Intestine** NC **9 Duodenum** NC **A Jejunum** NC Duodenojejunal flexure **B Ileum** NC **E Large Intestine** NC **F Large Intestine, Right** NC **G Large Intestine, Left** NC **H Cecum** NC **J Appendix** NC Vermiform appendix **K Ascending Colon** NC **L Transverse Colon** NC Hepatic flexure Splenic flexure **M Descending Colon** NC **N Sigmoid Colon** NC Rectosigmoid junction Sigmoid flexure **P Rectum** NC Anorectal junction **Q Anus** NC Anal orifice	**Ø Open** **3 Percutaneous** **4 Percutaneous Endoscopic** **7 Via Natural or Artificial Opening** **8 Via Natural or Artificial Opening Endoscopic** **X External**	**Z No Device**	**Z No Qualifier**

Non-OR ØDF[5,6,8,9,A,B,E,F,G,H,J,K,L,M,N,P,Q]XZZ
NC ØDF[5,6,8,9,A,B,E,F,G,H,J,K,L,M,N,P,Q]XZZ

Ø Medical and Surgical
D Gastrointestinal System
H Insertion Definition: Putting in a nonbiological appliance that monitors, assists, performs, or prevents a physiological function but does not physically take the place of a body part

Explanation: None

Body Part Character 4	Approach Character 5	Device Character 6	Qualifier Character 7
Ø Upper Intestinal Tract D Lower Intestinal Tract	Ø Open 3 Percutaneous 4 Percutaneous Endoscopic 7 Via Natural or Artificial Opening 8 Via Natural or Artificial Opening Endoscopic	Y Other Device	Z No Qualifier
5 Esophagus	Ø Open 3 Percutaneous 4 Percutaneous Endoscopic	1 Radioactive Element 2 Monitoring Device 3 Infusion Device D Intraluminal Device U Feeding Device Y Other Device	Z No Qualifier
5 Esophagus	7 Via Natural or Artificial Opening 8 Via Natural or Artificial Opening Endoscopic	1 Radioactive Element 2 Monitoring Device 3 Infusion Device B Intraluminal Device, Airway D Intraluminal Device U Feeding Device Y Other Device	Z No Qualifier
6 Stomach ⊞	Ø Open 3 Percutaneous 4 Percutaneous Endoscopic	1 Radioactive Element 2 Monitoring Device 3 Infusion Device D Intraluminal Device M Stimulator Lead U Feeding Device Y Other Device	Z No Qualifier
6 Stomach	7 Via Natural or Artificial Opening 8 Via Natural or Artificial Opening Endoscopic	1 Radioactive Element 2 Monitoring Device 3 Infusion Device D Intraluminal Device U Feeding Device Y Other Device	Z No Qualifier
8 Small Intestine 9 Duodenum A Jejunum Duodenojejunal flexure B Ileum	Ø Open 3 Percutaneous 4 Percutaneous Endoscopic 7 Via Natural or Artificial Opening 8 Via Natural or Artificial Opening Endoscopic	1 Radioactive Element 2 Monitoring Device 3 Infusion Device D Intraluminal Device U Feeding Device	Z No Qualifier
E Large Intestine P Rectum Anorectal junction	Ø Open 3 Percutaneous 4 Percutaneous Endoscopic 7 Via Natural or Artificial Opening 8 Via Natural or Artificial Opening Endoscopic	1 Radioactive Element D Intraluminal Device	Z No Qualifier
Q Anus Anal orifice	Ø Open 3 Percutaneous 4 Percutaneous Endoscopic	D Intraluminal Device L Artificial Sphincter	Z No Qualifier
Q Anus Anal orifice	7 Via Natural or Artificial Opening 8 Via Natural or Artificial Opening Endoscopic	D Intraluminal Device	Z No Qualifier
R Anal Sphincter External anal sphincter Internal anal sphincter	Ø Open 3 Percutaneous 4 Percutaneous Endoscopic	M Stimulator Lead	Z No Qualifier

Non-OR ØDH[Ø,D][Ø,3,4,7,8]YZ
Non-OR ØDH5[Ø,3,4][D,U]Z
Non-OR ØDH5[3,4]YZ
Non-OR ØDH5[7,8][2,3,B,D,U,Y]Z
Non-OR ØDH6[3,4][U,Y]Z
Non-OR ØDH6[7,8][2,3,D,U,Y]Z
Non-OR ØDH[8,9,A,B][Ø,3,4][D,U]Z
Non-OR ØDH[8,9,A,B][7,8][2,3,D,U]Z
Non-OR ØDH[E,P][Ø,3,4,7,8]DZ

See Appendix L for Procedure Combinations
⊞ ØDH6[Ø,3,4]MZ

Ø Medical and Surgical
D Gastrointestinal System
J Inspection Definition: Visually and/or manually exploring a body part

Explanation: Visual exploration may be performed with or without optical instrumentation. Manual exploration may be performed directly or through intervening body layers.

Body Part Character 4	Approach Character 5	Device Character 6	Qualifier Character 7
Ø Upper Intestinal Tract **6 Stomach** **D Lower Intestinal Tract**	**Ø Open** **3 Percutaneous** **4 Percutaneous Endoscopic** **7 Via Natural or Artificial Opening** **8 Via Natural or Artificial Opening Endoscopic** **X External**	**Z No Device**	**Z No Qualifier**
U Omentum Gastrocolic ligament Gastrocolic omentum Gastrohepatic omentum Gastrophrenic ligament Gastrosplenic ligament Greater Omentum Hepatogastric ligament Lesser Omentum **V Mesentery** Mesoappendix Mesocolon **W Peritoneum** Epiploic foramen	**Ø Open** **3 Percutaneous** **4 Percutaneous Endoscopic** **X External**	**Z No Device**	**Z No Qualifier**

Non-OR ØDJ[Ø,6,D][3,7,8,X]ZZ
Non-OR ØDJ[U,V,W][3,X]ZZ

Ø Medical and Surgical
D Gastrointestinal System
L Occlusion Definition: Completely closing an orifice or the lumen of a tubular body part
Explanation: The orifice can be a natural orifice or an artificially created orifice

Body Part Character 4		Approach Character 5	Device Character 6	Qualifier Character 7
1 Esophagus, Upper Cervical esophagus **2 Esophagus, Middle** Thoracic esophagus **3 Esophagus, Lower** Abdominal esophagus **4 Esophagogastric Junction** Cardia Cardioesophageal junction Gastroesophageal (GE) junction **5 Esophagus** **6 Stomach** **7 Stomach, Pylorus** Pyloric antrum Pyloric canal Pyloric sphincter **8 Small Intestine**	**9 Duodenum** **A Jejunum** Duodenojejunal flexure **B Ileum** **C Ileocecal Valve** **E Large Intestine** **F Large Intestine, Right** **G Large Intestine, Left** **H Cecum** **K Ascending Colon** **L Transverse Colon** Hepatic flexure Splenic flexure **M Descending Colon** **N Sigmoid Colon** Rectosigmoid junction Sigmoid flexure **P Rectum** Anorectal junction	**Ø Open** **3 Percutaneous** **4 Percutaneous Endoscopic**	**C Extraluminal Device** **D Intraluminal Device** **Z No Device**	**Z No Qualifier**
1 Esophagus, Upper Cervical esophagus **2 Esophagus, Middle** Thoracic esophagus **3 Esophagus, Lower** Abdominal esophagus **4 Esophagogastric Junction** Cardia Cardioesophageal junction Gastroesophageal (GE) junction **5 Esophagus** **6 Stomach** **7 Stomach, Pylorus** Pyloric antrum Pyloric canal Pyloric sphincter **8 Small Intestine**	**9 Duodenum** **A Jejunum** Duodenojejunal flexure **B Ileum** **C Ileocecal Valve** **E Large Intestine** **F Large Intestine, Right** **G Large Intestine, Left** **H Cecum** **K Ascending Colon** **L Transverse Colon** Hepatic flexure Splenic flexure **M Descending Colon** **N Sigmoid Colon** Rectosigmoid junction Sigmoid flexure **P Rectum** Anorectal junction	**7 Via Natural or Artificial Opening** **8 Via Natural or Artificial Opening Endoscopic**	**D Intraluminal Device** **Z No Device**	**Z No Qualifier**
Q Anus Anal orifice		**Ø Open** **3 Percutaneous** **4 Percutaneous Endoscopic** **X External**	**C Extraluminal Device** **D Intraluminal Device** **Z No Device**	**Z No Qualifier**
Q Anus Anal orifice		**7 Via Natural or Artificial Opening** **8 Via Natural or Artificial Opening Endoscopic**	**D Intraluminal Device** **Z No Device**	**Z No Qualifier**

Non-OR ØDL[1,2,3,4,5][Ø,3,4][C,D,Z]Z
Non-OR ØDL[1,2,3,4,5][7,8][D,Z]Z

Ø Medical and Surgical
D Gastrointestinal System
M Reattachment Definition: Putting back in or on all or a portion of a separated body part to its normal location or other suitable location
Explanation: Vascular circulation and nervous pathways may or may not be reestablished

Body Part Character 4	Approach Character 5	Device Character 6	Qualifier Character 7
5 Esophagus **6** Stomach **8** Small Intestine **9** Duodenum **A** Jejunum Duodenojejunal flexure **B** Ileum **E** Large Intestine **F** Large Intestine, Right **G** Large Intestine, Left **H** Cecum **K** Ascending Colon **L** Transverse Colon Hepatic flexure Splenic flexure **M** Descending Colon **N** Sigmoid Colon Rectosigmoid junction Sigmoid flexure **P** Rectum Anorectal junction	**Ø** Open **4** Percutaneous Endoscopic	**Z** No Device	**Z** No Qualifier

Ø Medical and Surgical
D Gastrointestinal System
N Release Definition: Freeing a body part from an abnormal physical constraint by cutting or by the use of force
Explanation: Some of the restraining tissue may be taken out but none of the body part is taken out

Body Part Character 4	Approach Character 5	Device Character 6	Qualifier Character 7
1 Esophagus, Upper Cervical esophagus **2** Esophagus, Middle Thoracic esophagus **3** Esophagus, Lower Abdominal esophagus **4** Esophagogastric Junction Cardia Cardioesophageal junction Gastroesophageal (GE) junction **5** Esophagus **6** Stomach **7** Stomach, Pylorus Pyloric antrum Pyloric canal Pyloric sphincter **8** Small Intestine **9** Duodenum **A** Jejunum Duodenojejunal flexure **B** Ileum **C** Ileocecal Valve **E** Large Intestine **F** Large Intestine, Right **G** Large Intestine, Left **H** Cecum **J** Appendix Vermiform appendix **K** Ascending Colon **L** Transverse Colon Hepatic flexure Splenic flexure **M** Descending Colon **N** Sigmoid Colon Rectosigmoid junction Sigmoid flexure **P** Rectum Anorectal junction	**Ø** Open **3** Percutaneous **4** Percutaneous Endoscopic **7** Via Natural or Artificial Opening **8** Via Natural or Artificial Opening Endoscopic	**Z** No Device	**Z** No Qualifier
Q Anus Anal orifice	**Ø** Open **3** Percutaneous **4** Percutaneous Endoscopic **7** Via Natural or Artificial Opening **8** Via Natural or Artificial Opening Endoscopic **X** External	**Z** No Device	**Z** No Qualifier
R Anal Sphincter External anal sphincter Internal anal sphincter **U** Omentum Gastrocolic ligament Gastrocolic omentum Gastrohepatic omentum Gastrophrenic ligament Gastrosplenic ligament Greater Omentum Hepatogastric ligament Lesser Omentum **V** Mesentery Mesoappendix Mesocolon **W** Peritoneum Epiploic foramen	**Ø** Open **3** Percutaneous **4** Percutaneous Endoscopic	**Z** No Device	**Z** No Qualifier

Non-OR ØDN[8,9,A,B,E,F,G,H,K,L,M,N][7,8]ZZ

Ø Medical and Surgical
D Gastrointestinal System
P Removal Definition: Taking out or off a device from a body part

Explanation: If a device is taken out and a similar device put in without cutting or puncturing the skin or mucous membrane, the procedure is coded to the root operation CHANGE. Otherwise, the procedure for taking out a device is coded to the root operation REMOVAL.

Body Part Character 4	Approach Character 5	Device Character 6	Qualifier Character 7
Ø Upper Intestinal Tract D Lower Intestinal Tract	Ø Open 3 Percutaneous 4 Percutaneous Endoscopic 7 Via Natural or Artificial Opening 8 Via Natural or Artificial Opening Endoscopic	Ø Drainage Device 2 Monitoring Device 3 Infusion Device 7 Autologous Tissue Substitute C Extraluminal Device D Intraluminal Device J Synthetic Substitute K Nonautologous Tissue Substitute U Feeding Device Y Other Device	Z No Qualifier
Ø Upper Intestinal Tract D Lower Intestinal Tract	X External	Ø Drainage Device 2 Monitoring Device 3 Infusion Device D Intraluminal Device U Feeding Device	Z No Qualifier
5 Esophagus	Ø Open 3 Percutaneous 4 Percutaneous Endoscopic	1 Radioactive Element 2 Monitoring Device 3 Infusion Device U Feeding Device Y Other Device	Z No Qualifier
5 Esophagus	7 Via Natural or Artificial Opening 8 Via Natural or Artificial Opening Endoscopic	1 Radioactive Element D Intraluminal Device Y Other Device	Z No Qualifier
5 Esophagus	X External	1 Radioactive Element 2 Monitoring Device 3 Infusion Device D Intraluminal Device U Feeding Device	Z No Qualifier
6 Stomach	Ø Open 3 Percutaneous 4 Percutaneous Endoscopic	Ø Drainage Device 2 Monitoring Device 3 Infusion Device 7 Autologous Tissue Substitute C Extraluminal Device D Intraluminal Device J Synthetic Substitute K Nonautologous Tissue Substitute M Stimulator Lead U Feeding Device Y Other Device	Z No Qualifier
6 Stomach	7 Via Natural or Artificial Opening 8 Via Natural or Artificial Opening Endoscopic	Ø Drainage Device 2 Monitoring Device 3 Infusion Device 7 Autologous Tissue Substitute C Extraluminal Device D Intraluminal Device J Synthetic Substitute K Nonautologous Tissue Substitute U Feeding Device Y Other Device	Z No Qualifier
6 Stomach	X External	Ø Drainage Device 2 Monitoring Device 3 Infusion Device D Intraluminal Device U Feeding Device	Z No Qualifier

Non-OR ØDP[Ø,D][3,4]YZ
Non-OR ØDP[Ø,D][7,8][Ø,2,3,D,U,Y]Z
Non-OR ØDP[Ø,D]X[Ø,2,3,D,U]Z
Non-OR ØDP5[3,4]YZ
Non-OR ØDP5[7,8][1,D,Y]Z
Non-OR ØDP5X[1,2,3,D,U]Z
Non-OR ØDP6[3,4]YZ
Non-OR ØDP6[7,8][Ø,2,3,D,U,Y]Z
Non-OR ØDP6X[Ø,2,3,D,U]Z

ØDP Continued on next page

Ø Medical and Surgical
D Gastrointestinal System
P Removal Definition: Taking out or off a device from a body part

ØDP Continued

Explanation: If a device is taken out and a similar device put in without cutting or puncturing the skin or mucous membrane, the procedure is coded to the root operation CHANGE. Otherwise, the procedure for taking out a device is coded to the root operation REMOVAL.

Body Part Character 4	Approach Character 5	Device Character 6	Qualifier Character 7
P Rectum Anorectal junction	**Ø Open** **3 Percutaneous** **4 Percutaneous Endoscopic** **7 Via Natural or Artificial Opening** **8 Via Natural or Artificial Opening Endoscopic** **X External**	**1 Radioactive Element**	**Z No Qualifier**
Q Anus Anal orifice	**Ø Open** **3 Percutaneous** **4 Percutaneous Endoscopic** **7 Via Natural or Artificial Opening** **8 Via Natural or Artificial Opening Endoscopic**	**L Artificial Sphincter**	**Z No Qualifier**
R Anal Sphincter External anal sphincter Internal anal sphincter	**Ø Open** **3 Percutaneous** **4 Percutaneous Endoscopic**	**M Stimulator Lead**	**Z No Qualifier**
U Omentum Gastrocolic ligament Gastrocolic omentum Gastrohepatic omentum Gastrophrenic ligament Gastrosplenic ligament Greater Omentum Hepatogastric ligament Lesser Omentum **V Mesentery** Mesoappendix Mesocolon **W Peritoneum** Epiploic foramen	**Ø Open** **3 Percutaneous** **4 Percutaneous Endoscopic**	**Ø Drainage Device** **1 Radioactive Element** **7 Autologous Tissue Substitute** **J Synthetic Substitute** **K Nonautologous Tissue Substitute**	**Z No Qualifier**

Non-OR ØDPP[7,8,X]1Z

Ø Medical and Surgical
D Gastrointestinal System
Q Repair Definition: Restoring, to the extent possible, a body part to its normal anatomic structure and function
Explanation: Used only when the method to accomplish the repair is not one of the other root operations

Body Part Character 4	Approach Character 5	Device Character 6	Qualifier Character 7
1 Esophagus, Upper Cervical esophagus **2 Esophagus, Middle** Thoracic esophagus **3 Esophagus, Lower** Abdominal esophagus **4 Esophagogastric Junction** Cardia, Cardioesophageal junction, Gastroesophageal (GE) junction **5 Esophagus** **6 Stomach** **7 Stomach, Pylorus** Pyloric antrum, Pyloric canal, Pyloric sphincter **8 Small Intestine** ⊞ **9 Duodenum** ⊞ **A Jejunum** ⊞ Duodenojejunal flexure **B Ileum** ⊞ **C Ileocecal Valve** **E Large Intestine** ⊞ **F Large Intestine, Right** ⊞ **G Large Intestine, Left** ⊞ **H Cecum** ⊞ **J Appendix** Vermiform appendix **K Ascending Colon** ⊞ **L Transverse Colon** ⊞ Hepatic flexure, Splenic flexure **M Descending Colon** ⊞ **N Sigmoid Colon** ⊞ Rectosigmoid junction, Sigmoid flexure **P Rectum** Anorectal junction	**Ø Open** **3 Percutaneous** **4 Percutaneous Endoscopic** **7 Via Natural or Artificial Opening** **8 Via Natural or Artificial Opening Endoscopic**	**Z No Device**	**Z No Qualifier**
Q Anus Anal orifice	**Ø Open** **3 Percutaneous** **4 Percutaneous Endoscopic** **7 Via Natural or Artificial Opening** **8 Via Natural or Artificial Opening Endoscopic** **X External**	**Z No Device**	**Z No Qualifier**
R Anal Sphincter External anal sphincter, Internal anal sphincter **U Omentum** Gastrocolic ligament, Gastrocolic omentum, Gastrohepatic omentum, Gastrophrenic ligament, Gastrosplenic ligament, Greater Omentum, Hepatogastric ligament, Lesser Omentum **V Mesentery** Mesoappendix, Mesocolon **W Peritoneum** Epiploic foramen	**Ø Open** **3 Percutaneous** **4 Percutaneous Endoscopic**	**Z No Device**	**Z No Qualifier**

Non-OR ØDQU[Ø,3,4]ZZ

See Appendix L for Procedure Combinations
⊞ ØDQ[8,9,A,B,E,F,G,H,K,L,M,N]ØZZ

Ø Medical and Surgical
D Gastrointestinal System
R Replacement Definition: Putting in or on biological or synthetic material that physically takes the place and/or function of all or a portion of a body part

Explanation: The body part may have been taken out or replaced, or may be taken out, physically eradicated, or rendered nonfunctional during the REPLACEMENT procedure. A REMOVAL procedure is coded for taking out the device used in a previous replacement procedure.

Body Part Character 4	Approach Character 5	Device Character 6	Qualifier Character 7
5 Esophagus	**Ø Open** **4 Percutaneous Endoscopic** **7 Via Natural or Artificial Opening** **8 Via Natural or Artificial Opening Endoscopic**	**7 Autologous Tissue Substitute** **J Synthetic Substitute** **K Nonautologous Tissue Substitute**	**Z No Qualifier**
R Anal Sphincter External anal sphincter Internal anal sphincter **U Omentum** Gastrocolic ligament Gastrocolic omentum Gastrohepatic omentum Gastrophrenic ligament Gastrosplenic ligament Greater Omentum Hepatogastric ligament Lesser Omentum **V Mesentery** Mesoappendix Mesocolon **W Peritoneum** Epiploic foramen	**Ø Open** **4 Percutaneous Endoscopic**	**7 Autologous Tissue Substitute** **J Synthetic Substitute** **K Nonautologous Tissue Substitute**	**Z No Qualifier**

Ø Medical and Surgical
D Gastrointestinal System
S Reposition Definition: Moving to its normal location, or other suitable location, all or a portion of a body part

Explanation: The body part is moved to a new location from an abnormal location, or from a normal location where it is not functioning correctly. The body part may or may not be cut out or off to be moved to the new location.

Body Part Character 4	Approach Character 5	Device Character 6	Qualifier Character 7
5 Esophagus **6 Stomach** **9 Duodenum** **A Jejunum** Duodenojejunal flexure **B Ileum** **H Cecum** **K Ascending Colon** **L Transverse Colon** Hepatic flexure Splenic flexure **M Descending Colon** **N Sigmoid Colon** Rectosigmoid junction Sigmoid flexure **P Rectum** Anorectal junction **Q Anus** Anal orifice	**Ø Open** **4 Percutaneous Endoscopic** **7 Via Natural or Artificial Opening** **8 Via Natural or Artificial Opening Endoscopic** **X External**	**Z No Device**	**Z No Qualifier**
8 Small Intestine **E Large Intestine**	**Ø Open** **4 Percutaneous Endoscopic** **7 Via Natural or Artificial Opening** **8 Via Natural or Artificial Opening Endoscopic**	**Z No Device**	**Z No Qualifier**

Non-OR ØDS[5,6,9,A,B,H,K,L,M,N,P,Q]XZZ

Ø Medical and Surgical
D Gastrointestinal System
T Resection Definition: Cutting out or off, without replacement, all of a body part
Explanation: None

Body Part Character 4	Approach Character 5	Device Character 6	Qualifier Character 7
1 Esophagus, Upper Cervical esophagus **2 Esophagus, Middle** Thoracic esophagus **3 Esophagus, Lower** Abdominal esophagus **4 Esophagogastric Junction** Cardia Cardioesophageal junction Gastroesophageal (GE) junction **5 Esophagus** **6 Stomach** **7 Stomach, Pylorus** Pyloric antrum Pyloric canal Pyloric sphincter **8 Small Intestine** **9 Duodenum** ⊞ **A Jejunum** Duodenojejunal flexure **B Ileum** **C Ileocecal Valve** **E Large Intestine** **F Large Intestine, Right** **H Cecum** **J Appendix** Vermiform appendix **K Ascending Colon** **P Rectum** Anorectal junction **Q Anus** Anal orifice	**Ø Open** **4 Percutaneous Endoscopic** **7 Via Natural or Artificial Opening** **8 Via Natural or Artificial Opening Endoscopic**	**Z No Device**	**Z No Qualifier**
G Large Intestine, Left **L Transverse Colon** Hepatic flexure Splenic flexure **M Descending Colon** **N Sigmoid Colon** Rectosigmoid junction Sigmoid flexure	**Ø Open** **4 Percutaneous Endoscopic** **7 Via Natural or Artificial Opening** **8 Via Natural or Artificial Opening Endoscopic** **F Via Natural or Artificial Opening with Percutaneous Endoscopic Assistance**	**Z No Device**	**Z No Qualifier**
R Anal Sphincter External anal sphincter Internal anal sphincter **U Omentum** Gastrocolic ligament Gastrocolic omentum Gastrohepatic omentum Gastrophrenic ligament Gastrosplenic ligament Greater Omentum Hepatogastric ligament Lesser Omentum	**Ø Open** **4 Percutaneous Endoscopic**	**Z No Device**	**Z No Qualifier**

See Appendix L for Procedure Combinations
⊞ ØDT9ØZZ

Ø Medical and Surgical
D Gastrointestinal System
U Supplement Definition: Putting in or on biological or synthetic material that physically reinforces and/or augments the function of a portion of a body part

Explanation: The biological material is non-living, or is living and from the same individual. The body part may have been previously replaced, and the SUPPLEMENT procedure is performed to physically reinforce and/or augment the function of the replaced body part.

Body Part Character 4	Approach Character 5	Device Character 6	Qualifier Character 7
1 Esophagus, Upper Cervical esophagus **2 Esophagus, Middle** Thoracic esophagus **3 Esophagus, Lower** Abdominal esophagus **4 Esophagogastric Junction** Cardia Cardioesophageal junction Gastroesophageal (GE) junction **5 Esophagus** **6 Stomach** **7 Stomach, Pylorus** Pyloric antrum Pyloric canal Pyloric sphincter **8 Small Intestine** **9 Duodenum** **A Jejunum** Duodenojejunal flexure **B Ileum** **C Ileocecal Valve** **E Large Intestine** **F Large Intestine, Right** **G Large Intestine, Left** **H Cecum** **K Ascending Colon** **L Transverse Colon** Hepatic flexure Splenic flexure **M Descending Colon** **N Sigmoid Colon** Rectosigmoid junction Sigmoid flexure **P Rectum** Anorectal junction	**Ø Open** **4 Percutaneous Endoscopic** **7 Via Natural or Artificial Opening** **8 Via Natural or Artificial Opening Endoscopic**	**7 Autologous Tissue Substitute** **J Synthetic Substitute** **K Nonautologous Tissue Substitute**	**Z No Qualifier**
Q Anus Anal orifice	**Ø Open** **4 Percutaneous Endoscopic** **7 Via Natural or Artificial Opening** **8 Via Natural or Artificial Opening Endoscopic** **X External**	**7 Autologous Tissue Substitute** **J Synthetic Substitute** **K Nonautologous Tissue Substitute**	**Z No Qualifier**
R Anal Sphincter External anal sphincter Internal anal sphincter **U Omentum** Gastrocolic ligament Gastrocolic omentum Gastrohepatic omentum Gastrophrenic ligament Gastrosplenic ligament Greater Omentum Hepatogastric ligament Lesser Omentum **V Mesentery** Mesoappendix Mesocolon **W Peritoneum** Epiploic foramen	**Ø Open** **4 Percutaneous Endoscopic**	**7 Autologous Tissue Substitute** **J Synthetic Substitute** **K Nonautologous Tissue Substitute**	**Z No Qualifier**

Ø Medical and Surgical
D Gastrointestinal System
V Restriction Definition: Partially closing an orifice or the lumen of a tubular body part
Explanation: The orifice can be a natural orifice or an artificially created orifice

Body Part Character 4		Approach Character 5	Device Character 6	Qualifier Character 7
1 Esophagus, Upper Cervical esophagus **2 Esophagus, Middle** Thoracic esophagus **3 Esophagus, Lower** Abdominal esophagus **4 Esophagogastric Junction** Cardia, Cardioesophageal junction, Gastroesophageal (GE) junction **5 Esophagus** **6 Stomach** **7 Stomach, Pylorus** Pyloric antrum, Pyloric canal, Pyloric sphincter **8 Small Intestine**	**9 Duodenum** **A Jejunum** Duodenojejunal flexure **B Ileum** **C Ileocecal Valve** **E Large Intestine** **F Large Intestine, Right** **G Large Intestine, Left** **H Cecum** **K Ascending Colon** **L Transverse Colon** Hepatic flexure, Splenic flexure **M Descending Colon** **N Sigmoid Colon** Rectosigmoid junction, Sigmoid flexure **P Rectum** Anorectal junction	**Ø Open** **3 Percutaneous** **4 Percutaneous Endoscopic**	**C Extraluminal Device** **D Intraluminal Device** **Z No Device**	**Z No Qualifier**
1 Esophagus, Upper Cervical esophagus **2 Esophagus, Middle** Thoracic esophagus **3 Esophagus, Lower** Abdominal esophagus **4 Esophagogastric Junction** Cardia, Cardioesophageal junction, Gastroesophageal (GE) junction **5 Esophagus** **6 Stomach** NC **7 Stomach, Pylorus** Pyloric antrum, Pyloric canal, Pyloric sphincter **8 Small Intestine**	**9 Duodenum** **A Jejunum** Duodenojejunal flexure **B Ileum** **C Ileocecal Valve** **E Large Intestine** **F Large Intestine, Right** **G Large Intestine, Left** **H Cecum** **K Ascending Colon** **L Transverse Colon** Hepatic flexure, Splenic flexure **M Descending Colon** **N Sigmoid Colon** Rectosigmoid junction, Sigmoid flexure **P Rectum** Anorectal junction	**7 Via Natural or Artificial Opening** **8 Via Natural or Artificial Opening Endoscopic**	**D Intraluminal Device** **Z No Device**	**Z No Qualifier**
Q Anus Anal orifice		**Ø Open** **3 Percutaneous** **4 Percutaneous Endoscopic** **X External**	**C Extraluminal Device** **D Intraluminal Device** **Z No Device**	**Z No Qualifier**
Q Anus Anal orifice		**7 Via Natural or Artificial Opening** **8 Via Natural or Artificial Opening Endoscopic**	**D Intraluminal Device** **Z No Device**	**Z No Qualifier**

Non-OR ØDV6[7,8]DZ
HAC ØDV64CZ when reported with PDx E66.Ø1 and SDx K68.11, K95.Ø1, K95.81, or T81.4Ø–T81.49 with 7th character A
NC ØDV6[7,8]DZ

Ø Medical and Surgical
D Gastrointestinal System
W Revision Definition: Correcting, to the extent possible, a portion of a malfunctioning device or the position of a displaced device

Explanation: Revision can include correcting a malfunctioning or displaced device by taking out or putting in components of the device such as a screw or pin

Body Part Character 4	Approach Character 5	Device Character 6	Qualifier Character 7
Ø Upper Intestinal Tract **D** Lower Intestinal Tract	**Ø** Open **3** Percutaneous **4** Percutaneous Endoscopic **7** Via Natural or Artificial Opening **8** Via Natural or Artificial Opening Endoscopic	**Ø** Drainage Device **2** Monitoring Device **3** Infusion Device **7** Autologous Tissue Substitute **C** Extraluminal Device **D** Intraluminal Device **J** Synthetic Substitute **K** Nonautologous Tissue Substitute **U** Feeding Device **Y** Other Device	**Z** No Qualifier
Ø Upper Intestinal Tract **D** Lower Intestinal Tract	**X** External	**Ø** Drainage Device **2** Monitoring Device **3** Infusion Device **7** Autologous Tissue Substitute **C** Extraluminal Device **D** Intraluminal Device **J** Synthetic Substitute **K** Nonautologous Tissue Substitute **U** Feeding Device	**Z** No Qualifier
5 Esophagus	**Ø** Open **3** Percutaneous **4** Percutaneous Endoscopic	**Y** Other Device	**Z** No Qualifier
5 Esophagus	**7** Via Natural or Artificial Opening **8** Via Natural or Artificial Opening Endoscopic	**D** Intraluminal Device **Y** Other Device	**Z** No Qualifier
5 Esophagus	**X** External	**D** Intraluminal Device	**Z** No Qualifier
6 Stomach	**Ø** Open **3** Percutaneous **4** Percutaneous Endoscopic	**Ø** Drainage Device **2** Monitoring Device **3** Infusion Device **7** Autologous Tissue Substitute **C** Extraluminal Device **D** Intraluminal Device **J** Synthetic Substitute **K** Nonautologous Tissue Substitute **M** Stimulator Lead **U** Feeding Device **Y** Other Device	**Z** No Qualifier
6 Stomach	**7** Via Natural or Artificial Opening **8** Via Natural or Artificial Opening Endoscopic	**Ø** Drainage Device **2** Monitoring Device **3** Infusion Device **7** Autologous Tissue Substitute **C** Extraluminal Device **D** Intraluminal Device **J** Synthetic Substitute **K** Nonautologous Tissue Substitute **U** Feeding Device **Y** Other Device	**Z** No Qualifier
6 Stomach	**X** External	**Ø** Drainage Device **2** Monitoring Device **3** Infusion Device **7** Autologous Tissue Substitute **C** Extraluminal Device **D** Intraluminal Device **J** Synthetic Substitute **K** Nonautologous Tissue Substitute **U** Feeding Device	**Z** No Qualifier

Non-OR ØDW[Ø,D][3,4,7,8]YZ
Non-OR ØDW[Ø,D]8UZ
Non-OR ØDW[Ø,D]X[Ø,2,3,7,C,D,J,K,U]Z
Non-OR ØDW5[Ø,3,4]YZ
Non-OR ØDW5[7,8]YZ
Non-OR ØDW5XDZ
Non-OR ØDW6[3,4]YZ
Non-OR ØDW68UZ
Non-OR ØDW6[7,8]YZ
Non-OR ØDW6X[Ø,2,3,7,C,D,J,K,U]Z

ØDW Continued on next page

ØDW Continued

Ø Medical and Surgical
D Gastrointestinal System
W Revision Definition: Correcting, to the extent possible, a portion of a malfunctioning device or the position of a displaced device

Explanation: Revision can include correcting a malfunctioning or displaced device by taking out or putting in components of the device such as a screw or pin

Body Part Character 4	Approach Character 5	Device Character 6	Qualifier Character 7
8 Small Intestine **E** Large Intestine	**Ø** Open **4** Percutaneous Endoscopic **7** Via Natural or Artificial Opening **8** Via Natural or Artificial Opening Endoscopic	**7** Autologous Tissue Substitute **J** Synthetic Substitute **K** Nonautologous Tissue Substitute	**Z** No Qualifier
Q Anus Anal orifice	**Ø** Open **3** Percutaneous **4** Percutaneous Endoscopic **7** Via Natural or Artificial Opening **8** Via Natural or Artificial Opening Endoscopic	**L** Artificial Sphincter	**Z** No Qualifier
R Anal Sphincter External anal sphincter Internal anal sphincter	**Ø** Open **3** Percutaneous **4** Percutaneous Endoscopic	**M** Stimulator Lead	**Z** No Qualifier
U Omentum Gastrocolic ligament Gastrocolic omentum Gastrohepatic omentum Gastrophrenic ligament Gastrosplenic ligament Greater Omentum Hepatogastric ligament Lesser Omentum **V** Mesentery Mesoappendix Mesocolon **W** Peritoneum Epiploic foramen	**Ø** Open **3** Percutaneous **4** Percutaneous Endoscopic	**Ø** Drainage Device **7** Autologous Tissue Substitute **J** Synthetic Substitute **K** Nonautologous Tissue Substitute	**Z** No Qualifier

Non-OR ØDW[U,V,W][Ø,3,4]ØZ

Ø Medical and Surgical
D Gastrointestinal System
X Transfer Definition: Moving, without taking out, all or a portion of a body part to another location to take over the function of all or a portion of a body part

Explanation: The body part transferred remains connected to its vascular and nervous supply

Body Part Character 4	Approach Character 5	Device Character 6	Qualifier Character 7
6 Stomach **8** Small Intestine	**Ø** Open **4** Percutaneous Endoscopic	**Z** No Device	**5** Esophagus
E Large Intestine	**Ø** Open **4** Percutaneous Endoscopic	**Z** No Device	**5** Esophagus **7** Vagina ♀

♀ ØDXE[Ø,4]Z7

Ø Medical and Surgical
D Gastrointestinal System
Y Transplantation Definition: Putting in or on all or a portion of a living body part taken from another individual or animal to physically take the place and/or function of all or a portion of a similar body part

Explanation: The native body part may or may not be taken out, and the transplanted body part may take over all or a portion of its function

Body Part Character 4	Approach Character 5	Device Character 6	Qualifier Character 7
5 Esophagus **6** Stomach **8** Small Intestine LC **E** Large Intestine LC	**Ø** Open	**Z** No Device	**Ø** Allogeneic **1** Syngeneic **2** Zooplastic

Non-OR ØDY5ØZ[Ø,1,2]
LC ØDY[8,E]ØZ[Ø,1,2]

Hepatobiliary System and Pancreas ØF1–ØFY

Character Meanings

This Character Meaning table is provided as a guide to assist the user in the identification of character members that may be found in this section of code tables. It **SHOULD NOT** be used to build a PCS code.

Operation–Character 3	Body Part–Character 4	Approach–Character 5	Device–Character 6	Qualifier–Character 7
1 Bypass	Ø Liver	Ø Open	Ø Drainage Device	Ø Allogeneic
2 Change	1 Liver, Right Lobe	3 Percutaneous	1 Radioactive Element	1 Syngeneic
5 Destruction	2 Liver, Left Lobe	4 Percutaneous Endoscopic	2 Monitoring Device	2 Zooplastic
7 Dilation	4 Gallbladder	7 Via Natural or Artificial Opening	3 Infusion Device	3 Duodenum
8 Division	5 Hepatic Duct, Right	8 Via Natural or Artificial Opening Endoscopic	7 Autologous Tissue Substitute	4 Stomach
9 Drainage	6 Hepatic Duct, Left	X External	C Extraluminal Device	5 Hepatic Duct, Right
B Excision	7 Hepatic Duct, Common		D Intraluminal Device	6 Hepatic Duct, Left
C Extirpation	8 Cystic Duct		J Synthetic Substitute	7 Hepatic Duct, Caudate
D Extraction	9 Common Bile Duct		K Nonautologous Tissue Substitute	8 Cystic Duct
F Fragmentation	B Hepatobiliary Duct		Y Other Device	9 Common Bile Duct
H Insertion	C Ampulla of Vater		Z No Device	B Small Intestine
J Inspection	D Pancreatic Duct			C Large Intestine
L Occlusion	F Pancreatic Duct, Accessory			F Irreversible Electroporation
M Reattachment	G Pancreas			X Diagnostic
N Release				Z No Qualifier
P Removal				
Q Repair				
R Replacement				
S Reposition				
T Resection				
U Supplement				
V Restriction				
W Revision				
Y Transplantation				

AHA Coding Clinic for table ØF5
2018, 4Q, 39 Irreversible electroporation

AHA Coding Clinic for table ØF7
2016, 3Q, 27 Endoscopic retrograde cholangiopancreatography with sphincterotomy and insertion of pancreatic stent
2016, 1Q, 25 Endoscopic retrograde cholangiopancreatography with brush biopsy of pancreatic and common bile ducts
2015, 1Q, 32 Percutaneous transhepatic biliary drainage catheter placement
2014, 3Q, 15 Drainage of pancreatic pseudocyst

AHA Coding Clinic for table ØF9
2015, 1Q, 32 Percutaneous transhepatic biliary drainage catheter placement
2014, 3Q, 15 Drainage of pancreatic pseudocyst

AHA Coding Clinic for table ØFB
2019, 1Q, 3-8 Whipple procedure
2016, 3Q, 41 Open cholecystectomy with needle biopsy of liver
2016, 1Q, 23 Endoscopic ultrasound with aspiration biopsy of common hepatic duct
2016, 1Q, 25 Endoscopic retrograde cholangiopancreatography with brush biopsy of pancreatic and common bile ducts
2014, 3Q, 32 Pyloric-sparing Whipple procedure

AHA Coding Clinic for table ØFC
2016, 3Q, 27 Endoscopic retrograde cholangiopancreatography with sphincterotomy and insertion of pancreatic stent

AHA Coding Clinic for table ØFQ
2016, 3Q, 27 Revision of common bile duct anastomosis
2013, 4Q, 109 Separating conjoined twins

AHA Coding Clinic for table ØFT
2019, 1Q, 3-8 Whipple Procedure
2012, 4Q, 99 Domino liver transplant

AHA Coding Clinic for table ØFY
2014, 3Q, 13 Orthotopic liver transplant with end to side cavoplasty
2012, 4Q, 99 Domino liver transplant

Liver

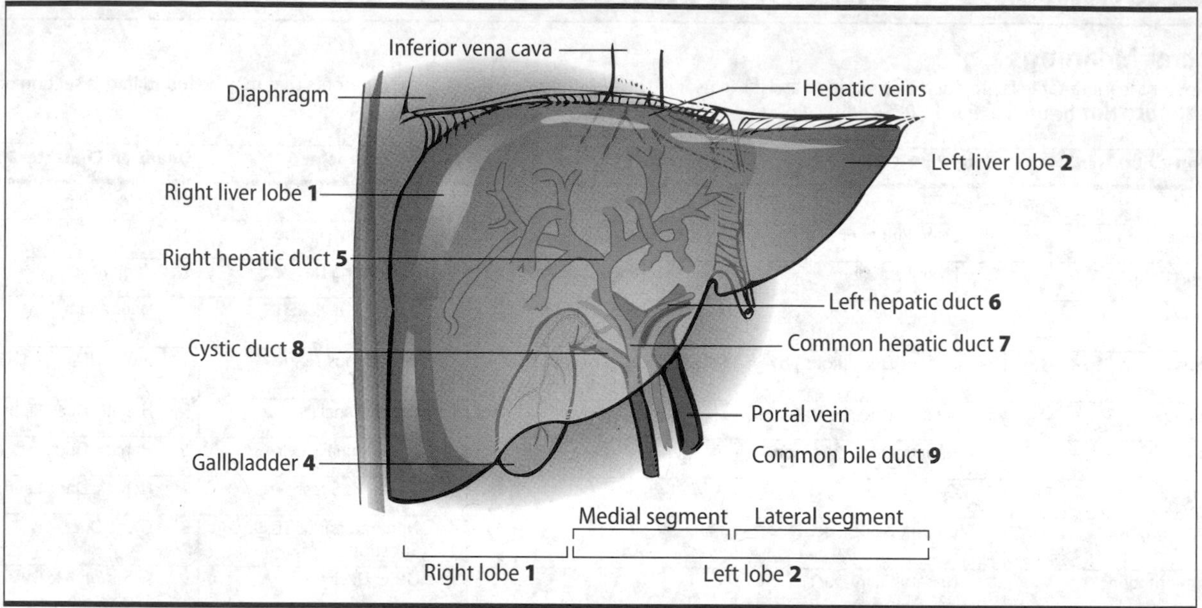

Pancreas

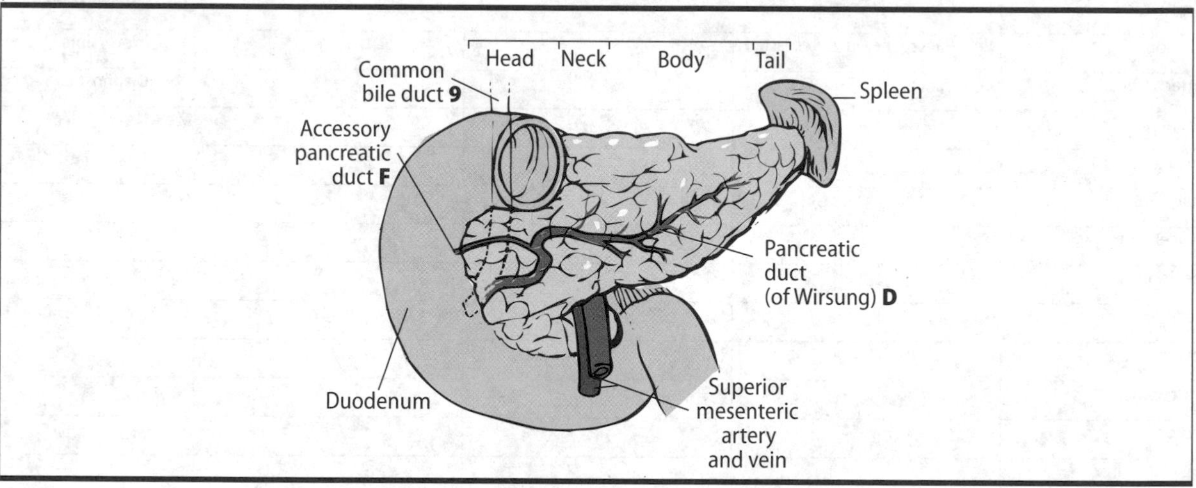

Gallbladder and Ducts

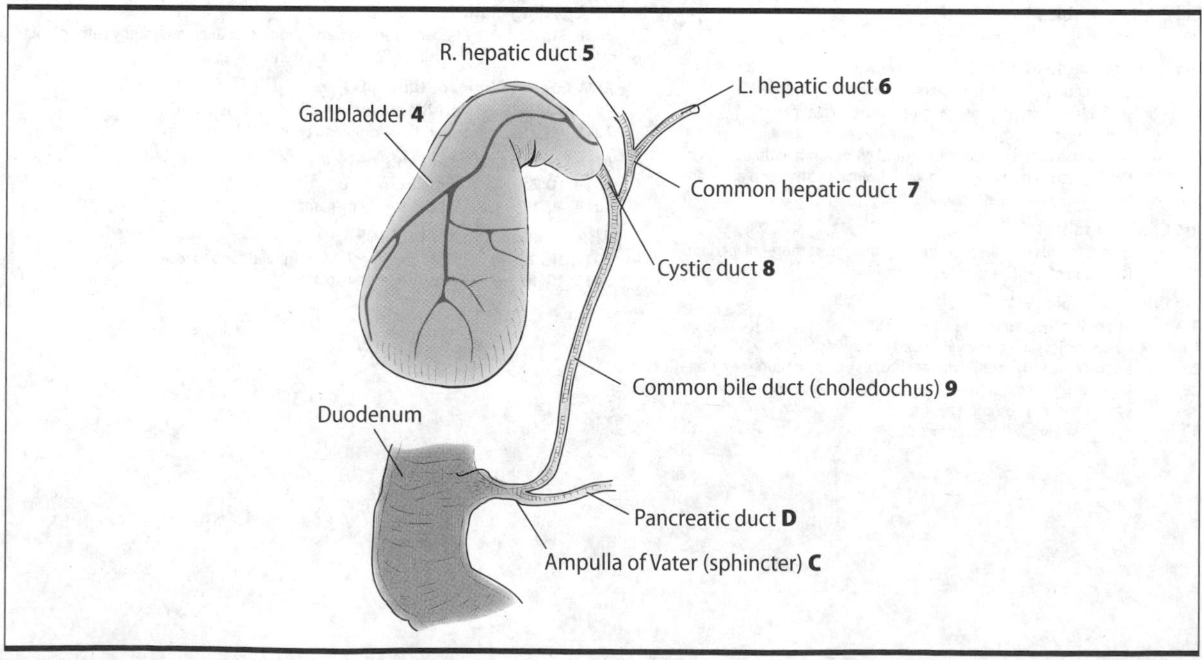

Ø Medical and Surgical
F Hepatobiliary System and Pancreas
1 Bypass Definition: Altering the route of passage of the contents of a tubular body part

Explanation: Rerouting contents of a body part to a downstream area of the normal route, to a similar route and body part, or to an abnormal route and dissimilar body part. Includes one or more anastomoses, with or without the use of a device.

Body Part Character 4	Approach Character 5	Device Character 6	Qualifier Character 7
4 Gallbladder 5 Hepatic Duct, Right 6 Hepatic Duct, Left 7 Hepatic Duct, Common 8 Cystic Duct 9 Common Bile Duct	Ø Open 4 Percutaneous Endoscopic	D Intraluminal Device Z No Device	3 Duodenum 4 Stomach 5 Hepatic Duct, Right 6 Hepatic Duct, Left 7 Hepatic Duct, Caudate 8 Cystic Duct 9 Common Bile Duct B Small Intestine
D Pancreatic Duct Duct of Wirsung	Ø Open 4 Percutaneous Endoscopic	D Intraluminal Device Z No Device	3 Duodenum 4 Stomach B Small Intestine C Large Intestine
F Pancreatic Duct, Accessory Duct of Santorini G Pancreas	Ø Open 4 Percutaneous Endoscopic	D Intraluminal Device Z No Device	3 Duodenum B Small Intestine C Large Intestine

Ø Medical and Surgical
F Hepatobiliary System and Pancreas
2 Change Definition: Taking out or off a device from a body part and putting back an identical or similar device in or on the same body part without cutting or puncturing the skin or a mucous membrane

Explanation: All CHANGE procedures are coded using the approach EXTERNAL

Body Part Character 4	Approach Character 5	Device Character 6	Qualifier Character 7
Ø Liver Quadrate lobe 4 Gallbladder B Hepatobiliary Duct D Pancreatic Duct Duct of Wirsung G Pancreas	X External	Ø Drainage Device Y Other Device	Z No Qualifier

Non-OR All body part, approach, device, and qualifier values

Ø Medical and Surgical
F Hepatobiliary System and Pancreas
5 Destruction Definition: Physical eradication of all or a portion of a body part by the direct use of energy, force, or a destructive agent

Explanation: None of the body part is physically taken out

Body Part Character 4	Approach Character 5	Device Character 6	Qualifier Character 7
Ø Liver Quadrate lobe 1 Liver, Right Lobe 2 Liver, Left Lobe	Ø Open 3 Percutaneous 4 Percutaneous Endoscopic	Z No Device	F Irreversible Electroporation Z No Qualifier
4 Gallbladder	Ø Open 3 Percutaneous 4 Percutaneous Endoscopic 8 Via Natural or Artificial Opening Endoscopic	Z No Device	Z No Qualifier
5 Hepatic Duct, Right 6 Hepatic Duct, Left 7 Hepatic Duct, Common 8 Cystic Duct 9 Common Bile Duct C Ampulla of Vater Duodenal ampulla Hepatopancreatic ampulla D Pancreatic Duct Duct of Wirsung F Pancreatic Duct, Accessory Duct of Santorini	Ø Open 3 Percutaneous 4 Percutaneous Endoscopic 7 Via Natural or Artificial Opening 8 Via Natural or Artificial Opening Endoscopic	Z No Device	Z No Qualifier
G Pancreas	Ø Open 3 Percutaneous 4 Percutaneous Endoscopic	Z No Device	F Irreversible Electroporation Z No Qualifier
G Pancreas	8 Via Natural or Artificial Opening Endoscopic	Z No Device	Z No Qualifier

Non-OR ØF5[5,6,7,8,9,C,D,F][4,8]ZZ
Non-OR ØF5G4Z[F,Z]
Non-OR ØF5G8ZZ

Ø Medical and Surgical
F Hepatobiliary System and Pancreas
7 Dilation Definition: Expanding an orifice or the lumen of a tubular body part

Explanation: The orifice can be a natural orifice or an artificially created orifice. Accomplished by stretching a tubular body part using intraluminal pressure or by cutting part of the orifice or wall of the tubular body part.

Body Part Character 4	Approach Character 5	Device Character 6	Qualifier Character 7
5 Hepatic Duct, Right 6 Hepatic Duct, Left 7 Hepatic Duct, Common 8 Cystic Duct 9 Common Bile Duct C Ampulla of Vater Duodenal ampulla Hepatopancreatic ampulla D Pancreatic Duct Duct of Wirsung F Pancreatic Duct, Accessory Duct of Santorini	Ø Open 3 Percutaneous 4 Percutaneous Endoscopic 7 Via Natural or Artificial Opening 8 Via Natural or Artificial Opening Endoscopic	D Intraluminal Device Z No Device	Z No Qualifier

Non-OR ØF7[5,6,7,8,9][3,4,8][D,Z]Z
Non-OR ØF7[5,6,7,8,9,D]]7DZ
Non-OR ØF7C8[D,Z]Z
Non-OR ØF7[D,F][4,8][D,Z]Z

Ø Medical and Surgical
F Hepatobiliary System and Pancreas
8 Division Definition: Cutting into a body part, without draining fluids and/or gases from the body part, in order to separate or transect a body part

Explanation: All or a portion of the body part is separated into two or more portions

Body Part Character 4	Approach Character 5	Device Character 6	Qualifier Character 7
G Pancreas	Ø Open 3 Percutaneous 4 Percutaneous Endoscopic	Z No Device	Z No Qualifier

Ø Medical and Surgical
F Hepatobiliary System and Pancreas
9 Drainage Definition: Taking or letting out fluids and/or gases from a body part
Explanation: The qualifier DIAGNOSTIC is used to identify drainage procedures that are biopsies

Body Part Character 4	Approach Character 5	Device Character 6	Qualifier Character 7
Ø Liver Quadrate lobe **1 Liver, Right Lobe** **2 Liver, Left Lobe**	**Ø Open** **3 Percutaneous** **4 Percutaneous Endoscopic**	**Ø Drainage Device**	**Z No Qualifier**
Ø Liver Quadrate lobe **1 Liver, Right Lobe** **2 Liver, Left Lobe**	**Ø Open** **3 Percutaneous** **4 Percutaneous Endoscopic**	**Z No Device**	**X Diagnostic** **Z No Qualifier**
4 Gallbladder **G Pancreas**	**Ø Open** **3 Percutaneous** **4 Percutaneous Endoscopic** **8 Via Natural or Artificial Opening Endoscopic**	**Ø Drainage Device**	**Z No Qualifier**
4 Gallbladder **G Pancreas**	**Ø Open** **3 Percutaneous** **4 Percutaneous Endoscopic** **8 Via Natural or Artificial Opening Endoscopic**	**Z No Device**	**X Diagnostic** **Z No Qualifier**
5 Hepatic Duct, Right **6 Hepatic Duct, Left** **7 Hepatic Duct, Common** **8 Cystic Duct** **9 Common Bile Duct** **C Ampulla of Vater** Duodenal ampulla Hepatopancreatic ampulla **D Pancreatic Duct** Duct of Wirsung **F Pancreatic Duct, Accessory** Duct of Santorini	**Ø Open** **3 Percutaneous** **4 Percutaneous Endoscopic** **7 Via Natural or Artificial Opening** **8 Via Natural or Artificial Opening Endoscopic**	**Ø Drainage Device**	**Z No Qualifier**
5 Hepatic Duct, Right **6 Hepatic Duct, Left** **7 Hepatic Duct, Common** **8 Cystic Duct** **9 Common Bile Duct** **C Ampulla of Vater** Duodenal ampulla Hepatopancreatic ampulla **D Pancreatic Duct** Duct of Wirsung **F Pancreatic Duct, Accessory** Duct of Santorini	**Ø Open** **3 Percutaneous** **4 Percutaneous Endoscopic** **7 Via Natural or Artificial Opening** **8 Via Natural or Artificial Opening Endoscopic**	**Z No Device**	**X Diagnostic** **Z No Qualifier**

Non-OR ØF9[Ø,1,2][3,4]ØZ
Non-OR ØF9[Ø,1,2][3,4]Z[X,Z]
Non-OR ØF9[4,G]8ØZ
Non-OR ØF9G3ØZ
Non-OR ØF9[4,G]8Z[X,Z]
Non-OR ØF9G3Z[XZ]
Non-OR ØF9G4ZX
Non-OR ØF9[5,6,8][3,8]ØZ
Non-OR ØF97[3,4,7,8]ØZ
Non-OR ØF99[3,8]ØZ
Non-OR ØF9C[3,4,8]ØZ
Non-OR ØF9[D,F][3,8]ØZ
Non-OR ØF9[5,6,8,9,C,D,F]3Z[X,Z]
Non-OR ØF9[5,6,8,9,C,D,F][4,7,8]ZX
Non-OR ØF9[5,6,8,D,F]8ZZ
Non-OR ØF97[3,4,7,8]Z[X,Z]
Non-OR ØF99[4,7,8]ZZ
Non-OR ØF9C[4,8]ZZ

Ø Medical and Surgical
F Hepatobiliary System and Pancreas
B Excision Definition: Cutting out or off, without replacement, a portion of a body part
Explanation: The qualifier DIAGNOSTIC is used to identify excision procedures that are biopsies

Body Part Character 4	Approach Character 5	Device Character 6	Qualifier Character 7
Ø Liver Quadrate lobe 1 Liver, Right Lobe 2 Liver, Left Lobe	Ø Open 3 Percutaneous 4 Percutaneous Endoscopic	Z No Device	X Diagnostic Z No Qualifier
4 Gallbladder G Pancreas	Ø Open 3 Percutaneous 4 Percutaneous Endoscopic 8 Via Natural or Artificial Opening Endoscopic	Z No Device	X Diagnostic Z No Qualifier
5 Hepatic Duct, Right 6 Hepatic Duct, Left 7 Hepatic Duct, Common 8 Cystic Duct 9 Common Bile Duct C Ampulla of Vater Duodenal ampulla Hepatopancreatic ampulla D Pancreatic Duct Duct of Wirsung F Pancreatic Duct, Accessory Duct of Santorini	Ø Open 3 Percutaneous 4 Percutaneous Endoscopic 7 Via Natural or Artificial Opening 8 Via Natural or Artificial Opening Endoscopic	Z No Device	X Diagnostic Z No Qualifier

Non-OR ØFB[Ø,1,2]3ZX
Non-OR ØFB[4,G][3,4,8]ZX
Non-OR ØFB[5,6,7,8,9,C,D,F][3,4,7,8]ZX
Non-OR ØFB[5,6,7,8,9,C,D,F][4,8]ZZ

Ø Medical and Surgical
F Hepatobiliary System and Pancreas
C Extirpation Definition: Taking or cutting out solid matter from a body part
Explanation: The solid matter may be an abnormal byproduct of a biological function or a foreign body; it may be imbedded in a body part or in the lumen of a tubular body part. The solid matter may or may not have been previously broken into pieces.

Body Part Character 4	Approach Character 5	Device Character 6	Qualifier Character 7
Ø Liver Quadrate lobe 1 Liver, Right Lobe 2 Liver, Left Lobe	Ø Open 3 Percutaneous 4 Percutaneous Endoscopic	Z No Device	Z No Qualifier
4 Gallbladder G Pancreas	Ø Open 3 Percutaneous 4 Percutaneous Endoscopic 8 Via Natural or Artificial Opening Endoscopic	Z No Device	Z No Qualifier
5 Hepatic Duct, Right 6 Hepatic Duct, Left 7 Hepatic Duct, Common 8 Cystic Duct 9 Common Bile Duct C Ampulla of Vater Duodenal ampulla Hepatopancreatic ampulla D Pancreatic Duct Duct of Wirsung F Pancreatic Duct, Accessory Duct of Santorini	Ø Open 3 Percutaneous 4 Percutaneous Endoscopic 7 Via Natural or Artificial Opening 8 Via Natural or Artificial Opening Endoscopic	Z No Device	Z No Qualifier

Non-OR ØFC[5,6,7,8,9][3,4,7,8]ZZ
Non-OR ØFCC[4,8]ZZ
Non-OR ØFC[D,F][3,4,8]ZZ

Ø Medical and Surgical
F Hepatobiliary System and Pancreas
D Extraction Definition: Pulling or stripping out or off all or a portion of a body part by the use of force

Explanation: The qualifier DIAGNOSTIC is used to identify extraction procedures that are biopsies

Body Part Character 4	Approach Character 5	Device Character 6	Qualifier Character 7
Ø Liver Quadrate lobe **1 Liver, Right Lobe** **2 Liver, Left Lobe**	**3 Percutaneous** **4 Percutaneous Endoscopic**	**Z No Device**	**X Diagnostic**
4 Gallbladder **5 Hepatic Duct, Right** **6 Hepatic Duct, Left** **7 Hepatic Duct, Common** **8 Cystic Duct** **9 Common Bile Duct** **C Ampulla of Vater** Duodenal ampulla Hepatopancreatic ampulla **D Pancreatic Duct** Duct of Wirsung **F Pancreatic Duct, Accessory** Duct of Santorini **G Pancreas**	**3 Percutaneous** **4 Percutaneous Endoscopic** **8 Via Natural or Artificial Opening Endoscopic**	**Z No Device**	**X Diagnostic**

Non-OR ØFD[Ø,1,2]3ZX
Non-OR ØFD[4,5,6,7,8,9,C,D,F,G][3,4,8]ZX

Ø Medical and Surgical
F Hepatobiliary System and Pancreas
F Fragmentation Definition: Breaking solid matter in a body part into pieces

Explanation: Physical force (e.g., manual, ultrasonic) applied directly or indirectly is used to break the solid matter into pieces. The solid matter may be an abnormal byproduct of a biological function or a foreign body. The pieces of solid matter are not taken out.

Body Part Character 4	Approach Character 5	Device Character 6	Qualifier Character 7
4 Gallbladder NC **5 Hepatic Duct, Right** NC **6 Hepatic Duct, Left** NC **7 Hepatic Duct, Common** **8 Cystic Duct** NC **9 Common Bile Duct** NC **C Ampulla of Vater** NC Duodenal ampulla Hepatopancreatic ampulla **D Pancreatic Duct** NC Duct of Wirsung **F Pancreatic Duct, Accessory** NC Duct of Santorini	**Ø Open** **3 Percutaneous** **4 Percutaneous Endoscopic** **7 Via Natural or Artificial Opening** **8 Via Natural or Artificial Opening Endoscopic** **X External**	**Z No Device**	**Z No Qualifier**

Non-OR ØFF[4,5,6,7,8,9,C,D,F][8,X]ZZ
NC ØFF[4,5,6,8,9,C,D,F]XZZ

Ø Medical and Surgical
F Hepatobiliary System and Pancreas
H Insertion Definition: Putting in a nonbiological appliance that monitors, assists, performs, or prevents a physiological function but does not physically take the place of a body part

Explanation: None

Body Part Character 4	Approach Character 5	Device Character 6	Qualifier Character 7
Ø Liver Quadrate lobe **4 Gallbladder** **G Pancreas**	**Ø Open** **3 Percutaneous** **4 Percutaneous Endoscopic**	**1 Radioactive Element** **2 Monitoring Device** **3 Infusion Device** **Y Other Device**	**Z No Qualifier**
1 Liver, Right Lobe **2 Liver, Left Lobe**	**Ø Open** **3 Percutaneous** **4 Percutaneous Endoscopic**	**2 Monitoring Device** **3 Infusion Device**	**Z No Qualifier**
B Hepatobiliary Duct ⊞ **D Pancreatic Duct** Duct of Wirsung	**Ø Open** **3 Percutaneous** **4 Percutaneous Endoscopic** **7 Via Natural or Artificial Opening** **8 Via Natural or Artificial Opening Endoscopic**	**1 Radioactive Element** **2 Monitoring Device** **3 Infusion Device** **D Intraluminal Device** **Y Other Device**	**Z No Qualifier**

Non-OR ØFH[Ø,4,G][Ø,3,4]3Z
Non-OR ØFH[Ø,4,G][3,4]YZ
Non-OR ØFH[1,2][Ø,3,4]3Z
Non-OR ØFH[B,D][Ø,3,4]3Z
Non-OR ØFH[B,D]4DZ
Non-OR ØFH[B,D][7,8][2,3]Z
Non-OR ØFH[B,D]8DZ
Non-OR ØFH[B,D][3,4,7,8]YZ

See Appendix L for Procedure Combinations
⊞ ØFHB7DZ

Ø Medical and Surgical
F Hepatobiliary System and Pancreas
J Inspection Definition: Visually and/or manually exploring a body part

Explanation: Visual exploration may be performed with or without optical instrumentation. Manual exploration may be performed directly or through intervening body layers.

Body Part Character 4	Approach Character 5	Device Character 6	Qualifier Character 7
Ø Liver Quadrate lobe	**Ø Open** **3 Percutaneous** **4 Percutaneous Endoscopic** **X External**	**Z No Device**	**Z No Qualifier**
4 Gallbladder **G Pancreas**	**Ø Open** **3 Percutaneous** **4 Percutaneous Endoscopic** **8 Via Natural or Artificial Opening Endoscopic** **X External**	**Z No Device**	**Z No Qualifier**
B Hepatobiliary Duct **D Pancreatic Duct** Duct of Wirsung	**Ø Open** **3 Percutaneous** **4 Percutaneous Endoscopic** **7 Via Natural or Artificial Opening** **8 Via Natural or Artificial Opening Endoscopic**	**Z No Device**	**Z No Qualifier**

Non-OR ØFJØ[3,X]ZZ
Non-OR ØFJ[4,G][3,8,X]ZZ
Non-OR ØFJ[B,D][3,7,8]ZZ

Ø Medical and Surgical
F Hepatobiliary System and Pancreas
L Occlusion Definition: Completely closing an orifice or the lumen of a tubular body part

Explanation: The orifice can be a natural orifice or an artificially created orifice

Body Part Character 4	Approach Character 5	Device Character 6	Qualifier Character 7
5 Hepatic Duct, Right **6 Hepatic Duct, Left** **7 Hepatic Duct, Common** **8 Cystic Duct** **9 Common Bile Duct** **C Ampulla of Vater** Duodenal ampulla Hepatopancreatic ampulla **D Pancreatic Duct** Duct of Wirsung **F Pancreatic Duct, Accessory** Duct of Santorini	**Ø Open** **3 Percutaneous** **4 Percutaneous Endoscopic**	**C Extraluminal Device** **D Intraluminal Device** **Z No Device**	**Z No Qualifier**
5 Hepatic Duct, Right **6 Hepatic Duct, Left** **7 Hepatic Duct, Common** **8 Cystic Duct** **9 Common Bile Duct** **C Ampulla of Vater** Duodenal ampulla Hepatopancreatic ampulla **D Pancreatic Duct** Duct of Wirsung **F Pancreatic Duct, Accessory** Duct of Santorini	**7 Via Natural or Artificial Opening** **8 Via Natural or Artificial Opening Endoscopic**	**D Intraluminal Device** **Z No Device**	**Z No Qualifier**

Non-OR ØFL[5,6,7,8,9][3,4][C,D,Z]Z
Non-OR ØFL[5,6,7,8,9][7,8][D,Z]Z

Ø Medical and Surgical
F Hepatobiliary System and Pancreas
M Reattachment Definition: Putting back in or on all or a portion of a separated body part to its normal location or other suitable location
Explanation: Vascular circulation and nervous pathways may or may not be reestablished

Body Part Character 4	Approach Character 5	Device Character 6	Qualifier Character 7
Ø Liver Quadrate lobe **1 Liver, Right Lobe** **2 Liver, Left Lobe** **4 Gallbladder** **5 Hepatic Duct, Right** **6 Hepatic Duct, Left** **7 Hepatic Duct, Common** **8 Cystic Duct** **9 Common Bile Duct** **C Ampulla of Vater** Duodenal ampulla Hepatopancreatic ampulla **D Pancreatic Duct** Duct of Wirsung **F Pancreatic Duct, Accessory** Duct of Santorini **G Pancreas**	**Ø Open** **4 Percutaneous Endoscopic**	**Z No Device**	**Z No Qualifier**

Non-OR ØFM[4,5,6,7,8,9]4ZZ

Ø Medical and Surgical
F Hepatobiliary System and Pancreas
N Release Definition: Freeing a body part from an abnormal physical constraint by cutting or by the use of force
Explanation: Some of the restraining tissue may be taken out but none of the body part is taken out

Body Part Character 4	Approach Character 5	Device Character 6	Qualifier Character 7
Ø Liver Quadrate lobe **1 Liver, Right Lobe** **2 Liver, Left Lobe**	**Ø Open** **3 Percutaneous** **4 Percutaneous Endoscopic**	**Z No Device**	**Z No Qualifier**
4 Gallbladder **G Pancreas**	**Ø Open** **3 Percutaneous** **4 Percutaneous Endoscopic** **8 Via Natural or Artificial Opening Endoscopic**	**Z No Device**	**Z No Qualifier**
5 Hepatic Duct, Right **6 Hepatic Duct, Left** **7 Hepatic Duct, Common** **8 Cystic Duct** **9 Common Bile Duct** **C Ampulla of Vater** Duodenal ampulla Hepatopancreatic ampulla **D Pancreatic Duct** Duct of Wirsung **F Pancreatic Duct, Accessory** Duct of Santorini	**Ø Open** **3 Percutaneous** **4 Percutaneous Endoscopic** **7 Via Natural or Artificial Opening** **8 Via Natural or Artificial Opening Endoscopic**	**Z No Device**	**Z No Qualifier**

Ø Medical and Surgical
F Hepatobiliary System and Pancreas
P Removal Definition: Taking out or off a device from a body part

Explanation: If a device is taken out and a similar device put in without cutting or puncturing the skin or mucous membrane, the procedure is coded to the root operation CHANGE. Otherwise, the procedure for taking out a device is coded to the root operation REMOVAL.

Body Part Character 4	Approach Character 5	Device Character 6	Qualifier Character 7
Ø Liver Quadrate lobe	**Ø Open** **3 Percutaneous** **4 Percutaneous Endoscopic**	**Ø Drainage Device** **2 Monitoring Device** **3 Infusion Device** **Y Other Device**	**Z No Qualifier**
Ø Liver Quadrate lobe	**X External**	**Ø Drainage Device** **2 Monitoring Device** **3 Infusion Device**	**Z No Qualifier**
4 Gallbladder **G Pancreas**	**Ø Open** **3 Percutaneous** **4 Percutaneous Endoscopic**	**Ø Drainage Device** **2 Monitoring Device** **3 Infusion Device** **D Intraluminal Device** **Y Other Device**	**Z No Qualifier**
4 Gallbladder **G Pancreas**	**X External**	**Ø Drainage Device** **2 Monitoring Device** **3 Infusion Device** **D Intraluminal Device**	**Z No Qualifier**
B Hepatobiliary Duct **D Pancreatic Duct** Duct of Wirsung	**Ø Open** **3 Percutaneous** **4 Percutaneous Endoscopic** **7 Via Natural or Artificial Opening** **8 Via Natural or Artificial Opening Endoscopic**	**Ø Drainage Device** **1 Radioactive Element** **2 Monitoring Device** **3 Infusion Device** **7 Autologous Tissue Substitute** **C Extraluminal Device** **D Intraluminal Device** **J Synthetic Substitute** **K Nonautologous Tissue Substitute** **Y Other Device**	**Z No Qualifier**
B Hepatobiliary Duct **D Pancreatic Duct** Duct of Wirsung	**X External**	**Ø Drainage Device** **1 Radioactive Element** **2 Monitoring Device** **3 Infusion Device** **D Intraluminal Device**	**Z No Qualifier**

Non-OR ØFPØ[3,4]YZ
Non-OR ØFPØX[Ø,2,3]Z
Non-OR ØFPG3ØZ
Non-OR ØFP[4,G][3,4]YZ
Non-OR ØFP4X[Ø,2,3,D]Z
Non-OR ØFPGX[Ø,2,3]Z
Non-OR ØFP[B,D][3,4]YZ
Non-OR ØFP[B,D][7,8][Ø,2,3,D,Y]Z
Non-OR ØFP[B,D]X[Ø,1,2,3,D]Z

See Appendix L for Procedure Combinations
Combo-only ØFP[B,D][7,8]DZ
Combo-only ØFP[B,D]XDZ

Ø Medical and Surgical
F Hepatobiliary System and Pancreas
Q Repair Definition: Restoring, to the extent possible, a body part to its normal anatomic structure and function
Explanation: Used only when the method to accomplish the repair is not one of the other root operations

Body Part Character 4	Approach Character 5	Device Character 6	Qualifier Character 7
Ø Liver Quadrate lobe 1 Liver, Right Lobe 2 Liver, Left Lobe	Ø Open 3 Percutaneous 4 Percutaneous Endoscopic	Z No Device	Z No Qualifier
4 Gallbladder G Pancreas	Ø Open 3 Percutaneous 4 Percutaneous Endoscopic 8 Via Natural or Artificial Opening Endoscopic	Z No Device	Z No Qualifier
5 Hepatic Duct, Right 6 Hepatic Duct, Left 7 Hepatic Duct, Common 8 Cystic Duct 9 Common Bile Duct C Ampulla of Vater Duodenal ampulla Hepatopancreatic ampulla D Pancreatic Duct Duct of Wirsung F Pancreatic Duct, Accessory Duct of Santorini	Ø Open 3 Percutaneous 4 Percutaneous Endoscopic 7 Via Natural or Artificial Opening 8 Via Natural or Artificial Opening Endoscopic	Z No Device	Z No Qualifier

Ø Medical and Surgical
F Hepatobiliary System and Pancreas
R Replacement Definition: Putting in or on biological or synthetic material that physically takes the place and/or function of all or a portion of a body part
Explanation: The body part may have been taken out or replaced, or may be taken out, physically eradicated, or rendered nonfunctional during the REPLACEMENT procedure. A REMOVAL procedure is coded for taking out the device used In a previous replacement procedure.

Body Part Character 4	Approach Character 5	Device Character 6	Qualifier Character 7
5 Hepatic Duct, Right 6 Hepatic Duct, Left 7 Hepatic Duct, Common 8 Cystic Duct 9 Common Bile Duct C Ampulla of Vater Duodenal ampulla Hepatopancreatic ampulla D Pancreatic Duct Duct of Wirsung F Pancreatic Duct, Accessory Duct of Santorini	Ø Open 4 Percutaneous Endoscopic 8 Via Natural or Artificial Opening Endoscopic	7 Autologous Tissue Substitute J Synthetic Substitute K Nonautologous Tissue Substitute	Z No Qualifier

Ø Medical and Surgical
F Hepatobiliary System and Pancreas
S Reposition Definition: Moving to its normal location, or other suitable location, all or a portion of a body part
Explanation: The body part is moved to a new location from an abnormal location, or from a normal location where it is not functioning correctly. The body part may or may not be cut out or off to be moved to the new location.

Body Part Character 4	Approach Character 5	Device Character 6	Qualifier Character 7
Ø Liver Quadrate lobe 4 Gallbladder 5 Hepatic Duct, Right 6 Hepatic Duct, Left 7 Hepatic Duct, Common 8 Cystic Duct 9 Common Bile Duct C Ampulla of Vater Duodenal ampulla Hepatopancreatic ampulla D Pancreatic Duct Duct of Wirsung F Pancreatic Duct, Accessory Duct of Santorini G Pancreas	Ø Open 4 Percutaneous Endoscopic	Z No Device	Z No Qualifier

Ø Medical and Surgical
F Hepatobiliary System and Pancreas
T Resection Definition: Cutting out or off, without replacement, all of a body part
Explanation: None

Body Part Character 4	Approach Character 5	Device Character 6	Qualifier Character 7
Ø Liver Quadrate lobe **1 Liver, Right Lobe** **2 Liver, Left Lobe** **4 Gallbladder** **G Pancreas** ⊞	**Ø Open** **4 Percutaneous Endoscopic**	**Z No Device**	**Z No Qualifier**
5 Hepatic Duct, Right **6 Hepatic Duct, Left** **7 Hepatic Duct, Common** **8 Cystic Duct** **9 Common Bile Duct** **C Ampulla of Vater** Duodenal ampulla Hepatopancreatic ampulla **D Pancreatic Duct** Duct of Wirsung **F Pancreatic Duct, Accessory** Duct of Santorini	**Ø Open** **4 Percutaneous Endoscopic** **7 Via Natural or Artificial Opening** **8 Via Natural or Artificial Opening Endoscopic**	**Z No Device**	**Z No Qualifier**

Non-OR ØFT[D,F][4,8]ZZ

See Appendix L for Procedure Combinations
⊞ ØFTGØZZ

Ø Medical and Surgical
F Hepatobiliary System and Pancreas
U Supplement Definition: Putting in or on biological or synthetic material that physically reinforces and/or augments the function of a portion of a body part
Explanation: The biological material is non-living, or is living and from the same individual. The body part may have been previously replaced, and the SUPPLEMENT procedure is performed to physically reinforce and/or augment the function of the replaced body part.

Body Part Character 4	Approach Character 5	Device Character 6	Qualifier Character 7
5 Hepatic Duct, Right **6 Hepatic Duct, Left** **7 Hepatic Duct, Common** **8 Cystic Duct** **9 Common Bile Duct** **C Ampulla of Vater** Duodenal ampulla Hepatopancreatic ampulla **D Pancreatic Duct** Duct of Wirsung **F Pancreatic Duct, Accessory** Duct of Santorini	**Ø Open** **3 Percutaneous** **4 Percutaneous Endoscopic** **8 Via Natural or Artificial Opening Endoscopic**	**7 Autologous Tissue Substitute** **J Synthetic Substitute** **K Nonautologous Tissue Substitute**	**Z No Qualifier**

Ø Medical and Surgical
F Hepatobiliary System and Pancreas
V Restriction Definition: Partially closing an orifice or the lumen of a tubular body part
Explanation: The orifice can be a natural orifice or an artificially created orifice

Body Part Character 4	Approach Character 5	Device Character 6	Qualifier Character 7
5 Hepatic Duct, Right 6 Hepatic Duct, Left 7 Hepatic Duct, Common 8 Cystic Duct 9 Common Bile Duct C Ampulla of Vater Duodenal ampulla Hepatopancreatic ampulla D Pancreatic Duct Duct of Wirsung F Pancreatic Duct, Accessory Duct of Santorini	Ø Open 3 Percutaneous 4 Percutaneous Endoscopic	C Extraluminal Device D Intraluminal Device Z No Device	Z No Qualifier
5 Hepatic Duct, Right 6 Hepatic Duct, Left 7 Hepatic Duct, Common 8 Cystic Duct 9 Common Bile Duct C Ampulla of Vater Duodenal ampulla Hepatopancreatic ampulla D Pancreatic Duct Duct of Wirsung F Pancreatic Duct, Accessory Duct of Santorini	7 Via Natural or Artificial Opening 8 Via Natural or Artificial Opening Endoscopic	D Intraluminal Device Z No Device	Z No Qualifier

Non-OR ØFV[5,6,7,8,9][3,4][C,D,Z]Z
Non-OR ØFV[5,6,7,8,9][7,8][D,Z]Z

Ø Medical and Surgical
F Hepatobiliary System and Pancreas
W Revision Definition: Correcting, to the extent possible, a portion of a malfunctioning device or the position of a displaced device

Explanation: Revision can include correcting a malfunctioning or displaced device by taking out or putting in components of the device such as a screw or pin

Body Part Character 4	Approach Character 5	Device Character 6	Qualifier Character 7
Ø Liver Quadrate lobe	Ø Open 3 Percutaneous 4 Percutaneous Endoscopic	Ø Drainage Device 2 Monitoring Device 3 Infusion Device Y Other Device	Z No Qualifier
Ø Liver Quadrate lobe	X External	Ø Drainage Device 2 Monitoring Device 3 Infusion Device	Z No Qualifier
4 Gallbladder G Pancreas	Ø Open 3 Percutaneous 4 Percutaneous Endoscopic	Ø Drainage Device 2 Monitoring Device 3 Infusion Device D Intraluminal Device Y Other Device	Z No Qualifier
4 Gallbladder G Pancreas	X External	Ø Drainage Device 2 Monitoring Device 3 Infusion Device D Intraluminal Device	Z No Qualifier
B Hepatobiliary Duct D Pancreatic Duct Duct of Wirsung	Ø Open 3 Percutaneous 4 Percutaneous Endoscopic 7 Via Natural or Artificial Opening 8 Via Natural or Artificial Opening Endoscopic	Ø Drainage Device 2 Monitoring Device 3 Infusion Device 7 Autologous Tissue Substitute C Extraluminal Device D Intraluminal Device J Synthetic Substitute K Nonautologous Tissue Substitute Y Other Device	Z No Qualifier
B Hepatobiliary Duct D Pancreatic Duct Duct of Wirsung	X External	Ø Drainage Device 2 Monitoring Device 3 Infusion Device 7 Autologous Tissue Substitute C Extraluminal Device D Intraluminal Device J Synthetic Substitute K Nonautologous Tissue Substitute	Z No Qualifier

Non-OR ØFWØ[3,4]YZ
Non-OR ØFWØX[Ø,2,3]Z
Non-OR ØFW[4,G][3,4]YZ
Non-OR ØFW[4,G]X[Ø,2,3,D]Z
Non-OR ØFW[B,D][3,4,7,8]YZ
Non-OR ØFW[B,D]X[Ø,2,3,7,C,D,J,K]Z

Ø Medical and Surgical
F Hepatobiliary System and Pancreas
Y Transplantation Definition: Putting in or on all or a portion of a living body part taken from another individual or animal to physically take the place and/or function of all or a portion of a similar body part

Explanation: The native body part may or may not be taken out, and the transplanted body part may take over all or a portion of its function

Body Part Character 4	Approach Character 5	Device Character 6	Qualifier Character 7
Ø Liver LC Quadrate lobe G Pancreas LC NC ⊞	Ø Open	Z No Device	Ø Allogeneic 1 Syngeneic 2 Zooplastic

LC ØFYØØZ[Ø,1,2]
LC ØFYGØZ[Ø,1]
NC ØFYGØZ2
NC ØFYGØZ[Ø,1] If reported alone without one of the following procedures ØTYØØZ[Ø,1,2], ØTY1ØZ[Ø,1,2] and without one of the following diagnoses E1Ø.1Ø-E1Ø.9, E89.1

See Appendix L for Procedure Combinations
⊞ ØFYGØZ[Ø,1,2]

Endocrine System ØG2–ØGW

Character Meanings

This Character Meaning table is provided as a guide to assist the user in the identification of character members that may be found in this section of code tables. It **SHOULD NOT** be used to build a PCS code.

Operation–Character 3	Body Part–Character 4	Approach–Character 5	Device–Character 6	Qualifier–Character 7
2 Change	Ø Pituitary Gland	Ø Open	Ø Drainage Device	X Diagnostic
5 Destruction	1 Pineal Body	3 Percutaneous	1 Radioactive Element	Z No Qualifier
8 Division	2 Adrenal Gland, Left	4 Percutaneous Endoscopic	2 Monitoring Device	
9 Drainage	3 Adrenal Gland, Right	X External	3 Infusion Device	
B Excision	4 Adrenal Glands, Bilateral		Y Other Device	
C Extirpation	5 Adrenal Gland		Z No Device	
H Insertion	6 Carotid Body, Left			
J Inspection	7 Carotid Body, Right			
M Reattachment	8 Carotid Bodies, Bilateral			
N Release	9 Para-aortic Body			
P Removal	B Coccygeal Glomus			
Q Repair	C Glomus Jugulare			
S Reposition	D Aortic Body			
T Resection	F Paraganglion Extremity			
W Revision	G Thyroid Gland Lobe, Left			
	H Thyroid Gland Lobe, Right			
	J Thyroid Gland Isthmus			
	K Thyroid Gland			
	L Superior Parathyroid Gland, Right			
	M Superior Parathyroid Gland, Left			
	N Inferior Parathyroid Gland, Right			
	P Inferior Parathyroid Gland, Left			
	Q Parathyroid Glands, Multiple			
	R Parathyroid Gland			
	S Endocrine Gland			

AHA Coding Clinic for table ØGB

2017, 2Q, 20 Near total thyroidectomy
2014, 3Q, 22 Transsphenoidal removal of pituitary tumor and fat graft placement

AHA Coding Clinic for table ØGT

2017, 2Q, 20 Near total thyroidectomy

Endocrine System

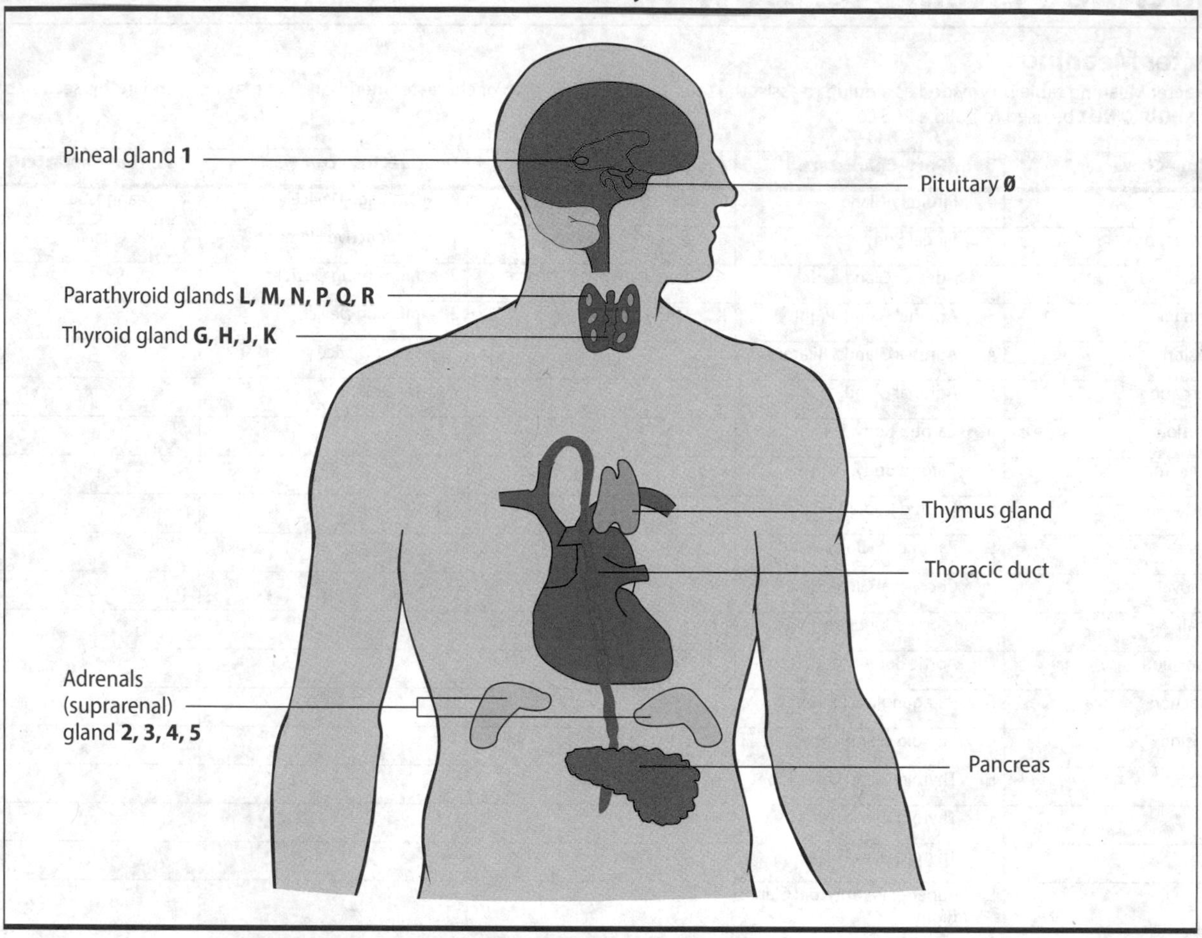

Pineal gland 1
Pituitary Ø
Parathyroid glands L, M, N, P, Q, R
Thyroid gland G, H, J, K
Thymus gland
Thoracic duct
Adrenals (suprarenal) gland 2, 3, 4, 5
Pancreas

Left Adrenal Gland

Left adrenal (suprarenal) gland 2
Fat and retroperitoneal wall
Renal pelvis
Ureter
Left kidney

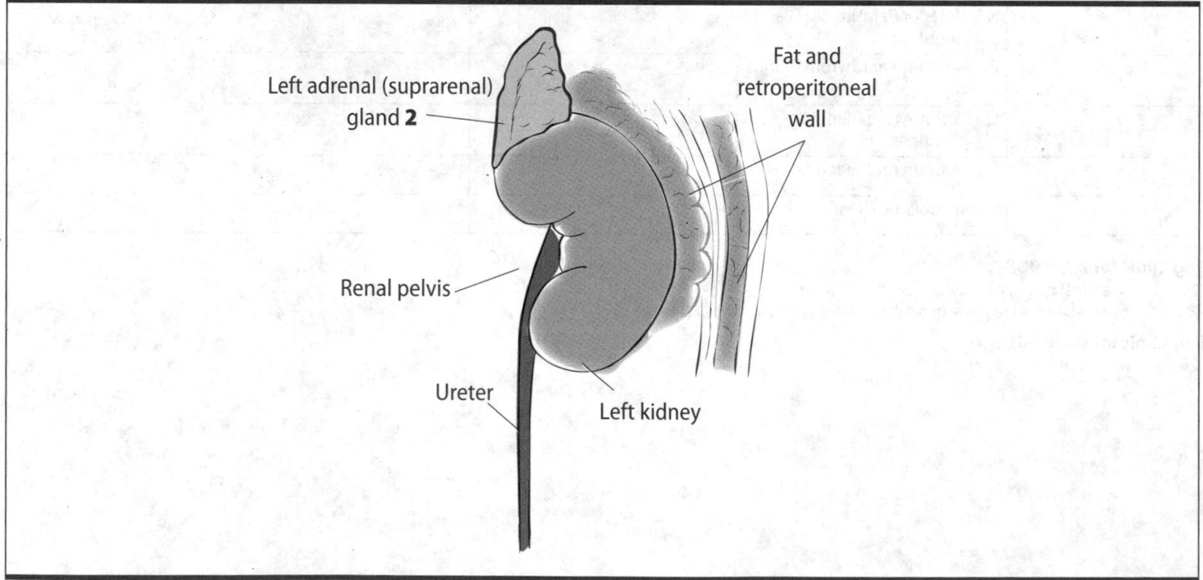

Thyroid

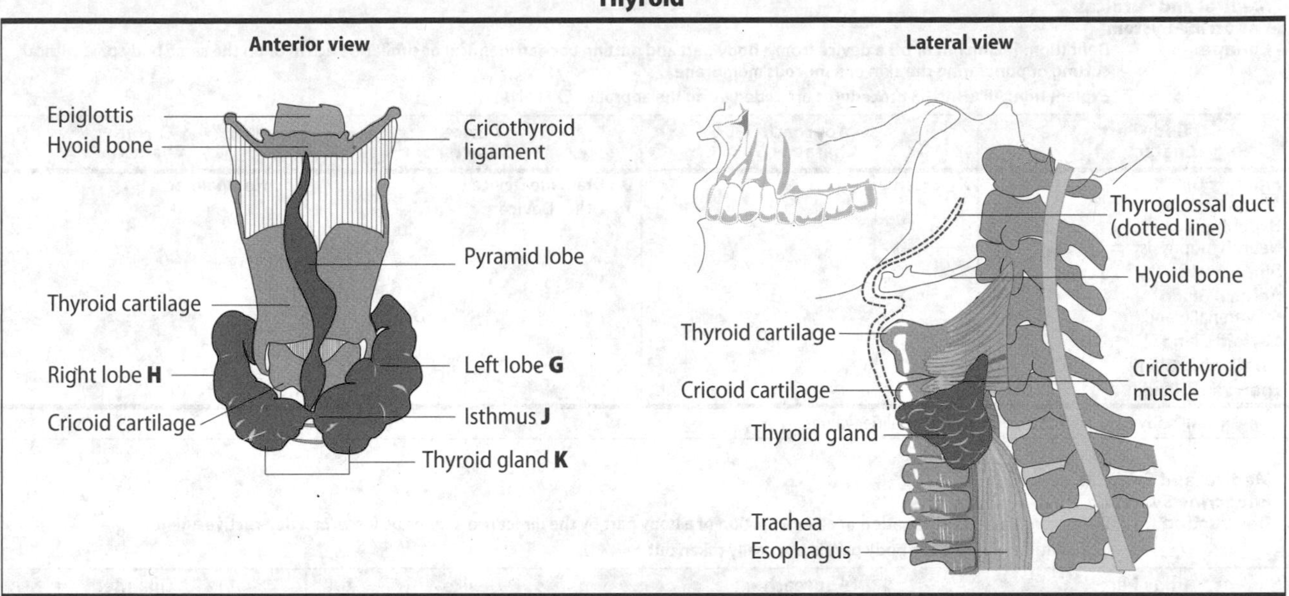

Thyroid and Parathyroid Glands

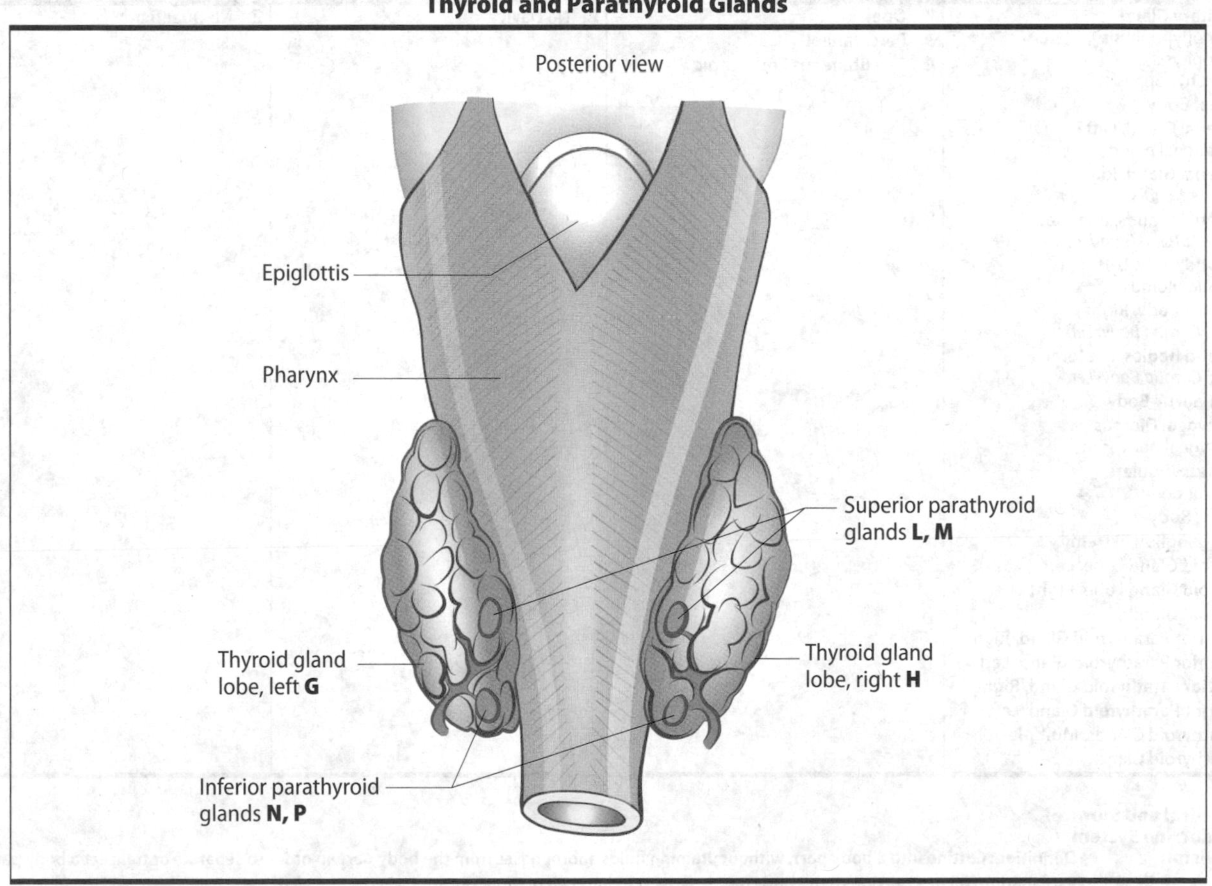

Ø Medical and Surgical
G Endocrine System
2 Change Definition: Taking out or off a device from a body part and putting back an identical or similar device in or on the same body part without cutting or puncturing the skin or a mucous membrane
Explanation: All CHANGE procedures are coded using the approach EXTERNAL

Body Part Character 4	Approach Character 5	Device Character 6	Qualifier Character 7
Ø Pituitary Gland Adenohypophysis Hypophysis Neurohypophysis 1 Pineal Body 5 Adrenal Gland Suprarenal gland K Thyroid Gland R Parathyroid Gland S Endocrine Gland	X External	Ø Drainage Device Y Other Device	Z No Qualifier

Non-OR All body part, approach, device, and qualifier values

Ø Medical and Surgical
G Endocrine System
5 Destruction Definition: Physical eradication of all or a portion of a body part by the direct use of energy, force, or a destructive agent
Explanation: None of the body part is physically taken out

Body Part Character 4	Approach Character 5	Device Character 6	Qualifier Character 7
Ø Pituitary Gland Adenohypophysis Hypophysis Neurohypophysis 1 Pineal Body 2 Adrenal Gland, Left Suprarenal gland 3 Adrenal Gland, Right *See 2 Adrenal Gland, Left* 4 Adrenal Glands, Bilateral *See 2 Adrenal Gland, Left* 6 Carotid Body, Left Carotid glomus 7 Carotid Body, Right *See 6 Carotid Body, Left* 8 Carotid Bodies, Bilateral *See 6 Carotid Body, Left* 9 Para-aortic Body B Coccygeal Glomus Coccygeal body C Glomus Jugulare Jugular body D Aortic Body F Paraganglion Extremity G Thyroid Gland Lobe, Left H Thyroid Gland Lobe, Right K Thyroid Gland L Superior Parathyroid Gland, Right M Superior Parathyroid Gland, Left N Inferior Parathyroid Gland, Right P Inferior Parathyroid Gland, Left Q Parathyroid Glands, Multiple R Parathyroid Gland	Ø Open 3 Percutaneous 4 Percutaneous Endoscopic	Z No Device	Z No Qualifier

Ø Medical and Surgical
G Endocrine System
8 Division Definition: Cutting into a body part, without draining fluids and/or gases from the body part, in order to separate or transect a body part
Explanation: All or a portion of the body part is separated into two or more portions

Body Part Character 4	Approach Character 5	Device Character 6	Qualifier Character 7
Ø Pituitary Gland Adenohypophysis Hypophysis Neurohypophysis J Thyroid Gland Isthmus	Ø Open 3 Percutaneous 4 Percutaneous Endoscopic	Z No Device	Z No Qualifier

Ø Medical and Surgical
G Endocrine System
9 Drainage Definition: Taking or letting out fluids and/or gases from a body part
Explanation: The qualifier DIAGNOSTIC is used to identify drainage procedures that are biopsies

Body Part Character 4	Approach Character 5	Device Character 6	Qualifier Character 7
Ø Pituitary Gland Adenohypophysis Hypophysis Neurohypophysis **1** Pineal Body **2** Adrenal Gland, Left Suprarenal gland **3** Adrenal Gland, Right *See 2 Adrenal Gland, Left* **4** Adrenal Glands, Bilateral *See 2 Adrenal Gland, Left* **6** Carotid Body, Left Carotid glomus **7** Carotid Body, Right *See 6 Carotid Body, Left* **8** Carotid Bodies, Bilateral *See 6 Carotid Body, Left* **9** Para-aortic Body **B** Coccygeal Glomus Coccygeal body **C** Glomus Jugulare Jugular body **D** Aortic Body **F** Paraganglion Extremity **G** Thyroid Gland Lobe, Left **H** Thyroid Gland Lobe, Right **K** Thyroid Gland **L** Superior Parathyroid Gland, Right **M** Superior Parathyroid Gland, Left **N** Inferior Parathyroid Gland, Right **P** Inferior Parathyroid Gland, Left **Q** Parathyroid Glands, Multiple **R** Parathyroid Gland	**Ø** Open **3** Percutaneous **4** Percutaneous Endoscopic	**Ø** Drainage Device	**Z** No Qualifier
Ø Pituitary Gland Adenohypophysis Hypophysis Neurohypophysis **1** Pineal Body **2** Adrenal Gland, Left Suprarenal gland **3** Adrenal Gland, Right *See 2 Adrenal Gland, Left* **4** Adrenal Glands, Bilateral *See 2 Adrenal Gland, Left* **6** Carotid Body, Left Carotid glomus **7** Carotid Body, Right *See 6 Carotid Body, Left* **8** Carotid Bodies, Bilateral *See 6 Carotid Body, Left* **9** Para-aortic Body **B** Coccygeal Glomus Coccygeal body **C** Glomus Jugulare Jugular body **D** Aortic Body **F** Paraganglion Extremity **G** Thyroid Gland Lobe, Left **H** Thyroid Gland Lobe, Right **K** Thyroid Gland **L** Superior Parathyroid Gland, Right **M** Superior Parathyroid Gland, Left **N** Inferior Parathyroid Gland, Right **P** Inferior Parathyroid Gland, Left **Q** Parathyroid Glands, Multiple **R** Parathyroid Gland	**Ø** Open **3** Percutaneous **4** Percutaneous Endoscopic	**Z** No Device	**X** Diagnostic **Z** No Qualifier

Non-OR ØG9[Ø,1,2,3,4,6,7,8,9,B,C,D,F,G,H,K,L,M,N,P,Q,R]3ØZ
Non-OR ØG9[G,H,K,L,M,N,P,Q,R]4ØZ
Non-OR ØG9[2,3,4,G,H,K][3,4]ZX
Non-OR ØG9[Ø,1,2,3,4,6,7,8,9,B,C,D,F,G,H,K,L,M,N,P,Q,R]3ZZ
Non-OR ØG9[G,H,K,L,M,N,P,Q,R]4ZZ

Ø Medical and Surgical
G Endocrine System
B Excision Definition: Cutting out or off, without replacement, a portion of a body part
Explanation: The qualifier DIAGNOSTIC is used to identify excision procedures that are biopsies

Body Part Character 4	Approach Character 5	Device Character 6	Qualifier Character 7
Ø Pituitary Gland Adenohypophysis Hypophysis Neurohypophysis **1 Pineal Body** **2 Adrenal Gland, Left** Suprarenal gland **3 Adrenal Gland, Right** *See 2 Adrenal Gland, Left* **4 Adrenal Glands, Bilateral** *See 2 Adrenal Gland, Left* **6 Carotid Body, Left** Carotid glomus **7 Carotid Body, Right** *See 6 Carotid Body, Left* **8 Carotid Bodies, Bilateral** *See 6 Carotid Body, Left* **9 Para-aortic Body** **B Coccygeal Glomus** Coccygeal body **C Glomus Jugulare** Jugular body **D Aortic Body** **F Paraganglion Extremity** **G Thyroid Gland Lobe, Left** **H Thyroid Gland Lobe, Right** **J Thyroid Gland Isthmus** **L Superior Parathyroid Gland, Right** **M Superior Parathyroid Gland, Left** **N Inferior Parathyroid Gland, Right** **P Inferior Parathyroid Gland, Left** **Q Parathyroid Glands, Multiple** **R Parathyroid Gland**	**Ø Open** **3 Percutaneous** **4 Percutaneous Endoscopic**	**Z No Device**	**X Diagnostic** **Z No Qualifier**

Non-OR ØGB[2,3,4,G,H,J][3,4]ZX

Ø Medical and Surgical
G Endocrine System
C Extirpation Definition: Taking or cutting out solid matter from a body part
Explanation: The solid matter may be an abnormal byproduct of a biological function or a foreign body; it may be imbedded in a body part or in the lumen of a tubular body part. The solid matter may or may not have been previously broken into pieces.

Body Part Character 4	Approach Character 5	Device Character 6	Qualifier Character 7
Ø Pituitary Gland Adenohypophysis Hypophysis Neurohypophysis **1 Pineal Body** **2 Adrenal Gland, Left** Suprarenal gland **3 Adrenal Gland, Right** *See 2 Adrenal Gland, Left* **4 Adrenal Glands, Bilateral** *See 2 Adrenal Gland, Left* **6 Carotid Body, Left** Carotid glomus **7 Carotid Body, Right** *See 6 Carotid Body, Left* **8 Carotid Bodies, Bilateral** *See 6 Carotid Body, Left* **9 Para-aortic Body** **B Coccygeal Glomus** Coccygeal body **C Glomus Jugulare** Jugular body **D Aortic Body** **F Paraganglion Extremity** **G Thyroid Gland Lobe, Left** **H Thyroid Gland Lobe, Right** **K Thyroid Gland** **L Superior Parathyroid Gland, Right** **M Superior Parathyroid Gland, Left** **N Inferior Parathyroid Gland, Right** **P Inferior Parathyroid Gland, Left** **Q Parathyroid Glands, Multiple** **R Parathyroid Gland**	**Ø Open** **3 Percutaneous** **4 Percutaneous Endoscopic**	**Z No Device**	**Z No Qualifier**

Ø Medical and Surgical
G Endocrine System
H Insertion Definition: Putting in a nonbiological appliance that monitors, assists, performs, or prevents a physiological function but does not physically take the place of a body part

Explanation: None

Body Part Character 4	Approach Character 5	Device Character 6	Qualifier Character 7
S Endocrine Gland	Ø Open 3 Percutaneous 4 Percutaneous Endoscopic	1 Radioactive Element 2 Monitoring Device 3 Infusion Device Y Other Device	Z No Qualifier

Non-OR ØGHS[3,4]YZ

Ø Medical and Surgical
G Endocrine System
J Inspection Definition: Visually and/or manually exploring a body part

Explanation: Visual exploration may be performed with or without optical instrumentation. Manual exploration may be performed directly or through intervening body layers.

Body Part Character 4	Approach Character 5	Device Character 6	Qualifier Character 7
Ø Pituitary Gland Adenohypophysis Hypophysis Neurohypophysis 1 Pineal Body 5 Adrenal Gland Suprarenal gland K Thyroid Gland R Parathyroid Gland S Endocrine Gland	Ø Open 3 Percutaneous 4 Percutaneous Endoscopic	Z No Device	Z No Qualifier

Non-OR ØGJ[Ø,1,5,K,R,S]3ZZ

Ø Medical and Surgical
G Endocrine System
M Reattachment Definition: Putting back in or on all or a portion of a separated body part to its normal location or other suitable location

Explanation: Vascular circulation and nervous pathways may or may not be reestablished

Body Part Character 4	Approach Character 5	Device Character 6	Qualifier Character 7
2 Adrenal Gland, Left Suprarenal gland 3 Adrenal Gland, Right *See 2 Adrenal Gland, Left* G Thyroid Gland Lobe, Left H Thyroid Gland Lobe, Right L Superior Parathyroid Gland, Right M Superior Parathyroid Gland, Left N Inferior Parathyroid Gland, Right P Inferior Parathyroid Gland, Left Q Parathyroid Glands, Multiple R Parathyroid Gland	Ø Open 4 Percutaneous Endoscopic	Z No Device	Z No Qualifier

Ø Medical and Surgical
G Endocrine System
N Release Definition: Freeing a body part from an abnormal physical constraint by cutting or by the use of force

Explanation: Some of the restraining tissue may be taken out but none of the body part is taken out

Body Part Character 4	Approach Character 5	Device Character 6	Qualifier Character 7
Ø Pituitary Gland Adenohypophysis Hypophysis Neurohypophysis **1 Pineal Body** **2 Adrenal Gland, Left** Suprarenal gland **3 Adrenal Gland, Right** *See 2 Adrenal Gland, Left* **4 Adrenal Glands, Bilateral** *See 2 Adrenal Gland, Left* **6 Carotid Body, Left** Carotid glomus **7 Carotid Body, Right** *See 6 Carotid Body, Left* **8 Carotid Bodies, Bilateral** *See 6 Carotid Body, Left* **9 Para-aortic Body** **B Coccygeal Glomus** Coccygeal body **C Glomus Jugulare** Jugular body **D Aortic Body** **F Paraganglion Extremity** **G Thyroid Gland Lobe, Left** **H Thyroid Gland Lobe, Right** **K Thyroid Gland** **L Superior Parathyroid Gland, Right** **M Superior Parathyroid Gland, Left** **N Inferior Parathyroid Gland, Right** **P Inferior Parathyroid Gland, Left** **Q Parathyroid Glands, Multiple** **R Parathyroid Gland**	**Ø Open** **3 Percutaneous** **4 Percutaneous Endoscopic**	**Z No Device**	**Z No Qualifier**

Non-OR ØGN[6,7,8,9,B,C,D,F][Ø,3,4]ZZ

Ø Medical and Surgical
G Endocrine System
P Removal Definition: Taking out or off a device from a body part

Explanation: If a device is taken out and a similar device put in without cutting or puncturing the skin or mucous membrane, the procedure is coded to the root operation CHANGE. Otherwise, the procedure for taking out a device is coded to the root operation REMOVAL.

Body Part Character 4	Approach Character 5	Device Character 6	Qualifier Character 7
Ø Pituitary Gland Adenohypophysis Hypophysis Neurohypophysis **1 Pineal Body** **5 Adrenal Gland** Suprarenal gland **K Thyroid Gland** **R Parathyroid Gland**	**Ø Open** **3 Percutaneous** **4 Percutaneous Endoscopic** **X External**	**Ø Drainage Device**	**Z No Qualifier**
S Endocrine Gland	**Ø Open** **3 Percutaneous** **4 Percutaneous Endoscopic**	**Ø Drainage Device** **2 Monitoring Device** **3 Infusion Device** **Y Other Device**	**Z No Qualifier**
S Endocrine Gland	**X External**	**Ø Drainage Device** **2 Monitoring Device** **3 Infusion Device**	**Z No Qualifier**

Non-OR ØGP[Ø,1,5,K,R]XØZ
Non-OR ØGPS[3,4]YZ
Non-OR ØGPSX[Ø,2,3]Z

Ø Medical and Surgical
G Endocrine System
Q Repair Definition: Restoring, to the extent possible, a body part to its normal anatomic structure and function

Explanation: Used only when the method to accomplish the repair is not one of the other root operations

Body Part Character 4	Approach Character 5	Device Character 6	Qualifier Character 7
Ø Pituitary Gland Adenohypophysis Hypophysis Neurohypophysis **1 Pineal Body** **2 Adrenal Gland, Left** Suprarenal gland **3 Adrenal Gland, Right** *See 2 Adrenal Gland, Left* **4 Adrenal Glands, Bilateral** *See 2 Adrenal Gland, Left* **6 Carotid Body, Left** Carotid glomus **7 Carotid Body, Right** *See 6 Carotid Body, Left* **8 Carotid Bodies, Bilateral** *See 6 Carotid Body, Left* **9 Para-aortic Body** **B Coccygeal Glomus** Coccygeal body **C Glomus Jugulare** Jugular body **D Aortic Body** **F Paraganglion Extremity** **G Thyroid Gland Lobe, Left** **H Thyroid Gland Lobe, Right** **J Thyroid Gland Isthmus** **K Thyroid Gland** **L Superior Parathyroid Gland, Right** **M Superior Parathyroid Gland, Left** **N Inferior Parathyroid Gland, Right** **P Inferior Parathyroid Gland, Left** **Q Parathyroid Glands, Multiple** **R Parathyroid Gland**	**Ø Open** **3 Percutaneous** **4 Percutaneous Endoscopic**	**Z No Device**	**Z No Qualifier**

Ø Medical and Surgical
G Endocrine System
S Reposition Definition: Moving to its normal location, or other suitable location, all or a portion of a body part

Explanation: The body part is moved to a new location from an abnormal location, or from a normal location where it is not functioning correctly. The body part may or may not be cut out or off to be moved to the new location.

Body Part Character 4	Approach Character 5	Device Character 6	Qualifier Character 7
2 Adrenal Gland, Left Suprarenal gland **3 Adrenal Gland, Right** *See 2 Adrenal Gland, Left* **G Thyroid Gland Lobe, Left** **H Thyroid Gland Lobe, Right** **L Superior Parathyroid Gland, Right** **M Superior Parathyroid Gland, Left** **N Inferior Parathyroid Gland, Right** **P Inferior Parathyroid Gland, Left** **Q Parathyroid Glands, Multiple** **R Parathyroid Gland**	**Ø Open** **4 Percutaneous Endoscopic**	**Z No Device**	**Z No Qualifier**

Ø Medical and Surgical
G Endocrine System
T Resection Definition: Cutting out or off, without replacement, all of a body part
Explanation: None

Body Part Character 4	Approach Character 5	Device Character 6	Qualifier Character 7
Ø Pituitary Gland Adenohypophysis Hypophysis Neurohypophysis **1 Pineal Body** **2 Adrenal Gland, Left** Suprarenal gland **3 Adrenal Gland, Right** *See 2 Adrenal Gland, Left* **4 Adrenal Glands, Bilateral** *See 2 Adrenal Gland, Left* **6 Carotid Body, Left** Carotid glomus **7 Carotid Body, Right** *See 6 Carotid Body, Left* **8 Carotid Bodies, Bilateral** *See 6 Carotid Body, Left* **9 Para-aortic Body** **B Coccygeal Glomus** Coccygeal body **C Glomus Jugulare** Jugular body **D Aortic Body** **F Paraganglion Extremity** **G Thyroid Gland Lobe, Left** **H Thyroid Gland Lobe, Right** **J Thyroid Gland Isthmus** **K Thyroid Gland** **L Superior Parathyroid Gland, Right** **M Superior Parathyroid Gland, Left** **N Inferior Parathyroid Gland, Right** **P Inferior Parathyroid Gland, Left** **Q Parathyroid Glands, Multiple** **R Parathyroid Gland**	**Ø Open** **4 Percutaneous Endoscopic**	**Z No Device**	**Z No Qualifier**

Non-OR ØGT[6,7,8,9,B,C,D,F][Ø,4]ZZ

Ø Medical and Surgical
G Endocrine System
W Revision Definition: Correcting, to the extent possible, a portion of a malfunctioning device or the position of a displaced device
Explanation: Revision can include correcting a malfunctioning or displaced device by taking out or putting in components of the device such as a screw or pin

Body Part Character 4	Approach Character 5	Device Character 6	Qualifier Character 7
Ø Pituitary Gland Adenohypophysis Hypophysis Neurohypophysis **1 Pineal Body** **5 Adrenal Gland** Suprarenal gland **K Thyroid Gland** **R Parathyroid Gland**	**Ø Open** **3 Percutaneous** **4 Percutaneous Endoscopic** **X External**	**Ø Drainage Device**	**Z No Qualifier**
S Endocrine Gland	**Ø Open** **3 Percutaneous** **4 Percutaneous Endoscopic**	**Ø Drainage Device** **2 Monitoring Device** **3 Infusion Device** **Y Other Device**	**Z No Qualifier**
S Endocrine Gland	**X External**	**Ø Drainage Device** **2 Monitoring Device** **3 Infusion Device**	**Z No Qualifier**

Non-OR ØGW[Ø,1,5,K,R]XØZ
Non-OR ØGWS[3,4]YZ
Non-OR ØGWSX[Ø,2,3]Z

Skin and Breast ØHØ–ØHX

Character Meanings*

This Character Meaning table is provided as a guide to assist the user in the identification of character members that may be found in this section of code tables. It **SHOULD NOT** be used to build a PCS code.

Operation–Character 3	Body Part–Character 4	Approach–Character 5	Device–Character 6	Qualifier–Character 7
Ø Alteration	Ø Skin, Scalp	Ø Open	Ø Drainage Device	2 Cell Suspension Technique
2 Change	1 Skin, Face	3 Percutaneous	1 Radioactive Element	3 Full Thickness
5 Destruction	2 Skin, Right Ear	7 Via Natural or Artificial Opening	7 Autologous Tissue Substitute	4 Partial Thickness
8 Division	3 Skin, Left Ear	8 Via Natural or Artificial Opening Endoscopic	J Synthetic Substitute	5 Latissimus Dorsi Myocutaneous Flap
9 Drainage	4 Skin, Neck	X External	K Nonautologous Tissue Substitute	6 Transverse Rectus Abdominis Myocutaneous Flap
B Excision	5 Skin, Chest		N Tissue Expander	7 Deep Inferior Epigastric Artery Perforator Flap
C Extirpation	6 Skin, Back		Y Other Device	8 Superficial Inferior Epigastric Artery Flap
D Extraction	7 Skin, Abdomen		Z No Device	9 Gluteal Artery Perforator Flap
H Insertion	8 Skin, Buttock			D Multiple
J Inspection	9 Skin, Perineum			X Diagnostic
M Reattachment	A Skin, Inguinal			Z No Qualifier
N Release	B Skin, Right Upper Arm			
P Removal	C Skin, Left Upper Arm			
Q Repair	D Skin, Right Lower Arm			
R Replacement	E Skin, Left Lower Arm			
S Reposition	F Skin, Right Hand			
T Resection	G Skin, Left Hand			
U Supplement	H Skin, Right Upper Leg			
W Revision	J Skin, Left Upper Leg			
X Transfer	K Skin, Right Lower Leg			
	L Skin, Left Lower Leg			
	M Skin, Right Foot			
	N Skin, Left Foot			
	P Skin			
	Q Finger Nail			
	R Toe Nail			
	S Hair			
	T Breast, Right			
	U Breast, Left			
	V Breast, Bilateral			
	W Nipple, Right			
	X Nipple, Left			
	Y Supernumerary Breast			

* Includes skin and breast glands and ducts.

AHA Coding Clinic for table ØHØ

2019, 4Q, 30-31 Breast procedures

AHA Coding Clinic for table ØH5

2019, 4Q, 30-31 Breast procedures

AHA Coding Clinic for table ØH9

2019, 4Q, 30-31 Breast procedures

AHA Coding Clinic for table ØHB

2020, 1Q, 31 Repair of buried penis
2019, 4Q, 30-31 Breast procedures
2018, 1Q, 14 Excisional debridement of breast tissue and skin
2016, 3Q, 29 Closure of bilateral alveolar clefts
2015, 3Q, 3-8 Excisional and nonexcisional debridement

AHA Coding Clinic for table ØHC

2019, 4Q, 30-31 Breast procedures

AHA Coding Clinic for table ØHD

2019, 4Q, 30-31 Breast procedures
2016, 1Q, 40 Nonexcisional debridement of skin and subcutaneous tissue
2015, 3Q, 3-8 Excisional and nonexcisional debridement

AHA Coding Clinic for table ØHH

2019, 4Q, 30-31 Breast procedures
2017, 4Q, 67 New qualifier values - Pedicle flap procedures
2014, 2Q, 12 Pedicle latissimus myocutaneous flap with placement of breast tissue expanders
2013, 4Q, 107 Breast tissue expander placement using acellular dermal matrix

AHA Coding Clinic for table ØHJ

2019, 4Q, 30-31 Breast procedures

AHA Coding Clinic for table ØHN

2019, 4Q, 30-31 Breast procedures

AHA Coding Clinic for table ØHP

2019, 4Q, 30-31 Breast procedures
2018, 3Q, 13 Deep inferior epigastric artery perforator flap breast reconstruction
2016, 2Q, 27 Removal of nonviable transverse rectus abdominis myocutaneous (TRAM) flaps

AHA Coding Clinic for table ØHQ

2019, 4Q, 30-31 Breast procedures
2018, 2Q, 25 Third and fourth degree obstetric lacerations
2016, 1Q, 7 Obstetrical perineal laceration repair
2014, 4Q, 31 Delayed wound closure following fracture treatment

AHA Coding Clinic for table ØHR

2020, 1Q, 27 Delayed reconstruction following mastectomy using gracilis musculocutaneous free flap
2020, 1Q, 28 Free flap microvascular breast reconstruction
2020, 1Q, 30 Polarity Skin TE™ application
2019, 4Q, 30-31 Breast procedures
2019, 4Q, 32 Cell suspension epithelial autograft
2019, 3Q, 32 Breast reconstruction with neurotization
2018, 3Q, 13 Deep inferior epigastric artery perforator flap breast reconstruction
2017, 1Q, 35 Epifix® allograft
2014, 3Q, 14 Application of TheraSkin® and excisional debridement

AHA Coding Clinic for table ØHT

2018, 3Q, 13 Deep inferior epigastric artery perforator flap breast reconstruction
2014, 4Q, 34 Skin-sparing mastectomy

AHA Coding Clinic for table ØHU

2019, 4Q, 30-31 Breast procedures

AHA Coding Clinic for table ØHW

2019, 4Q, 30-31 Breast procedures

Integumentary Anatomy

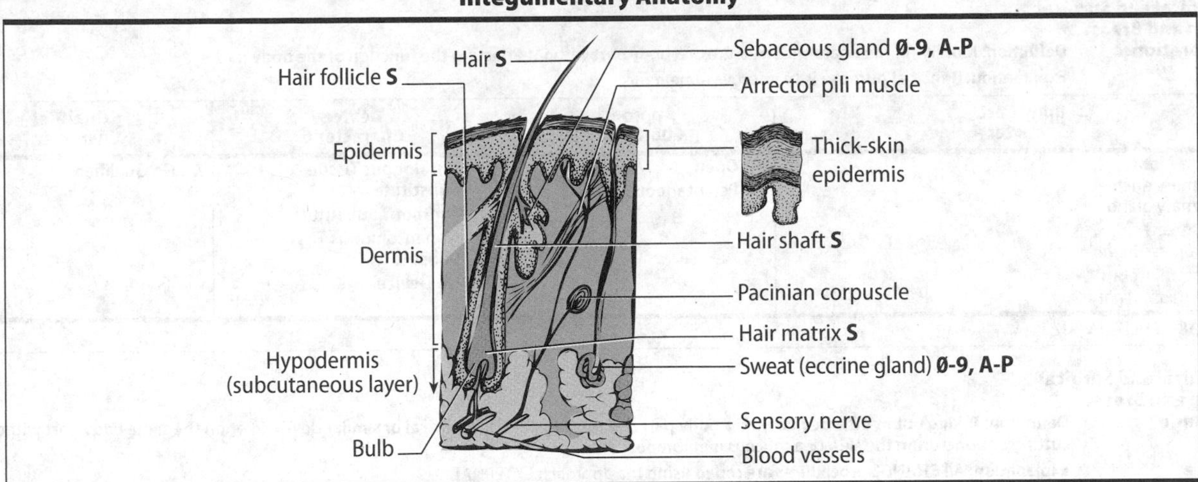

Nail Anatomy

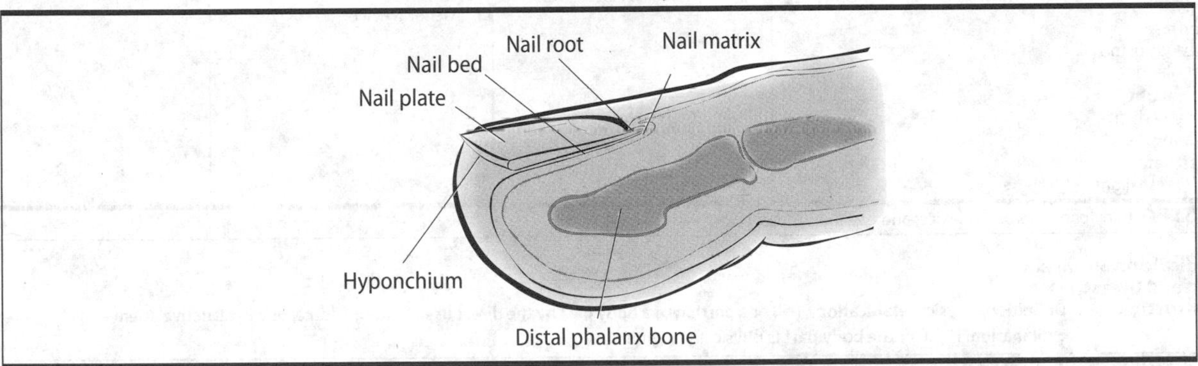

Breast

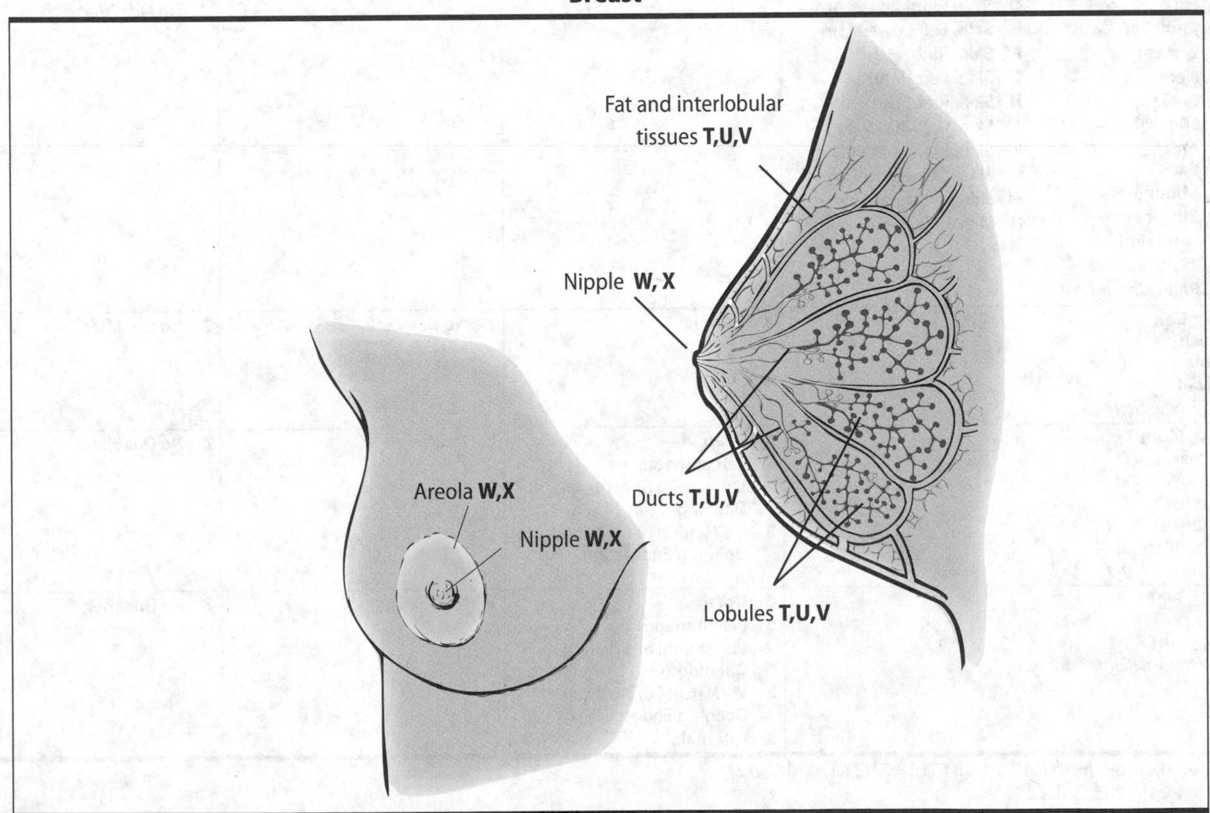

Ø Medical and Surgical
H Skin and Breast
Ø Alteration Definition: Modifying the anatomic structure of a body part without affecting the function of the body part
Explanation: Principal purpose is to improve appearance

Body Part Character 4	Approach Character 5	Device Character 6	Qualifier Character 7
T Breast, Right Mammary duct Mammary gland U Breast, Left *See T Breast, Right* V Breast, Bilateral *See T Breast, Right*	Ø Open 3 Percutaneous	7 Autologous Tissue Substitute J Synthetic Substitute K Nonautologous Tissue Substitute Z No Device	Z No Qualifier

Non-OR ØHØ[T,U,V]3JZ

Ø Medical and Surgical
H Skin and Breast
2 Change Definition: Taking out or off a device from a body part and putting back an identical or similar device in or on the same body part without cutting or puncturing the skin or a mucous membrane
Explanation: All CHANGE procedures are coded using the approach EXTERNAL

Body Part Character 4	Approach Character 5	Device Character 6	Qualifier Character 7
P Skin Dermis Epidermis Sebaceous gland Sweat gland T Breast, Right Mammary duct Mammary gland U Breast, Left *See T Breast, Right*	X External	Ø Drainage Device Y Other Device	Z No Qualifier

Non-OR All body part, approach, device, and qualifier values

Ø Medical and Surgical
H Skin and Breast
5 Destruction Definition: Physical eradication of all or a portion of a body part by the direct use of energy, force, or a destructive agent
Explanation: None of the body part is physically taken out

Body Part Character 4	Approach Character 5	Device Character 6	Qualifier Character 7
Ø Skin, Scalp 1 Skin, Face 2 Skin, Right Ear 3 Skin, Left Ear 4 Skin, Neck 5 Skin, Chest Breast procedures, skin only 6 Skin, Back 7 Skin, Abdomen 8 Skin, Buttock 9 Skin, Perineum A Skin, Inguinal B Skin, Right Upper Arm C Skin, Left Upper Arm D Skin, Right Lower Arm E Skin, Left Lower Arm F Skin, Right Hand G Skin, Left Hand H Skin, Right Upper Leg J Skin, Left Upper Leg K Skin, Right Lower Leg L Skin, Left Lower Leg M Skin, Right Foot N Skin, Left Foot	X External	Z No Device	D Multiple Z No Qualifier
Q Finger Nail Nail bed Nail plate R Toe Nail *See Q Finger Nail*	X External	Z No Device	Z No Qualifier
T Breast, Right Mammary duct Mammary gland U Breast, Left *See T Breast, Right* V Breast, Bilateral *See T Breast, Right*	Ø Open 3 Percutaneous 7 Via Natural or Artificial Opening 8 Via Natural or Artificial Opening Endoscopic	Z No Device	Z No Qualifier
W Nipple, Right Areola X Nipple, Left *See W Nipple, Right*	Ø Open 3 Percutaneous 7 Via Natural or Artificial Opening 8 Via Natural or Artificial Opening Endoscopic X External	Z No Device	Z No Qualifier

DRG Non-OR ØH5[Ø,1,4,5,6,7,8,9,A,B,C,D,E,F,G,H,J,K,L,M,N]XZ[D,Z]
DRG Non-OR ØH5[Q,R]XZZ
Non-OR ØH5[2,3]XZ[D,Z]

Ø Medical and Surgical
H Skin and Breast
8 Division Definition: Cutting into a body part, without draining fluids and/or gases from the body part, in order to separate or transect a body part
Explanation: All or a portion of the body part is separated into two or more portions

Body Part Character 4	Approach Character 5	Device Character 6	Qualifier Character 7
Ø Skin, Scalp 1 Skin, Face 2 Skin, Right Ear 3 Skin, Left Ear 4 Skin, Neck 5 Skin, Chest Breast procedures, skin only 6 Skin, Back 7 Skin, Abdomen 8 Skin, Buttock 9 Skin, Perineum A Skin, Inguinal B Skin, Right Upper Arm C Skin, Left Upper Arm D Skin, Right Lower Arm E Skin, Left Lower Arm F Skin, Right Hand G Skin, Left Hand H Skin, Right Upper Leg J Skin, Left Upper Leg K Skin, Right Lower Leg L Skin, Left Lower Leg M Skin, Right Foot N Skin, Left Foot	X External	Z No Device	Z No Qualifier

Non-OR All body part, approach, device, and qualifier values

Ø Medical and Surgical
H Skin and Breast
9 Drainage Definition: Taking or letting out fluids and/or gases from a body part
Explanation: The qualifier DIAGNOSTIC is used to identify drainage procedures that are biopsies

Body Part Character 4		Approach Character 5	Device Character 6	Qualifier Character 7
Ø Skin, Scalp **1** Skin, Face **2** Skin, Right Ear **3** Skin, Left Ear **4** Skin, Neck **5** Skin, Chest Breast procedures, skin only **6** Skin, Back **7** Skin, Abdomen **8** Skin, Buttock **9** Skin, Perineum **A** Skin, Inguinal **B** Skin, Right Upper Arm **C** Skin, Left Upper Arm **D** Skin, Right Lower Arm	**E** Skin, Left Lower Arm **F** Skin, Right Hand **G** Skin, Left Hand **H** Skin, Right Upper Leg **J** Skin, Left Upper Leg **K** Skin, Right Lower Leg **L** Skin, Left Lower Leg **M** Skin, Right Foot **N** Skin, Left Foot **Q** Finger Nail Nail bed Nail plate **R** Toe Nail *See Q Finger Nail*	**X** External	**Ø** Drainage Device	**Z** No Qualifier
Ø Skin, Scalp **1** Skin, Face **2** Skin, Right Ear **3** Skin, Left Ear **4** Skin, Neck **5** Skin, Chest Breast procedures, skin only **6** Skin, Back **7** Skin, Abdomen **8** Skin, Buttock **9** Skin, Perineum **A** Skin, Inguinal **B** Skin, Right Upper Arm **C** Skin, Left Upper Arm **D** Skin, Right Lower Arm	**E** Skin, Left Lower Arm **F** Skin, Right Hand **G** Skin, Left Hand **H** Skin, Right Upper Leg **J** Skin, Left Upper Leg **K** Skin, Right Lower Leg **L** Skin, Left Lower Leg **M** Skin, Right Foot **N** Skin, Left Foot **Q** Finger Nail Nail bed Nail plate **R** Toe Nail *See Q Finger Nail*	**X** External	**Z** No Device	**X** Diagnostic **Z** No Qualifier
T Breast, Right Mammary duct Mammary gland **U** Breast, Left *See T Breast, Right* **V** Breast, Bilateral *See T Breast, Right*		**Ø** Open **3** Percutaneous **7** Via Natural or Artificial Opening **8** Via Natural or Artificial Opening Endoscopic	**Ø** Drainage Device	**Z** No Qualifier
T Breast, Right Mammary duct Mammary gland **U** Breast, Left *See T Breast, Right* **V** Breast, Bilateral *See T Breast, Right*		**Ø** Open **3** Percutaneous **7** Via Natural or Artificial Opening **8** Via Natural or Artificial Opening Endoscopic	**Z** No Device	**X** Diagnostic **Z** No Qualifier
W Nipple, Right Areola **X** Nipple, Left *See W Nipple, Right*		**Ø** Open **3** Percutaneous **7** Via Natural or Artificial Opening **8** Via Natural or Artificial Opening Endoscopic **X** External	**Ø** Drainage Device	**Z** No Qualifier
W Nipple, Right Areola **X** Nipple, Left *See W Nipple, Right*		**Ø** Open **3** Percutaneous **7** Via Natural or Artificial Opening **8** Via Natural or Artificial Opening Endoscopic **X** External	**Z** No Device	**X** Diagnostic **Z** No Qualifier

Non-OR ØH9[Ø,1,2,3,4,5,6,7,8,A,B,C,D,E,F,G,H,J,K,L,M,N,Q,R]XØZ
Non-OR ØH9[Ø,1,2,3,4,5,6,7,8,A,B,C,D,E,F,G,H,J,K,L,M,N,Q,R]XZ[X,Z]
Non-OR ØH99XZX
Non-OR ØH9[T,U,V][Ø,3,7,8]ØZ
Non-OR ØH9[T,U,V][3,7,8]Z[X,Z]
Non-OR ØH9[W,X][Ø,3,7,8,X]ØZ
Non-OR ØH9[W,X][3,7,8,X]Z[X,Z]

Ø Medical and Surgical
H Skin and Breast
B Excision Definition: Cutting out or off, without replacement, a portion of a body part
Explanation: The qualifier DIAGNOSTIC is used to identify excision procedures that are biopsies

Body Part Character 4	Approach Character 5	Device Character 6	Qualifier Character 7
Ø Skin, Scalp **1 Skin, Face** **2 Skin, Right Ear** **3 Skin, Left Ear** **4 Skin, Neck** **5 Skin, Chest** Breast procedures, skin only **6 Skin, Back** **7 Skin, Abdomen** **8 Skin, Buttock** **9 Skin, Perineum** **A Skin, Inguinal** **B Skin, Right Upper Arm** **C Skin, Left Upper Arm** **D Skin, Right Lower Arm** **E Skin, Left Lower Arm** **F Skin, Right Hand** **G Skin, Left Hand** **H Skin, Right Upper Leg** **J Skin, Left Upper Leg** **K Skin, Right Lower Leg** **L Skin, Left Lower Leg** **M Skin, Right Foot** **N Skin, Left Foot** **Q Finger Nail** Nail bed Nail plate **R Toe Nail** *See Q Finger Nail*	**X External**	**Z No Device**	**X Diagnostic** **Z No Qualifier**
T Breast, Right Mammary duct Mammary gland **U Breast, Left** *See T Breast, Right* **V Breast, Bilateral** *See T Breast, Right* **Y Supernumerary Breast**	**Ø Open** **3 Percutaneous** **7 Via Natural or Artificial Opening** **8 Via Natural or Artificial Opening Endoscopic**	**Z No Device**	**X Diagnostic** **Z No Qualifier**
W Nipple, Right Areola **X Nipple, Left** *See W Nipple, Right*	**Ø Open** **3 Percutaneous** **7 Via Natural or Artificial Opening** **8 Via Natural or Artificial Opening Endoscopic** **X External**	**Z No Device**	**X Diagnostic** **Z No Qualifier**

DRG Non-OR	ØHB9XZZ
Non-OR	ØHB[Ø,1,2,3,4,5,6,7,8,A,B,C,D,E,F,G,H,J,K,L,M,N,Q,R]XZ[X,Z]
Non-OR	ØHB9XZX
Non-OR	ØHB[T,U,V,Y][3,7,8]ZX
Non-OR	ØHB[W,X][3,7,8,X]ZX

Ø Medical and Surgical
H Skin and Breast
C Extirpation Definition: Taking or cutting out solid matter from a body part

Explanation: The solid matter may be an abnormal byproduct of a biological function or a foreign body; it may be imbedded in a body part or in the lumen of a tubular body part. The solid matter may or may not have been previously broken into pieces.

Body Part Character 4	Approach Character 5	Device Character 6	Qualifier Character 7
Ø Skin, Scalp **1** Skin, Face **2** Skin, Right Ear **3** Skin, Left Ear **4** Skin, Neck **5** Skin, Chest Breast procedures, skln only **6** Skin, Back **7** Skin, Abdomen **8** Skin, Buttock **9** Skin, Perineum **A** Skin, Inguinal **B** Skin, Right Upper Arm **C** Skin, Left Upper Arm **D** Skin, Right Lower Arm **E** Skin, Left Lower Arm **F** Skin, Right Hand **G** Skin, Left Hand **H** Skin, Right Upper Leg **J** Skin, Left Upper Leg **K** Skin, Right Lower Leg **L** Skin, Left Lower Leg **M** Skin, Right Foot **N** Skin, Left Foot **Q** Finger Nail Nail bed Nail plate **R** Toe Nail *See Q Finger Nail*	**X** External	**Z** No Device	**Z** No Qualifier
T Breast, Right Mammary duct Mammary gland **U** Breast, Left *See T Breast, Right* **V** Breast, Bilateral *See T Breast, Right*	**Ø** Open **3** Percutaneous **7** Via Natural or Artificial Opening **8** Via Natural or Artificial Opening Endoscopic	**Z** No Device	**Z** No Qualifier
W Nipple, Right Areola **X** Nipple, Left *See W Nipple, Right*	**Ø** Open **3** Percutaneous **7** Via Natural or Artificial Opening **8** Via Natural or Artificial Opening Endoscopic **X** External	**Z** No Device	**Z** No Qualifier

Non-OR ØHC[Ø,1,2,3,4,5,6,7,8,9,A,B,C,D,E,F,G,H,J,K,L,M,N,Q,R]XZZ
Non-OR ØHC[T,U,V][3,7,8]ZZ
Non-OR ØHC[W,X][3,7,8,X]ZZ

Ø Medical and Surgical
H Skin and Breast
D Extraction Definition: Pulling or stripping out or off all or a portion of a body part by the use of force
Explanation: The qualifier DIAGNOSTIC is used to identify extraction procedures that are biopsies

Body Part Character 4	Approach Character 5	Device Character 6	Qualifier Character 7
Ø Skin, Scalp 1 Skin, Face 2 Skin, Right Ear 3 Skin, Left Ear 4 Skin, Neck 5 Skin, Chest Breast procedures, skin only 6 Skin, Back 7 Skin, Abdomen 8 Skin, Buttock 9 Skin, Perineum A Skin, Inguinal B Skin, Right Upper Arm C Skin, Left Upper Arm D Skin, Right Lower Arm E Skin, Left Lower Arm F Skin, Right Hand G Skin, Left Hand H Skin, Right Upper Leg J Skin, Left Upper Leg K Skin, Right Lower Leg L Skin, Left Lower Leg M Skin, Right Foot N Skin, Left Foot Q Finger Nail Nail bed Nail plate R Toe Nail *See Q Finger Nail* S Hair	X External	Z No Device	Z No Qualifier
T Breast, Right Mammary duct Mammary gland U Breast, Left *See T Breast, Right* V Breast, Bilateral *See T Breast, Right* Y Supernumerary Breast	Ø Open	Z No Device	Z No Qualifier

Non-OR All body part, approach, device, and qualifier values

Ø Medical and Surgical
H Skin and Breast
H Insertion Definition: Putting in a nonbiological appliance that monitors, assists, performs, or prevents a physiological function but does not physically take the place of a body part

Explanation: None

Body Part Character 4	Approach Character 5	Device Character 6	Qualifier Character 7
P Skin	**X External**	**Y Other Device**	**Z No Qualifier**
T Breast, Right Mammary duct Mammary gland **U Breast, Left** *See T Breast, Right*	**Ø Open** **3 Percutaneous** **7 Via Natural or Artificial Opening** **8 Via Natural or Artificial Opening Endoscopic**	**1 Radioactive Element** **N Tissue Expander** **Y Other Device**	**Z No Qualifier**
V Breast, Bilateral Mammary duct Mammary gland	**Ø Open** **3 Percutaneous** **7 Via Natural or Artificial Opening** **8 Via Natural or Artificial Opening Endoscopic**	**1 Radioactive Element** **N Tissue Expander**	**Z No Qualifier**
W Nipple, Right Areola **X Nipple, Left** *See W Nipple, Right*	**Ø Open** **3 Percutaneous** **7 Via Natural or Artificial Opening** **8 Via Natural or Artificial Opening Endoscopic**	**1 Radioactive Element** **N Tissue Expander**	**Z No Qualifier**
W Nipple, Right Areola **X Nipple, Left** *See W Nipple, Right*	**X External**	**1 Radioactive Element**	**Z No Qualifier**

Non-OR ØHHPXYZ
Non-OR ØHH[T,U][3,7,8]YZ

Ø Medical and Surgical
H Skin and Breast
J Inspection Definition: Visually and/or manually exploring a body part

Explanation: Visual exploration may be performed with or without optical instrumentation. Manual exploration may be performed directly or through intervening body layers.

Body Part Character 4	Approach Character 5	Device Character 6	Qualifier Character 7
P Skin Dermis Epidermis Sebaceous gland Sweat gland **Q Finger Nail** Nail bed Nail plate **R Toe Nail** *See Q Finger Nail*	**X External**	**Z No Device**	**Z No Qualifier**
T Breast, Right Mammary duct Mammary gland **U Breast, Left** *See T Breast, Right*	**Ø Open** **3 Percutaneous** **7 Via Natural or Artificial Opening** **8 Via Natural or Artificial Opening Endoscopic**	**Z No Device**	**Z No Qualifier**

Non-OR All body part, approach, device and qualifier values

Ø Medical and Surgical
H Skin and Breast
M Reattachment Definition: Putting back in or on all or a portion of a separated body part to its normal location or other suitable location
Explanation: Vascular circulation and nervous pathways may or may not be reestablished

Body Part Character 4	Approach Character 5	Device Character 6	Qualifier Character 7
Ø Skin, Scalp **1 Skin, Face** **2 Skin, Right Ear** **3 Skin, Left Ear** **4 Skin, Neck** **5 Skin, Chest** Breast procedures, skin only **6 Skin, Back** **7 Skin, Abdomen** **8 Skin, Buttock** **9 Skin, Perineum** **A Skin, Inguinal** **B Skin, Right Upper Arm** **C Skin, Left Upper Arm** **D Skin, Right Lower Arm** **E Skin, Left Lower Arm** **F Skin, Right Hand** **G Skin, Left Hand** **H Skin, Right Upper Leg** **J Skin, Left Upper Leg** **K Skin, Right Lower Leg** **L Skin, Left Lower Leg** **M Skin, Right Foot** **N Skin, Left Foot** **T Breast, Right** Mammary duct Mammary gland **U Breast, Left** *See T Breast, Right* **V Breast, Bilateral** *See T Breast, Right* **W Nipple, Right** Areola **X Nipple, Left** *See W Nipple, Right*	**X External**	**Z No Device**	**Z No Qualifier**

Non-OR ØHMØXZZ

Ø Medical and Surgical
H Skin and Breast
N Release Definition: Freeing a body part from an abnormal physical constraint by cutting or by the use of force
Explanation: Some of the restraining tissue may be taken out but none of the body part is taken out

Body Part Character 4	Approach Character 5	Device Character 6	Qualifier Character 7
Ø Skin, Scalp **1** Skin, Face **2** Skin, Right Ear **3** Skin, Left Ear **4** Skin, Neck **5** Skin, Chest Breast procedures, skin only **6** Skin, Back **7** Skin, Abdomen **8** Skin, Buttock **9** Skin, Perineum **A** Skin, Inguinal **B** Skin, Right Upper Arm **C** Skin, Left Upper Arm **D** Skin, Right Lower Arm **E** Skin, Left Lower Arm **F** Skin, Right Hand **G** Skin, Left Hand **H** Skin, Right Upper Leg **J** Skin, Left Upper Leg **K** Skin, Right Lower Leg **L** Skin, Left Lower Leg **M** Skin, Right Foot **N** Skin, Left Foot **Q** Finger Nail Nail bed Nail plate **R** Toe Nail *See Q Finger Nail*	**X** External	**Z** No Device	**Z** No Qualifier
T Breast, Right Mammary duct Mammary gland **U** Breast, Left *See T Breast, Right* **V** Breast, Bilateral *See T Breast, Right*	**Ø** Open **3** Percutaneous **7** Via Natural or Artificial Opening **8** Via Natural or Artificial Opening Endoscopic	**Z** No Device	**Z** No Qualifier
W Nipple, Right Areola **X** Nipple, Left *See W Nipple, Right*	**Ø** Open **3** Percutaneous **7** Via Natural or Artificial Opening **8** Via Natural or Artificial Opening Endoscopic **X** External	**Z** No Device	**Z** No Qualifier

Ø Medical and Surgical
H Skin and Breast
P Removal Definition: Taking out or off a device from a body part

Explanation: If a device is taken out and a similar device put in without cutting or puncturing the skin or mucous membrane, the procedure is coded to the root operation CHANGE. Otherwise, the procedure for taking out a device is coded to the root operation REMOVAL.

Body Part Character 4	Approach Character 5	Device Character 6	Qualifier Character 7
P Skin Dermis Epidermis Sebaceous gland Sweat gland	**X External**	**Ø Drainage Device** **7 Autologous Tissue Substitute** **J Synthetic Substitute** **K Nonautologous Tissue Substitute** **Y Other Device**	**Z No Qualifier**
Q Finger Nail Nail bed Nail plate **R Toe Nail** *See Q Finger Nail*	**X External**	**Ø Drainage Device** **7 Autologous Tissue Substitute** **J Synthetic Substitute** **K Nonautologous Tissue Substitute**	**Z No Qualifier**
S Hair	**X External**	**7 Autologous Tissue Substitute** **J Synthetic Substitute** **K Nonautologous Tissue Substitute**	**Z No Qualifier**
T Breast, Right Mammary duct Mammary gland **U Breast, Left** *See T Breast, Right*	**Ø Open** **3 Percutaneous** **7 Via Natural or Artificial Opening** **8 Via Natural or Artificial Opening Endoscopic**	**Ø Drainage Device** **1 Radioactive Element** **7 Autologous Tissue Substitute** **J Synthetic Substitute** **K Nonautologous Tissue Substitute** **N Tissue Expander** **Y Other Device**	**Z No Qualifier**

Non-OR ØHPPX[Ø,7,J,K,Y]Z
Non-OR ØHP[Q,R]X[Ø,7,J,K]Z
Non-OR ØHPSX[7,J,K]Z
Non-OR ØHP[T,U]Ø[Ø,1,7,K]Z
Non-OR ØHP[T,U]3[Ø,1,7,K,Y]Z
Non-OR ØHP[T,U][7,8][Ø,1,7,J,K,N,Y]Z

Ø Medical and Surgical
H Skin and Breast
Q Repair Definition: Restoring, to the extent possible, a body part to its normal anatomic structure and function
Explanation: Used only when the method to accomplish the repair is not one of the other root operations

Body Part Character 4	Approach Character 5	Device Character 6	Qualifier Character 7
Ø Skin, Scalp **1 Skin, Face** **2 Skin, Right Ear** **3 Skin, Left Ear** **4 Skin, Neck** **5 Skin, Chest** Breast procedures, skin only **6 Skin, Back** **7 Skin, Abdomen** **8 Skin, Buttock** **9 Skin, Perineum** **A Skin, Inguinal** **B Skin, Right Upper Arm** **C Skin, Left Upper Arm** **D Skin, Right Lower Arm** **E Skin, Left Lower Arm** **F Skin, Right Hand** **G Skin, Left Hand** **H Skin, Right Upper Leg** **J Skin, Left Upper Leg** **K Skin, Right Lower Leg** **L Skin, Left Lower Leg** **M Skin, Right Foot** **N Skin, Left Foot** **Q Finger Nail** Nail bed Nail plate **R Toe Nail** *See Q Finger Nail*	**X External**	**Z No Device**	**Z No Qualifier**
T Breast, Right Mammary duct Mammary gland **U Breast, Left** *See T Breast, Right* **V Breast, Bilateral** *See T Breast, Right* **Y Supernumerary Breast**	**Ø Open** **3 Percutaneous** **7 Via Natural or Artificial Opening** **8 Via Natural or Artificial Opening Endoscopic**	**Z No Device**	**Z No Qualifier**
W Nipple, Right Areola **X Nipple, Left** *See W Nipple, Right*	**Ø Open** **3 Percutaneous** **7 Via Natural or Artificial Opening** **8 Via Natural or Artificial Opening Endoscopic** **X External**	**Z No Device**	**Z No Qualifier**

DRG Non-OR ØHQ9XZZ
Non-OR ØHQ[Ø,1,2,3,4,5,6,7,8,A,B,C,D,E,F,G,H,J,K,L,M,N]XZZ

Ø Medical and Surgical
H Skin and Breast
R Replacement Definition: Putting in or on biological or synthetic material that physically takes the place and/or function of all or a portion of a body part

Explanation: The body part may have been taken out or replaced, or may be taken out, physically eradicated, or rendered nonfunctional during the REPLACEMENT procedure. A REMOVAL procedure is coded for taking out the device used in a previous replacement procedure.

Body Part Character 4	Approach Character 5	Device Character 6	Qualifier Character 7
Ø Skin, Scalp **1 Skin, Face** **2 Skin, Right Ear** **3 Skin, Left Ear** **4 Skin, Neck** **5 Skin, Chest** Breast procedures, skin only **6 Skin, Back** **7 Skin, Abdomen** **8 Skin, Buttock** **9 Skin, Perineum** **A Skin, Inguinal** **B Skin, Right Upper Arm** **C Skin, Left Upper Arm** **D Skin, Right Lower Arm** **E Skin, Left Lower Arm** **F Skin, Right Hand** **G Skin, Left Hand** **H Skin, Right Upper Leg** **J Skin, Left Upper Leg** **K Skin, Right Lower Leg** **L Skin, Left Lower Leg** **M Skin, Right Foot** **N Skin, Left Foot**	**X External**	**7 Autologous Tissue Substitute**	**2 Cell Suspension Technique** **3 Full Thickness** **4 Partial Thickness**
Ø Skin, Scalp **1 Skin, Face** **2 Skin, Right Ear** **3 Skin, Left Ear** **4 Skin, Neck** **5 Skin, Chest** Breast procedures, skin only **6 Skin, Back** **7 Skin, Abdomen** **8 Skin, Buttock** **9 Skin, Perineum** **A Skin, Inguinal** **B Skin, Right Upper Arm** **C Skin, Left Upper Arm** **D Skin, Right Lower Arm** **E Skin, Left Lower Arm** **F Skin, Right Hand** **G Skin, Left Hand** **H Skin, Right Upper Leg** **J Skin, Left Upper Leg** **K Skin, Right Lower Leg** **L Skin, Left Lower Leg** **M Skin, Right Foot** **N Skin, Left Foot**	**X External**	**J Synthetic Substitute**	**3 Full Thickness** **4 Partial Thickness** **Z No Qualifier**
Ø Skin, Scalp **1 Skin, Face** **2 Skin, Right Ear** **3 Skin, Left Ear** **4 Skin, Neck** **5 Skin, Chest** Breast procedures, skin only **6 Skin, Back** **7 Skin, Abdomen** **8 Skin Buttock** **9 Skin, Perineum** **A Skin, Inguinal** **B Skin, Right Upper Arm** **C Skin, Left Upper Arm** **D Skin, Right Lower Arm** **E Skin, Left Lower Arm** **F Skin, Right Hand** **G Skin, Left Hand** **H Skin, Right Upper Leg** **J Skin, Left Upper Leg** **K Skin, Right Lower Leg** **L Skin, Left Lower Leg** **M Skin, Right Foot** **N Skin, Left Foot**	**X External**	**K Nonautologous Tissue Substitute**	**3 Full Thickness** **4 Partial Thickness**
Q Finger Nail Nail bed Nail plate **R Toe Nail** *See Q Finger Nail* **S Hair**	**X External**	**7 Autologous Tissue Substitute** **J Synthetic Substitute** **K Nonautologous Tissue Substitute**	**Z No Qualifier**
T Breast, Right Mammary duct Mammary gland **U Breast, Left** *See T Breast, Right* **V Breast, Bilateral** *See T Breast, Right*	**Ø Open**	**7 Autologous Tissue Substitute**	**5 Latissimus Dorsi Myocutaneous Flap** **6 Transverse Rectus Abdominis Myocutaneous Flap** **7 Deep Inferior Epigastric Artery Perforator Flap** **8 Superficial Inferior Epigastric Artery Flap** **9 Gluteal Artery Perforator Flap** **Z No Qualifier**
T Breast, Right Mammary duct Mammary gland **U Breast, Left** *See T Breast, Right* **V Breast, Bilateral** *See T Breast, Right*	**Ø Open**	**J Synthetic Substitute** **K Nonautologous Tissue Substitute**	**Z No Qualifier**
T Breast, Right ⊞ Mammary duct Mammary gland **U Breast, Left** ⊞ *See T Breast, Right* **V Breast, Bilateral** ⊞ *See T Breast, Right*	**3 Percutaneous**	**7 Autologous Tissue Substitute** **J Synthetic Substitute** **K Nonautologous Tissue Substitute**	**Z No Qualifier**
W Nipple, Right Areola **X Nipple, Left** *See W Nipple, Right*	**Ø Open** **3 Percutaneous** **X External**	**7 Autologous Tissue Substitute** **J Synthetic Substitute** **K Nonautologous Tissue Substitute**	**Z No Qualifier**

Non-OR ØHRSX7Z

See Appendix L for Procedure Combinations
⊞ ØHR[T,U,V]37Z

Ø Medical and Surgical
H Skin and Breast
S Reposition Definition: Moving to its normal location, or other suitable location, all or a portion of a body part

Explanation: The body part is moved to a new location from an abnormal location, or from a normal location where it is not functioning correctly. The body part may or may not be cut out or off to be moved to the new location.

Body Part Character 4	Approach Character 5	Device Character 6	Qualifier Character 7
S Hair **W** Nipple, Right Areola **X** Nipple, Left *See W Nipple, Right*	**X** External	**Z** No Device	**Z** No Qualifier
T Breast, Right Mammary duct Mammary gland **U** Breast, Left *See T Breast, Right* **V** Breast, Bilateral *See T Breast, Right*	**Ø** Open	**Z** No Device	**Z** No Qualifier

Non-OR ØHSSXZZ

Ø Medical and Surgical
H Skin and Breast
T Resection Definition: Cutting out or off, without replacement, all of a body part

Explanation: None

Body Part Character 4	Approach Character 5	Device Character 6	Qualifier Character 7
Q Finger Nail Nail bed Nail plate **R** Toe Nail *See Q Finger Nail* **W** Nipple, Right Areola **X** Nipple, Left *See W Nipple, Right*	**X** External	**Z** No Device	**Z** No Qualifier
T Breast, Right ⊞ Mammary duct Mammary gland **U** Breast, Left ⊞ *See T Breast, Right* **V** Breast, Bilateral ⊞ *See T Breast, Right* **Y** Supernumerary Breast	**Ø** Open	**Z** No Device	**Z** No Qualifier

Non-OR ØHT[Q,R]XZZ

See Appendix L for Procedure Combinations
⊞ ØHT[T,U,V]ØZZ

Ø Medical and Surgical
H Skin and Breast
U Supplement Definition: Putting in or on biological or synthetic material that physically reinforces and/or augments the function of a portion of a body part

Explanation: The biological material is non-living, or is living and from the same individual. The body part may have been previously replaced, and the SUPPLEMENT procedure is performed to physically reinforce and/or augment the function of the replaced body part.

Body Part Character 4	Approach Character 5	Device Character 6	Qualifier Character 7
T Breast, Right Mammary duct Mammary gland **U** Breast, Left *See T Breast, Right* **V** Breast, Bilateral *See T Breast, Right*	**Ø** Open **3** Percutaneous **7** Via Natural or Artificial Opening **8** Via Natural or Artificial Opening Endoscopic	**7** Autologous Tissue Substitute **J** Synthetic Substitute **K** Nonautologous Tissue Substitute	**Z** No Qualifier
W Nipple, Right Areola **X** Nipple, Left *See W Nipple, Right*	**Ø** Open **3** Percutaneous **7** Via Natural or Artificial Opening **8** Via Natural or Artificial Opening Endoscopic **X** External	**7** Autologous Tissue Substitute **J** Synthetic Substitute **K** Nonautologous Tissue Substitute	**Z** No Qualifier

Non-OR ØHU[T,U,V]3JZ

Ø Medical and Surgical
H Skin and Breast
W Revision Definition: Correcting, to the extent possible, a portion of a malfunctioning device or the position of a displaced device

Explanation: Revision can include correcting a malfunctioning or displaced device by taking out or putting in components of the device such as a screw or pin

Body Part Character 4	Approach Character 5	Device Character 6	Qualifier Character 7
P Skin Dermis Epidermis Sebaceous gland Sweat gland	X External	Ø Drainage Device 7 Autologous Tissue Substitute J Synthetic Substitute K Nonautologous Tissue Substitute Y Other Device	Z No Qualifier
Q Finger Nail Nail bed Nail plate R Toe Nail *See Q Finger Nail*	X External	Ø Drainage Device 7 Autologous Tissue Substitute J Synthetic Substitute K Nonautologous Tissue Substitute	Z No Qualifier
S Hair	X External	7 Autologous Tissue Substitute J Synthetic Substitute K Nonautologous Tissue Substitute	Z No Qualifier
T Breast, Right Mammary duct Mammary gland U Breast, Left *See T Breast, Right*	Ø Open 3 Percutaneous 7 Via Natural or Artificial Opening 8 Via Natural or Artificial Opening Endoscopic	Ø Drainage Device 7 Autologous Tissue Substitute J Synthetic Substitute K Nonautologous Tissue Substitute N Tissue Expander Y Other Device	Z No Qualifier

Non-OR ØHWPX[Ø,7,J,K,Y]Z
Non-OR ØHW[Q,R]X[Ø,7,J,K]Z
Non-OR ØHWSX[7,J,K]Z
Non-OR ØHW[T,U]Ø[Ø,7,K,N]Z
Non-OR ØHW[T,U]3[Ø,7,K,N,Y]Z
Non-OR ØHW[T,U][7,8][Ø,7,J,K,N,Y]Z

Ø Medical and Surgical
H Skin and Breast
X Transfer Definition: Moving, without taking out, all or a portion of a body part to another location to take over the function of all or a portion of a body part

Explanation: The body part transferred remains connected to its vascular and nervous supply

Body Part Character 4	Approach Character 5	Device Character 6	Qualifier Character 7
Ø Skin, Scalp 1 Skin, Face 2 Skin, Right Ear 3 Skin, Left Ear 4 Skin, Neck 5 Skin, Chest Breast procedures, skin only 6 Skin, Back 7 Skin, Abdomen 8 Skin, Buttock 9 Skin, Perineum A Skin, Inguinal B Skin, Right Upper Arm C Skin, Left Upper Arm D Skin, Right Lower Arm E Skin, Left Lower Arm F Skin, Right Hand G Skin, Left Hand H Skin, Right Upper Leg J Skin, Left Upper Leg K Skin, Right Lower Leg L Skin, Left Lower Leg M Skin, Right Foot N Skin, Left Foot	X External	Z No Device	Z No Qualifier

Subcutaneous Tissue and Fascia ØJØ–ØJX

Character Meanings

This Character Meaning table is provided as a guide to assist the user in the identification of character members that may be found in this section of code tables. It **SHOULD NOT** be used to build a PCS code.

Operation–Character 3	Body Part–Character 4	Approach–Character 5	Device–Character 6	Qualifier–Character 7
Ø Alteration	Ø Subcutaneous Tissue and Fascia, Scalp	Ø Open	Ø Drainage Device OR Monitoring Device, Hemodynamic	B Skin and Subcutaneous Tissue
2 Change	1 Subcutaneous Tissue and Fascia, Face	3 Percutaneous	1 Radioactive Element	C Skin, Subcutaneous Tissue and Fascia
5 Destruction	4 Subcutaneous Tissue and Fascia, Right Neck	X External	2 Monitoring Device	X Diagnostic
8 Division	5 Subcutaneous Tissue and Fascia, Left Neck		3 Infusion Device	Z No Qualifier
9 Drainage	6 Subcutaneous Tissue and Fascia, Chest		4 Pacemaker, Single Chamber	
B Excision	7 Subcutaneous Tissue and Fascia, Back		5 Pacemaker, Single Chamber Rate Responsive	
C Extirpation	8 Subcutaneous Tissue and Fascia, Abdomen		6 Pacemaker, Dual Chamber	
D Extraction	9 Subcutaneous Tissue and Fascia, Buttock		7 Autologous Tissue Substitute OR Cardiac Resynchronization Pacemaker Pulse Generator	
H Insertion	B Subcutaneous Tissue and Fascia, Perineum		8 Defibrillator Generator	
J Inspection	C Subcutaneous Tissue and Fascia, Pelvic Region		9 Cardiac Resynchronization Defibrillator Pulse Generator	
N Release	D Subcutaneous Tissue and Fascia, Right Upper Arm		A Contractility Modulation Device	
P Removal	F Subcutaneous Tissue and Fascia, Left Upper Arm		B Stimulator Generator, Single Array	
Q Repair	G Subcutaneous Tissue and Fascia, Right Lower Arm		C Stimulator Generator, Single Array Rechargeable	
R Replacement	H Subcutaneous Tissue and Fascia, Left Lower Arm		D Stimulator Generator, Multiple Array	
U Supplement	J Subcutaneous Tissue and Fascia, Right Hand		E Stimulator Generator, Multiple Array Rechargeable	
W Revision	K Subcutaneous Tissue and Fascia, Left Hand		F Subcutaneous Defibrillator Lead	
X Transfer	L Subcutaneous Tissue and Fascia, Right Upper Leg		H Contraceptive Device	
	M Subcutaneous Tissue and Fascia, Left Upper Leg		J Synthetic Substitute	
	N Subcutaneous Tissue and Fascia, Right Lower Leg		K Nonautologous Tissue Substitute	
	P Subcutaneous Tissue and Fascia, Left Lower Leg		M Stimulator Generator	
	Q Subcutaneous Tissue and Fascia, Right Foot		N Tissue Expander	
	R Subcutaneous Tissue and Fascia, Left Foot		P Cardiac Rhythm Related Device	
	S Subcutaneous Tissue and Fascia, Head and Neck		V Infusion Device, Pump	
	T Subcutaneous Tissue and Fascia, Trunk		W Vascular Access Device, Totally Implantable	
	V Subcutaneous Tissue and Fascia, Upper Extremity		X Vascular Access Device, Tunneled	
	W Subcutaneous Tissue and Fascia, Lower Extremity		Y Other Device	
			Z No Device	

AHA Coding Clinic for table ØJ2
2018, 3Q, 10 Disruption of perma-catheter fibrin sheath via angioplasty of superior vena cava
2017, 2Q, 26 Exchange of tunneled catheter

AHA Coding Clinic for table ØJ5
2019, 3Q, 25 Endoscopic removal of pilonidal sinus and cyst

AHA Coding Clinic for table ØJ8
2017, 3Q, 11 Bilateral escharotomy of leg, thigh and foot

AHA Coding Clinic for table ØJ9
2018, 3Q, 16 Incision and drainage of submandibular space
2018, 3Q, 16 Incision and drainage of neck abscess
2015, 3Q, 23 Incision and drainage of multiple abscess cavities using vessel loop

AHA Coding Clinic for table ØJB
2020, 1Q, 31 Repair of buried penis
2019, 3Q, 25 Endoscopic removal of pilonidal sinus and cyst
2018, 3Q, 17 Excisional debridement of periosteum
2018, 1Q, 7 Placement of fat graft following lumbar decompression surgery
2015, 3Q, 3-8 Excisional and nonexcisional debridement
2015, 2Q, 13 Transfer of free flap to reconstruct orbital defect
2015, 1Q, 29 Fistulectomy with placement of seton
2014, 4Q, 38 Abdominoplasty and abdominal wall plication for hernia repair
2014, 3Q, 22 Transsphenoidal removal of pituitary tumor and fat graft placement

AHA Coding Clinic for table ØJC
2017, 3Q, 22 Replacement of native skull bone flap

AHA Coding Clinic for table ØJD
2016, 3Q, 20 VersaJet™ nonexcisional debridement of leg muscle
2016, 3Q, 21 Nonexcisional debridement of infected lumbar wound
2016, 3Q, 21 Nonexcisional pulsed lavage debridement
2016, 3Q, 22 Debridement of bone and tendon using Tenex ultrasound device
2016, 1Q, 40 Nonexcisional debridement of skin and subcutaneous tissue
2015, 3Q, 3-8 Excisional and nonexcisional debridement
2015, 1Q, 23 Non-Excisional debridement with lavage of wound

AHA Coding Clinic for table ØJH
2020, 2Q, 15 Ommaya Reservoir with Ventricular Catheter Placement
2020, 2Q, 16 Ommaya Reservoir Placement for Cerebrospinal Fluid Infusion Therapy
2019, 4Q, 33 Subcutaneous implantable cardioverter defibrillator lead
2017, 4Q, 63-64 Added and revised device values - Vascular access reservoir
2017, 2Q, 24 Tunneled catheter versus totally implantable catheter
2017, 2Q, 26 Exchange of tunneled catheter
2016, 4Q, 97-98 Phrenic neurostimulator
2016, 2Q, 14 Insertion of peritoneal totally implantable venous access device
2016, 2Q, 15 Removal and replacement of tunneled internal jugular catheter
2015, 4Q, 14 New Section X codes—New Technology procedures
2015, 4Q, 30-31 Vascular access devices
2015, 2Q, 33 Totally implantable central venous access device (Port-a-Cath)
2014, 3Q, 19 End of life replacement of Baclofen pump
2013, 4Q, 116 Device character for Port-A-Cath placement
2012, 4Q, 104 Placement of subcutaneous implantable cardioverter defibrillator

AHA Coding Clinic for table ØJN
2017, 3Q, 11 Bilateral escharotomy of leg, thigh and foot

AHA Coding Clinic for table ØJP
2019, 4Q, 33 Subcutaneous implantable cardioverter defibrillator lead
2018, 4Q, 86 Placement of lumboatrial shunt
2018, 3Q, 29 Decommissioning of left ventricular assist device with exploration of mediastinum
2016, 2Q, 15 Removal and replacement of tunneled internal jugular catheter
2015, 4Q, 31 Vascular access devices
2014, 3Q, 19 End of life replacement of Baclofen pump
2013, 4Q, 109 Separating conjoined twins
2012, 4Q, 104 Placement of subcutaneous implantable cardioverter defibrillator

AHA Coding Clinic for table ØJQ
2017, 3Q, 19 Anterior repair of cystocele
2014, 4Q, 44 Posterior colporrhaphy/rectocele repair

AHA Coding Clinic for table ØJR
2015, 2Q, 13 Transfer of free flap to reconstruct orbital defect

AHA Coding Clinic for table ØJU
2018, 2Q, 20 Prelaminated free flap graft using Alloderm™
2018, 1Q, 7 Placement of fat graft following lumbar decompression surgery

AHA Coding Clinic for table ØJW
2019, 4Q, 33 Subcutaneous implantable cardioverter defibrillator lead
2018, 1Q, 8 Ventricular peritoneal shunt ligation
2015, 4Q, 33 Externalization of peritoneal dialysis catheter
2015, 2Q, 9 Revision of ventriculoperitoneal (VP) shunt
2012, 4Q, 104 Placement of subcutaneous implantable cardioverter defibrillator

AHA Coding Clinic for table ØJX
2018, 1Q, 10 Complex wound closure using pericranial flap
2014, 3Q, 18 Placement of reverse sural fasciocutaneous pedicle flap
2013, 4Q, 109 Separating conjoined twins

Ø Medical and Surgical
J Subcutaneous Tissue and Fascia
Ø Alteration Definition: Modifying the anatomic structure of a body part without affecting the function of the body part

Explanation: Principal purpose is to improve appearance

Body Part Character 4		Approach Character 5	Device Character 6	Qualifier Character 7
1 Subcutaneous Tissue and Fascia, Face Masseteric fascia Orbital fascia Submandibular space **4 Subcutaneous Tissue and Fascia, Right Neck** Deep cervical fascia Pretracheal fascia Prevertebral fascia **5 Subcutaneous Tissue and Fascia, Left Neck** ***See*** *4 Subcutaneous Tissue and Fascia, Right Neck* **6 Subcutaneous Tissue and Fascia, Chest** Pectoral fascia **7 Subcutaneous Tissue and Fascia, Back** **8 Subcutaneous Tissue and Fascia, Abdomen** **9 Subcutaneous Tissue and Fascia, Buttock** **D Subcutaneous Tissue and Fascia, Right Upper Arm** Axillary fascia Deltoid fascia Infraspinatus fascia Subscapular aponeurosis Supraspinatus fascia	**F Subcutaneous Tissue and Fascia, Left Upper Arm** ***See*** *D Subcutaneous Tissue and Fascia, Right Upper Arm* **G Subcutaneous Tissue and Fascia, Right Lower Arm** Antebrachial fascia Bicipital aponeurosis **H Subcutaneous Tissue and Fascia, Left Lower Arm** ***See*** *G Subcutaneous Tissue and Fascia, Right Lower Arm* **L Subcutaneous Tissue and Fascia, Right Upper Leg** Crural fascia Fascia lata Iliac fascia Iliotibial tract (band) **M Subcutaneous Tissue and Fascia, Left Upper Leg** ***See*** *L Subcutaneous Tissue and Fascia, Right Upper Leg* **N Subcutaneous Tissue and Fascia, Right Lower Leg** **P Subcutaneous Tissue and Fascia, Left Lower Leg**	**Ø Open** **3 Percutaneous**	**Z No Device**	**Z No Qualifier**

Ø Medical and Surgical
J Subcutaneous Tissue and Fascia
2 Change Definition: Taking out or off a device from a body part and putting back an identical or similar device in or on the same body part without cutting or puncturing the skin or a mucous membrane

Explanation: All CHANGE procedures are coded using the approach EXTERNAL

Body Part Character 4	Approach Character 5	Device Character 6	Qualifier Character 7
S Subcutaneous Tissue and Fascia, Head and Neck **T Subcutaneous Tissue and Fascia, Trunk** External oblique aponeurosis Transversalis fascia **V Subcutaneous Tissue and Fascia, Upper Extremity** **W Subcutaneous Tissue and Fascia, Lower Extremity**	**X External**	**Ø Drainage Device** **Y Other Device**	**Z No Qualifier**

Non-OR All body part, approach, device, and qualifier values

Ø Medical and Surgical
J Subcutaneous Tissue and Fascia
5 Destruction Definition: Physical eradication of all or a portion of a body part by the direct use of energy, force, or a destructive agent
Explanation: None of the body part is physically taken out

Body Part Character 4		Approach Character 5	Device Character 6	Qualifier Character 7
Ø Subcutaneous Tissue and Fascia, Scalp Galea aponeurotica 1 Subcutaneous Tissue and Fascia, Face Masseteric fascia Orbital fascia Submandibular space 4 Subcutaneous Tissue and Fascia, Right Neck Deep cervical fascia Pretracheal fascia Prevertebral fascia 5 Subcutaneous Tissue and Fascia, Left Neck *See 4 Subcutaneous Tissue and Fascia, Right Neck* 6 Subcutaneous Tissue and Fascia, Chest Pectoral fascia 7 Subcutaneous Tissue and Fascia, Back 8 Subcutaneous Tissue and Fascia, Abdomen 9 Subcutaneous Tissue and Fascia, Buttock B Subcutaneous Tissue and Fascia, Perineum C Subcutaneous Tissue and Fascia, Pelvic Region D Subcutaneous Tissue and Fascia, Right Upper Arm Axillary fascia Deltoid fascia Infraspinatus fascia Subscapular aponeurosis Supraspinatus fascia F Subcutaneous Tissue and Fascia, Left Upper Arm *See D Subcutaneous Tissue and Fascia, Right Upper Arm*	G Subcutaneous Tissue and Fascia, Right Lower Arm Antebrachial fascia Bicipital aponeurosis H Subcutaneous Tissue and Fascia, Left Lower Arm *See G Subcutaneous Tissue and Fascia, Right Lower Arm* J Subcutaneous Tissue and Fascia, Right Hand Palmar fascia (aponeurosis) K Subcutaneous Tissue and Fascia, Left Hand *See J Subcutaneous Tissue and Fascia, Right Hand* L Subcutaneous Tissue and Fascia, Right Upper Leg Crural fascia Fascia lata Iliac fascia Iliotibial tract (band) M Subcutaneous Tissue and Fascia, Left Upper Leg *See L Subcutaneous Tissue and Fascia, Right Upper Leg* N Subcutaneous Tissue and Fascia, Right Lower Leg P Subcutaneous Tissue and Fascia, Left Lower Leg Q Subcutaneous Tissue and Fascia, Right Foot Plantar fascia (aponeurosis) R Subcutaneous Tissue and Fascia, Left Foot *See Q Subcutaneous Tissue and Fascia, Right Foot*	Ø Open 3 Percutaneous	Z No Device	Z No Qualifier

DRG Non-OR All body part, approach, device, and qualifier values

Ø Medical and Surgical
J Subcutaneous Tissue and Fascia
8 Division Definition: Cutting into a body part, without draining fluids and/or gases from the body part, in order to separate or transect a body part

Explanation: All or a portion of the body part is separated into two or more portions

Body Part Character 4	Approach Character 5	Device Character 6	Qualifier Character 7
Ø Subcutaneous Tissue and Fascia, Scalp Galea aponeurotica **1 Subcutaneous Tissue and Fascia, Face** Masseteric fascia Orbital fascia Submandibular space **4 Subcutaneous Tissue and Fascia, Right Neck** Deep cervical fascia Pretracheal fascia Prevertebral fascia **5 Subcutaneous Tissue and Fascia, Left Neck** *See 4 Subcutaneous Tissue and Fascia, Right Neck* **6 Subcutaneous Tissue and Fascia, Chest** Pectoral fascia **7 Subcutaneous Tissue and Fascia, Back** **8 Subcutaneous Tissue and Fascia, Abdomen** **9 Subcutaneous Tissue and Fascia, Buttock** **B Subcutaneous Tissue and Fascia, Perineum** **C Subcutaneous Tissue and Fascia, Pelvic Region** **D Subcutaneous Tissue and Fascia, Right Upper Arm** Axillary fascia Deltoid fascia Infraspinatus fascia Subscapular aponeurosis Supraspinatus fascia **F Subcutaneous Tissue and Fascia, Left Upper Arm** *See D Subcutaneous Tissue and Fascia, Right Upper Arm* **G Subcutaneous Tissue and Fascia, Right Lower Arm** Antebrachial fascia Bicipital aponeurosis **H Subcutaneous Tissue and Fascia, Left Lower Arm** *See G Subcutaneous Tissue and Fascia, Right Lower Arm* **J Subcutaneous Tissue and Fascia, Right Hand** Palmar fascia (aponeurosis) **K Subcutaneous Tissue and Fascia, Left Hand** *See J Subcutaneous Tissue and Fascia, Right Hand* **L Subcutaneous Tissue and Fascia, Right Upper Leg** Crural fascia Fascia lata Iliac fascia Iliotibial tract (band) **M Subcutaneous Tissue and Fascia, Left Upper Leg** *See L Subcutaneous Tissue and Fascia, Right Upper Leg* **N Subcutaneous Tissue and Fascia, Right Lower Leg** **P Subcutaneous Tissue and Fascia, Left Lower Leg** **Q Subcutaneous Tissue and Fascia, Right Foot** Plantar fascia (aponeurosis) **R Subcutaneous Tissue and Fascia, Left Foot** *See Q Subcutaneous Tissue and Fascia, Right Foot* **S Subcutaneous Tissue and Fascia, Head and Neck** **T Subcutaneous Tissue and Fascia, Trunk** External oblique aponeurosis Transversalis fascia **V Subcutaneous Tissue and Fascia, Upper Extremity** **W Subcutaneous Tissue and Fascia, Lower Extremity**	**Ø Open** **3 Percutaneous**	**Z No Device**	**Z No Qualifier**

Ø Medical and Surgical
J Subcutaneous Tissue and Fascia
9 Drainage Definition: Taking or letting out fluids and/or gases from a body part
Explanation: The qualifier DIAGNOSTIC is used to identify drainage procedures that are biopsies

Body Part Character 4		Approach Character 5	Device Character 6	Qualifier Character 7
Ø Subcutaneous Tissue and Fascia, Scalp Galea aponeurotica **1 Subcutaneous Tissue and Fascia, Face** Masseteric fascia Orbital fascia Submandibular space **4 Subcutaneous Tissue and Fascia, Right Neck** Deep cervical fascia Pretracheal fascia Prevertebral fascia **5 Subcutaneous Tissue and Fascia, Left Neck** *See 4 Subcutaneous Tissue and Fascia, Right Neck* **6 Subcutaneous Tissue and Fascia, Chest** Pectoral fascia **7 Subcutaneous Tissue and Fascia, Back** **8 Subcutaneous Tissue and Fascia, Abdomen** **9 Subcutaneous Tissue and Fascia, Buttock** **B Subcutaneous Tissue and Fascia, Perineum** **C Subcutaneous Tissue and Fascia, Pelvic Region** **D Subcutaneous Tissue and Fascia, Right Upper Arm** Axillary fascia Deltoid fascia Infraspinatus fascia Subscapular aponeurosis Supraspinatus fascia **F Subcutaneous Tissue and Fascia, Left Upper Arm** *See D Subcutaneous Tissue and Fascia, Right Upper Arm*	**G Subcutaneous Tissue and Fascia, Right Lower Arm** Antebrachial fascia Bicipital aponeurosis **H Subcutaneous Tissue and Fascia, Left Lower Arm** *See G Subcutaneous Tissue and Fascia, Right Lower Arm* **J Subcutaneous Tissue and Fascia, Right Hand** Palmar fascia (aponeurosis) **K Subcutaneous Tissue and Fascia, Left Hand** *See J Subcutaneous Tissue and Fascia, Right Hand* **L Subcutaneous Tissue and Fascia, Right Upper Leg** Crural fascia Fascia lata Iliac fascia Iliotibial tract (band) **M Subcutaneous Tissue and Fascia, Left Upper Leg** *See L Subcutaneous Tissue and Fascia, Right Upper Leg* **N Subcutaneous Tissue and Fascia, Right Lower Leg** **P Subcutaneous Tissue and Fascia, Left Lower Leg** **Q Subcutaneous Tissue and Fascia, Right Foot** Plantar fascia (aponeurosis) **R Subcutaneous Tissue and Fascia, Left Foot** *See Q Subcutaneous Tissue and Fascia, Right Foot*	**Ø Open** **3 Percutaneous**	**Ø Drainage Device**	**Z No Qualifier**

Non-OR ØJ9[Ø,1,4,5,6,7,8,9,B,C,D,F,G,H,J,K,L,M,N,P,Q,R][Ø,3]ØZ

ØJ9 Continued on next page

ØJ9 Continued

Ø Medical and Surgical
J Subcutaneous Tissue and Fascia
9 Drainage Definition: Taking or letting out fluids and/or gases from a body part
Explanation: The qualifier DIAGNOSTIC is used to identify drainage procedures that are biopsies

Body Part Character 4		Approach Character 5	Device Character 6	Qualifier Character 7
Ø Subcutaneous Tissue and Fascia, Scalp Galea aponeurotica **1 Subcutaneous Tissue and Fascia, Face** Masseteric fascia Orbital fascia Submandibular space **4 Subcutaneous Tissue and Fascia, Right Neck** Deep cervical fascia Pretracheal fascia Prevertebral fascia **5 Subcutaneous Tissue and Fascia, Left Neck** **See** *4 Subcutaneous Tissue and Fascia, Right Neck* **6 Subcutaneous Tissue and Fascia, Chest** Pectoral fascia **7 Subcutaneous Tissue and Fascia, Back** **8 Subcutaneous Tissue and Fascia, Abdomen** **9 Subcutaneous Tissue and Fascia, Buttock** **B Subcutaneous Tissue and Fascia, Perineum** **C Subcutaneous Tissue and Fascia, Pelvic Region** **D Subcutaneous Tissue and Fascia, Right Upper Arm** Axillary fascia Deltoid fascia Infraspinatus fascia Subscapular aponeurosis Supraspinatus fascia **F Subcutaneous Tissue and Fascia, Left Upper Arm** **See** *D Subcutaneous Tissue and Fascia, Right Upper Arm*	**G Subcutaneous Tissue and Fascia, Right Lower Arm** Antebrachial fascia Bicipital aponeurosis **H Subcutaneous Tissue and Fascia, Left Lower Arm** **See** *G Subcutaneous Tissue and Fascia, Right Lower Arm* **J Subcutaneous Tissue and Fascia, Right Hand** Palmar fascia (aponeurosis) **K Subcutaenous Tissue and Fascia, Left Hand** **See** *J Subcutaneous Tissue and Fascia, Right Hand* **L Subcutaneous Tissue and Fascia, Right Upper Leg** Crural fascia Fascia lata Iliac fascia Iliotibial tract (band) **M Subcutaneous Tissue and Fascia, Left Upper Leg** **See** *L Subcutaneous Tissue and Fascia, Right Upper Leg* **N Subcutaneous TIssue and Fascia, Right Lower Leg** **P Subcutaneous Tissue and Fascia, Left Lower Leg** **Q Subcutaneous Tissue and Fascia, Right Foot** Plantar fascia (aponeurosis) **R Subcutaneous Tissue and Fascia, Left Foot** **See** *Q Subcutaneous Tissue and Fascia, Right Foot*	**Ø Open** **3 Percutaneous**	**Z No Device**	**X Diagnostic** **Z No Qualifier**

Non-OR ØJ9[Ø,1,4,5,6,7,8,9,B,C,D,F,G,H,J,K,L,M,N,P,Q,R][Ø,3]ZX
Non-OR ØJ9[Ø,1,4,5,6,7,8,9,B,C,D,F,G,H,J,K,L,M,N,P,Q,R]3ZZ

Ø Medical and Surgical
J Subcutaneous Tissue and Fascia
B Excision Definition: Cutting out or off, without replacement, a portion of a body part
Explanation: The qualifier DIAGNOSTIC is used to identify excision procedures that are biopsies

Body Part Character 4		Approach Character 5	Device Character 6	Qualifier Character 7
Ø Subcutaneous Tissue and Fascia, Scalp Galea aponeurotica **1 Subcutaneous Tissue and Fascia, Face** Masseteric fascia Orbital fascia Submandibular space **4 Subcutaneous Tissue and Fascia, Right Neck** Deep cervical fascia Pretracheal fascia Prevertebral fascia **5 Subcutaneous Tissue and Fascia, Left Neck** ***See*** *4 Subcutaneous Tissue and Fascia, Right Neck* **6 Subcutaneous Tissue and Fascia, Chest** Pectoral fascia **7 Subcutaneous Tissue and Fascia, Back** **8 Subcutaneous Tissue and Fascia, Abdomen** **9 Subcutaneous Tissue and Fascia, Buttock** **B Subcutaneous Tissue and Fascia, Perineum** **C Subcutaneous Tissue and Fascia, Pelvic Region** **D Subcutaneous Tissue and Fascia, Right Upper Arm** Axillary fascia Deltoid fascia Infraspinatus fascia Subscapular aponeurosis Supraspinatus fascia **F Subcutaneous Tissue and Fascia, Left Upper Arm** ***See*** *D Subcutaneous Tissue and Fascia, Right Upper Arm*	**G Subcutaneous Tissue and Fascia, Right Lower Arm** Antebrachial fascia Bicipital aponeurosis **H Subcutaneous Tissue and Fascia, Left Lower Arm** ***See*** *G Subcutaneous Tissue and Fascia, Right Lower Arm* **J Subcutaneous Tissue and Fascia, Right Hand** Palmar fascia (aponeurosis) **K Subcutaneous Tissue and Fascia, Left Hand** ***See*** *J Subcutaneous Tissue and Fascia, Right Hand* **L Subcutaneous Tissue and Fascia, Right Upper Leg** Crural fascia Fascia lata Iliac fascia Iliotibial tract (band) **M Subcutaneous Tissue and Fascia, Left Upper Leg** ***See*** *L Subcutaneous Tissue and Fascia, Right Upper Leg* **N Subcutaneous Tissue and Fascia, Right Lower Leg** **P Subcutaneous Tissue and Fascia, Left Lower Leg** **Q Subcutaneous Tissue and Fascia, Right Foot** Plantar fascia (aponeurosis) **R Subcutaneous Tissue and Fascia, Left Foot** ***See*** *Q Subcutaneous Tissue and Fascia, Right Foot*	**Ø Open** **3 Percutaneous**	**Z No Device**	**X Diagnostic** **Z No Qualifier**

DRG Non-OR ØJB[Ø,4,5,6,7,8,9,B,C,D,F,G,H,L,M,N,P,Q,R]3ZZ
Non-OR ØJB[Ø,1,4,5,6,7,8,9,B,C,D,F,G,H,J,K,L,M,N,P,Q,R][Ø,3]ZX

Ø Medical and Surgical
J Subcutaneous Tissue and Fascia
C Extirpation Definition: Taking or cutting out solid matter from a body part

Explanation: The solid matter may be an abnormal byproduct of a biological function or a foreign body; it may be imbedded in a body part or in the lumen of a tubular body part. The solid matter may or may not have been previously broken into pieces.

Body Part Character 4	Approach Character 5	Device Character 6	Qualifier Character 7
Ø Subcutaneous Tissue and Fascia, Scalp Galea aponeurotica **1 Subcutaneous Tissue and Fascia, Face** Masseteric fascia Orbital fascia Submandibular space **4 Subcutaneous Tissue and Fascia, Right Neck** Deep cervical fascia Pretracheal fascia Prevertebral fascia **5 Subcutaneous Tissue and Fascia, Left Neck** ***See*** *4 Subcutaneous Tissue and Fascia, Right Neck* **6 Subcutaneous Tissue and Fascia, Chest** Pectoral fascia **7 Subcutaneous Tissue and Fascia, Back** **8 Subcutaneous Tissue and Fascia, Abdomen** **9 Subcutaneous Tissue and Fascia, Buttock** **B Subcutaneous Tissue and Fascia, Perineum** **C Subcutaneous Tissue and Fascia, Pelvic Region** **D Subcutaneous Tissue and Fascia, Right Upper Arm** Axillary fascia Deltoid fascia Infraspinatus fascia Subscapular aponeurosis Supraspinatus fascia **F Subcutaneous Tissue and Fascia, Left Upper Arm** ***See*** *D Subcutaneous Tissue and Fascia, Right Upper Arm* **G Subcutaneous Tissue and Fascia, Right Lower Arm** Antebrachial fascia Bicipital aponeurosis **H Subcutaneous Tissue and Fascia, Left Lower Arm** ***See*** *G Subcutaneous Tissue and Fascia, Right Lower Arm* **J Subcutaneous Tissue and Fascia, Right Hand** Palmar fascia (aponeurosis) **K Subcutaneous Tissue and Fascia, Left Hand** ***See*** *J Subcutaneous Tissue and Fascia, Right Hand* **L Subcutaneous Tissue and Fascia, Right Upper Leg** Crural fascia Fascia lata Iliac fascia Iliotibial tract (band) **M Subcutaneous Tissue and Fascia, Left Upper Leg** ***See*** *L Subcutaneous Tissue and Fascia, Right Upper Leg* **N Subcutaneous Tissue and Fascia, Right Lower Leg** **P Subcutaneous Tissue and Fascia, Left Lower Leg** **Q Subcutaneous Tissue and Fascia, Right Foot** Plantar fascia (aponeurosis) **R Subcutaneous Tissue and Fascia, Left Foot** ***See*** *Q Subcutaneous Tissue and Fascia, Right Foot*	**Ø** Open **3** Percutaneous	**Z** No Device	**Z** No Qualifier

Non-OR All body part, approach, device, and qualifier values

Ø Medical and Surgical
J Subcutaneous Tissue and Fascia
D Extraction Definition: Pulling or stripping out or off all or a portion of a body part by the use of force
Explanation: The qualifier DIAGNOSTIC is used to identify extraction procedures that are biopsies

Body Part Character 4	Body Part Character 4 (cont.)	Approach Character 5	Device Character 6	Qualifier Character 7
Ø Subcutaneous Tissue and Fascia, Scalp Galea aponeurotica **1 Subcutaneous Tissue and Fascia, Face** Masseteric fascia Orbital fascia Submandibular space **4 Subcutaneous Tissue and Fascia, Right Neck** Deep cervical fascia Pretracheal fascia Prevertebral fascia **5 Subcutaneous Tissue and Fascia, Left Neck** ***See*** *4 Subcutaneous Tissue and Fascia, Right Neck* **6 Subcutaneous Tissue and Fascia, Chest** Pectoral fascia **7 Subcutaneous Tissue and Fascia, Back** **8 Subcutaneous Tissue and Fascia, Abdomen** **9 Subcutaneous Tissue and Fascia, Buttock** **B Subcutaneous Tissue and Fascia, Perineum** **C Subcutaneous Tissue and Fascia, Pelvic Region** **D Subcutaneous Tissue and Fascia, Right Upper Arm** Axillary fascia Deltoid fascia Infraspinatus fascia Subscapular aponeurosis Supraspinatus fascia **F Subcutaneous Tissue and Fascia, Left Upper Arm** ***See*** *D Subcutaneous Tissue and Fascia, Right Upper Arm*	**G Subcutaneous Tissue and Fascia, Right Lower Arm** Antebrachial fascia Bicipital aponeurosis **H Subcutaneous Tissue and Fascia, Left Lower Arm** ***See*** *G Subcutaneous Tissue and Fascia, Right Lower Arm* **J Subcutaneous Tissue and Fascia, Right Hand** Palmar fascia (aponeurosis) **K Subcutaneous Tissue and Fascia, Left Hand** ***See*** *J Subcutaneous Tissue and Fascia, Right Hand* **L Subcutaneous Tissue and Fascia, Right Upper Leg** Crural fascia Fascia lata Iliac fascia Iliotibial tract (band) **M Subcutaneous Tissue and Fascia, Left Upper Leg** ***See*** *L Subcutaneous Tissue and Fascia, Right Upper Leg* **N Subcutaneous Tissue and Fascia, Right Lower Leg** **P Subcutaneous Tissue and Fascia, Left Lower Leg** **Q Subcutaneous Tissue and Fascia, Right Foot** Plantar fascia (aponeurosis) **R Subcutaneous Tissue and Fascia, Left Foot** ***See*** *Q Subcutaneous Tissue and Fascia, Right Foot*	**Ø Open** **3 Percutaneous**	**Z No Device**	**Z No Qualifier**

Non-OR ØJD[Ø,1,4,5,B,C,D,F,G,H,J,K,N,P,Q,R]3ZZ

See Appendix L for Procedure Combinations
Combo-only ØJD[6,7,8,9,L,M]3ZZ

Ø Medical and Surgical
J Subcutaneous Tissue and Fascia
H Insertion Definition: Putting in a nonbiological appliance that monitors, assists, performs, or prevents a physiological function but does not physically take the place of a body part

Explanation: None

Body Part Character 4		Approach Character 5	Device Character 6	Qualifier Character 7
Ø Subcutaneous Tissue and Fascia, Scalp Galea aponeurotica **1 Subcutaneous Tissue and Fascia, Face** Masseteric fascia, Orbital fascia, Submandibular space **4 Subcutaneous Tissue and Fascia, Right Neck** Deep cervical fascia, Pretracheal fascia, Prevertebral fascia **5 Subcutaneous Tissue and Fascia, Left Neck** *See 4 Subcutaneous Tissue and Fascia, Right Neck* **9 Subcutaneous Tissue and Fascia, Buttock** **B Subcutaneous Tissue and Fascia, Perineum**	**C Subcutaneous Tissue and Fascia, Pelvic Region** **J Subcutaneous Tissue and Fascia, Right Hand** Palmar fascia (aponeurosis) **K Subcutaneous Tissue and Fascia, Left Hand** *See J Subcutaneous Tissue and Fascia, Right Hand* **Q Subcutaneous Tissue and Fascia, Right Foot** Plantar fascia (aponeurosis) **R Subcutaneous Tissue and Fascia, Left Foot** *See Q Subcutaneous Tissue and Fascia, Right Foot*	Ø Open 3 Percutaneous	N Tissue Expander	Z No Qualifier
6 Subcutaneous Tissue and Fascia, Chest ⊞ Pectoral fascia		Ø Open 3 Percutaneous	Ø Monitoring Device, Hemodynamic 2 Monitoring Device 4 Pacemaker, Single Chamber 5 Pacemaker, Single Chamber Rate Responsive 6 Pacemaker, Dual Chamber 7 Cardiac Resynchronization Pacemaker Pulse Generator 8 Defibrillator Generator 9 Cardiac Resynchronization Defibrillator Pulse Generator A Contractility Modulation Device B Stimulator Generator, Single Array C Stimulator Generator, Single Array Rechargeable D Stimulator Generator, Multiple Array E Stimulator Generator, Multiple Array Rechargeable F Subcutaneous Defibrillator Lead H Contraceptive Device M Stimulator Generator N Tissue Expander P Cardiac Rhythm Related Device V Infusion Device, Pump W Vascular Access Device, Totally Implantable X Vascular Access Device, Tunneled Y Other Device	Z No Qualifier
7 Subcutaneous Tissue and Fascia, Back NC ⊞		Ø Open 3 Percutaneous	B Stimulator Generator, Single Array C Stimulator Generator, Single Array Rechargeable D Stimulator Generator, Multiple Array E Stimulator Generator, Multiple Array Rechargeable M Stimulator Generator N Tissue Expander V Infusion Device, Pump Y Other Device	Z No Qualifier

DRG Non-OR ØJH6[Ø,3][4,5,6,7,H,P,X]Z
DRG Non-OR ØJH63WX
HAC ØJH6[Ø,3][4,5,6,7,8,9,P]Z when reported with SDx K68.11 or T81.4Ø-T81.49, T82.6-T82.7 with 7th character A
HAC ØJH63XZ when reported with SDx J95.811
NC ØJH7[Ø,3]MZ

See Appendix L for Procedure Combinations
⊞ ØJH6[Ø,3][4,5,6,7,8,9,A,B,C,D,E,F,P]Z
⊞ ØJH7[Ø,3][B,C,D,E]Z

ØJH Continued on next page

Subcutaneous Tissue and Fascia

Ø Medical and Surgical
J Subcutaneous Tissue and Fascia
H Insertion Definition: Putting in a nonbiological appliance that monitors, assists, performs, or prevents a physiological function but does not physically take the place of a body part
Explanation: None

ØJH Continued

Body Part Character 4	Approach Character 5	Device Character 6	Qualifier Character 7
8 Subcutaneous Tissue and Fascia, Abdomen NC ⊞	Ø Open 3 Percutaneous	Ø Monitoring Device, Hemodynamic 2 Monitoring Device 4 Pacemaker, Single Chamber 5 Pacemaker, Single Chamber Rate Responsive 6 Pacemaker, Dual Chamber 7 Cardiac Resynchronization Pacemaker Pulse Generator 8 Defibrillator Generator 9 Cardiac Resynchronization Defibrillator Pulse Generator A Contractility Modulation Device B Stimulator Generator, Single Array C Stimulator Generator, Single Array Rechargeable D Stimulator Generator, Multiple Array E Stimulator Generator, Multiple Array Rechargeable H Contraceptive Device M Stimulator Generator N Tissue Expander P Cardiac Rhythm Related Device V Infusion Device, Pump W Vascular Access Device, Totally Implantable X Vascular Access Device, Tunneled Y Other Device	Z No Qualifier
D Subcutaneous Tissue and Fascia, Right Upper Arm Axillary fascia Deltoid fascia Infraspinatus fascia Subscapular aponeurosis Supraspinatus fascia F Subcutaneous Tissue and Fascia, Left Upper Arm *See* *D Subcutaneous Tissue and Fascia, Right Upper Arm* G Subcutaneous Tissue and Fascia, Right Lower Arm Antebrachial fascia Bicipital aponeurosis H Subcutaneous Tissue and Fascia, Left Lower Arm *See* *G Subcutaneous Tissue and Fascia, Right Lower Arm* L Subcutaneous Tissue and Fascia, Right Upper Leg Crural fascia Fascia lata Iliac fascia Iliotibial tract (band) M Subcutaneous Tissue and Fascia, Left Upper Leg *See* *L Subcutaneous Tissue and Fascia, Right Upper Leg* N Subcutaneous Tissue and Fascia, Right Lower Leg P Subcutaneous Tissue and Fascia, Left Lower Leg	Ø Open 3 Percutaneous	H Contraceptive Device N Tissue Expander V Infusion Device, Pump W Vascular Access Device, Totally Implantable X Vascular Access Device, Tunneled	Z No Qualifier
S Subcutaneous Tissue and Fascia, Head and Neck V Subcutaneous Tissue and Fascia, Upper Extremity W Subcutaneous Tissue and Fascia, Lower Extremity	Ø Open 3 Percutaneous	1 Radioactive Element 3 Infusion Device Y Other Device	Z No Qualifier
T Subcutaneous Tissue and Fascia, Trunk External oblique aponeurosis Transversalis fascia	Ø Open 3 Percutaneous	1 Radioactive Element 3 Infusion Device V Infusion Device, Pump Y Other Device	Z No Qualifier

DRG Non-OR ØJH8[Ø,3][2,4,5,6,7,H,P,X]Z
DRG Non-OR ØJH83WX
DRG Non-OR ØJH[D,F,G,H,L,M,N,P]ØXZ
DRG Non-OR ØJH[D,F,G,H,L,M,N,P]3[W,X]Z
DRG Non-OR ØJHN3HZ
DRG Non-OR ØJHP[Ø,3]HZ

Non-OR ØJH[D,F,G,H,L,M][Ø,3]HZ
Non-OR ØJHNØHZ
Non-OR ØJH[S,V,W]Ø3Z
Non-OR ØJH[S,V,W]3[3,Y]Z
Non-OR ØJHTØ3Z
Non-OR ØJHT3[3,Y]Z

HAC ØJH8[Ø,3][4,5,6,7,8,9,P]Z when reported with SDx K68.11 or T81.4Ø-T81.49, T82.6-T82.7 with 7th character A
NC ØJH8[Ø,3]MZ
See Appendix L for Procedure Combinations
⊞ ØJH8[Ø,3][4,5,6,7,8,9,A,B,C,D,E,P]Z

Ø Medical and Surgical
J Subcutaneous Tissue and Fascia
J Inspection Definition: Visually and/or manually exploring a body part

Explanation: Visual exploration may be performed with or without optical instrumentation. Manual exploration may be performed directly or through intervening body layers.

Body Part Character 4	Approach Character 5	Device Character 6	Qualifier Character 7
S Subcutaneous Tissue and Fascia, Head and Neck **T** Subcutaneous Tissue and Fascia, Trunk External oblique aponeurosis Transversalis fascia **V** Subcutaneous Tissue and Fascia, Upper Extremity **W** Subcutaneous Tissue and Fascia, Lower Extremity	**Ø** Open **3** Percutaneous **X** External	**Z** No Device	**Z** No Qualifier

Non-OR All body part, approach, device, and qualifier values

Ø Medical and Surgical
J Subcutaneous Tissue and Fascia
N Release Definition: Freeing a body part from an abnormal physical constraint by cutting or by the use of force

Explanation: Some of the restraining tissue may be taken out but none of the body part is taken out

Body Part Character 4	Approach Character 5	Device Character 6	Qualifier Character 7
Ø Subcutaneous Tissue and Fascia, Scalp Galea aponeurotica **1** Subcutaneous Tissue and Fascia, Face Masseteric fascia Orbital fascia Submandibular space **4** Subcutaneous Tissue and Fascia, Right Neck Deep cervical fascia Pretracheal fascia Prevertebral fascia **5** Subcutaneous Tissue and Fascia, Left Neck **See** *4 Subcutaneous Tissue and Fascia, Right Neck* **6** Subcutaneous Tissue and Fascia, Chest Pectoral fascia **7** Subcutaneous Tissue and Fascia, Back **8** Subcutaneous Tissue and Fascia, Abdomen **9** Subcutaneous Tissue and Fascia, Buttock **B** Subcutaneous Tissue and Fascia, Perineum **C** Subcutaneous Tissue and Fascia, Pelvic Region **D** Subcutaneous Tissue and Fascia, Right Upper Arm Axillary fascia Deltoid fascia Infraspinatus fascia Subscapular aponeurosis Supraspinatus fascia **F** Subcutaneous Tissue and Fascia, Left Upper Arm **See** *D Subcutaneous Tissue and Fascia, Right Upper Arm* **G** Subcutaneous Tissue and Fascia, Right Lower Arm Antebrachial fascia Bicipital aponeurosis **H** Subcutaneous Tissue and Fascia, Left Lower Arm **See** *G Subcutaneous Tissue and Fascia, Right Lower Arm* **J** Subcutaneous Tissue and Fascia, Right Hand Palmar fascia (aponeurosis) **K** Subcutaneous Tissue and Fascia, Left Hand **See** *J Subcutaneous Tissue and Fascia, Right Hand* **L** Subcutaneous Tissue and Fascia, Right Upper Leg Crural fascia Fascia lata Iliac fascia Iliotibial tract (band) **M** Subcutaneous Tissue and Fascia, Left Upper Leg **See** *L Subcutaneous Tissue and Fascia, Right Upper Leg* **N** Subcutaneous Tissue and Fascia, Right Lower Leg **P** Subcutaneous Tissue and Fascia, Left Lower Leg **Q** Subcutaneous Tissue and Fascia, Right Foot Plantar fascia (aponeurosis) **R** Subcutaneous Tissue and Fascia, Left Foot **See** *Q Subcutaneous Tissue and Fascia, Right Foot*	**Ø** Open **3** Percutaneous **X** External	**Z** No Device	**Z** No Qualifier

Non-OR ØJN[Ø,1,4,5,6,7,8,9,B,C,D,F,G,H,J,K,L,M,N,P,Q,R]XZZ

Ø Medical and Surgical
J Subcutaneous Tissue and Fascia
P Removal Definition: Taking out or off a device from a body part

Explanation: If a device is taken out and a similar device put in without cutting or puncturing the skin or mucous membrane, the procedure is coded to the root operation CHANGE. Otherwise, the procedure for taking out a device is coded to the root operation REMOVAL.

Body Part Character 4	Approach Character 5	Device Character 6	Qualifier Character 7
S Subcutaneous Tissue and Fascia, Head and Neck	Ø Open 3 Percutaneous	Ø Drainage Device 1 Radioactive Element 3 Infusion Device 7 Autologous Tissue Substitute J Synthetic Substitute K Nonautologous Tissue Substitute N Tissue Expander Y Other Device	Z No Qualifier
S Subcutaneous Tissue and Fascia, Head and Neck	X External	Ø Drainage Device 1 Radioactive Element 3 Infusion Device	Z No Qualifier
T Subcutaneous Tissue and Fascia, Trunk External oblique aponeurosis Transversalis fascia	Ø Open 3 Percutaneous	Ø Drainage Device 1 Radioactive Element 2 Monitoring Device 3 Infusion Device 7 Autologous Tissue Substitute F Subcutaneous Defibrillator Lead H Contraceptive Device J Synthetic Substitute K Nonautologous Tissue Substitute M Stimulator Generator N Tissue Expander P Cardiac Rhythm Related Device V Infusion Device, Pump W Vascular Access Device, Totally Implantable X Vascular Access Device, Tunneled Y Other Device	Z No Qualifier
T Subcutaneous Tissue and Fascia, Trunk External oblique aponeurosis Transversalis fascia	X External	Ø Drainage Device 1 Radioactive Element 2 Monitoring Device 3 Infusion Device H Contraceptive Device V Infusion Device, Pump X Vascular Access Device, Tunneled	Z No Qualifier
V Subcutaneous Tissue and Fascia, Upper Extremity W Subcutaneous Tissue and Fascia, Lower Extremity	Ø Open 3 Percutaneous	Ø Drainage Device 1 Radioactive Element 3 Infusion Device 7 Autologous Tissue Substitute H Contraceptive Device J Synthetic Substitute K Nonautologous Tissue Substitute N Tissue Expander V Infusion Device, Pump W Vascular Access Device, Totally Implantable X Vascular Access Device, Tunneled Y Other Device	Z No Qualifier
V Subcutaneous Tissue and Fascia, Upper Extremity W Subcutaneous Tissue and Fascia, Lower Extremity	X External	Ø Drainage Device 1 Radioactive Element 3 Infusion Device H Contraceptive Device V Infusion Device, Pump X Vascular Access Device, Tunneled	Z No Qualifier

Non-OR ØJPS[Ø,3][Ø,1,3,7,J,K,N,Y]Z
Non-OR ØJPSX[Ø,1,3]Z
Non-OR ØJPT[Ø,3][Ø,1,2,3,7,H,J,K,M,N,V,W,X,Y]Z
Non-OR ØJPTX[Ø,1,2,3,H,V,X]Z
Non-OR ØJP[V,W][Ø,3][Ø,1,3,7,H,J,K,N,V,W,X,Y]Z
Non-OR ØJP[V,W]X[Ø,1,3,H,V,X]Z
HAC ØJPT[Ø,3][F,P]Z when reported with SDx K68.11 or T81.4Ø-T81.49, T82.6-T82.7 with 7th character A

Ø Medical and Surgical
J Subcutaneous Tissue and Fascia
Q Repair Definition: Restoring, to the extent possible, a body part to its normal anatomic structure and function
Explanation: Used only when the method to accomplish the repair is not one of the other root operations

Body Part Character 4		Approach Character 5	Device Character 6	Qualifier Character 7
Ø Subcutaneous Tissue and Fascia, Scalp Galea aponeurotica **1** Subcutaneous Tissue and Fascia, Face Masseteric fascia Orbital fascia Submandibular space **4** Subcutaneous Tissue and Fascia, Right Neck Deep cervical fascia Pretracheal fascia Prevertebral fascia **5** Subcutaneous Tissue and Fascia, Left Neck ***See*** *4 Subcutaneous Tissue and Fascia, Right Neck* **6** Subcutaneous Tissue and Fascia, Chest Pectoral fascia **7** Subcutaneous Tissue and Fascia, Back **8** Subcutaneous Tissue and Fascia, Abdomen **9** Subcutaneous Tissue and Fascia, Buttock **B** Subcutaneous Tissue and Fascia, Perineum **C** Subcutaneous Tissue and Fascia, Pelvic Region **D** Subcutaneous Tissue and Fascia, Right Upper Arm Axillary fascia Deltoid fascia Infraspinatus fascia Subscapular aponeurosis Supraspinatus fascia **F** Subcutaneous Tissue and Fascia, Left Upper Arm ***See*** *D Subcutaneous Tissue and Fascia, Right Upper Arm*	**G** Subcutaneous Tissue and Fascia, Right Lower Arm Antebrachial fascia Bicipital aponeurosis **H** Subcutaneous Tissue and Fascia, Left Lower Arm ***See*** *G Subcutaneous Tissue and Fascia, Right Lower Arm* **J** Subcutaneous Tissue and Fascia, Right Hand Palmar fascia (aponeurosis) **K** Subcutaneous Tissue and Fascia, Left Hand ***See*** *J Subcutaneous Tissue and Fascia, Right Hand* **L** Subcutaneous Tissue and Fascia, Right Upper Leg Crural fascia Fascia lata Iliac fascia Iliotibial tract (band) **M** Subcutaneous Tissue and Fascia, Left Upper Leg ***See*** *L Subcutaneous Tissue and Fascia, Right Upper Leg* **N** Subcutaneous Tissue and Fascia, Right Lower Leg **P** Subcutaneous Tissue and Fascia, Left Lower Leg **Q** Subcutaneous Tissue and Fascia, Right Foot Plantar fascia (aponeurosis) **R** Subcutaneous Tissue and Fascia, Left Foot ***See*** *Q Subcutaneous Tissue and Fascia, Right Foot*	**Ø** Open **3** Percutaneous	**Z** No Device	**Z** No Qualifier

Non-OR ØJQ[Ø,1,4,5,6,7,8,9,B,C,D,F,G,H,J,K,L,M,N,P,Q,R]3ZZ

Ø Medical and Surgical
J Subcutaneous Tissue and Fascia
R Replacement Definition: Putting in or on biological or synthetic material that physically takes the place and/or function of all or a portion of a body part

Explanation: The body part may have been taken out or replaced, or may be taken out, physically eradicated, or rendered nonfunctional during the REPLACEMENT procedure. A REMOVAL procedure is coded for taking out the device used in a previous replacement procedure.

Body Part Character 4	Approach Character 5	Device Character 6	Qualifier Character 7
Ø Subcutaneous Tissue and Fascia, Scalp Galea aponeurotica **1 Subcutaneous Tissue and Fascia, Face** Masseteric fascia Orbital fascia Submandibular space **4 Subcutaneous Tissue and Fascia, Right Neck** Deep cervical fascia Pretracheal fascia Prevertebral fascia **5 Subcutaneous Tissue and Fascia, Left Neck** ***See*** *4 Subcutaneous Tissue and Fascia, Right Neck* **6 Subcutaneous Tissue and Fascia, Chest** Pectoral fascia **7 Subcutaneous Tissue and Fascia, Back** **8 Subcutaneous Tissue and Fascia, Abdomen** **9 Subcutaneous Tissue and Fascia, Buttock** **B Subcutaneous Tissue and Fascia, Perineum** **C Subcutaneous Tissue and Fascia, Pelvic Region** **D Subcutaneous Tissue and Fascia, Right Upper Arm** Axillary fascia Deltoid fascia Infraspinatus fascia Subscapular aponeurosis Supraspinatus fascia **F Subcutaneous Tissue and Fascia, Left Upper Arm** ***See*** *D Subcutaneous Tissue and Fascia, Right Upper Arm* **G Subcutaneous Tissue and Fascia, Right Lower Arm** Antebrachial fascia Bicipital aponeurosis **H Subcutaneous Tissue and Fascia, Left Lower Arm** ***See*** *G Subcutaneous Tissue and Fascia, Right Lower Arm* **J Subcutaneous Tissue and Fascia, Right Hand** Palmar fascia (aponeurosis) **K Subcutaneous Tissue and Fascia, Left Hand** ***See*** *J Subcutaneous Tissue and Fascia, Right Hand* **L Subcutaneous Tissue and Fascia, Right Upper Leg** Crural fascia Fascia lata Iliac fascia Iliotibial tract (band) **M Subcutaneous Tissue and Fascia, Left Upper Leg** ***See*** *L Subcutaneous Tissue and Fascia, Right Upper Leg* **N Subcutaneous Tissue and Fascia, Right Lower Leg** **P Subcutaneous Tissue and Fascia, Left Lower Leg** **Q Subcutaneous Tissue and Fascia, Right Foot** Plantar fascia (aponeurosis) **R Subcutaneous Tissue and Fascia, Left Foot** ***See*** *Q Subcutaneous Tissue and Fascia, Right Foot*	**Ø Open** **3 Percutaneous**	**7 Autologous Tissue Substitute** **J Synthetic Substitute** **K Nonautologous Tissue Substitute**	**Z No Qualifier**

Ø Medical and Surgical
J Subcutaneous Tissue and Fascia
U Supplement: Definition: Putting in or on biological or synthetic material that physically reinforces and/or augments the function of a portion of a body part

Explanation: The biological material is non-living, or is living and from the same individual. The body part may have been previously replaced, and the SUPPLEMENT procedure is performed to physically reinforce and/or augment the function of the replaced body part.

Body Part Character 4	Approach Character 5	Device Character 6	Qualifier Character 7
Ø Subcutaneous Tissue and Fascia, Scalp Galea aponeurotica **1 Subcutaneous Tissue and Fascia, Face** Masseteric fascia Orbital fascia Submandibular space **4 Subcutaneous Tissue and Fascia, Right Neck** Deep cervical fascia Pretracheal fascia Prevertebral fascia **5 Subcutaneous Tissue and Fascia, Left Neck** *See 4 Subcutaneous Tissue and Fascia, Right Neck* **6 Subcutaneous Tissue and Fascia, Chest** Pectoral fascia **7 Subcutaneous Tissue and Fascia, Back** **8 Subcutaneous Tissue and Fascia, Abdomen** **9 Subcutaneous Tissue and Fascia, Buttock** **B Subcutaneous Tissue and Fascia, Perineum** **C Subcutaneous Tissue and Fascia, Pelvic Region** **D Subcutaneous Tissue and Fascia, Right Upper Arm** Axillary fascia Deltoid fascia Infraspinatus fascia Subscapular aponeurosis Supraspinatus fascia **F Subcutaneous Tissue and Fascia, Left Upper Arm** *See D Subcutaneous Tissue and Fascia, Right Upper Arm* **G Subcutaneous Tissue and Fascia, Right Lower Arm** Antebrachial fascia Bicipital aponeurosis **H Subcutaneous Tissue and Fascia, Left Lower Arm** *See G Subcutaneous Tissue and Fascia, Right Lower Arm* **J Subcutaneous Tissue and Fascia, Right Hand** Palmar fascia (aponeurosis) **K Subcutaneous Tissue and Fascia, Left Hand** *See J Subcutaneous Tissue and Fascia, Right Hand* **L Subcutaneous Tissue and Fascia, Right Upper Leg** Crural fascia Fascia lata Iliac fascia Iliotibial tract (band) **M Subcutaneous Tissue and Fascia, Left Upper Leg** *See L Subcutaneous Tissue and Fascia, Right Upper Leg* **N Subcutaneous Tissue and Fascia, Right Lower Leg** **P Subcutaneous Tissue and Fascia, Left Lower Leg** **Q Subcutaneous Tissue and Fascia, Right Foot** Plantar fascia (aponeurosis) **R Subcutaneous Tissue and Fascia, Left Foot** *See Q Subcutaneous Tissue and Fascia, Right Foot*	**Ø Open** **3 Percutaneous**	**7 Autologous Tissue Substitute** **J Synthetic Substitute** **K Nonautologous Tissue Substitute**	**Z No Qualifier**

Ø Medical and Surgical
J Subcutaneous Tissue and Fascia
W Revision Definition: Correcting, to the extent possible, a portion of a malfunctioning device or the position of a displaced device

Explanation: Revision can include correcting a malfunctioning or displaced device by taking out or putting in components of the device such as a screw or pin

Body Part Character 4	Approach Character 5	Device Character 6	Qualifier Character 7
S Subcutaneous Tissue and Fascia, Head and Neck	Ø Open 3 Percutaneous	Ø Drainage Device 3 Infusion Device 7 Autologous Tissue Substitute J Synthetic Substitute K Nonautologous Tissue Substitute N Tissue Expander Y Other Device	Z No Qualifier
S Subcutaneous Tissue and Fascia, Head and Neck	X External	Ø Drainage Device 3 Infusion Device 7 Autologous Tissue Substitute J Synthetic Substitute K Nonautologous Tissue Substitute N Tissue Expander	Z No Qualifier
T Subcutaneous Tissue and Fascia, Trunk External oblique aponeurosis Transversalis fascia	Ø Open 3 Percutaneous	Ø Drainage Device 2 Monitoring Device 3 Infusion Device 7 Autologous Tissue Substitute F Subcutaneous Defibrillator Lead H Contraceptive Device J Synthetic Substitute K Nonautologous Tissue Substitute M Stimulator Generator N Tissue Expander P Cardiac Rhythm Related Device V Infusion Device, Pump W Vascular Access Device, Totally Implantable X Vascular Access Device, Tunneled Y Other Device	Z No Qualifier
T Subcutaneous Tissue and Fascia, Trunk External oblique aponeurosis Transversalis fascia	X External	Ø Drainage Device 2 Monitoring Device 3 Infusion Device 7 Autologous Tissue Substitute F Subcutaneous Defibrillator Lead H Contraceptive Device J Synthetic Substitute K Nonautologous Tissue Substitute M Stimulator Generator N Tissue Expander P Cardiac Rhythm Related Device V Infusion Device, Pump W Vascular Access Device, Totally Implantable X Vascular Access Device, Tunneled	Z No Qualifier
V Subcutaneous Tissue and Fascia, Upper Extremity W Subcutaneous Tissue and Fascia, Lower Extremity	Ø Open 3 Percutaneous	Ø Drainage Device 3 Infusion Device 7 Autologous Tissue Substitute H Contraceptive Device J Synthetic Substitute K Nonautologous Tissue Substitute N Tissue Expander V Infusion Device, Pump W Vascular Access Device, Totally Implantable X Vascular Access Device, Tunneled Y Other Device	Z No Qualifier
V Subcutaneous Tissue and Fascia, Upper Extremity W Subcutaneous Tissue and Fascia, Lower Extremity	X External	Ø Drainage Device 3 Infusion Device 7 Autologous Tissue Substitute H Contraceptive Device J Synthetic Substitute K Nonautologous Tissue Substitute N Tissue Expander V Infusion Device, Pump W Vascular Access Device, Totally Implantable X Vascular Access Device, Tunneled	Z No Qualifier

DRG Non-OR ØJWS[Ø,3][Ø,3,7,J,K,N,Y]Z
DRG Non-OR ØJWT[Ø,3][Ø,3,7,H,J,K,M,N,V,W,X]Z
DRG Non-OR ØJWTXMZ
DRG Non-OR ØJW[V,W][Ø,3][Ø,3,7,H,J,K,N,V,W,X,Y]Z
Non-OR ØJWSX[Ø,3,7,J,K,N]Z
Non-OR ØJWT3YZ
Non-OR ØJWTX[Ø,2,3,7,F,H,J,K,N,P,V,W,X]Z
Non-OR ØJW[V,W]X[Ø,3,7,H,J,K,N,V,W,X]Z

HAC ØJWT[Ø,3][F,P]Z when reported with SDx K68.11 or T81.4Ø-T81.49, T82.6-T82.7 with 7th character A

Ø Medical and Surgical
J Subcutaneous Tissue and Fascia
X Transfer Definition: Moving, without taking out, all or a portion of a body part to another location to take over the function of all or a portion of a body part
Explanation: The body part transferred remains connected to its vascular and nervous supply

Body Part Character 4	Approach Character 5	Device Character 6	Qualifier Character 7
Ø Subcutaneous Tissue and Fascia, Scalp Galea aponeurotica **1 Subcutaneous Tissue and Fascia, Face** Masseteric fascia Orbital fascia Submandibular space **4 Subcutaneous Tissue and Fascia, Right Neck** Deep cervical fascia Pretracheal fascia Prevertebral fascia **5 Subcutaneous Tissue and Fascia, Left Neck** ***See*** *4 Subcutaneous Tissue and Fascia, Right Neck* **6 Subcutaneous Tissue and Fascia, Chest** Pectoral fascia **7 Subcutaneous Tissue and Fascia, Back** **8 Subcutaneous Tissue and Fascia, Abdomen** **9 Subcutaneous Tissue and Fascia, Buttock** **B Subcutaneous Tissue and Fascia, Perineum** **C Subcutaneous Tissue and Fascia, Pelvic Region** **D Subcutaneous Tissue and Fascia, Right Upper Arm** Axillary fascia Deltoid fascia Infraspinatus fascia Subscapular aponeurosis Supraspinatus fascia **F Subcutaneous Tissue and Fascia, Left Upper Arm** ***See*** *D Subcutaneous Tissue and Fascia, Right Upper Arm* **G Subcutaneous Tissue and Fascia, Right Lower Arm** Antebrachial fascia Bicipital aponeurosis **H Subcutaneous Tissue and Fascia, Left Lower Arm** ***See*** *G Subcutaneous Tissue and Fascia, Right Lower Arm* **J Subcutaneous Tissue and Fascia, Right Hand** Palmar fascia (aponeurosis) **K Subcutaneous Tissue and Fascia, Left Hand** ***See*** *J Subcutaneous Tissue and Fascia, Right Hand* **L Subcutaneous Tissue and Fascia, Right Upper Leg** Crural fascia Fascia lata Iliac fascia Iliotibial tract (band) **M Subcutaneous Tissue and Fascia, Left Upper Leg** ***See*** *L Subcutaneous Tissue and Fascia, Right Upper Leg* **N Subcutaneous Tissue and Fascia, Right Lower Leg** **P Subcutaneous Tissue and Fascia, Left Lower Leg** **Q Subcutaneous Tissue and Fascia, Right Foot** Plantar fascia (aponeurosis) **R Subcutaneous Tissue and Fascia, Left Foot** ***See*** *Q Subcutaneous Tissue and Fascia, Right Foot*	**Ø Open** **3 Percutaneous**	**Z No Device**	**B Skin and Subcutaneous Tissue** **C Skin, Subcutaneous Tissue and Fascia** **Z No Qualifier**

Muscles ØK2–ØKX

Character Meanings

This Character Meaning table is provided as a guide to assist the user in the identification of character members that may be found in this section of code tables. It **SHOULD NOT** be used to build a PCS code.

Operation–Character 3	Body Part–Character 4	Approach–Character 5	Device–Character 6	Qualifier–Character 7
2 Change	Ø Head Muscle	Ø Open	Ø Drainage Device	Ø Skin
5 Destruction	1 Facial Muscle	3 Percutaneous	7 Autologous Tissue Substitute	1 Subcutaneous Tissue
8 Division	2 Neck Muscle, Right	4 Percutaneous Endoscopic	J Synthetic Substitute	2 Skin and Subcutaneous Tissue
9 Drainage	3 Neck Muscle, Left	X External	K Nonautologous Tissue Substitute	5 Latissimus Dorsi Myocutaneous Flap
B Excision	4 Tongue, Palate, Pharynx Muscle		M Stimulator Lead	6 Transverse Rectus Abdominis Myocutaneous Flap
C Extirpation	5 Shoulder Muscle, Right		Y Other Device	7 Deep Inferior Epigastric Artery Perforator Flap
D Extraction	6 Shoulder Muscle, Left		Z No Device	8 Superficial Inferior Epigastric Artery Flap
H Insertion	7 Upper Arm Muscle, Right			9 Gluteal Artery Perforator Flap
J Inspection	8 Upper Arm Muscle, Left			X Diagnostic
M Reattachment	9 Lower Arm and Wrist Muscle, Right			Z No Qualifier
N Release	B Lower Arm and Wrist Muscle, Left			
P Removal	C Hand Muscle, Right			
Q Repair	D Hand Muscle, Left			
R Replacement	F Trunk Muscle, Right			
S Reposition	G Trunk Muscle, Left			
T Resection	H Thorax Muscle, Right			
U Supplement	J Thorax Muscle, Left			
W Revision	K Abdomen Muscle, Right			
X Transfer	L Abdomen Muscle, Left			
	M Perineum Muscle			
	N Hip Muscle, Right			
	P Hip Muscle, Left			
	Q Upper Leg Muscle, Right			
	R Upper Leg Muscle, Left			
	S Lower Leg Muscle, Right			
	T Lower Leg Muscle, Left			
	V Foot Muscle, Right			
	W Foot Muscle, Left			
	X Upper Muscle			
	Y Lower Muscle			

AHA Coding Clinic for table ØK8

2020, 2Q, 25 Endoscopic Stapling of Zenker's Diverticulum

AHA Coding Clinic for table ØKB

2020, 1Q, 27 Delayed reconstruction following mastectomy using gracilis musculocutaneous free flap
2016, 3Q, 20 Excisional debridement of sacrum
2015, 3Q, 3-8 Excisional and nonexcisional debridement

AHA Coding Clinic for table ØKD

2017, 4Q, 41-42 Extraction procedures

AHA Coding Clinic for table ØKN

2017, 2Q, 12 Compartment syndrome and fasciotomy of foot
2017, 2Q, 13 Compartment syndrome and fasciotomy of leg
2015, 2Q, 22 Arthroscopic subacromial decompression
2014, 4Q, 39 Abdominal component release with placement of mesh for hernia repair

AHA Coding Clinic for table ØKQ

2018, 2Q, 25 Third and fourth degree obstetric lacerations
2016, 2Q, 34 Assisted vaginal delivery
2016, 1Q, 7 Obstetrical perineal laceration repair
2014, 4Q, 43 Second degree obstetric perineal laceration
2013, 4Q, 120 Repair of second degree perineum obstetric laceration

AHA Coding Clinic for table ØKS

2017, 1Q, 41 Manual reduction of hernia

AHA Coding Clinic for table ØKT

2016, 2Q, 12 Resection of malignant neoplasm of infratemporal fossa
2015, 1Q, 38 Abdominoperineal resection with flap closure of the perineum and colostomy

AHA Coding Clinic for table ØKX

2018, 2Q, 18 Transverse rectus abdominis myocutaneous (TRAM) delay
2017, 4Q, 67 New qualifier values - Pedicle flap procedures
2016, 3Q, 30 Resection of femur with interposition arthroplasty
2015, 3Q, 33 Cleft lip repair using Millard rotation advancement
2015, 2Q, 26 Pharyngeal flap to soft palate
2014, 4Q, 41 Abdominoperineal resection (APR) with flap closure of perineum and colostomy
2014, 2Q, 10 Transverse abdominomyocutaneous (TRAM) breast reconstruction
2014, 2Q, 12 Pedicle latissimus myocutaneous flap with placement of breast tissue expanders

Muscles

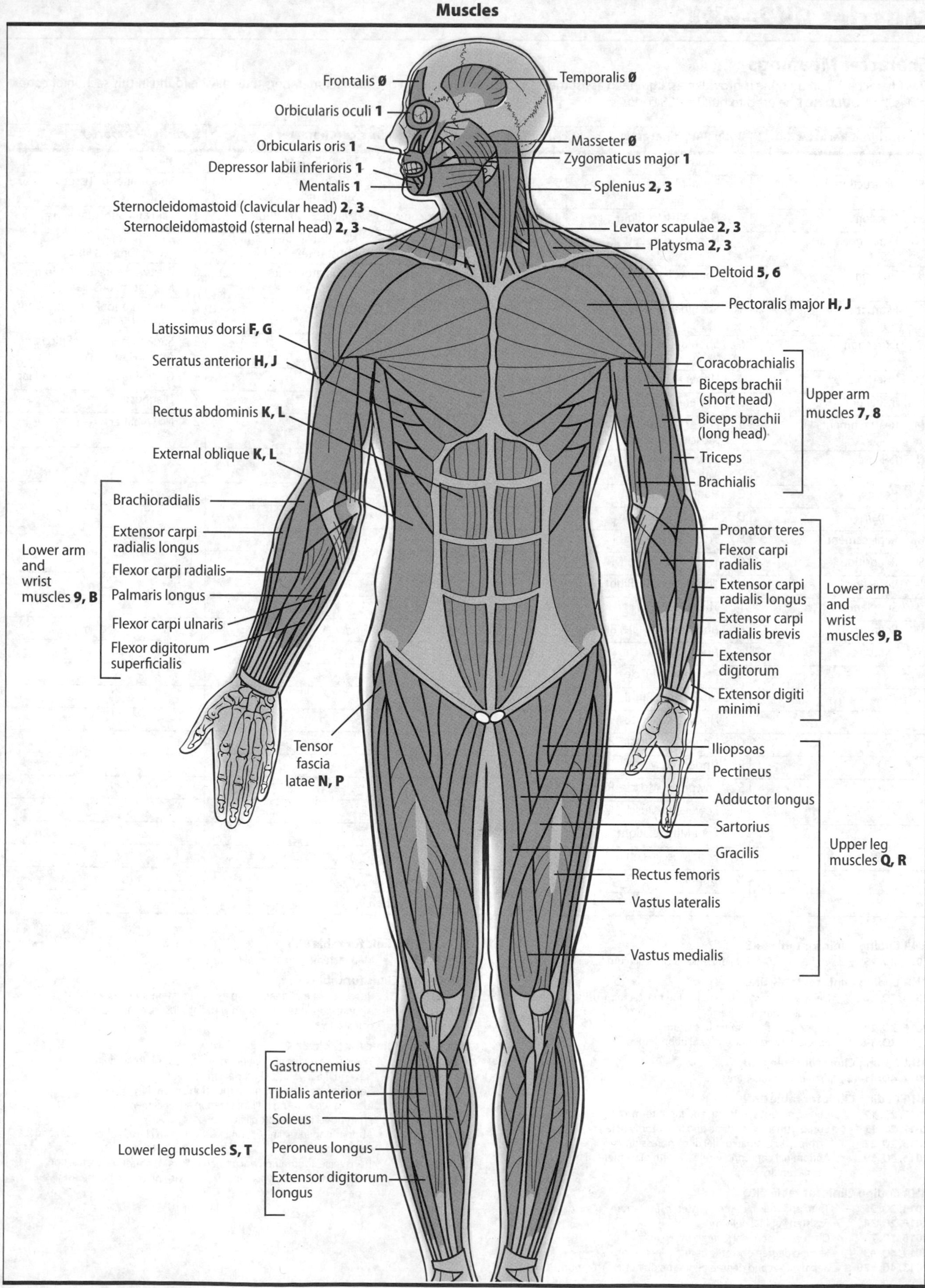
Frontalis Ø
Temporalis Ø
Orbicularis oculi 1
Orbicularis oris 1
Masseter Ø
Zygomaticus major 1
Depressor labii inferioris 1
Mentalis 1
Splenius 2, 3
Sternocleidomastoid (clavicular head) 2, 3
Sternocleidomastoid (sternal head) 2, 3
Levator scapulae 2, 3
Platysma 2, 3
Deltoid 5, 6
Pectoralis major H, J
Latissimus dorsi F, G
Serratus anterior H, J
Coracobrachialis
Biceps brachii (short head)
Upper arm muscles 7, 8
Biceps brachii (long head)
Rectus abdominis K, L
External oblique K, L
Triceps
Brachialis
Brachioradialis
Extensor carpi radialis longus
Flexor carpi radialis
Lower arm and wrist muscles 9, B
Palmaris longus
Flexor carpi ulnaris
Flexor digitorum superficialis
Pronator teres
Flexor carpi radialis
Extensor carpi radialis longus
Extensor carpi radialis brevis
Lower arm and wrist muscles 9, B
Extensor digitorum
Extensor digiti minimi
Tensor fascia latae N, P
Iliopsoas
Pectineus
Adductor longus
Sartorius
Gracilis
Upper leg muscles Q, R
Rectus femoris
Vastus lateralis
Vastus medialis
Gastrocnemius
Tibialis anterior
Soleus
Lower leg muscles S, T
Peroneus longus
Extensor digitorum longus

Ø Medical and Surgical
K Muscles
2 Change Definition: Taking out or off a device from a body part and putting back an identical or similar device in or on the same body part without cutting or puncturing the skin or a mucous membrane
Explanation: All CHANGE procedures are coded using the approach EXTERNAL

Body Part Character 4	Approach Character 5	Device Character 6	Qualifier Character 7
X Upper Muscle Y Lower Muscle	X External	Ø Drainage Device Y Other Device	Z No Qualifier

Non-OR All body part, approach, device, and qualifier values

Ø Medical and Surgical
K Muscles
5 Destruction Definition: Physical eradication of all or a portion of a body part by the direct use of energy, force, or a destructive agent
Explanation: None of the body part is physically taken out

Body Part Character 4	Approach Character 5	Device Character 6	Qualifier Character 7
Ø Head Muscle Auricularis muscle Masseter muscle Pterygoid muscle Splenius capitis muscle Temporalis muscle Temporoparietalis muscle	Ø Open 3 Percutaneous 4 Percutaneous Endoscopic	Z No Device	Z No Qualifier
1 Facial Muscle Buccinator muscle Corrugator supercilii muscle Depressor anguli oris muscle Depressor labii inferioris muscle Depressor septi nasi muscle Depressor supercilii muscle Levator anguli oris muscle Levator labii superioris alaeque nasi muscle Levator labii superioris muscle Mentalis muscle Nasalis muscle Occipitofrontalis muscle Orbicularis oris muscle Procerus muscle Risorius muscle Zygomaticus muscle			
2 Neck Muscle, Right Anterior vertebral muscle Arytenoid muscle Cricothyroid muscle Infrahyoid muscle Levator scapulae muscle Platysma muscle Scalene muscle Splenius cervicis muscle Sternocleidomastoid muscle Suprahyoid muscle Thyroarytenoid muscle			
3 Neck Muscle, Left *See 2 Neck Muscle, Right*			
4 Tongue, Palate, Pharynx Muscle Chondroglossus muscle Genioglossus muscle Hyoglossus muscle Inferior longitudinal muscle Levator veli palatini muscle Palatoglossal muscle Palatopharyngeal muscle Pharyngeal constrictor muscle Salpingopharyngeus muscle Styloglossus muscle Stylopharyngeus muscle Superior longitudinal muscle Tensor veli palatini muscle			
5 Shoulder Muscle, Right Deltoid muscle Infraspinatus muscle Subscapularis muscle Supraspinatus muscle Teres major muscle Teres minor muscle			
6 Shoulder Muscle, Left *See 5 Shoulder Muscle, Right*			
7 Upper Arm Muscle, Right Biceps brachii muscle Brachialis muscle Coracobrachialis muscle Triceps brachii muscle			
8 Upper Arm Muscle, Left *See 7 Upper Arm Muscle, Right*			
9 Lower Arm and Wrist Muscle, Right Anatomical snuffbox Brachioradialis muscle Extensor carpi radialis muscle Extensor carpi ulnaris muscle Flexor carpi radialis muscle Flexor carpi ulnaris muscle Flexor pollicis longus muscle Palmaris longus muscle Pronator quadratus muscle Pronator teres muscle			
B Lower Arm and Wrist Muscle, Left *See 9 Lower Arm and Wrist Muscle, Right*			
C Hand Muscle, Right Hypothenar muscle Palmar interosseous muscle Thenar muscle			
D Hand Muscle, Left *See C Hand Muscle, Right*			
F Trunk Muscle, Right Coccygeus muscle Erector spinae muscle Interspinalis muscle Intertransversarius muscle Latissimus dorsi muscle Quadratus lumborum muscle Rhomboid major muscle Rhomboid minor muscle Serratus posterior muscle Transversospinalis muscle Trapezius muscle			
G Trunk Muscle, Left *See F Trunk Muscle, Right*			
H Thorax Muscle, Right Intercostal muscle Levatores costarum muscle Pectoralis major muscle Pectoralis minor muscle Serratus anterior muscle Subclavius muscle Subcostal muscle Transverse thoracis muscle			
J Thorax Muscle, Left *See H Thorax Muscle, Right*			
K Abdomen Muscle, Right External oblique muscle Internal oblique muscle Pyramidalis muscle Rectus abdominis muscle Transversus abdominis muscle			
L Abdomen Muscle, Left *See K Abdomen Muscle, Right*			
M Perineum Muscle Bulbospongiosus muscle Cremaster muscle Deep transverse perineal muscle Ischiocavernosus muscle Levator ani muscle Superficial transverse perineal muscle			
N Hip Muscle, Right Gemellus muscle Gluteus maximus muscle Gluteus medius muscle Gluteus minimus muscle Iliacus muscle Obturator muscle Piriformis muscle Psoas muscle Quadratus femoris muscle Tensor fasciae latae muscle			
P Hip Muscle, Left *See N Hip Muscle, Right*			
Q Upper Leg Muscle, Right Adductor brevis muscle Adductor longus muscle Adductor magnus muscle Biceps femoris muscle Gracilis muscle Pectineus muscle Quadriceps (femoris) Rectus femoris muscle Sartorius muscle Semimembranosus muscle Semitendinosus muscle Vastus intermedius muscle Vastus lateralis muscle Vastus medialis muscle			
R Upper Leg Muscle, Left *See Q Upper Leg Muscle, Right*			
S Lower Leg Muscle, Right Extensor digitorum longus muscle Extensor hallucis longus muscle Fibularis brevis muscle Fibularis longus muscle Flexor digitorum longus muscle Flexor hallucis longus muscle Gastrocnemius muscle Peroneus brevis muscle Peroneus longus muscle Popliteus muscle Soleus muscle Tibialis anterior muscle Tibialis posterior muscle			
T Lower Leg Muscle, Left *See S Lower Leg Muscle, Right*			
V Foot Muscle, Right Abductor hallucis muscle Adductor hallucis muscle Extensor digitorum brevis muscle Extensor hallucis brevis muscle Flexor digitorum brevis muscle Flexor hallucis brevis muscle Quadratus plantae muscle			
W Foot Muscle, Left *See V Foot Muscle, Right*			

Ø Medical and Surgical
K Muscles
8 Division

Definition: Cutting into a body part, without draining fluids and/or gases from the body part, in order to separate or transect a body part

Explanation: All or a portion of the body part is separated into two or more portions

Body Part Character 4	Approach Character 5	Device Character 6	Qualifier Character 7
Ø Head Muscle Auricularis muscle Masseter muscle Pterygoid muscle Splenius capitis muscle Temporalis muscle Temporoparietalis muscle **1 Facial Muscle** Buccinator muscle Corrugator supercilii muscle Depressor anguli oris muscle Depressor labii inferioris muscle Depressor septi nasi muscle Depressor supercilii muscle Levator anguli oris muscle Levator labii superioris alaeque nasi muscle Levator labii superioris muscle Mentalis muscle Nasalis muscle Occipitofrontalis muscle Orbicularis oris muscle Procerus muscle Risorius muscle Zygomaticus muscle **2 Neck Muscle, Right** Anterior vertebral muscle Arytenoid muscle Cricothyroid muscle Infrahyoid muscle Levator scapulae muscle Platysma muscle Scalene muscle Splenius cervicis muscle Sternocleidomastoid muscle Suprahyoid muscle Thyroarytenoid muscle **3 Neck Muscle, Left** *See 2 Neck Muscle, Right* **4 Tongue, Palate, Pharynx Muscle** Chondroglossus muscle Genioglossus muscle Hyoglossus muscle Inferior longitudinal muscle Levator veli palatini muscle Palatoglossal muscle Palatopharyngeal muscle Pharyngeal constrictor muscle Salpingopharyngeus muscle Styloglossus muscle Stylopharyngeus muscle Superior longitudinal muscle Tensor veli palatini muscle **5 Shoulder Muscle, Right** Deltoid muscle Infraspinatus muscle Subscapularis muscle Supraspinatus muscle Teres major muscle Teres minor muscle **6 Shoulder Muscle, Left** *See 5 Shoulder Muscle, Right* **7 Upper Arm Muscle, Right** Biceps brachii muscle Brachialis muscle Coracobrachialis muscle Triceps brachii muscle **8 Upper Arm Muscle, Left** *See 7 Upper Arm Muscle, Right* **9 Lower Arm and Wrist Muscle, Right** Anatomical snuffbox Brachioradialis muscle Extensor carpi radialis muscle Extensor carpi ulnaris muscle Flexor carpi radialis muscle Flexor carpi ulnaris muscle Flexor pollicis longus muscle Palmaris longus muscle Pronator quadratus muscle Pronator teres muscle **B Lower Arm and Wrist Muscle, Left** *See 9 Lower Arm and Wrist Muscle, Right* **C Hand Muscle, Right** Hypothenar muscle Palmar interosseous muscle Thenar muscle **D Hand Muscle, Left** *See C Hand Muscle, Right* **F Trunk Muscle, Right** Coccygeus muscle Erector spinae muscle Interspinalis muscle Intertransversarius muscle Latissimus dorsi muscle Quadratus lumborum muscle Rhomboid major muscle Rhomboid minor muscle Serratus posterior muscle Transversospinalis muscle Trapezius muscle **G Trunk Muscle, Left** *See F Trunk Muscle, Right* **H Thorax Muscle, Right** Intercostal muscle Levatores costarum muscle Pectoralis major muscle Pectoralis minor muscle Serratus anterior muscle Subclavius muscle Subcostal muscle Transverse thoracis muscle **J Thorax Muscle, Left** *See H Thorax Muscle, Right* **K Abdomen Muscle, Right** External oblique muscle Internal oblique muscle Pyramidalis muscle Rectus abdominis muscle Transversus abdominis muscle **L Abdomen Muscle, Left** *See K Abdomen Muscle, Right* **M Perineum Muscle** Bulbospongiosus muscle Cremaster muscle Deep transverse perineal muscle Ischiocavernosus muscle Levator ani muscle Superficial transverse perineal muscle **N Hip Muscle, Right** Gemellus muscle Gluteus maximus muscle Gluteus medius muscle Gluteus minimus muscle Iliacus muscle Obturator muscle Piriformis muscle Psoas muscle Quadratus femoris muscle Tensor fasciae latae muscle **P Hip Muscle, Left** *See N Hip Muscle, Right* **Q Upper Leg Muscle, Right** Adductor brevis muscle Adductor longus muscle Adductor magnus muscle Biceps femoris muscle Gracilis muscle Pectineus muscle Quadriceps (femoris) Rectus femoris muscle Sartorius muscle Semimembranosus muscle Semitendinosus muscle Vastus intermedius muscle Vastus lateralis muscle Vastus medialis muscle **R Upper Leg Muscle, Left** *See Q Upper Leg Muscle, Right* **S Lower Leg Muscle, Right** Extensor digitorum longus muscle Extensor hallucis longus muscle Fibularis brevis muscle Fibularis longus muscle Flexor digitorum longus muscle Flexor hallucis longus muscle Gastrocnemius muscle Peroneus brevis muscle Peroneus longus muscle Popliteus muscle Soleus muscle Tibialis anterior muscle Tibialis posterior muscle **T Lower Leg Muscle, Left** *See S Lower Leg Muscle, Right* **V Foot Muscle, Right** Abductor hallucis muscle Adductor hallucis muscle Extensor digitorum brevis muscle Extensor hallucis brevis muscle Flexor digitorum brevis muscle Flexor hallucis brevis muscle Quadratus plantae muscle **W Foot Muscle, Left** *See V Foot Muscle, Right*	**Ø Open** **3 Percutaneous** **4 Percutaneous Endoscopic**	**Z** No Device	**Z** No Qualifier

Ø Medical and Surgical
K Muscles
9 Drainage Definition: Taking or letting out fluids and/or gases from a body part

Explanation: The qualifier DIAGNOSTIC is used to identify drainage procedures that are biopsies

Body Part Character 4	Approach Character 5	Device Character 6	Qualifier Character 7
Ø **Head Muscle** Auricularis muscle Masseter muscle Pterygoid muscle Splenius capitis muscle Temporalis muscle Temporoparietalis muscle 1 **Facial Muscle** Buccinator muscle Corrugator supercilii muscle Depressor anguli oris muscle Depressor labii inferioris muscle Depressor septi nasi muscle Depressor supercilii muscle Levator anguli oris muscle Levator labii superioris alaeque nasi muscle Levator labii superioris muscle Mentalis muscle Nasalis muscle Occipitofrontalis muscle Orbicularis oris muscle Procerus muscle Risorius muscle Zygomaticus muscle 2 **Neck Muscle, Right** Anterior vertebral muscle Arytenoid muscle Cricothyroid muscle Infrahyoid muscle Levator scapulae muscle Platysma muscle Scalene muscle Splenius cervicis muscle Sternocleidomastoid muscle Suprahyoid muscle Thyroarytenoid muscle 3 **Neck Muscle, Left** *See 2 Neck Muscle, Right* 4 **Tongue, Palate, Pharynx Muscle** Chondroglossus muscle Genioglossus muscle Hyoglossus muscle Inferior longitudinal muscle Levator veli palatini muscle Palatoglossal muscle Palatopharyngeal muscle Pharyngeal constrictor muscle Salpingopharyngeus muscle Styloglossus muscle Stylopharyngeus muscle Superior longitudinal muscle Tensor veli palatini muscle 5 **Shoulder Muscle, Right** Deltoid muscle Infraspinatus muscle Subscapularis muscle Supraspinatus muscle Teres major muscle Teres minor muscle 6 **Shoulder Muscle, Left** *See 5 Shoulder Muscle, Right* 7 **Upper Arm Muscle, Right** Biceps brachii muscle Brachialis muscle Coracobrachialis muscle Triceps brachii muscle 8 **Upper Arm Muscle, Left** *See 7 Upper Arm Muscle, Right* 9 **Lower Arm and Wrist Muscle, Right** Anatomical snuffbox Brachioradialis muscle Extensor carpi radialis muscle Extensor carpi ulnaris muscle Flexor carpi radialis muscle Flexor carpi ulnaris muscle Flexor pollicis longus muscle Palmaris longus muscle Pronator quadratus muscle Pronator teres muscle B **Lower Arm and Wrist Muscle, Left** *See 9 Lower Arm and Wrist Muscle, Right* C **Hand Muscle, Right** Hypothenar muscle Palmar interosseous muscle Thenar muscle D **Hand Muscle, Left** *See C Hand Muscle, Right* F **Trunk Muscle, Right** Coccygeus muscle Erector spinae muscle Interspinalis muscle Intertransversarius muscle Latissimus dorsi muscle Quadratus lumborum muscle Rhomboid major muscle Rhomboid minor muscle Serratus posterior muscle Transversospinalis muscle Trapezius muscle G **Trunk Muscle, Left** *See F Trunk Muscle, Right* H **Thorax Muscle, Right** Intercostal muscle Levatores costarum muscle Pectoralis major muscle Pectoralis minor muscle Serratus anterior muscle Subclavius muscle Subcostal muscle Transverse thoracis muscle J **Thorax Muscle, Left** *See H Thorax Muscle, Right* K **Abdomen Muscle, Right** External oblique muscle Internal oblique muscle Pyramidalis muscle Rectus abdominis muscle Transversus abdominis muscle L **Abdomen Muscle, Left** *See K Abdomen Muscle, Right* M **Perineum Muscle** Bulbospongiosus muscle Cremaster muscle Deep transverse perineal muscle Ischiocavernosus muscle Levator ani muscle Superficial transverse perineal muscle N **Hip Muscle, Right** Gemellus muscle Gluteus maximus muscle Gluteus medius muscle Gluteus minimus muscle Iliacus muscle Obturator muscle Piriformis muscle Psoas muscle Quadratus femoris muscle Tensor fasciae latae muscle P **Hip Muscle, Left** *See N Hip Muscle, Right* Q **Upper Leg Muscle, Right** Adductor brevis muscle Adductor longus muscle Adductor magnus muscle Biceps femoris muscle Gracilis muscle Pectineus muscle Quadriceps (femoris) Rectus femoris muscle Sartorius muscle Semimembranosus muscle Semitendinosus muscle Vastus intermedius muscle Vastus lateralis muscle Vastus medialis muscle R **Upper Leg Muscle, Left** *See Q Upper Leg Muscle, Right* S **Lower Leg Muscle, Right** Extensor digitorum longus muscle Extensor hallucis longus muscle Fibularis brevis muscle Fibularis longus muscle Flexor digitorum longus muscle Flexor hallucis longus muscle Gastrocnemius muscle Peroneus brevis muscle Peroneus longus muscle Popliteus muscle Soleus muscle Tibialis anterior muscle Tibialis posterior muscle T **Lower Leg Muscle, Left** *See S Lower Leg Muscle, Right* V **Foot Muscle, Right** Abductor hallucis muscle Adductor hallucis muscle Extensor digitorum brevis muscle Extensor hallucis brevis muscle Flexor digitorum brevis muscle Flexor hallucis brevis muscle Quadratus plantae muscle W **Foot Muscle, Left** *See V Foot Muscle, Right*	Ø Open 3 Percutaneous 4 Percutaneous Endoscopic	Ø Drainage Device	Z No Qualifier

Non-OR ØK9[Ø,1,2,3,4,5,6,7,8,9,B,C,D,F,G,H,J,K,L,M,N,P,Q,R,S,T,V,W]3ØZ

ØK9 Continued on next page

Ø Medical and Surgical
K Muscles
9 Drainage Definition: Taking or letting out fluids and/or gases from a body part
Explanation: The qualifier DIAGNOSTIC is used to identify drainage procedures that are biopsies

ØK9 Continued

Body Part Character 4	Approach Character 5	Device Character 6	Qualifier Character 7
Ø **Head Muscle** Auricularis muscle Masseter muscle Pterygoid muscle Splenius capitis muscle Temporalis muscle Temporoparietalis muscle 1 **Facial Muscle** Buccinator muscle Corrugator supercilii muscle Depressor anguli oris muscle Depressor labii inferioris muscle Depressor septi nasi muscle Depressor supercilii muscle Levator anguli oris muscle Levator labii superioris alaeque nasi muscle Levator labii superioris muscle Mentalis muscle Nasalis muscle Occipitofrontalis muscle Orbicularis oris muscle Procerus muscle Risorius muscle Zygomaticus muscle 2 **Neck Muscle, Right** Anterior vertebral muscle Arytenoid muscle Cricothyroid muscle Infrahyoid muscle Levator scapulae muscle Platysma muscle Scalene muscle Splenius cervicis muscle Sternocleidomastoid muscle Suprahyoid muscle Thyroarytenoid muscle 3 **Neck Muscle, Left** *See 2 Neck Muscle, Right* 4 **Tongue, Palate, Pharynx Muscle** Chondroglossus muscle Genioglossus muscle Hyoglossus muscle Inferior longitudinal muscle Levator veli palatini muscle Palatoglossal muscle Palatopharyngeal muscle Pharyngeal constrictor muscle Salpingopharyngeus muscle Styloglossus muscle Stylopharyngeus muscle Superior longitudinal muscle Tensor veli palatini muscle 5 **Shoulder Muscle, Right** Deltoid muscle Infraspinatus muscle Subscapularis muscle Supraspinatus muscle Teres major muscle Teres minor muscle 6 **Shoulder Muscle, Left** *See 5 Shoulder Muscle, Right* 7 **Upper Arm Muscle, Right** Biceps brachii muscle Brachialis muscle Coracobrachialis muscle Triceps brachii muscle 8 **Upper Arm Muscle, Left** *See 7 Upper Arm Muscle, Right* 9 **Lower Arm and Wrist Muscle, Right** Anatomical snuffbox Brachioradialis muscle Extensor carpi radialis muscle Extensor carpi ulnaris muscle Flexor carpi radialis muscle Flexor carpi ulnaris muscle Flexor pollicis longus muscle Palmaris longus muscle Pronator quadratus muscle Pronator teres muscle B **Lower Arm and Wrist Muscle, Left** *See 9 Lower Arm and Wrist Muscle, Right* C **Hand Muscle, Right** Hypothenar muscle Palmar interosseous muscle Thenar muscle D **Hand Muscle, Left** *See C Hand Muscle, Right* F **Trunk Muscle, Right** Coccygeus muscle Erector spinae muscle Interspinalis muscle Intertransversarius muscle Latissimus dorsi muscle Quadratus lumborum muscle Rhomboid major muscle Rhomboid minor muscle Serratus posterior muscle Transversospinalis muscle Trapezius muscle G **Trunk Muscle, Left** *See F Trunk Muscle, Right* H **Thorax Muscle, Right** Intercostal muscle Levatores costarum muscle Pectoralis major muscle Pectoralis minor muscle Serratus anterior muscle Subclavius muscle Subcostal muscle Transverse thoracis muscle J **Thorax Muscle, Left** *See H Thorax Muscle, Right* K **Abdomen Muscle, Right** External oblique muscle Internal oblique muscle Pyramidalis muscle Rectus abdominis muscle Transversus abdominis muscle L **Abdomen Muscle, Left** *See K Abdomen Muscle, Right* M **Perineum Muscle** Bulbospongiosus muscle Cremaster muscle Deep transverse perineal muscle Ischiocavernosus muscle Levator ani muscle Superficial transverse perineal muscle N **Hip Muscle, Right** Gemellus muscle Gluteus maximus muscle Gluteus medius muscle Gluteus minimus muscle Iliacus muscle Obturator muscle Piriformis muscle Psoas muscle Quadratus femoris muscle Tensor fasciae latae muscle P **Hip Muscle, Left** *See N Hip Muscle, Right* Q **Upper Leg Muscle, Right** Adductor brevis muscle Adductor longus muscle Adductor magnus muscle Biceps femoris muscle Gracilis muscle Pectineus muscle Quadriceps (femoris) Rectus femoris muscle Sartorius muscle Semimembranosus muscle Semitendinosus muscle Vastus intermedius muscle Vastus lateralis muscle Vastus medialis muscle R **Upper Leg Muscle, Left** *See Q Upper Leg Muscle, Right* S **Lower Leg Muscle, Right** Extensor digitorum longus muscle Extensor hallucis longus muscle Fibularis brevis muscle Fibularis longus muscle Flexor digitorum longus muscle Flexor hallucis longus muscle Gastrocnemius muscle Peroneus brevis muscle Peroneus longus muscle Popliteus muscle Soleus muscle Tibialis anterior muscle Tibialis posterior muscle T **Lower Leg Muscle, Left** *See S Lower Leg Muscle, Right* V **Foot Muscle, Right** Abductor hallucis muscle Adductor hallucis muscle Extensor digitorum brevis muscle Extensor hallucis brevis muscle Flexor digitorum brevis muscle Flexor hallucis brevis muscle Quadratus plantae muscle W **Foot Muscle, Left** *See V Foot Muscle, Right*	Ø **Open** 3 **Percutaneous** 4 **Percutaneous Endoscopic**	Z **No Device**	X **Diagnostic** Z **No Qualifier**

Non-OR ØK9[Ø,1,2,3,4,5,6,7,8,9,B,F,G,H,J,K,L,M,N,P,Q,R,S,T,V,W]3ZZ
Non-OR ØK9[C,D][3,4]ZZ

Ø Medical and Surgical
K Muscles
B Excision **Definition: Cutting out or off, without replacement, a portion of a body part**
Explanation: The qualifier DIAGNOSTIC is used to identify excision procedures that are biopsies

Body Part Character 4	Approach Character 5	Device Character 6	Qualifier Character 7
Ø Head Muscle Auricularis muscle Masseter muscle Pterygoid muscle Splenius capitis muscle Temporalis muscle Temporoparietalis muscle **1 Facial Muscle** Buccinator muscle Corrugator supercilii muscle Depressor anguli oris muscle Depressor labii inferioris muscle Depressor septi nasi muscle Depressor supercilii muscle Levator anguli oris muscle Levator labii superioris alaeque nasi muscle Levator labii superioris muscle Mentalis muscle Nasalis muscle Occipitofrontalis muscle Orbicularis oris muscle Procerus muscle Risorius muscle Zygomaticus muscle **2 Neck Muscle, Right** Anterior vertebral muscle Arytenoid muscle Cricothyroid muscle Infrahyoid muscle Levator scapulae muscle Platysma muscle Scalene muscle Splenius cervicis muscle Sternocleidomastoid muscle Suprahyoid muscle Thyroarytenoid muscle **3 Neck Muscle, Left** *See 2 Neck Muscle, Right* **4 Tongue, Palate, Pharynx Muscle** Chondroglossus muscle Genioglossus muscle Hyoglossus muscle Inferior longitudinal muscle Levator veli palatini muscle Palatoglossal muscle Palatopharyngeal muscle Pharyngeal constrictor muscle Salpingopharyngeus muscle Styloglossus muscle Stylopharyngeus muscle Superior longitudinal muscle Tensor veli palatini muscle **5 Shoulder Muscle, Right** Deltoid muscle Infraspinatus muscle Subscapularis muscle Supraspinatus muscle Teres major muscle Teres minor muscle **6 Shoulder Muscle, Left** *See 5 Shoulder Muscle, Right* **7 Upper Arm Muscle, Right** Biceps brachii muscle Brachialis muscle Coracobrachialis muscle Triceps brachii muscle **8 Upper Arm Muscle, Left** *See 7 Upper Arm Muscle, Right* **9 Lower Arm and Wrist Muscle, Right** Anatomical snuffbox Brachioradialis muscle Extensor carpi radialis muscle Extensor carpi ulnaris muscle Flexor carpi radialis muscle Flexor carpi ulnaris muscle Flexor pollicis longus muscle Palmaris longus muscle Pronator quadratus muscle Pronator teres muscle **B Lower Arm and Wrist Muscle, Left** *See 9 Lower Arm and Wrist Muscle, Right* **C Hand Muscle, Right** Hypothenar muscle Palmar interosseous muscle Thenar muscle **D Hand Muscle, Left** *See C Hand Muscle, Right* **F Trunk Muscle, Right** Coccygeus muscle Erector spinae muscle Interspinalis muscle Intertransversarius muscle Latissimus dorsi muscle Quadratus lumborum muscle Rhomboid major muscle Rhomboid minor muscle Serratus posterior muscle Transversospinalis muscle Trapezius muscle **G Trunk Muscle, Left** *See F Trunk Muscle, Right* **H Thorax Muscle, Right** Intercostal muscle Levatores costarum muscle Pectoralis major muscle Pectoralis minor muscle Serratus anterior muscle Subclavius muscle Subcostal muscle Transverse thoracis muscle **J Thorax Muscle, Left** *See H Thorax Muscle, Right* **K Abdomen Muscle, Right** External oblique muscle Internal oblique muscle Pyramidalis muscle Rectus abdominis muscle Transversus abdominis muscle **L Abdomen Muscle, Left** *See K Abdomen Muscle, Right* **M Perineum Muscle** Bulbospongiosus muscle Cremaster muscle Deep transverse perineal muscle Ischiocavernosus muscle Levator ani muscle Superficial transverse perineal muscle **N Hip Muscle, Right** Gemellus muscle Gluteus maximus muscle Gluteus medius muscle Gluteus minimus muscle Iliacus muscle Obturator muscle Piriformis muscle Psoas muscle Quadratus femoris muscle Tensor fasciae latae muscle **P Hip Muscle, Left** *See N Hip Muscle, Right* **Q Upper Leg Muscle, Right** Adductor brevis muscle Adductor longus muscle Adductor magnus muscle Biceps femoris muscle Gracilis muscle Pectineus muscle Quadriceps (femoris) Rectus femoris muscle Sartorius muscle Semimembranosus muscle Semitendinosus muscle Vastus intermedius muscle Vastus lateralis muscle Vastus medialis muscle **R Upper Leg Muscle, Left** *See Q Upper Leg Muscle, Right* **S Lower Leg Muscle, Right** Extensor digitorum longus muscle Extensor hallucis longus muscle Fibularis brevis muscle Fibularis longus muscle Flexor digitorum longus muscle Flexor hallucis longus muscle Gastrocnemius muscle Peroneus brevis muscle Peroneus longus muscle Popliteus muscle Soleus muscle Tibialis anterior muscle Tibialis posterior muscle **T Lower Leg Muscle, Left** *See S Lower Leg Muscle, Right* **V Foot Muscle, Right** Abductor hallucis muscle Adductor hallucis muscle Extensor digitorum brevis muscle Extensor hallucis brevis muscle Flexor digitorum brevis muscle Flexor hallucis brevis muscle Quadratus plantae muscle **W Foot Muscle, Left** *See V Foot Muscle, Right*	**Ø Open** **3 Percutaneous** **4 Percutaneous Endoscopic**	**Z No Device**	**X Diagnostic** **Z No Qualifier**

Ø Medical and Surgical
K Muscles
C Extirpation Definition: Taking or cutting out solid matter from a body part

Explanation: The solid matter may be an abnormal byproduct of a biological function or a foreign body; it may be imbedded in a body part or in the lumen of a tubular body part. The solid matter may or may not have been previously broken into pieces.

Body Part Character 4	Approach Character 5	Device Character 6	Qualifier Character 7
Ø Head Muscle Auricularis muscle Masseter muscle Pterygoid muscle Splenius capitis muscle Temporalis muscle Temporoparietalis muscle **1 Facial Muscle** Buccinator muscle Corrugator supercilii muscle Depressor anguli oris muscle Depressor labii inferioris muscle Depressor septi nasi muscle Depressor supercilii muscle Levator anguli oris muscle Levator labii superioris alaeque nasi muscle Levator labii superioris muscle Mentalis muscle Nasalis muscle Occipitofrontalis muscle Orbicularis oris muscle Procerus muscle Risorius muscle Zygomaticus muscle **2 Neck Muscle, Right** Anterior vertebral muscle Arytenoid muscle Cricothyroid muscle Infrahyoid muscle Levator scapulae muscle Platysma muscle Scalene muscle Splenius cervicis muscle Sternocleidomastoid muscle Suprahyoid muscle Thyroarytenoid muscle **3 Neck Muscle, Left** *See 2 Neck Muscle, Right* **4 Tongue, Palate, Pharynx Muscle** Chondroglossus muscle Genioglossus muscle Hyoglossus muscle Inferior longitudinal muscle Levator veli palatini muscle Palatoglossal muscle Palatopharyngeal muscle Pharyngeal constrictor muscle Salpingopharyngeus muscle Styloglossus muscle Stylopharyngeus muscle Superior longitudinal muscle Tensor veli palatini muscle **5 Shoulder Muscle, Right** Deltoid muscle Infraspinatus muscle Subscapularis muscle Supraspinatus muscle Teres major muscle Teres minor muscle **6 Shoulder Muscle, Left** *See 5 Shoulder Muscle, Right* **7 Upper Arm Muscle, Right** Biceps brachii muscle Brachialis muscle Coracobrachialis muscle Triceps brachii muscle **8 Upper Arm Muscle, Left** *See 7 Upper Arm Muscle, Right* **9 Lower Arm and Wrist Muscle, Right** Anatomical snuffbox Brachioradialis muscle Extensor carpi radialis muscle Extensor carpi ulnaris muscle Flexor carpi radialis muscle Flexor carpi ulnaris muscle Flexor pollicis longus muscle Palmaris longus muscle Pronator quadratus muscle Pronator teres muscle **B Lower Arm and Wrist Muscle, Left** *See 9 Lower Arm and Wrist Muscle, Right* **C Hand Muscle, Right** Hypothenar muscle Palmar interosseous muscle Thenar muscle **D Hand Muscle, Left** *See C Hand Muscle, Right* **F Trunk Muscle, Right** Coccygeus muscle Erector spinae muscle Interspinalis muscle Intertransversarius muscle Latissimus dorsi muscle Quadratus lumborum muscle Rhomboid major muscle Rhomboid minor muscle Serratus posterior muscle Transversospinalis muscle Trapezius muscle **G Trunk Muscle, Left** *See F Trunk Muscle, Right* **H Thorax Muscle, Right** Intercostal muscle Levatores costarum muscle Pectoralis major muscle Pectoralis minor muscle Serratus anterior muscle Subclavius muscle Subcostal muscle Transverse thoracis muscle **J Thorax Muscle, Left** *See H Thorax Muscle, Right* **K Abdomen Muscle, Right** External oblique muscle Internal oblique muscle Pyramidalis muscle Rectus abdominis muscle Transversus abdominis muscle **L Abdomen Muscle, Left** *See K Abdomen Muscle, Right* **M Perineum Muscle** Bulbospongiosus muscle Cremaster muscle Deep transverse perineal muscle Ischiocavernosus muscle Levator ani muscle Superficial transverse perineal muscle **N Hip Muscle, Right** Gemellus muscle Gluteus maximus muscle Gluteus medius muscle Gluteus minimus muscle Iliacus muscle Obturator muscle Piriformis muscle Psoas muscle Quadratus femoris muscle Tensor fasciae latae muscle **P Hip Muscle, Left** *See N Hip Muscle, Right* **Q Upper Leg Muscle, Right** Adductor brevis muscle Adductor longus muscle Adductor magnus muscle Biceps femoris muscle Gracilis muscle Pectineus muscle Quadriceps (femoris) Rectus femoris muscle Sartorius muscle Semimembranosus muscle Semitendinosus muscle Vastus intermedius muscle Vastus lateralis muscle Vastus medialis muscle **R Upper Leg Muscle, Left** *See Q Upper Leg Muscle, Right* **S Lower Leg Muscle, Right** Extensor digitorum longus muscle Extensor hallucis longus muscle Fibularis brevis muscle Fibularis longus muscle Flexor digitorum longus muscle Flexor hallucis longus muscle Gastrocnemius muscle Peroneus brevis muscle Peroneus longus muscle Popliteus muscle Soleus muscle Tibialis anterior muscle Tibialis posterior muscle **T Lower Leg Muscle, Left** *See S Lower Leg Muscle, Right* **V Foot Muscle, Right** Abductor hallucis muscle Adductor hallucis muscle Extensor digitorum brevis muscle Extensor hallucis brevis muscle Flexor digitorum brevis muscle Flexor hallucis brevis muscle Quadratus plantae muscle **W Foot Muscle, Left** *See V Foot Muscle, Right*	**Ø Open** **3 Percutaneous** **4 Percutaneous Endoscopic**	**Z No Device**	**Z No Qualifier**

LC Limited Coverage NC Noncovered ⊞ Combination Member HAC associated procedure Combination Only DRG Non-OR Non-OR New/Revised in GREEN

Ø Medical and Surgical
K Muscles
D Extraction Definition: Pulling or stripping out or off all or a portion of a body part by the use of force
Explanation: The qualifier DIAGNOSTIC is used to identify extraction procedures that are biopsies

Body Part Character 4	Approach Character 5	Device Character 6	Qualifier Character 7
Ø Head Muscle Auricularis muscle Masseter muscle Pterygoid muscle Splenius capitis muscle Temporalis muscle Temporoparietalis muscle **1 Facial Muscle** Buccinator muscle Corrugator supercilii muscle Depressor anguli oris muscle Depressor labii inferioris muscle Depressor septi nasi muscle Depressor supercilii muscle Levator anguli oris muscle Levator labii superioris alaeque nasi muscle Levator labii superioris muscle Mentalis muscle Nasalis muscle Occipitofrontalis muscle Orbicularis oris muscle Procerus muscle Risorius muscle Zygomaticus muscle **2 Neck Muscle, Right** Anterior vertebral muscle Arytenoid muscle Cricothyroid muscle Infrahyoid muscle Levator scapulae muscle Platysma muscle Scalene muscle Splenius cervicis muscle Sternocleidomastoid muscle Suprahyoid muscle Thyroarytenoid muscle **3 Neck Muscle, Left** **See** *2 Neck Muscle, Right* **4 Tongue, Palate, Pharynx Muscle** Chondroglossus muscle Genioglossus muscle Hyoglossus muscle Inferior longitudinal muscle Levator veli palatini muscle Palatoglossal muscle Palatopharyngeal muscle Pharyngeal constrictor muscle Salpingopharyngeus muscle Styloglossus muscle Stylopharyngeus muscle Superior longitudinal muscle Tensor veli palatini muscle **5 Shoulder Muscle, Right** Deltoid muscle Infraspinatus muscle Subscapularis muscle Supraspinatus muscle Teres major muscle Teres minor muscle **6 Shoulder Muscle, Left** **See** *5 Shoulder Muscle, Right* **7 Upper Arm Muscle, Right** Biceps brachii muscle Brachialis muscle Coracobrachialis muscle Triceps brachii muscle **8 Upper Arm Muscle, Left** **See** *7 Upper Arm Muscle, Right* **9 Lower Arm and Wrist Muscle, Right** Anatomical snuffbox Brachioradialis muscle Extensor carpi radialis muscle Extensor carpi ulnaris muscle Flexor carpi radialis muscle Flexor carpi ulnaris muscle Flexor pollicis longus muscle Palmaris longus muscle Pronator quadratus muscle Pronator teres muscle **B Lower Arm and Wrist Muscle, Left** **See** *9 Lower Arm and Wrist Muscle, Right* **C Hand Muscle, Right** Hypothenar muscle Palmar interosseous muscle Thenar muscle **D Hand Muscle, Left** **See** *C Hand Muscle, Right* **F Trunk Muscle, Right** Coccygeus muscle Erector spinae muscle Interspinalis muscle Intertransversarius muscle Latissimus dorsi muscle Quadratus lumborum muscle Rhomboid major muscle Rhomboid minor muscle Serratus posterior muscle Transversospinalis muscle Trapezius muscle **G Trunk Muscle, Left** **See** *F Trunk Muscle, Right* **H Thorax Muscle, Right** Intercostal muscle Levatores costarum muscle Pectoralis major muscle Pectoralis minor muscle Serratus anterior muscle Subclavius muscle Subcostal muscle Transverse thoracis muscle **J Thorax Muscle, Left** **See** *H Thorax Muscle, Right* **K Abdomen Muscle, Right** External oblique muscle Internal oblique muscle Pyramidalis muscle Rectus abdominis muscle Transversus abdominis muscle **L Abdomen Muscle, Left** **See** *K Abdomen Muscle, Right* **M Perineum Muscle** Bulbospongiosus muscle Cremaster muscle Deep transverse perineal muscle Ischiocavernosus muscle Levator ani muscle Superficial transverse perineal muscle **N Hip Muscle, Right** Gemellus muscle Gluteus maximus muscle Gluteus medius muscle Gluteus minimus muscle Iliacus muscle Obturator muscle Piriformis muscle Psoas muscle Quadratus femoris muscle Tensor fasciae latae muscle **P Hip Muscle, Left** **See** *N Hip Muscle, Right* **Q Upper Leg Muscle, Right** Adductor brevis muscle Adductor longus muscle Adductor magnus muscle Biceps femoris muscle Gracilis muscle Pectineus muscle Quadriceps (femoris) Rectus femoris muscle Sartorius muscle Semimembranosus muscle Semitendinosus muscle Vastus intermedius muscle Vastus lateralis muscle Vastus medialis muscle **R Upper Leg Muscle, Left** **See** *Q Upper Leg Muscle, Right* **S Lower Leg Muscle, Right** Extensor digitorum longus muscle Extensor hallucis longus muscle Fibularis brevis muscle Fibularis longus muscle Flexor digitorum longus muscle Flexor hallucis longus muscle Gastrocnemius muscle Peroneus brevis muscle Peroneus longus muscle Popliteus muscle Soleus muscle Tibialis anterior muscle Tibialis posterior muscle **T Lower Leg Muscle, Left** **See** *S Lower Leg Muscle, Right* **V Foot Muscle, Right** Abductor hallucis muscle Adductor hallucis muscle Extensor digitorum brevis muscle Extensor hallucis brevis muscle Flexor digitorum brevis muscle Flexor hallucis brevis muscle Quadratus plantae muscle **W Foot Muscle, Left** **See** *V Foot Muscle, Right*	**Ø** Open	**Z** No Device	**Z** No Qualifier

Ø Medical and Surgical
K Muscles
H Insertion

Definition: Putting in a nonbiological appliance that monitors, assists, performs, or prevents a physiological function but does not physically take the place of a body part

Explanation: None

Body Part Character 4	Approach Character 5	Device Character 6	Qualifier Character 7
X Upper Muscle Y Lower Muscle	Ø Open 3 Percutaneous 4 Percutaneous Endoscopic	M Stimulator Lead Y Other Device	Z No Qualifier

Non-OR ØKH[X,Y][3,4]YZ

Ø Medical and Surgical
K Muscles
J Inspection

Definition: Visually and/or manually exploring a body part

Explanation: Visual exploration may be performed with or without optical instrumentation. Manual exploration may be performed directly or through intervening body layers.

Body Part Character 4	Approach Character 5	Device Character 6	Qualifier Character 7
X Upper Muscle Y Lower Muscle	Ø Open 3 Percutaneous 4 Percutaneous Endoscopic X External	Z No Device	Z No Qualifier

Non-OR ØKJ[X,Y][3,X]ZZ

Ø Medical and Surgical
K Muscles
M Reattachment Definition: Putting back in or on all or a portion of a separated body part to its normal location or other suitable location
Explanation: Vascular circulation and nervous pathways may or may not be reestablished

Body Part Character 4	Approach Character 5	Device Character 6	Qualifier Character 7
Ø Head Muscle Auricularis muscle Masseter muscle Pterygoid muscle Splenius capitis muscle Temporalis muscle Temporoparietalis muscle **1 Facial Muscle** Buccinator muscle Corrugator supercilii muscle Depressor anguli oris muscle Depressor labii inferioris muscle Depressor septi nasi muscle Depressor supercilii muscle Levator anguli oris muscle Levator labii superioris alaeque nasi muscle Levator labii superioris muscle Mentalis muscle Nasalis muscle Occipitofrontalis muscle Orbicularis oris muscle Procerus muscle Risorius muscle Zygomaticus muscle **2 Neck Muscle, Right** Anterior vertebral muscle Arytenoid muscle Cricothyroid muscle Infrahyoid muscle Levator scapulae muscle Platysma muscle Scalene muscle Splenius cervicis muscle Sternocleidomastoid muscle Suprahyoid muscle Thyroarytenoid muscle **3 Neck Muscle, Left** *See 2 Neck Muscle, Right* **4 Tongue, Palate, Pharynx Muscle** Chondroglossus muscle Genioglossus muscle Hyoglossus muscle Inferior longitudinal muscle Levator veli palatini muscle Palatoglossal muscle Palatopharyngeal muscle Pharyngeal constrictor muscle Salpingopharyngeus muscle Styloglossus muscle Stylopharyngeus muscle Superior longitudinal muscle Tensor veli palatini muscle **5 Shoulder Muscle, Right** Deltoid muscle Infraspinatus muscle Subscapularis muscle Supraspinatus muscle Teres major muscle Teres minor muscle **6 Shoulder Muscle, Left** *See 5 Shoulder Muscle, Right* **7 Upper Arm Muscle, Right** Biceps brachii muscle Brachialis muscle Coracobrachialis muscle Triceps brachii muscle **8 Upper Arm Muscle, Left** *See 7 Upper Arm Muscle, Right* **9 Lower Arm and Wrist Muscle, Right** Anatomical snuffbox Brachioradialis muscle Extensor carpi radialis muscle Extensor carpi ulnaris muscle Flexor carpi radialis muscle Flexor carpi ulnaris muscle Flexor pollicis longus muscle Palmaris longus muscle Pronator quadratus muscle Pronator teres muscle **B Lower Arm and Wrist Muscle, Left** *See 9 Lower Arm and Wrist Muscle, Right* **C Hand Muscle, Right** Hypothenar muscle Palmar interosseous muscle Thenar muscle **D Hand Muscle, Left** *See C Hand Muscle, Right* **F Trunk Muscle, Right** Coccygeus muscle Erector spinae muscle Interspinalis muscle Intertransversarius muscle Latissimus dorsi muscle Quadratus lumborum muscle Rhomboid major muscle Rhomboid minor muscle Serratus posterior muscle Transversospinalis muscle Trapezius muscle **G Trunk Muscle, Left** *See F Trunk Muscle, Right* **H Thorax Muscle, Right** Intercostal muscle Levatores costarum muscle Pectoralis major muscle Pectoralis minor muscle Serratus anterior muscle Subclavius muscle Subcostal muscle Transverse thoracis muscle **J Thorax Muscle, Left** *See H Thorax Muscle, Right* **K Abdomen Muscle, Right** External oblique muscle Internal oblique muscle Pyramidalis muscle Rectus abdominis muscle Transversus abdominis muscle **L Abdomen Muscle, Left** *See K Abdomen Muscle, Right* **M Perineum Muscle** Bulbospongiosus muscle Cremaster muscle Deep transverse perineal muscle Ischiocavernosus muscle Levator ani muscle Superficial transverse perineal muscle **N Hip Muscle, Right** Gemellus muscle Gluteus maximus muscle Gluteus medius muscle Gluteus minimus muscle Iliacus muscle Obturator muscle Piriformis muscle Psoas muscle Quadratus femoris muscle Tensor fasciae latae muscle **P Hip Muscle, Left** *See N Hip Muscle, Right* **Q Upper Leg Muscle, Right** Adductor brevis muscle Adductor longus muscle Adductor magnus muscle Biceps femoris muscle Gracilis muscle Pectineus muscle Quadriceps (femoris) Rectus femoris muscle Sartorius muscle Semimembranosus muscle Semitendinosus muscle Vastus intermedius muscle Vastus lateralis muscle Vastus medialis muscle **R Upper Leg Muscle, Left** *See Q Upper Leg Muscle, Right* **S Lower Leg Muscle, Right** Extensor digitorum longus muscle Extensor hallucis longus muscle Fibularis brevis muscle Fibularis longus muscle Flexor digitorum longus muscle Flexor hallucis longus muscle Gastrocnemius muscle Peroneus brevis muscle Peroneus longus muscle Popliteus muscle Soleus muscle Tibialis anterior muscle Tibialis posterior muscle **T Lower Leg Muscle, Left** *See S Lower Leg Muscle, Right* **V Foot Muscle, Right** Abductor hallucis muscle Adductor hallucis muscle Extensor digitorum brevis muscle Extensor hallucis brevis muscle Flexor digitorum brevis muscle Flexor hallucis brevis muscle Quadratus plantae muscle **W Foot Muscle, Left** *See V Foot Muscle, Right*	**Ø Open** **4 Percutaneous Endoscopic**	**Z No Device**	**Z No Qualifier**

Ø Medical and Surgical
K Muscles
N Release Definition: Freeing a body part from an abnormal physical constraint by cutting or by the use of force
Explanation: Some of the restraining tissue may be taken out but none of the body part is taken out

Body Part Character 4	Approach Character 5	Device Character 6	Qualifier Character 7
Ø Head Muscle Auricularis muscle, Masseter muscle, Pterygoid muscle, Splenius capitis muscle, Temporalis muscle, Temporoparietalis muscle **1 Facial Muscle** Buccinator muscle, Corrugator supercilii muscle, Depressor anguli oris muscle, Depressor labii inferioris muscle, Depressor septi nasi muscle, Depressor supercilii muscle, Levator anguli oris muscle, Levator labii superioris alaeque nasi muscle, Levator labii superioris muscle, Mentalis muscle, Nasalis muscle, Occipitofrontalis muscle, Orbicularis oris muscle, Procerus muscle, Risorius muscle, Zygomaticus muscle **2 Neck Muscle, Right** Anterior vertebral muscle, Arytenoid muscle, Cricothyroid muscle, Infrahyoid muscle, Levator scapulae muscle, Platysma muscle, Scalene muscle, Splenius cervicis muscle, Sternocleidomastoid muscle, Suprahyoid muscle, Thyroarytenoid muscle **3 Neck Muscle, Left** *See 2 Neck Muscle, Right* **4 Tongue, Palate, Pharynx Muscle** Chondroglossus muscle, Genioglossus muscle, Hyoglossus muscle, Inferior longitudinal muscle, Levator veli palatini muscle, Palatoglossal muscle, Palatopharyngeal muscle, Pharyngeal constrictor muscle, Salpingopharyngeus muscle, Styloglossus muscle, Stylopharyngeus muscle, Superior longitudinal muscle, Tensor veli palatini muscle **5 Shoulder Muscle, Right** Deltoid muscle, Infraspinatus muscle, Subscapularis muscle, Supraspinatus muscle, Teres major muscle, Teres minor muscle **6 Shoulder Muscle, Left** *See 5 Shoulder Muscle, Right* **7 Upper Arm Muscle, Right** Biceps brachii muscle, Brachialis muscle, Coracobrachialis muscle, Triceps brachii muscle **8 Upper Arm Muscle, Left** *See 7 Upper Arm Muscle, Right* **9 Lower Arm and Wrist Muscle, Right** Anatomical snuffbox, Brachioradialis muscle, Extensor carpi radialis muscle, Extensor carpi ulnaris muscle, Flexor carpi radialis muscle, Flexor carpi ulnaris muscle, Flexor pollicis longus muscle, Palmaris longus muscle, Pronator quadratus muscle, Pronator teres muscle **B Lower Arm and Wrist Muscle, Left** *See 9 Lower Arm and Wrist Muscle, Right* **C Hand Muscle, Right** Hypothenar muscle, Palmar interosseous muscle, Thenar muscle **D Hand Muscle, Left** *See C Hand Muscle, Right* **F Trunk Muscle, Right** Coccygeus muscle, Erector spinae muscle, Interspinalis muscle, Intertransversarius muscle, Latissimus dorsi muscle, Quadratus lumborum muscle, Rhomboid major muscle, Rhomboid minor muscle, Serratus posterior muscle, Transversospinalis muscle, Trapezius muscle **G Trunk Muscle, Left** *See F Trunk Muscle, Right* **H Thorax Muscle, Right** Intercostal muscle, Levatores costarum muscle, Pectoralis major muscle, Pectoralis minor muscle, Serratus anterior muscle, Subclavius muscle, Subcostal muscle, Transverse thoracis muscle **J Thorax Muscle, Left** *See H Thorax Muscle, Right* **K Abdomen Muscle, Right** External oblique muscle, Internal oblique muscle, Pyramidalis muscle, Rectus abdominis muscle, Transversus abdominis muscle **L Abdomen Muscle, Left** *See K Abdomen Muscle, Right* **M Perineum Muscle** Bulbospongiosus muscle, Cremaster muscle, Deep transverse perineal muscle, Ischiocavernosus muscle, Levator ani muscle, Superficial transverse perineal muscle **N Hip Muscle, Right** Gemellus muscle, Gluteus maximus muscle, Gluteus medius muscle, Gluteus minimus muscle, Iliacus muscle, Obturator muscle, Piriformis muscle, Psoas muscle, Quadratus femoris muscle, Tensor fasciae latae muscle **P Hip Muscle, Left** *See N Hip Muscle, Right* **Q Upper Leg Muscle, Right** Adductor brevis muscle, Adductor longus muscle, Adductor magnus muscle, Biceps femoris muscle, Gracilis muscle, Pectineus muscle, Quadriceps (femoris), Rectus femoris muscle, Sartorius muscle, Semimembranosus muscle, Semitendinosus muscle, Vastus intermedius muscle, Vastus lateralis muscle, Vastus medialis muscle **R Upper Leg Muscle, Left** *See Q Upper Leg Muscle, Right* **S Lower Leg Muscle, Right** Extensor digitorum longus muscle, Extensor hallucis longus muscle, Fibularis brevis muscle, Fibularis longus muscle, Flexor digitorum longus muscle, Flexor hallucis longus muscle, Gastrocnemius muscle, Peroneus brevis muscle, Peroneus longus muscle, Popliteus muscle, Soleus muscle, Tibialis anterior muscle, Tibialis posterior muscle **T Lower Leg Muscle, Left** *See S Lower Leg Muscle, Right* **V Foot Muscle, Right** Abductor hallucis muscle, Adductor hallucis muscle, Extensor digitorum brevis muscle, Extensor hallucis brevis muscle, Flexor digitorum brevis muscle, Flexor hallucis brevis muscle, Quadratus plantae muscle **W Foot Muscle, Left** *See V Foot Muscle, Right*	Ø Open 3 Percutaneous 4 Percutaneous Endoscopic X External	Z No Device	Z No Qualifier

Non-OR ØKN[Ø,1,2,3,4,5,6,7,8,9,B,C,D,F,G,H,J,K,L,M,N,P,Q,R,S,T,V,W]XZZ

Ø Medical and Surgical
K Muscles
P Removal

Definition: Taking out or off a device from a body part

Explanation: If a device is taken out and a similar device put in without cutting or puncturing the skin or mucous membrane, the procedure is coded to the root operation CHANGE. Otherwise, the procedure for taking out a device is coded to the root operation REMOVAL.

Body Part Character 4	Approach Character 5	Device Character 6	Qualifier Character 7
X Upper Muscle Y Lower Muscle	Ø Open 3 Percutaneous 4 Percutaneous Endoscopic	Ø Drainage Device 7 Autologous Tissue Substitute J Synthetic Substitute K Nonautologous Tissue Substitute M Stimulator Lead Y Other Device	Z No Qualifier
X Upper Muscle Y Lower Muscle	X External	Ø Drainage Device M Stimulator Lead	Z No Qualifier

Non-OR ØKP[X,Y][3,4]YZ
Non-OR ØKP[X,Y]X[Ø,M]Z

Ø Medical and Surgical
K Muscles
Q Repair Definition: Restoring, to the extent possible, a body part to its normal anatomic structure and function
Explanation: Used only when the method to accomplish the repair is not one of the other root operations

Body Part Character 4			Approach Character 5	Device Character 6	Qualifier Character 7
Ø Head Muscle Auricularis muscle Masseter muscle Pterygoid muscle Splenius capitis muscle Temporalis muscle Temporoparietalis muscle **1 Facial Muscle** Buccinator muscle Corrugator supercilii muscle Depressor anguli oris muscle Depressor labii inferioris muscle Depressor septi nasi muscle Depressor supercilii muscle Levator anguli oris muscle Levator labii superioris alaeque nasi muscle Levator labii superioris muscle Mentalis muscle Nasalis muscle Occipitofrontalis muscle Orbicularis oris muscle Procerus muscle Risorius muscle Zygomaticus muscle **2 Neck Muscle, Right** Anterior vertebral muscle Arytenoid muscle Cricothyroid muscle Infrahyoid muscle Levator scapulae muscle Platysma muscle Scalene muscle Splenius cervicis muscle Sternocleidomastoid muscle Suprahyoid muscle Thyroarytenoid muscle **3 Neck Muscle, Left** *See 2 Neck Muscle, Right* **4 Tongue, Palate, Pharynx Muscle** Chondroglossus muscle Genioglossus muscle Hyoglossus muscle Inferior longitudinal muscle Levator veli palatini muscle Palatoglossal muscle Palatopharyngeal muscle Pharyngeal constrictor muscle Salpingopharyngeus muscle Styloglossus muscle Stylopharyngeus muscle Superior longitudinal muscle Tensor veli palatini muscle **5 Shoulder Muscle, Right** Deltoid muscle Infraspinatus muscle Subscapularis muscle Supraspinatus muscle Teres major muscle Teres minor muscle **6 Shoulder Muscle, Left** *See 5 Shoulder Muscle, Right*	**7 Upper Arm Muscle, Right** Biceps brachii muscle Brachialis muscle Coracobrachialis muscle Triceps brachii muscle **8 Upper Arm Muscle, Left** *See 7 Upper Arm Muscle, Right* **9 Lower Arm and Wrist Muscle, Right** Anatomical snuffbox Brachioradialis muscle Extensor carpi radialis muscle Extensor carpi ulnaris muscle Flexor carpi radialis muscle Flexor carpi ulnaris muscle Flexor pollicis longus muscle Palmaris longus muscle Pronator quadratus muscle Pronator teres muscle **B Lower Arm and Wrist Muscle, Left** *See 9 Lower Arm and Wrist Muscle, Right* **C Hand Muscle, Right** Hypothenar muscle Palmar interosseous muscle Thenar muscle **D Hand Muscle, Left** *See C Hand Muscle, Right* **F Trunk Muscle, Right** Coccygeus muscle Erector spinae muscle Interspinalis muscle Intertransversarius muscle Latissimus dorsi muscle Quadratus lumborum muscle Rhomboid major muscle Rhomboid minor muscle Serratus posterior muscle Transversospinalis muscle Trapezius muscle **G Trunk Muscle, Left** *See F Trunk Muscle, Right* **H Thorax Muscle, Right** Intercostal muscle Levatores costarum muscle Pectoralis major muscle Pectoralis minor muscle Serratus anterior muscle Subclavius muscle Subcostal muscle Transverse thoracis muscle **J Thorax Muscle, Left** *See H Thorax Muscle, Right* **K Abdomen Muscle, Right** External oblique muscle Internal oblique muscle Pyramidalis muscle Rectus abdominis muscle Transversus abdominis muscle **L Abdomen Muscle, Left** *See K Abdomen Muscle, Right*	**M Perineum Muscle** Bulbospongiosus muscle Cremaster muscle Deep transverse perineal muscle Ischiocavernosus muscle Levator ani muscle Superficial transverse perineal muscle **N Hip Muscle, Right** Gemellus muscle Gluteus maximus muscle Gluteus medius muscle Gluteus minimus muscle Iliacus muscle Obturator muscle Piriformis muscle Psoas muscle Quadratus femoris muscle Tensor fasciae latae muscle **P Hip Muscle, Left** *See N Hip Muscle, Right* **Q Upper Leg Muscle, Right** Adductor brevis muscle Adductor longus muscle Adductor magnus muscle Biceps femoris muscle Gracilis muscle Pectineus muscle Quadriceps (femoris) Rectus femoris muscle Sartorius muscle Semimembranosus muscle Semitendinosus muscle Vastus intermedius muscle Vastus lateralis muscle Vastus medialis muscle **R Upper Leg Muscle, Left** *See Q Upper Leg Muscle, Right* **S Lower Leg Muscle, Right** Extensor digitorum longus muscle Extensor hallucis longus muscle Fibularis brevis muscle Fibularis longus muscle Flexor digitorum longus muscle Flexor hallucis longus muscle Gastrocnemius muscle Peroneus brevis muscle Peroneus longus muscle Popliteus muscle Soleus muscle Tibialis anterior muscle Tibialis posterior muscle **T Lower Leg Muscle, Left** *See S Lower Leg Muscle, Right* **V Foot Muscle, Right** Abductor hallucis muscle Adductor hallucis muscle Extensor digitorum brevis muscle Extensor hallucis brevis muscle Flexor digitorum brevis muscle Flexor hallucis brevis muscle Quadratus plantae muscle **W Foot Muscle, Left** *See V Foot Muscle, Right*	**Ø Open** **3 Percutaneous** **4 Percutaneous Endoscopic**	**Z No Device**	**Z No Qualifier**

Ø Medical and Surgical
K Muscles
R Replacement Definition: Putting in or on biological or synthetic material that physically takes the place and/or function of all or a portion of a body part

Explanation: The body part may have been taken out or replaced, or may be taken out, physically eradicated, or rendered nonfunctional during the REPLACEMENT procedure. A REMOVAL procedure is coded for taking out the device used in a previous replacement procedure.

Body Part Character 4	Approach Character 5	Device Character 6	Qualifier Character 7
Ø Head Muscle Auricularis muscle Masseter muscle Pterygoid muscle Splenius capitis muscle Temporalis muscle Temporoparietalis muscle **1 Facial Muscle** Buccinator muscle Corrugator supercilii muscle Depressor anguli oris muscle Depressor labii inferioris muscle Depressor septi nasi muscle Depressor supercilii muscle Levator anguli oris muscle Levator labii superioris alaeque nasi muscle Levator labii superioris muscle Mentalis muscle Nasalis muscle Occipitofrontalis muscle Orbicularis oris muscle Procerus muscle Risorius muscle Zygomaticus muscle **2 Neck Muscle, Right** Anterior vertebral muscle Arytenoid muscle Cricothyroid muscle Infrahyoid muscle Levator scapulae muscle Platysma muscle Scalene muscle Splenius cervicis muscle Sternocleidomastoid muscle Suprahyoid muscle Thyroarytenoid muscle **3 Neck Muscle, Left** *See 2 Neck Muscle, Right* **4 Tongue, Palate, Pharynx Muscle** Chondroglossus muscle Genioglossus muscle Hyoglossus muscle Inferior longitudinal muscle Levator veli palatini muscle Palatoglossal muscle Palatopharyngeal muscle Pharyngeal constrictor muscle Salpingopharyngeus muscle Styloglossus muscle Stylopharyngeus muscle Superior longitudinal muscle Tensor veli palatini muscle **5 Shoulder Muscle, Right** Deltoid muscle Infraspinatus muscle Subscapularis muscle Supraspinatus muscle Teres major muscle Teres minor muscle **6 Shoulder Muscle, Left** *See 5 Shoulder Muscle, Right* **7 Upper Arm Muscle, Right** Biceps brachii muscle Brachialis muscle Coracobrachialis muscle Triceps brachii muscle **8 Upper Arm Muscle, Left** *See 7 Upper Arm Muscle, Right* **9 Lower Arm and Wrist Muscle, Right** Anatomical snuffbox Brachioradialis muscle Extensor carpi radialis muscle Extensor carpi ulnaris muscle Flexor carpi radialis muscle Flexor carpi ulnaris muscle Flexor pollicis longus muscle Palmaris longus muscle Pronator quadratus muscle Pronator teres muscle **B Lower Arm and Wrist Muscle, Left** *See 9 Lower Arm and Wrist Muscle, Right* **C Hand Muscle, Right** Hypothenar muscle Palmar interosseous muscle Thenar muscle **D Hand Muscle, Left** *See C Hand Muscle, Right* **F Trunk Muscle, Right** Coccygeus muscle Erector spinae muscle Interspinalis muscle Intertransversarius muscle Latissimus dorsi muscle Quadratus lumborum muscle Rhomboid major muscle Rhomboid minor muscle Serratus posterior muscle Transversospinalis muscle Trapezius muscle **G Trunk Muscle, Left** *See F Trunk Muscle, Right* **H Thorax Muscle, Right** Intercostal muscle Levatores costarum muscle Pectoralis major muscle Pectoralis minor muscle Serratus anterior muscle Subclavius muscle Subcostal muscle Transverse thoracis muscle **J Thorax Muscle, Left** *See H Thorax Muscle, Right* **K Abdomen Muscle, Right** External oblique muscle Internal oblique muscle Pyramidalis muscle Rectus abdominis muscle Transversus abdominis muscle **L Abdomen Muscle, Left** *See K Abdomen Muscle, Right* **M Perineum Muscle** Bulbospongiosus muscle Cremaster muscle Deep transverse perineal muscle Ischiocavernosus muscle Levator ani muscle Superficial transverse perineal muscle **N Hip Muscle, Right** Gemellus muscle Gluteus maximus muscle Gluteus medius muscle Gluteus minimus muscle Iliacus muscle Obturator muscle Piriformis muscle Psoas muscle Quadratus femoris muscle Tensor fasciae latae muscle **P Hip Muscle, Left** *See N Hip Muscle, Right* **Q Upper Leg Muscle, Right** Adductor brevis muscle Adductor longus muscle Adductor magnus muscle Biceps femoris muscle Gracilis muscle Pectineus muscle Quadriceps (femoris) Rectus femoris muscle Sartorius muscle Semimembranosus muscle Semitendinosus muscle Vastus intermedius muscle Vastus lateralis muscle Vastus medialis muscle **R Upper Leg Muscle, Left** *See Q Upper Leg Muscle, Right* **S Lower Leg Muscle, Right** Extensor digitorum longus muscle Extensor hallucis longus muscle Fibularis brevis muscle Fibularis longus muscle Flexor digitorum longus muscle Flexor hallucis longus muscle Gastrocnemius muscle Peroneus brevis muscle Peroneus longus muscle Popliteus muscle Soleus muscle Tibialis anterior muscle Tibialis posterior muscle **T Lower Leg Muscle, Left** *See S Lower Leg Muscle, Right* **V Foot Muscle, Right** Abductor hallucis muscle Adductor hallucis muscle Extensor digitorum brevis muscle Extensor hallucis brevis muscle Flexor digitorum brevis muscle Flexor hallucis brevis muscle Quadratus plantae muscle **W Foot Muscle, Left** *See V Foot Muscle, Right*	**Ø Open** **4 Percutaneous Endoscopic**	**7 Autologous Tissue Substitute** **J Synthetic Substitute** **K Nonautologous Tissue Substitute**	**Z No Qualifier**

Ø Medical and Surgical
K Muscles
S Reposition Definition: Moving to its normal location, or other suitable location, all or a portion of a body part

Explanation: The body part is moved to a new location from an abnormal location, or from a normal location where it is not functioning correctly. The body part may or may not be cut out or off to be moved to the new location.

Body Part Character 4			Approach Character 5	Device Character 6	Qualifier Character 7
Ø Head Muscle Auricularis muscle Masseter muscle Pterygoid muscle Splenius capitis muscle Temporalis muscle Temporoparietalis muscle **1 Facial Muscle** Buccinator muscle Corrugator supercilii muscle Depressor anguli oris muscle Depressor labii inferioris muscle Depressor septi nasi muscle Depressor supercilii muscle Levator anguli oris muscle Levator labii superioris alaeque nasi muscle Levator labii superioris muscle Mentalis muscle Nasalis muscle Occipitofrontalis muscle Orbicularis oris muscle Procerus muscle Risorius muscle Zygomaticus muscle **2 Neck Muscle, Right** Anterior vertebral muscle Arytenoid muscle Cricothyroid muscle Infrahyoid muscle Levator scapulae muscle Platysma muscle Scalene muscle Splenius cervicis muscle Sternocleidomastoid muscle Suprahyoid muscle Thyroarytenoid muscle **3 Neck Muscle, Left** *See 2 Neck Muscle, Right* **4 Tongue, Palate, Pharynx Muscle** Chondroglossus muscle Genioglossus muscle Hyoglossus muscle Inferior longitudinal muscle Levator veli palatini muscle Palatoglossal muscle Palatopharyngeal muscle Pharyngeal constrictor muscle Salpingopharyngeus muscle Styloglossus muscle Stylopharyngeus muscle Superior longitudinal muscle Tensor veli palatini muscle **5 Shoulder Muscle, Right** Deltoid muscle Infraspinatus muscle Subscapularis muscle Supraspinatus muscle Teres major muscle Teres minor muscle **6 Shoulder Muscle, Left** *See 5 Shoulder Muscle, Right*	**7 Upper Arm Muscle, Right** Biceps brachii muscle Brachialis muscle Coracobrachialis muscle Triceps brachii muscle **8 Upper Arm Muscle, Left** *See 7 Upper Arm Muscle, Right* **9 Lower Arm and Wrist Muscle, Right** Anatomical snuffbox Brachioradialis muscle Extensor carpi radialis muscle Extensor carpi ulnaris muscle Flexor carpi radialis muscle Flexor carpi ulnaris muscle Flexor pollicis longus muscle Palmaris longus muscle Pronator quadratus muscle Pronator teres muscle **B Lower Arm and Wrist Muscle, Left** *See 9 Lower Arm and Wrist Muscle, Right* **C Hand Muscle, Right** Hypothenar muscle Palmar interosseous muscle Thenar muscle **D Hand Muscle, Left** *See C Hand Muscle, Right* **F Trunk Muscle, Right** Coccygeus muscle Erector spinae muscle Interspinalis muscle Intertransversarius muscle Latissimus dorsi muscle Quadratus lumborum muscle Rhomboid major muscle Rhomboid minor muscle Serratus posterior muscle Transversospinalis muscle Trapezius muscle **G Trunk Muscle, Left** *See F Trunk Muscle, Right* **H Thorax Muscle, Right** Intercostal muscle Levatores costarum muscle Pectoralis major muscle Pectoralis minor muscle Serratus anterior muscle Subclavius muscle Subcostal muscle Transverse thoracis muscle **J Thorax Muscle, Left** *See H Thorax Muscle, Right* **K Abdomen Muscle, Right** External oblique muscle Internal oblique muscle Pyramidalis muscle Rectus abdominis muscle Transversus abdominis muscle **L Abdomen Muscle, Left** *See K Abdomen Muscle, Right*	**M Perineum Muscle** Bulbospongiosus muscle Cremaster muscle Deep transverse perineal muscle Ischiocavernosus muscle Levator ani muscle Superficial transverse perineal muscle **N Hip Muscle, Right** Gemellus muscle Gluteus maximus muscle Gluteus medius muscle Gluteus minimus muscle Iliacus muscle Obturator muscle Piriformis muscle Psoas muscle Quadratus femoris muscle Tensor fasciae latae muscle **P Hip Muscle, Left** *See N Hip Muscle, Right* **Q Upper Leg Muscle, Right** Adductor brevis muscle Adductor longus muscle Adductor magnus muscle Biceps femoris muscle Gracilis muscle Pectineus muscle Quadriceps (femoris) Rectus femoris muscle Sartorius muscle Semimembranosus muscle Semitendinosus muscle Vastus intermedius muscle Vastus lateralis muscle Vastus medialis muscle **R Upper Leg Muscle, Left** *See Q Upper Leg Muscle, Right* **S Lower Leg Muscle, Right** Extensor digitorum longus muscle Extensor hallucis longus muscle Fibularis brevis muscle Fibularis longus muscle Flexor digitorum longus muscle Flexor hallucis longus muscle Gastrocnemius muscle Peroneus brevis muscle Peroneus longus muscle Popliteus muscle Soleus muscle Tibialis anterior muscle Tibialis posterior muscle **T Lower Leg Muscle, Left** *See S Lower Leg Muscle, Right* **V Foot Muscle, Right** Abductor hallucis muscle Adductor hallucis muscle Extensor digitorum brevis muscle Extensor hallucis brevis muscle Flexor digitorum brevis muscle Flexor hallucis brevis muscle Quadratus plantae muscle **W Foot Muscle, Left** *See V Foot Muscle, Right*	**Ø Open** **4 Percutaneous Endoscopic**	**Z No Device**	**Z No Qualifier**

Ø Medical and Surgical
K Muscles
T Resection Definition: Cutting out or off, without replacement, all of a body part
Explanation: None

Body Part Character 4	Approach Character 5	Device Character 6	Qualifier Character 7
Ø Head Muscle Auricularis muscle Masseter muscle Pterygoid muscle Splenius capitis muscle Temporalis muscle Temporoparietalis muscle **1 Facial Muscle** Buccinator muscle Corrugator supercilii muscle Depressor anguli oris muscle Depressor labii inferioris muscle Depressor septi nasi muscle Depressor supercilii muscle Levator anguli oris muscle Levator labii superioris alaeque nasi muscle Levator labii superioris muscle Mentalis muscle Nasalis muscle Occipitofrontalis muscle Orbicularis oris muscle Procerus muscle Risorius muscle Zygomaticus muscle **2 Neck Muscle, Right** Anterior vertebral muscle Arytenoid muscle Cricothyroid muscle Infrahyoid muscle Levator scapulae muscle Platysma muscle Scalene muscle Splenius cervicis muscle Sternocleidomastoid muscle Suprahyoid muscle Thyroarytenoid muscle **3 Neck Muscle, Left** ***See*** *2 Neck Muscle, Right* **4 Tongue, Palate, Pharynx Muscle** Chondroglossus muscle Genioglossus muscle Hyoglossus muscle Inferior longitudinal muscle Levator veli palatini muscle Palatoglossal muscle Palatopharyngeal muscle Pharyngeal constrictor muscle Salpingopharyngeus muscle Styloglossus muscle Stylopharyngeus muscle Superior longitudinal muscle Tensor veli palatini muscle **5 Shoulder Muscle, Right** Deltoid muscle Infraspinatus muscle Subscapularis muscle Supraspinatus muscle Teres major muscle Teres minor muscle **6 Shoulder Muscle, Left** ***See*** *5 Shoulder Muscle, Right* **7 Upper Arm Muscle, Right** Biceps brachii muscle Brachialis muscle Coracobrachialis muscle Triceps brachii muscle **8 Upper Arm Muscle, Left** ***See*** *7 Upper Arm Muscle, Right* **9 Lower Arm and Wrist Muscle, Right** Anatomical snuffbox Brachioradialis muscle Extensor carpi radialis muscle Extensor carpi ulnaris muscle Flexor carpi radialis muscle Flexor carpi ulnaris muscle Flexor pollicis longus muscle Palmaris longus muscle Pronator quadratus muscle Pronator teres muscle **B Lower Arm and Wrist Muscle, Left** ***See*** *9 Lower Arm and Wrist Muscle, Right* **C Hand Muscle, Right** Hypothenar muscle Palmar interosseous muscle Thenar muscle **D Hand Muscle, Left** ***See*** *C Hand Muscle, Right* **F Trunk Muscle, Right** Coccygeus muscle Erector spinae muscle Interspinalis muscle Intertransversarius muscle Latissimus dorsi muscle Quadratus lumborum muscle Rhomboid major muscle Rhomboid minor muscle Serratus posterior muscle Transversospinalis muscle Trapezius muscle **G Trunk Muscle, Left** ***See*** *F Trunk Muscle, Right* **H Thorax Muscle, Right** ⊞ Intercostal muscle Levatores costarum muscle Pectoralis major muscle Pectoralis minor muscle Serratus anterior muscle Subclavius muscle Subcostal muscle Transverse thoracis muscle **J Thorax Muscle, Left** ⊞ ***See*** *H Thorax Muscle, Right* **K Abdomen Muscle, Right** External oblique muscle Internal oblique muscle Pyramidalis muscle Rectus abdominis muscle Transversus abdominis muscle **L Abdomen Muscle, Left** ***See*** *K Abdomen Muscle, Right* **M Perineum Muscle** Bulbospongiosus muscle Cremaster muscle Deep transverse perineal muscle Ischiocavernosus muscle Levator ani muscle Superficial transverse perineal muscle **N Hip Muscle, Right** Gemellus muscle Gluteus maximus muscle Gluteus medius muscle Gluteus minimus muscle Iliacus muscle Obturator muscle Piriformis muscle Psoas muscle Quadratus femoris muscle Tensor fasciae latae muscle **P Hip Muscle, Left** ***See*** *N Hip Muscle, Right* **Q Upper Leg Muscle, Right** Adductor brevis muscle Adductor longus muscle Adductor magnus muscle Biceps femoris muscle Gracilis muscle Pectineus muscle Quadriceps (femoris) Rectus femoris muscle Sartorius muscle Semimembranosus muscle Semitendinosus muscle Vastus intermedius muscle Vastus lateralis muscle Vastus medialis muscle **R Upper Leg Muscle, Left** ***See*** *Q Upper Leg Muscle, Right* **S Lower Leg Muscle, Right** Extensor digitorum longus muscle Extensor hallucis longus muscle Fibularis brevis muscle Fibularis longus muscle Flexor digitorum longus muscle Flexor hallucis longus muscle Gastrocnemius muscle Peroneus brevis muscle Peroneus longus muscle Popliteus muscle Soleus muscle Tibialis anterior muscle Tibialis posterior muscle **T Lower Leg Muscle, Left** ***See*** *S Lower Leg Muscle, Right* **V Foot Muscle, Right** Abductor hallucis muscle Adductor hallucis muscle Extensor digitorum brevis muscle Extensor hallucis brevis muscle Flexor digitorum brevis muscle Flexor hallucis brevis muscle Quadratus plantae muscle **W Foot Muscle, Left** ***See*** *V Foot Muscle, Right*	**Ø Open** **4 Percutaneous Endoscopic**	**Z No Device**	**Z No Qualifier**

See Appendix L for Procedure Combinations
⊞ ØKT[H,J]ØZZ

Ø Medical and Surgical
K Muscles
U Supplement

Definition: Putting in or on biological or synthetic material that physically reinforces and/or augments the function of a portion of a body part

Explanation: The biological material is non-living, or is living and from the same individual. The body part may have been previously replaced, and the SUPPLEMENT procedure is performed to physically reinforce and/or augment the function of the replaced body part.

Body Part Character 4	Approach Character 5	Device Character 6	Qualifier Character 7
Ø Head Muscle Auricularis muscle; Masseter muscle; Pterygoid muscle; Splenius capitis muscle; Temporalis muscle; Temporoparietalis muscle **1 Facial Muscle** Buccinator muscle; Corrugator supercilii muscle; Depressor anguli oris muscle; Depressor labii inferioris muscle; Depressor septi nasi muscle; Depressor supercilii muscle; Levator anguli oris muscle; Levator labii superioris alaeque nasi muscle; Levator labii superioris muscle; Mentalis muscle; Nasalis muscle; Occipitofrontalis muscle; Orbicularis oris muscle; Procerus muscle; Risorius muscle; Zygomaticus muscle **2 Neck Muscle, Right** Anterior vertebral muscle; Arytenoid muscle; Cricothyroid muscle; Infrahyoid muscle; Levator scapulae muscle; Platysma muscle; Scalene muscle; Splenius cervicis muscle; Sternocleidomastoid muscle; Suprahyoid muscle; Thyroarytenoid muscle **3 Neck Muscle, Left** *See 2 Neck Muscle, Right* **4 Tongue, Palate, Pharynx Muscle** Chondroglossus muscle; Genioglossus muscle; Hyoglossus muscle; Inferior longitudinal muscle; Levator veli palatini muscle; Palatoglossal muscle; Palatopharyngeal muscle; Pharyngeal constrictor muscle; Salpingopharyngeus muscle; Styloglossus muscle; Stylopharyngeus muscle; Superior longitudinal muscle; Tensor veli palatini muscle **5 Shoulder Muscle, Right** Deltoid muscle; Infraspinatus muscle; Subscapularis muscle; Supraspinatus muscle; Teres major muscle; Teres minor muscle **6 Shoulder Muscle, Left** *See 5 Shoulder Muscle, Right* **7 Upper Arm Muscle, Right** Biceps brachii muscle; Brachialis muscle; Coracobrachialis muscle; Triceps brachii muscle **8 Upper Arm Muscle, Left** *See 7 Upper Arm Muscle, Right* **9 Lower Arm and Wrist Muscle, Right** Anatomical snuffbox; Brachioradialis muscle; Extensor carpi radialis muscle; Extensor carpi ulnaris muscle; Flexor carpi radialis muscle; Flexor carpi ulnaris muscle; Flexor pollicis longus muscle; Palmaris longus muscle; Pronator quadratus muscle; Pronator teres muscle **B Lower Arm and Wrist Muscle, Left** *See 9 Lower Arm and Wrist Muscle, Right* **C Hand Muscle, Right** Hypothenar muscle; Palmar interosseous muscle; Thenar muscle **D Hand Muscle, Left** *See C Hand Muscle, Right* **F Trunk Muscle, Right** Coccygeus muscle; Erector spinae muscle; Interspinalis muscle; Intertransversarius muscle; Latissimus dorsi muscle; Quadratus lumborum muscle; Rhomboid major muscle; Rhomboid minor muscle; Serratus posterior muscle; Transversospinalis muscle; Trapezius muscle **G Trunk Muscle, Left** *See F Trunk Muscle, Right* **H Thorax Muscle, Right** Intercostal muscle; Levatores costarum muscle; Pectoralis major muscle; Pectoralis minor muscle; Serratus anterior muscle; Subclavius muscle; Subcostal muscle; Transverse thoracis muscle **J Thorax Muscle, Left** *See H Thorax Muscle, Right* **K Abdomen Muscle, Right** External oblique muscle; Internal oblique muscle; Pyramidalis muscle; Rectus abdominis muscle; Transversus abdominis muscle **L Abdomen Muscle, Left** *See K Abdomen Muscle, Right* **M Perineum Muscle** Bulbospongiosus muscle; Cremaster muscle; Deep transverse perineal muscle; Ischiocavernosus muscle; Levator ani muscle; Superficial transverse perineal muscle **N Hip Muscle, Right** Gemellus muscle; Gluteus maximus muscle; Gluteus medius muscle; Gluteus minimus muscle; Iliacus muscle; Obturator muscle; Piriformis muscle; Psoas muscle; Quadratus femoris muscle; Tensor fasciae latae muscle **P Hip Muscle, Left** *See N Hip Muscle, Right* **Q Upper Leg Muscle, Right** Adductor brevis muscle; Adductor longus muscle; Adductor magnus muscle; Biceps femoris muscle; Gracilis muscle; Pectineus muscle; Quadriceps (femoris); Rectus femoris muscle; Sartorius muscle; Semimembranosus muscle; Semitendinosus muscle; Vastus intermedius muscle; Vastus lateralis muscle; Vastus medialis muscle **R Upper Leg Muscle, Left** *See Q Upper Leg Muscle, Right* **S Lower Leg Muscle, Right** Extensor digitorum longus muscle; Extensor hallucis longus muscle; Fibularis brevis muscle; Fibularis longus muscle; Flexor digitorum longus muscle; Flexor hallucis longus muscle; Gastrocnemius muscle; Peroneus brevis muscle; Peroneus longus muscle; Popliteus muscle; Soleus muscle; Tibialis anterior muscle; Tibialis posterior muscle **T Lower Leg Muscle, Left** *See S Lower Leg Muscle, Right* **V Foot Muscle, Right** Abductor hallucis muscle; Adductor hallucis muscle; Extensor digitorum brevis muscle; Extensor hallucis brevis muscle; Flexor digitorum brevis muscle; Flexor hallucis brevis muscle; Quadratus plantae muscle **W Foot Muscle, Left** *See V Foot Muscle, Right*	**Ø Open** **4 Percutaneous Endoscopic**	**7 Autologous Tissue Substitute** **J Synthetic Substitute** **K Nonautologous Tissue Substitute**	**Z No Qualifier**

Ø Medical and Surgical
K Muscles
W Revision Definition: Correcting, to the extent possible, a portion of a malfunctioning device or the position of a displaced device

Explanation: Revision can include correcting a malfunctioning or displaced device by taking out or putting in components of the device such as a screw or pin

Body Part Character 4	Approach Character 5	Device Character 6	Qualifier Character 7
X Upper Muscle Y Lower Muscle	Ø Open 3 Percutaneous 4 Percutaneous Endoscopic	Ø Drainage Device 7 Autologous Tissue Substitute J Synthetic Substitute K Nonautologous Tissue Substitute M Stimulator Lead Y Other Device	Z No Qualifier
X Upper Muscle Y Lower Muscle	X External	Ø Drainage Device 7 Autologous Tissue Substitute J Synthetic Substitute K Nonautologous Tissue Substitute M Stimulator Lead	Z No Qualifier

Non-OR ØKW[X,Y][3,4]YZ
Non-OR ØKW[X,Y]X[Ø,7,J,K,M]Z

Ø Medical and Surgical
K Muscles
X Transfer Definition: Moving, without taking out, all or a portion of a body part to another location to take over the function of all or a portion of a body part
Explanation: The body part transferred remains connected to its vascular and nervous supply

Body Part Character 4	Approach Character 5	Device Character 6	Qualifier Character 7
Ø Head Muscle Auricularis muscle Masseter muscle Pterygoid muscle Splenius capitis muscle Temporalis muscle Temporoparietalis muscle **1 Facial Muscle** Buccinator muscle Corrugator supercilii muscle Depressor anguli oris muscle Depressor labii inferioris muscle Depressor septi nasi muscle Depressor supercilii muscle Levator anguli oris muscle Levator labii superioris alaeque nasi muscle Levator labii superioris muscle Mentalis muscle Nasalis muscle Occipitofrontalis muscle Orbicularis oris muscle Procerus muscle Risorius muscle Zygomaticus muscle **2 Neck Muscle, Right** Anterior vertebral muscle Arytenoid muscle Cricothyroid muscle Infrahyoid muscle Levator scapulae muscle Platysma muscle Scalene muscle Splenius cervicis muscle Sternocleidomastoid muscle Suprahyoid muscle Thyroarytenoid muscle **3 Neck Muscle, Left** ***See*** *2 Neck Muscle, Right* **4 Tongue, Palate, Pharynx Muscle** Chondroglossus muscle Genioglossus muscle Hyoglossus muscle Inferior longitudinal muscle Levator veli palatini muscle Palatoglossal muscle Palatopharyngeal muscle Pharyngeal constrictor muscle Salpingopharyngeus muscle Styloglossus muscle Stylopharyngeus muscle Superior longitudinal muscle Tensor veli palatini muscle **5 Shoulder Muscle, Right** Deltoid muscle Infraspinatus muscle Subscapularis muscle Supraspinatus muscle Teres major muscle Teres minor muscle **6 Shoulder Muscle, Left** ***See*** *5 Shoulder Muscle, Right* **7 Upper Arm Muscle, Right** Biceps brachii muscle Brachialis muscle Coracobrachialis muscle Triceps brachii muscle **8 Upper Arm Muscle, Left** ***See*** *7 Upper Arm Muscle, Right* **9 Lower Arm and Wrist Muscle, Right** Anatomical snuffbox Brachioradialis muscle Extensor carpi radialis muscle Extensor carpi ulnaris muscle Flexor carpi radialis muscle Flexor carpi ulnaris muscle Flexor pollicis longus muscle Palmaris longus muscle Pronator quadratus muscle Pronator teres muscle **B Lower Arm and Wrist Muscle, Left** ***See*** *9 Lower Arm and Wrist Muscle, Right* **C Hand Muscle, Right** Hypothenar muscle Palmar interosseous muscle Thenar muscle **D Hand Muscle, Left** ***See*** *C Hand Muscle, Right* **H Thorax Muscle, Right** Intercostal muscle Levatores costarum muscle Pectoralis major muscle Pectoralis minor muscle Serratus anterior muscle Subclavius muscle Subcostal muscle Transverse thoracis muscle **J Thorax Muscle, Left** ***See*** *H Thorax Muscle, Right* **M Perineum Muscle** Bulbospongiosus muscle Cremaster muscle Deep transverse perineal muscle Ischiocavernosus muscle Levator ani muscle Superficial transverse perineal muscle **N Hip Muscle, Right** Gemellus muscle Gluteus maximus muscle Gluteus medius muscle Gluteus minimus muscle Iliacus muscle Obturator muscle Piriformis muscle Psoas muscle Quadratus femoris muscle Tensor fasciae latae muscle **P Hip Muscle, Left** ***See*** *N Hip Muscle, Right* **Q Upper Leg Muscle, Right** Adductor brevis muscle Adductor longus muscle Adductor magnus muscle Biceps femoris muscle Gracilis muscle Pectineus muscle Quadriceps (femoris) Rectus femoris muscle Sartorius muscle Semimembranosus muscle Semitendinosus muscle Vastus intermedius muscle Vastus lateralis muscle Vastus medialis muscle **R Upper Leg Muscle, Left** ***See*** *Q Upper Leg Muscle, Right* **S Lower Leg Muscle, Right** Extensor digitorum longus muscle Extensor hallucis longus muscle Fibularis brevis muscle Fibularis longus muscle Flexor digitorum longus muscle Flexor hallucis longus muscle Gastrocnemius muscle Peroneus brevis muscle Peroneus longus muscle Popliteus muscle Soleus muscle Tibialis anterior muscle Tibialis posterior muscle **T Lower Leg Muscle, Left** ***See*** *S Lower Leg Muscle, Right* **V Foot Muscle, Right** Abductor hallucis muscle Adductor hallucis muscle Extensor digitorum brevis muscle Extensor hallucis brevis muscle Flexor digitorum brevis muscle Flexor hallucis brevis muscle Quadratus plantae muscle **W Foot Muscle, Left** ***See*** *V Foot Muscle, Right*	**Ø** Open **4** Percutaneous Endoscopic	**Z** No Device	**Ø** Skin **1** Subcutaneous Tissue **2** Skin and Subcutaneous Tissue **Z** No Qualifier

ØKX Continued on next page

Ø Medical and Surgical
K Muscles
X Transfer

ØKX Continued

Definition: Moving, without taking out, all or a portion of a body part to another location to take over the function of all or a portion of a body part

Explanation: The body part transferred remains connected to its vascular and nervous supply

Body Part Character 4	Approach Character 5	Device Character 6	Qualifier Character 7
F Trunk Muscle, Right Coccygeus muscle Erector spinae muscle Interspinalis muscle Intertransversarius muscle Latissimus dorsi muscle Quadratus lumborum muscle Rhomboid major muscle Rhomboid minor muscle Serratus posterior muscle Transversospinalis muscle Trapezius muscle **G Trunk Muscle, Left** *See F Trunk Muscle, Right*	**Ø Open** **4 Percutaneous Endoscopic**	**Z No Device**	**Ø Skin** **1 Subcutaneous Tissue** **2 Skin and Subcutaneous Tissue** **5 Latissimus Dorsi Myocutaneous Flap** **7 Deep Inferior Epigastric Artery Perforator Flap** **8 Superficial Inferior Epigastric Artery Flap** **9 Gluteal Artery Perforator Flap** **Z No Qualifier**
K Abdomen Muscle, Right External oblique muscle Internal oblique muscle Pyramidalis muscle Rectus abdominis muscle Transversus abdominis muscle **L Abdomen Muscle, Left** *See K Abdomen Muscle, Right*	**Ø Open** **4 Percutaneous Endoscopic**	**Z No Device**	**Ø Skin** **1 Subcutaneous Tissue** **2 Skin and Subcutaneous Tissue** **6 Transverse Rectus Abdominis Myocutaneous Flap** **Z No Qualifier**

Tendons ØL2–ØLX

Character Meanings*

This Character Meaning table is provided as a guide to assist the user in the identification of character members that may be found in this section of code tables. It **SHOULD NOT** be used to build a PCS code.

Operation–Character 3	Body Part–Character 4	Approach–Character 5	Device–Character 6	Qualifier–Character 7
2 Change	Ø Head and Neck Tendon	Ø Open	Ø Drainage Device	X Diagnostic
5 Destruction	1 Shoulder Tendon, Right	3 Percutaneous	7 Autologous Tissue Substitute	Z No Qualifier
8 Division	2 Shoulder Tendon, Left	4 Percutaneous Endoscopic	J Synthetic Substitute	
9 Drainage	3 Upper Arm Tendon, Right	X External	K Nonautologous Tissue Substitute	
B Excision	4 Upper Arm Tendon, Left		Y Other Device	
C Extirpation	5 Lower Arm and Wrist Tendon, Right		Z No Device	
D Extraction	6 Lower Arm and Wrist Tendon, Left			
H Insertion	7 Hand Tendon, Right			
J Inspection	8 Hand Tendon, Left			
M Reattachment	9 Trunk Tendon, Right			
N Release	B Trunk Tendon, Left			
P Removal	C Thorax Tendon, Right			
Q Repair	D Thorax Tendon, Left			
R Replacement	F Abdomen Tendon, Right			
S Reposition	G Abdomen Tendon, Left			
T Resection	H Perineum Tendon			
U Supplement	J Hip Tendon, Right			
W Revision	K Hip Tendon, Left			
X Transfer	L Upper Leg Tendon, Right			
	M Upper Leg Tendon, Left			
	N Lower Leg Tendon, Right			
	P Lower Leg Tendon, Left			
	Q Knee Tendon, Right			
	R Knee Tendon, Left			
	S Ankle Tendon, Right			
	T Ankle Tendon, Left			
	V Foot Tendon, Right			
	W Foot Tendon, Left			
	X Upper Tendon			
	Y Lower Tendon			

* Includes synovial membrane.

AHA Coding Clinic for table ØL8
2016, 3Q, 30 Resection of femur with interposition arthroplasty

AHA Coding Clinic for table ØLB
2017, 2Q, 21 Arthroscopic anterior cruciate ligament revision using autograft with anterolateral ligament reconstruction
2015, 3Q, 26 Thumb arthroplasty with resection of trapezium
2014, 3Q, 14 Application of TheraSkin® and excisional debridement
2014, 3Q, 18 Placement of reverse sural fasciocutaneous pedicle flap

AHA Coding Clinic for table ØLD
2017, 4Q, 41 Extraction procedures

AHA Coding Clinic for table ØLQ
2016, 3Q, 32 Rotator cuff repair, tenodesis, decompression, acromioplasty and coracoplasty
2015, 2Q, 11 Repair of patellar and quadriceps tendons with allograft
2013, 3Q, 20 Superior labrum anterior posterior (SLAP) repair and subacromial decompression

AHA Coding Clinic for table ØLS
2016, 3Q, 32 Rotator cuff repair, tenodesis, decompression, acromioplasty and coracoplasty
2015, 3Q, 14 Endoprosthetic replacement of humerus and tendon reattachment

AHA Coding Clinic for table ØLU
2015, 2Q, 11 Repair of patellar and quadriceps tendons with allograft

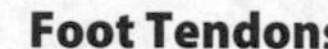

Foot Tendons

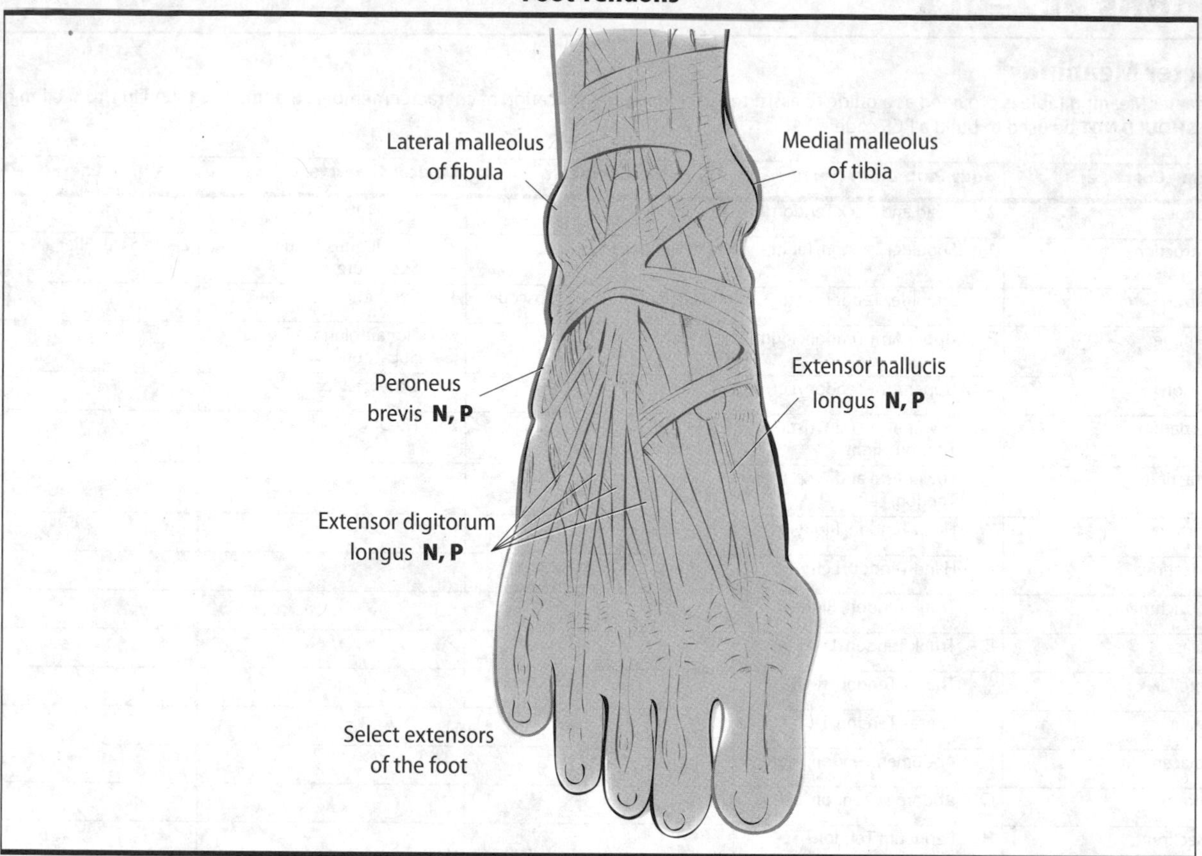

Shoulder Tendons

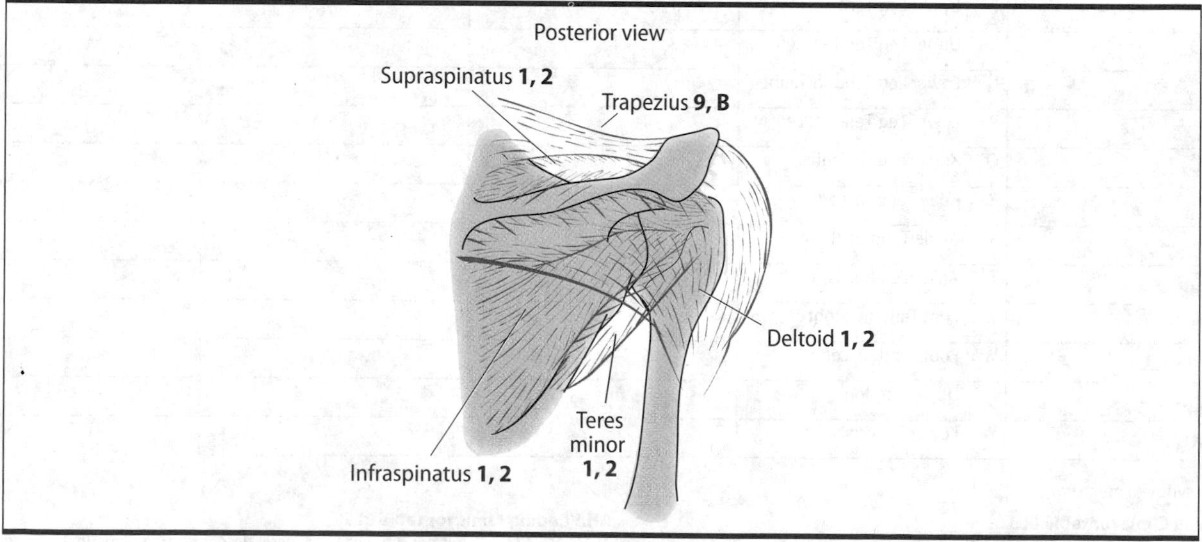

Tendons of Wrist and Hand

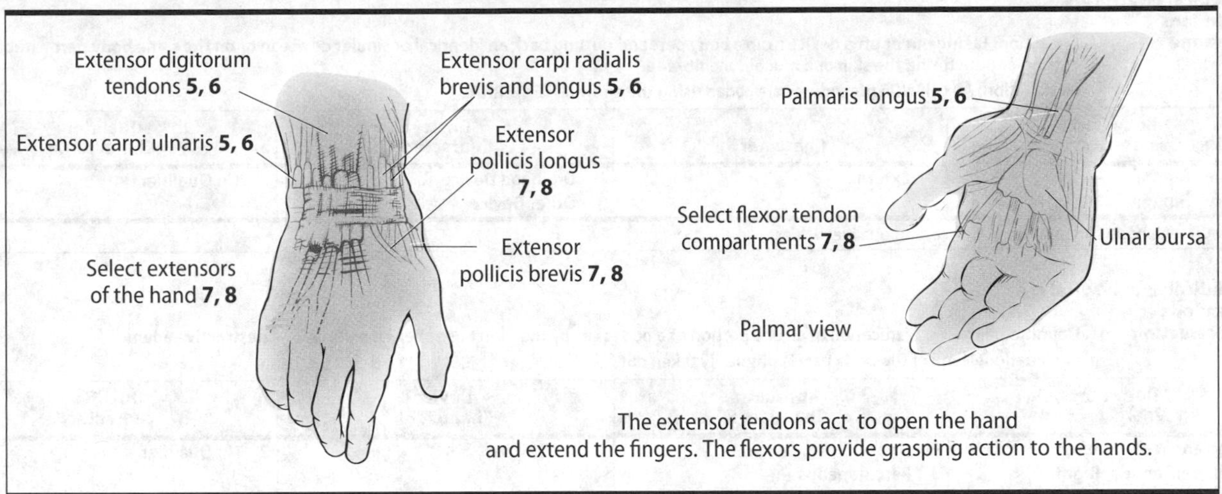

The extensor tendons act to open the hand and extend the fingers. The flexors provide grasping action to the hands.

Leg Muscles and Tendons

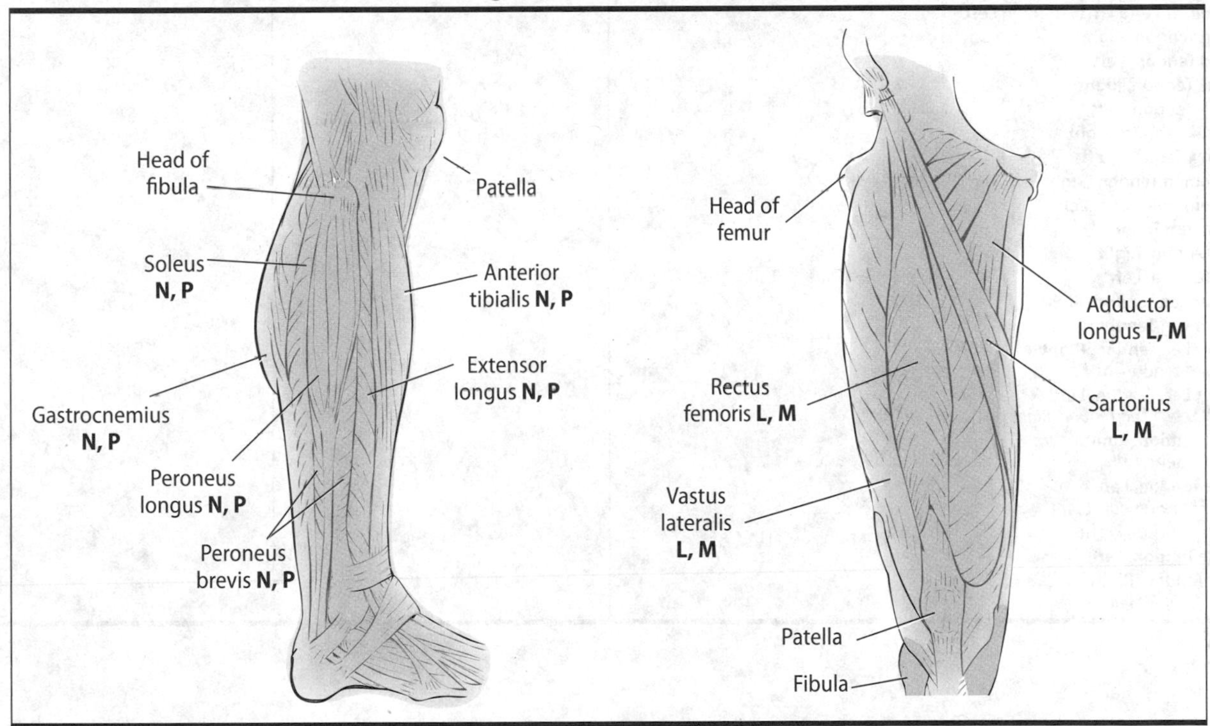

Ø Medical and Surgical
L Tendons
2 Change

Definition: Taking out or off a device from a body part and putting back an identical or similar device in or on the same body part without cutting or puncturing the skin or a mucous membrane

Explanation: All CHANGE procedures are coded using the approach EXTERNAL

Body Part Character 4	Approach Character 5	Device Character 6	Qualifier Character 7
X Upper Tendon Y Lower Tendon	X External	Ø Drainage Device Y Other Device	Z No Qualifier

Non-OR All body part, approach, device, and qualifier values

Ø Medical and Surgical
L Tendons
5 Destruction

Definition: Physical eradication of all or a portion of a body part by the direct use of energy, force, or a destructive agent

Explanation: None of the body part is physically taken out

Body Part Character 4	Approach Character 5	Device Character 6	Qualifier Character 7
Ø Head and Neck Tendon 1 Shoulder Tendon, Right 2 Shoulder Tendon, Left 3 Upper Arm Tendon, Right 4 Upper Arm Tendon, Left 5 Lower Arm and Wrist Tendon, Right 6 Lower Arm and Wrist Tendon, Left 7 Hand Tendon, Right 8 Hand Tendon, Left 9 Trunk Tendon, Right B Trunk Tendon, Left C Thorax Tendon, Right D Thorax Tendon, Left F Abdomen Tendon, Right G Abdomen Tendon, Left H Perineum Tendon J Hip Tendon, Right K Hip Tendon, Left L Upper Leg Tendon, Right M Upper Leg Tendon, Left N Lower Leg Tendon, Right Achilles tendon P Lower Leg Tendon, Left *See N Lower Leg Tendon, Right* Q Knee Tendon, Right Patellar tendon R Knee Tendon, Left *See Q Knee Tendon, Right* S Ankle Tendon, Right T Ankle Tendon, Left V Foot Tendon, Right W Foot Tendon, Left	Ø Open 3 Percutaneous 4 Percutaneous Endoscopic	Z No Device	Z No Qualifier

Ø Medical and Surgical
L Tendons
8 Division Definition: Cutting into a body part, without draining fluids and/or gases from the body part, in order to separate or transect a body part
Explanation: All or a portion of the body part is separated into two or more portions

Body Part Character 4	Approach Character 5	Device Character 6	Qualifier Character 7
Ø Head and Neck Tendon 1 Shoulder Tendon, Right 2 Shoulder Tendon, Left 3 Upper Arm Tendon, Right 4 Upper Arm Tendon, Left 5 Lower Arm and Wrist Tendon, Right 6 Lower Arm and Wrist Tendon, Left 7 Hand Tendon, Right 8 Hand Tendon, Left 9 Trunk Tendon, Right B Trunk Tendon, Left C Thorax Tendon, Right D Thorax Tendon, Left F Abdomen Tendon, Right G Abdomen Tendon, Left H Perineum Tendon J Hip Tendon, Right K Hip Tendon, Left L Upper Leg Tendon, Right M Upper Leg Tendon, Left N Lower Leg Tendon, Right Achilles tendon P Lower Leg Tendon, Left *See* *N Lower Leg Tendon, Right* Q Knee Tendon, Right Patellar tendon R Knee Tendon, Left *See* *Q Knee Tendon, Right* S Ankle Tendon, Right T Ankle Tendon, Left V Foot Tendon, Right W Foot Tendon, Left	Ø Open 3 Percutaneous 4 Percutaneous Endoscopic	Z No Device	Z No Qualifier

Ø Medical and Surgical
L Tendons
9 Drainage Definition: Taking or letting out fluids and/or gases from a body part
Explanation: The qualifier DIAGNOSTIC is used to identify drainage procedures that are biopsies

Body Part Character 4	Approach Character 5	Device Character 6	Qualifier Character 7
Ø Head and Neck Tendon **1** Shoulder Tendon, Right **2** Shoulder Tendon, Left **3** Upper Arm Tendon, Right **4** Upper Arm Tendon, Left **5** Lower Arm and Wrist Tendon, Right **6** Lower Arm and Wrist Tendon, Left **7** Hand Tendon, Right **8** Hand Tendon, Left **9** Trunk Tendon, Right **B** Trunk Tendon, Left **C** Thorax Tendon, Right **D** Thorax Tendon, Left **F** Abdomen Tendon, Right **G** Abdomen Tendon, Left **H** Perineum Tendon **J** Hip Tendon, Right **K** Hip Tendon, Left **L** Upper Leg Tendon, Right **M** Upper Leg Tendon, Left **N** Lower Leg Tendon, Right Achilles tendon **P** Lower Leg Tendon, Left *See N Lower Leg Tendon, Right* **Q** Knee Tendon, Right Patellar tendon **R** Knee Tendon, Left *See Q Knee Tendon, Right* **S** Ankle Tendon, Right **T** Ankle Tendon, Left **V** Foot Tendon, Right **W** Foot Tendon, Left	**Ø** Open **3** Percutaneous **4** Percutaneous Endoscopic	**Ø** Drainage Device	**Z** No Qualifier
Ø Head and Neck Tendon **1** Shoulder Tendon, Right **2** Shoulder Tendon, Left **3** Upper Arm Tendon, Right **4** Upper Arm Tendon, Left **5** Lower Arm and Wrist Tendon, Right **6** Lower Arm and Wrist Tendon, Left **7** Hand Tendon, Right **8** Hand Tendon, Left **9** Trunk Tendon, Right **B** Trunk Tendon, Left **C** Thorax Tendon, Right **D** Thorax Tendon, Left **F** Abdomen Tendon, Right **G** Abdomen Tendon, Left **H** Perineum Tendon **J** Hip Tendon, Right **K** Hip Tendon, Left **L** Upper Leg Tendon, Right **M** Upper Leg Tendon, Left **N** Lower Leg Tendon, Right Achilles tendon **P** Lower Leg Tendon, Left *See N Lower Leg Tendon, Right* **Q** Knee Tendon, Right Patellar tendon **R** Knee Tendon, Left *See Q Knee Tendon, Right* **S** Ankle Tendon, Right **T** Ankle Tendon, Left **V** Foot Tendon, Right **W** Foot Tendon, Left	**Ø** Open **3** Percutaneous **4** Percutaneous Endoscopic	**Z** No Device	**X** Diagnostic **Z** No Qualifier

Non-OR ØL9[Ø,1,2,3,4,5,6,7,8,9,B,C,D,F,G,H,J,K,L,M,N,P,Q,R,S,T,V,W]3ØZ
Non-OR ØL9[Ø,1,2,3,4,5,6,7,8,9,B,C,D,F,G,H,J,K,L,M,N,P,Q,R,S,T,V,W]3ZZ
Non-OR ØL9[7,8]4ZZ

Ø Medical and Surgical
L Tendons
B Excision Definition: Cutting out or off, without replacement, a portion of a body part
Explanation: The qualifier DIAGNOSTIC is used to identify excision procedures that are biopsies

Body Part Character 4	Approach Character 5	Device Character 6	Qualifier Character 7
Ø Head and Neck Tendon **1 Shoulder Tendon, Right** **2 Shoulder Tendon, Left** **3 Upper Arm Tendon, Right** **4 Upper Arm Tendon, Left** **5 Lower Arm and Wrist Tendon, Right** **6 Lower Arm and Wrist Tendon, Left** **7 Hand Tendon, Right** **8 Hand Tendon, Left** **9 Trunk Tendon, Right** **B Trunk Tendon, Left** **C Thorax Tendon, Right** **D Thorax Tendon, Left** **F Abdomen Tendon, Right** **G Abdomen Tendon, Left** **H Perineum Tendon** **J Hip Tendon, Right** **K Hip Tendon, Left** **L Upper Leg Tendon, Right** **M Upper Leg Tendon, Left** **N Lower Leg Tendon, Right** Achilles tendon **P Lower Leg Tendon, Left** ***See*** *N Lower Leg Tendon, Right* **Q Knee Tendon, Right** Patellar tendon **R Knee Tendon, Left** ***See*** *Q Knee Tendon, Right* **S Ankle Tendon, Right** **T Ankle Tendon, Left** **V Foot Tendon, Right** **W Foot Tendon, Left**	**Ø Open** **3 Percutaneous** **4 Percutaneous Endoscopic**	**Z No Device**	**X Diagnostic** **Z No Qualifier**

Ø Medical and Surgical
L Tendons
C Extirpation Definition: Taking or cutting out solid matter from a body part

Explanation: The solid matter may be an abnormal byproduct of a biological function or a foreign body; it may be imbedded in a body part or in the lumen of a tubular body part. The solid matter may or may not have been previously broken into pieces.

Body Part Character 4	Approach Character 5	Device Character 6	Qualifier Character 7
Ø Head and Neck Tendon **1 Shoulder Tendon, Right** **2 Shoulder Tendon, Left** **3 Upper Arm Tendon, Right** **4 Upper Arm Tendon, Left** **5 Lower Arm and Wrist Tendon, Right** **6 Lower Arm and Wrist Tendon, Left** **7 Hand Tendon, Right** **8 Hand Tendon, Left** **9 Trunk Tendon, Right** **B Trunk Tendon, Left** **C Thorax Tendon, Right** **D Thorax Tendon, Left** **F Abdomen Tendon, Right** **G Abdomen Tendon, Left** **H Perineum Tendon** **J Hip Tendon, Right** **K Hip Tendon, Left** **L Upper Leg Tendon, Right** **M Upper Leg Tendon, Left** **N Lower Leg Tendon, Right** Achilles tendon **P Lower Leg Tendon, Left** *See N Lower Leg Tendon, Right* **Q Knee Tendon, Right** Patellar tendon **R Knee Tendon, Left** *See Q Knee Tendon, Right* **S Ankle Tendon, Right** **T Ankle Tendon, Left** **V Foot Tendon, Right** **W Foot Tendon, Left**	**Ø Open** **3 Percutaneous** **4 Percutaneous Endoscopic**	**Z No Device**	**Z No Qualifier**

Ø Medical and Surgical
L Tendons
D Extraction Definition: Pulling or stripping out or off all or a portion of a body part by the use of force

Explanation: The qualifier DIAGNOSTIC is used to identify extraction procedures that are biopsies

Body Part Character 4	Approach Character 5	Device Character 6	Qualifier Character 7
Ø Head and Neck Tendon 1 Shoulder Tendon, Right 2 Shoulder Tendon, Left 3 Upper Arm Tendon, Right 4 Upper Arm Tendon, Left 5 Lower Arm and Wrist Tendon, Right 6 Lower Arm and Wrist Tendon, Left 7 Hand Tendon, Right 8 Hand Tendon, Left 9 Trunk Tendon, Right B Trunk Tendon, Left C Thorax Tendon, Right D Thorax Tendon, Left F Abdomen Tendon, Right G Abdomen Tendon, Left H Perineum Tendon J Hip Tendon, Right K Hip Tendon, Left L Upper Leg Tendon, Right M Upper Leg Tendon, Left N Lower Leg Tendon, Right Achilles tendon P Lower Leg Tendon, Left *See N Lower Leg Tendon, Right* Q Knee Tendon, Right Patellar tendon R Knee Tendon, Left *See Q Knee Tendon, Right* S Ankle Tendon, Right T Ankle Tendon, Left V Foot Tendon, Right W Foot Tendon, Left	Ø Open	Z No Device	Z No Qualifier

Ø Medical and Surgical
L Tendons
H Insertion Definition: Putting in a nonbiological appliance that monitors, assists, performs, or prevents a physiological function but does not physically take the place of a body part

Explanation: None

Body Part Character 4	Approach Character 5	Device Character 6	Qualifier Character 7
X Upper Tendon Y Lower Tendon	Ø Open 3 Percutaneous 4 Percutaneous Endoscopic	Y Other Device	Z No Qualifier

Non-OR ØLH[X,Y][3,4]YZ

Ø Medical and Surgical
L Tendons
J Inspection Definition: Visually and/or manually exploring a body part

Explanation: Visual exploration may be performed with or without optical instrumentation. Manual exploration may be performed directly or through intervening body layers.

Body Part Character 4	Approach Character 5	Device Character 6	Qualifier Character 7
X Upper Tendon Y Lower Tendon	Ø Open 3 Percutaneous 4 Percutaneous Endoscopic X External	Z No Device	Z No Qualifier

Non-OR ØLJ[X,Y][3,X]ZZ

Ø Medical and Surgical
L Tendons
M Reattachment Definition: Putting back in or on all or a portion of a separated body part to its normal location or other suitable location
Explanation: Vascular circulation and nervous pathways may or may not be reestablished

Body Part Character 4	Approach Character 5	Device Character 6	Qualifier Character 7
Ø Head and Neck Tendon 1 Shoulder Tendon, Right 2 Shoulder Tendon, Left 3 Upper Arm Tendon, Right 4 Upper Arm Tendon, Left 5 Lower Arm and Wrist Tendon, Right 6 Lower Arm and Wrist Tendon, Left 7 Hand Tendon, Right 8 Hand Tendon, Left 9 Trunk Tendon, Right B Trunk Tendon, Left C Thorax Tendon, Right D Thorax Tendon, Left F Abdomen Tendon, Right G Abdomen Tendon, Left H Perineum Tendon J Hip Tendon, Right K Hip Tendon, Left L Upper Leg Tendon, Right M Upper Leg Tendon, Left N Lower Leg Tendon, Right Achilles tendon P Lower Leg Tendon, Left *See N Lower Leg Tendon, Right* Q Knee Tendon, Right Patellar tendon R Knee Tendon, Left *See Q Knee Tendon, Right* S Ankle Tendon, Right T Ankle Tendon, Left V Foot Tendon, Right W Foot Tendon, Left	Ø Open 4 Percutaneous Endoscopic	Z No Device	Z No Qualifier

Ø Medical and Surgical
L Tendons
N Release Definition: Freeing a body part from an abnormal physical constraint by cutting or by the use of force
Explanation: Some of the restraining tissue may be taken out but none of the body part is taken out

Body Part Character 4	Approach Character 5	Device Character 6	Qualifier Character 7
Ø Head and Neck Tendon 1 Shoulder Tendon, Right 2 Shoulder Tendon, Left 3 Upper Arm Tendon, Right 4 Upper Arm Tendon, Left 5 Lower Arm and Wrist Tendon, Right 6 Lower Arm and Wrist Tendon, Left 7 Hand Tendon, Right 8 Hand Tendon, Left 9 Trunk Tendon, Right B Trunk Tendon, Left C Thorax Tendon, Right D Thorax Tendon, Left F Abdomen Tendon, Right G Abdomen Tendon, Left H Perineum Tendon J Hip Tendon, Right K Hip Tendon, Left L Upper Leg Tendon, Right M Upper Leg Tendon, Left N Lower Leg Tendon, Right Achilles tendon P Lower Leg Tendon, Left *See N Lower Leg Tendon, Right* Q Knee Tendon, Right Patellar tendon R Knee Tendon, Left *See Q Knee Tendon, Right* S Ankle Tendon, Right T Ankle Tendon, Left V Foot Tendon, Right W Foot Tendon, Left	Ø Open 3 Percutaneous 4 Percutaneous Endoscopic X External	Z No Device	Z No Qualifier

Non-OR ØLN[Ø,1,2,3,4,5,6,7,8,9,B,C,D,F,G,H,J,K,L,M,N,P,Q,R,S,T,V,W]XZZ

Ø Medical and Surgical
L Tendons
P Removal Definition: Taking out or off a device from a body part

Explanation: If a device is taken out and a similar device put in without cutting or puncturing the skin or mucous membrane, the procedure is coded to the root operation CHANGE. Otherwise, the procedure for taking out a device is coded to the root operation REMOVAL.

Body Part Character 4	Approach Character 5	Device Character 6	Qualifier Character 7
X Upper Tendon Y Lower Tendon	Ø Open 3 Percutaneous 4 Percutaneous Endoscopic	Ø Drainage Device 7 Autologous Tissue Substitute J Synthetic Substitute K Nonautologous Tissue Substitute Y Other Device	Z No Qualifier
X Upper Tendon Y Lower Tendon	X External	Ø Drainage Device	Z No Qualifier

Non-OR ØLP[X,Y]3ØZ
Non-OR ØLP[X,Y][3,4]YZ
Non-OR ØLP[X,Y]XØZ

Ø Medical and Surgical
L Tendons
Q Repair Definition: Restoring, to the extent possible, a body part to its normal anatomic structure and function

Explanation: Used only when the method to accomplish the repair is not one of the other root operations

Body Part Character 4	Approach Character 5	Device Character 6	Qualifier Character 7
Ø Head and Neck Tendon 1 Shoulder Tendon, Right 2 Shoulder Tendon, Left 3 Upper Arm Tendon, Right 4 Upper Arm Tendon, Left 5 Lower Arm and Wrist Tendon, Right 6 Lower Arm and Wrist Tendon, Left 7 Hand Tendon, Right 8 Hand Tendon, Left 9 Trunk Tendon, Right B Trunk Tendon, Left C Thorax Tendon, Right D Thorax Tendon, Left F Abdomen Tendon, Right G Abdomen Tendon, Left H Perineum Tendon J Hip Tendon, Right K Hip Tendon, Left L Upper Leg Tendon, Right M Upper Leg Tendon, Left N Lower Leg Tendon, Right Achilles tendon P Lower Leg Tendon, Left *See N Lower Leg Tendon, Right* Q Knee Tendon, Right Patellar tendon R Knee Tendon, Left *See Q Knee Tendon, Right* S Ankle Tendon, Right T Ankle Tendon, Left V Foot Tendon, Right W Foot Tendon, Left	Ø Open 3 Percutaneous 4 Percutaneous Endoscopic	Z No Device	Z No Qualifier

Ø Medical and Surgical
L Tendons
R Replacement Definition: Putting in or on biological or synthetic material that physically takes the place and/or function of all or a portion of a body part

Explanation: The body part may have been taken out or replaced, or may be taken out, physically eradicated, or rendered nonfunctional during the REPLACEMENT procedure. A REMOVAL procedure is coded for taking out the device used in a previous replacement procedure.

Body Part Character 4	Approach Character 5	Device Character 6	Qualifier Character 7
Ø Head and Neck Tendon 1 Shoulder Tendon, Right 2 Shoulder Tendon, Left 3 Upper Arm Tendon, Right 4 Upper Arm Tendon, Left 5 Lower Arm and Wrist Tendon, Right 6 Lower Arm and Wrist Tendon, Left 7 Hand Tendon, Right 8 Hand Tendon, Left 9 Trunk Tendon, Right B Trunk Tendon, Left C Thorax Tendon, Right D Thorax Tendon, Left F Abdomen Tendon, Right G Abdomen Tendon, Left H Perineum Tendon J Hip Tendon, Right K Hip Tendon, Left L Upper Leg Tendon, Right M Upper Leg Tendon, Left N Lower Leg Tendon, Right Achilles tendon P Lower Leg Tendon, Left *See N Lower Leg Tendon, Right* Q Knee Tendon, Right Patellar tendon R Knee Tendon, Left *See Q Knee Tendon, Right* S Ankle Tendon, Right T Ankle Tendon, Left V Foot Tendon, Right W Foot Tendon, Left	Ø Open 4 Percutaneous Endoscopic	7 Autologous Tissue Substitute J Synthetic Substitute K Nonautologous Tissue Substitute	Z No Qualifier

Ø Medical and Surgical
L Tendons
S Reposition Definition: Moving to its normal location, or other suitable location, all or a portion of a body part

Explanation: The body part is moved to a new location from an abnormal location, or from a normal location where it is not functioning correctly. The body part may or may not be cut out or off to be moved to the new location.

Body Part Character 4	Approach Character 5	Device Character 6	Qualifier Character 7
Ø Head and Neck Tendon 1 Shoulder Tendon, Right 2 Shoulder Tendon, Left 3 Upper Arm Tendon, Right 4 Upper Arm Tendon, Left 5 Lower Arm and Wrist Tendon, Right 6 Lower Arm and Wrist Tendon, Left 7 Hand Tendon, Right 8 Hand Tendon, Left 9 Trunk Tendon, Right B Trunk Tendon, Left C Thorax Tendon, Right D Thorax Tendon, Left F Abdomen Tendon, Right G Abdomen Tendon, Left H Perineum Tendon J Hip Tendon, Right K Hip Tendon, Left L Upper Leg Tendon, Right M Upper Leg Tendon, Left N Lower Leg Tendon, Right Achilles tendon P Lower Leg Tendon, Left *See N Lower Leg Tendon, Right* Q Knee Tendon, Right Patellar tendon R Knee Tendon, Left *See Q Knee Tendon, Right* S Ankle Tendon, Right T Ankle Tendon, Left V Foot Tendon, Right W Foot Tendon, Left	Ø Open 4 Percutaneous Endoscopic	Z No Device	Z No Qualifier

Ø Medical and Surgical
L Tendons
T Resection Definition: Cutting out or off, without replacement, all of a body part

Explanation: None

Body Part Character 4	Approach Character 5	Device Character 6	Qualifier Character 7
Ø Head and Neck Tendon 1 Shoulder Tendon, Right 2 Shoulder Tendon, Left 3 Upper Arm Tendon, Right 4 Upper Arm Tendon, Left 5 Lower Arm and Wrist Tendon, Right 6 Lower Arm and Wrist Tendon, Left 7 Hand Tendon, Right 8 Hand Tendon, Left 9 Trunk Tendon, Right B Trunk Tendon, Left C Thorax Tendon, Right D Thorax Tendon, Left F Abdomen Tendon, Right G Abdomen Tendon, Left H Perineum Tendon J Hip Tendon, Right K Hip Tendon, Left L Upper Leg Tendon, Right M Upper Leg Tendon, Left N Lower Leg Tendon, Right Achilles tendon P Lower Leg Tendon, Left *See N Lower Leg Tendon, Right* Q Knee Tendon, Right Patellar tendon R Knee Tendon, Left *See Q Knee Tendon, Right* S Ankle Tendon, Right T Ankle Tendon, Left V Foot Tendon, Right W Foot Tendon, Left	Ø Open 4 Percutaneous Endoscopic	Z No Device	Z No Qualifier

Ø Medical and Surgical
L Tendons
U Supplement Definition: Putting in or on biological or synthetic material that physically reinforces and/or augments the function of a portion of a body part

Explanation: The biological material is non-living, or is living and from the same individual. The body part may have been previously replaced, and the SUPPLEMENT procedure is performed to physically reinforce and/or augment the function of the replaced body part.

Body Part Character 4	Approach Character 5	Device Character 6	Qualifier Character 7
Ø Head and Neck Tendon 1 Shoulder Tendon, Right 2 Shoulder Tendon, Left 3 Upper Arm Tendon, Right 4 Upper Arm Tendon, Left 5 Lower Arm and Wrist Tendon, Right 6 Lower Arm and Wrist Tendon, Left 7 Hand Tendon, Right 8 Hand Tendon, Left 9 Trunk Tendon, Right B Trunk Tendon, Left C Thorax Tendon, Right D Thorax Tendon, Left F Abdomen Tendon, Right G Abdomen Tendon, Left H Perineum Tendon J Hip Tendon, Right K Hip Tendon, Left L Upper Leg Tendon, Right M Upper Leg Tendon, Left N Lower Leg Tendon, Right Achilles tendon P Lower Leg Tendon, Left *See N Lower Leg Tendon, Right* Q Knee Tendon, Right Patellar tendon R Knee Tendon, Left *See Q Knee Tendon, Right* S Ankle Tendon, Right T Ankle Tendon, Left V Foot Tendon, Right W Foot Tendon, Left	Ø Open 4 Percutaneous Endoscopic	7 Autologous Tissue Substitute J Synthetic Substitute K Nonautologous Tissue Substitute	Z No Qualifier

Tendons

ØLW–ØLX

Ø Medical and Surgical
L Tendons
W Revision

Definition: Correcting, to the extent possible, a portion of a malfunctioning device or the position of a displaced device

Explanation: Revision can include correcting a malfunctioning or displaced device by taking out or putting in components of the device such as a screw or pin

Body Part Character 4	Approach Character 5	Device Character 6	Qualifier Character 7
X Upper Tendon Y Lower Tendon	Ø Open 3 Percutaneous 4 Percutaneous Endoscopic	Ø Drainage Device 7 Autologous Tissue Substitute J Synthetic Substitute K Nonautologous Tissue Substitute Y Other Device	Z No Qualifier
X Upper Tendon Y Lower Tendon	X External	Ø Drainage Device 7 Autologous Tissue Substitute J Synthetic Substitute K Nonautologous Tissue Substitute	Z No Qualifier

Non-OR ØLW[X,Y][3,4]YZ
Non-OR ØLW[X,Y]X[Ø,7,J,K]Z

Ø Medical and Surgical
L Tendons
X Transfer

Definition: Moving, without taking out, all or a portion of a body part to another location to take over the function of all or a portion of a body part

Explanation: The body part transferred remains connected to its vascular and nervous supply

Body Part Character 4	Approach Character 5	Device Character 6	Qualifier Character 7
Ø Head and Neck Tendon 1 Shoulder Tendon, Right 2 Shoulder Tendon, Left 3 Upper Arm Tendon, Right 4 Upper Arm Tendon, Left 5 Lower Arm and Wrist Tendon, Right 6 Lower Arm and Wrist Tendon, Left 7 Hand Tendon, Right 8 Hand Tendon, Left 9 Trunk Tendon, Right B Trunk Tendon, Left C Thorax Tendon, Right D Thorax Tendon, Left F Abdomen Tendon, Right G Abdomen Tendon, Left H Perineum Tendon J Hip Tendon, Right K Hip Tendon, Left L Upper Leg Tendon, Right M Upper Leg Tendon, Left N Lower Leg Tendon, Right Achilles tendon P Lower Leg Tendon, Left *See N Lower Leg Tendon, Right* Q Knee Tendon, Right Patellar tendon R Knee Tendon, Left *See Q Knee Tendon, Right* S Ankle Tendon, Right T Ankle Tendon, Left V Foot Tendon, Right W Foot Tendon, Left	Ø Open 4 Percutaneous Endoscopic	Z No Device	Z No Qualifier

Bursae and Ligaments ØM2–ØMX

Character Meanings*

This Character Meaning table is provided as a guide to assist the user in the identification of character members that may be found in this section of code tables. It **SHOULD NOT** be used to build a PCS code.

Operation–Character 3		Body Part–Character 4		Approach–Character 5		Device–Character 6		Qualifier–Character 7	
2	Change	Ø	Head and Neck Bursa and Ligament	Ø	Open	Ø	Drainage Device	X	Diagnostic
5	Destruction	1	Shoulder Bursa and Ligament, Right	3	Percutaneous	7	Autologous Tissue Substitute	Z	No Qualifier
8	Division	2	Shoulder Bursa and Ligament, Left	4	Percutaneous Endoscopic	J	Synthetic Substitute		
9	Drainage	3	Elbow Bursa and Ligament, Right	X	External	K	Nonautologous Tissue Substitute		
B	Excision	4	Elbow Bursa and Ligament, Left			Y	Other Device		
C	Extirpation	5	Wrist Bursa and Ligament, Right			Z	No Device		
D	Extraction	6	Wrist Bursa and Ligament, Left						
H	Insertion	7	Hand Bursa and Ligament, Right						
J	Inspection	8	Hand Bursa and Ligament, Left						
M	Reattachment	9	Upper Extremity Bursa and Ligament, Right						
N	Release	B	Upper Extremity Bursa and Ligament, Left						
P	Removal	C	Upper Spine Bursa and Ligament						
Q	Repair	D	Lower Spine Bursa and Ligament						
R	Replacement	F	Sternum Bursa and Ligament						
S	Reposition	G	Rib(s) Bursa and Ligament						
T	Resection	H	Abdomen Bursa and Ligament, Right						
U	Supplement	J	Abdomen Bursa and Ligament, Left						
W	Revision	K	Perineum Bursa and Ligament						
X	Transfer	L	Hip Bursa and Ligament, Right						
		M	Hip Bursa and Ligament, Left						
		N	Knee Bursa and Ligament, Right						
		P	Knee Bursa and Ligament, Left						
		Q	Ankle Bursa and Ligament, Right						
		R	Ankle Bursa and Ligament, Left						
		S	Foot Bursa and Ligament, Right						
		T	Foot Bursa and Ligament, Left						
		V	Lower Extremity Bursa and Ligament, Right						
		W	Lower Extremity Bursa and Ligament, Left						
		X	Upper Bursa and Ligament						
		Y	Lower Bursa and Ligament						

* Includes synovial membrane.

AHA Coding Clinic for table ØMB
2018, 3Q, 17 Excisional debridement of periosteum

AHA Coding Clinic for table ØMM
2013, 3Q, 20 Superior labrum anterior posterior (SLAP) repair and subacromial decompression

AHA Coding Clinic for table ØMQ
2014, 3Q, 9 Interspinous ligamentoplasty

AHA Coding Clinic for table ØMT
2017, 2Q, 21 Arthroscopic anterior cruciate ligament revision using autograft with anterolateral ligament reconstruction

AHA Coding Clinic for table ØMU
2017, 2Q, 21 Arthroscopic anterior cruciate ligament revision using autograft with anterolateral ligament reconstruction

Shoulder Ligaments

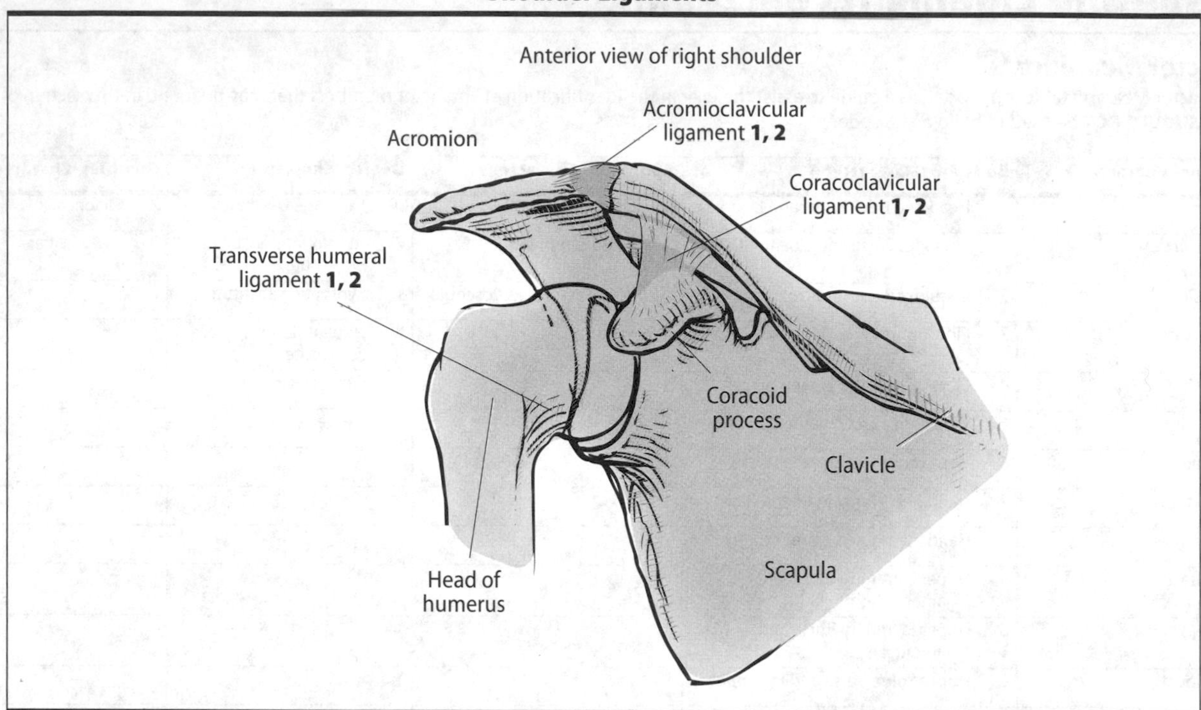

Knee Bursae

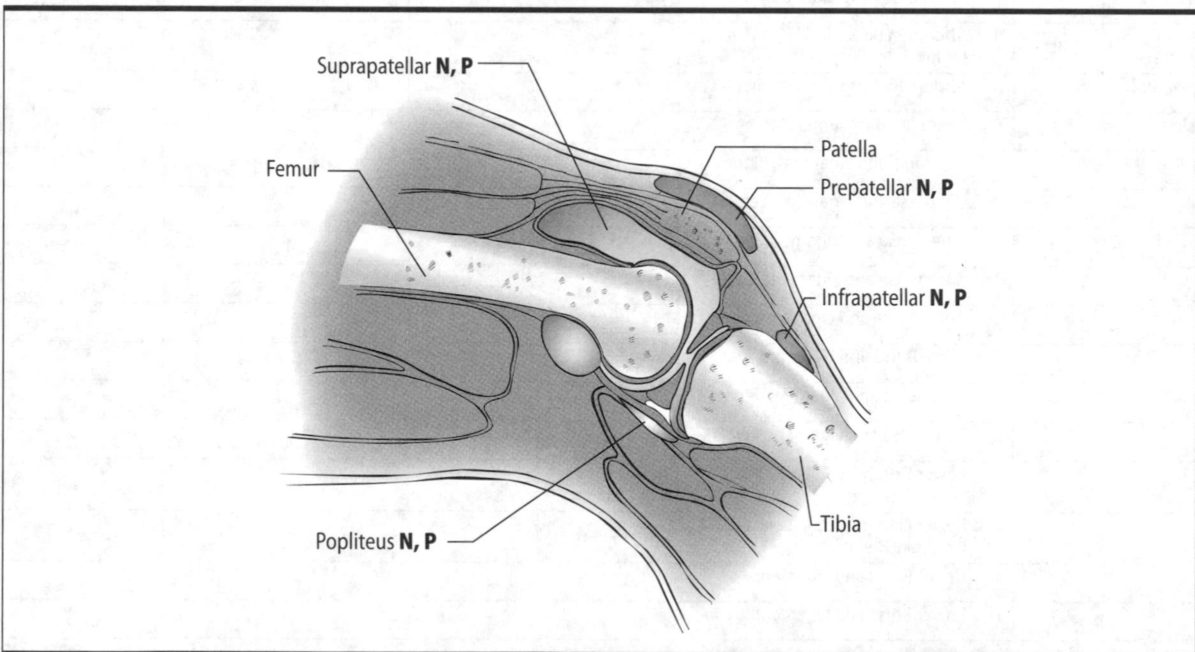

Knee Ligaments

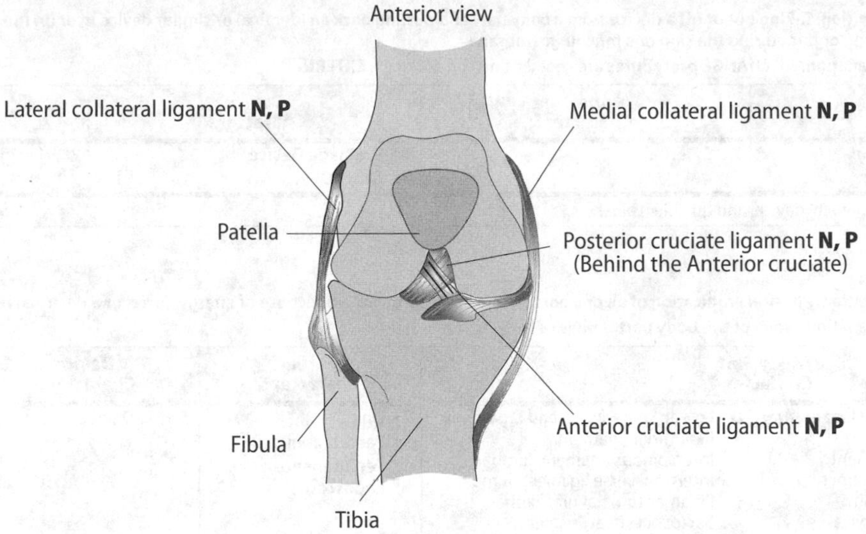

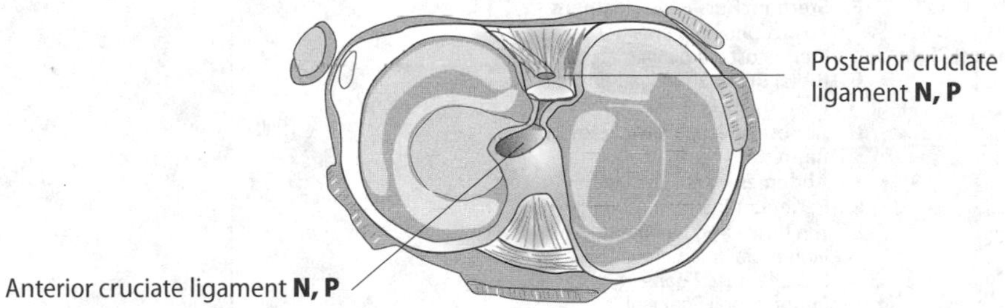

Anterior view
Lateral collateral ligament N, P
Medial collateral ligament N, P
Patella
Posterior cruciate ligament N, P
(Behind the Anterior cruciate)
Fibula
Anterior cruciate ligament N, P
Tibia

Posterior cruciate
ligament N, P
Anterior cruciate ligament N, P

Wrist Ligaments

Palmar view
5
4
3
2
1
Flexor carpi
ulnaris 5, 6
Radial collateral
carpal 5, 6
Ulnar collateral
carpal 5, 6
Palmar radiocarpal 5, 6

Dorsal view
1
2
3
4
5
Ulnar collateral
carpal 5, 6
Radial collateral
carpal 5, 6
Dorsal
radiocarpal 5, 6
Ulnocarpal 5, 6

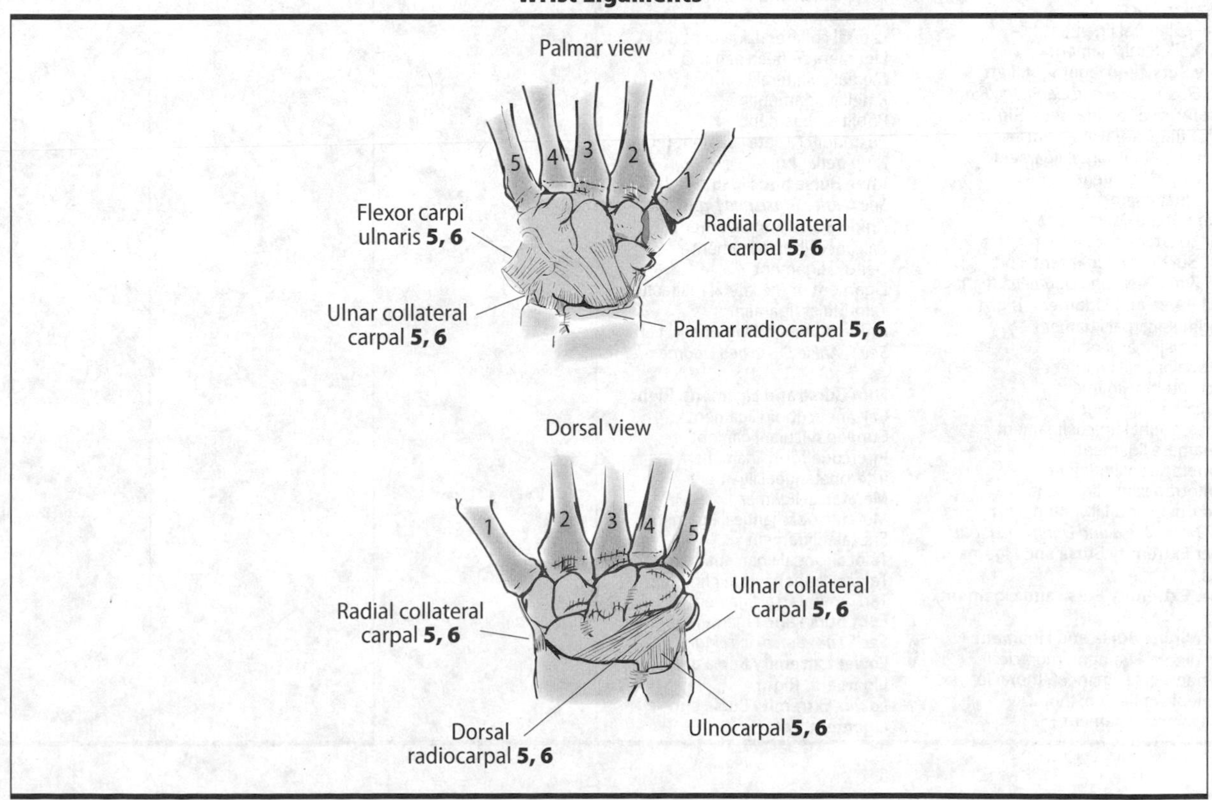

Ø Medical and Surgical
M Bursae and Ligaments
2 Change Definition: Taking out or off a device from a body part and putting back an identical or similar device in or on the same body part without cutting or puncturing the skin or a mucous membrane

Explanation: All CHANGE procedures are coded using the approach EXTERNAL

Body Part Character 4	Approach Character 5	Device Character 6	Qualifier Character 7
X Upper Bursa and Ligament Y Lower Bursa and Ligament	X External	Ø Drainage Device Y Other Device	Z No Qualifier

Non-OR All body part, approach, device, and qualifier values

Ø Medical and Surgical
M Bursae and Ligaments
5 Destruction Definition: Physical eradication of all or a portion of a body part by the direct use of energy, force, or a destructive agent

Explanation: None of the body part is physically taken out

Body Part Character 4		Approach Character 5	Device Character 6	Qualifier Character 7
Ø Head and Neck Bursa and Ligament Alar ligament of axis Cervical interspinous ligament Cervical intertransverse ligament Cervical ligamentum flavum Interspinous ligament, cervical Intertransverse ligament, cervical Lateral temporomandibular ligament Ligamentum flavum, cervical Sphenomandibular ligament Stylomandibular ligament Transverse ligament of atlas **1 Shoulder Bursa and Ligament, Right** Acromioclavicular ligament Coracoacromial ligament Coracoclavicular ligament Coracohumeral ligament Costoclavicular ligament Glenohumeral ligament Interclavicular ligament Sternoclavicular ligament Subacromial bursa Transverse humeral ligament Transverse scapular ligament **2 Shoulder Bursa and Ligament, Left** *See 1 Shoulder Bursa and Ligament, Right* **3 Elbow Bursa and Ligfament, Right** Annular ligament Olecranon bursa Radial collateral ligament Ulnar collateral ligament **4 Elbow Bursa and Ligament, Left** *See 3 Elbow Bursa and Ligament, Right* **5 Wrist Bursa and Ligament, Right** Palmar ulnocarpal ligament Radial collateral carpal ligament Radiocarpal ligament Radioulnar ligament Scapholunate ligament Ulnar collateral carpal ligament **6 Wrist Bursa and Ligament, Left** *See 5 Wrist Bursa and Ligament, Right* **7 Hand Bursa and Ligament, Right** Carpometacarpal ligament Intercarpal ligament Interphalangeal ligament Lunotriquetral ligament Metacarpal ligament Metacarpophalangeal ligament Pisohamate ligament Pisometacarpal ligament Scaphotrapezium ligament **8 Hand Bursa and Ligament, Left** *See 7 Hand Bursa and Ligament, Right* **9 Upper Extremity Bursa and Ligament, Right** **B Upper Extremity Bursa and Ligament, Left** **C Upper Spine Bursa and Ligament** Interspinous ligament, thoracic Intertransverse ligament, thoracic Ligamentum flavum, thoracic Supraspinous ligament	**D Lower Spine Bursa and Ligament** Iliolumbar ligament Interspinous ligament, lumbar Intertransverse ligament, lumbar Ligamentum flavum, lumbar Sacrococcygeal ligament Sacroiliac ligament Sacrospinous ligament Sacrotuberous ligament Supraspinous ligament **F Sternum Bursa and Ligament** Costoxiphoid ligament Sternocostal ligament **G Rib(s) Bursa and Ligament** Costotransverse ligament **H Abdomen Bursa and Ligament, Right** **J Abdomen Bursa and Ligament, Left** **K Perineum Bursa and Ligament** **L Hip Bursa and Ligament, Right** Iliofemoral ligament Ischiofemoral ligament Pubofemoral ligament Transverse acetabular ligament Trochanteric bursa **M Hip Bursa and Ligament, Left** *See L Hip Bursa and Ligament, Right* **N Knee Bursa and Ligament, Right** Anterior cruciate ligament (ACL) Lateral collateral ligament (LCL) Ligament of head of fibula Medial collateral ligament (MCL) Patellar ligament Popliteal ligament Posterior cruciate ligament (PCL) Prepatellar bursa **P Knee Bursa and Ligament, Left** *See N Knee Bursa and Ligament, Right* **Q Ankle Bursa and Ligament, Right** Calcaneofibular ligament Deltoid ligament Ligament of the lateral malleolus Talofibular ligament **R Ankle Bursa and Ligament, Left** *See Q Ankle Bursa and Ligament, Right* **S Foot Bursa and Ligament, Right** Calcaneocuboid ligament Cuneonavicular ligament Intercuneiform ligament Interphalangeal ligament Metatarsal ligament Metatarsophalangeal ligament Subtalar ligament Talocalcaneal ligament Talocalcaneonavicular ligament Tarsometatarsal ligament **T Foot Bursa and Ligament, Left** *See S Foot Bursa and Ligament, Right* **V Lower Extremity Bursa and Ligament, Right** **W Lower Extremity Bursa and Ligament, Left**	Ø Open 3 Percutaneous 4 Percutaneous Endoscopic	Z No Device	Z No Qualifier

Ø Medical and Surgical
M Bursae and Ligaments
8 Division Definition: Cutting into a body part, without draining fluids and/or gases from the body part, in order to separate or transect a body part

Explanation: All or a portion of the body part is separated into two or more portions

Body Part Character 4	Approach Character 5	Device Character 6	Qualifier Character 7
Ø Head and Neck Bursa and Ligament Alar ligament of axis Cervical interspinous ligament Cervical intertransverse ligament Cervical ligamentum flavum Interspinous ligament, cervical Intertransverse ligament, cervical Lateral temporomandibular ligament Ligamentum flavum, cervical Sphenomandibular ligament Stylomandibular ligament Transverse ligament of atlas **1 Shoulder Bursa and Ligament, Right** Acromioclavicular ligament Coracoacromial ligament Coracoclavicular ligament Coracohumeral ligament Costoclavicular ligament Glenohumeral ligament Interclavicular ligament Sternoclavicular ligament Subacromial bursa Transverse humeral ligament Transverse scapular ligament **2 Shoulder Bursa and Ligament, Left** **See** *1 Shoulder Bursa and Ligament, Right* **3 Elbow Bursa and Ligament, Right** Annular ligament Olecranon bursa Radial collateral ligament Ulnar collateral ligament **4 Elbow Bursa and Ligament, Left** **See** *3 Elbow Bursa and Ligament, Right* **5 Wrist Bursa and Ligament, Right** Palmar ulnocarpal ligament Radial collateral carpal ligament Radiocarpal ligament Radioulnar ligament Scapholunate ligament Ulnar collateral carpal ligament **6 Wrist Bursa and Ligament, Left** **See** *5 Wrist Bursa and Ligament, Right* **7 Hand Bursa and Ligament, Right** Carpometacarpal ligament Intercarpal ligament Interphalangeal ligament Lunotriquetral ligament Metacarpal ligament Metacarpophalangeal ligament Pisohamate ligament Pisometacarpal ligament Scaphotrapezium ligament **8 Hand Bursa and Ligament, Left** **See** *7 Hand Bursa and Ligament, Right* **9 Upper Extremity Bursa and Ligament, Right** **B Upper Extremity Bursa and Ligament, Left** **C Upper Spine Bursa and Ligament** Interspinous ligament, thoracic Intertransverse ligament, thoracic Ligamentum flavum, thoracic Supraspinous ligament **D Lower Spine Bursa and Ligament** Iliolumbar ligament Interspinous ligament, lumbar Intertransverse ligament, lumbar Ligamentum flavum, lumbar Sacrococcygeal ligament Sacroiliac ligament Sacrospinous ligament Sacrotuberous ligament Supraspinous ligament **F Sternum Bursa and Ligament** Costoxiphoid ligament Sternocostal ligament **G Rib(s) Bursa and Ligament** Costotransverse ligament **H Abdomen Bursa and Ligament, Right** **J Abdomen Bursa and Ligament, Left** **K Perineum Bursa and Ligament** **L Hip Bursa and Ligament, Right** Iliofemoral ligament Ischiofemoral ligament Pubofemoral ligament Transverse acetabular ligament Trochanteric bursa **M Hip Bursa and Ligament, Left** **See** *L Hip Bursa and Ligament, Right* **N Knee Bursa and Ligament, Right** Anterior cruciate ligament (ACL) Lateral collateral ligament (LCL) Ligament of head of fibula Medial collateral ligament (MCL) Patellar ligament Popliteal ligament Posterior cruciate ligament (PCL) Prepatellar bursa **P Knee Bursa and Ligament, Left** **See** *N Knee Bursa and Ligament, Right* **Q Ankle Bursa and Ligament, Right** Calcaneofibular ligament Deltoid ligament Ligament of the lateral malleolus Talofibular ligament **R Ankle Bursa and Ligament, Left** **See** *Q Ankle Bursa and Ligament, Right* **S Foot Bursa and Ligament, Right** Calcaneocuboid ligament Cuneonavicular ligament Intercuneiform ligament Interphalangeal ligament Metatarsal ligament Metatarsophalangeal ligament Subtalar ligament Talocalcaneal ligament Talocalcaneonavicular ligament Tarsometatarsal ligament **T Foot Bursa and Ligament, Left** **See** *S Foot Bursa and Ligament, Right* **V Lower Extremity Bursa and Ligament, Right** **W Lower Extremity Bursa and Ligament, Left**	**Ø Open** **3 Percutaneous** **4 Percutaneous Endoscopic**	**Z No Device**	**Z No Qualifier**

Ø Medical and Surgical
M Bursae and Ligaments
9 Drainage Definition: Taking or letting out fluids and/or gases from a body part
Explanation: The qualifier DIAGNOSTIC is used to identify drainage procedures that are biopsies

Body Part Character 4	Body Part Character 4 (cont.)	Approach Character 5	Device Character 6	Qualifier Character 7
Ø **Head and Neck Bursa and Ligament** Alar ligament of axis Cervical interspinous ligament Cervical intertransverse ligament Cervical ligamentum flavum Interspinous ligament, cervical Intertransverse ligament, cervical Lateral temporomandibular ligament Ligamentum flavum, cervical Sphenomandibular ligament Stylomandibular ligament Transverse ligament of atlas 1 **Shoulder Bursa and Ligament, Right** Acromioclavicular ligament Coracoacromial ligament Coracoclavicular ligament Coracohumeral ligament Costoclavicular ligament Glenohumeral ligament Interclavicular ligament Sternoclavicular ligament Subacromial bursa Transverse humeral ligament Transverse scapular ligament 2 **Shoulder Bursa and Ligament, Left** *See 1 Shoulder Bursa and Ligament, Right* 3 **Elbow Bursa and Ligament, Right** Annular ligament Olecranon bursa Radial collateral ligament Ulnar collateral ligament 4 **Elbow Bursa and Ligament, Left** *See 3 Elbow Bursa and Ligament, Right* 5 **Wrist Bursa and Ligament, Right** Palmar ulnocarpal ligament Radial collateral carpal ligament Radiocarpal ligament Radioulnar ligament Scapholunate ligament Ulnar collateral carpal ligament 6 **Wrist Bursa and Ligament, Left** *See 5 Wrist Bursa and Ligament, Right* 7 **Hand Bursa and Ligament, Right** Carpometacarpal ligament Intercarpal ligament Interphalangeal ligament Lunotriquetral ligament Metacarpal ligament Metacarpophalangeal ligament Pisohamate ligament Pisometacarpal ligament Scaphotrapezium ligament 8 **Hand Bursa and Ligament, Left** *See 7 Hand Bursa and Ligament, Right* 9 **Upper Extremity Bursa and Ligament, Right** B **Upper Extremity Bursa and Ligament, Left** C **Upper Spine Bursa and Ligament** Interspinous ligament, thoracic Intertransverse ligament, thoracic Ligamentum flavum, thoracic Supraspinous ligament	D **Lower Spine Bursa and Ligament** Iliolumbar ligament Interspinous ligament, lumbar Intertransverse ligament, lumbar Ligamentum flavum, lumbar Sacrococcygeal ligament Sacroiliac ligament Sacrospinous ligament Sacrotuberous ligament Supraspinous ligament F **Sternum Bursa and Ligament** Costoxiphoid ligament Sternocostal ligament G **Rib(s) Bursa and Ligament** Costotransverse ligament H **Abdomen Bursa and Ligament, Right** J **Abdomen Bursa and Ligament, Left** K **Perineum Bursa and Ligament** L **Hip Bursa and Ligament, Right** Iliofemoral ligament Ischiofemoral ligament Pubofemoral ligament Transverse acetabular ligament Trochanteric bursa M **Hip Bursa and Ligament, Left** *See L Hip Bursa and Ligament, Right* N **Knee Bursa and Ligament, Right** Anterior cruciate ligament (ACL) Lateral collateral ligament (LCL) Ligament of head of fibula Medial collateral ligament (MCL) Patellar ligament Popliteal ligament Posterior cruciate ligament (PCL) Prepatellar bursa P **Knee Bursa and Ligament, Left** *See N Knee Bursa and Ligament, Right* Q **Ankle Bursa and Ligament, Right** Calcaneofibular ligament Deltoid ligament Ligament of the lateral malleolus Talofibular ligament R **Ankle Bursa and Ligament, Left** *See Q Ankle Bursa and Ligament, Right* S **Foot Bursa and Ligament, Right** Calcaneocuboid ligament Cuneonavicular ligament Intercuneiform ligament Interphalangeal ligament Metatarsal ligament Metatarsophalangeal ligament Subtalar ligament Talocalcaneal ligament Talocalcaneonavicular ligament Tarsometatarsal ligament T **Foot Bursa and Ligament, Left** *See S Foot Bursa and Ligament, Right* V **Lower Extremity Bursa and Ligament, Right** W **Lower Extremity Bursa and Ligament, Left**	Ø Open 3 Percutaneous 4 Percutaneous Endoscopic	Ø Drainage Device	Z No Qualifier

Non-OR ØM9[Ø,1,2,3,4,5,6,7,8,9,B,C,D,F,G,H,J,K,L,M,N,P,Q,R,S,T,V,W]3ØZ
Non-OR ØM9[1,2,3,4,7,8,9,B,C,D,F,G,H,J,K,L,M,V,W]4ØZ

ØM9 Continued on next page

ØM9 Continued

Ø Medical and Surgical
M Bursae and Ligaments
9 Drainage Definition: Taking or letting out fluids and/or gases from a body part
Explanation: The qualifier DIAGNOSTIC is used to identify drainage procedures that are biopsies

Body Part Character 4	Approach Character 5	Device Character 6	Qualifier Character 7
Ø Head and Neck Bursa and Ligament Alar ligament of axis Cervical interspinous ligament Cervical intertransverse ligament Cervical ligamentum flavum Interspinous ligament, cervical Intertransverse ligament, cervical Lateral temporomandibular ligament Ligamentum flavum, cervical Sphenomandibular ligament Stylomandibular ligament Transverse ligament of atlas **1 Shoulder Bursa and Ligament, Right** Acromioclavicular ligament Coracoacromial ligament Coracoclavicular ligament Coracohumeral ligament Costoclavicular ligament Glenohumeral ligament Interclavicular ligament Sternoclavicular ligament Subacromial bursa Transverse humeral ligament Transverse scapular ligament **2 Shoulder Bursa and Ligament, Left** *See 1 Shoulder Bursa and Ligament, Right* **3 Elbow Bursa and Ligament, Right** Annular ligament Olecranon bursa Radial collateral ligament Ulnar collateral ligament **4 Elbow Bursa and Ligament, Left** *See 3 Elbow Bursa and Ligament, Right* **5 Wrist Bursa and Ligament, Right** Palmar ulnocarpal ligament Radial collateral carpal ligament Radiocarpal ligament Radioulnar ligament Scapholunate ligament Ulnar collateral carpal ligament **6 Wrist Bursa and Ligament, Left** *See 5 Wrist Bursa and Ligament, Right* **7 Hand Bursa and Ligament, Right** Carpometacarpal ligament Intercarpal ligament Interphalangeal ligament Lunotriquetral ligament Metacarpal ligament Metacarpophalangeal ligament Pisohamate ligament Pisometacarpal ligament Scaphotrapezium ligament **8 Hand Bursa and Ligament, Left** *See 7 Hand Bursa and Ligament, Right* **9 Upper Extremity Bursa and Ligament, Right** **B Upper Extremity Bursa and Ligament, Left** **C Upper Spine Bursa and Ligament** Interspinous ligament, thoracic Intertransverse ligament, thoracic Ligamentum flavum, thoracic Supraspinous ligament **D Lower Spine Bursa and Ligament** Iliolumbar ligament Interspinous ligament, lumbar Intertransverse ligament, lumbar Ligamentum flavum, lumbar Sacrococcygeal ligament Sacroiliac ligament Sacrospinous ligament Sacrotuberous ligament Supraspinous ligament **F Sternum Bursa and Ligament** Costoxiphoid ligament Sternocostal ligament **G Rib(s) Bursa and Ligament** Costotransverse ligament **H Abdomen Bursa and Ligament, Right** **J Abdomen Bursa and Ligament, Left** **K Perineum Bursa and Ligament** **L Hip Bursa and Ligament, Right** Iliofemoral ligament Ischiofemoral ligament Pubofemoral ligament Transverse acetabular ligament Trochanteric bursa **M Hip Bursa and Ligament, Left** *See L Hip Bursa and Ligament, Right* **N Knee Bursa and Ligament, Right** Anterior cruciate ligament (ACL) Lateral collateral ligament (LCL) Ligament of head of fibula Medial collateral ligament (MCL) Patellar ligament Popliteal ligament Posterior cruciate ligament (PCL) Prepatellar bursa **P Knee Bursa and Ligament, Left** *See N Knee Bursa and Ligament, Right* **Q Ankle Bursa and Ligament, Right** Calcaneofibular ligament Deltoid ligament Ligament of the lateral malleolus Talofibular ligament **R Ankle Bursa and Ligament, Left** *See Q Ankle Bursa and Ligament, Right* **S Foot Bursa and Ligament, Right** Calcaneocuboid ligament Cuneonavicular ligament Intercuneiform ligament Interphalangeal ligament Metatarsal ligament Metatarsophalangeal ligament Subtalar ligament Talocalcaneal ligament Talocalcaneonavicular ligament Tarsometatarsal ligament **T Foot Bursa and Ligament, Left** *See S Foot Bursa and Ligament, Right* **V Lower Extremity Bursa and Ligament, Right** **W Lower Extremity Bursa and Ligament, Left**	**Ø** Open **3** Percutaneous **4** Percutaneous Endoscopic	**Z** No Device	**X** Diagnostic **Z** No Qualifier

Non-OR ØM9[Ø,1,2,3,4,5,6,7,8,C,D,F,G,L,M,N,P,Q,R,S,T][Ø,3,4]ZX
Non-OR ØM9[Ø,1,2,3,4,5,6,7,8,9,B,C,D,F,G,H,J,K,L,M,N,P,Q,R,S,T,V,W]3ZZ
Non-OR ØM9[Ø,5,6,7,8,9,B,C,D,F,G,H,J,K,N,P,Q,R,S,T,V,W]4ZZ

Ø Medical and Surgical
M Bursae and Ligaments
B Excision Definition: Cutting out or off, without replacement, a portion of a body part
Explanation: The qualifier DIAGNOSTIC is used to identify excision procedures that are biopsies

Body Part Character 4	Approach Character 5	Device Character 6	Qualifier Character 7
Ø Head and Neck Bursa and Ligament Alar ligament of axis Cervical interspinous ligament Cervical intertransverse ligament Cervical ligamentum flavum Interspinous ligament, cervical Intertransverse ligament, cervical Lateral temporomandibular ligament Ligamentum flavum, cervical Sphenomandibular ligament Stylomandibular ligament Transverse ligament of atlas **1 Shoulder Bursa and Ligament, Right** Acromioclavicular ligament Coracoacromial ligament Coracoclavicular ligament Coracohumeral ligament Costoclavicular ligament Glenohumeral ligament Interclavicular ligament Sternoclavicular ligament Subacromial bursa Transverse humeral ligament Transverse scapular ligament **2 Shoulder Bursa and Ligament, Left** **See** *1 Shoulder Bursa and Ligament, Right* **3 Elbow Bursa and Ligament, Right** Annular ligament Olecranon bursa Radial collateral ligament Ulnar collateral ligament **4 Elbow Bursa and Ligament, Left** **See** *3 Elbow Bursa and Ligament, Right* **5 Wrist Bursa and Ligament, Right** Palmar ulnocarpal ligament Radial collateral carpal ligament Radiocarpal ligament Radioulnar ligament Scapholunate ligament Ulnar collateral carpal ligament **6 Wrist Bursa and Ligament, Left** **See** *5 Wrist Bursa and Ligament, Right* **7 Hand Bursa and Ligament, Right** Carpometacarpal ligament Intercarpal ligament Interphalangeal ligament Lunotriquetral ligament Metacarpal ligament Metacarpophalangeal ligament Pisohamate ligament Pisometacarpal ligament Scaphotrapezium ligament **8 Hand Bursa and Ligament, Left** **See** *7 Hand Bursa and Ligament, Right* **9 Upper Extremity Bursa and Ligament, Right** **B Upper Extremity Bursa and Ligament, Left** **C Upper Spine Bursa and Ligament** Interspinous ligament, thoracic Intertransverse ligament, thoracic Ligamentum flavum, thoracic Supraspinous ligament **D Lower Spine Bursa and Ligament** Iliolumbar ligament Interspinous ligament, lumbar Intertransverse ligament, lumbar Ligamentum flavum, lumbar Sacrococcygeal ligament Sacroiliac ligament Sacrospinous ligament Sacrotuberous ligament Supraspinous ligament **F Sternum Bursa and Ligament** Costoxiphoid ligament Sternocostal ligament **G Rib(s) Bursa and Ligament** Costotransverse ligament **H Abdomen Bursa and Ligament, Right** **J Abdomen Bursa and Ligament, Left** **K Perineum Bursa and Ligament** **L Hip Bursa and Ligament, Right** Iliofemoral ligament Ischiofemoral ligament Pubofemoral ligament Transverse acetabular ligament Trochanteric bursa **M Hip Bursa and Ligament, Left** **See** *L Hip Bursa and Ligament, Right* **N Knee Bursa and Ligament, Right** Anterior cruciate ligament (ACL) Lateral collateral ligament (LCL) Ligament of head of fibula Medial collateral ligament (MCL) Patellar ligament Popliteal ligament Posterior cruciate ligament (PCL) Prepatellar bursa **P Knee Bursa and Ligament, Left** **See** *N Knee Bursa and Ligament, Right* **Q Ankle Bursa and Ligament, Right** Calcaneofibular ligament Deltoid ligament Ligament of the lateral malleolus Talofibular ligament **R Ankle Bursa and Ligament, Left** **See** *Q Ankle Bursa and Ligament, Right* **S Foot Bursa and Ligament, Right** Calcaneocuboid ligament Cuneonavicular ligament Intercuneiform ligament Interphalangeal ligament Metatarsal ligament Metatarsophalangeal ligament Subtalar ligament Talocalcaneal ligament Talocalcaneonavicular ligament Tarsometatarsal ligament **T Foot Bursa and Ligament, Left** **See** *S Foot Bursa and Ligament, Right* **V Lower Extremity Bursa and Ligament, Right** **W Lower Extremity Bursa and Ligament, Left**	**Ø Open** **3 Percutaneous** **4 Percutaneous Endoscopic**	**Z No Device**	**X Diagnostic** **Z No Qualifier**

Non-OR ØMB[Ø,1,2,3,4,5,6,7,8,B,C,D,F,G,L,M,N,P,Q,R,S,T][Ø,3,4]ZX
Non-OR ØMB94ZX

Ø Medical and Surgical
M Bursae and Ligaments
C Extirpation Definition: Taking or cutting out solid matter from a body part

Explanation: The solid matter may be an abnormal byproduct of a biological function or a foreign body; it may be imbedded in a body part or in the lumen of a tubular body part. The solid matter may or may not have been previously broken into pieces.

Body Part Character 4	Approach Character 5	Device Character 6	Qualifier Character 7
Ø Head and Neck Bursa and Ligament Alar ligament of axis Cervical interspinous ligament Cervical intertransverse ligament Cervical ligamentum flavum Interspinous ligament, cervical Intertransverse ligament, cervical Lateral temporomandibular ligament Ligamentum flavum, cervical Sphenomandibular ligament Stylomandibular ligament Transverse ligament of atlas **1 Shoulder Bursa and Ligament, Right** Acromioclavicular ligament Coracoacromial ligament Coracoclavicular ligament Coracohumeral ligament Costoclavicular ligament Glenohumeral ligament Interclavicular ligament Sternoclavicular ligament Subacromial bursa Transverse humeral ligament Transverse scapular ligament **2 Shoulder Bursa and Ligament, Left** *See 1 Shoulder Bursa and Ligament, Right* **3 Elbow Bursa and Ligament, Right** Annular ligament Olecranon bursa Radial collateral ligament Ulnar collateral ligament **4 Elbow Bursa and Ligament, Left** *See 3 Elbow Bursa and Ligament, Right* **5 Wrist Bursa and Ligament, Right** Palmar ulnocarpal ligament Radial collateral carpal ligament Radiocarpal ligament Radioulnar ligament Scapholunate ligament Ulnar collateral carpal ligament **6 Wrist Bursa and Ligament, Left** *See 5 Wrist Bursa and Ligament, Right* **7 Hand Bursa and Ligament, Right** Carpometacarpal ligament Intercarpal ligament Interphalangeal ligament Lunotriquetral ligament Metacarpal ligament Metacarpophalangeal ligament Pisohamate ligament Pisometacarpal ligament Scaphotrapezium ligament **8 Hand Bursa and Ligament, Left** *See 7 Hand Bursa and Ligament, Right* **9 Upper Extremity Bursa and Ligament, Right** **B Upper Extremity Bursa and Ligament, Left** **C Upper Spine Bursa and Ligament** Interspinous ligament, thoracic Intertransverse ligament, thoracic Ligamentum flavum, thoracic Supraspinous ligament **D Lower Spine Bursa and Ligament** Iliolumbar ligament Interspinous ligament, lumbar Intertransverse ligament, lumbar Ligamentum flavum, lumbar Sacrococcygeal ligament Sacroiliac ligament Sacrospinous ligament Sacrotuberous ligament Supraspinous ligament **F Sternum Bursa and Ligament** Costoxiphoid ligament Sternocostal ligament **G Rib(s) Bursa and Ligament** Costotransverse ligament **H Abdomen Bursa and Ligament, Right** **J Abdomen Bursa and Ligament, Left** **K Perineum Bursa and Ligament** **L Hip Bursa and Ligament, Right** Iliofemoral ligament Ischiofemoral ligament Pubofemoral ligament Transverse acetabular ligament Trochanteric bursa **M Hip Bursa and Ligament, Left** *See L Hip Bursa and Ligament, Right* **N Knee Bursa and Ligament, Right** Anterior cruciate ligament (ACL) Lateral collateral ligament (LCL) Ligament of head of fibula Medial collateral ligament (MCL) Patellar ligament Popliteal ligament Posterior cruciate ligament (PCL) Prepatellar bursa **P Knee Bursa and Ligament, Left** *See N Knee Bursa and Ligament, Right* **Q Ankle Bursa and Ligament, Right** Calcaneofibular ligament Deltoid ligament Ligament of the lateral malleolus Talofibular ligament **R Ankle Bursa and Ligament, Left** *See Q Ankle Bursa and Ligament, Right* **S Foot Bursa and Ligament, Right** Calcaneocuboid ligament Cuneonavicular ligament Intercuneiform ligament Interphalangeal ligament Metatarsal ligament Metatarsophalangeal ligament Subtalar ligament Talocalcaneal ligament Talocalcaneonavicular ligament Tarsometatarsal ligament **T Foot Bursa and Ligament, Left** *See S Foot Bursa and Ligament, Right* **V Lower Extremity Bursa and Ligament, Right** **W Lower Extremity Bursa and Ligament, Left**	**Ø Open** **3 Percutaneous** **4 Percutaneous Endoscopic**	**Z No Device**	**Z No Qualifier**

Ø Medical and Surgical
M Bursae and Ligaments
D Extraction Definition: Pulling or stripping out or off all or a portion of a body part by the use of force
Explanation: The qualifier DIAGNOSTIC is used to identify extraction procedures that are biopsies

Body Part Character 4	Approach Character 5	Device Character 6	Qualifier Character 7
Ø Head and Neck Bursa and Ligament Alar ligament of axis Cervical interspinous ligament Cervical intertransverse ligament Cervical ligamentum flavum Interspinous ligament, cervical Intertransverse ligament, cervical Lateral temporomandibular ligament Ligamentum flavum, cervical Sphenomandibular ligament Stylomandibular ligament Transverse ligament of atlas **1 Shoulder Bursa and Ligament, Right** Acromioclavicular ligament Coracoacromial ligament Coracoclavicular ligament Coracohumeral ligament Costoclavicular ligament Glenohumeral ligament Interclavicular ligament Sternoclavicular ligament Subacromial bursa Transverse humeral ligament Transverse scapular ligament **2 Shoulder Bursa and Ligament, Left** **See** *1 Shoulder Bursa and Ligament, Right* **3 Elbow Bursa and Ligament, Right** Annular ligament Olecranon bursa Radial collateral ligament Ulnar collateral ligament **4 Elbow Bursa and Ligament, Left** **See** *3 Elbow Bursa and Ligament, Right* **5 Wrist Bursa and Ligament, Right** Palmar ulnocarpal ligament Radial collateral carpal ligament Radiocarpal ligament Radioulnar ligament Scapholunate ligament Ulnar collateral carpal ligament **6 Wrist Bursa and Ligament, Left** **See** *5 Wrist Bursa and Ligament, Right* **7 Hand Bursa and Ligament, Right** Carpometacarpal ligament Intercarpal ligament Interphalangeal ligament Lunotriquetral ligament Metacarpal ligament Metacarpophalangeal ligament Pisohamate ligament Pisometacarpal ligament Scaphotrapezium ligament **8 Hand Bursa and Ligament, Left** **See** *7 Hand Bursa and Ligament, Right* **9 Upper Extremity Bursa and Ligament, Right** **B Upper Extremity Bursa and Ligament, Left** **C Upper Spine Bursa and Ligament** Interspinous ligament, thoracic Intertransverse ligament, thoracic Ligamentum flavum, thoracic Supraspinous ligament **D Lower Spine Bursa and Ligament** Iliolumbar ligament Interspinous ligament, lumbar Intertransverse ligament, lumbar Ligamentum flavum, lumbar Sacrococcygeal ligament Sacroiliac ligament Sacrospinous ligament Sacrotuberous ligament Supraspinous ligament **F Sternum Bursa and Ligament** Costoxiphoid ligament Sternocostal ligament **G Rib(s) Bursa and Ligament** Costotransverse ligament **H Abdomen Bursa and Ligament, Right** **J Abdomen Bursa and Ligament, Left** **K Perineum Bursa and Ligament** **L Hip Bursa and Ligament, Right** Iliofemoral ligament Ischiofemoral ligament Pubofemoral ligament Transverse acetabular ligament Trochanteric bursa **M Hip Bursa and Ligament, Left** **See** *L Hip Bursa and Ligament, Right* **N Knee Bursa and Ligament, Right** Anterior cruciate ligament (ACL) Lateral collateral ligament (LCL) Ligament of head of fibula Medial collateral ligament (MCL) Patellar ligament Popliteal ligament Posterior cruciate ligament (PCL) Prepatellar bursa **P Knee Bursa and Ligament, Left** **See** *N Knee Bursa and Ligament, Right* **Q Ankle Bursa and Ligament, Right** Calcaneofibular ligament Deltoid ligament Ligament of the lateral malleolus Talofibular ligament **R Ankle Bursa and Ligament, Left** **See** *Q Ankle Bursa and Ligament, Right* **S Foot Bursa and Ligament, Right** Calcaneocuboid ligament Cuneonavicular ligament Intercuneiform ligament Interphalangeal ligament Metatarsal ligament Metatarsophalangeal ligament Subtalar ligament Talocalcaneal ligament Talocalcaneonavicular ligament Tarsometatarsal ligament **T Foot Bursa and Ligament, Left** **See** *S Foot Bursa and Ligament, Right* **V Lower Extremity Bursa and Ligament, Right** **W Lower Extremity Bursa and Ligament, Left**	**Ø Open** **3 Percutaneous** **4 Percutaneous Endoscopic**	**Z No Device**	**Z No Qualifier**

LC Limited Coverage NC Noncovered ⊞ Combination Member HAC associated procedure Combination Only DRG Non-OR Non-OR New/Revised in GREEN

Ø Medical and Surgical
M Bursae and Ligaments
H Insertion Definition: Putting in a nonbiological appliance that monitors, assists, performs, or prevents a physiological function but does not physically take the place of a body part

Explanation: None

Body Part Character 4	Approach Character 5	Device Character 6	Qualifier Character 7
X Upper Bursa and Ligament Y Lower Bursa and Ligament	Ø Open 3 Percutaneous 4 Percutaneous Endoscopic	Y Other Device	Z No Qualifier

Non-OR ØMH[X,Y][3,4]YZ

Ø Medical and Surgical
M Bursae and Ligaments
J Inspection Definition: Visually and/or manually exploring a body part

Explanation: Visual exploration may be performed with or without optical instrumentation. Manual exploration may be performed directly or through intervening body layers.

Body Part Character 4	Approach Character 5	Device Character 6	Qualifier Character 7
X Upper Bursa and Ligament Y Lower Bursa and Ligament	Ø Open 3 Percutaneous 4 Percutaneous Endoscopic X External	Z No Device	Z No Qualifier

Non-OR ØMJ[X,Y][3,X]ZZ

Ø Medical and Surgical
M Bursae and Ligaments
M Reattachment Definition: Putting back in or on all or a portion of a separated body part to its normal location or other suitable location

Explanation: Vascular circulation and nervous pathways may or may not be reestablished

Body Part Character 4		Approach Character 5	Device Character 6	Qualifier Character 7
Ø Head and Neck Bursa and Ligament Alar ligament of axis Cervical interspinous ligament Cervical intertransverse ligament Cervical ligamentum flavum Interspinous ligament, cervical Intertransverse ligament, cervical Lateral temporomandibular ligament Ligamentum flavum, cervical Sphenomandibular ligament Stylomandibular ligament Transverse ligament of atlas **1 Shoulder Bursa and Ligament, Right** Acromioclavicular ligament Coracoacromial ligament Coracoclavicular ligament Coracohumeral ligament Costoclavicular ligament Glenohumeral ligament Interclavicular ligament Sternoclavicular ligament Subacromial bursa Transverse humeral ligament Transverse scapular ligament **2 Shoulder Bursa and Ligament, Left** ***See*** *1 Shoulder Bursa and Ligament, Right* **3 Elbow Bursa and Ligament, Right** Annular ligament Olecranon bursa Radial collateral ligament Ulnar collateral ligament **4 Elbow Bursa and Ligament, Left** ***See*** *3 Elbow Bursa and Ligament, Right* **5 Wrist Bursa and Ligament, Right** Palmar ulnocarpal ligament Radial collateral carpal ligament Radiocarpal ligament Radioulnar ligament Scapholunate ligament Ulnar collateral carpal ligament **6 Wrist Bursa and Ligament, Left** ***See*** *5 Wrist Bursa and Ligament, Right* **7 Hand Bursa and Ligament, Right** Carpometacarpal ligament Intercarpal ligament Interphalangeal ligament Lunotriquetral ligament Metacarpal ligament Metacarpophalangeal ligament Pisohamate ligament Pisometacarpal ligament Scaphotrapezium ligament **8 Hand Bursa and Ligament, Left** ***See*** *7 Hand Bursa and Ligament, Right* **9 Upper Extremity Bursa and Ligament, Right** **B Upper Extremity Bursa and Ligament, Left** **C Upper Spine Bursa and Ligament** Interspinous ligament, thoracic Intertransverse ligament, thoracic Ligamentum flavum, thoracic Supraspinous ligament	**D Lower Spine Bursa and Ligament** Iliolumbar ligament Interspinous ligament, lumbar Intertransverse ligament, lumbar Ligamentum flavum, lumbar Sacrococcygeal ligament Sacroiliac ligament Sacrospinous ligament Sacrotuberous ligament Supraspinous ligament **F Sternum Bursa and Ligament** Costoxiphoid ligament Sternocostal ligament **G Rib(s) Bursa and Ligament** Costotransverse ligament **H Abdomen Bursa and Ligament, Right** **J Abdomen Bursa and Ligament, Left** **K Perineum Bursa and Ligament** **L Hip Bursa and Ligament, Right** Iliofemoral ligament Ischiofemoral ligament Pubofemoral ligament Transverse acetabular ligament Trochanteric bursa **M Hip Bursa and Ligament, Left** ***See*** *L Hip Bursa and Ligament, Right* **N Knee Bursa and Ligament, Right** Anterior cruciate ligament (ACL) Lateral collateral ligament (LCL) Ligament of head of fibula Medial collateral ligament (MCL) Patellar ligament Popliteal ligament Posterior cruciate ligament (PCL) Prepatellar bursa **P Knee Bursa and Ligament, Left** ***See*** *N Knee Bursa and Ligament, Right* **Q Ankle Bursa and Ligament, Right** Calcaneofibular ligament Deltoid ligament Ligament of the lateral malleolus Talofibular ligament **R Ankle Bursa and Ligament, Left** ***See*** *Q Ankle Bursa and Ligament, Right* **S Foot Bursa and Ligament, Right** Calcaneocuboid ligament Cuneonavicular ligament Intercuneiform ligament Interphalangeal ligament Metatarsal ligament Metatarsophalangeal ligament Subtalar ligament Talocalcaneal ligament Talocalcaneonavicular ligament Tarsometatarsal ligament **T Foot Bursa and Ligament, Left** ***See*** *S Foot Bursa and Ligament, Right* **V Lower Extremity Bursa and Ligament, Right** **W Lower Extremity Bursa and Ligament, Left**	**Ø Open** **4 Percutaneous Endoscopic**	**Z No Device**	**Z No Qualifier**

Ø Medical and Surgical
M Bursae and Ligaments
N Release Definition: Freeing a body part from an abnormal physical constraint by cutting or by the use of force
Explanation: Some of the restraining tissue may be taken out but none of the body part is taken out

Body Part Character 4	Approach Character 5	Device Character 6	Qualifier Character 7
Ø Head and Neck Bursa and Ligament Alar ligament of axis Cervical interspinous ligament Cervical intertransverse ligament Cervical ligamentum flavum Interspinous ligament, cervical Intertransverse ligament, cervical Lateral temporomandibular ligament Ligamentum flavum, cervical Sphenomandibular ligament Stylomandibular ligament Transverse ligament of atlas 1 Shoulder Bursa and Ligament, Right Acromioclavicular ligament Coracoacromial ligament Coracoclavicular ligament Coracohumeral ligament Costoclavicular ligament Glenohumeral ligament Interclavicular ligament Sternoclavicular ligament Subacromial bursa Transverse humeral ligament Transverse scapular ligament 2 Shoulder Bursa and Ligament, Left *See 1 Shoulder Bursa and Ligament, Right* 3 Elbow Bursa and Ligament, Right Annular ligament Olecranon bursa Radial collateral ligament Ulnar collateral ligament 4 Elbow Bursa and Ligament, Left *See 3 Elbow Bursa and Ligament, Right* 5 Wrist Bursa and Ligament, Right Palmar ulnocarpal ligament Radial collateral carpal ligament Radiocarpal ligament Radioulnar ligament Scapholunate ligament Ulnar collateral carpal ligament 6 Wrist Bursa and Ligament, Left *See 5 Wrist Bursa and Ligament, Right* 7 Hand Bursa and Ligament, Right Carpometacarpal ligament Intercarpal ligament Interphalangeal ligament Lunotriquetral ligament Metacarpal ligament Metacarpophalangeal ligament Pisohamate ligament Pisometacarpal ligament Scaphotrapezium ligament 8 Hand Bursa and Ligament, Left *See 7 Hand Bursa and Ligament, Right* 9 Upper Extremity Bursa and Ligament, Right B Upper Extremity Bursa and Ligament, Left C Upper Spine Bursa and Ligament Interspinous ligament, thoracic Intertransverse ligament, thoracic Ligamentum flavum, thoracic Supraspinous ligament D Lower Spine Bursa and Ligament Iliolumbar ligament Interspinous ligament, lumbar Intertransverse ligament, lumbar Ligamentum flavum, lumbar Sacrococcygeal ligament Sacroiliac ligament Sacrospinous ligament Sacrotuberous ligament Supraspinous ligament F Sternum Bursa and Ligament Costoxiphoid ligament Sternocostal ligament G Rib(s) Bursa and Ligament Costotransverse ligament H Abdomen Bursa and Ligament, Right J Abdomen Bursa and Ligament, Left K Perineum Bursa and Ligament L Hip Bursa and Ligament, Right Iliofemoral ligament Ischiofemoral ligament Pubofemoral ligament Transverse acetabular ligament Trochanteric bursa M Hip Bursa and Ligament, Left *See L Hip Bursa and Ligament, Right* N Knee Bursa and Ligament, Right Anterior cruciate ligament (ACL) Lateral collateral ligament (LCL) Ligament of head of fibula Medial collateral ligament (MCL) Patellar ligament Popliteal ligament Posterior cruciate ligament (PCL) Prepatellar bursa P Knee Bursa and Ligament, Left *See N Knee Bursa and Ligament, Right* Q Ankle Bursa and Ligament, Right Calcaneofibular ligament Deltoid ligament Ligament of the lateral malleolus Talofibular ligament R Ankle Bursa and Ligament, Left *See Q Ankle Bursa and Ligament, Right* S Foot Bursa and Ligament, Right Calcaneocuboid ligament Cuneonavicular ligament Intercuneiform ligament Interphalangeal ligament Metatarsal ligament Metatarsophalangeal ligament Subtalar ligament Talocalcaneal ligament Talocalcaneonavicular ligament Tarsometatarsal ligament T Foot Bursa and Ligament, Left *See S Foot Bursa and Ligament, Right* V Lower Extremity Bursa and Ligament, Right W Lower Extremity Bursa and Ligament, Left	Ø Open 3 Percutaneous 4 Percutaneous Endoscopic X External	Z No Device	Z No Qualifier

Non-OR ØMN[Ø,1,2,3,4,5,6,7,8,9,B,C,D,F,G,H,J,K,L,M,N,P,Q,R,S,T,V,W]XZZ

Ø Medical and Surgical
M Bursae and Ligaments
P Removal Definition: Taking out or off a device from a body part

Explanation: If a device is taken out and a similar device put in without cutting or puncturing the skin or mucous membrane, the procedure is coded to the root operation CHANGE. Otherwise, the procedure for taking out a device is coded to the root operation REMOVAL.

Body Part Character 4	Approach Character 5	Device Character 6	Qualifier Character 7
X Upper Bursa and Ligament Y Lower Bursa and Ligament	Ø Open 3 Percutaneous 4 Percutaneous Endoscopic	Ø Drainage Device 7 Autologous Tissue Substitute J Synthetic Substitute K Nonautologous Tissue Substitute Y Other Device	Z No Qualifier
X Upper Bursa and Ligament Y Lower Bursa and Ligament	X External	Ø Drainage Device	Z No Qualifier

Non-OR ØMP[X,Y]3ØZ
Non-OR ØMP[X,Y][3,4]YZ
Non-OR ØMP[X,Y]XØZ

Ø Medical and Surgical
M Bursae and Ligaments
Q Repair Definition: Restoring, to the extent possible, a body part to its normal anatomic structure and function
Explanation: Used only when the method to accomplish the repair is not one of the other root operations

Body Part Character 4	Approach Character 5	Device Character 6	Qualifier Character 7
Ø Head and Neck Bursa and Ligament Alar ligament of axis Cervical interspinous ligament Cervical intertransverse ligament Cervical ligamentum flavum Interspinous ligament, cervical Intertransverse ligament, cervical Lateral temporomandibular ligament Ligamentum flavum, cervical Sphenomandibular ligament Stylomandibular ligament Transverse ligament of atlas **1 Shoulder Bursa and Ligament, Right** Acromioclavicular ligament Coracoacromial ligament Coracoclavicular ligament Coracohumeral ligament Costoclavicular ligament Glenohumeral ligament Interclavicular ligament Sternoclavicular ligament Subacromial bursa Transverse humeral ligament Transverse scapular ligament **2 Shoulder Bursa and Ligament, Left** *See 1 Shoulder Bursa and Ligament, Right* **3 Elbow Bursa and Ligament, Right** Annular ligament Olecranon bursa Radial collateral ligament Ulnar collateral ligament **4 Elbow Bursa and Ligament, Left** *See 3 Elbow Bursa and Ligament, Right* **5 Wrist Bursa and Ligament, Right** Palmar ulnocarpal ligament Radial collateral carpal ligament Radiocarpal ligament Radioulnar ligament Scapholunate ligament Ulnar collateral carpal ligament **6 Wrist Bursa and Ligament, Left** *See 5 Wrist Bursa and Ligament, Right* **7 Hand Bursa and Ligament, Right** Carpometacarpal ligament Intercarpal ligament Interphalangeal ligament Lunotriquetral ligament Metacarpal ligament Metacarpophalangeal ligament Pisohamate ligament Pisometacarpal ligament Scaphotrapezium ligament **8 Hand Bursa and Ligament, Left** *See 7 Hand Bursa and Ligament, Right* **9 Upper Extremity Bursa and Ligament, Right** **B Upper Extremity Bursa and Ligament, Left** **C Upper Spine Bursa and Ligament** Interspinous ligament, thoracic Intertransverse ligament, thoracic Ligamentum flavum, thoracic Supraspinous ligament **D Lower Spine Bursa and Ligament** Iliolumbar ligament Interspinous ligament, lumbar Intertransverse ligament, lumbar Ligamentum flavum, lumbar Sacrococcygeal ligament Sacroiliac ligament Sacrospinous ligament Sacrotuberous ligament Supraspinous ligament **F Sternum Bursa and Ligament** Costoxiphoid ligament Sternocostal ligament **G Rib(s) Bursa and Ligament** Costotransverse ligament **H Abdomen Bursa and Ligament, Right** **J Abdomen Bursa and Ligament, Left** **K Perineum Bursa and Ligament** **L Hip Bursa and Ligament, Right** Iliofemoral ligament Ischiofemoral ligament Pubofemoral ligament Transverse acetabular ligament Trochanteric bursa **M Hip Bursa and Ligament, Left** *See L Hip Bursa and Ligament, Right* **N Knee Bursa and Ligament, Right** Anterior cruciate ligament (ACL) Lateral collateral ligament (LCL) Ligament of head of fibula Medial collateral ligament (MCL) Patellar ligament Popliteal ligament Posterior cruciate ligament (PCL) Prepatellar bursa **P Knee Bursa and Ligament, Left** *See N Knee Bursa and Ligament, Right* **Q Ankle Bursa and Ligament, Right** Calcaneofibular ligament Deltoid ligament Ligament of the lateral malleolus Talofibular ligament **R Ankle Bursa and Ligament, Left** *See Q Ankle Bursa and Ligament, Right* **S Foot Bursa and Ligament, Right** Calcaneocuboid ligament Cuneonavicular ligament Intercuneiform ligament Interphalangeal ligament Metatarsal ligament Metatarsophalangeal ligament Subtalar ligament Talocalcaneal ligament Talocalcaneonavicular ligament Tarsometatarsal ligament **T Foot Bursa and Ligament, Left** *See S Foot Bursa and Ligament, Right* **V Lower Extremity Bursa and Ligament, Right** **W Lower Extremity Bursa and Ligament, Left**	**Ø Open** **3 Percutaneous** **4 Percutaneous Endoscopic**	**Z No Device**	**Z No Qualifier**

Ø Medical and Surgical
M Bursae and Ligaments
R Replacement Definition: Putting in or on biological or synthetic material that physically takes the place and/or function of all or a portion of a body part

Explanation: The body part may have been taken out or replaced, or may be taken out, physically eradicated, or rendered nonfunctional during the REPLACEMENT procedure. A REMOVAL procedure is coded for taking out the device used in a previous replacement procedure.

Body Part Character 4	Approach Character 5	Device Character 6	Qualifier Character 7
Ø Head and Neck Bursa and Ligament Alar ligament of axis Cervical interspinous ligament Cervical intertransverse ligament Cervical ligamentum flavum Interspinous ligament, cervical Intertransverse ligament, cervical Lateral temporomandibular ligament Ligamentum flavum, cervical Sphenomandibular ligament Stylomandibular ligament Transverse ligament of atlas **1 Shoulder Bursa and Ligament, Right** Acromioclavicular ligament Coracoacromial ligament Coracoclavicular ligament Coracohumeral ligament Costoclavicular ligament Glenohumeral ligament Interclavicular ligament Sternoclavicular ligament Subacromial bursa Transverse humeral ligament Transverse scapular ligament **2 Shoulder Bursa and Ligament, Left** *See 1 Shoulder Bursa and Ligament, Right* **3 Elbow Bursa and Ligament, Right** Annular ligament Olecranon bursa Radial collateral ligament Ulnar collateral ligament **4 Elbow Bursa and Ligament, Left** *See 3 Elbow Bursa and Ligament, Right* **5 Wrist Bursa and Ligament, Right** Palmar ulnocarpal ligament Radial collateral carpal ligament Radiocarpal ligament Radioulnar ligament Scapholunate ligament Ulnar collateral carpal ligament **6 Wrist Bursa and Ligament, Left** *See 5 Wrist Bursa and Ligament, Right* **7 Hand Bursa and Ligament, Right** Carpometacarpal ligament Intercarpal ligament Interphalangeal ligament Lunotriquetral ligament Metacarpal ligament Metacarpophalangeal ligament Pisohamate ligament Pisometacarpal ligament Scaphotrapezium ligament **8 Hand Bursa and Ligament, Left** *See 7 Hand Bursa and Ligament, Right* **9 Upper Extremity Bursa and Ligament, Right** **B Upper Extremity Bursa and Ligament, Left** **C Upper Spine Bursa and Ligament** Interspinous ligament, thoracic Intertransverse ligament, thoracic Ligamentum flavum, thoracic Supraspinous ligament **D Lower Spine Bursa and Ligament** Iliolumbar ligament Interspinous ligament, lumbar Intertransverse ligament, lumbar Ligamentum flavum, lumbar Sacrococcygeal ligament Sacroiliac ligament Sacrospinous ligament Sacrotuberous ligament Supraspinous ligament **F Sternum Bursa and Ligament** Costoxiphoid ligament Sternocostal ligament **G Rib(s) Bursa and Ligament** Costotransverse ligament **H Abdomen Bursa and Ligament, Right** **J Abdomen Bursa and Ligament, Left** **K Perineum Bursa and Ligament** **L Hip Bursa and Ligament, Right** Iliofemoral ligament Ischiofemoral ligament Pubofemoral ligament Transverse acetabular ligament Trochanteric bursa **M Hip Bursa and Ligament, Left** *See L Hip Bursa and Ligament, Right* **N Knee Bursa and Ligament, Right** Anterior cruciate ligament (ACL) Lateral collateral ligament (LCL) Ligament of head of fibula Medial collateral ligament (MCL) Patellar ligament Popliteal ligament Posterior cruciate ligament (PCL) Prepatellar bursa **P Knee Bursa and Ligament, Left** *See N Knee Bursa and Ligament, Right* **Q Ankle Bursa and Ligament, Right** Calcaneofibular ligament Deltoid ligament Ligament of the lateral malleolus Talofibular ligament **R Ankle Bursa and Ligament, Left** *See Q Ankle Bursa and Ligament, Right* **S Foot Bursa and Ligament, Right** Calcaneocuboid ligament Cuneonavicular ligament Intercuneiform ligament Interphalangeal ligament Metatarsal ligament Metatarsophalangeal ligament Subtalar ligament Talocalcaneal ligament Talocalcaneonavicular ligament Tarsometatarsal ligament **T Foot Bursa and Ligament, Left** *See S Foot Bursa and Ligament, Right* **V Lower Extremity Bursa and Ligament, Right** **W Lower Extremity Bursa and Ligament, Left**	**Ø Open** **4 Percutaneous Endoscopic**	**7 Autologous Tissue Substitute** **J Synthetic Substitute** **K Nonautologous Tissue Substitute**	**Z No Qualifier**

Ø Medical and Surgical
M Bursae and Ligaments
S Reposition Definition: Moving to its normal location, or other suitable location, all or a portion of a body part

Explanation: The body part is moved to a new location from an abnormal location, or from a normal location where it is not functioning correctly. The body part may or may not be cut out or off to be moved to the new location.

Body Part Character 4	Approach Character 5	Device Character 6	Qualifier Character 7
Ø Head and Neck Bursa and Ligament Alar ligament of axis Cervical interspinous ligament Cervical intertransverse ligament Cervical ligamentum flavum Interspinous ligament, cervical Intertransverse ligament, cervical Lateral temporomandibular ligament Ligamentum flavum, cervical Sphenomandibular ligament Stylomandibular ligament Transverse ligament of atlas **1 Shoulder Bursa and Ligament, Right** Acromioclavicular ligament Coracoacromial ligament Coracoclavicular ligament Coracohumeral ligament Costoclavicular ligament Glenohumeral ligament Interclavicular ligament Sternoclavicular ligament Subacromial bursa Transverse humeral ligament Transverse scapular ligament **2 Shoulder Bursa and Ligament, Left** *See 1 Shoulder Bursa and Ligament, Right* **3 Elbow Bursa and Ligament, Right** Annular ligament Olecranon bursa Radial collateral ligament Ulnar collateral ligament **4 Elbow Bursa and Ligament, Left** *See 3 Elbow Bursa and Ligament, Right* **5 Wrist Bursa and Ligament, Right** Palmar ulnocarpal ligament Radial collateral carpal ligament Radiocarpal ligament Radioulnar ligament Scapholunate ligament Ulnar collateral carpal ligament **6 Wrist Bursa and Ligament, Left** *See 5 Wrist Bursa and Ligament, Right* **7 Hand Bursa and Ligament, Right** Carpometacarpal ligament Intercarpal ligament Interphalangeal ligament Lunotriquetral ligament Metacarpal ligament Metacarpophalangeal ligament Pisohamate ligament Pisometacarpal ligament Scaphotrapezium ligament **8 Hand Bursa and Ligament, Left** *See 7 Hand Bursa and Ligament, Right* **9 Upper Extremity Bursa and Ligament, Right** **B Upper Extremity Bursa and Ligament, Left** **C Upper Spine Bursa and Ligament** Interspinous ligament, thoracic Intertransverse ligament, thoracic Ligamentum flavum, thoracic Supraspinous ligament **D Lower Spine Bursa and Ligament** Iliolumbar ligament Interspinous ligament, lumbar Intertransverse ligament, lumbar Ligamentum flavum, lumbar Sacrococcygeal ligament Sacroiliac ligament Sacrospinous ligament Sacrotuberous ligament Supraspinous ligament **F Sternum Bursa and Ligament** Costoxiphoid ligament Sternocostal ligament **G Rib(s) Bursa and Ligament** Costotransverse ligament **H Abdomen Bursa and Ligament, Right** **J Abdomen Bursa and Ligament, Left** **K Perineum Bursa and Ligament** **L Hip Bursa and Ligament, Right** Iliofemoral ligament Ischiofemoral ligament Pubofemoral ligament Transverse acetabular ligament Trochanteric bursa **M Hip Bursa and Ligament, Left** *See L Hip Bursa and Ligament, Right* **N Knee Bursa and Ligament, Right** Anterior cruciate ligament (ACL) Lateral collateral ligament (LCL) Ligament of head of fibula Medial collateral ligament (MCL) Patellar ligament Popliteal ligament Posterior cruciate ligament (PCL) Prepatellar bursa **P Knee Bursa and Ligament, Left** *See N Knee Bursa and Ligament, Right* **Q Ankle Bursa and Ligament, Right** Calcaneofibular ligament Deltoid ligament Ligament of the lateral malleolus Talofibular ligament **R Ankle Bursa and Ligament, Left** *See Q Ankle Bursa and Ligament, Right* **S Foot Bursa and Ligament, Right** Calcaneocuboid ligament Cuneonavicular ligament Intercuneiform ligament Interphalangeal ligament Metatarsal ligament Metatarsophalangeal ligament Subtalar ligament Talocalcaneal ligament Talocalcaneonavicular ligament Tarsometatarsal ligament **T Foot Bursa and Ligament, Left** *See S Foot Bursa and Ligament, Right* **V Lower Extremity Bursa and Ligament, Right** **W Lower Extremity Bursa and Ligament, Left**	**Ø Open** **4 Percutaneous Endoscopic**	**Z No Device**	**Z No Qualifier**

Ø Medical and Surgical
M Bursae and Ligaments
T Resection Definition: Cutting out or off, without replacement, all of a body part
Explanation: None

Body Part Character 4		Approach Character 5	Device Character 6	Qualifier Character 7
Ø Head and Neck Bursa and Ligament Alar ligament of axis Cervical interspinous ligament Cervical intertransverse ligament Cervical ligamentum flavum Interspinous ligament, cervical Intertransverse ligament, cervical Lateral temporomandibular ligament Ligamentum flavum, cervical Sphenomandibular ligament Stylomandibular ligament Transverse ligament of atlas **1 Shoulder Bursa and Ligament, Right** Acromioclavicular ligament Coracoacromial ligament Coracoclavicular ligament Coracohumeral ligament Costoclavicular ligament Glenohumeral ligament Interclavicular ligament Sternoclavicular ligament Subacromial bursa Transverse humeral ligament Transverse scapular ligament **2 Shoulder Bursa and Ligament, Left** *See 1 Shoulder Bursa and Ligament, Right* **3 Elbow Bursa and Ligament, Right** Annular ligament Olecranon bursa Radial collateral ligament Ulnar collateral ligament **4 Elbow Bursa and Ligament, Left** *See 3 Elbow Bursa and Ligament, Right* **5 Wrist Bursa and Ligament, Right** Palmar ulnocarpal ligament Radial collateral carpal ligament Radiocarpal ligament Radioulnar ligament Scapholunate ligament Ulnar collateral carpal ligament **6 Wrist Bursa and Ligament, Left** *See 5 Wrist Bursa and Ligament, Right* **7 Hand Bursa and Ligament, Right** Carpometacarpal ligament Intercarpal ligament Interphalangeal ligament Lunotriquetral ligament Metacarpal ligament Metacarpophalangeal ligament Pisohamate ligament Pisometacarpal ligament Scaphotrapezium ligament **8 Hand Bursa and Ligament, Left** *See 7 Hand Bursa and Ligament, Right* **9 Upper Extremity Bursa and Ligament, Right** **B Upper Extremity Bursa and Ligament, Left** **C Upper Spine Bursa and Ligament** Interspinous ligament, thoracic Intertransverse ligament, thoracic Ligamentum flavum, thoracic Supraspinous ligament	**D Lower Spine Bursa and Ligament** Iliolumbar ligament Interspinous ligament, lumbar Intertransverse ligament, lumbar Ligamentum flavum, lumbar Sacrococcygeal ligament Sacroiliac ligament Sacrospinous ligament Sacrotuberous ligament Supraspinous ligament **F Sternum Bursa and Ligament** Costoxiphoid ligament Sternocostal ligament **G Rib(s) Bursa and Ligament** Costotransverse ligament **H Abdomen Bursa and Ligament, Right** **J Abdomen Bursa and Ligament, Left** **K Perineum Bursa and Ligament** **L Hip Bursa and Ligament, Right** Iliofemoral ligament Ischiofemoral ligament Pubofemoral ligament Transverse acetabular ligament Trochanteric bursa **M Hip Bursa and Ligament, Left** *See L Hip Bursa and Ligament, Right* **N Knee Bursa and Ligament, Right** Anterior cruciate ligament (ACL) Lateral collateral ligament (LCL) Ligament of head of fibula Medial collateral ligament (MCL) Patellar ligament Popliteal ligament Posterior cruciate ligament (PCL) Prepatellar bursa **P Knee Bursa and Ligament, Left** *See N Knee Bursa and Ligament, Right* **Q Ankle Bursa and Ligament, Right** Calcaneofibular ligament Deltoid ligament Ligament of the lateral malleolus Talofibular ligament **R Ankle Bursa and Ligament, Left** *See Q Ankle Bursa and Ligament, Right* **S Foot Bursa and Ligament, Right** Calcaneocuboid ligament Cuneonavicular ligament Intercuneiform ligament Interphalangeal ligament Metatarsal ligament Metatarsophalangeal ligament Subtalar ligament Talocalcaneal ligament Talocalcaneonavicular ligament Tarsometatarsal ligament **T Foot Bursa and Ligament, Left** *See S Foot Bursa and Ligament, Right* **V Lower Extremity Bursa and Ligament, Right** **W Lower Extremity Bursa and Ligament, Left**	**Ø Open** **4 Percutaneous Endoscopic**	**Z No Device**	**Z No Qualifier**

Ø Medical and Surgical
M Bursae and Ligaments
U Supplement Definition: Putting in or on biological or synthetic material that physically reinforces and/or augments the function of a portion of a body part

Explanation: The biological material is non-living, or is living and from the same individual. The body part may have been previously replaced, and the SUPPLEMENT procedure is performed to physically reinforce and/or augment the function of the replaced body part.

Body Part Character 4		Approach Character 5	Device Character 6	Qualifier Character 7
Ø Head and Neck Bursa and Ligament Alar ligament of axis Cervical interspinous ligament Cervical intertransverse ligament Cervical ligamentum flavum Interspinous ligament, cervical Intertransverse ligament, cervical Lateral temporomandibular ligament Ligamentum flavum, cervical Sphenomandibular ligament Stylomandibular ligament Transverse ligament of atlas **1 Shoulder Bursa and Ligament, Right** Acromioclavicular ligament Coracoacromial ligament Coracoclavicular ligament Coracohumeral ligament Costoclavicular ligament Glenohumeral ligament Interclavicular ligament Sternoclavicular ligament Subacromial bursa Transverse humeral ligament Transverse scapular ligament **2 Shoulder Bursa and Ligament, Left** *See 1 Shoulder Bursa and Ligament, Right* **3 Elbow Bursa and Ligament, Right** Annular ligament Olecranon bursa Radial collateral ligament Ulnar collateral ligament **4 Elbow Bursa and Ligament, Left** *See 3 Elbow Bursa and Ligament, Right* **5 Wrist Bursa and Ligament, Right** Palmar ulnocarpal ligament Radial collateral carpal ligament Radiocarpal ligament Radioulnar ligament Scapholunate ligament Ulnar collateral carpal ligament **6 Wrist Bursa and Ligament, Left** *See 5 Wrist Bursa and Ligament, Right* **7 Hand Bursa and Ligament, Right** Carpometacarpal ligament Intercarpal ligament Interphalangeal ligament Lunotriquetral ligament Metacarpal ligament Metacarpophalangeal ligament Pisohamate ligament Pisometacarpal ligament Scaphotrapezium ligament **8 Hand Bursa and Ligament, Left** *See 7 Hand Bursa and Ligament, Right* **9 Upper Extremity Bursa and Ligament, Right** **B Upper Extremity Bursa and Ligament, Left** **C Upper Spine Bursa and Ligament** Interspinous ligament, thoracic Intertransverse ligament, thoracic Ligamentum flavum, thoracic Supraspinous ligament	**D Lower Spine Bursa and Ligament** Iliolumbar ligament Interspinous ligament, lumbar Intertransverse ligament, lumbar Ligamentum flavum, lumbar Sacrococcygeal ligament Sacroiliac ligament Sacrospinous ligament Sacrotuberous ligament Supraspinous ligament **F Sternum Bursa and Ligament** Costoxiphoid ligament Sternocostal ligament **G Rib(s) Bursa and Ligament** Costotransverse ligament **H Abdomen Bursa and Ligament, Right** **J Abdomen Bursa and Ligament, Left** **K Perineum Bursa and Ligament** **L Hip Bursa and Ligament, Right** Iliofemoral ligament Ischiofemoral ligament Pubofemoral ligament Transverse acetabular ligament Trochanteric bursa **M Hip Bursa and Ligament, Left** *See L Hip Bursa and Ligament, Right* **N Knee Bursa and Ligament, Right** Anterior cruciate ligament (ACL) Lateral collateral ligament (LCL) Ligament of head of fibula Medial collateral ligament (MCL) Patellar ligament Popliteal ligament Posterior cruciate ligament (PCL) Prepatellar bursa **P Knee Bursa and Ligament, Left** *See N Knee Bursa and Ligament, Right* **Q Ankle Bursa and Ligament, Right** Calcaneofibular ligament Deltoid ligament Ligament of the lateral malleolus Talofibular ligament **R Ankle Bursa and Ligament, Left** *See Q Ankle Bursa and Ligament, Right* **S Foot Bursa and Ligament, Right** Calcaneocuboid ligament Cuneonavicular ligament Intercuneiform ligament Interphalangeal ligament Metatarsal ligament Metatarsophalangeal ligament Subtalar ligament Talocalcaneal ligament Talocalcaneonavicular ligament Tarsometatarsal ligament **T Foot Bursa and Ligament, Left** *See S Foot Bursa and Ligament, Right* **V Lower Extremity Bursa and Ligament, Right** **W Lower Extremity Bursa and Ligament, Left**	**Ø Open** **4 Percutaneous Endoscopic**	**7 Autologous Tissue Substitute** **J Synthetic Substitute** **K Nonautologous Tissue Substitute**	**Z No Qualifier**

Ø Medical and Surgical
M Bursae and Ligaments
W Revision Definition: Correcting, to the extent possible, a portion of a malfunctioning device or the position of a displaced device

Explanation: Revision can include correcting a malfunctioning or displaced device by taking out or putting in components of the device such as a screw or pin

Body Part Character 4	Approach Character 5	Device Character 6	Qualifier Character 7
X Upper Bursa and Ligament Y Lower Bursa and Ligament	Ø Open 3 Percutaneous 4 Percutaneous Endoscopic	Ø Drainage Device 7 Autologous Tissue Substitute J Synthetic Substitute K Nonautologous Tissue Substitute Y Other Device	Z No Qualifier
X Upper Bursa and Ligament Y Lower Bursa and Ligament	X External	Ø Drainage Device 7 Autologous Tissue Substitute J Synthetic Substitute K Nonautologous Tissue Substitute	Z No Qualifier

Non-OR ØMW[X,Y][3,4]YZ
Non-OR ØMW[X,Y]X[Ø,7,J,K]Z

Ø Medical and Surgical
M Bursae and Ligaments
X Transfer Definition: Moving, without taking out, all or a portion of a body part to another location to take over the function of all or a portion of a body part

Explanation: The body part transferred remains connected to its vascular and nervous supply

Body Part Character 4	Approach Character 5	Device Character 6	Qualifier Character 7
Ø Head and Neck Bursa and Ligament Alar ligament of axis Cervical interspinous ligament Cervical intertransverse ligament Cervical ligamentum flavum Interspinous ligament, cervical Intertransverse ligament, cervical Lateral temporomandibular ligament Ligamentum flavum, cervical Sphenomandibular ligament Stylomandibular ligament Transverse ligament of atlas **1 Shoulder Bursa and Ligament, Right** Acromioclavicular ligament Coracoacromial ligament Coracoclavicular ligament Coracohumeral ligament Costoclavicular ligament Glenohumeral ligament Interclavicular ligament Sternoclavicular ligament Subacromial bursa Transverse humeral ligament Transverse scapular ligament **2 Shoulder Bursa and Ligament, Left** ***See*** *1 Shoulder Bursa and Ligament, Right* **3 Elbow Bursa and Ligament, Right** Annular ligament Olecranon bursa Radial collateral ligament Ulnar collateral ligament **4 Elbow Bursa and Ligament, Left** ***See*** *3 Elbow Bursa and Ligament, Right* **5 Wrist Bursa and Ligament, Right** Palmar ulnocarpal ligament Radial collateral carpal ligament Radiocarpal ligament Radioulnar ligament Scapholunate ligament Ulnar collateral carpal ligament **6 Wrist Bursa and Ligament, Left** ***See*** *5 Wrist Bursa and Ligament, Right* **7 Hand Bursa and Ligament, Right** Carpometacarpal ligament Intercarpal ligament Interphalangeal ligament Lunotriquetral ligament Metacarpal ligament Metacarpophalangeal ligament Pisohamate ligament Pisometacarpal ligament Scaphotrapezium ligament **8 Hand Bursa and Ligament, Left** ***See*** *7 Hand Bursa and Ligament, Right* **9 Upper Extremity Bursa and Ligament, Right** **B Upper Extremity Bursa and Ligament, Left** **C Upper Spine Bursa and Ligament** Interspinous ligament, thoracic Intertransverse ligament, thoracic Ligamentum flavum, thoracic Supraspinous ligament **D Lower Spine Bursa and Ligament** Iliolumbar ligament Interspinous ligament, lumbar Intertransverse ligament, lumbar Ligamentum flavum, lumbar Sacrococcygeal ligament Sacroiliac ligament Sacrospinous ligament Sacrotuberous ligament Supraspinous ligament **F Sternum Bursa and Ligament** Costoxiphoid ligament Sternocostal ligament **G Rib(s) Bursa and Ligament** Costotransverse ligament **H Abdomen Bursa and Ligament, Right** **J Abdomen Bursa and Ligament, Left** **K Perineum Bursa and Ligament** **L Hip Bursa and Ligament, Right** Iliofemoral ligament Ischiofemoral ligament Pubofemoral ligament Transverse acetabular ligament Trochanteric bursa **M Hip Bursa and Ligament, Left** ***See*** *L Hip Bursa and Ligament, Right* **N Knee Bursa and Ligament, Right** Anterior cruciate ligament (ACL) Lateral collateral ligament (LCL) Ligament of head of fibula Medial collateral ligament (MCL) Patellar ligament Popliteal ligament Posterior cruciate ligament (PCL) Prepatellar bursa **P Knee Bursa and Ligament, Left** ***See*** *N Knee Bursa and Ligament, Right* **Q Ankle Bursa and Ligament, Right** Calcaneofibular ligament Deltoid ligament Ligament of the lateral malleolus Talofibular ligament **R Ankle Bursa and Ligament, Left** ***See*** *Q Ankle Bursa and Ligament, Right* **S Foot Bursa and Ligament, Right** Calcaneocuboid ligament Cuneonavicular ligament Intercuneiform ligament Interphalangeal ligament Metatarsal ligament Metatarsophalangeal ligament Subtalar ligament Talocalcaneal ligament Talocalcaneonavicular ligament Tarsometatarsal ligament **T Foot Bursa and Ligament, Left** ***See*** *S Foot Bursa and Ligament, Right* **V Lower Extremity Bursa and Ligament, Right** **W Lower Extremity Bursa and Ligament, Left**	**Ø Open** **4 Percutaneous Endoscopic**	**Z No Device**	**Z No Qualifier**

Head and Facial Bones ØN2–ØNW

Character Meanings

This Character Meaning table is provided as a guide to assist the user in the identification of character members that may be found in this section of code tables. It **SHOULD NOT** be used to build a PCS code.

Operation–Character 3	Body Part–Character 4	Approach–Character 5	Device–Character 6	Qualifier–Character 7
2 Change	Ø Skull	Ø Open	Ø Drainage Device	X Diagnostic
5 Destruction	1 Frontal Bone	3 Percutaneous	4 Internal Fixation Device	Z No Qualifier
8 Division	3 Parietal Bone, Right	4 Percutaneous Endoscopic	5 External Fixation Device	
9 Drainage	4 Parietal Bone, Left	X External	7 Autologous Tissue Substitute	
B Excision	5 Temporal Bone, Right		J Synthetic Substitute	
C Extirpation	6 Temporal Bone, Left		K Nonautologous Tissue Substitute	
D Extraction	7 Occipital Bone		M Bone Growth Stimulator	
H Insertion	B Nasal Bone		N Neurostimulator Generator	
J Inspection	C Sphenoid Bone		S Hearing Device	
N Release	F Ethmoid Bone, Right		Y Other Device	
P Removal	G Ethmoid Bone, Left		Z No Device	
Q Repair	H Lacrimal Bone, Right			
R Replacement	J Lacrimal Bone, Left			
S Reposition	K Palatine Bone, Right			
T Resection	L Palatine Bone, Left			
U Supplement	M Zygomatic Bone, Right			
W Revision	N Zygomatic Bone, Left			
	P Orbit, Right			
	Q Orbit, Left			
	R Maxilla			
	T Mandible, Right			
	V Mandible, Left			
	W Facial Bone			
	X Hyoid Bone			

AHA Coding Clinic for table ØNB
2017, 1Q, 20 Preparatory nasal adhesion repair before definitive cleft palate repair
2015, 3Q, 3-8 Excisional and nonexcisional debridement
2015, 2Q, 12 Orbital exenteration

AHA Coding Clinic for table ØND
2017, 4Q, 41 Extraction procedures

AHA Coding Clinic for table ØNH
2015, 3Q, 13 Nonexcisional debridement of cranial wound with removal and replacement of hardware

AHA Coding Clinic for table ØNP
2015, 3Q, 13 Nonexcisional debridement of cranial wound with removal and replacement of hardware

AHA Coding Clinic for table ØNQ
2016, 3Q, 29 Closure of bilateral alveolar clefts

AHA Coding Clinic for table ØNR
2017, 3Q, 17 Resection of schwannoma and placement of DuraGen and Lorenz cranial plating system
2017, 3Q, 22 Replacement of native skull bone flap
2017, 1Q, 23 Reconstruction of mandible using titanium and bone
2014, 3Q, 7 Hemi-cranioplasty for repair of cranial defect

AHA Coding Clinic for table ØNS
2017, 3Q, 22 Replacement of native skull bone flap
2017, 1Q, 20 Preparatory nasal adhesion repair before definitive cleft palate repair
2016, 2Q, 30 Clipping (occlusion) of cerebral artery, decompressive craniectomy and storage of bone flap in abdominal wall
2015, 3Q, 17 Craniosynostosis with cranial vault reconstruction
2015, 3Q, 27 Moyamoya disease and hemispheric pial synagiosis with craniotomy
2014, 3Q, 23 Le Fort I osteotomy
2013, 3Q, 24 Distraction osteogenesis
2013, 3Q, 25 Fracture of frontal bone with repair and coagulation for hemostasis

AHA Coding Clinic for table ØNU
2016, 3Q, 29 Closure of bilateral alveolar clefts
2013, 3Q, 24 Distraction osteogenesis

Head and Facial Bones

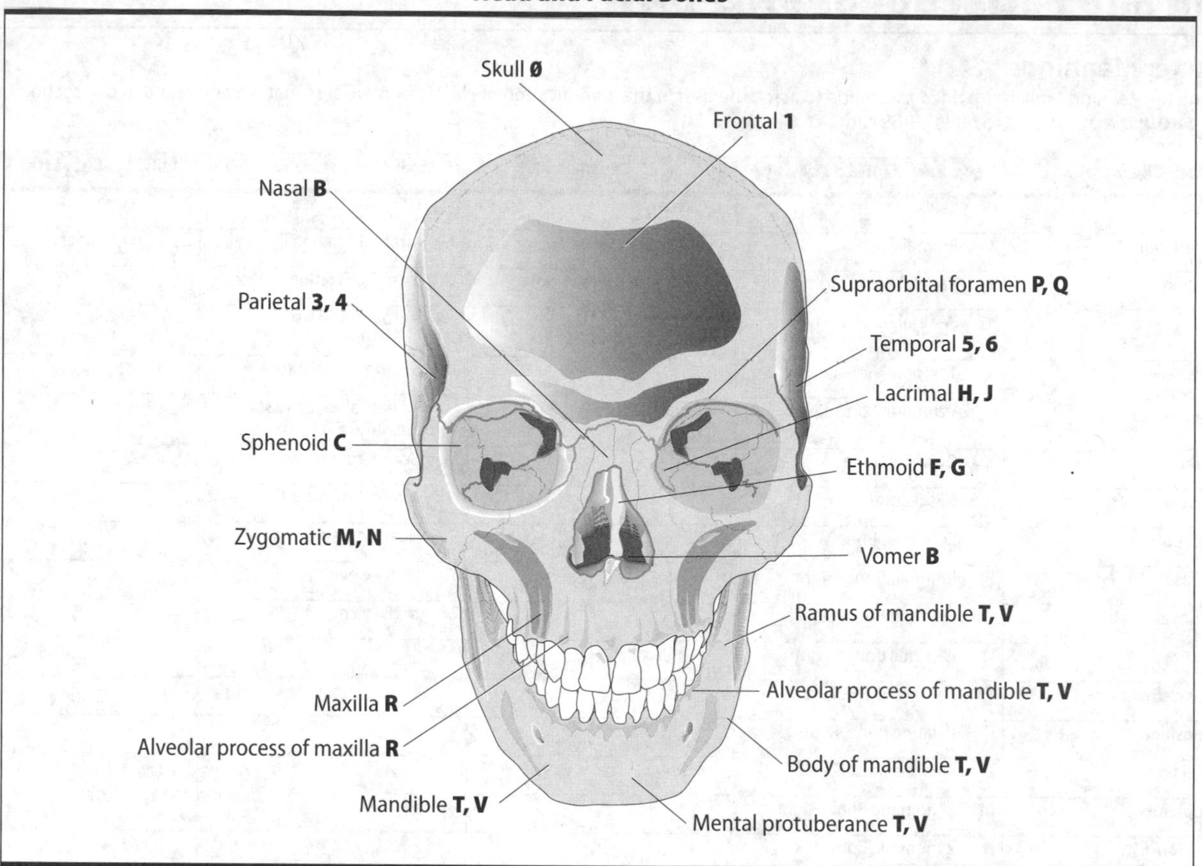

Skull Bones

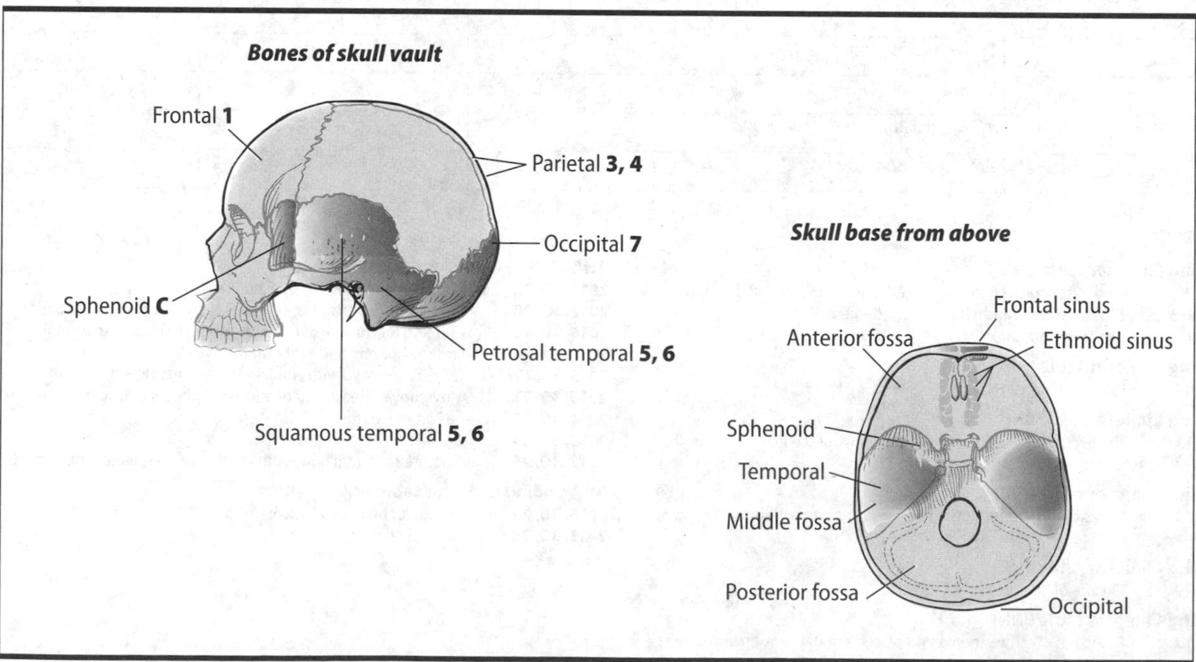

Ø Medical and Surgical
N Head and Facial Bones
2 Change Definition: Taking out or off a device from a body part and putting back an identical or similar device in or on the same body part without cutting or puncturing the skin or a mucous membrane
Explanation: All CHANGE procedures are coded using the approach EXTERNAL

Body Part Character 4	Approach Character 5	Device Character 6	Qualifier Character 7
Ø Skull B Nasal Bone Vomer of nasal septum W Facial Bone	X External	Ø Drainage Device Y Other Device	Z No Qualifier
Non-OR All body part, approach, device, and qualifier values			

Ø Medical and Surgical
N Head and Facial Bones
5 Destruction Definition: Physical eradication of all or a portion of a body part by the direct use of energy, force, or a destructive agent
Explanation: None of the body part is physically taken out

Body Part Character 4	Approach Character 5	Device Character 6	Qualifier Character 7
Ø Skull 1 Frontal Bone Zygomatic process of frontal bone 3 Parietal Bone, Right 4 Parietal Bone, Left 5 Temporal Bone, Right Mastoid process Petrous part of temporal bone Tympanic part of temporal bone Zygomatic process of temporal bone 6 Temporal Bone, Left *See 5 Temporal Bone, Right* 7 Occipital Bone Foramen magnum B Nasal Bone Vomer of nasal septum C Sphenoid Bone Greater wing Lesser wing Optic foramen Pterygoid process Sella turcica F Ethmoid Bone, Right Cribriform plate G Ethmoid Bone, Left *See F Ethmoid Bone, Right* H Lacrimal Bone, Right J Lacrimal Bone, Left K Palatine Bone, Right L Palatine Bone, Left M Zygomatic Bone, Right N Zygomatic Bone, Left P Orbit, Right Bony orbit Orbital portion of ethmoid bone Orbital portion of frontal bone Orbital portion of lacrimal bone Orbital portion of maxilla Orbital portion of palatine bone Orbital portion of sphenoid bone Orbital portion of zygomatic bone Q Orbit, Left *See P Orbit, Right* R Maxilla Alveolar process of maxilla T Mandible, Right Alveolar process of mandible Condyloid process Mandibular notch Mental foramen V Mandible, Left *See T Mandible, Right* X Hyoid Bone	Ø Open 3 Percutaneous 4 Percutaneous Endoscopic	Z No Device	Z No Qualifier

Ø Medical and Surgical
N Head and Facial Bones
8 Division Definition: Cutting into a body part, without draining fluids and/or gases from the body part, in order to separate or transect a body part

Explanation: All or a portion of the body part is separated into two or more portions

Body Part Character 4	Approach Character 5	Device Character 6	Qualifier Character 7
Ø Skull **1 Frontal Bone** Zygomatic process of frontal bone **3 Parietal Bone, Right** **4 Parietal Bone, Left** **5 Temporal Bone, Right** Mastoid process Petrous part of temporal bone Tympanic part of temporal bone Zygomatic process of temporal bone **6 Temporal Bone, Left** *See 5 Temporal Bone, Right* **7 Occipital Bone** Foramen magnum **B Nasal Bone** Vomer of nasal septum **C Sphenoid Bone** Greater wing Lesser wing Optic foramen Pterygoid process Sella turcica **F Ethmoid Bone, Right** Cribriform plate **G Ethmoid Bone, Left** *See F Ethmoid Bone, Right* **H Lacrimal Bone, Right** **J Lacrimal Bone, Left** **K Palatine Bone, Right** **L Palatine Bone, Left** **M Zygomatic Bone, Right** **N Zygomatic Bone, Left** **P Orbit, Right** Bony orbit Orbital portion of ethmoid bone Orbital portion of frontal bone Orbital portion of lacrimal bone Orbital portion of maxilla Orbital portion of palatine bone Orbital portion of sphenoid bone Orbital portion of zygomatic bone **Q Orbit, Left** *See P Orbit, Right* **R Maxilla** Alveolar process of maxilla **T Mandible, Right** Alveolar process of mandible Condyloid process Mandibular notch Mental foramen **V Mandible, Left** *See T Mandible, Right* **X Hyoid Bone**	**Ø Open** **3 Percutaneous** **4 Percutaneous Endoscopic**	**Z No Device**	**Z No Qualifier**

Non-OR ØN8B[Ø,3,4]ZZ

Ø **Medical and Surgical**
N **Head and Facial Bones**
9 **Drainage** Definition: Taking or letting out fluids and/or gases from a body part
Explanation: The qualifier DIAGNOSTIC is used to identify drainage procedures that are biopsies

Body Part Character 4	Approach Character 5	Device Character 6	Qualifier Character 7
Ø Skull **1** Frontal Bone Zygomatic process of frontal bone **3** Parietal Bone, Right **4** Parietal Bone, Left **5** Temporal Bone, Right Mastoid process Petrous part of temporal bone Tympanic part of temporal bone Zygomatic process of temporal bone **6** Temporal Bone, Left *See 5 Temporal Bone, Right* **7** Occipital Bone Foramen magnum **B** Nasal Bone Vomer of nasal septum **C** Sphenoid Bone Greater wing Lesser wing Optic foramen Pterygoid process Sella turcica **F** Ethmoid Bone, Right Cribriform plate **G** Ethmoid Bone, Left *See F Ethmoid Bone, Right* **H** Lacrimal Bone, Right **J** Lacrimal Bone, Left **K** Palatine Bone, Right **L** Palatine Bone, Left **M** Zygomatic Bone, Right **N** Zygomatic Bone, Left **P** Orbit, Right Bony orbit Orbital portion of ethmoid bone Orbital portion of frontal bone Orbital portion of lacrimal bone Orbital portion of maxilla Orbital portion of palatine bone Orbital portion of sphenoid bone Orbital portion of zygomatic bone **Q** Orbit, Left *See P Orbit, Right* **R** Maxilla Alveolar process of maxilla **T** Mandible, Right Alveolar process of mandible Condyloid process Mandibular notch Mental foramen **V** Mandible, Left *See T Mandible, Right* **X** Hyoid Bone	**Ø** Open **3** Percutaneous **4** Percutaneous Endoscopic	**Ø** Drainage Device	**Z** No Qualifier

Non-OR ØN9[Ø,1,3,4,5,6,7,C,F,G,H,J,K,L,M,N,P,Q,X]3ØZ
Non-OR ØN9[B,R,T,V][Ø,3,4]ØZ

ØN9 Continued on next page

Ø Medical and Surgical
N Head and Facial Bones
9 Drainage Definition: Taking or letting out fluids and/or gases from a body part
Explanation: The qualifier DIAGNOSTIC is used to identify drainage procedures that are biopsies

ØN9 Continued

Body Part Character 4	Approach Character 5	Device Character 6	Qualifier Character 7
Ø Skull **1 Frontal Bone** Zygomatic process of frontal bone **3 Parietal Bone, Right** **4 Parietal Bone, Left** **5 Temporal Bone, Right** Mastoid process Petrous part of temporal bone Tympanic part of temporal bone Zygomatic process of temporal bone **6 Temporal Bone, Left** ***See*** *5 Temporal Bone, Right* **7 Occipital Bone** Foramen magnum **B Nasal Bone** Vomer of nasal septum **C Sphenoid Bone** Greater wing Lesser wing Optic foramen Pterygoid process Sella turcica **F Ethmoid Bone, Right** Cribriform plate **G Ethmoid Bone, Left** ***See*** *F Ethmoid Bone, Right* **H Lacrimal Bone, Right** **J Lacrimal Bone, Left** **K Palatine Bone, Right** **L Palatine Bone, Left** **M Zygomatic Bone, Right** **N Zygomatic Bone, Left** **P Orbit, Right** Bony orbit Orbital portion of ethmoid bone Orbital portion of frontal bone Orbital portion of lacrimal bone Orbital portion of maxilla Orbital portion of palatine bone Orbital portion of sphenoid bone Orbital portion of zygomatic bone **Q Orbit, Left** ***See*** *P Orbit, Right* **R Maxilla** Alveolar process of maxilla **T Mandible, Right** Alveolar process of mandible Condyloid process Mandibular notch Mental foramen **V Mandible, Left** ***See*** *T Mandible, Right* **X Hyoid Bone**	**Ø Open** **3 Percutaneous** **4 Percutaneous Endoscopic**	**Z No Device**	**X Diagnostic** **Z No Qualifier**

Non-OR ØN9[Ø,1,3,4,5,6,7,C,F,G,H,J,K,L,M,N,P,Q,X]3ZZ
Non-OR ØN9B[Ø,3,4]Z[X,Z]
Non-OR ØN9[R,T,V][Ø,3,4]ZZ

Ø Medical and Surgical
N Head and Facial Bones
B Excision Definition: Cutting out or off, without replacement, a portion of a body part
Explanation: The qualifier DIAGNOSTIC is used to identify excision procedures that are biopsies

Body Part Character 4	Approach Character 5	Device Character 6	Qualifier Character 7
Ø Skull **1 Frontal Bone** Zygomatic process of frontal bone **3 Parietal Bone, Right** **4 Parietal Bone, Left** **5 Temporal Bone, Right** Mastoid process Petrous part of temporal bone Tympanic part of temporal bone Zygomatic process of temporal bone **6 Temporal Bone, Left** *See 5 Temporal Bone, Right* **7 Occipital Bone** Foramen magnum **B Nasal Bone** Vomer of nasal septum **C Sphenoid Bone** Greater wing Lesser wing Optic foramen Pterygoid process Sella turcica **F Ethmoid Bone, Right** Cribriform plate **G Ethmoid Bone, Left** *See F Ethmoid Bone, Right* **H Lacrimal Bone, Right** **J Lacrimal Bone, Left** **K Palatine Bone, Right** **L Palatine Bone, Left** **M Zygomatic Bone, Right** **N Zygomatic Bone, Left** **P Orbit, Right** Bony orbit Orbital portion of ethmoid bone Orbital portion of frontal bone Orbital portion of lacrimal bone Orbital portion of maxilla Orbital portion of palatine bone Orbital portion of sphenoid bone Orbital portion of zygomatic bone **Q Orbit, Left** *See P Orbit, Right* **R Maxilla** Alveolar process of maxilla **T Mandible, Right** Alveolar process of mandible Condyloid process Mandibular notch Mental foramen **V Mandible, Left** *See T Mandible, Right* **X Hyoid Bone**	**Ø Open** **3 Percutaneous** **4 Percutaneous Endoscopic**	**Z No Device**	**X Diagnostic** **Z No Qualifier**

Non-OR ØNB[B,R,T,V][Ø,3,4]ZX

Ø Medical and Surgical
N Head and Facial Bones
C Extirpation Definition: Taking or cutting out solid matter from a body part

Explanation: The solid matter may be an abnormal byproduct of a biological function or a foreign body; it may be imbedded in a body part or in the lumen of a tubular body part. The solid matter may or may not have been previously broken into pieces.

Body Part Character 4	Approach Character 5	Device Character 6	Qualifier Character 7
1 Frontal Bone Zygomatic process of frontal bone **3 Parietal Bone, Right** **4 Parietal Bone, Left** **5 Temporal Bone, Right** Mastoid process Petrous part of temporal bone Tympanic part of temporal bone Zygomatic process of temporal bone **6 Temporal Bone, Left** *See 5 Temporal Bone, Right* **7 Occipital Bone** Foramen magnum **B Nasal Bone** Vomer of nasal septum **C Sphenoid Bone** Greater wing Lesser wing Optic foramen Pterygoid process Sella turcica **F Ethmoid Bone, Right** Cribriform plate **G Ethmoid Bone, Left** *See F Ethmoid Bone, Right* **H Lacrimal Bone, Right** **J Lacrimal Bone, Left** **K Palatine Bone, Right** **L Palatine Bone, Left** **M Zygomatic Bone, Right** **N Zygomatic Bone, Left** **P Orbit, Right** Bony orbit Orbital portion of ethmoid bone Orbital portion of frontal bone Orbital portion of lacrimal bone Orbital portion of maxilla Orbital portion of palatine bone Orbital portion of sphenoid bone Orbital portion of zygomatic bone **Q Orbit, Left** *See P Orbit, Right* **R Maxilla** Alveolar process of maxilla **T Mandible, Right** Alveolar process of mandible Condyloid process Mandibular notch Mental foramen **V Mandible, Left** *See T Mandible, Right* **X Hyoid Bone**	**Ø Open** **3 Percutaneous** **4 Percutaneous Endoscopic**	**Z No Device**	**Z No Qualifier**

Non-OR ØNC[B,R,T,V][Ø,3,4]ZZ

Ø Medical and Surgical
N Head and Facial Bones
D Extraction Definition: Pulling or stripping out or off all or a portion of a body part by the use of force
Explanation: The qualifier DIAGNOSTIC is used to identify extraction procedures that are biopsies

Body Part Character 4	Approach Character 5	Device Character 6	Qualifier Character 7
Ø Skull **1 Frontal Bone** Zygomatic process of frontal bone **3 Parietal Bone, Right** **4 Parietal Bone, Left** **5 Temporal Bone, Right** Mastoid process Petrous part of temporal bone Tympanic part of temporal bone Zygomatic process of temporal bone **6 Temporal Bone, Left** *See 5 Temporal Bone, Right* **7 Occipital Bone** Foramen magnum **B Nasal Bone** Vomer of nasal septum **C Sphenoid Bone** Greater wing Lesser wing Optic foramen Pterygoid process Sella turcica **F Ethmoid Bone, Right** Cribriform plate **G Ethmoid Bone, Left** *See F Ethmoid Bone, Right* **H Lacrimal Bone, Right** **J Lacrimal Bone, Left** **K Palatine Bone, Right** **L Palatine Bone, Left** **M Zygomatic Bone, Right** **N Zygomatic Bone, Left** **P Orbit, Right** Bony orbit Orbital portion of ethmoid bone Orbital portion of frontal bone Orbital portion of lacrimal bone Orbital portion of maxilla Orbital portion of palatine bone Orbital portion of sphenoid bone Orbital portion of zygomatic bone **Q Orbit, Left** *See P Orbit, Right* **R Maxilla** Alveolar process of maxilla **T Mandible, Right** Alveolar process of mandible Condyloid process Mandibular notch Mental foramen **V Mandible, Left** *See T Mandible, Right* **X Hyoid Bone**	Ø Open	Z No Device	Z No Qualifier

Ø Medical and Surgical
N Head and Facial Bones
H Insertion Definition: Putting in a nonbiological appliance that monitors, assists, performs, or prevents a physiological function but does not physically take the place of a body part

Explanation: None

Body Part Character 4	Approach Character 5	Device Character 6	Qualifier Character 7
Ø Skull ⊞	**Ø Open**	**4 Internal Fixation Device** **5 External Fixation Device** **M Bone Growth Stimulator** **N Neurostimulator Generator**	**Z No Qualifier**
Ø Skull	**3 Percutaneous** **4 Percutaneous Endoscopic**	**4 Internal Fixation Device** **5 External Fixation Device** **M Bone Growth Stimulator**	**Z No Qualifier**
1 Frontal Bone Zygomatic process of frontal bone **3 Parietal Bone, Right** **4 Parietal Bone, Left** **7 Occipital Bone** Foramen magnum **C Sphenoid Bone** Greater wing Lesser wing Optic foramen Pterygoid process Sella turcica **F Ethmoid Bone, Right** Cribriform plate **G Ethmoid Bone, Left** *See F Ethmoid Bone, Right* **H Lacrimal Bone, Right** **J Lacrimal Bone, Left** **K Palatine Bone, Right** **L Palatine Bone, Left** **M Zygomatic Bone, Right** **N Zygomatic Bone, Left** **P Orbit, Right** Bony orbit Orbital portion of ethmoid bone Orbital portion of frontal bone Orbital portion of lacrimal bone Orbital portion of maxilla Orbital portion of palatine bone Orbital portion of sphenoid bone Orbital portion of zygomatic bone **Q Orbit, Left** *See P Orbit, Right* **X Hyoid Bone**	**Ø Open** **3 Percutaneous** **4 Percutaneous Endoscopic**	**4 Internal Fixation Device**	**Z No Qualifier**
5 Temporal Bone, Right Mastoid process Petrous part of temporal bone Tympanic part of temporal bone Zygomatic process of temporal bone **6 Temporal Bone, Left** *See 5 Temporal Bone, Right*	**Ø Open** **3 Percutaneous** **4 Percutaneous Endoscopic**	**4 Internal Fixation Device** **S Hearing Device**	**Z No Qualifier**
B Nasal Bone Vomer of nasal septum	**Ø Open** **3 Percutaneous** **4 Percutaneous Endoscopic**	**4 Internal Fixation Device** **M Bone Growth Stimulator**	**Z No Qualifier**
R Maxilla Alveolar process of maxilla **T Mandible, Right** Alveolar process of mandible Condyloid process Mandibular notch Mental foramen **V Mandible, Left** *See T Mandible, Right*	**Ø Open** **3 Percutaneous** **4 Percutaneous Endoscopic**	**4 Internal Fixation Device** **5 External Fixation Device**	**Z No Qualifier**
W Facial Bone	**Ø Open** **3 Percutaneous** **4 Percutaneous Endoscopic**	**M Bone Growth Stimulator**	**Z No Qualifier**

Non-OR ØNHØØ5Z
Non-OR ØNHØ[3,4]5Z
Non-OR ØNHB[Ø,3,4][4,M]Z

See Appendix L for Procedure Combinations
⊞ ØNHØØNZ

Ø Medical and Surgical
N Head and Facial Bones
J Inspection Definition: Visually and/or manually exploring a body part

Explanation: Visual exploration may be performed with or without optical instrumentation. Manual exploration may be performed directly or through intervening body layers.

Body Part Character 4	Approach Character 5	Device Character 6	Qualifier Character 7
Ø Skull **B Nasal Bone** Vomer of nasal septum **W Facial Bone**	**Ø Open** **3 Percutaneous** **4 Percutaneous Endoscopic** **X External**	**Z No Device**	**Z No Qualifier**

Non-OR ØNJ[Ø,B,W][3,X]ZZ

Ø Medical and Surgical
N Head and Facial Bones
N Release Definition: Freeing a body part from an abnormal physical constraint by cutting or by the use of force

Explanation: Some of the restraining tissue may be taken out but none of the body part is taken out

Body Part Character 4	Approach Character 5	Device Character 6	Qualifier Character 7
1 Frontal Bone Zygomatic process of frontal bone **3 Parietal Bone, Right** **4 Parietal Bone, Left** **5 Temporal Bone, Right** Mastoid process Petrous part of temporal bone Tympanic part of temporal bone Zygomatic process of temporal bone **6 Temporal Bone, Left** *See 5 Temporal Bone, Right* **7 Occipital Bone** Foramen magnum **B Nasal Bone** Vomer of nasal septum **C Sphenoid Bone** Greater wing Lesser wing Optic foramen Pterygoid process Sella turcica **F Ethmoid Bone, Right** Cribriform plate **G Ethmoid Bone, Left** *See F Ethmoid Bone, Right* **H Lacrimal Bone, Right** **J Lacrimal Bone, Left** **K Palatine Bone, Right** **L Palatine Bone, Left** **M Zygomatic Bone, Right** **N Zygomatic Bone, Left** **P Orbit, Right** Bony orbit Orbital portion of ethmoid bone Orbital portion of frontal bone Orbital portion of lacrimal bone Orbital portion of maxilla Orbital portion of palatine bone Orbital portion of sphenoid bone Orbital portion of zygomatic bone **Q Orbit, Left** *See P Orbit, Right* **R Maxilla** Alveolar process of maxilla **T Mandible, Right** Alveolar process of mandible Condyloid process Mandibular notch Mental foramen **V Mandible, Left** *See T Mandible, Right* **X Hyoid Bone**	**Ø Open** **3 Percutaneous** **4 Percutaneous Endoscopic**	**Z No Device**	**Z No Qualifier**

Non-OR ØNNB[Ø,3,4]ZZ

Head and Facial Bones

ØNJ–ØNN

Ø Medical and Surgical
N Head and Facial Bones
P Removal Definition: Taking out or off a device from a body part

Explanation: If a device is taken out and a similar device put in without cutting or puncturing the skin or mucous membrane, the procedure is coded to the root operation CHANGE. Otherwise, the procedure for taking out a device is coded to the root operation REMOVAL.

Body Part Character 4	Approach Character 5	Device Character 6	Qualifier Character 7
Ø Skull	Ø Open	Ø Drainage Device 4 Internal Fixation Device 5 External Fixation Device 7 Autologous Tissue Substitute J Synthetic Substitute K Nonautologous Tissue Substitute M Bone Growth Stimulator N Neurostimulator Generator S Hearing Device	Z No Qualifier
Ø Skull	3 Percutaneous 4 Percutaneous Endoscopic	Ø Drainage Device 4 Internal Fixation Device 5 External Fixation Device 7 Autologous Tissue Substitute J Synthetic Substitute K Nonautologous Tissue Substitute M Bone Growth Stimulator S Hearing Device	Z No Qualifier
Ø Skull	X External	Ø Drainage Device 4 Internal Fixation Device 5 External Fixation Device M Bone Growth Stimulator S Hearing Device	Z No Qualifier
B Nasal Bone Vomer of nasal septum W Facial Bone	Ø Open 3 Percutaneous 4 Percutaneous Endoscopic	Ø Drainage Device 4 Internal Fixation Device 7 Autologous Tissue Substitute J Synthetic Substitute K Nonautologous Tissue Substitute M Bone Growth Stimulator	Z No Qualifier
B Nasal Bone Vomer of nasal septum W Facial Bone	X External	Ø Drainage Device 4 Internal Fixation Device M Bone Growth Stimulator	Z No Qualifier

Non-OR ØNPØ[3,4]5Z
Non-OR ØNPØX[Ø,5]Z
Non-OR ØNPB[Ø,3,4][Ø,4,7,J,K,M]Z
Non-OR ØNPBX[Ø,4,M]Z
Non-OR ØNPWX[Ø,M]Z

Ø Medical and Surgical
N Head and Facial Bones
Q Repair Definition: Restoring, to the extent possible, a body part to its normal anatomic structure and function
Explanation: Used only when the method to accomplish the repair is not one of the other root operations

Body Part Character 4	Approach Character 5	Device Character 6	Qualifier Character 7
Ø Skull **1 Frontal Bone** Zygomatic process of frontal bone **3 Parietal Bone, Right** **4 Parietal Bone, Left** **5 Temporal Bone, Right** Mastoid process Petrous part of temporal bone Tympanic part of temporal bone Zygomatic process of temporal bone **6 Temporal Bone, Left** *See 5 Temporal Bone, Right* **7 Occipital Bone** Foramen magnum **B Nasal Bone** Vomer of nasal septum **C Sphenoid Bone** Greater wing Lesser wing Optic foramen Pterygoid process Sella turcica **F Ethmoid Bone, Right** Cribriform plate **G Ethmoid Bone, Left** *See F Ethmoid Bone, Right* **H Lacrimal Bone, Right** **J Lacrimal Bone, Left** **K Palatine Bone, Right** **L Palatine Bone, Left** **M Zygomatic Bone, Right** **N Zygomatic Bone, Left** **P Orbit, Right** Bony orbit Orbital portion of ethmoid bone Orbital portion of frontal bone Orbital portion of lacrimal bone Orbital portion of maxilla Orbital portion of palatine bone Orbital portion of sphenoid bone Orbital portion of zygomatic bone **Q Orbit, Left** *See P Orbit, Right* **R Maxilla** Alveolar process of maxilla **T Mandible, Right** Alveolar process of mandible Condyloid process Mandibular notch Mental foramen **V Mandible, Left** *See T Mandible, Right* **X Hyoid Bone**	**Ø Open** **3 Percutaneous** **4 Percutaneous Endoscopic** **X External**	**Z No Device**	**Z No Qualifier**

Non-OR ØNQ[Ø,1,3,4,5,6,7,B,C,F,G,H,J,K,L,M,N,P,Q,R,T,V,X]XZZ

Ø Medical and Surgical
N Head and Facial Bones
R Replacement Definition: Putting in or on biological or synthetic material that physically takes the place and/or function of all or a portion of a body part

Explanation: The body part may have been taken out or replaced, or may be taken out, physically eradicated, or rendered nonfunctional during the REPLACEMENT procedure. A REMOVAL procedure is coded for taking out the device used in a previous replacement procedure.

Body Part Character 4	Approach Character 5	Device Character 6	Qualifier Character 7
Ø Skull **1 Frontal Bone** Zygomatic process of frontal bone **3 Parietal Bone, Right** **4 Parietal Bone, Left** **5 Temporal Bone, Right** Mastoid process Petrous part of temporal bone Tympanic part of temporal bone Zygomatic process of temporal bone **6 Temporal Bone, Left** *See 5 Temporal Bone, Right* **7 Occipital Bone** Foramen magnum **B Nasal Bone** Vomer of nasal septum **C Sphenoid Bone** Greater wing Lesser wing Optic foramen Pterygoid process Sella turcica **F Ethmoid Bone, Right** Cribriform plate **G Ethmoid Bone, Left** *See F Ethmoid Bone, Right* **H Lacrimal Bone, Right** **J Lacrimal Bone, Left** **K Palatine Bone, Right** **L Palatine Bone, Left** **M Zygomatic Bone, Right** **N Zygomatic Bone, Left** **P Orbit, Right** Bony orbit Orbital portion of ethmoid bone Orbital portion of frontal bone Orbital portion of lacrimal bone Orbital portion of maxilla Orbital portion of palatine bone Orbital portion of sphenoid bone Orbital portion of zygomatic bone **Q Orbit, Left** *See P Orbit, Right* **R Maxilla** Alveolar process of maxilla **T Mandible, Right** Alveolar process of mandible Condyloid process Mandibular notch Mental foramen **V Mandible, Left** *See T Mandible, Right* **X Hyoid Bone**	**Ø Open** **3 Percutaneous** **4 Percutaneous Endoscopic**	**7 Autologous Tissue Substitute** **J Synthetic Substitute** **K Nonautologous Tissue Substitute**	**Z No Qualifier**

Ø Medical and Surgical
N Head and Facial Bones
S Reposition Definition: Moving to its normal location, or other suitable location, all or a portion of a body part

Explanation: The body part is moved to a new location from an abnormal location, or from a normal location where it is not functioning correctly. The body part may or may not be cut out or off to be moved to the new location.

Body Part Character 4	Approach Character 5	Device Character 6	Qualifier Character 7
Ø Skull **R Maxilla** Alveolar process of maxilla **T Mandible, Right** Alveolar process of mandible Condyloid process Mandibular notch Mental foramen **V Mandible, Left** *See T Mandible, Right*	**Ø Open** **3 Percutaneous** **4 Percutaneous Endoscopic**	**4 Internal Fixation Device** **5 External Fixation Device** **Z No Device**	**Z No Qualifier**
Ø Skull **R Maxilla** Alveolar process of maxilla **T Mandible, Right** Alveolar process of mandible Condyloid process Mandibular notch Mental foramen **V Mandible, Left** *See T Mandible, Right*	**X External**	**Z No Device**	**Z No Qualifier**
1 Frontal Bone Zygomatic process of frontal bone **3 Parietal Bone, Right** **4 Parietal Bone, Left** **5 Temporal Bone, Right** Mastoid process Petrous part of temporal bone Tympanic part of temporal bone Zygomatic process of temporal bone **6 Temporal Bone, Left** *See 5 Temporal Bone, Right* **7 Occipital Bone** Foramen magnum **B Nasal Bone** Vomer of nasal septum **C Sphenoid Bone** Greater wing Lesser wing Optic foramen Pterygoid process Sella turcica **F Ethmoid Bone, Right** Cribriform plate **G Ethmoid Bone, Left** *See F Ethmoid Bone, Right* **H Lacrimal Bone, Right** **J Lacrimal Bone, Left** **K Palatine Bone, Right** **L Palatine Bone, Left** **M Zygomatic Bone, Right** **N Zygomatic Bone, Left** **P Orbit, Right** Bony orbit Orbital portion of ethmoid bone Orbital portion of frontal bone Orbital portion of lacrimal bone Orbital portion of maxilla Orbital portion of palatine bone Orbital portion of sphenoid bone Orbital portion of zygomatic bone **Q Orbit, Left** *See P Orbit, Right* **X Hyoid Bone**	**Ø Open** **3 Percutaneous** **4 Percutaneous Endoscopic**	**4 Internal Fixation Device** **Z No Device**	**Z No Qualifier**

Non-OR ØNS[R,T,V][3,4][4,5,Z]Z
Non-OR ØNS[Ø,R,T,V]XZZ
Non-OR ØNS[B,C,F,G,H,J,K,L,M,N,P,Q,X][3,4][4,Z]Z

ØNS Continued on next page

ØNS Continued

Ø Medical and Surgical
N Head and Facial Bones
S Reposition Definition: Moving to its normal location, or other suitable location, all or a portion of a body part

Explanation: The body part is moved to a new location from an abnormal location, or from a normal location where it is not functioning correctly. The body part may or may not be cut out or off to be moved to the new location.

Body Part Character 4	Approach Character 5	Device Character 6	Qualifier Character 7
1 Frontal Bone Zygomatic process of frontal bone **3 Parietal Bone, Right** **4 Parietal Bone, Left** **5 Temporal Bone, Right** Mastoid process Petrous part of temporal bone Tympanic part of temporal bone Zygomatic process of temporal bone **6 Temporal Bone, Left** *See 5 Temporal Bone, Right* **7 Occipital Bone** Foramen magnum **B Nasal Bone** Vomer of nasal septum **C Sphenoid Bone** Greater wing Lesser wing Optic foramen Pterygoid process Sella turcica **F Ethmoid Bone, Right** Cribriform plate **G Ethmoid Bone, Left** *See F Ethmoid Bone, Right* **H Lacrimal Bone, Right** **J Lacrimal Bone, Left** **K Palatine Bone, Right** **L Palatine Bone, Left** **M Zygomatic Bone, Right** **N Zygomatic Bone, Left** **P Orbit, Right** Bony orbit Orbital portion of ethmoid bone Orbital portion of frontal bone Orbital portion of lacrimal bone Orbital portion of maxilla Orbital portion of palatine bone Orbital portion of sphenoid bone Orbital portion of zygomatic bone **Q Orbit, Left** *See P Orbit, Right* **X Hyoid Bone**	**X External**	**Z No Device**	**Z No Qualifier**

Non-OR ØNS[1,3,4,5,6,7,B,C,F,G,H,J,K,L,M,N,P,Q,X]XZZ

Ø Medical and Surgical
N Head and Facial Bones
T Resection Definition: Cutting out or off, without replacement, all of a body part

Explanation: None

Body Part Character 4	Approach Character 5	Device Character 6	Qualifier Character 7
1 Frontal Bone Zygomatic process of frontal bone **3 Parietal Bone, Right** **4 Parietal Bone, Left** **5 Temporal Bone, Right** Mastoid process Petrous part of temporal bone Tympanic part of temporal bone Zygomatic process of temporal bone **6 Temporal Bone, Left** *See 5 Temporal Bone, Right* **7 Occipital Bone** Foramen magnum **B Nasal Bone** Vomer of nasal septum **C Sphenoid Bone** Greater wing Lesser wing Optic foramen Pterygoid process Sella turcica **F Ethmoid Bone, Right** Cribriform plate **G Ethmoid Bone, Left** *See F Ethmoid Bone, Right* **H Lacrimal Bone, Right** **J Lacrimal Bone, Left** **K Palatine Bone, Right** **L Palatine Bone, Left** **M Zygomatic Bone, Right** **N Zygomatic Bone, Left** **P Orbit, Right** Bony orbit Orbital portion of ethmoid bone Orbital portion of frontal bone Orbital portion of lacrimal bone Orbital portion of maxilla Orbital portion of palatine bone Orbital portion of sphenoid bone Orbital portion of zygomatic bone **Q Orbit, Left** *See P Orbit, Right* **R Maxilla** Alveolar process of maxilla **T Mandible, Right** Alveolar process of mandible Condyloid process Mandibular notch Mental foramen **V Mandible, Left** *See T Mandible, Right* **X Hyoid Bone**	**Ø Open**	**Z No Device**	**Z No Qualifier**

Ø Medical and Surgical
N Head and Facial Bones
U Supplement Definition: Putting in or on biological or synthetic material that physically reinforces and/or augments the function of a portion of a body part

Explanation: The biological material is non-living, or is living and from the same individual. The body part may have been previously replaced, and the SUPPLEMENT procedure is performed to physically reinforce and/or augment the function of the replaced body part.

Body Part Character 4	Approach Character 5	Device Character 6	Qualifier Character 7
Ø Skull **1 Frontal Bone** Zygomatic process of frontal bone **3 Parietal Bone, Right** **4 Parietal Bone, Left** **5 Temporal Bone, Right** Mastoid process Petrous part of temporal bone Tympanic part of temporal bone Zygomatic process of temporal bone **6 Temporal Bone, Left** *See 5 Temporal Bone, Right* **7 Occipital Bone** Foramen magnum **B Nasal Bone** Vomer of nasal septum **C Sphenoid Bone** Greater wing Lesser wing Optic foramen Pterygoid process Sella turcica **F Ethmoid Bone, Right** Cribriform plate **G Ethmoid Bone, Left** *See F Ethmoid Bone, Right* **H Lacrimal Bone, Right** **J Lacrimal Bone, Left** **K Palatine Bone, Right** **L Palatine Bone, Left** **M Zygomatic Bone, Right** **N Zygomatic Bone, Left** **P Orbit, Right** Bony orbit Orbital portion of ethmoid bone Orbital portion of frontal bone Orbital portion of lacrimal bone Orbital portion of maxilla Orbital portion of palatine bone Orbital portion of sphenoid bone Orbital portion of zygomatic bone **Q Orbit, Left** *See P Orbit, Right* **R Maxilla** Alveolar process of maxilla **T Mandible, Right** Alveolar process of mandible Condyloid process Mandibular notch Mental foramen **V Mandible, Left** *See T Mandible, Right* **X Hyoid Bone**	**Ø Open** **3 Percutaneous** **4 Percutaneous Endoscopic**	**7 Autologous Tissue Substitute** **J Synthetic Substitute** **K Nonautologous Tissue Substitute**	**Z No Qualifier**

Ø Medical and Surgical
N Head and Facial Bones
W Revision

Definition: Correcting, to the extent possible, a portion of a malfunctioning device or the position of a displaced device

Explanation: Revision can include correcting a malfunctioning or displaced device by taking out or putting in components of the device such as a screw or pin

Body Part Character 4	Approach Character 5	Device Character 6	Qualifier Character 7
Ø Skull	**Ø** Open	**Ø** Drainage Device **4** Internal Fixation Device **5** External Fixation Device **7** Autologous Tissue Substitute **J** Synthetic Substitute **K** Nonautologous Tissue Substitute **M** Bone Growth Stimulator **N** Neurostimulator Generator **S** Hearing Device	**Z** No Qualifier
Ø Skull	**3** Percutaneous **4** Percutaneous Endoscopic **X** External	**Ø** Drainage Device **4** Internal Fixation Device **5** External Fixation Device **7** Autologous Tissue Substitute **J** Synthetic Substitute **K** Nonautologous Tissue Substitute **M** Bone Growth Stimulator **S** Hearing Device	**Z** No Qualifier
B Nasal Bone Vomer of nasal septum **W** Facial Bone	**Ø** Open **3** Percutaneous **4** Percutaneous Endoscopic **X** External	**Ø** Drainage Device **4** Internal Fixation Device **7** Autologous Tissue Substitute **J** Synthetic Substitute **K** Nonautologous Tissue Substitute **M** Bone Growth Stimulator	**Z** No Qualifier

Non-OR ØNWØX[Ø,4,5,7,J,K,M,S]Z
Non-OR ØNWB[Ø,3,4,X][Ø,4,7,J,K,M]Z
Non-OR ØNWWX[Ø,4,7,J,K,M]Z

Upper Bones ØP2–ØPW

Character Meanings

This Character Meaning table is provided as a guide to assist the user in the identification of character members that may be found in this section of code tables. It **SHOULD NOT** be used to build a PCS code.

Operation–Character 3	Body Part–Character 4	Approach–Character 5	Device–Character 6	Qualifier–Character 7
2 Change	Ø Sternum	Ø Open	Ø Drainage Device OR Internal Fixation Device, Rigid Plate	X Diagnostic
5 Destruction	1 Ribs, 1 to 2	3 Percutaneous	4 Internal Fixation Device	Z No Qualifier
8 Division	2 Ribs, 3 or more	4 Percutaneous Endoscopic	5 External Fixation Device	
9 Drainage	3 Cervical Vertebra	X External	6 Internal Fixation Device, Intramedullary	
B Excision	4 Thoracic Vertebra		7 Autologous Tissue Substitute OR Internal Fixation Device, Intramedullary Limb Lengthening	
C Extirpation	5 Scapula, Right		8 External Fixation Device, Limb Lengthening	
D Extraction	6 Scapula, Left		B External Fixation Device, Monoplanar	
H Insertion	7 Glenoid Cavity, Right		C External Fixation Device, Ring	
J Inspection	8 Glenoid Cavity, Left		D External Fixation Device, Hybrid	
N Release	9 Clavicle, Right		J Synthetic Substitute	
P Removal	B Clavicle, Left		K Nonautologous TIssue Substitute	
Q Repair	C Humeral Head, Right		M Bone Growth Stimulator	
R Replacement	D Humeral Head, Left		Y Other Device	
S Reposition	F Humeral Shaft, Right		Z No Device	
T Resection	G Humeral Shaft, Left			
U Supplement	H Radius, Right			
W Revision	J Radius, Left			
	K Ulna, Right			
	L Ulna, Left			
	M Carpal, Right			
	N Carpal, Left			
	P Metacarpal, Right			
	Q Metacarpal, Left			
	R Thumb Phalanx, Right			
	S Thumb Phalanx, Left			
	T Finger Phalanx, Right			
	V Finger Phalanx, Left			
	Y Upper Bone			

AHA Coding Clinic for table ØPB
2015, 3Q, 3-8 Excisional and nonexcisional debridement
2015, 2Q, 34 Decompressive laminectomy
2013, 4Q, 109 Separating conjoined twins
2013, 4Q, 116 Spinal decompression
2013, 3Q, 20 Superior labrum anterior posterior (SLAP) repair and subacromialdecompression
2012, 4Q, 101 Rib resection with reconstruction of anterior chest wall
2012, 2Q, 19 Multiple decompressive cervical laminectomies

AHA Coding Clinic for table ØPC
2019, 3Q, 19 Removal of sternal wire

AHA Coding Clinic for table ØPD
2017, 4Q, 41 Extraction procedures

AHA Coding Clinic for table ØPH
2020, 1Q, 29 Repair of sternal dehiscence using Sternal Talon® device
2019, 4Q, 34 Intramedullary limb lengthening internal fixation device
2019, 2Q, 40 Decompression of spinal cord and placement of instrumentation
2018, 3Q, 26 Anterior vertebral tethering using Dynesys Tethering System
2017, 2Q, 20 Exchange of intramedullary antibiotic impregnated spacer
2016, 4Q, 117 Placement of magnetic growth rods
2014, 4Q, 28 Removal and replacement of displaced growing rods

AHA Coding Clinic for table ØPP
2019, 3Q, 19 Removal of sternal wire
2017, 2Q, 20 Exchange of intramedullary antibiotic impregnated spacer
2016, 4Q, 117 Placement of magnetic growth rods
2014, 4Q, 28 Removal and replacement of displaced growing rods

AHA Coding Clinic for table ØPR
2018, 4Q, 92 Radial head arthroplasty

AHA Coding Clinic for table ØPS
2020, 1Q, 33 Spinal fusion without use of bone graft
2018, 3Q, 26 Anterior vertebral tethering using Dynesys Tethering System
2017, 4Q, 53 New and revised body part values - Ribs
2016, 1Q, 21 Elongation derotation flexion casting
2015, 4Q, 33 Ravitch operation
2015, 2Q, 35 Application of tongs to reduce and stabilize cervical fracture
2014, 4Q, 26 Placement of vertical expandable prosthetic titanium rib (VEPTR)
2014, 4Q, 32 Open reduction internal fixation of fracture with debridement
2014, 3Q, 33 Radial fracture treatment with open reduction internal fixation, and release of carpal ligament

AHA Coding Clinic for table ØPT
2015, 3Q, 26 Thumb arthroplasty with resection of trapezium

AHA Coding Clinic for table ØPU
2015, 2Q, 20 Cervical laminoplasty
2013, 4Q, 109 Separating conjoined twins

AHA Coding Clinic for table ØPW
2014, 4Q, 26 Adjustment of VEPTR lengthening mechanism
2014, 4Q, 27 Bilateral lengthening of growing rods

Upper Bones

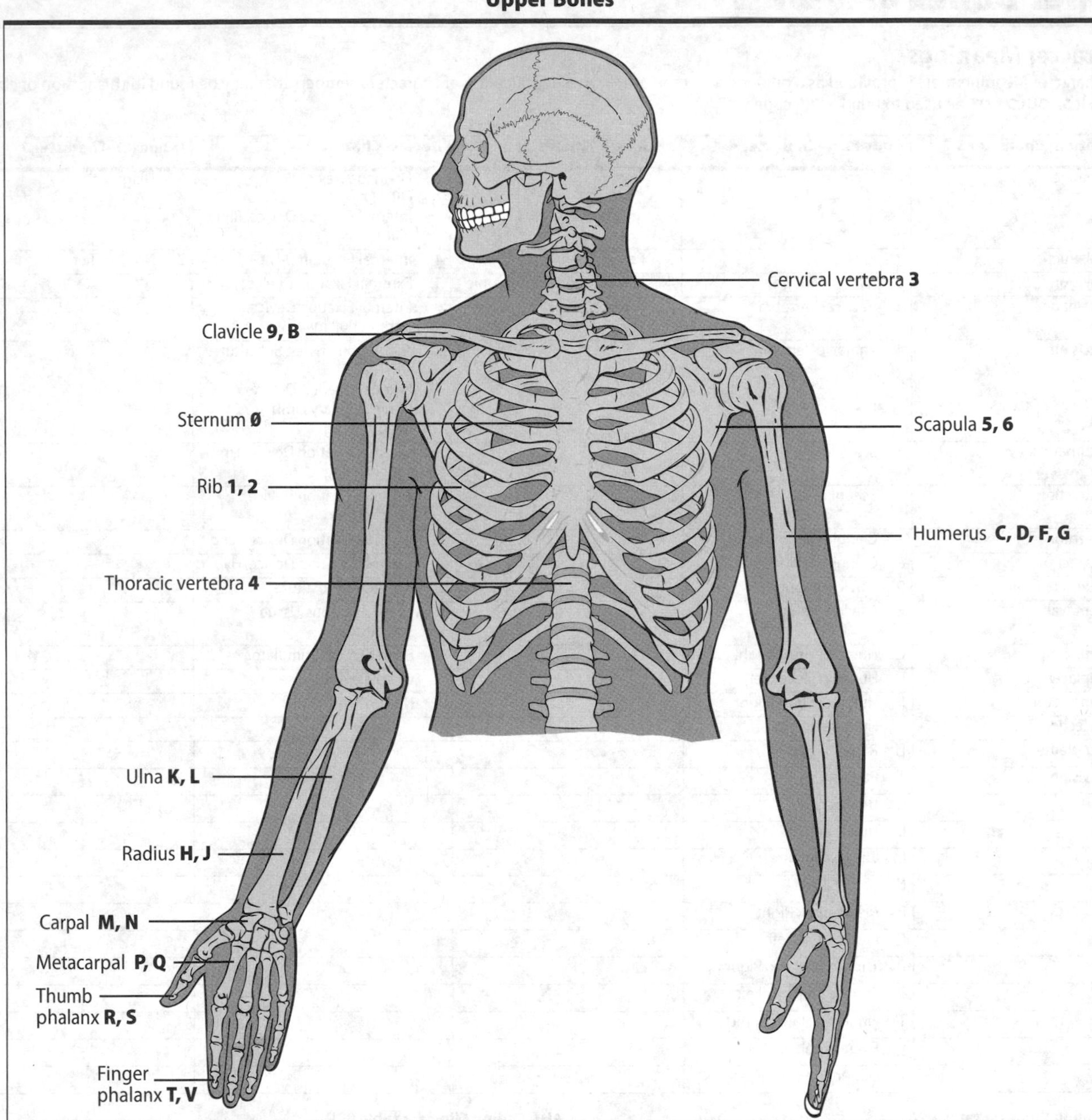
Cervical vertebra 3
Clavicle 9, B
Sternum Ø
Scapula 5, 6
Rib 1, 2
Humerus C, D, F, G
Thoracic vertebra 4
Ulna K, L
Radius H, J
Carpal M, N
Metacarpal P, Q
Thumb phalanx R, S
Finger phalanx T, V

Humerus and Scapula

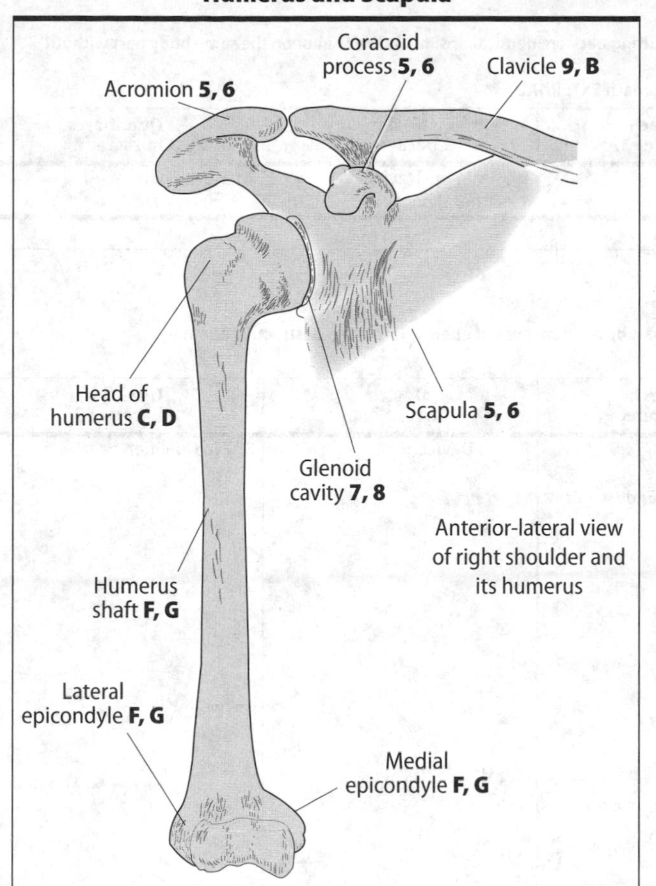

Radius and Ulna

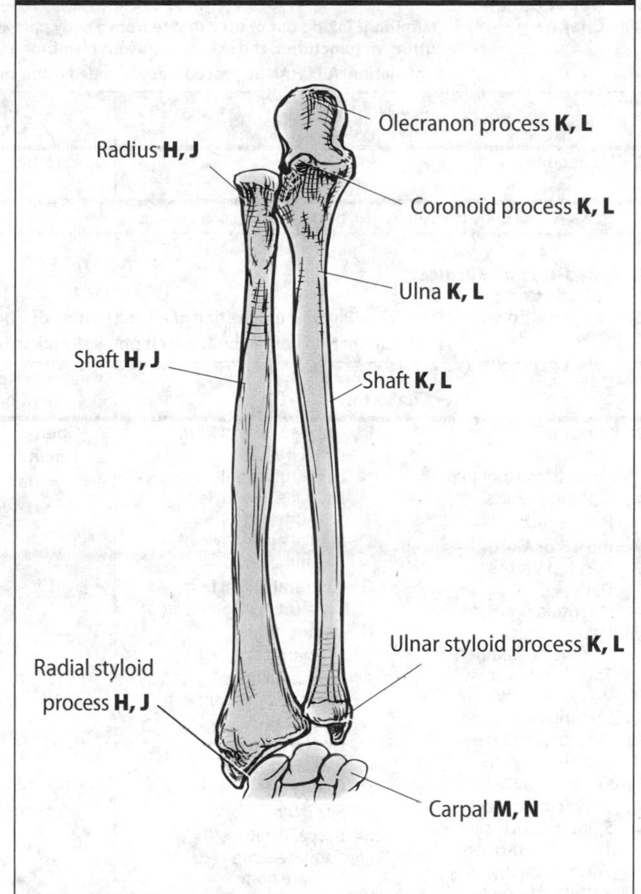

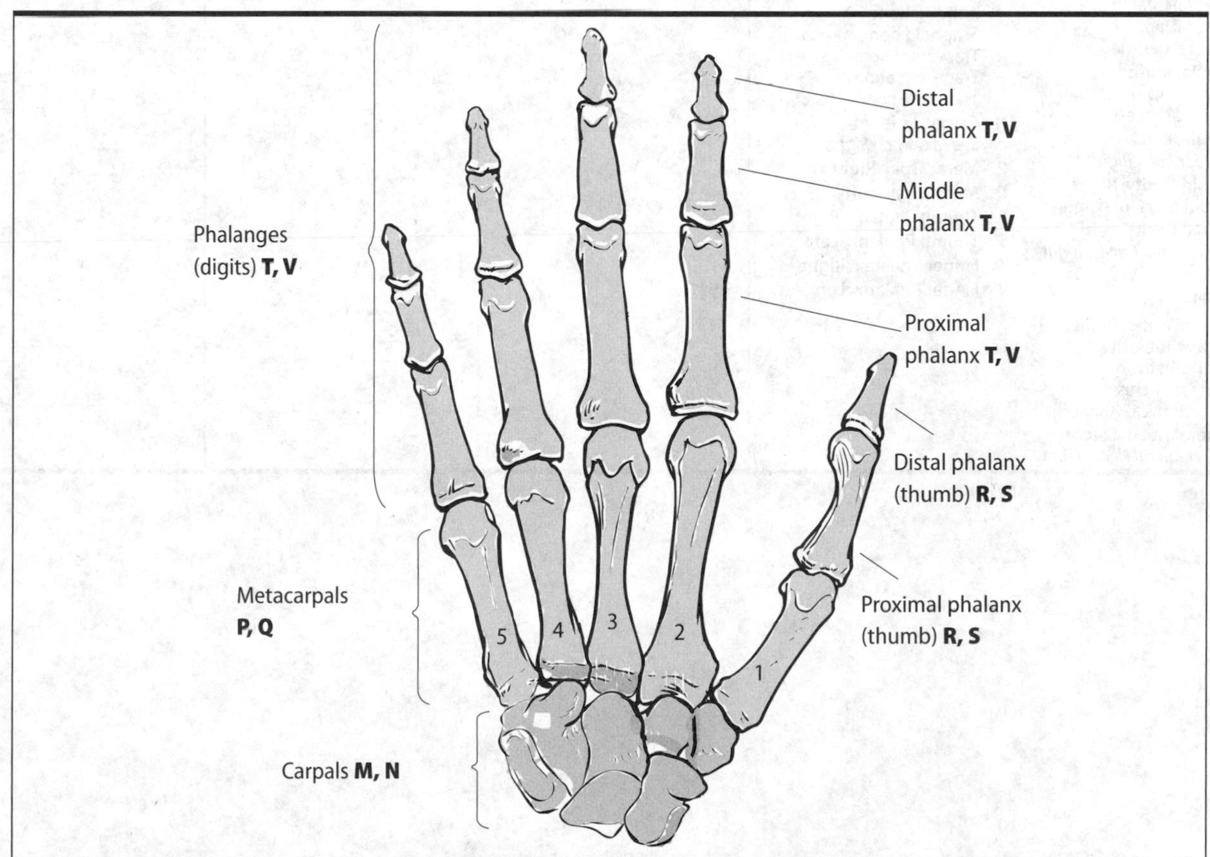

Ø Medical and Surgical
P Upper Bones
2 Change Definition: Taking out or off a device from a body part and putting back an identical or similar device in or on the same body part without cutting or puncturing the skin or a mucous membrane
Explanation: All CHANGE procedures are coded using the approach EXTERNAL

Body Part Character 4	Approach Character 5	Device Character 6	Qualifier Character 7
Y Upper Bone	X External	Ø Drainage Device Y Other Device	Z No Qualifier

Non-OR All body part, approach, device, and qualifier values

Ø Medical and Surgical
P Upper Bones
5 Destruction Definition: Physical eradication of all or a portion of a body part by the direct use of energy, force, or a destructive agent
Explanation: None of the body part is physically taken out

Body Part Character 4		Approach Character 5	Device Character 6	Qualifier Character 7
Ø Sternum Manubrium Suprasternal notch Xiphoid process **1 Ribs, 1 to 2** **2 Ribs, 3 or More** **3 Cervical Vertebra** Dens Odontoid process Spinous process Transverse foramen Transverse process Vertebral arch Vertebral body Vertebral foramen Vertebral lamina Vertebral pedicle **4 Thoracic Vertebra** Spinous process Transverse process Vertebral arch Vertebral body Vertebral foramen Vertebral lamina Vertebral pedicle **5 Scapula, Right** Acromion (process) Coracoid process **6 Scapula, Left** *See 5 Scapula, Right* **7 Glenoid Cavity, Right** Glenoid fossa (of scapula) **8 Glenoid Cavity, Left** *See 7 Glenoid Cavity, Right* **9 Clavicle, Right** **B Clavicle, Left** **C Humeral Head, Right** Greater tuberosity Lesser tuberosity Neck of humerus (anatomical)(surgical) **D Humeral Head, Left** *See C Humeral Head, Right*	**F Humeral Shaft, Right** Distal humerus Humerus, distal Lateral epicondyle of humerus Medial epicondyle of humerus **G Humeral Shaft, Left** *See F Humeral Shaft, Right* **H Radius, Right** Ulnar notch **J Radius, Left** *See H Radius, Right* **K Ulna, Right** Olecranon process Radial notch **L Ulna, Left** *See K Ulna, Right* **M Carpal, Right** Capitate bone Hamate bone Lunate bone Pisiform bone Scaphoid bone Trapezium bone Trapezoid bone Triquetral bone **N Carpal, Left** *See M Carpal, Right* **P Metacarpal, Right** **Q Metacarpal, Left** **R Thumb Phalanx, Right** **S Thumb Phalanx, Left** **T Finger Phalanx, Right** **V Finger Phalanx, Left**	Ø Open 3 Percutaneous 4 Percutaneous Endoscopic	Z No Device	Z No Qualifier

Ø Medical and Surgical
P Upper Bones
8 Division Definition: Cutting into a body part, without draining fluids and/or gases from the body part, in order to separate or transect a body part
Explanation: All or a portion of the body part is separated into two or more portions

Body Part Character 4		Approach Character 5	Device Character 6	Qualifier Character 7
Ø Sternum Manubrium Suprasternal notch Xiphoid process **1 Ribs, 1 to 2** **2 Ribs, 3 or More** **3 Cervical Vertebra** Dens Odontoid process Spinous process Transverse foramen Transverse process Vertebral arch Vertebral body Vertebral foramen Vertebral lamina Vertebral pedicle **4 Thoracic Vertebra** Spinous process Transverse process Vertebral arch Vertebral body Vertebral foramen Vertebral lamina Vertebral pedicle **5 Scapula, Right** Acromion (process) Coracoid process **6 Scapula, Left** *See 5 Scapula, Right* **7 Glenoid Cavity, Right** Glenoid fossa (of scapula) **8 Glenoid Cavity, Left** *See 7 Glenoid Cavity, Right* **9 Clavicle, Right** **B Clavicle, Left** **C Humeral Head, Right** Greater tuberosity Lesser tuberosity Neck of humerus (anatomical)(surgical) **D Humeral Head, Left** *See C Humeral Head, Right*	**F Humeral Shaft, Right** Distal humerus Humerus, distal Lateral epicondyle of humerus Medial epicondyle of humerus **G Humeral Shaft, Left** *See F Humeral Shaft, Right* **H Radius, Right** Ulnar notch **J Radius, Left** *See H Radius, Right* **K Ulna, Right** Olecranon process Radial notch **L Ulna, Left** *See K Ulna, Right* **M Carpal, Right** Capitate bone Hamate bone Lunate bone Pisiform bone Scaphoid bone Trapezium bone Trapezoid bone Triquetral bone **N Carpal, Left** *See M Carpal, Right* **P Metacarpal, Right** **Q Metacarpal, Left** **R Thumb Phalanx, Right** **S Thumb Phalanx, Left** **T Finger Phalanx, Right** **V Finger Phalanx, Left**	**Ø Open** **3 Percutaneous** **4 Percutaneous Endoscopic**	**Z No Device**	**Z No Qualifier**

Ø Medical and Surgical
P Upper Bones
9 Drainage Definition: Taking or letting out fluids and/or gases from a body part
Explanation: The qualifier DIAGNOSTIC is used to identify drainage procedures that are biopsies

Body Part Character 4	Approach Character 5	Device Character 6	Qualifier Character 7
Ø Sternum Manubrium Suprasternal notch Xiphoid process **1 Ribs, 1 to 2** **2 Ribs, 3 or More** **3 Cervical Vertebra** Dens Odontoid process Spinous process Transverse foramen Transverse process Vertebral arch Vertebral body Vertebral foramen Vertebral lamina Vertebral pedicle **4 Thoracic Vertebra** Spinous process Transverse process Vertebral arch Vertebral body Vertebral foramen Vertebral lamina Vertebral pedicle **5 Scapula, Right** Acromion (process) Coracoid process **6 Scapula, Left** *See 5 Scapula, Right* **7 Glenoid Cavity, Right** Glenoid fossa (of scapula) **8 Glenoid Cavity, Left** *See 7 Glenoid Cavity, Right* **9 Clavicle, Right** **B Clavicle, Left** **C Humeral Head, Right** Greater tuberosity Lesser tuberosity Neck of humerus (anatomical)(surgical) **D Humeral Head, Left** *See C Humeral Head, Right* **F Humeral Shaft, Right** Distal humerus Humerus, distal Lateral epicondyle of humerus Medial epicondyle of humerus **G Humeral Shaft, Left** *See F Humeral Shaft, Right* **H Radius, Right** Ulnar notch **J Radius, Left** *See H Radius, Right* **K Ulna, Right** Olecranon process Radial notch **L Ulna, Left** *See K Ulna, Right* **M Carpal, Right** Capitate bone Hamate bone Lunate bone Pisiform bone Scaphoid bone Trapezium bone Trapezoid bone Triquetral bone **N Carpal, Left** *See M Carpal, Right* **P Metacarpal, Right** **Q Metacarpal, Left** **R Thumb Phalanx, Right** **S Thumb Phalanx, Left** **T Finger Phalanx, Right** **V Finger Phalanx, Left**	**Ø Open** **3 Percutaneous** **4 Percutaneous Endoscopic**	**Ø Drainage Device**	**Z No Qualifier**

Non-OR ØP9[Ø,1,2,3,4,5,6,7,8,9,B,C,D,F,G,H,J,K,L,M,N,P,Q,R,S,T,V]3ØZ

ØP9 Continued on next page

ØP9 Continued

Ø Medical and Surgical
P Upper Bones
9 Drainage Definition: Taking or letting out fluids and/or gases from a body part
Explanation: The qualifier DIAGNOSTIC is used to identify drainage procedures that are biopsies

Body Part Character 4		Approach Character 5	Device Character 6	Qualifier Character 7
Ø Sternum Manubrium Suprasternal notch Xiphoid process **1 Ribs, 1 to 2** **2 Ribs, 3 or More** **3 Cervical Vertebra** Dens Odontoid process Spinous process Transverse foramen Transverse process Vertebral arch Vertebral body Vertebral foramen Vertebral lamina Vertebral pedicle **4 Thoracic Vertebra** Spinous process Transverse process Vertebral arch Vertebral body Vertebral foramen Vertebral lamina Vertebral pedicle **5 Scapula, Right** Acromion (process) Coracoid process **6 Scapula, Left** ***See** 5 Scapula, Right* **7 Glenoid Cavity, Right** Glenoid fossa (of scapula) **8 Glenoid Cavity, Left** ***See** 7 Glenoid Cavity, Right* **9 Clavicle, Right** **B Clavicle, Left** **C Humeral Head, Right** Greater tuberosity Lesser tuberosity Neck of humerus (anatomical)(surgical)	**D Humeral Head, Left** ***See** C Humeral Head, Right* **F Humeral Shaft, Right** Distal humerus Humerus, distal Lateral epicondyle of humerus Medial epicondyle of humerus **G Humeral Shaft, Left** ***See** F Humeral Shaft, Right* **H Radius, Right** Ulnar notch **J Radius, Left** ***See** H Radius, Right* **K Ulna, Right** Olecranon process Radial notch **L Ulna, Left** ***See** K Ulna, Right* **M Carpal, Right** Capitate bone Hamate bone Lunate bone Pisiform bone Scaphoid bone Trapezium bone Trapezoid bone Triquetral bone **N Carpal, Left** ***See** M Carpal, Right* **P Metacarpal, Right** **Q Metacarpal, Left** **R Thumb Phalanx, Right** **S Thumb Phalanx, Left** **T Finger Phalanx, Right** **V Finger Phalanx, Left**	**Ø Open** **3 Percutaneous** **4 Percutaneous Endoscopic**	**Z No Device**	**X Diagnostic** **Z No Qualifier**

Non-OR ØP9[Ø,1,2,3,4,5,6,7,8,9,B,C,D,F,G,H,J,K,L,M,N,P,Q,R,S,T,V]3ZZ

Ø Medical and Surgical
P Upper Bones
B Excision

Definition: Cutting out or off, without replacement, a portion of a body part
Explanation: The qualifier DIAGNOSTIC is used to identify excision procedures that are biopsies

Body Part Character 4	Approach Character 5	Device Character 6	Qualifier Character 7
Ø Sternum Manubrium Suprasternal notch Xiphoid process **1 Ribs, 1 to 2** **2 Ribs, 3 or More** **3 Cervical Vertebra** Dens Odontoid process Spinous process Transverse foramen Transverse process Vertebral arch Vertebral body Vertebral foramen Vertebral lamina Vertebral pedicle **4 Thoracic Vertebra** Spinous process Transverse process Vertebral arch Vertebral body Vertebral foramen Vertebral lamina Vertebral pedicle **5 Scapula, Right** Acromion (process) Coracoid process **6 Scapula, Left** *See 5 Scapula, Right* **7 Glenoid Cavity, Right** Glenoid fossa (of scapula) **8 Glenoid Cavity, Left** *See 7 Glenoid Cavity, Right* **9 Clavicle, Right** **B Clavicle, Left** **C Humeral Head, Right** Greater tuberosity Lesser tuberosity Neck of humerus (anatomical)(surgical) **D Humeral Head, Left** *See C Humeral Head, Right* **F Humeral Shaft, Right** Distal humerus Humerus, distal Lateral epicondyle of humerus Medial epicondyle of humerus **G Humeral Shaft, Left** *See F Humeral Shaft, Right* **H Radius, Right** Ulnar notch **J Radius, Left** *See H Radius, Right* **K Ulna, Right** Olecranon process Radial notch **L Ulna, Left** *See K Ulna, Right* **M Carpal, Right** Capitate bone Hamate bone Lunate bone Pisiform bone Scaphoid bone Trapezium bone Trapezoid bone Triquetral bone **N Carpal, Left** *See M Carpal, Right* **P Metacarpal, Right** **Q Metacarpal, Left** **R Thumb Phalanx, Right** **S Thumb Phalanx, Left** **T Finger Phalanx, Right** **V Finger Phalanx, Left**	**Ø Open** **3 Percutaneous** **4 Percutaneous Endoscopic**	**Z No Device**	**X Diagnostic** **Z No Qualifier**

Ø Medical and Surgical
P Upper Bones
C Extirpation Definition: Taking or cutting out solid matter from a body part

Explanation: The solid matter may be an abnormal byproduct of a biological function or a foreign body; it may be imbedded in a body part or in the lumen of a tubular body part. The solid matter may or may not have been previously broken into pieces.

Body Part Character 4		Approach Character 5	Device Character 6	Qualifier Character 7
Ø Sternum Manubrium Suprasternal notch Xiphoid process **1 Ribs, 1 to 2** **2 Ribs, 3 or More** **3 Cervical Vertebra** Dens Odontoid process Spinous process Transverse foramen Transverse process Vertebral arch Vertebral body Vertebral foramen Vertebral lamina Vertebral pedicle **4 Thoracic Vertebra** Spinous process Transverse process Vertebral arch Vertebral body Vertebral foramen Vertebral lamina Vertebral pedicle **5 Scapula, Right** Acromion (process) Coracoid process **6 Scapula, Left** *See 5 Scapula, Right* **7 Glenoid Cavity, Right** Glenoid fossa (of scapula) **8 Glenoid Cavity, Left** *See 7 Glenoid Cavity, Right* **9 Clavicle, Right** **B Clavicle, Left** **C Humeral Head, Right** Greater tuberosity Lesser tuberosity Neck of humerus (anatomical)(surgical) **D Humeral Head, Left** *See C Humeral Head, Right*	**F Humeral Shaft, Right** Distal humerus Humerus, distal Lateral epicondyle of humerus Medial epicondyle of humerus **G Humeral Shaft, Left** *See F Humeral Shaft, Right* **H Radius, Right** Ulnar notch **J Radius, Left** *See H Radius, Right* **K Ulna, Right** Olecranon process Radial notch **L Ulna, Left** *See K Ulna, Right* **M Carpal, Right** Capitate bone Hamate bone Lunate bone Pisiform bone Scaphoid bone Trapezium bone Trapezoid bone Triquetral bone **N Carpal, Left** *See M Carpal, Right* **P Metacarpal, Right** **Q Metacarpal, Left** **R Thumb Phalanx, Right** **S Thumb Phalanx, Left** **T Finger Phalanx, Right** **V Finger Phalanx, Left**	**Ø Open** **3 Percutaneous** **4 Percutaneous Endoscopic**	**Z No Device**	**Z No Qualifier**

Ø Medical and Surgical
P Upper Bones
D Extraction Definition: Pulling or stripping out or off all or a portion of a body part by the use of force
Explanation: The qualifier DIAGNOSTIC is used to identify extraction procedures that are biopsies

Body Part Character 4		Approach Character 5	Device Character 6	Qualifier Character 7
Ø Sternum Manubrium Suprasternal notch Xiphoid process **1 Ribs, 1 to 2** **2 Ribs, 3 or More** **3 Cervical Vertebra** Dens Odontoid process Spinous process Transverse foramen Transverse process Vertebral arch Vertebral body Vertebral foramen Vertebral lamina Vertebral pedicle **4 Thoracic Vertebra** Spinous process Transverse process Vertebral arch Vertebral body Vertebral foramen Vertebral lamina Vertebral pedicle **5 Scapula, Right** Acromion (process) Coracoid process **6 Scapula, Left** *See 5 Scapula, Right* **7 Glenoid Cavity, Right** Glenoid fossa (of scapula) **8 Glenoid Cavity, Left** *See 7 Glenoid Cavity, Right* **9 Clavicle, Right** **B Clavicle, Left** **C Humeral Head, Right** Greater tuberosity Lesser tuberosity Neck of humerus (anatomical)(surgical) **D Humeral Head, Left** *See C Humeral Head, Right*	**F Humeral Shaft, Right** Distal humerus Humerus, distal Lateral epicondyle of humerus Medial epicondyle of humerus **G Humeral Shaft, Left** *See F Humeral Shaft, Right* **H Radius, Right** Ulnar notch **J Radius, Left** *See H Radius, Right* **K Ulna, Right** Olecranon process Radial notch **L Ulna, Left** *See K Ulna, Right* **M Carpal, Right** Capitate bone Hamate bone Lunate bone Pisiform bone Scaphoid bone Trapezium bone Trapezoid bone Triquetral bone **N Carpal, Left** *See M Carpal, Right* **P Metacarpal, Right** **Q Metacarpal, Left** **R Thumb Phalanx, Right** **S Thumb Phalanx, Left** **T Finger Phalanx, Right** **V Finger Phalanx, Left**	**Ø Open**	**Z No Device**	**Z No Qualifier**

Ø Medical and Surgical
P Upper Bones
H Insertion

Definition: Putting in a nonbiological appliance that monitors, assists, performs, or prevents a physiological function but does not physically take the place of a body part

Explanation: None

Body Part Character 4		Approach Character 5	Device Character 6	Qualifier Character 7
Ø Sternum Manubrium Suprasternal notch Xiphoid process		**Ø Open** **3 Percutaneous** **4 Percutaneous Endoscopic**	**Ø Internal Fixation Device, Rigid Plate** **4 Internal Fixation Device**	**Z No Qualifier**
1 Ribs, 1 to 2 **2 Ribs, 3 or More** **3 Cervical Vertebra** Dens Odontoid process Spinous process Transverse foramen Transverse process Vertebral arch Vertebral body Vertebral foramen Vertebral lamina Vertebral pedicle **4 Thoracic Vertebra** Spinous process Transverse process Vertebral arch Vertebral body Vertebral foramen Vertebral lamina Vertebral pedicle	**5 Scapula, Right** Acromion (process) Coracoid process **6 Scapula, Left** *See 5 Scapula, Right* **7 Glenoid Cavity, Right** Glenoid fossa (of scapula) **8 Glenoid Cavity, Left** *See 7 Glenoid Cavity, Right* **9 Clavicle, Right** **B Clavicle, Left**	**Ø Open** **3 Percutaneous** **4 Percutaneous Endoscopic**	**4 Internal Fixation Device**	**Z No Qualifier**
C Humeral Head, Right Greater tuberosity Lesser tuberosity Neck of humerus (anatomical)(surgical) **D Humeral Head, Left** *See C Humeral Head, Right*	**H Radius, Right** Ulnar notch **J Radius, Left** *See H Radius, Right* **K Ulna, Right** Olecranon process Radial notch **L Ulna, Left** *See K Ulna, Right*	**Ø Open** **3 Percutaneous** **4 Percutaneous Endoscopic**	**4 Internal Fixation Device** **5 External Fixation Device** **6 Internal Fixation Device, Intramedullary** **8 External Fixation Device, Limb Lengthening** **B External Fixation Device, Monoplanar** **C External Fixation Device, Ring** **D External Fixation Device, Hybrid**	**Z No Qualifier**
F Humeral Shaft, Right Distal humerus Humerus, distal Lateral epicondyle of humerus Medial epicondyle of humerus	**G Humeral Shaft, Left** *See F Humeral Shaft, Right*	**Ø Open** **3 Percutaneous** **4 Percutaneous Endoscopic**	**4 Internal Fixation Device** **5 External Fixation Device** **6 Internal Fixation Device, Intramedullary** **7 Internal Fixation Device, Intramedullary Limb Lengthening** **8 External Fixation Device, Limb Lengthening** **B External Fixation Device, Monoplanar** **C External Fixation Device, Ring** **D External Fixation Device, Hybrid**	**Z No Qualifier**
M Carpal, Right Capitate bone Hamate bone Lunate bone Pisiform bone Scaphoid bone Trapezium bone Trapezoid bone Triquetral bone **N Carpal, Left** *See M Carpal, Right*	**P Metacarpal, Right** **Q Metacarpal, Left** **R Thumb Phalanx, Right** **S Thumb Phalanx, Left** **T Finger Phalanx, Right** **V Finger Phalanx, Left**	**Ø Open** **3 Percutaneous** **4 Percutaneous Endoscopic**	**4 Internal Fixation Device** **5 External Fixation Device**	**Z No Qualifier**
Y Upper Bone		**Ø Open** **3 Percutaneous** **4 Percutaneous Endoscopic**	**M Bone Growth Stimulator**	**Z No Qualifier**

Non-OR ØPH[C,D,H,J,K,L][Ø,3,4]8Z
Non-OR ØPH[F,G][Ø,3,4]8Z

Ø Medical and Surgical
P Upper Bones
J Inspection Definition: Visually and/or manually exploring a body part

Explanation: Visual exploration may be performed with or without optical instrumentation. Manual exploration may be performed directly or through intervening body layers.

Body Part Character 4	Approach Character 5	Device Character 6	Qualifier Character 7
Y Upper Bone	**Ø** Open **3** Percutaneous **4** Percutaneous Endoscopic **X** External	**Z** No Device	**Z** No Qualifier

Non-OR ØPJY[3,X]ZZ

Ø Medical and Surgical
P Upper Bones
N Release Definition: Freeing a body part from an abnormal physical constraint by cutting or by the use of force

Explanation: Some of the restraining tissue may be taken out but none of the body part is taken out

Body Part Character 4	Approach Character 5	Device Character 6	Qualifier Character 7
Ø Sternum Manubrium Suprasternal notch Xiphoid process **1** Ribs, 1 to 2 **2** Ribs, 3 or More **3** Cervical Vertebra Dens Odontoid process Spinous process Transverse foramen Transverse process Vertebral arch Vertebral body Vertebral foramen Vertebral lamina Vertebral pedicle **4** Thoracic Vertebra Spinous process Transverse process Vertebral arch Vertebral body Vertebral foramen Vertebral lamina Vertebral pedicle **5** Scapula, Right Acromion (process) Coracoid process **6** Scapula, Left *See 5 Scapula, Right* **7** Glenoid Cavity, Right Glenoid fossa (of scapula) **8** Glenoid Cavity, Left *See 7 Glenoid Cavity, Right* **9** Clavicle, Right **B** Clavicle, Left **C** Humeral Head, Right Greater tuberosity Lesser tuberosity Neck of humerus (anatomical) (surgical) **D** Humeral Head, Left *See C Humeral Head, Right* **F** Humeral Shaft, Right Distal humerus Humerus, distal Lateral epicondyle of humerus Medial epicondyle of humerus **G** Humeral Shaft, Left *See F Humeral Shaft, Right* **H** Radius, Right Ulnar notch **J** Radius, Left *See H Radius, Right* **K** Ulna, Right Olecranon process Radial notch **L** Ulna, Left *See K Ulna, Right* **M** Carpal, Right Capitate bone Hamate bone Lunate bone Pisiform bone Scaphoid bone Trapezium bone Trapezoid bone Triquetral bone **N** Carpal, Left *See M Carpal, Right* **P** Metacarpal, Right **Q** Metacarpal, Left **R** Thumb Phalanx, Right **S** Thumb Phalanx, Left **T** Finger Phalanx, Right **V** Finger Phalanx, Left	**Ø** Open **3** Percutaneous **4** Percutaneous Endoscopic	**Z** No Device	**Z** No Qualifier

Ø Medical and Surgical
P Upper Bones
P Removal Definition: Taking out or off a device from a body part

Explanation: If a device is taken out and a similar device put in without cutting or puncturing the skin or mucous membrane, the procedure is coded to the root operation CHANGE. Otherwise, the procedure for taking out a device is coded to the root operation REMOVAL.

Body Part Character 4		Approach Character 5	Device Character 6	Qualifier Character 7
Ø Sternum Manubrium Suprasternal notch Xiphoid process **1 Ribs, 1 to 2** **2 Ribs, 3 or More** **3 Cervical Vertebra** Dens Odontoid process Spinous process Transverse foramen Transverse process Vertebral arch Vertebral body Vertebral foramen Vertebral lamina Vertebral pedicle	**4 Thoracic Vertebra** Spinous process Transverse process Vertebral arch Vertebral body Vertebral foramen Vertebral lamina Vertebral pedicle **5 Scapula, Right** Acromion (process) Coracoid process **6 Scapula, Left** *See 5 Scapula, Right* **7 Glenoid Cavity, Right** Glenoid fossa (of scapula) **8 Glenoid Cavity, Left** *See 7 Glenoid Cavity, Right* **9 Clavicle, Right** **B Clavicle, Left**	**Ø Open** **3 Percutaneous** **4 Percutaneous Endoscopic**	**4 Internal Fixation Device** **7 Autologous Tissue Substitute** **J Synthetic Substitute** **K Nonautologous Tissue Substitute**	**Z No Qualifier**
Ø Sternum Manubrium Suprasternal notch Xiphoid process **1 Ribs, 1 to 2** **2 Ribs, 3 or More** **3 Cervical Vertebra** Dens Odontoid process Spinous process Transverse foramen Transverse process Vertebral arch Vertebral body Vertebral foramen Vertebral lamina Vertebral pedicle	**4 Thoracic Vertebra** Spinous process Transverse process Vertebral arch Vertebral body Vertebral foramen Vertebral lamina Vertebral pedicle **5 Scapula, Right** Acromion (process) Coracoid process **6 Scapula, Left** *See 5 Scapula, Right* **7 Glenoid Cavity, Right** Glenoid fossa (of scapula) **8 Glenoid Cavity, Left** *See 7 Glenoid Cavity, Right* **9 Clavicle, Right** **B Clavicle, Left**	**X External**	**4 Internal Fixation Device**	**Z No Qualifier**
C Humeral Head, Right Greater tuberosity Lesser tuberosity Neck of humerus (anatomical) (surgical) **D Humeral Head, Left** *See C Humeral Head, Right* **F Humeral Shaft, Right** Distal humerus Humerus, distal Lateral epicondyle of humerus Medial epicondyle of humerus **G Humeral Shaft, Left** *See F Humeral Shaft, Right* **H Radius, Right** Ulnar notch **J Radius, Left** *See H Radius, Right* **K Ulna, Right** Olecranon process Radial notch	**L Ulna, Left** *See K Ulna, Right* **M Carpal, Right** Capitate bone Hamate bone Lunate bone Pisiform bone Scaphoid bone Trapezium bone Trapezoid bone Triquetral bone **N Carpal, Left** *See M Carpal, Right* **P Metacarpal, Right** **Q Metacarpal, Left** **R Thumb Phalanx, Right** **S Thumb Phalanx, Left** **T Finger Phalanx, Right** **V Finger Phalanx, Left**	**Ø Open** **3 Percutaneous** **4 Percutaneous Endoscopic**	**4 Internal Fixation Device** **5 External Fixation Device** **7 Autologous Tissue Substitute** **J Synthetic Substitute** **K Nonautologous Tissue Substitute**	**Z No Qualifier**

Non-OR ØPP[Ø,1,2,3,4,5,6,7,8,9,B]X4Z

ØPP Continued on next page

Ø Medical and Surgical
P Upper Bones
P Removal Definition: Taking out or off a device from a body part

ØPP Continued

Explanation: If a device is taken out and a similar device put in without cutting or puncturing the skin or mucous membrane, the procedure is coded to the root operation CHANGE. Otherwise, the procedure for taking out a device is coded to the root operation REMOVAL.

Body Part Character 4	Approach Character 5	Device Character 6	Qualifier Character 7
C Humeral Head, Right Greater tuberosity Lesser tuberosity Neck of humerus (anatomical) (surgical) **D Humeral Head, Left** *See C Humeral Head, Right* **F Humeral Shaft, Right** Distal humerus Humerus, distal Lateral epicondyle of humerus Medial epicondyle of humerus **G Humeral Shaft, Left** *See F Humeral Shaft, Right* **H Radius, Right** Ulnar notch **J Radius, Left** *See H Radius, Right* **K Ulna, Right** Olecranon process Radial notch **L Ulna, Left** *See K Ulna, Right* **M Carpal, Right** Capitate bone Hamate bone Lunate bone Pisiform bone Scaphoid bone Trapezium bone Trapezoid bone Triquetral bone **N Carpal, Left** *See M Carpal, Right* **P Metacarpal, Right** **Q Metacarpal, Left** **R Thumb Phalanx, Right** **S Thumb Phalanx, Left** **T Finger Phalanx, Right** **V Finger Phalanx, Left**	**X External**	**4 Internal Fixation Device** **5 External Fixation Device**	**Z No Qualifier**
Y Upper Bone	**Ø Open** **3 Percutaneous** **4 Percutaneous Endoscopic** **X External**	**Ø Drainage Device** **M Bone Growth Stimulator**	**Z No Qualifier**

Non-OR ØPP[C,D,F,G,H,J,K,L,M,N,P,Q,R,S,T,V]X[4,5]Z
Non-OR ØPPY3ØZ
Non-OR ØPPYX[Ø,M]Z

Ø Medical and Surgical
P Upper Bones
Q Repair Definition: Restoring, to the extent possible, a body part to its normal anatomic structure and function
Explanation: Used only when the method to accomplish the repair is not one of the other root operations

Body Part Character 4		Approach Character 5	Device Character 6	Qualifier Character 7
Ø Sternum Manubrium Suprasternal notch Xiphoid process **1 Ribs, 1 to 2** **2 Ribs, 3 or More** **3 Cervical Vertebra** Dens Odontoid process Spinous process Transverse foramen Transverse process Vertebral arch Vertebral body Vertebral foramen Vertebral lamina Vertebral pedicle **4 Thoracic Vertebra** Spinous process Transverse process Vertebral arch Vertebral body Vertebral foramen Vertebral lamina Vertebral pedicle **5 Scapula, Right** Acromion (process) Coracoid process **6 Scapula, Left** *See 5 Scapula, Right* **7 Glenoid Cavity, Right** Glenoid fossa (of scapula) **8 Glenoid Cavity, Left** *See 7 Glenoid Cavity, Right* **9 Clavicle, Right** **B Clavicle, Left** **C Humeral Head, Right** Greater tuberosity Lesser tuberosity Neck of humerus (anatomical)(surgical) **D Humeral Head, Left** *See C Humeral Head, Right*	**F Humeral Shaft, Right** Distal humerus Humerus, distal Lateral epicondyle of humerus Medial epicondyle of humerus **G Humeral Shaft, Left** *See F Humeral Shaft, Right* **H Radius, Right** Ulnar notch **J Radius, Left** *See H Radius, Right* **K Ulna, Right** Olecranon process Radial notch **L Ulna, Left** *See K Ulna, Right* **M Carpal, Right** Capitate bone Hamate bone Lunate bone Pisiform bone Scaphoid bone Trapezium bone Trapezold bone Triquetral bone **N Carpal, Left** *See M Carpal, Right* **P Metacarpal, Right** **Q Metacarpal, Left** **R Thumb Phalanx, Right** **S Thumb Phalanx, Left** **T Finger Phalanx, Right** **V Finger Phalanx, Left**	**Ø Open** **3 Percutaneous** **4 Percutaneous Endoscopic** **X External**	**Z No Device**	**Z No Qualifier**

Non-OR ØPQ[Ø,1,2,3,4,5,6,7,8,9,B,C,D,F,G,H,J,K,L,M,N,P,Q,R,S,T,V]XZZ

Ø Medical and Surgical
P Upper Bones
R Replacement Definition: Putting in or on biological or synthetic material that physically takes the place and/or function of all or a portion of a body part

Explanation: The body part may have been taken out or replaced, or may be taken out, physically eradicated, or rendered nonfunctional during the REPLACEMENT procedure. A REMOVAL procedure is coded for taking out the device used in a previous replacement procedure.

Body Part Character 4	Approach Character 5	Device Character 6	Qualifier Character 7
Ø Sternum Manubrium, Suprasternal notch, Xiphoid process **1 Ribs, 1 to 2** **2 Ribs, 3 or More** **3 Cervical Vertebra** Dens, Odontoid process, Spinous process, Transverse foramen, Transverse process, Vertebral arch, Vertebral body, Vertebral foramen, Vertebral lamina, Vertebral pedicle **4 Thoracic Vertebra** Spinous process, Transverse process, Vertebral arch, Vertebral body, Vertebral foramen, Vertebral lamina, Vertebral pedicle **5 Scapula, Right** Acromion (process), Coracoid process **6 Scapula, Left** *See 5 Scapula, Right* **7 Glenoid Cavity, Right** Glenoid fossa (of scapula) **8 Glenoid Cavity, Left** *See 7 Glenoid Cavity, Right* **9 Clavicle, Right** **B Clavicle, Left** **C Humeral Head, Right** Greater tuberosity, Lesser tuberosity, Neck of humerus (anatomical)(surgical) **D Humeral Head, Left** *See C Humeral Head, Right* **F Humeral Shaft, Right** Distal humerus, Humerus, distal, Lateral epicondyle of humerus, Medial epicondyle of humerus **G Humeral Shaft, Left** *See F Humeral Shaft, Right* **H Radius, Right** Ulnar notch **J Radius, Left** *See H Radius, Right* **K Ulna, Right** Olecranon process, Radial notch **L Ulna, Left** *See K Ulna, Right* **M Carpal, Right** Capitate bone, Hamate bone, Lunate bone, Pisiform bone, Scaphoid bone, Trapezium bone, Trapezoid bone, Triquetral bone **N Carpal, Left** *See M Carpal, Right* **P Metacarpal, Right** **Q Metacarpal, Left** **R Thumb Phalanx, Right** **S Thumb Phalanx, Left** **T Finger Phalanx, Right** **V Finger Phalanx, Left**	**Ø Open** **3 Percutaneous** **4 Percutaneous Endoscopic**	**7 Autologous Tissue Substitute** **J Synthetic Substitute** **K Nonautologous Tissue Substitute**	**Z No Qualifier**

Ø Medical and Surgical
P Upper Bones
S Reposition

Definition: Moving to its normal location, or other suitable location, all or a portion of a body part

Explanation: The body part is moved to a new location from an abnormal location, or from a normal location where it is not functioning correctly. The body part may or may not be cut out or off to be moved to the new location.

Body Part Character 4	Approach Character 5	Device Character 6	Qualifier Character 7
Ø Sternum Manubrium Suprasternal notch Xiphoid process	**Ø Open** **3 Percutaneous** **4 Percutaneous Endoscopic**	**Ø Internal Fixation Device, Rigid Plate** **4 Internal Fixation Device** **Z No Device**	**Z No Qualifier**
Ø Sternum Manubrium Suprasternal notch Xiphoid process	**X External**	**Z No Device**	**Z No Qualifier**
1 Ribs, 1 to 2 **2 Ribs, 3 or More** **3 Cervical Vertebra** ⊞ Dens Odontoid process Spinous process Transverse foramen Transverse process Vertebral arch Vertebral body Vertebral foramen Vertebral lamina Vertebral pedicle **4 Thoracic Vertebra** ⊞ Spinous process Transverse process Vertebral arch Vertebral body Vertebral foramen Vertebral lamina Vertebral pedicle **5 Scapula, Right** Acromion (process) Coracoid process **6 Scapula, Left** *See 5 Scapula, Right* **7 Glenoid Cavity, Right** Glenoid fossa (of scapula) **8 Glenoid Cavity, Left** *See 7 Glenoid Cavity, Right* **9 Clavicle, Right** **B Clavicle, Left**	**Ø Open** **3 Percutaneous** **4 Percutaneous Endoscopic**	**4 Internal Fixation Device** **Z No Device**	**Z No Qualifier**
1 Ribs, 1 to 2 **2 Ribs, 3 or More** **3 Cervical Vertebra** Dens Odontoid process Spinous process Transverse foramen Transverse process Vertebral arch Vertebral body Vertebral foramen Vertebral lamina Vertebral pedicle **4 Thoracic Vertebra** Spinous process Transverse process Vertebral arch Vertebral body Vertebral foramen Vertebral lamina Vertebral pedicle **5 Scapula, Right** Acromion (process) Coracoid process **6 Scapula, Left** *See 5 Scapula, Right* **7 Glenoid Cavity, Right** Glenoid fossa (of scapula) **8 Glenoid Cavity, Left** *See 7 Glenoid Cavity, Right* **9 Clavicle, Right** **B Clavicle, Left**	**X External**	**Z No Device**	**Z No Qualifier**
C Humeral Head, Right Greater tuberosity Lesser tuberosity Neck of humerus (anatomical)(surgical) **D Humeral Head, Left** *See C Humeral Head, Right* **F Humeral Shaft, Right** Distal humerus Humerus, distal Lateral epicondyle of humerus Medial epicondyle of humerus **G Humeral Shaft, Left** *See F Humeral Shaft, Right* **H Radius, Right** Ulnar notch **J Radius, Left** *See H Radius, Right* **K Ulna, Right** Olecranon process Radial notch **L Ulna, Left** *See K Ulna, Right*	**Ø Open** **3 Percutaneous** **4 Percutaneous Endoscopic**	**4 Internal Fixation Device** **5 External Fixation Device** **6 Internal Fixation Device, Intramedullary** **B External Fixation Device, Monoplanar** **C External Fixation Device, Ring** **D External Fixation Device, Hybrid** **Z No Device**	**Z No Qualifier**

Non-OR ØPSØ[3,4]ZZ
Non-OR ØPSØXZZ
Non-OR ØPS[1,2,5,6,7,8,9,B][3,4]ZZ
Non-OR ØPS[1,2,3,4,5,6,7,8,9,B]XZZ
Non-OR ØPS[C,D,F,G,H,J,K,L][3,4]ZZ

See Appendix L for Procedure Combinations
⊞ ØPS[3,4]3ZZ

ØPS Continued on next page

ØPS Continued

Ø Medical and Surgical
P Upper Bones
S Reposition

Definition: Moving to its normal location, or other suitable location, all or a portion of a body part

Explanation: The body part is moved to a new location from an abnormal location, or from a normal location where it is not functioning correctly. The body part may or may not be cut out or off to be moved to the new location.

Body Part Character 4		Approach Character 5	Device Character 6	Qualifier Character 7
C Humeral Head, Right Greater tuberosity Lesser tuberosity Neck of humerus (anatomical)(surgical) **D Humeral Head, Left** *See C Humeral Head, Right* **F Humeral Shaft, Right** Distal humerus Humerus, distal Lateral epicondyle of humerus Medial epicondyle of humerus	**G Humeral Shaft, Left** *See F Humeral Shaft, Right* **H Radius, Right** Ulnar notch **J Radius, Left** *See H Radius, Right* **K Ulna, Right** Olecranon process Radial notch **L Ulna, Left** *See K Ulna, Right*	**X External**	**Z No Device**	**Z No Qualifier**
M Carpal, Right Capitate bone Hamate bone Lunate bone Pisiform bone Scaphoid bone Trapezium bone Trapezoid bone Triquetral bone	**N Carpal, Left** *See M Carpal, Right* **P Metacarpal, Right** **Q Metacarpal, Left** **R Thumb Phalanx, Right** **S Thumb Phalanx, Left** **T Finger Phalanx, Right** **V Finger Phalanx, Left**	**Ø Open** **3 Percutaneous** **4 Percutaneous Endoscopic**	**4 Internal Fixation Device** **5 External Fixation Device** **Z No Device**	**Z No Qualifier**
M Carpal, Right Capitate bone Hamate bone Lunate bone Pisiform bone Scaphoid bone Trapezium bone Trapezoid bone Triquetral bone	**N Carpal, Left** *See M Carpal, Right* **P Metacarpal, Right** **Q Metacarpal, Left** **R Thumb Phalanx, Right** **S Thumb Phalanx, Left** **T Finger Phalanx, Right** **V Finger Phalanx, Left**	**X External**	**Z No Device**	**Z No Qualifier**

Non-OR ØPS[C,D,F,G,H,J,K,L]XZZ
Non-OR ØPS[M,N,P,Q,R,S,T,V][3,4]ZZ
Non-OR ØPS[M,N,P,Q,R,S,T,V]XZZ

Ø Medical and Surgical
P Upper Bones
T Resection

Definition: Cutting out or off, without replacement, all of a body part

Explanation: None

Body Part Character 4		Approach Character 5	Device Character 6	Qualifier Character 7
Ø Sternum Manubrium Suprasternal notch Xiphoid process **1 Ribs, 1 to 2** **2 Ribs, 3 or More** **5 Scapula, Right** Acromion (process) Coracoid process **6 Scapula, Left** *See 5 Scapula, Right* **7 Glenoid Cavity, Right** Glenoid fossa (of scapula) **8 Glenoid Cavity, Left** *See 7 Glenoid Cavity, Right* **9 Clavicle, Right** **B Clavicle, Left** **C Humeral Head, Right** Greater tuberosity Lesser tuberosity Neck of humerus (anatomical) (surgical) **D Humeral Head, Left** *See C Humeral Head, Right* **F Humeral Shaft, Right** Distal humerus Humerus, distal Lateral epicondyle of humerus Medial epicondyle of humerus	**G Humeral Shaft, Left** *See F Humeral Shaft, Right* **H Radius, Right** Ulnar notch **J Radius, Left** *See H Radius, Right* **K Ulna, Right** Olecranon process Radial notch **L Ulna, Left** *See K Ulna, Right* **M Carpal, Right** Capitate bone Hamate bone Lunate bone Pisiform bone Scaphoid bone Trapezium bone Trapezoid bone Triquetral bone **N Carpal, Left** *See M Carpal, Right* **P Metacarpal, Right** **Q Metacarpal, Left** **R Thumb Phalanx, Right** **S Thumb Phalanx, Left** **T Finger Phalanx, Right** **V Finger Phalanx, Left**	**Ø Open**	**Z No Device**	**Z No Qualifier**

Ø Medical and Surgical
P Upper Bones
U Supplement

Definition: Putting in or on biological or synthetic material that physically reinforces and/or augments the function of a portion of a body part

Explanation: The biological material is non-living, or is living and from the same individual. The body part may have been previously replaced, and the SUPPLEMENT procedure is performed to physically reinforce and/or augment the function of the replaced body part.

Body Part Character 4		Approach Character 5	Device Character 6	Qualifier Character 7
Ø Sternum Manubrium Suprasternal notch Xiphoid process **1 Ribs, 1 to 2** **2 Ribs, 3 or More** **3 Cervical Vertebra** ⊞ Dens Odontoid process Spinous process Transverse foramen Transverse process Vertebral arch Vertebral body Vertebral foramen Vertebral lamina Vertebral pedicle **4 Thoracic Vertebra** ⊞ Spinous process Transverse process Vertebral arch Vertebral body Vertebral foramen Vertebral lamina Vertebral pedicle **5 Scapula, Right** Acromion (process) Coracoid process **6 Scapula, Left** *See 5 Scapula, Right* **7 Glenoid Cavity, Right** Glenoid fossa (of scapula) **8 Glenoid Cavity, Left** *See 7 Glenoid Cavity, Right* **9 Clavicle, Right** **B Clavicle, Left** **C Humeral Head, Right** Greater tuberosity Lesser tuberosity Neck of humerus (anatomical) (surgical)	**D Humeral Head, Left** *See C Humeral Head, Right* **F Humeral Shaft, Right** Distal humerus Humerus, distal Lateral epicondyle of humerus Medial epicondyle of humerus **G Humeral Shaft, Left** *See F Humeral Shaft, Right* **H Radius, Right** Ulnar notch **J Radius, Left** *See H Radius, Right* **K Ulna, Right** Olecranon process Radial notch **L Ulna, Left** *See K Ulna, Right* **M Carpal, Right** Capitate bone Hamate bone Lunate bone Pisiform bone Scaphoid bone Trapezium bone Trapezoid bone Triquetral bone **N Carpal, Left** *See M Carpal, Right* **P Metacarpal, Right** **Q Metacarpal, Left** **R Thumb Phalanx, Right** **S Thumb Phalanx, Left** **T Finger Phalanx, Right** **V Finger Phalanx, Left**	**Ø Open** **3 Percutaneous** **4 Percutaneous Endoscopic**	**7 Autologous Tissue Substitute** **J Synthetic Substitute** **K Nonautologous Tissue Substitute**	**Z No Qualifier**

See Appendix L for Procedure Combinations

⊞ ØPU[3,4]3JZ

Ø Medical and Surgical
P Upper Bones
W Revision

Definition: Correcting, to the extent possible, a portion of a malfunctioning device or the position of a displaced device

Explanation: Revision can include correcting a malfunctioning or displaced device by taking out or putting in components of the device such as a screw or pin

Body Part Character 4		Approach Character 5	Device Character 6	Qualifier Character 7
Ø Sternum Manubrium Suprasternal notch Xiphoid process **1 Ribs, 1 to 2** **2 Ribs, 3 or More** **3 Cervical Vertebra** Dens Odontoid process Spinous process Transverse foramen Transverse process Vertebral arch Vertebral body Vertebral foramen Vertebral lamina Vertebral pedicle **4 Thoracic Vertebra** Spinous process Transverse process Vertebral arch Vertebral body Vertebral foramen Vertebral lamina Vertebral pedicle	**5 Scapula, Right** Acromion (process) Coracoid process **6 Scapula, Left** *See 5 Scapula, Right* **7 Glenoid Cavity, Right** Glenoid fossa (of scapula) **8 Glenoid Cavity, Left** *See 7 Glenoid Cavity, Right* **9 Clavicle, Right** **B Clavicle, Left**	**Ø Open** **3 Percutaneous** **4 Percutaneous Endoscopic** **X External**	**4 Internal Fixation Device** **7 Autologous Tissue Substitute** **J Synthetic Substitute** **K Nonautologous Tissue Substitute**	**Z No Qualifier**
C Humeral Head, Right Greater tuberosity Lesser tuberosity Neck of humerus (anatomical)(surgical) **D Humeral Head, Left** *See C Humeral Head, Right* **F Humeral Shaft, Right** Distal humerus Humerus, distal Lateral epicondyle of humerus Medial epicondyle of humerus **G Humeral Shaft, Left** *See F Humeral Shaft, Right* **H Radius, Right** Ulnar notch **J Radius, Left** *See H Radius, Right* **K Ulna, Right** Olecranon process Radial notch	**L Ulna, Left** *See K Ulna, Right* **M Carpal, Right** Capitate bone Hamate bone Lunate bone Pisiform bone Scaphoid bone Trapezium bone Trapezoid bone Triquetral bone **N Carpal, Left** *See M Carpal, Right* **P Metacarpal, Right** **Q Metacarpal, Left** **R Thumb Phalanx, Right** **S Thumb Phalanx, Left** **T Finger Phalanx, Right** **V Finger Phalanx, Left**	**Ø Open** **3 Percutaneous** **4 Percutaneous Endoscopic** **X External**	**4 Internal Fixation Device** **5 External Fixation Device** **7 Autologous Tissue Substitute** **J Synthetic Substitute** **K Nonautologous Tissue Substitute**	**Z No Qualifier**
Y Upper Bone		**Ø Open** **3 Percutaneous** **4 Percutaneous Endoscopic** **X External**	**Ø Drainage Device** **M Bone Growth Stimulator**	**Z No Qualifier**

Non-OR ØPW[Ø,1,2,3,4,5,6,7,8,9,B]X[4,7,J,K]Z
Non-OR ØPW[C,D,F,G,H,J,K,L,M,N,P,Q,R,S,T,V]X[4,5,7,J,K]Z
Non-OR ØPWYX[Ø,M]Z

Lower Bones ØQ2–ØQW

Character Meanings

This Character Meaning table is provided as a guide to assist the user in the identification of character members that may be found in this section of code tables. It **SHOULD NOT** be used to build a PCS code.

Operation–Character 3	Body Part–Character 4	Approach–Character 5	Device–Character 6	Qualifier–Character 7
2 Change	Ø Lumbar Vertebra	Ø Open	Ø Drainage Device	2 Sesamoid Bone(s) 1st Toe
5 Destruction	1 Sacrum	3 Percutaneous	4 Internal Fixation Device	X Diagnostic
8 Division	2 Pelvic Bone, Right	4 Percutaneous Endoscopic	5 External Fixation Device	Z No Qualifier
9 Drainage	3 Pelvic Bone, Left	X External	6 Internal Fixation Device, Intramedullary	
B Excision	4 Acetabulum, Right		7 Autologous Tissue Substitute OR Internal Fixation Device, Intramedullary Limb Lengthening	
C Extirpation	5 Acetabulum, Left		8 External Fixation Device, Limb Lengthening	
D Extraction	6 Upper Femur, Right		B External Fixation Device, Monoplanar	
H Insertion	7 Upper Femur, Left		C External Fixation Device, Ring	
J Inspection	8 Femoral Shaft, Right		D External Fixation Device, Hybrid	
N Release	9 Femoral Shaft, Left		J Synthetic Substitute	
P Removal	B Lower Femur, Right		K Nonautologous Tissue Substitute	
Q Repair	C Lower Femur, Left		M Bone Growth Stimulator	
R Replacement	D Patella, Right		Y Other Device	
S Reposition	F Patella, Left		Z No Device	
T Resection	G Tibia, Right			
U Supplement	H Tibia, Left			
W Revision	J Fibula, Right			
	K Fibula, Left			
	L Tarsal, Right			
	M Tarsal, Left			
	N Metatarsal, Right			
	P Metatarsal, Left			
	Q Toe Phalanx, Right			
	R Toe Phalanx, Left			
	S Coccyx			
	Y Lower Bone			

AHA Coding Clinic for table ØQ8

2018, 1Q, 25 Periacetabular osteotomy for repair of congenital hip dysplasia
2016, 2Q, 31 Periacetabular ostectomy for repair of congenital hip dysplasia

AHA Coding Clinic for table ØQB

2020, 2Q, 26 Sacral Pressure Ulcer with Excisional and Nonexcisional Debridement of Same Site
2019, 2Q, 19 Cervical spinal fusion, decompression and placement of interfacet stabilization device
2018, 3Q, 17 Excisional debridement of periosteum
2017, 1Q, 23 Reconstruction of mandible using titanium and bone
2016, 3Q, 30 Resection of femur with interposition arthroplasty
2015, 3Q, 3-8 Excisional and nonexcisional debridement
2015, 3Q, 26 Femoral head resection
2015, 2Q, 34 Decompressive laminectomy
2014, 4Q, 25 Femoroacetabular impingement and labral tear with repair
2014, 2Q, 6 Posterior lumbar fusion with discectomy
2013, 4Q, 116 Spinal decompression
2013, 2Q, 39 Ankle fusion, osteotomy, and removal of hardware
2012, 2Q, 19 Multiple decompressive cervical laminectomies

AHA Coding Clinic for table ØQD

2017, 4Q, 41 Extraction procedures

AHA Coding Clinic for table ØQH

2019, 4Q, 34 Intramedullary limb lengthening internal fixation device
2017, 1Q, 21 Staged scoliosis surgery with iliac fixation and spinal fusion
2016, 3Q, 34 Tibial/fibula epiphysiodesis

AHA Coding Clinic for table ØQP

2017, 4Q, 74-75 Magnetic growth rods
2015, 2Q, 6 Planned implant break

AHA Coding Clinic for table ØQQ

2018, 1Q, 15 Pubic symphysis fusion
2014, 3Q, 24 Repair of lipomyelomeningocele and tethered cord

AHA Coding Clinic for table ØQR

2017, 1Q, 22 Total knee replacement and patellar component
2016, 3Q, 30 Resection of femur with interposition arthroplasty

AHA Coding Clinic for table ØQS

2020, 1Q, 33 Spinal fusion without use of bone graft
2019, 3Q, 26 Open reduction with internal fixation and placement of strut allograft
2018, 1Q, 13 Bilateral cuboid osteotomy for repair of congenital talipes equinovarus
2018, 1Q, 25 Periacetabular osteotomy for repair of congenital hip dysplasia
2016, 3Q, 34 Tibial/fibula epiphysiodesis
2014, 4Q, 29 Rotational osteosynthesis
2014, 4Q, 31 Reposition of femur for correction of valgus and recurvatum deformities

AHA Coding Clinic for table ØQT

2017, 1Q, 22 Chopart amputation of foot
2016, 3Q, 30 Resection of femur with interposition arthroplasty
2015, 3Q, 26 Femoral head resection
2014, 4Q, 29 Rotational osteosynthesis

AHA Coding Clinic for table ØQU

2019, 3Q, 26 Open reduction with internal fixation and placement of strut allograft
2019, 2Q, 35 Kiva® kyphoplasty
2015, 3Q, 18 Total hip replacement with acetabular reconstruction
2014, 4Q, 31 Reposition of femur for correction of valgus and recurvatum deformities
2014, 2Q, 12 Percutaneous vertebroplasty using cement
2013, 2Q, 35 Use of bone void filler in grafting

AHA Coding Clinic for table ØQW

2017, 4Q, 74-75 Magnetic growth rods

Lower Bones

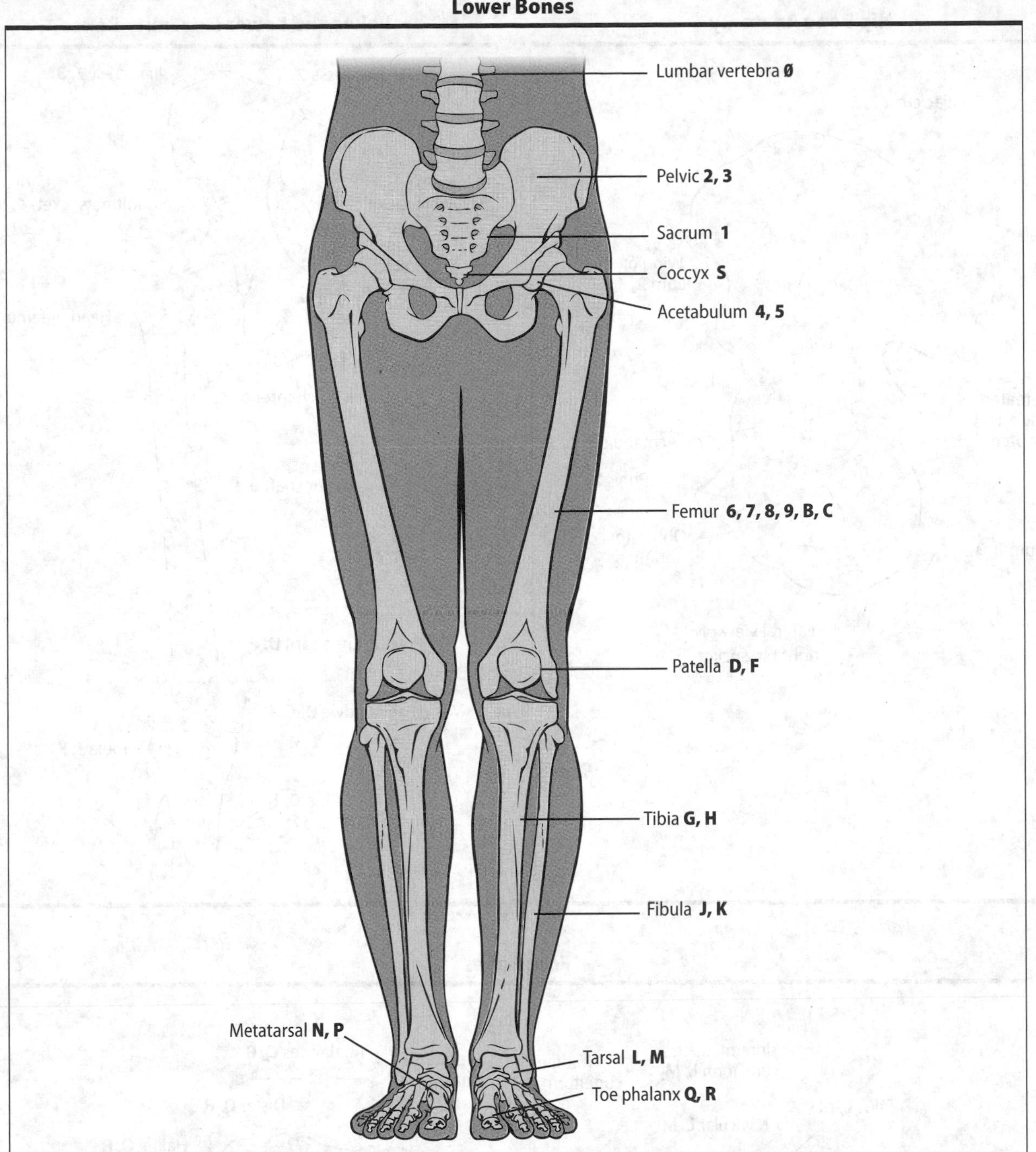
Lumbar vertebra Ø
Pelvic 2, 3
Sacrum 1
Coccyx S
Acetabulum 4, 5
Femur 6, 7, 8, 9, B, C
Patella D, F
Tibia G, H
Fibula J, K
Metatarsal N, P
Tarsal L, M
Toe phalanx Q, R

Hip Bone Anatomy

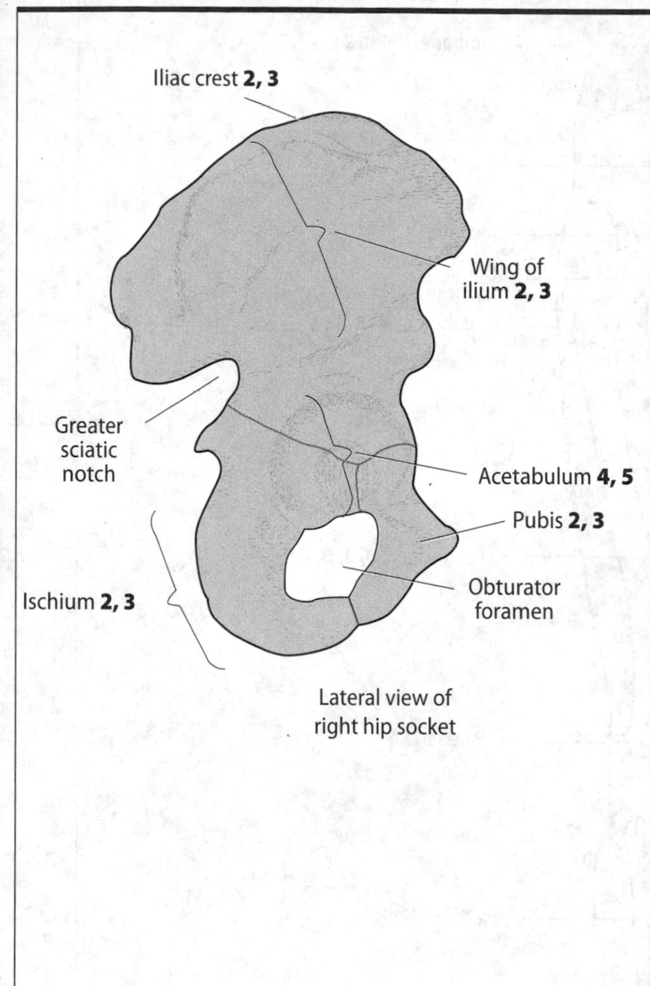

Pelvic and Lower Extremity Bones

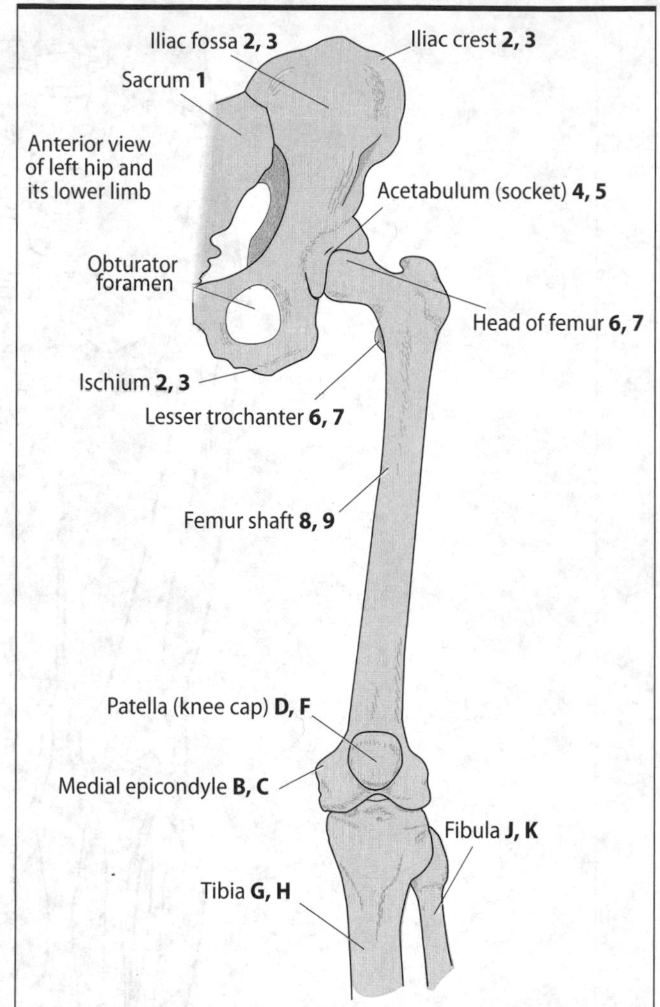

Foot Bones

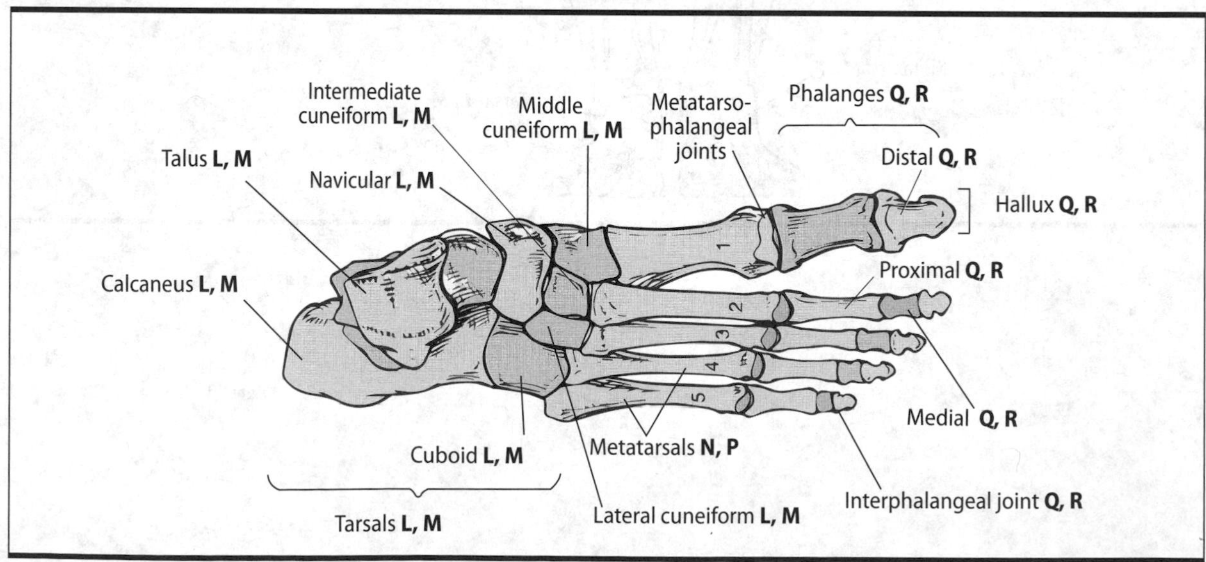

Ø Medical and Surgical
Q Lower Bones
2 Change

Definition: Taking out or off a device from a body part and putting back an identical or similar device in or on the same body part without cutting or puncturing the skin or a mucous membrane

Explanation: All CHANGE procedures are coded using the approach EXTERNAL

Body Part Character 4	Approach Character 5	Device Character 6	Qualifier Character 7
Y Lower Bone	X External	Ø Drainage Device Y Other Device	Z No Qualifier

Non-OR All body part, approach, device, and qualifier values

Ø Medical and Surgical
Q Lower Bones
5 Destruction

Definition: Physical eradication of all or a portion of a body part by the direct use of energy, force, or a destructive agent

Explanation: None of the body part is physically taken out

Body Part Character 4	Body Part Character 4	Approach Character 5	Device Character 6	Qualifier Character 7
Ø Lumbar Vertebra Spinous process Transverse process Vertebral arch Vertebral body Vertebral foramen Vertebral lamina Vertebral pedicle **1 Sacrum** **2 Pelvic Bone, Right** Iliac crest Ilium Ischium Pubis **3 Pelvic Bone, Left** *See 2 Pelvic Bone, Right* **4 Acetabulum, Right** **5 Acetabulum, Left** **6 Upper Femur, Right** Femoral head Greater trochanter Lesser trochanter Neck of femur **7 Upper Femur, Left** *See 6 Upper Femur, Right* **8 Femoral Shaft, Right** Body of femur **9 Femoral Shaft, Left** *See 8 Femoral Shaft, Right* **B Lower Femur, Right** Lateral condyle of femur Lateral epicondyle of femur Medial condyle of femur Medial epicondyle of femur **C Lower Femur, Left** *See B Lower Femur, Right*	**D Patella, Right** **F Patella, Left** **G Tibia, Right** Lateral condyle of tibia Medial condyle of tibia Medial malleolus **H Tibia, Left** *See G Tibia, Right* **J Fibula, Right** Body of fibula Head of fibula Lateral malleolus **K Fibula, Left** *See J Fibula, Right* **L Tarsal, Right** Calcaneus Cuboid bone Intermediate cuneiform bone Lateral cuneiform bone Medial cuneiform bone Navicular bone Talus bone **M Tarsal, Left** *See L Tarsal, Right* **N Metatarsal, Right** **P Metatarsal, Left** **Q Toe Phalanx, Right** **R Toe Phalanx, Left** **S Coccyx**	Ø Open 3 Percutaneous 4 Percutaneous Endoscopic	Z No Device	Z No Qualifier

Ø Medical and Surgical
Q Lower Bones
8 Division Definition: Cutting into a body part, without draining fluids and/or gases from the body part, in order to separate or transect a body part
Explanation: All or a portion of the body part is separated into two or more portions

Body Part Character 4	Approach Character 5	Device Character 6	Qualifier Character 7
Ø Lumbar Vertebra Spinous process Transverse process Vertebral arch Vertebral body Vertebral foramen Vertebral lamina Vertebral pedicle **1 Sacrum** **2 Pelvic Bone, Right** Iliac crest Ilium Ischium Pubis **3 Pelvic Bone, Left** *See 2 Pelvic Bone, Right* **4 Acetabulum, Right** **5 Acetabulum, Left** **6 Upper Femur, Right** Femoral head Greater trochanter Lesser trochanter Neck of femur **7 Upper Femur, Left** *See 6 Upper Femur, Right* **8 Femoral Shaft, Right** Body of femur **9 Femoral Shaft, Left** *See 8 Femoral Shaft, Right* **B Lower Femur, Right** Lateral condyle of femur Lateral epicondyle of femur Medial condyle of femur Medial epicondyle of femur **C Lower Femur, Left** *See B Lower Femur, Right* **D Patella, Right** **F Patella, Left** **G Tibia, Right** Lateral condyle of tibia Medial condyle of tibia Medial malleolus **H Tibia, Left** *See G Tibia, Right* **J Fibula, Right** Body of fibula Head of fibula Lateral malleolus **K Fibula, Left** *See J Fibula, Right* **L Tarsal, Right** Calcaneus Cuboid bone Intermediate cuneiform bone Lateral cuneiform bone Medial cuneiform bone Navicular bone Talus bone **M Tarsal, Left** *See L Tarsal, Right* **N Metatarsal, Right** **P Metatarsal, Left** **Q Toe Phalanx, Right** **R Toe Phalanx, Left** **S Coccyx**	**Ø Open** **3 Percutaneous** **4 Percutaneous Endoscopic**	**Z No Device**	**Z No Qualifier**

Ø Medical and Surgical
Q Lower Bones
9 Drainage Definition: Taking or letting out fluids and/or gases from a body part
Explanation: The qualifier DIAGNOSTIC is used to identify drainage procedures that are biopsies

Body Part Character 4	Approach Character 5	Device Character 6	Qualifier Character 7
Ø Lumbar Vertebra Spinous process Transverse process Vertebral arch Vertebral body Vertebral foramen Vertebral lamina Vertebral pedicle **1 Sacrum** **2 Pelvic Bone, Right** Iliac crest Ilium Ischium Pubis **3 Pelvic Bone, Left** *See 2 Pelvic Bone, Right* **4 Acetabulum, Right** **5 Acetabulum, Left** **6 Upper Femur, Right** Femoral head Greater trochanter Lesser trochanter Neck of femur **7 Upper Femur, Left** *See 6 Upper Femur, Right* **8 Femoral Shaft, Right** Body of femur **9 Femoral Shaft, Left** *See 8 Femoral Shaft, Right* **B Lower Femur, Right** Lateral condyle of femur Lateral epicondyle of femur Medial condyle of femur Medial epicondyle of femur **C Lower Femur, Left** *See B Lower Femur, Right* **D Patella, Right** **F Patella, Left** **G Tibia, Right** Lateral condyle of tibia Medial condyle of tibia Medial malleolus **H Tibia, Left** *See G Tibia, Right* **J Fibula, Right** Body of fibula Head of fibula Lateral malleolus **K Fibula, Left** *See J Fibula, Right* **L Tarsal, Right** Calcaneus Cuboid bone Intermediate cuneiform bone Lateral cuneiform bone Medial cuneiform bone Navicular bone Talus bone **M Tarsal, Left** *See L Tarsal, Right* **N Metatarsal, Right** **P Metatarsal, Left** **Q Toe Phalanx, Right** **R Toe Phalanx, Left** **S Coccyx**	**Ø Open** **3 Percutaneous** **4 Percutaneous Endoscopic**	**Ø Drainage Device**	**Z No Qualifier**
Ø Lumbar Vertebra Spinous process Transverse process Vertebral arch Vertebral body Vertebral foramen Vertebral lamina Vertebral pedicle **1 Sacrum** **2 Pelvic Bone, Right** Iliac crest Ilium Ischium Pubis **3 Pelvic Bone, Left** *See 2 Pelvic Bone, Right* **4 Acetabulum, Right** **5 Acetabulum, Left** **6 Upper Femur, Right** Femoral head Greater trochanter Lesser trochanter Neck of femur **7 Upper Femur, Left** *See 6 Upper Femur, Right* **8 Femoral Shaft, Right** Body of femur **9 Femoral Shaft, Left** *See 8 Femoral Shaft, Right* **B Lower Femur, Right** Lateral condyle of femur Lateral epicondyle of femur Medial condyle of femur Medial epicondyle of femur **C Lower Femur, Left** *See B Lower Femur, Right* **D Patella, Right** **F Patella, Left** **G Tibia, Right** Lateral condyle of tibia Medial condyle of tibia Medial malleolus **H Tibia, Left** *See G Tibia, Right* **J Fibula, Right** Body of fibula Head of fibula Lateral malleolus **K Fibula, Left** *See J Fibula, Right* **L Tarsal, Right** Calcaneus Cuboid bone Intermediate cuneiform bone Lateral cuneiform bone Medial cuneiform bone Navicular bone Talus bone **M Tarsal, Left** *See L Tarsal, Right* **N Metatarsal, Right** **P Metatarsal, Left** **Q Toe Phalanx, Right** **R Toe Phalanx, Left** **S Coccyx**	**Ø Open** **3 Percutaneous** **4 Percutaneous Endoscopic**	**Z No Device**	**X Diagnostic** **Z No Qualifier**

Non-OR ØQ9[Ø,1,2,3,4,5,6,7,8,9,B,C,D,F,G,H,J,K,L,M,P,Q,R,S]3ØZ
Non-OR ØQ9[Ø,1,2,3,4,5,6,7,8,9,B,C,D,F,G,H,J,K,L,M,P,Q,R,S]3ZZ

Ø Medical and Surgical
Q Lower Bones
B Excision Definition: Cutting out or off, without replacement, a portion of a body part
Explanation: The qualifier DIAGNOSTIC is used to identify excision procedures that are biopsies

Body Part Character 4	Approach Character 5	Device Character 6	Qualifier Character 7
Ø Lumbar Vertebra Spinous process Transverse process Vertebral arch Vertebral body Vertebral foramen Vertebral lamina Vertebral pedicle **1 Sacrum** **2 Pelvic Bone, Right** Iliac crest Ilium Ischium Pubis **3 Pelvic Bone, Left** *See 2 Pelvic Bone, Right* **4 Acetabulum, Right** **5 Acetabulum, Left** **6 Upper Femur, Right** Femoral head Greater trochanter Lesser trochanter Neck of femur **7 Upper Femur, Left** *See 6 Upper Femur, Right* **8 Femoral Shaft, Right** Body of femur **9 Femoral Shaft, Left** *See 8 Femoral Shaft, Right* **B Lower Femur, Right** Lateral condyle of femur Lateral epicondyle of femur Medial condyle of femur Medial epicondyle of femur **C Lower Femur, Left** *See B Lower Femur, Right* **D Patella, Right** **F Patella, Left** **G Tibia, Right** Lateral condyle of tibia Medial condyle of tibia Medial malleolus **H Tibia, Left** *See G Tibia, Right* **J Fibula, Right** Body of fibula Head of fibula Lateral malleolus **K Fibula, Left** *See J Fibula, Right* **L Tarsal, Right** Calcaneus Cuboid bone Intermediate cuneiform bone Lateral cuneiform bone Medial cuneiform bone Navicular bone Talus bone **M Tarsal, Left** *See L Tarsal, Right* **N Metatarsal, Right** **P Metatarsal, Left** **Q Toe Phalanx, Right** **R Toe Phalanx, Left** **S Coccyx**	**Ø Open** **3 Percutaneous** **4 Percutaneous Endoscopic**	**Z No Device**	**X Diagnostic** **Z No Qualifier**

Ø Medical and Surgical
Q Lower Bones
C Extirpation Definition: Taking or cutting out solid matter from a body part

Explanation: The solid matter may be an abnormal byproduct of a biological function or a foreign body; it may be imbedded in a body part or in the lumen of a tubular body part. The solid matter may or may not have been previously broken into pieces.

Body Part Character 4		Approach Character 5	Device Character 6	Qualifier Character 7
Ø Lumbar Vertebra Spinous process Transverse process Vertebral arch Vertebral body Vertebral foramen Vertebral lamina Vertebral pedicle **1 Sacrum** **2 Pelvic Bone, Right** Iliac crest Ilium Ischium Pubis **3 Pelvic Bone, Left** *See 2 Pelvic Bone, Right* **4 Acetabulum, Right** **5 Acetabulum, Left** **6 Upper Femur, Right** Femoral head Greater trochanter Lesser trochanter Neck of femur **7 Upper Femur, Left** *See 6 Upper Femur, Right* **8 Femoral Shaft, Right** Body of femur **9 Femoral Shaft, Left** *See 8 Femoral Shaft, Right* **B Lower Femur, Right** Lateral condyle of femur Lateral epicondyle of femur Medial condyle of femur Medial epicondyle of femur	**C Lower Femur, Left** *See B Lower Femur, Right* **D Patella, Right** **F Patella, Left** **G Tibia, Right** Lateral condyle of tibia Medial condyle of tibia Medial malleolus **H Tibia, Left** *See G Tibia, Right* **J Fibula, Right** Body of fibula Head of fibula Lateral malleolus **K Fibula, Left** *See J Fibula, Right* **L Tarsal, Right** Calcaneus Cuboid bone Intermediate cuneiform bone Lateral cuneiform bone Medial cuneiform bone Navicular bone Talus bone **M Tarsal, Left** *See L Tarsal, Right* **N Metatarsal, Right** **P Metatarsal, Left** **Q Toe Phalanx, Right** **R Toe Phalanx, Left** **S Coccyx**	**Ø Open** **3 Percutaneous** **4 Percutaneous Endoscopic**	**Z No Device**	**Z No Qualifier**

Ø Medical and Surgical
Q Lower Bones
D Extraction Definition: Pulling or stripping out or off all or a portion of a body part by the use of force

Explanation: The qualifier DIAGNOSTIC is used to identify extraction procedures that are biopsies

Body Part Character 4		Approach Character 5	Device Character 6	Qualifier Character 7
Ø Lumbar Vertebra Spinous process Transverse process Vertebral arch Vertebral body Vertebral foramen Vertebral lamina Vertebral pedicle **1 Sacrum** **2 Pelvic Bone, Right** Iliac crest Ilium Ischium Pubis **3 Pelvic Bone, Left** *See 2 Pelvic Bone, Right* **4 Acetabulum, Right** **5 Acetabulum, Left** **6 Upper Femur, Right** Femoral head Greater trochanter Lesser trochanter Neck of femur **7 Upper Femur, Left** *See 6 Upper Femur, Right* **8 Femoral Shaft, Right** Body of femur **9 Femoral Shaft, Left** *See 8 Femoral Shaft, Right* **B Lower Femur, Right** Lateral condyle of femur Lateral epicondyle of femur Medial condyle of femur Medial epicondyle of femur	**C Lower Femur, Left** *See B Lower Femur, Right* **D Patella, Right** **F Patella, Left** **G Tibia, Right** Lateral condyle of tibia Medial condyle of tibia Medial malleolus **H Tibia, Left** *See G Tibia, Right* **J Fibula, Right** Body of fibula Head of fibula Lateral malleolus **K Fibula, Left** *See J Fibula, Right* **L Tarsal, Right** Calcaneus Cuboid bone Intermediate cuneiform bone Lateral cuneiform bone Medial cuneiform bone Navicular bone Talus bone **M Tarsal, Left** *See L Tarsal, Right* **N Metatarsal, Right** **P Metatarsal, Left** **Q Toe Phalanx, Right** **R Toe Phalanx, Left** **S Coccyx**	**Ø Open**	**Z No Device**	**Z No Qualifier**

Ø Medical and Surgical
Q Lower Bones
H Insertion Definition: Putting in a nonbiological appliance that monitors, assists, performs, or prevents a physiological function but does not physically take the place of a body part

Explanation: None

Body Part Character 4		Approach Character 5	Device Character 6	Qualifier Character 7
Ø Lumbar Vertebra Spinous process Transverse process Vertebral arch Vertebral body Vertebral foramen Vertebral lamina Vertebral pedicle **1 Sacrum** **2 Pelvic Bone, Right** Iliac crest Ilium Ischium Pubis **3 Pelvic Bone, Left** *See 2 Pelvic Bone, Right* **4 Acetabulum, Right** **5 Acetabulum, Left**	**D Patella, Right** **F Patella, Left** **L Tarsal, Right** Calcaneus Cuboid bone Intermediate cuneiform bone Lateral cuneiform bone Medial cuneiform bone Navicular bone Talus bone **M Tarsal, Left** *See L Tarsal, Right* **N Metatarsal, Right** **P Metatarsal, Left** **Q Toe Phalanx, Right** **R Toe Phalanx, Left** **S Coccyx**	**Ø Open** **3 Percutaneous** **4 Percutaneous Endoscopic**	**4 Internal Fixation Device** **5 External Fixation Device**	**Z No Qualifier**
6 Upper Femur, Right Femoral head Greater trochanter Lesser trochanter Neck of femur **7 Upper Femur, Left** *See 6 Upper Femur, Right* **B Lower Femur, Right** Lateral condyle of femur Lateral epicondyle of femur Medial condyle of femur Medial epicondyle of femur	**C Lower Femur, Left** *See B Lower Femur, Right* **J Fibula, Right** Body of fibula Head of fibula Lateral malleolus **K Fibula, Left** *See J Fibula, Right*	**Ø Open** **3 Percutaneous** **4 Percutaneous Endoscopic**	**4 Internal Fixation Device** **5 External Fixation Device** **6 Internal Fixation Device, Intramedullary** **8 External Fixation Device, Limb Lengthening** **B External Fixation Device, Monoplanar** **C External Fixation Device, Ring** **D External Fixation Device, Hybrid**	**Z No Qualifier**
8 Femoral Shaft, Right Body of femur **9 Femoral Shaft, Left** *See 8 Femoral Shaft, Right*	**G Tibia, Right** Lateral condyle of tibia Medial condyle of tibia Medial malleolus **H Tibia, Left** *See G Tibia, Right*	**Ø Open** **3 Percutaneous** **4 Percutaneous Endoscopic**	**4 Internal Fixation Device** **5 External Fixation Device** **6 Internal Fixation Device, Intramedullary** **7 Internal Fixation Device, Intramedullary Limb Lengthening** **8 External Fixation Device, Limb Lengthening** **B External Fixation Device, Monoplanar** **C External Fixation Device, Ring** **D External Fixation Device, Hybrid**	**Z No Qualifier**
Y Lower Bone		**Ø Open** **3 Percutaneous** **4 Percutaneous Endoscopic**	**M Bone Growth Stimulator**	**Z No Qualifier**

Non-OR ØQH[6,7,B,C,J,K][Ø,3,4]8Z
Non-OR ØQH[8,9,G,H][Ø,3,4]8Z

Ø Medical and Surgical
Q Lower Bones
J Inspection Definition: Visually and/or manually exploring a body part

Explanation: Visual exploration may be performed with or without optical instrumentation. Manual exploration may be performed directly or through intervening body layers.

Body Part Character 4	Approach Character 5	Device Character 6	Qualifier Character 7
Y Lower Bone	**Ø Open** **3 Percutaneous** **4 Percutaneous Endoscopic** **X External**	**Z No Device**	**Z No Qualifier**

Non-OR ØQJY[3,X]ZZ

Ø Medical and Surgical
Q Lower Bones
N Release Definition: Freeing a body part from an abnormal physical constraint by cutting or by the use of force
Explanation: Some of the restraining tissue may be taken out but none of the body part is taken out

Body Part Character 4		Approach Character 5	Device Character 6	Qualifier Character 7
Ø Lumbar Vertebra Spinous process Transverse process Vertebral arch Vertebral body Vertebral foramen Vertebral lamina Vertebral pedicle **1 Sacrum** **2 Pelvic Bone, Right** Iliac crest Ilium Ischium Pubis **3 Pelvic Bone, Left** *See 2 Pelvic Bone, Right* **4 Acetabulum, Right** **5 Acetabulum, Left** **6 Upper Femur, Right** Femoral head Greater trochanter Lesser trochanter Neck of femur **7 Upper Femur, Left** *See 6 Upper Femur, Right* **8 Femoral Shaft, Right** Body of femur **9 Femoral Shaft, Left** *See 8 Femoral Shaft, Right* **B Lower Femur, Right** Lateral condyle of femur Lateral epicondyle of femur Medial condyle of femur Medial epicondyle of femur	**C Lower Femur, Left** *See B Lower Femur, Right* **D Patella, Right** **F Patella, Left** **G Tibia, Right** Lateral condyle of tibia Medial condyle of tibia Medial malleolus **H Tibia, Left** *See G Tibia, Right* **J Fibula, Right** Body of fibula Head of fibula Lateral malleolus **K Fibula, Left** *See J Fibula, Right* **L Tarsal, Right** Calcaneus Cuboid bone Intermediate cuneiform bone Lateral cuneiform bone Medial cuneiform bone Navicular bone Talus bone **M Tarsal, Left** *See L Tarsal, Right* **N Metatarsal, Right** **P Metatarsal, Left** **Q Toe Phalanx, Right** **R Toe Phalanx, Left** **S Coccyx**	**Ø Open** **3 Percutaneous** **4 Percutaneous Endoscopic**	**Z No Device**	**Z No Qualifier**

Ø Medical and Surgical
Q Lower Bones
P Removal Definition: Taking out or off a device from a body part

Explanation: If a device is taken out and a similar device put in without cutting or puncturing the skin or mucous membrane, the procedure is coded to the root operation CHANGE. Otherwise, the procedure for taking out a device is coded to the root operation REMOVAL.

Body Part Character 4		Approach Character 5	Device Character 6	Qualifier Character 7
Ø Lumbar Vertebra Spinous process, Transverse process, Vertebral arch, Vertebral body, Vertebral foramen, Vertebral lamina, Vertebral pedicle **1 Sacrum** **2 Pelvic Bone, Right** Iliac crest, Ilium, Ischium, Pubis **3 Pelvic Bone, Left** *See 2 Pelvic Bone, Right* **4 Acetabulum, Right** **5 Acetabulum, Left** **6 Upper Femur, Right** Femoral head, Greater trochanter, Lesser trochanter, Neck of femur **7 Upper Femur, Left** *See 6 Upper Femur, Right* **8 Femoral Shaft, Right** Body of femur **9 Femoral Shaft, Left** *See 8 Femoral Shaft, Right* **B Lower Femur, Right** Lateral condyle of femur, Lateral epicondyle of femur, Medial condyle of femur, Medial epicondyle of femur	**C Lower Femur, Left** *See B Lower Femur, Right* **D Patella, Right** **F Patella, Left** **G Tibia, Right** Lateral condyle of tibia, Medial condyle of tibia, Medial malleolus **H Tibia, Left** *See G Tibia, Right* **J Fibula, Right** Body of fibula, Head of fibula, Lateral malleolus **K Fibula, Left** *See J Fibula, Right* **L Tarsal, Right** Calcaneus, Cuboid bone, Intermediate cuneiform bone, Lateral cuneiform bone, Medial cuneiform bone, Navicular bone, Talus bone **M Tarsal, Left** *See L Tarsal, Right* **N Metatarsal, Right** **P Metatarsal, Left** **Q Toe Phalanx, Right** **R Toe Phalanx, Left** **S Coccyx**	**Ø Open** **3 Percutaneous** **4 Percutaneous Endoscopic**	**4 Internal Fixation Device** **5 External Fixation Device** **7 Autologous Tissue Substitute** **J Synthetic Substitute** **K Nonautologous Tissue Substitute**	**Z No Qualifier**
Ø Lumbar Vertebra Spinous process, Transverse process, Vertebral arch, Vertebral body, Vertebral foramen, Vertebral lamina, Vertebral pedicle **1 Sacrum** **2 Pelvic Bone, Right** Iliac crest, Ilium, Ischium, Pubis **3 Pelvic Bone, Left** *See 2 Pelvic Bone, Right* **4 Acetabulum, Right** **5 Acetabulum, Left** **6 Upper Femur, Right** Femoral head, Greater trochanter, Lesser trochanter, Neck of femur **7 Upper Femur, Left** *See 6 Upper Femur, Right* **8 Femoral Shaft, Right** Body of femur **9 Femoral Shaft, Left** *See 8 Femoral Shaft, Right* **B Lower Femur, Right** Lateral condyle of femur, Lateral epicondyle of femur, Medial condyle of femur, Medial epicondyle of femur	**C Lower Femur, Left** *See B Lower Femur, Right* **D Patella, Right** **F Patella, Left** **G Tibia, Right** Lateral condyle of tibia, Medial condyle of tibia, Medial malleolus **H Tibia, Left** *See G Tibia, Right* **J Fibula, Right** Body of fibula, Head of fibula, Lateral malleolus **K Fibula, Left** *See J Fibula, Right* **L Tarsal, Right** Calcaneus, Cuboid bone, Intermediate cuneiform bone, Lateral cuneiform bone, Medial cuneiform bone, Navicular bone, Talus bone **M Tarsal, Left** *See L Tarsal, Right* **N Metatarsal, Right** **P Metatarsal, Left** **Q Toe Phalanx, Right** **R Toe Phalanx, Left** **S Coccyx**	**X External**	**4 Internal Fixation Device** **5 External Fixation Device**	**Z No Qualifier**
Y Lower Bone		**Ø Open** **3 Percutaneous** **4 Percutaneous Endoscopic** **X External**	**Ø Drainage Device** **M Bone Growth Stimulator**	**Z No Qualifier**

Non-OR ØQP[Ø,1,4,5,S]X4Z
Non-OR ØQP[2,3,6,7,8,9,B,C,D,F,G,H,J,K,L,M,N,P,Q,R]X[4,5]Z
Non-OR ØQPY3ØZ
Non-OR ØQPYX[Ø,M]Z

Ø Medical and Surgical
Q Lower Bones
Q Repair Definition: Restoring, to the extent possible, a body part to its normal anatomic structure and function
Explanation: Used only when the method to accomplish the repair is not one of the other root operations

Body Part Character 4	Approach Character 5	Device Character 6	Qualifier Character 7
Ø Lumbar Vertebra Spinous process Transverse process Vertebral arch Vertebral body Vertebral foramen Vertebral lamina Vertebral pedicle **1 Sacrum** **2 Pelvic Bone, Right** Iliac crest Ilium Ischium Pubis **3 Pelvic Bone, Left** ***See*** *2 Pelvic Bone, Right* **4 Acetabulum, Right** **5 Acetabulum, Left** **6 Upper Femur, Right** Femoral head Greater trochanter Lesser trochanter Neck of femur **7 Upper Femur, Left** ***See*** *6 Upper Femur, Right* **8 Femoral Shaft, Right** Body of femur **9 Femoral Shaft, Left** ***See*** *8 Femoral Shaft, Right* **B Lower Femur, Right** Lateral condyle of femur Lateral epicondyle of femur Medial condyle of femur Medial epicondyle of femur **C Lower Femur, Left** ***See*** *B Lower Femur, Right* **D Patella, Right** **F Patella, Left** **G Tibia, Right** Lateral condyle of tibia Medial condyle of tibia Medial malleolus **H Tibia, Left** ***See*** *G Tibia, Right* **J Fibula, Right** Body of fibula Head of fibula Lateral malleolus **K Fibula, Left** ***See*** *J Fibula, Right* **L Tarsal, Right** Calcaneus Cuboid bone Intermediate cuneiform bone Lateral cuneiform bone Medial cuneiform bone Navicular bone Talus bone **M Tarsal, Left** ***See*** *L Tarsal, Right* **N Metatarsal, Right** **P Metatarsal, Left** **Q Toe Phalanx, Right** **R Toe Phalanx, Left** **S Coccyx**	**Ø Open** **3 Percutaneous** **4 Percutaneous Endoscopic** **X External**	**Z No Device**	**Z No Qualifier**

Non-OR ØQQ[Ø,1,2,3,4,5,6,7,8,9,B,C,D,F,G,H,J,K,L,M,N,P,Q,R,S]XZZ

Ø Medical and Surgical
Q Lower Bones
R Replacement Definition: Putting in or on biological or synthetic material that physically takes the place and/or function of all or a portion of a body part

Explanation: The body part may have been taken out or replaced, or may be taken out, physically eradicated, or rendered nonfunctional during the REPLACEMENT procedure. A REMOVAL procedure is coded for taking out the device used in a previous replacement procedure.

Body Part Character 4	Approach Character 5	Device Character 6	Qualifier Character 7
Ø Lumbar Vertebra Spinous process Transverse process Vertebral arch Vertebral body Vertebral foramen Vertebral lamina Vertebral pedicle **1 Sacrum** **2 Pelvic Bone, Right** Iliac crest Ilium Ischium Pubis **3 Pelvic Bone, Left** *See 2 Pelvic Bone, Right* **4 Acetabulum, Right** **5 Acetabulum, Left** **6 Upper Femur, Right** Femoral head Greater trochanter Lesser trochanter Neck of femur **7 Upper Femur, Left** *See 6 Upper Femur, Right* **8 Femoral Shaft, Right** Body of femur **9 Femoral Shaft, Left** *See 8 Femoral Shaft, Right* **B Lower Femur, Right** Lateral condyle of femur Lateral epicondyle of femur Medial condyle of femur Medial epicondyle of femur **C Lower Femur, Left** *See B Lower Femur, Right* **D Patella, Right** **F Patella, Left** **G Tibia, Right** Lateral condyle of tibia Medial condyle of tibia Medial malleolus **H Tibia, Left** *See G Tibia, Right* **J Fibula, Right** Body of fibula Head of fibula Lateral malleolus **K Fibula, Left** *See J Fibula, Right* **L Tarsal, Right** Calcaneus Cuboid bone Intermediate cuneiform bone Lateral cuneiform bone Medial cuneiform bone Navicular bone Talus bone **M Tarsal, Left** *See L Tarsal, Right* **N Metatarsal, Right** **P Metatarsal, Left** **Q Toe Phalanx, Right** **R Toe Phalanx, Left** **S Coccyx**	**Ø Open** **3 Percutaneous** **4 Percutaneous Endoscopic**	**7 Autologous Tissue Substitute** **J Synthetic Substitute** **K Nonautologous Tissue Substitute**	**Z No Qualifier**

Ø Medical and Surgical
Q Lower Bones
S Reposition Definition: Moving to its normal location, or other suitable location, all or a portion of a body part

Explanation: The body part is moved to a new location from an abnormal location, or from a normal location where it is not functioning correctly. The body part may or may not be cut out or off to be moved to the new location.

Body Part Character 4	Approach Character 5	Device Character 6	Qualifier Character 7
Ø Lumbar Vertebra ⊞ Spinous process Transverse process Vertebral arch Vertebral body Vertebral foramen Vertebral lamina Vertebral pedicle **1 Sacrum** ⊞ **4 Acetabulum, Right** **5 Acetabulum, Left** **S Coccyx** ⊞	**Ø Open** **3 Percutaneous** **4 Percutaneous Endoscopic**	**4 Internal Fixation Device** **Z No Device**	**Z No Qualifier**
Ø Lumbar Vertebra Spinous process Transverse process Vertebral arch Vertebral body Vertebral foramen Vertebral lamina Vertebral pedicle **1 Sacrum** **4 Acetabulum, Right** **5 Acetabulum, Left** **S Coccyx**	**X External**	**Z No Device**	**Z No Qualifier**
2 Pelvic Bone, Right Iliac crest Ilium Ischium Pubis **3 Pelvic Bone, Left** *See 2 Pelvic Bone, Right* **D Patella, Right** **F Patella, Left** **L Tarsal, Right** Calcaneus Cuboid bone Intermediate cuneiform bone Lateral cuneiform bone Medial cuneiform bone Navicular bone Talus bone **M Tarsal, Left** *See L Tarsal, Right* **Q Toe Phalanx, Right** **R Toe Phalanx, Left**	**Ø Open** **3 Percutaneous** **4 Percutaneous Endoscopic**	**4 Internal Fixation Device** **5 External Fixation Device** **Z No Device**	**Z No Qualifier**
2 Pelvic Bone, Right Iliac crest Ilium Ischium Pubis **3 Pelvic Bone, Left** *See 2 Pelvic Bone, Right* **D Patella, Right** **F Patella, Left** **L Tarsal, Right** Calcaneus Cuboid bone Intermediate cuneiform bone Lateral cuneiform bone Medial cuneiform bone Navicular bone Talus bone **M Tarsal, Left** *See L Tarsal, Right* **Q Toe Phalanx, Right** **R Toe Phalanx, Left**	**X External**	**Z No Device**	**Z No Qualifier**

Non-OR ØQS[4,5][3,4]ZZ
Non-OR ØQS[Ø,1,4,5,S]XZZ
Non-OR ØQS[2,3,D,F,L,M,Q,R][3,4]ZZ
Non-OR ØQS[2,3,D,F,L,M,Q,R]XZZ

See Appendix L for Procedure Combinations
⊞ ØQS[Ø,1,S]3ZZ

ØQS Continued on next page

Ø Medical and Surgical
Q Lower Bones
S Reposition Definition: Moving to its normal location, or other suitable location, all or a portion of a body part

Explanation: The body part is moved to a new location from an abnormal location, or from a normal location where it is not functioning correctly. The body part may or may not be cut out or off to be moved to the new location.

ØQS Continued

Body Part Character 4	Approach Character 5	Device Character 6	Qualifier Character 7
6 Upper Femur, Right Femoral head Greater trochanter Lesser trochanter Neck of femur **7 Upper Femur, Left** *See 6 Upper Femur, Right* **8 Femoral Shaft, Right** Body of femur **9 Femoral Shaft, Left** *See 8 Femoral Shaft, Right* **B Lower Femur, Right** Lateral condyle of femur Lateral epicondyle of femur Medial condyle of femur Medial epicondyle of femur **C Lower Femur, Left** *See B Lower Femur, Right* **G Tibia, Right** Lateral condyle of tibia Medial condyle of tibia Medial malleolus **H Tibia, Left** *See G Tibia, Right* **J Fibula, Right** Body of fibula Head of fibula Lateral malleolus **K Fibula, Left** *See J Fibula, Right*	**Ø Open** **3 Percutaneous** **4 Percutaneous Endoscopic**	**4 Internal Fixation Device** **5 External Fixation Device** **6 Internal Fixation Device, Intramedullary** **B External Fixation Device, Monoplanar** **C External Fixation Device, Ring** **D External Fixation Device, Hybrid** **Z No Device**	**Z No Qualifier**
6 Upper Femur, Right Femoral head Greater trochanter Lesser trochanter Neck of femur **7 Upper Femur, Left** *See 6 Upper Femur, Right* **8 Femoral Shaft, Right** Body of femur **9 Femoral Shaft, Left** *See 8 Femoral Shaft, Right* **B Lower Femur, Right** Lateral condyle of femur Lateral epicondyle of femur Medial condyle of femur Medial epicondyle of femur **C Lower Femur, Left** *See B Lower Femur, Right* **G Tibia, Right** Lateral condyle of tibia Medial condyle of tibia Medial malleolus **H Tibia, Left** *See G Tibia, Right* **J Fibula, Right** Body of fibula Head of fibula Lateral malleolus **K Fibula, Left** *See J Fibula, Right*	**X External**	**Z No Device**	**Z No Qualifier**
N Metatarsal, Right **P Metatarsal, Left**	**Ø Open** **3 Percutaneous** **4 Percutaneous Endoscopic**	**4 Internal Fixation Device** **5 External Fixation Device** **Z No Device**	**2 Sesamoid Bone(s) 1st Toe** **Z No Qualifier**
N Metatarsal, Right **P Metatarsal, Left**	**X External**	**Z No Device**	**2 Sesamoid Bone(s) 1st Toe** **Z No Qualifier**

Non-OR ØQS[6,7,8,9,B,C,G,H,J,K][3,4]ZZ
Non-OR ØQS[6,7,8,9,B,C,G,H,J,K]XZZ
Non-OR ØQS[N,P][3,4]Z[2,Z]
Non-OR ØQS[N,P]XZ[2,Z]

Ø Medical and Surgical
Q Lower Bones
T Resection Definition: Cutting out or off, without replacement, all of a body part
Explanation: None

Body Part Character 4		Approach Character 5	Device Character 6	Qualifier Character 7
2 Pelvic Bone, Right Iliac crest Ilium Ischium Pubis **3 Pelvic Bone, Left** *See 2 Pelvic Bone, Right* **4 Acetabulum, Right** **5 Acetabulum, Left** **6 Upper Femur, Right** Femoral head Greater trochanter Lesser trochanter Neck of femur **7 Upper Femur, Left** *See 6 Upper Femur, Right* **8 Femoral Shaft, Right** Body of femur **9 Femoral Shaft, Left** *See 8 Femoral Shaft, Right* **B Lower Femur, Right** Lateral condyle of femur Lateral epicondyle of femur Medial condyle of femur Medial epicondyle of femur **C Lower Femur, Left** *See B Lower Femur, Right* **D Patella, Right**	**F Patella, Left** **G Tibia, Right** Lateral condyle of tibia Medial condyle of tibia Medial malleolus **H Tibia, Left** *See G Tibia, Right* **J Fibula, Right** Body of fibula Head of fibula Lateral malleolus **K Fibula, Left** *See J Fibula, Right* **L Tarsal, Right** Calcaneus Cuboid bone Intermediate cuneiform bone Lateral cuneiform bone Medial cuneiform bone Navicular bone Talus bone **M Tarsal, Left** *See L Tarsal, Right* **N Metatarsal, Right** **P Metatarsal, Left** **Q Toe Phalanx, Right** **R Toe Phalanx, Left** **S Coccyx**	**Ø Open**	**Z No Device**	**Z No Qualifier**

Ø Medical and Surgical
Q Lower Bones
U Supplement Definition: Putting in or on biological or synthetic material that physically reinforces and/or augments the function of a portion of a body part
Explanation: The biological material is non-living, or is living and from the same individual. The body part may have been previously replaced, and the SUPPLEMENT procedure is performed to physically reinforce and/or augment the function of the replaced body part.

Body Part Character 4		Approach Character 5	Device Character 6	Qualifier Character 7
Ø Lumbar Vertebra ⊞ Spinous process Transverse process Vertebral arch Vertebral body Vertebral foramen Vertebral lamina Vertebral pedicle **1 Sacrum** ⊞ **2 Pelvic Bone, Right** Iliac crest Ilium Ischium Pubis **3 Pelvic Bone, Left** *See 2 Pelvic Bone, Right* **4 Acetabulum, Right** **5 Acetabulum, Left** **6 Upper Femur, Right** Femoral head Greater trochanter Lesser trochanter Neck of femur **7 Upper Femur, Left** *See 6 Upper Femur, Right* **8 Femoral Shaft, Right** Body of femur **9 Femoral Shaft, Left** *See 8 Femoral Shaft, Right* **B Lower Femur, Right** Lateral condyle of femur Lateral epicondyle of femur Medial condyle of femur Medial epicondyle of femur	**C Lower Femur, Left** *See B Lower Femur, Right* **D Patella, Right** **F Patella, Left** **G Tibia, Right** Lateral condyle of tibia Medial condyle of tibia Medial malleolus **H Tibia, Left** *See G Tibia, Right* **J Fibula, Right** Body of fibula Head of fibula Lateral malleolus **K Fibula, Left** *See J Fibula, Right* **L Tarsal, Right** Calcaneus Cuboid bone Intermediate cuneiform bone Lateral cuneiform bone Medial cuneiform bone Navicular bone Talus bone **M Tarsal, Left** *See L Tarsal, Right* **N Metatarsal, Right** **P Metatarsal, Left** **Q Toe Phalanx, Right** **R Toe Phalanx, Left** **S Coccyx** ⊞	**Ø Open** **3 Percutaneous** **4 Percutaneous Endoscopic**	**7 Autologous Tissue Substitute** **J Synthetic Substitute** **K Nonautologous Tissue Substitute**	**Z No Qualifier**

See Appendix L for Procedure Combinations
⊞ ØQU[Ø,1,S]3JZ

Ø Medical and Surgical
Q Lower Bones
W Revision

Definition: Correcting, to the extent possible, a portion of a malfunctioning device or the position of a displaced device

Explanation: Revision can include correcting a malfunctioning or displaced device by taking out or putting in components of the device such as a screw or pin

Body Part Character 4	Approach Character 5	Device Character 6	Qualifier Character 7
Ø Lumbar Vertebra Spinous process Transverse process Vertebral arch Vertebral body Vertebral foramen Vertebral lamina Vertebral pedicle **1 Sacrum** **4 Acetabulum, Right** **5 Acetabulum, Left** **S Coccyx**	**Ø Open** **3 Percutaneous** **4 Percutaneous Endoscopic** **X External**	**4 Internal Fixation Device** **7 Autologous Tissue Substitute** **J Synthetic Substitute** **K Nonautologous Tissue Substitute**	**Z No Qualifier**
2 Pelvic Bone, Right Iliac crest Ilium Ischium Pubis **3 Pelvic Bone, Left** *See 2 Pelvic Bone, Right* **6 Upper Femur, Right** Femoral head Greater trochanter Lesser trochanter Neck of femur **7 Upper Femur, Left** *See 6 Upper Femur, Right* **8 Femoral Shaft, Right** Body of femur **9 Femoral Shaft, Left** *See 8 Femoral Shaft, Right* **B Lower Femur, Right** Lateral condyle of femur Lateral epicondyle of femur Medial condyle of femur Medial epicondyle of femur **C Lower Femur, Left** *See B Lower Femur, Right* **D Patella, Right** **F Patella, Left** **G Tibia, Right** Lateral condyle of tibia Medial condyle of tibia Medial malleolus **H Tibia, Left** *See G Tibia, Right* **J Fibula, Right** Body of fibula Head of fibula Lateral malleolus **K Fibula, Left** *See J Fibula, Right* **L Tarsal, Right** Calcaneus Cuboid bone Intermediate cuneiform bone Lateral cuneiform bone Medial cuneiform bone Navicular bone Talus bone **M Tarsal, Left** *See L Tarsal, Right* **N Metatarsal, Right** **P Metatarsal, Left** **Q Toe Phalanx, Right** **R Toe Phalanx, Left**	**Ø Open** **3 Percutaneous** **4 Percutaneous Endoscopic** **X External**	**4 Internal Fixation Device** **5 External Fixation Device** **7 Autologous Tissue Substitute** **J Synthetic Substitute** **K Nonautologous Tissue Substitute**	**Z No Qualifier**
Y Lower Bone	**Ø Open** **3 Percutaneous** **4 Percutaneous Endoscopic** **X External**	**Ø Drainage Device** **M Bone Growth Stimulator**	**Z No Qualifier**

Non-OR ØQW[Ø,1,4,5,S]X[4,7,J,K]Z
Non-OR ØQW[2,3,6,7,8,9,B,C,D,F,G,H,J,K,L,M,N,P,Q,R]X[4,5,7,J,K]Z
Non-OR ØQWYX[Ø,M]Z

Upper Joints ØR2–ØRW

Character Meanings*

This Character Meaning table is provided as a guide to assist the user in the identification of character members that may be found in this section of code tables. It **SHOULD NOT** be used to build a PCS code.

Operation–Character 3	Body Part–Character 4	Approach–Character 5	Device–Character 6	Qualifier–Character 7
2 Change	Ø Occipital-cervical Joint	Ø Open	Ø Drainage Device OR Synthetic Substitute, Reverse Ball and Socket	Ø Anterior Approach, Anterior Column
5 Destruction	1 Cervical Vertebral Joint	3 Percutaneous	3 Infusion Device OR Internal Fixation Device, Sustained Compression	1 Posterior Approach, Posterior Column
9 Drainage	2 Cervical Vertebral Joint, 2 or more	4 Percutaneous Endoscopic	4 Internal Fixation Device	6 Humeral Surface
B Excision	3 Cervical Vertebral Disc	X External	5 External Fixation Device	7 Glenoid Surface
C Extirpation	4 Cervicothoracic Vertebral Joint		7 Autologous Tissue Substitute	J Posterior Approach, Anterior Column
G Fusion	5 Cervicothoracic Vertebral Disc		8 Spacer	X Diagnostic
H Insertion	6 Thoracic Vertebral Joint		A Interbody Fusion Device	Z No Qualifier
J Inspection	7 Thoracic Vertebral Joint, 2 to 7		B Spinal Stabilization Device, Interspinous Process	
N Release	8 Thoracic Vertebral Joint, 8 or more		C Spinal Stabilization Device, Pedicle-Based	
P Removal	9 Thoracic Vertebral Disc		D Spinal Stabilization Device, Facet Replacement	
Q Repair	A Thoracolumbar Vertebral Joint		J Synthetic Substitute	
R Replacement	B Thoracolumbar Vertebral Disc		K Nonautologous Tissue Substitute	
S Reposition	C Temporomandibular Joint, Right		Y Other Device	
T Resection	D Temporomandibular Joint, Left		Z No Device	
U Supplement	E Sternoclavicular Joint, Right			
W Revision	F Sternoclavicular Joint, Left			
	G Acromioclavicular Joint, Right			
	H Acromioclavicular Joint, Left			
	J Shoulder Joint, Right			
	K Shoulder Joint, Left			
	L Elbow Joint, Right			
	M Elbow Joint, Left			
	N Wrist Joint, Right			
	P Wrist Joint, Left			
	Q Carpal Joint, Right			
	R Carpal Joint, Left			
	S Carpometacarpal Joint, Right			
	T Carpometacarpal Joint, Left			
	U Metacarpophalangeal Joint, Right			
	V Metacarpophalangeal Joint, Left			
	W Finger Phalangeal Joint, Right			
	X Finger Phalangeal Joint, Left			
	Y Upper Joint			

* Includes synovial membrane.

AHA Coding Clinic for table ØRB

2019, 3Q, 26 Acromioclavicular joint reconstruction using allograft

AHA Coding Clinic for table ØRG

2020, 2Q, 27 Spinal Fusion with NuVasive® VersaTie®
2020, 1Q, 33 Spinal fusion without use of bone graft
2019, 3Q, 28 Use of VERTE-STACK™ implant with fusion
2019, 3Q, 35 Fusion procedures of the spine (guideline B3.1Øc)
2019, 2Q, 19 Cervical spinal fusion, decompression and placement of interfacet stabilization device
2019, 1Q, 30 Spinal fusion performed at same level as decompressive laminectomy
2018, 4Q, 43 Joint fusion device value
2018, 1Q, 22 Spinal fusion procedures without bone graft
2017, 4Q, 62 Added and revised device values - Nerve substitutes
2017, 4Q, 76 Radiolucent porous interbody fusion device
2017, 2Q, 23 Decompression of spinal cord and placement of instrumentation
2014, 3Q, 30 Spinal fusion and fixation instrumentation
2014, 2Q, 7 Anterior cervical thoracic fusion with total discectomy
2013, 1Q, 21-23 Spinal fusion of thoracic and lumbar vertebrae
2013, 1Q, 29 Cervical and thoracic spinal fusion

AHA Coding Clinic for table ØRH

2019, 2Q, 40 Decompression of spinal cord and placement of instrumentation
2018, 3Q, 26 Anterior vertebral tethering using Dynesys Tethering System
2017, 2Q, 23 Decompression of spinal cord and placement of instrumentation
2016, 3Q, 32 Rotator cuff repair, tenodesis, decompression, acromioplasty and coracoplasty

AHA Coding Clinic for table ØRN

2019, 1Q, 30 Spinal fusion performed at same level as decompressive laminectomy
2016, 3Q, 32 Rotator cuff repair, tenodesis, decompression, acromioplasty and coracoplasty
2015, 2Q, 22 Arthroscopic subacromial decompression
2015, 2Q, 23 Arthroscopic release of shoulder joint

AHA Coding Clinic for table ØRP

2017, 4Q, 107 Total ankle replacement versus revision

AHA Coding Clinic for table ØRQ

2016, 1Q, 30 Thermal capsulorrhapy of shoulder

AHA Coding Clinic for table ØRR

2018, 4Q, 92 Radial head arthroplasty
2017, 4Q, 107 Total ankle replacement versus revision
2015, 3Q, 14 Endoprosthetic replacement of humerus and tendon reattachment
2015, 1Q, 27 Reverse total shoulder arthroplasty

AHA Coding Clinic for table ØRS

2019, 3Q, 26 Acromioclavicular joint reconstruction using allograft
2018, 3Q, 26 Anterior vertebral tethering using Dynesys Tethering System
2015, 2Q, 35 Application of tongs to reduce and stabilize cervical fracture
2014, 4Q, 32 Open reduction internal fixation of fracture with debridement
2014, 3Q, 33 Radial fracture treatment with open reduction internal fixation, and release of carpal ligament
2013, 2Q, 39 Application of cervical tongs for reduction of cervical fracture

AHA Coding Clinic for table ØRT

2019, 3Q, 26 Acromioclavicular joint reconstruction using allograft
2014, 2Q, 7 Anterior cervical thoracic fusion with total discectomy

AHA Coding Clinic for table ØRU

2019, 3Q, 26 Acromioclavicular joint reconstruction using allograft
2015, 3Q, 26 Thumb arthroplasty with resection of trapezium

AHA Coding Clinic for table ØRW

2017, 4Q, 107 Total ankle replacement versus revision

Upper Joints

Temporomandibular **C, D**
Acromioclavicular **G, H**
Sternoclavicular **E, F**
Shoulder **J, K**
Elbow **L, M**
Wrist: Radiocarpal **N, P**
Wrist: Midcarpal **N, P**
Carpometacarpal **S, T**
Metacarpophalangeal **U, V**

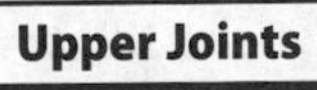

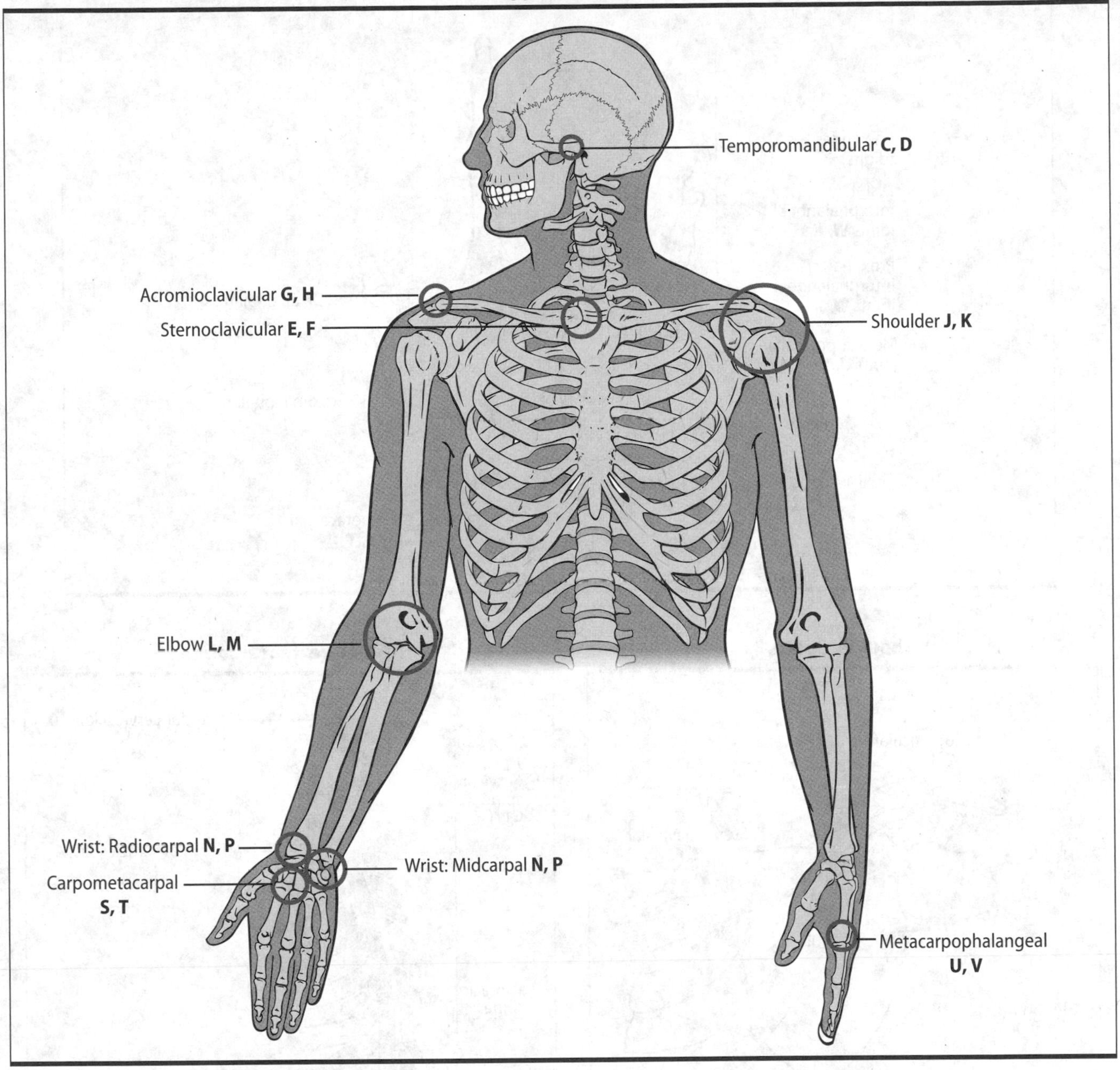

Hand Joints

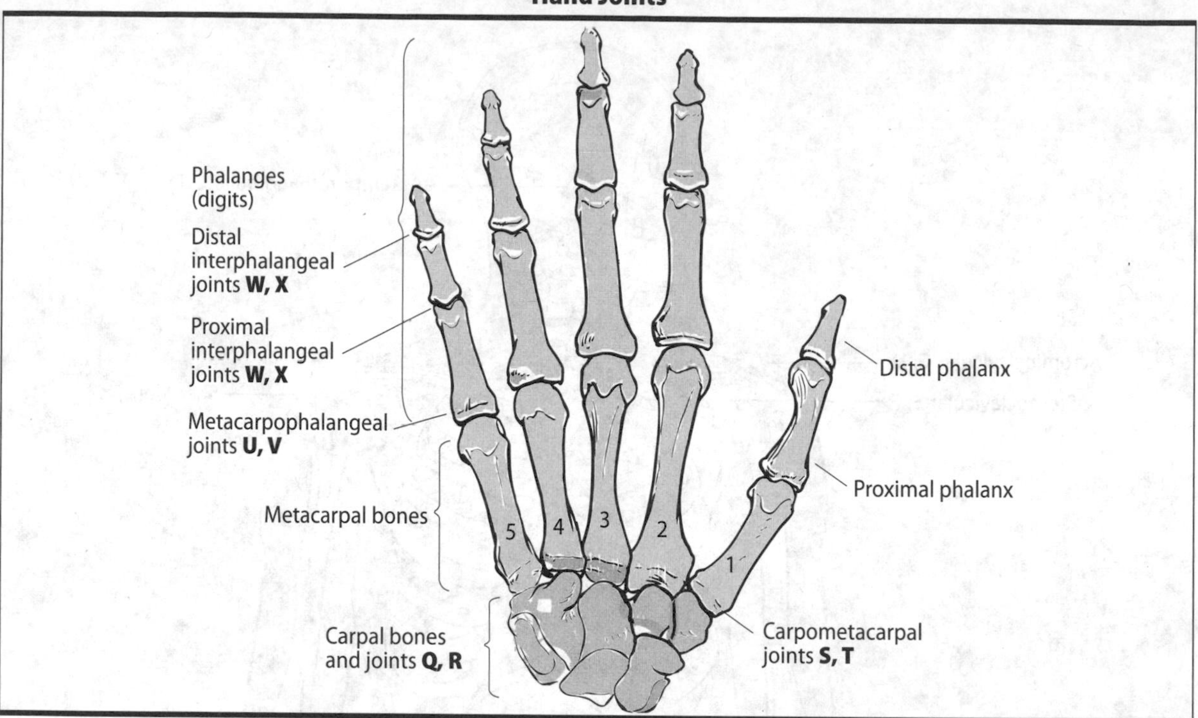

Shoulder Joints

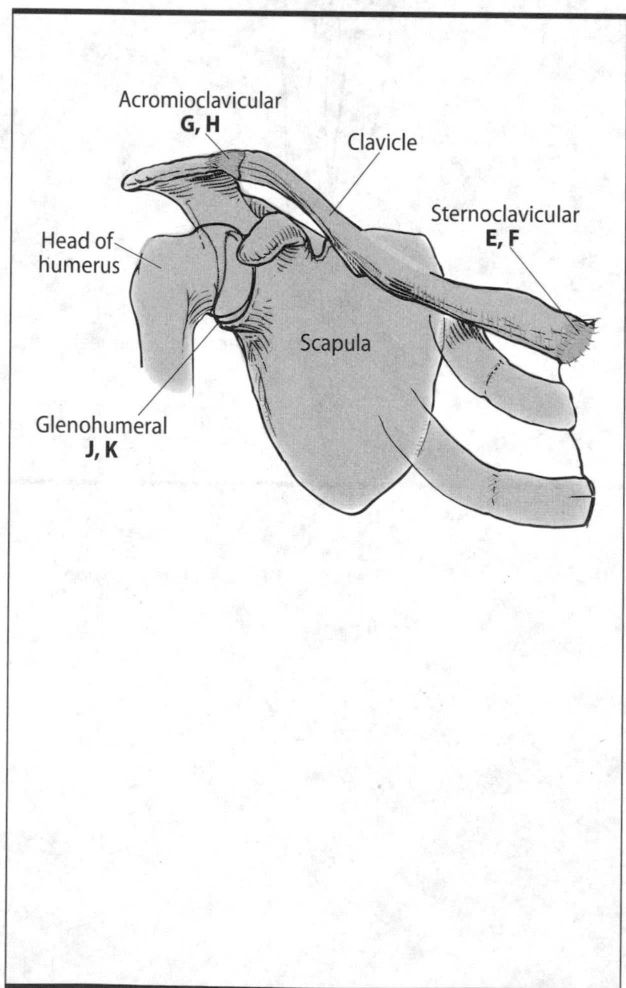

Upper Vertebral Joints

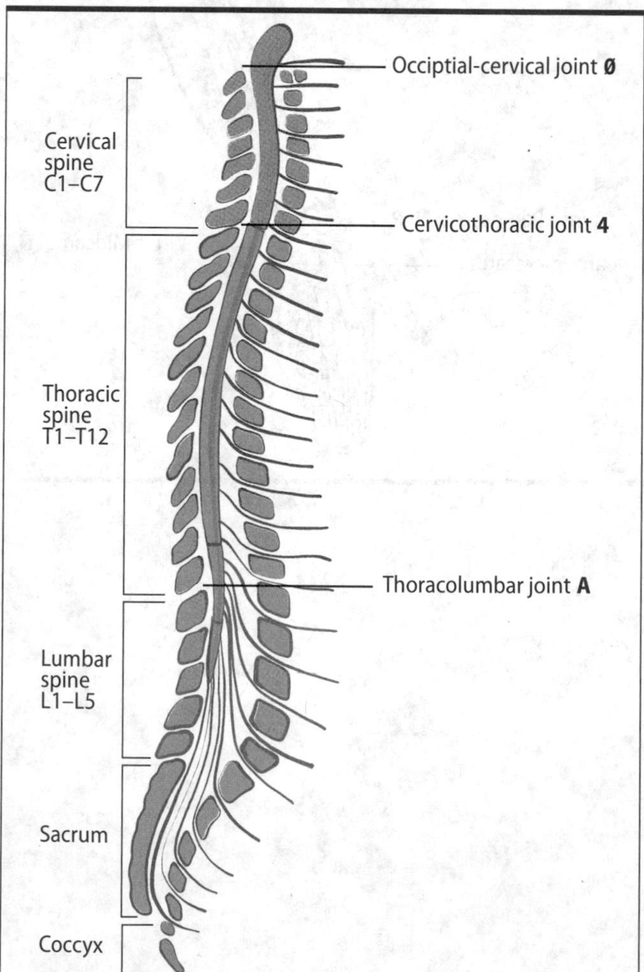

Ø Medical and Surgical
R Upper Joints
2 Change Definition: Taking out or off a device from a body part and putting back an identical or similar device in or on the same body part without cutting or puncturing the skin or a mucous membrane

Explanation: All CHANGE procedures are coded using the approach EXTERNAL

Body Part Character 4	Approach Character 5	Device Character 6	Qualifier Character 7
Y Upper Joint	X External	Ø Drainage Device Y Other Device	Z No Qualifier

Non-OR All body part, approach, device, and qualifier values

Ø Medical and Surgical
R Upper Joints
5 Destruction Definition: Physical eradication of all or a portion of a body part by the direct use of energy, force, or a destructive agent

Explanation: None of the body part is physically taken out

Body Part Character 4	Approach Character 5	Device Character 6	Qualifier Character 7
Ø Occipital-cervical Joint **1 Cervical Vertebral Joint** Atlantoaxial joint Cervical facet joint **3 Cervical Vertebral Disc** **4 Cervicothoracic Vertebral Joint** Cervicothoracic facet joint **5 Cervicothoracic Vertebral Disc** **6 Thoracic Vertebral Joint** Costotransverse joint Costovertebral joint Thoracic facet joint **9 Thoracic Vertebral Disc** **A Thoracolumbar Vertebral Joint** Thoracolumbar facet joint **B Thoracolumbar Vertebral Disc** **C Temporomandibular Joint, Right** **D Temporomandibular Joint, Left** **E Sternoclavicular Joint, Right** **F Sternoclavicular Joint, Left** **G Acromioclavicular Joint, Right** **H Acromioclavicular Joint, Left** **J Shoulder Joint, Right** Glenohumeral joint Glenoid ligament (labrum) **K Shoulder Joint, Left** *See J Shoulder Joint, Right* **L Elbow Joint, Right** Distal humerus, involving joint Humeroradial joint Humeroulnar joint Proximal radioulnar joint **M Elbow Joint, Left** *See L Elbow Joint, Right* **N Wrist Joint, Right** Distal radioulnar joint Radiocarpal joint **P Wrist Joint, Left** *See N Wrist Joint, Right* **Q Carpal Joint, Right** Intercarpal joint Midcarpal joint **R Carpal Joint, Left** *See Q Carpal Joint, Right* **S Carpometacarpal Joint, Right** **T Carpometacarpal Joint, Left** **U Metacarpophalangeal Joint, Right** **V Metacarpophalangeal Joint, Left** **W Finger Phalangeal Joint, Right** Interphalangeal (IP) joint **X Finger Phalangeal Joint, Left** *See W Finger Phalangeal Joint, Right*	Ø Open 3 Percutaneous 4 Percutaneous Endoscopic	Z No Device	Z No Qualifier

Non-OR ØR5[3,5,9,B][3,4]ZZ

Ø Medical and Surgical
R Upper Joints
9 Drainage Definition: Taking or letting out fluids and/or gases from a body part
Explanation: The qualifier DIAGNOSTIC is used to identify drainage procedures that are biopsies

Body Part Character 4		Approach Character 5	Device Character 6	Qualifier Character 7
Ø Occipital-cervical Joint 1 Cervical Vertebral Joint Atlantoaxial joint Cervical facet joint 3 Cervical Vertebral Disc 4 Cervicothoracic Vertebral Joint Cervicothoracic facet joint 5 Cervicothoracic Vertebral Disc 6 Thoracic Vertebral Joint Costotransverse joint Costovertebral joint Thoracic facet joint 9 Thoracic Vertebral Disc A Thoracolumbar Vertebral Joint Thoracolumbar facet joint B Thoracolumbar Vertebral Disc C Temporomandibular Joint, Right D Temporomandibular Joint, Left E Sternoclavicular Joint, Right F Sternoclavicular Joint, Left G Acromioclavicular Joint, Right H Acromioclavicular Joint, Left J Shoulder Joint, Right Glenohumeral joint Glenoid ligament (labrum) K Shoulder Joint, Left *See J Shoulder Joint, Right*	L Elbow Joint, Right Distal humerus, involving joint Humeroradial joint Humeroulnar joint Proximal radioulnar joint M Elbow Joint, Left *See L Elbow Joint, Right* N Wrist Joint, Right Distal radioulnar joint Radiocarpal joint P Wrist Joint, Left *See N Wrist Joint, Right* Q Carpal Joint, Right Intercarpal joint Midcarpal joint R Carpal Joint, Left *See Q Carpal Joint, Right* S Carpometacarpal Joint, Right T Carpometacarpal Joint, Left U Metacarpophalangeal Joint, Right V Metacarpophalangeal Joint, Left W Finger Phalangeal Joint, Right Interphalangeal (IP) joint X Finger Phalangeal Joint, Left *See W Finger Phalangeal Joint, Right*	Ø Open 3 Percutaneous 4 Percutaneous Endoscopic	Ø Drainage Device	Z No Qualifier
Ø Occipital-cervical Joint 1 Cervical Vertebral Joint Atlantoaxial joint Cervical facet joint 3 Cervical Vertebral Disc 4 Cervicothoracic Vertebral Joint Cervicothoracic facet joint 5 Cervicothoracic Vertebral Disc 6 Thoracic Vertebral Joint Costotransverse joint Costovertebral joint Thoracic facet joint 9 Thoracic Vertebral Disc A Thoracolumbar Vertebral Joint Thoracolumbar facet joint B Thoracolumbar Vertebral Disc C Temporomandibular Joint, Right D Temporomandibular Joint, Left E Sternoclavicular Joint, Right F Sternoclavicular Joint, Left G Acromioclavicular Joint, Right H Acromioclavicular Joint, Left J Shoulder Joint, Right Glenohumeral joint Glenoid ligament (labrum) K Shoulder Joint, Left *See J Shoulder Joint, Right*	L Elbow Joint, Right Distal humerus, involving joint Humeroradial joint Humeroulnar joint Proximal radioulnar joint M Elbow Joint, Left *See L Elbow Joint, Right* N Wrist Joint, Right Distal radioulnar joint Radiocarpal joint P Wrist Joint, Left *See N Wrist Joint, Right* Q Carpal Joint, Right Intercarpal joint Midcarpal joint R Carpal Joint, Left *See Q Carpal Joint, Right* S Carpometacarpal Joint, Right T Carpometacarpal Joint, Left U Metacarpophalangeal Joint, Right V Metacarpophalangeal Joint, Left W Finger Phalangeal Joint, Right Interphalangeal (IP) joint X Finger Phalangeal Joint, Left *See W Finger Phalangeal Joint, Right*	Ø Open 3 Percutaneous 4 Percutaneous Endoscopic	Z No Device	X Diagnostic Z No Qualifier

Non-OR ØR9[Ø,1,3,4,5,6,9,A,B,E,F,G,H,J,K,L,M,N,P,Q,R,S,T,U,V,W,X][3,4]ØZ
Non-OR ØR9[C,D]3ØZ
Non-OR ØR9[Ø,1,3,4,5,6,9,A,B,E,F,G,H,J,K,L,M,N,P,Q,R,S,T,U,V,W,X][Ø,3,4]ZX
Non-OR ØR9[Ø,1,3,4,5,6,9,A,B,E,F,G,H,J,K,L,M,N,P,Q,R,S,T,U,V,W,X][3,4]ZZ
Non-OR ØR9[C,D]3ZZ

Ø Medical and Surgical
R Upper Joints
B Excision Definition: Cutting out or off, without replacement, a portion of a body part
Explanation: The qualifier DIAGNOSTIC is used to identify excision procedures that are biopsies

Body Part Character 4	Approach Character 5	Device Character 6	Qualifier Character 7
Ø Occipital-cervical Joint 1 Cervical Vertebral Joint Atlantoaxial joint Cervical facet joint 3 Cervical Vertebral Disc 4 Cervicothoracic Vertebral Joint Cervicothoracic facet joint 5 Cervicothoracic Vertebral Disc 6 Thoracic Vertebral Joint Costotransverse joint Costovertebral joint Thoracic facet joint 9 Thoracic Vertebral Disc A Thoracolumbar Vertebral Joint Thoracolumbar facet joint B Thoracolumbar Vertebral Disc C Temporomandibular Joint, Right D Temporomandibular Joint, Left E Sternoclavicular Joint, Right F Sternoclavicular Joint, Left G Acromioclavicular Joint, Right H Acromioclavicular Joint, Left J Shoulder Joint, Right Glenohumeral joint Glenoid ligament (labrum) K Shoulder Joint, Left *See J Shoulder Joint, Right* L Elbow Joint, Right Distal humerus, involving joint Humeroradial joint Humeroulnar joint Proximal radioulnar joint M Elbow Joint, Left *See L Elbow Joint, Right* N Wrist Joint, Right Distal radioulnar joint Radiocarpal joint P Wrist Joint, Left *See N Wrist Joint, Right* Q Carpal Joint, Right Intercarpal joint Midcarpal joint R Carpal Joint, Left *See Q Carpal Joint, Right* S Carpometacarpal Joint, Right T Carpometacarpal Joint, Left U Metacarpophalangeal Joint, Right V Metacarpophalangeal Joint, Left W Finger Phalangeal Joint, Right Interphalangeal (IP) joint X Finger Phalangeal Joint, Left *See W Finger Phalangeal Joint, Right*	Ø Open 3 Percutaneous 4 Percutaneous Endoscopic	Z No Device	X Diagnostic Z No Qualifier

Non-OR ØRB[Ø,1,3,4,5,6,9,A,B,E,F,G,H,J,K,L,M,N,P,Q,R,S,T,U,V,W,X][Ø,3,4]ZX

Ø Medical and Surgical
R Upper Joints
C Extirpation Definition: Taking or cutting out solid matter from a body part

Explanation: The solid matter may be an abnormal byproduct of a biological function or a foreign body; it may be imbedded in a body part or in the lumen of a tubular body part. The solid matter may or may not have been previously broken into pieces.

Body Part Character 4	Approach Character 5	Device Character 6	Qualifier Character 7
Ø Occipital-cervical Joint **1 Cervical Vertebral Joint** Atlantoaxial joint Cervical facet joint **3 Cervical Vertebral Disc** **4 Cervicothoracic Vertebral Joint** Cervicothoracic facet joint **5 Cervicothoracic Vertebral Disc** **6 Thoracic Vertebral Joint** Costotransverse joint Costovertebral joint Thoracic facet joint **9 Thoracic Vertebral Disc** **A Thoracolumbar Vertebral Joint** Thoracolumbar facet joint **B Thoracolumbar Vertebral Disc** **C Temporomandibular Joint, Right** **D Temporomandibular Joint, Left** **E Sternoclavicular Joint, Right** **F Sternoclavicular Joint, Left** **G Acromioclavicular Joint, Right** **H Acromioclavicular Joint, Left** **J Shoulder Joint, Right** Glenohumeral joint Glenoid ligament (labrum) **K Shoulder Joint, Left** *See J Shoulder Joint, Right* **L Elbow Joint, Right** Distal humerus, involving joint Humeroradial joint Humeroulnar joint Proximal radioulnar joint **M Elbow Joint, Left** *See L Elbow Joint, Right* **N Wrist Joint, Right** Distal radioulnar joint Radiocarpal joint **P Wrist Joint, Left** *See N Wrist Joint, Right* **Q Carpal Joint, Right** Intercarpal joint Midcarpal joint **R Carpal Joint, Left** *See Q Carpal Joint, Right* **S Carpometacarpal Joint, Right** **T Carpometacarpal Joint, Left** **U Metacarpophalangeal Joint, Right** **V Metacarpophalangeal Joint, Left** **W Finger Phalangeal Joint, Right** Interphalangeal (IP) joint **X Finger Phalangeal Joint, Left** *See W Finger Phalangeal Joint, Right*	**Ø Open** **3 Percutaneous** **4 Percutaneous Endoscopic**	**Z No Device**	**Z No Qualifier**

Ø Medical and Surgical
R Upper Joints
G Fusion Definition: Joining together portions of an articular body part rendering the articular body part immobile
Explanation: The body part is joined together by fixation device, bone graft, or other means

Body Part Character 4	Approach Character 5	Device Character 6	Qualifier Character 7
Ø Occipital-cervical Joint **1** Cervical Vertebral Joint Atlantoaxial joint Cervical facet joint **2** Cervical Vertebral Joints, 2 or more Cervical facet joint **4** Cervicothoracic Vertebral Joint Cervicothoracic facet joint **6** Thoracic Vertebral Joint Costotransverse joint Costovertebral joint Thoracic facet joint **7** Thoracic Vertebral Joints, 2 to 7 ⊞ **8** Thoracic Vertebral Joints, 8 or more **A** Thoracolumbar Vertebral Joint Thoracolumbar facet joint	**Ø** Open **3** Percutaneous **4** Percutaneous Endoscopic	**7** Autologous Tissue Substitute **J** Synthetic Substitute **K** Nonautologous Tissue Substitute	**Ø** Anterior Approach, Anterior Column **1** Posterior Approach, Posterior Column **J** Posterior Approach, Anterior Column
Ø Occipital-cervical Joint **1** Cervical Vertebral Joint Atlantoaxial joint Cervical facet joint **2** Cervical Vertebral Joints, 2 or more Cervical facet joint **4** Cervicothoracic Vertebral Joint Cervicothoracic facet joint **6** Thoracic Vertebral Joint Costotransverse joint Costovertebral joint Thoracic facet joint **7** Thoracic Vertebral Joints, 2 to 7 ⊞ **8** Thoracic Vertebral Joints, 8 or more **A** Thoracolumbar Vertebral Joint Thoracolumbar facet joint	**Ø** Open **3** Percutaneous **4** Percutaneous Endoscopic	**A** Interbody Fusion Device	**Ø** Anterior Approach, Anterior Column **J** Posterior Approach, Anterior Column
C Temporomandibular Joint, Right **D** Temporomandibular Joint, Left **E** Sternoclavicular Joint, Right **F** Sternoclavicular Joint, Left **G** Acromioclavicular Joint, Right **H** Acromioclavicular Joint, Left **J** Shoulder Joint, Right Glenohumeral joint Glenoid ligament (labrum) **K** Shoulder Joint, Left *See J Shoulder Joint, Right*	**Ø** Open **3** Percutaneous **4** Percutaneous Endoscopic	**4** Internal Fixation Device **7** Autologous Tissue Substitute **J** Synthetic Substitute **K** Nonautologous Tissue Substitute	**Z** No Qualifier
L Elbow Joint, Right Distal humerus, involving joint Humeroradial joint Humeroulnar joint Proximal radioulnar joint **M** Elbow Joint, Left *See L Elbow Joint, Right* **N** Wrist Joint, Right Distal radioulnar joint Radiocarpal joint **P** Wrist Joint, Left *See N Wrist Joint, Right* **Q** Carpal Joint, Right Intercarpal joint Midcarpal joint **R** Carpal Joint, Left *See Q Carpal Joint, Right* **S** Carpometacarpal Joint, Right **T** Carpometacarpal Joint, Left **U** Metacarpophalangeal Joint, Right **V** Metacarpophalangeal Joint, Left **W** Finger Phalangeal Joint, Right Interphalangeal (IP) joint **X** Finger Phalangeal Joint, Left *See W Finger Phalangeal Joint, Right*	**Ø** Open **3** Percutaneous **4** Percutaneous Endoscopic	**3** Internal Fixation Device, Sustained Compression **4** Internal Fixation Device **5** External Fixation Device **7** Autologous Tissue Substitute **J** Synthetic Substitute **K** Nonautologous Tissue Substitute	**Z** No Qualifier

HAC ØRG[Ø,1,2,4,6,7,8,A][Ø,3,4][7,J,K][Ø,1,J] when reported with SDx K68.11 or T81.4Ø–T81.49, T84.6Ø-T84.619, T84.63-T84.7 with 7th character A

HAC ØRG[Ø,1,2,4,6,7,8,A][Ø,3,4]A[Ø,J] when reported with SDx K68.11 or T81.4Ø–T81.49, T84.6Ø-T84.619, T84.63-T84.7 with 7th character A

HAC ØRG[E,F,G,H,J,K][Ø,3,4][4,7,J,K]Z when reported with SDx K68.11 or T81.4Ø–T81.49, T84.6Ø-T84.619, T84.63-T84.7 with 7th character A

HAC ØRG[L,M][Ø,3,4][4,5,7,J,K]Z when reported with SDx K68.11 or T81.4Ø–T81.49, T84.6Ø-T84.619, T84.63-T84.7 with 7th character A

See Appendix L for Procedure Combinations
⊞ ØRG7[Ø,3,4][7,J,K][Ø,1,J]
⊞ ØRG7[Ø,3,4]A[Ø,J]

Ø Medical and Surgical
R Upper Joints
H Insertion Definition: Putting in a nonbiological appliance that monitors, assists, performs, or prevents a physiological function but does not physically take the place of a body part

Explanation: None

Body Part Character 4	Approach Character 5	Device Character 6	Qualifier Character 7
Ø Occipital-cervical Joint **1** Cervical Vertebral Joint Atlantoaxial joint Cervical facet joint **4** Cervicothoracic Vertebral Joint Cervicothoracic facet joint **6** Thoracic Vertebral Joint Costotransverse joint Costovertebral joint Thoracic facet joint **A** Thoracolumbar Vertebral Joint Thoracolumbar facet joint	**Ø** Open **3** Percutaneous **4** Percutaneous Endoscopic	**3** Infusion Device **4** Internal Fixation Device **8** Spacer **B** Spinal Stabilization Device, Interspinous Process **C** Spinal Stabilization Device, Pedicle-Based **D** Spinal Stabilization Device, Facet Replacement	**Z** No Qualifier
3 Cervical Vertebral Disc **5** Cervicothoracic Vertebral Disc **9** Thoracic Vertebral Disc **B** Thoracolumbar Vertebral Disc	**Ø** Open **3** Percutaneous **4** Percutaneous Endoscopic	**3** Infusion Device	**Z** No Qualifier
C Temporomandibular Joint, Right **D** Temporomandibular Joint, Left **E** Sternoclavicular Joint, Right **F** Sternoclavicular Joint, Left **G** Acromioclavicular Joint, Right **H** Acromioclavicular Joint, Left **J** Shoulder Joint, Right Glenohumeral joint Glenoid ligament (labrum) **K** Shoulder Joint, Left *See J Shoulder Joint, Right*	**Ø** Open **3** Percutaneous **4** Percutaneous Endoscopic	**3** Infusion Device **4** Internal Fixation Device **8** Spacer	**Z** No Qualifier
L Elbow Joint, Right Distal humerus, involving joint Humeroradial joint Humeroulnar joint Proximal radioulnar joint **M** Elbow Joint, Left *See L Elbow Joint, Right* **N** Wrist Joint, Right Distal radioulnar joint Radiocarpal joint **P** Wrist Joint, Left *See N Wrist Joint, Right* **Q** Carpal Joint, Right Intercarpal joint Midcarpal joint **R** Carpal Joint, Left *See Q Carpal Joint, Right* **S** Carpometacarpal Joint, Right **T** Carpometacarpal Joint, Left **U** Metacarpophalangeal Joint, Right **V** Metacarpophalangeal Joint, Left **W** Finger Phalangeal Joint, Right Interphalangeal (IP) joint **X** Finger Phalangeal Joint, Left *See W Finger Phalangeal Joint, Right*	**Ø** Open **3** Percutaneous **4** Percutaneous Endoscopic	**3** Infusion Device **4** Internal Fixation Device **5** External Fixation Device **8** Spacer	**Z** No Qualifier

Non-OR ØRH[Ø,1,4,6,A][Ø,3,4][3,8]Z
Non-OR ØRH[3,5,9,B][Ø,3,4]3Z
Non-OR ØRH[C,D][Ø,4]8Z
Non-OR ØRH[C,D]3[3,8]Z
Non-OR ØRH[E,F,G,H,J,K][Ø,3,4][3,8]Z
Non-OR ØRH[L,M,N,P,Q,R,S,T,U,V,W,X][Ø,3,4][3,8]Z

Ø Medical and Surgical
R Upper Joints
J Inspection

Definition: Visually and/or manually exploring a body part

Explanation: Visual exploration may be performed with or without optical instrumentation. Manual exploration may be performed directly or through intervening body layers.

Body Part Character 4	Approach Character 5	Device Character 6	Qualifier Character 7
Ø Occipital-cervical Joint **1 Cervical Vertebral Joint** Atlantoaxial joint Cervical facet joint **3 Cervical Vertebral Disc** **4 Cervicothoracic Vertebral Joint** Cervicothoracic facet joint **5 Cervicothoracic Vertebral Disc** **6 Thoracic Vertebral Joint** Costotransverse joint Costovertebral joint Thoracic facet joint **9 Thoracic Vertebral Disc** **A Thoracolumbar Vertebral Joint** Thoracolumbar facet joint **B Thoracolumbar Vertebral Disc** **C Temporomandibular Joint, Right** **D Temporomandibular Joint, Left** **E Sternoclavicular Joint, Right** **F Sternoclavicular Joint, Left** **G Acromioclavicular Joint, Right** **H Acromioclavicular Joint, Left** **J Shoulder Joint, Right** Glenohumeral joint Glenoid ligament (labrum) **K Shoulder Joint, Left** *See J Shoulder Joint, Right* **L Elbow Joint, Right** Distal humerus, involving joint Humeroradial joint Humeroulnar joint Proximal radioulnar joint **M Elbow Joint, Left** *See L Elbow Joint, Right* **N Wrist Joint, Right** Distal radioulnar joint Radiocarpal joint **P Wrist Joint, Left** *See N Wrist Joint, Right* **Q Carpal Joint, Right** Intercarpal joint Midcarpal joint **R Carpal Joint, Left** *See Q Carpal Joint, Right* **S Carpometacarpal Joint, Right** **T Carpometacarpal Joint, Left** **U Metacarpophalangeal Joint, Right** **V Metacarpophalangeal Joint, Left** **W Finger Phalangeal Joint, Right** Interphalangeal (IP) joint **X Finger Phalangeal Joint, Left** *See W Finger Phalangeal Joint, Right*	**Ø** Open **3** Percutaneous **4** Percutaneous Endoscopic **X** External	**Z** No Device	**Z** No Qualifier

Non-OR ØRJ[Ø,1,3,4,5,6,9,A,B,C,D,E,F,G,H,J,K,L,M,N,P,Q,R,S,T,U,V,W,X][3,X]ZZ

Ø Medical and Surgical
R Upper Joints
N Release Definition: Freeing a body part from an abnormal physical constraint by cutting or by the use of force
Explanation: Some of the restraining tissue may be taken out but none of the body part is taken out

Body Part Character 4	Approach Character 5	Device Character 6	Qualifier Character 7
Ø Occipital-cervical Joint 1 Cervical Vertebral Joint Atlantoaxial joint Cervical facet joint 3 Cervical Vertebral Disc 4 Cervicothoracic Vertebral Joint Cervicothoracic facet joint 5 Cervicothoracic Vertebral Disc 6 Thoracic Vertebral Joint Costotransverse joint Costovertebral joint Thoracic facet joint 9 Thoracic Vertebral Disc A Thoracolumbar Vertebral Joint Thoracolumbar facet joint B Thoracolumbar Vertebral Disc C Temporomandibular Joint, Right D Temporomandibular Joint, Left E Sternoclavicular Joint, Right F Sternoclavicular Joint, Left G Acromioclavicular Joint, Right H Acromioclavicular Joint, Left J Shoulder Joint, Right Glenohumeral joint Glenoid ligament (labrum) K Shoulder Joint, Left *See J Shoulder Joint, Right* L Elbow Joint, Right Distal humerus, involving joint Humeroradial joint Humeroulnar joint Proximal radioulnar joint M Elbow Joint, Left *See L Elbow Joint, Right* N Wrist Joint, Right Distal radioulnar joint Radiocarpal joint P Wrist Joint, Left *See N Wrist Joint, Right* Q Carpal Joint, Right Intercarpal joint Midcarpal joint R Carpal Joint, Left *See Q Carpal Joint, Right* S Carpometacarpal Joint, Right T Carpometacarpal Joint, Left U Metacarpophalangeal Joint, Right V Metacarpophalangeal Joint, Left W Finger Phalangeal Joint, Right Interphalangeal (IP) joint X Finger Phalangeal Joint, Left *See W Finger Phalangeal Joint, Right*	Ø Open 3 Percutaneous 4 Percutaneous Endoscopic X External	Z No Device	Z No Qualifier

Non-OR ØRN[Ø,1,3,4,5,6,9,A,B,C,D,E,F,G,H,J,K,L,M,N,P,Q,R,S,T,U,V,W,X]XZZ

Ø Medical and Surgical
R Upper Joints
P Removal Definition: Taking out or off a device from a body part

Explanation: If a device is taken out and a similar device put in without cutting or puncturing the skin or mucous membrane, the procedure is coded to the root operation CHANGE. Otherwise, the procedure for taking out the device is coded to the root operation REMOVAL.

Body Part Character 4	Approach Character 5	Device Character 6	Qualifier Character 7
Ø Occipital-cervical Joint **1 Cervical Vertebral Joint** Atlantoaxial joint Cervical facet joint **4 Cervicothoracic Vertebral Joint** Cervicothoracic facet joint **6 Thoracic Vertebral Joint** Costotransverse joint Costovertebral joint Thoracic facet joint **A Thoracolumbar Vertebral Joint** Thoracolumbar facet joint	**Ø** Open **3** Percutaneous **4** Percutaneous Endoscopic	**Ø** Drainage Device **3** Infusion Device **4** Internal Fixation Device **7** Autologous Tissue Substitute **8** Spacer **A** Interbody Fusion Device **J** Synthetic Substitute **K** Nonautologous Tissue Substitute	**Z** No Qualifier
Ø Occipital-cervical Joint **1 Cervical Vertebral Joint** Atlantoaxial joint Cervical facet joint **4 Cervicothoracic Vertebral Joint** Cervicothoracic facet joint **6 Thoracic Vertebral Joint** Costotransverse joint Costovertebral joint Thoracic facet joint **A Thoracolumbar Vertebral Joint** Thoracolumbar facet joint	**X** External	**Ø** Drainage Device **3** Infusion Device **4** Internal Fixation Device	**Z** No Qualifier
3 Cervical Vertebral Disc **5 Cervicothoracic Vertebral Disc** **9 Thoracic Vertebral Disc** **B Thoracolumbar Vertebral Disc**	**Ø** Open **3** Percutaneous **4** Percutaneous Endoscopic	**Ø** Drainage Device **3** Infusion Device **7** Autologous Tissue Substitute **J** Synthetic Substitute **K** Nonautologous Tissue Substitute	**Z** No Qualifier
3 Cervical Vertebral Disc **5 Cervicothoracic Vertebral Disc** **9 Thoracic Vertebral Disc** **B Thoracolumbar Vertebral Disc**	**X** External	**Ø** Drainage Device **3** Infusion Device	**Z** No Qualifier
C Temporomandibular Joint, Right **D Temporomandibular Joint, Left** **E Sternoclavicular Joint, Right** **F Sternoclavicular Joint, Left** **G Acromioclavicular Joint, Right** **H Acromioclavicular Joint, Left** **J Shoulder Joint, Right** Glenohumeral joint Glenoid ligament (labrum) **K Shoulder Joint, Left** *See J Shoulder Joint, Right*	**Ø** Open **3** Percutaneous **4** Percutaneous Endoscopic	**Ø** Drainage Device **3** Infusion Device **4** Internal Fixation Device **7** Autologous Tissue Substitute **8** Spacer **J** Synthetic Substitute **K** Nonautologous Tissue Substitute	**Z** No Qualifier
C Temporomandibular Joint, Right **D Temporomandibular Joint, Left** **E Sternoclavicular Joint, Right** **F Sternoclavicular Joint, Left** **G Acromioclavicular Joint, Right** **H Acromioclavicular Joint, Left** **J Shoulder Joint, Right** Glenohumeral joint Glenoid ligament (labrum) **K Shoulder Joint, Left** *See J Shoulder Joint, Right*	**X** External	**Ø** Drainage Device **3** Infusion Device **4** Internal Fixation Device	**Z** No Qualifier

Non-OR ØRP[Ø,1,4,6,A]3[Ø,3,8]Z
Non-OR ØRP[Ø,1,4,6,A][Ø,4]8Z
Non-OR ØRP[Ø,1,4,6,A]X[Ø,3,4]Z
Non-OR ØRP[3,5,9,B]3[Ø,3]Z
Non-OR ØRP[3,5,9,B]X[Ø,3]Z
Non-OR ØRP[C,D,E,F,G,H,J,K]3[Ø,3,8]Z
Non-OR ØRP[C,D,E,F,G,H,J,K][Ø,4]8Z
Non-OR ØRP[C,D]X[Ø,3]Z
Non-OR ØRP[E,F,G,H,J,K]X[Ø,3,4]Z

ØRP Continued on next page

Ø Medical and Surgical
R Upper Joints
P Removal Definition: Taking out or off a device from a body part

ØRP Continued

Explanation: If a device is taken out and a similar device put in without cutting or puncturing the skin or mucous membrane, the procedure is coded to the root operation CHANGE. Otherwise, the procedure for taking out the device is coded to the root operation REMOVAL.

Body Part Character 4	Approach Character 5	Device Character 6	Qualifier Character 7
L Elbow Joint, Right Distal humerus, involving joint Humeroradial joint Humeroulnar joint Proximal radioulnar joint **M Elbow Joint, Left** *See L Elbow Joint, Right* **N Wrist Joint, Right** Distal radioulnar joint Radiocarpal joint **P Wrist Joint, Left** *See N Wrist Joint, Right* **Q Carpal Joint, Right** Intercarpal joint Midcarpal joint **R Carpal Joint, Left** *See Q Carpal Joint, Right* **S Carpometacarpal Joint, Right** **T Carpometacarpal Joint, Left** **U Metacarpophalangeal Joint, Right** **V Metacarpophalangeal Joint, Left** **W Finger Phalangeal Joint, Right** Interphalangeal (IP) joint **X Finger Phalangeal Joint, Left** *See W Finger Phalangeal Joint, Right*	**Ø Open** **3 Percutaneous** **4 Percutaneous Endoscopic**	**Ø Drainage Device** **3 Infusion Device** **4 Internal Fixation Device** **5 External Fixation Device** **7 Autologous Tissue Substitute** **8 Spacer** **J Synthetic Substitute** **K Nonautologous Tissue Substitute**	**Z No Qualifier**
L Elbow Joint, Right Distal humerus, involving joint Humeroradial joint Humeroulnar joint Proximal radioulnar joint **M Elbow Joint, Left** *See L Elbow Joint, Right* **N Wrist Joint, Right** Distal radioulnar joint Radiocarpal joint **P Wrist Joint, Left** *See N Wrist Joint, Right* **Q Carpal Joint, Right** Intercarpal joint Midcarpal joint **R Carpal Joint, Left** *See Q Carpal Joint, Right* **S Carpometacarpal Joint, Right** **T Carpometacarpal Joint, Left** **U Metacarpophalangeal Joint, Right** **V Metacarpophalangeal Joint, Left** **W Finger Phalangeal Joint, Right** Interphalangeal (IP) joint **X Finger Phalangeal Joint, Left** *See W Finger Phalangeal Joint, Right*	**X External**	**Ø Drainage Device** **3 Infusion Device** **4 Internal Fixation Device** **5 External Fixation Device**	**Z No Qualifier**

Non-OR ØRP[L,M,N,P,Q,R,S,T,U,V,W,X]3[Ø,3,8]Z
Non-OR ØRP[L,M,N,P,Q,R,S,T,U,V,W,X][Ø,4]8Z
Non-OR ØRP[L,M,N,P,Q,R,S,T,U,V,W,X]X[Ø,3,4,5]Z

Ø Medical and Surgical
R Upper Joints
Q Repair Definition: Restoring, to the extent possible, a body part to its normal anatomic structure and function

Explanation: Used only when the method to accomplish the repair is not one of the other root operations

Body Part Character 4	Approach Character 5	Device Character 6	Qualifier Character 7
Ø Occipital-cervical Joint 1 Cervical Vertebral Joint Atlantoaxial joint Cervical facet joint 3 Cervical Vertebral Disc 4 Cervicothoracic Vertebral Joint Cervicothoracic facet joint 5 Cervicothoracic Vertebral Disc 6 Thoracic Vertebral Joint Costotransverse joint Costovertebral joint Thoracic facet joint 9 Thoracic Vertebral Disc A Thoracolumbar Vertebral Joint Thoracolumbar facet joint B Thoracolumbar Vertebral Disc C Temporomandibular Joint, Right D Temporomandibular Joint, Left E Sternoclavicular Joint, Right F Sternoclavicular Joint, Left G Acromioclavicular Joint, Right H Acromioclavicular Joint, Left J Shoulder Joint, Right Glenohumeral joint Glenoid ligament (labrum) K Shoulder Joint, Left *See J Shoulder Joint, Right* L Elbow Joint, Right Distal humerus, involving joint Humeroradial joint Humeroulnar joint Proximal radioulnar joint M Elbow Joint, Left *See L Elbow Joint, Right* N Wrist Joint, Right Distal radioulnar joint Radiocarpal joint P Wrist Joint, Left *See N Wrist Joint, Right* Q Carpal Joint, Right Intercarpal joint Midcarpal joint R Carpal Joint, Left *See Q Carpal Joint, Right* S Carpometacarpal Joint, Right T Carpometacarpal Joint, Left U Metacarpophalangeal Joint, Right V Metacarpophalangeal Joint, Left W Finger Phalangeal Joint, Right Interphalangeal (IP) joint X Finger Phalangeal Joint, Left *See W Finger Phalangeal Joint, Right*	Ø Open 3 Percutaneous 4 Percutaneous Endoscopic X External	Z No Device	Z No Qualifier

Non-OR ØRQ[Ø,1,3,4,5,6,9,A,B,C,D,E,F,G,H,J,K,L,M,N,P,Q,R,S,T,U,V,W,X]XZZ

HAC ØRQ[E,F,G,H,J,K,L,M][Ø,3,4,X]ZZ when reported with SDx K68.11 or T81.4Ø–T81.49, T84.6Ø-T84.619, T84.63-T84.7 with 7th character A

Ø Medical and Surgical
R Upper Joints
R Replacement Definition: Putting in or on biological or synthetic material that physically takes the place and/or function of all or a portion of a body part

Explanation: The body part may have been taken out or replaced, or may be taken out, physically eradicated, or rendered nonfunctional during the REPLACEMENT procedure. A REMOVAL procedure is coded for taking out the device used in a previous replacement procedure.

Body Part Character 4	Approach Character 5	Device Character 6	Qualifier Character 7
Ø Occipital-cervical Joint **1 Cervical Vertebral Joint** Atlantoaxial joint Cervical facet joint **3 Cervical Vertebral Disc** **4 Cervicothoracic Vertebral Joint** Cervicothoracic facet joint **5 Cervicothoracic Vertebral Disc** **6 Thoracic Vertebral Joint** Costotransverse joint Costovertebral joint Thoracic facet joint **9 Thoracic Vertebral Disc** **A Thoracolumbar Vertebral Joint** Thoracolumbar facet joint **B Thoracolumbar Vertebral Disc** **C Temporomandibular Joint, Right** **D Temporomandibular Joint, Left** **E Sternoclavicular Joint, Right** **F Sternoclavicular Joint, Left** **G Acromioclavicular Joint, Right** **H Acromioclavicular Joint, Left** **L Elbow Joint, Right** Distal humerus, involving joint Humeroradial joint Humeroulnar joint Proximal radioulnar joint **M Elbow Joint, Left** *See L Elbow Joint, Right* **N Wrist Joint, Right** Distal radioulnar joint Radiocarpal joint **P Wrist Joint, Left** *See N Wrist Joint, Right* **Q Carpal Joint, Right** Intercarpal joint Midcarpal joint **R Carpal Joint, Left** *See Q Carpal Joint, Right* **S Carpometacarpal Joint, Right** **T Carpometacarpal Joint, Left** **U Metacarpophalangeal Joint, Right** **V Metacarpophalangeal Joint, Left** **W Finger Phalangeal Joint, Right** Interphalangeal (IP) joint **X Finger Phalangeal Joint, Left** *See W Finger Phalangeal Joint, Right*	**Ø Open**	**7 Autologous Tissue Substitute** **J Synthetic Substitute** **K Nonautologous Tissue Substitute**	**Z No Qualifier**
J Shoulder Joint, Right Glenohumeral joint Glenoid ligament (labrum) **K Shoulder Joint, Left** *See J Shoulder Joint, Right*	**Ø Open**	**Ø Synthetic Substitute, Reverse Ball and Socket** **7 Autologous Tissue Substitute** **K Nonautologous Tissue Substitute**	**Z No Qualifier**
J Shoulder Joint, Right Glenohumeral joint Glenoid ligament (labrum) **K Shoulder Joint, Left** *See J Shoulder Joint, Right*	**Ø Open**	**J Synthetic Substitute**	**6 Humeral Surface** **7 Glenoid Surface** **Z No Qualifier**

Ø **Medical and Surgical**
R **Upper Joints**
S **Reposition** Definition: Moving to its normal location, or other suitable location, all or a portion of a body part

Explanation: The body part is moved to a new location from an abnormal location, or from a normal location where it is not functioning correctly. The body part may or may not be cut out or off to be moved to the new location.

Body Part Character 4	Approach Character 5	Device Character 6	Qualifier Character 7
Ø Occipital-cervical Joint **1 Cervical Vertebral Joint** Atlantoaxial joint Cervical facet joint **4 Cervicothoracic Vertebral Joint** Cervicothoracic facet joint **6 Thoracic Vertebral Joint** Costotransverse joint Costovertebral joint Thoracic facet joint **A Thoracolumbar Vertebral Joint** Thoracolumbar facet joint **C Temporomandibular Joint, Right** **D Temporomandibular Joint, Left** **E Sternoclavicular Joint, Right** **F Sternoclavicular Joint, Left** **G Acromioclavicular Joint, Right** **H Acromioclavicular Joint, Left** **J Shoulder Joint, Right** Glenohumeral joint Glenoid ligament (labrum) **K Shoulder Joint, Left** ***See*** *J Shoulder Joint, Right*	**Ø Open** **3 Percutaneous** **4 Percutaneous Endoscopic** **X External**	**4 Internal Fixation Device** **Z No Device**	**Z No Qualifier**
L Elbow Joint, Right Distal humerus, involving joint Humeroradial joint Humeroulnar joint Proximal radioulnar joint **M Elbow Joint, Left** ***See*** *L Elbow Joint, Right* **N Wrist Joint, Right** Distal radioulnar joint Radiocarpal joint **P Wrist Joint, Left** ***See*** *N Wrist Joint, Right* **Q Carpal Joint, Right** Intercarpal joint Midcarpal joint **R Carpal Joint, Left** ***See*** *Q Carpal Joint, Right* **S Carpometacarpal Joint, Right** **T Carpometacarpal Joint, Left** **U Metacarpophalangeal Joint, Right** **V Metacarpophalangeal Joint, Left** **W Finger Phalangeal Joint, Right** Interphalangeal (IP) joint **X Finger Phalangeal Joint, Left** ***See*** *W Finger Phalangeal Joint, Right*	**Ø Open** **3 Percutaneous** **4 Percutaneous Endoscopic** **X External**	**4 Internal Fixation Device** **5 External Fixation Device** **Z No Device**	**Z No Qualifier**

Non-OR ØRS[Ø,1,4,6,A,C,D,E,F,G,H,J,K][3,4,X][4,Z]Z
Non-OR ØRS[L,M,N,P,Q,R,S,T,U,V,W,X][3,4,X][4,5,Z]Z

Ø Medical and Surgical
R Upper Joints
T Resection Definition: Cutting out or off, without replacement, all of a body part
Explanation: None

Body Part Character 4	Approach Character 5	Device Character 6	Qualifier Character 7
3 Cervical Vertebral Disc **4 Cervicothoracic Vertebral Joint** Cervicothoracic facet joint **5 Cervicothoracic Vertebral Disc** **9 Thoracic Vertebral Disc** **B Thoracolumbar Vertebral Disc** **C Temporomandibular Joint, Right** **D Temporomandibular Joint, Left** **E Sternoclavicular Joint, Right** **F Sternoclavicular Joint, Left** **G Acromioclavicular Joint, Right** **H Acromioclavicular Joint, Left** **J Shoulder Joint, Right** Glenohumeral joint Glenoid ligament (labrum) **K Shoulder Joint, Left** *See J Shoulder Joint, Right* **L Elbow Joint, Right** Distal humerus, involving joint Humeroradial joint Humeroulnar joint Proximal radioulnar joint **M Elbow Joint, Left** *See L Elbow Joint, Right* **N Wrist Joint, Right** Distal radioulnar joint Radiocarpal joint **P Wrist Joint, Left** *See N Wrist Joint, Right* **Q Carpal Joint, Right** Intercarpal joint Midcarpal joint **R Carpal Joint, Left** *See Q Carpal Joint, Right* **S Carpometacarpal Joint, Right** **T Carpometacarpal Joint, Left** **U Metacarpophalangeal Joint, Right** **V Metacarpophalangeal Joint, Left** **W Finger Phalangeal Joint, Right** Interphalangeal (IP) joint **X Finger Phalangeal Joint, Left** *See W Finger Phalangeal Joint, Right*	**Ø Open**	**Z No Device**	**Z No Qualifier**

Ø Medical and Surgical
R Upper Joints
U Supplement Definition: Putting in or on biological or synthetic material that physically reinforces and/or augments the function of a portion of a body part

Explanation: The biological material is non-living, or is living and from the same individual. The body part may have been previously replaced, and the SUPPLEMENT procedure is performed to physically reinforce and/or augment the function of the replaced body part.

Body Part Character 4	Approach Character 5	Device Character 6	Qualifier Character 7
Ø Occipital-cervical Joint **1 Cervical Vertebral Joint** Atlantoaxial joint Cervical facet joint **3 Cervical Vertebral Disc** **4 Cervicothoracic Vertebral Joint** Cervicothoracic facet joint **5 Cervicothoracic Vertebral Disc** **6 Thoracic Vertebral Joint** Costotransverse joint Costovertebral joint Thoracic facet joint **9 Thoracic Vertebral Disc** **A Thoracolumbar Vertebral Joint** Thoracolumbar facet joint **B Thoracolumbar Vertebral Disc** **C Temporomandibular Joint, Right** **D Temporomandibular Joint, Left** **E Sternoclavicular Joint, Right** **F Sternoclavicular Joint, Left** **G Acromioclavicular Joint, Right** **H Acromioclavicular Joint, Left** **J Shoulder Joint, Right** Glenohumeral joint Glenoid ligament (labrum) **K Shoulder Joint, Left** *See J Shoulder Joint, Right* **L Elbow Joint, Right** Distal humerus, involving joint Humeroradial joint Humeroulnar joint Proximal radioulnar joint **M Elbow Joint, Left** *See L Elbow Joint, Right* **N Wrist Joint, Right** Distal radioulnar joint Radiocarpal joint **P Wrist Joint, Left** *See N Wrist Joint, Right* **Q Carpal Joint, Right** Intercarpal joint Midcarpal joint **R Carpal Joint, Left** *See Q Carpal Joint, Right* **S Carpometacarpal Joint, Right** **T Carpometacarpal Joint, Left** **U Metacarpophalangeal Joint, Right** **V Metacarpophalangeal Joint, Left** **W Finger Phalangeal Joint, Right** Interphalangeal (IP) joint **X Finger Phalangeal Joint, Left** *See W Finger Phalangeal Joint, Right*	**Ø Open** **3 Percutaneous** **4 Percutaneous Endoscopic**	**7 Autologous Tissue Substitute** **J Synthetic Substitute** **K Nonautologous Tissue Substitute**	**Z No Qualifier**

HAC ØRU[E,F,G,H,J,K,L,M][Ø,3,4][7,J,K]Z when reported with SDx K68.11 or T81.4Ø–T81.49, T84.6Ø-T84.619, T84.63-T84.7 with 7th character A

Ø Medical and Surgical
R Upper Joints
W Revision Definition: Correcting, to the extent possible, a portion of a malfunctioning device or the position of a displaced device

Explanation: Revision can include correcting a malfunctioning or displaced device by taking out or putting in components of the device such as a screw or pin

Body Part Character 4	Approach Character 5	Device Character 6	Qualifier Character 7
Ø Occipital-cervical Joint **1** Cervical Vertebral Joint Atlantoaxial joint Cervical facet joint **4** Cervicothoracic Vertebral Joint Cervicothoracic facet joint **6** Thoracic Vertebral Joint Costotransverse joint Costovertebral joint Thoracic facet joint **A** Thoracolumbar Vertebral Joint Thoracolumbar facet joint	**Ø** Open **3** Percutaneous **4** Percutaneous Endoscopic **X** External	**Ø** Drainage Device **3** Infusion Device **4** Internal Fixation Device **7** Autologous Tissue Substitute **8** Spacer **A** Interbody Fusion Device **J** Synthetic Substitute **K** Nonautologous Tissue Substitute	**Z** No Qualifier
3 Cervical Vertebral Disc **5** Cervicothoracic Vertebral Disc **9** Thoracic Vertebral Disc **B** Thoracolumbar Vertebral Disc	**Ø** Open **3** Percutaneous **4** Percutaneous Endoscopic **X** External	**Ø** Drainage Device **3** Infusion Device **7** Autologous Tissue Substitute **J** Synthetic Substitute **K** Nonautologous Tissue Substitute	**Z** No Qualifier
C Temporomandibular Joint, Right **D** Temporomandibular Joint, Left **E** Sternoclavicular Joint, Right **F** Sternoclavicular Joint, Left **G** Acromioclavicular Joint, Right **H** Acromioclavicular Joint, Left **J** Shoulder Joint, Right Glenohumeral joint Glenoid ligament (labrum) **K** Shoulder Joint, Left *See J Shoulder Joint, Right*	**Ø** Open **3** Percutaneous **4** Percutaneous Endoscopic **X** External	**Ø** Drainage Device **3** Infusion Device **4** Internal Fixation Device **7** Autologous Tissue Substitute **8** Spacer **J** Synthetic Substitute **K** Nonautologous Tissue Substitute	**Z** No Qualifier
L Elbow Joint, Right Distal humerus, involving joint Humeroradial joint Humeroulnar joint Proximal radioulnar joint **M** Elbow Joint, Left *See L Elbow Joint, Right* **N** Wrist Joint, Right Distal radioulnar joint Radiocarpal joint **P** Wrist Joint, Left *See N Wrist Joint, Right* **Q** Carpal Joint, Right Intercarpal joint Midcarpal joint **R** Carpal Joint, Left *See Q Carpal Joint, Right* **S** Carpometacarpal Joint, Right **T** Carpometacarpal Joint, Left **U** Metacarpophalangeal Joint, Right **V** Metacarpophalangeal Joint, Left **W** Finger Phalangeal Joint, Right Interphalangeal (IP) joint **X** Finger Phalangeal Joint, Left *See W Finger Phalangeal Joint, Right*	**Ø** Open **3** Percutaneous **4** Percutaneous Endoscopic **X** External	**Ø** Drainage Device **3** Infusion Device **4** Internal Fixation Device **5** External Fixation Device **7** Autologous Tissue Substitute **8** Spacer **J** Synthetic Substitute **K** Nonautologous Tissue Substitute	**Z** No Qualifier

Non-OR ØRW[Ø,1,4,6,A]X[Ø,3,4,7,8,A,J,K]Z
Non-OR ØRW[3,5,9,B]X[Ø,3,7,J,K]Z
Non-OR ØRW[C,D,E,F,G,H,J,K]X[Ø,3,4,7,8,J,K]Z
Non-OR ØRW[L,M,N,P,Q,R,S,T,U,V,W,X]X[Ø,3,4,5,7,8,J,K]Z

Lower Joints ØS2–ØSW

Character Meanings*

This Character Meaning table is provided as a guide to assist the user in the identification of character members that may be found in this section of code tables. It **SHOULD NOT** be used to build a PCS code.

Operation–Character 3	Body Part–Character 4	Approach–Character 5	Device–Character 6	Qualifier–Character 7
2 Change	Ø Lumbar Vertebral Joint	Ø Open	Ø Drainage Device OR Synthetic Substitute, Polyethylene	Ø Anterior Approach, Anterior Column
5 Destruction	1 Lumbar Vertebral Joint, 2 or more	3 Percutaneous	1 Synthetic Substitute, Metal	1 Posterior Approach, Posterior Column
9 Drainage	2 Lumbar Vertebral Disc	4 Percutaneous Endoscopic	2 Synthetic Substitute, Metal on Polyethylene	9 Cemented
B Excision	3 Lumbosacral Joint	X External	3 Infusion Device OR Internal Fixation Device, Sustained Compression OR Synthetic Substitute, Ceramic	A Uncemented
C Extirpation	4 Lumbosacral Disc		4 Internal Fixation Device OR Synthetic Substitute, Ceramic on Polyethylene	C Patellar Surface
G Fusion	5 Sacrococcygeal Joint		5 External Fixation Device	J Posterior Approach, Anterior Column
H Insertion	6 Coccygeal Joint		6 Synthetic Substitute, Oxidized Zirconium on Polyethylene	X Diagnostic
J Inspection	7 Sacroiliac Joint, Right		7 Autologous Tissue Substitute	Z No Qualifier
N Release	8 Sacroiliac Joint, Left		8 Spacer	
P Removal	9 Hip Joint, Right		9 Liner	
Q Repair	A Hip Joint, Acetabular Surface, Right		A Interbody Fusion Device	
R Replacement	B Hip Joint, Left		B Resurfacing Device OR Spinal Stabilization Device, Interspinous Process	
S Reposition	C Knee Joint, Right		C Spinal Stabilization Device, Pedicle-Based	
T Resection	D Knee Joint, Left		D Spinal Stabilization Device, Facet Replacement	
U Supplement	E Hip Joint, Acetabular Surface, Left		E Articulating Spacer	
W Revision	F Ankle Joint, Right		J Synthetic Substitute	
	G Ankle Joint, Left		K Nonautologous Tissue Substitute	
	H Tarsal Joint, Right		L Synthetic Substitute, Unicondylar Medial	
	J Tarsal Joint, Left		M Synthetic Substitute, Unicondylar Lateral	
	K Tarsometatarsal Joint, Right		N Synthetic Substitute, Patellofemoral	
	L Tarsometatarsal Joint, Left		Y Other Device	
	M Metatarsal-Phalangeal Joint, Right		Z No Device	
	N Metatarsal-Phalangeal Joint, Left			
	P Toe Phalangeal Joint, Right			
	Q Toe Phalangeal Joint, Left			
	R Hip Joint, Femoral Surface, Right			
	S Hip Joint, Femoral Surface, Left			
	T Knee Joint, Femoral Surface, Right			
	U Knee Joint, Femoral Surface, Left			
	V Knee Joint, Tibial Surface, Right			
	W Knee Joint, Tibial Surface, Left			
	Y Lower Joint			

* Includes synovial membrane.

AHA Coding Clinic for table ØS9

2018, 2Q, 17 Arthroscopic drainage of knee and nonexcisional debridement
2017, 1Q, 50 Dry aspiration of ankle joint

AHA Coding Clinic for table ØSB

2017, 4Q, 76 Radiolucent porous interbody fusion device
2016, 2Q, 16 Decompressive laminectomy/foraminotomy and lumbar discectomy
2016, 1Q, 20 Metatarsophalangeal joint resection arthroplasty
2015, 1Q, 34 Arthroscopic meniscectomy with debridement and abrasion chondroplasty
2014, 2Q, 6 Posterior lumbar fusion with discectomy

AHA Coding Clinic for table ØSG

2020, 2Q, 27 Spinal Fusion with NuVasive® VersaTie®
2020, 1Q, 33 Spinal fusion without use of bone graft
2019, 3Q, 35 Fusion procedures of the spine (guideline B3.1Øc)
2019, 1Q, 30 Spinal fusion performed at same level as decompressive laminectomy
2018, 4Q, 43 Joint fusion device value
2018, 1Q, 22 Spinal fusion procedures without bone graft
2017, 4Q, 76 Radiolucent porous interbody fusion device
2017, 2Q, 23 Decompression of spinal cord and placement of instrumentation
2014, 3Q, 30 Spinal fusion and fixation instrumentation
2014, 3Q, 36 Lumbar interbody fusion of two vertebral levels
2014, 2Q, 6 Posterior lumbar fusion with discectomy
2013, 3Q, 25 36Ø-degree spinal fusion
2013, 2Q, 39 Ankle fusion, osteotomy, and removal of hardware
2013, 1Q, 21-23 Spinal fusion of thoracic and lumbar vertebrae

AHA Coding Clinic for table ØSH

2017, 2Q, 23 Decompression of spinal cord and placement of instrumentation

AHA Coding Clinic for table ØSJ

2017, 1Q, 50 Dry aspiration of ankle joint

AHA Coding Clinic for table ØSN

2020, 2Q, 26 Arthroscopic Manipulation and Nonexcisional Debridement of Knee Joint
2019, 1Q, 30 Spinal fusion performed at same level as decompressive laminectomy

AHA Coding Clinic for table ØSP

2018, 4Q, 43 Articulating spacer for hip and knee joint
2018, 2Q, 16 Exchange of tibial polyethylene component with stabilizing insert (tibial tray)
2017, 4Q, 107 Total ankle replacement versus revision
2016, 4Q, 110-112 Removal and revision of hip and knee devices
2015, 2Q, 18 Total knee revision
2015, 2Q, 19 Revision of femoral head and acetabular liner
2013, 2Q, 39 Ankle fusion, osteotomy, and removal of hardware

AHA Coding Clinic for table ØSQ

2014, 4Q, 25 Femoroacetabular impingement and labral tear with repair

AHA Coding Clinic for table ØSR

2018, 4Q, 43 Articulating spacer for hip and knee joint
2018, 2Q, 16 Exchange of tibial polyethylene component with stabilizing insert (tibial tray)
2017, 4Q, 38-39 Oxidized zirconium on polyethylene bearing surface
2017, 4Q, 107 Total ankle replacement versus revision
2017, 1Q, 22 Total knee replacement and patellar component
2016, 4Q, 110-111 Partial (unicondylar) knee replacement
2016, 4Q, 111-112 Removal and revision of hip and knee devices
2016, 3Q, 35 Use of cemented versus uncemented qualifier for joint replacement
2015, 3Q, 18 Total hip replacement with acetabular reconstruction
2015, 2Q, 18 Total knee revision
2015, 2Q, 19 Revision of femoral head and acetabular liner

AHA Coding Clinic for table ØSS

2016, 2Q, 31 Periacetabular ostectomy for repair of congenital hip dysplasia

AHA Coding Clinic for table ØST

2016, 1Q, 20 Metatarsophalangeal joint resection arthroplasty
2014, 4Q, 29 Rotational osteosynthesis

AHA Coding Clinic for table ØSU

2018, 2Q, 16 Exchange of tibial polyethylene component with stabilizing insert (tibial tray)
2016, 4Q, 111 Removal and revision of hip and knee devices
2015, 2Q, 19 Revision of femoral head and acetabular liner

AHA Coding Clinic for table ØSW

2017, 4Q, 107 Total ankle replacement versus revision
2016, 4Q, 110-112 Removal and revision of hip and knee devices
2015, 2Q, 18 Total knee revision
2015, 2Q, 19 Revision of femoral head and acetabular liner

Lower Joints

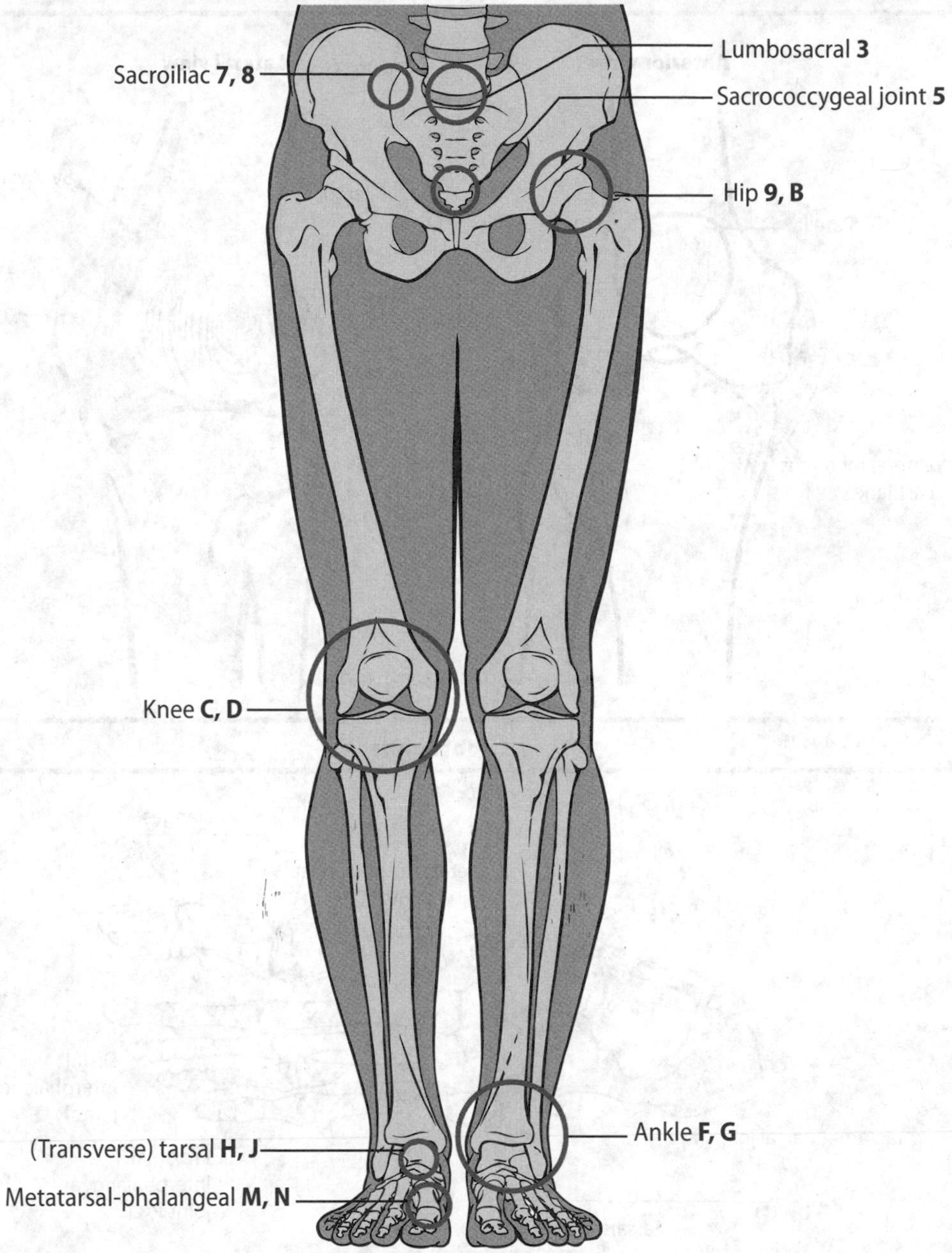

Lumbosacral **3**
Sacroiliac **7, 8**
Sacrococcygeal joint **5**
Hip **9, B**
Knee **C, D**
Ankle **F, G**
(Transverse) tarsal **H, J**
Metatarsal-phalangeal **M, N**

Hip Joint

Ilium
Sacroiliac joint **7, 8**
Sacrum
Acetabulofemoral joint **9, B**
Head of femur
Ischium

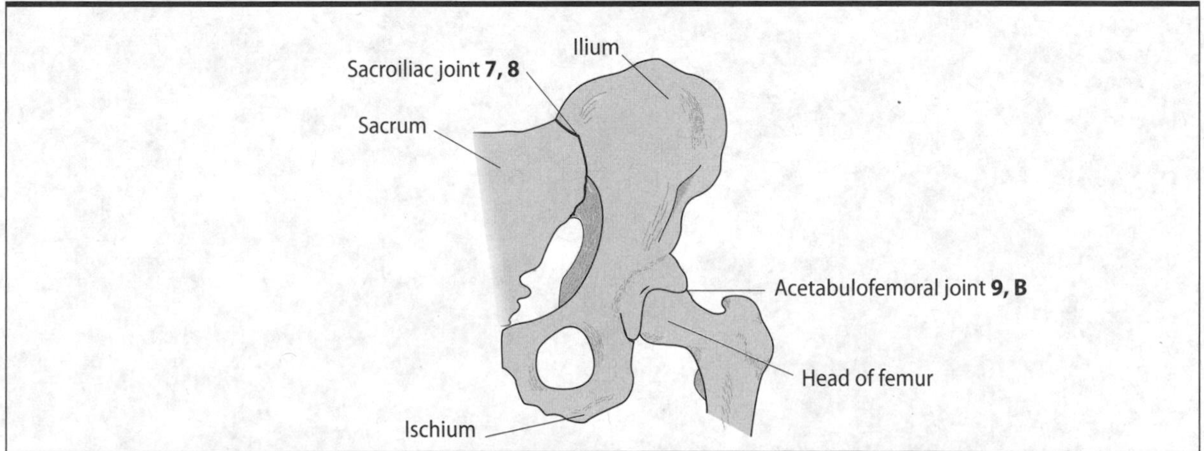

Knee Joint

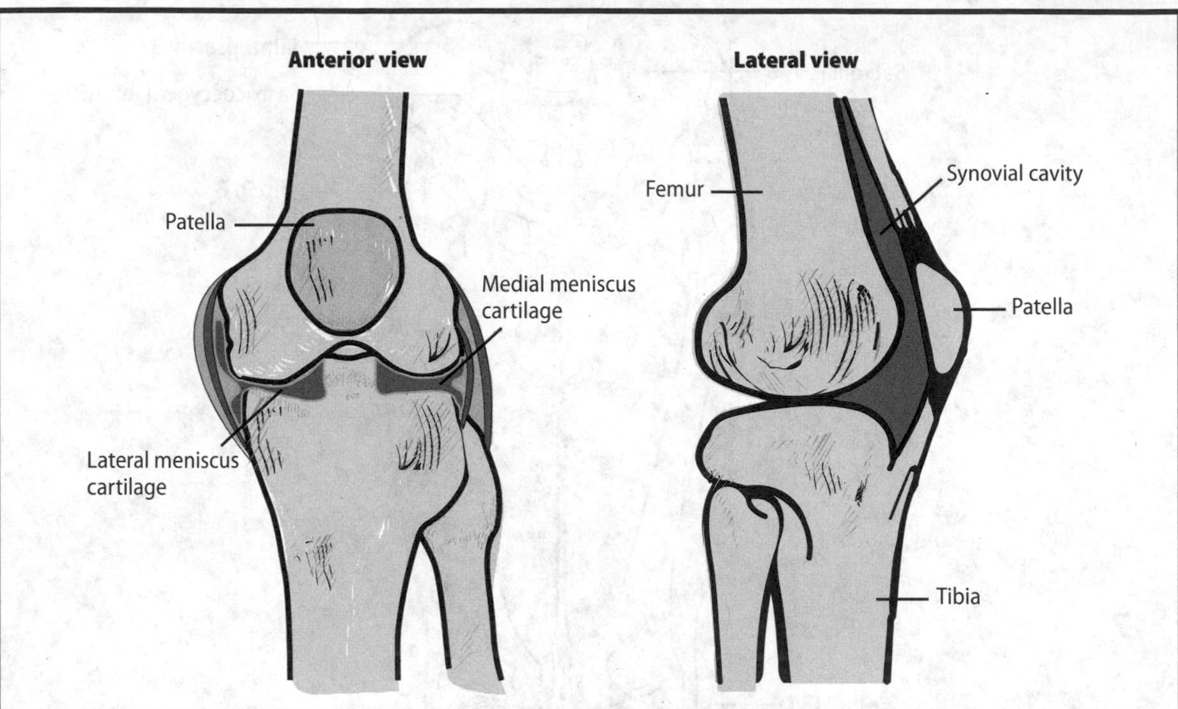

Foot Joints

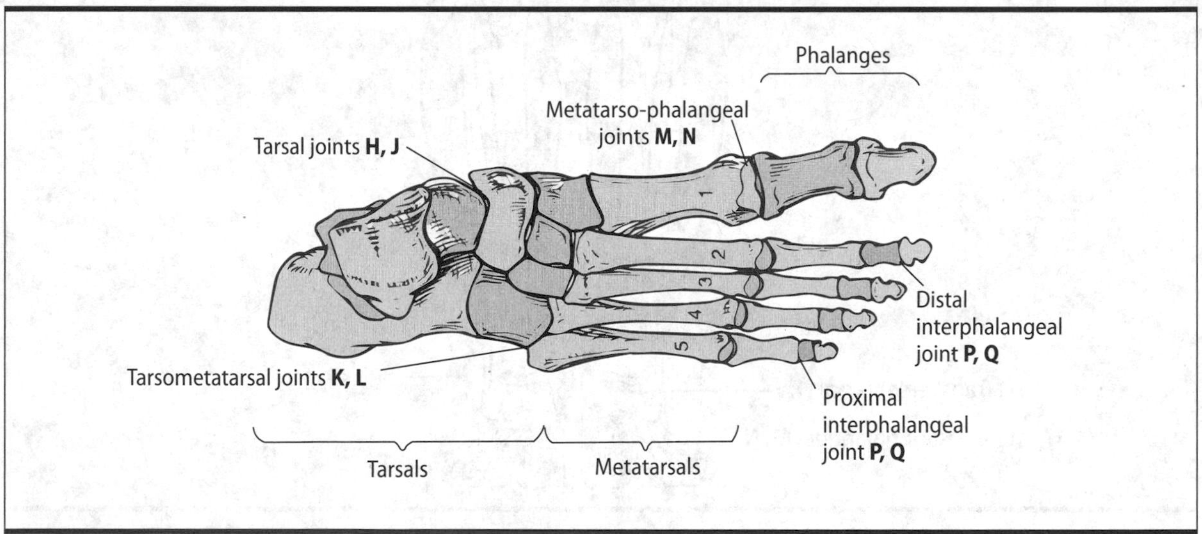

Ø Medical and Surgical
S Lower Joints
2 Change Definition: Taking out or off a device from a body part and putting back an identical or similar device in or on the same body part without cutting or puncturing the skin or a mucous membrane

Explanation: All CHANGE procedures are coded using the approach EXTERNAL

Body Part Character 4	Approach Character 5	Device Character 6	Qualifier Character 7
Y Lower Joint	X External	Ø Drainage Device Y Other Device	Z No Qualifier

Non-OR All body part, approach, device, and qualifier values

Ø Medical and Surgical
S Lower Joints
5 Destruction Definition: Physical eradication of all or a portion of a body part by the direct use of energy, force, or a destructive agent

Explanation: None of the body part is physically taken out

Body Part Character 4	Approach Character 5	Device Character 6	Qualifier Character 7
Ø **Lumbar Vertebral Joint** Lumbar facet joint 2 **Lumbar Vertebral Disc** 3 **Lumbosacral Joint** Lumbosacral facet joint 4 **Lumbosacral Disc** 5 **Sacrococcygeal Joint** Sacrococcygeal symphysis 6 **Coccygeal Joint** 7 **Sacroiliac Joint, Right** 8 **Sacroiliac Joint, Left** 9 **Hip Joint, Right** Acetabulofemoral joint B **Hip Joint, Left** *See 9 Hip Joint, Right* C **Knee Joint, Right** Femoropatellar joint Femorotibial joint Lateral meniscus Medial meniscus Patellofemoral joint Tibiofemoral joint D **Knee Joint, Left** *See C Knee Joint, Right* F **Ankle Joint, Right** Inferior tibiofibular joint Talocrural joint G **Ankle Joint, Left** *See F Ankle Joint, Right* H **Tarsal Joint, Right** Calcaneocuboid joint Cuboideonavicular joint Cuneonavicular joint Intercuneiform joint Subtalar (talocalcaneal) joint Talocalcaneal (subtalar) joint Talocalcaneonavicular joint J **Tarsal Joint, Left** *See H Tarsal Joint, Right* K **Tarsometatarsal Joint, Right** L **Tarsometatarsal Joint, Left** M **Metatarsal-Phalangeal Joint, Right** Metatarsophalangeal (MTP) joint N **Metatarsal-Phalangeal Joint, Left** *See M Metatarsal-Phalangeal Joint, Right* P **Toe Phalangeal Joint, Right** Interphalangeal (IP) joint Q **Toe Phalangeal Joint, Left** *See P Toe Phalangeal Joint, Right*	Ø Open 3 Percutaneous 4 Percutaneous Endoscopic	Z No Device	Z No Qualifier

Ø Medical and Surgical
S Lower Joints
9 Drainage Definition: Taking or letting out fluids and/or gases from a body part
Explanation: The qualifier DIAGNOSTIC is used to identify drainage procedures that are biopsies

Body Part Character 4		Approach Character 5	Device Character 6	Qualifier Character 7
Ø Lumbar Vertebral Joint Lumbar facet joint **2 Lumbar Vertebral Disc** **3 Lumbosacral Joint** Lumbosacral facet joint **4 Lumbosacral Disc** **5 Sacrococcygeal Joint** Sacrococcygeal symphysis **6 Coccygeal Joint** **7 Sacroiliac Joint, Right** **8 Sacroiliac Joint, Left** **9 Hip Joint, Right** Acetabulofemoral joint **B Hip Joint, Left** *See 9 Hip Joint, Right* **C Knee Joint, Right** Femoropatellar joint Femorotibial joint Lateral meniscus Medial meniscus Patellofemoral joint Tibiofemoral joint **D Knee Joint, Left** *See C Knee Joint, Right* **F Ankle Joint, Right** Inferior tibiofibular joint Talocrural joint **G Ankle Joint, Left** *See F Ankle Joint, Right*	**H Tarsal Joint, Right** Calcaneocuboid joint Cuboideonavicular joint Cuneonavicular joint Intercuneiform joint Subtalar (talocalcaneal) joint Talocalcaneal (subtalar) joint Talocalcaneonavicular joint **J Tarsal Joint, Left** *See H Tarsal Joint, Right* **K Tarsometatarsal Joint, Right** **L Tarsometatarsal Joint, Left** **M Metatarsal-Phalangeal Joint, Right** Metatarsophalangeal (MTP) joint **N Metatarsal-Phalangeal Joint, Left** *See M Metatarsal-Phalangeal Joint, Right* **P Toe Phalangeal Joint, Right** Interphalangeal (IP) joint **Q Toe Phalangeal Joint, Left** *See P Toe Phalangeal Joint, Right*	**Ø Open** **3 Percutaneous** **4 Percutaneous Endoscopic**	**Ø Drainage Device**	**Z No Qualifier**
Ø Lumbar Vertebral Joint Lumbar facet joint **2 Lumbar Vertebral Disc** **3 Lumbosacral Joint** Lumbosacral facet joint **4 Lumbosacral Disc** **5 Sacrococcygeal Joint** Sacrococcygeal symphysis **6 Coccygeal Joint** **7 Sacroiliac Joint, Right** **8 Sacroiliac Joint, Left** **9 Hip Joint, Right** Acetabulofemoral joint **B Hip Joint, Left** *See 9 Hip Joint, Right* **C Knee Joint, Right** Femoropatellar joint Femorotibial joint Lateral meniscus Medial meniscus Patellofemoral joint Tibiofemoral joint **D Knee Joint, Left** *See C Knee Joint, Right* **F Ankle Joint, Right** Inferior tibiofibular joint Talocrural joint **G Ankle Joint, Left** *See F Ankle Joint, Right*	**H Tarsal Joint, Right** Calcaneocuboid joint Cuboideonavicular joint Cuneonavicular joint Intercuneiform joint Subtalar (talocalcaneal) joint Talocalcaneal (subtalar) joint Talocalcaneonavicular joint **J Tarsal Joint, Left** *See H Tarsal Joint, Right* **K Tarsometatarsal Joint, Right** **L Tarsometatarsal Joint, Left** **M Metatarsal-Phalangeal Joint, Right** Metatarsophalangeal (MTP) joint **N Metatarsal-Phalangeal Joint, Left** *See M Metatarsal-Phalangeal Joint, Right* **P Toe Phalangeal Joint, Right** Interphalangeal (IP) joint **Q Toe Phalangeal Joint, Left** *See P Toe Phalangeal Joint, Right*	**Ø Open** **3 Percutaneous** **4 Percutaneous Endoscopic**	**Z No Device**	**X Diagnostic** **Z No Qualifier**

Non-OR ØS9[Ø,2,3,4,5,6,7,8,9,B,C,D,F,G,H,J,K,L,M,N,P,Q][3,4]ØZ
Non-OR ØS9[Ø,2,3,4,5,6,7,8,9,B,C,D,F,G,H,J,K,L,M,N,P,Q][Ø,3,4]ZX
Non-OR ØS9[Ø,2,3,4,5,6,7,8,9,B,C,D,F,G,H,J,K,L,M,N,P,Q][3,4]ZZ

Ø Medical and Surgical
S Lower Joints
B Excision Definition: Cutting out or off, without replacement, a portion of a body part
Explanation: The qualifier DIAGNOSTIC is used to identify excision procedures that are biopsies

Body Part Character 4		Approach Character 5	Device Character 6	Qualifier Character 7
Ø Lumbar Vertebral Joint Lumbar facet joint **2 Lumbar Vertebral Disc** **3 Lumbosacral Joint** Lumbosacral facet joint **4 Lumbosacral Disc** **5 Sacrococcygeal Joint** Sacrococcygeal symphysis **6 Coccygeal Joint** **7 Sacroiliac Joint, Right** **8 Sacroiliac Joint, Left** **9 Hip Joint, Right** Acetabulofemoral joint **B Hip Joint, Left** *See 9 Hip Joint, Right* **C Knee Joint, Right** Femoropatellar joint Femorotibial joint Lateral meniscus Medial meniscus Patellofemoral joint Tibiofemoral joint **D Knee Joint, Left** *See C Knee Joint, Right* **F Ankle Joint, Right** Inferior tibiofibular joint Talocrural joint **G Ankle Joint, Left** *See F Ankle Joint, Right*	**H Tarsal Joint, Right** Calcaneocuboid joint Cuboideonavicular joint Cuneonavicular joint Intercuneiform joint Subtalar (talocalcaneal) joint Talocalcaneal (subtalar) joint Talocalcaneonavicular joint **J Tarsal Joint, Left** *See H Tarsal Joint, Right* **K Tarsometatarsal Joint, Right** **L Tarsometatarsal Joint, Left** **M Metatarsal-Phalangeal Joint, Right** Metatarsophalangeal (MTP) joint **N Metatarsal-Phalangeal Joint, Left** *See M Metatarsal-Phalangeal Joint, Right* **P Toe Phalangeal Joint, Right** Interphalangeal (IP) joint **Q Toe Phalangeal Joint, Left** *See P Toe Phalangeal Joint, Right*	**Ø Open** **3 Percutaneous** **4 Percutaneous Endoscopic**	**Z No Device**	**X Diagnostic** **Z No Qualifier**

Non-OR ØSB[Ø,2,3,4,5,6,7,8,9,B,C,D,F,G,H,J,K,L,M,N,P,Q][Ø,3,4]ZX

Ø Medical and Surgical
S Lower Joints
C Extirpation Definition: Taking or cutting out solid matter from a body part
Explanation: The solid matter may be an abnormal byproduct of a biological function or a foreign body; it may be imbedded in a body part or in the lumen of a tubular body part. The solid matter may or may not have been previously broken into pieces.

Body Part Character 4		Approach Character 5	Device Character 6	Qualifier Character 7
Ø Lumbar Vertebral Joint Lumbar facet joint **2 Lumbar Vertebral Disc** **3 Lumbosacral Joint** Lumbosacral facet joint **4 Lumbosacral Disc** **5 Sacrococcygeal Joint** Sacrococcygeal symphysis **6 Coccygeal Joint** **7 Sacroiliac Joint, Right** **8 Sacroiliac Joint, Left** **9 Hip Joint, Right** Acetabulofemoral joint **B Hip Joint, Left** *See 9 Hip Joint, Right* **C Knee Joint, Right** Femoropatellar joint Femorotibial joint Lateral meniscus Medial meniscus Patellofemoral joint Tibiofemoral joint **D Knee Joint, Left** *See C Knee Joint, Right* **F Ankle Joint, Right** Inferior tibiofibular joint Talocrural joint **G Ankle Joint, Left** *See F Ankle Joint, Right*	**H Tarsal Joint, Right** Calcaneocuboid joint Cuboideonavicular joint Cuneonavicular joint Intercuneiform joint Subtalar (talocalcaneal) joint Talocalcaneal (subtalar) joint Talocalcaneonavicular joint **J Tarsal Joint, Left** *See H Tarsal Joint, Right* **K Tarsometatarsal Joint, Right** **L Tarsometatarsal Joint, Left** **M Metatarsal-Phalangeal Joint, Right** Metatarsophalangeal (MTP) joint **N Metatarsal-Phalangeal Joint, Left** *See M Metatarsal-Phalangeal Joint, Right* **P Toe Phalangeal Joint, Right** Interphalangeal (IP) joint **Q Toe Phalangeal Joint, Left** *See P Toe Phalangeal Joint, Right*	**Ø Open** **3 Percutaneous** **4 Percutaneous Endoscopic**	**Z No Device**	**Z No Qualifier**

Ø Medical and Surgical
S Lower Joints
G Fusion Definition: Joining together portions of an articular body part rendering the articular body part immobile
Explanation: The body part is joined together by fixation device, bone graft, or other means

Body Part Character 4	Approach Character 5	Device Character 6	Qualifier Character 7
Ø Lumbar Vertebral Joint Lumbar facet joint 1 Lumbar Vertebral Joints, 2 or more ⊞ 3 Lumbosacral Joint Lumbosacral facet joint	Ø Open 3 Percutaneous 4 Percutaneous Endoscopic	7 Autologous Tissue Substitute J Synthetic Substitute K Nonautologous Tissue Substitute	Ø Anterior Approach, Anterior Column 1 Posterior Approach, Posterior Column J Posterior Approach, Anterior Column
Ø Lumbar Vertebral Joint Lumbar facet joint 1 Lumbar Vertebral Joints, 2 or more ⊞ 3 Lumbosacral Joint Lumbosacral facet joint	Ø Open 3 Percutaneous 4 Percutaneous Endoscopic	A Interbody Fusion Device	Ø Anterior Approach, Anterior Column J Posterior Approach, Anterior Column
5 Sacrococcygeal Joint Sacrococcygeal symphysis 6 Coccygeal Joint 7 Sacroiliac Joint, Right 8 Sacroiliac Joint, Left	Ø Open 3 Percutaneous 4 Percutaneous Endoscopic	4 Internal Fixation Device 7 Autologous Tissue Substitute J Synthetic Substitute K Nonautologous Tissue Substitute	Z No Qualifier
9 Hip Joint, Right Acetabulofemoral joint B Hip Joint, Left *See 9 Hip Joint, Right* C Knee Joint, Right Femoropatellar joint Femorotibial joint Lateral meniscus Medial meniscus Patellofemoral joint Tibiofemoral joint D Knee Joint, Left *See C Knee Joint, Right* F Ankle Joint, Right Inferior tibiofibular joint Talocrural joint G Ankle Joint, Left *See F Ankle Joint, Right* H Tarsal Joint, Right Calcaneocuboid joint Cuboideonavicular joint Cuneonavicular joint Intercuneiform joint Subtalar (talocalcaneal) joint Talocalcaneal (subtalar) joint Talocalcaneonavicular joint J Tarsal Joint, Left *See H Tarsal Joint, Right* K Tarsometatarsal Joint, Right L Tarsometatarsal Joint, Left M Metatarsal-Phalangeal Joint, Right Metatarsophalangeal (MTP) joint N Metatarsal-Phalangeal Joint, Left *See M Metatarsal-Phalangeal Joint, Right* P Toe Phalangeal Joint, Right Interphalangeal (IP) joint Q Toe Phalangeal Joint, Left *See P Toe Phalangeal Joint, Right*	Ø Open 3 Percutaneous 4 Percutaneous Endoscopic	3 Internal Fixation Device, Sustained Compression 4 Internal Fixation Device 5 External Fixation Device 7 Autologous Tissue Substitute J Synthetic Substitute K Nonautologous Tissue Substitute	Z No Qualifier

HAC ØSG[Ø,1,3][Ø,3,4][7,J,K][Ø,1,J] when reported with SDx K68.11 or T81.4Ø–T81.49, T84.6Ø-T84.619, T84.63-T84.7 with 7th character A
HAC ØSG[Ø,1,3][Ø,3,4]A[Ø,J] when reported with SDx K68.11 or T81.4Ø–T81.49, T84.6Ø-T84.619, T84.63-T84.7 with 7th character A
HAC ØSG[7,8][Ø,3,4][4,7,J,K]Z when reported with SDx K68.11 or T81.4Ø–T81.49, T84.6Ø-T84.619, T84.63-T84.7 with 7th character A

See Appendix L for Procedure Combinations
⊞ ØSG1[Ø,3,4][7,J,K][Ø,1,J]
⊞ ØSG1[Ø,3,4]A[Ø,J]

Ø Medical and Surgical
S Lower Joints
H Insertion Definition: Putting in a nonbiological appliance that monitors, assists, performs, or prevents a physiological function but does not physically take the place of a body part

Explanation: None

Body Part Character 4	Approach Character 5	Device Character 6	Qualifier Character 7
Ø Lumbar Vertebral Joint Lumbar facet joint **3 Lumbosacral Joint** Lumbosacral facet joint	**Ø Open** **3 Percutaneous** **4 Percutaneous Endoscopic**	**3 Infusion Device** **4 Internal Fixation Device** **8 Spacer** **B Spinal Stabilization Device, Interspinous Process** **C Spinal Stabilization Device, Pedicle-Based** **D Spinal Stabilization Device, Facet Replacement**	**Z No Qualifier**
2 Lumbar Vertebral Disc **4 Lumbosacral Disc**	**Ø Open** **3 Percutaneous** **4 Percutaneous Endoscopic**	**3 Infusion Device** **8 Spacer**	**Z No Qualifier**
5 Sacrococcygeal Joint Sacrococcygeal symphysis **6 Coccygeal Joint** **7 Sacroiliac Joint, Right** **8 Sacroiliac Joint, Left**	**Ø Open** **3 Percutaneous** **4 Percutaneous Endoscopic**	**3 Infusion Device** **4 Internal Fixation Device** **8 Spacer**	**Z No Qualifier**
9 Hip Joint, Right Acetabulofemoral joint **B Hip Joint, Left** *See 9 Hip Joint, Right* **C Knee Joint, Right** Femoropatellar joint Femorotibial joint Lateral meniscus Medial meniscus Patellofemoral joint Tibiofemoral joint **D Knee Joint, Left** *See C Knee Joint, Right* **F Ankle Joint, Right** Inferior tibiofibular joint Talocrural joint **G Ankle Joint, Left** *See F Ankle Joint, Right* **H Tarsal Joint, Right** Calcaneocuboid joint Cuboideonavicular joint Cuneonavicular joint Intercuneiform joint Subtalar (talocalcaneal) joint Talocalcaneal (subtalar) joint Talocalcaneonavicular joint **J Tarsal Joint, Left** *See H Tarsal Joint, Right* **K Tarsometatarsal Joint, Right** **L Tarsometatarsal Joint, Left** **M Metatarsal-Phalangeal Joint, Right** Metatarsophalangeal (MTP) joint **N Metatarsal-Phalangeal Joint, Left** *See M Metatarsal-Phalangeal Joint, Right* **P Toe Phalangeal Joint, Right** Interphalangeal (IP) joint **Q Toe Phalangeal Joint, Left** *See P Toe Phalangeal Joint, Right*	**Ø Open** **3 Percutaneous** **4 Percutaneous Endoscopic**	**3 Infusion Device** **4 Internal Fixation Device** **5 External Fixation Device** **8 Spacer**	**Z No Qualifier**

Non-OR ØSH[Ø,3][Ø,3,4][3,8]Z
Non-OR ØSH[2,4][Ø,3,4][3,8]Z
Non-OR ØSH[5,6,7,8][Ø,3,4][3,8]Z
Non-OR ØSH[9,B,C,D][Ø,3,4]3Z
Non-OR ØSH[9,B,C,D][3,4]8Z
Non-OR ØSH[F,G,H,J,K,L,M,N,P,Q][Ø,3,4][3,8]Z

Ø Medical and Surgical
S Lower Joints
J Inspection Definition: Visually and/or manually exploring a body part

Explanation: Visual exploration may be performed with or without optical instrumentation. Manual exploration may be performed directly or through intervening body layers.

Body Part Character 4		Approach Character 5	Device Character 6	Qualifier Character 7
Ø Lumbar Vertebral Joint Lumbar facet joint 2 Lumbar Vertebral Disc 3 Lumbosacral Joint Lumbosacral facet joint 4 Lumbosacral Disc 5 Sacrococcygeal Joint Sacrococcygeal symphysis 6 Coccygeal Joint 7 Sacroiliac Joint, Right 8 Sacroiliac Joint, Left 9 Hip Joint, Right Acetabulofemoral joint B Hip Joint, Left *See 9 Hip Joint, Right* C Knee Joint, Right Femoropatellar joint Femorotibial joint Lateral meniscus Medial meniscus Patellofemoral joint Tibiofemoral joint D Knee Joint, Left *See C Knee Joint, Right* F Ankle Joint, Right Inferior tibiofibular joint Talocrural joint G Ankle Joint, Left *See F Ankle Joint, Right*	H Tarsal Joint, Right Calcaneocuboid joint Cuboideonavicular joint Cuneonavicular joint Intercuneiform joint Subtalar (talocalcaneal) joint Talocalcaneal (subtalar) joint Talocalcaneonavicular joint J Tarsal Joint, Left *See H Tarsal Joint, Right* K Tarsometatarsal Joint, Right L Tarsometatarsal Joint, Left M Metatarsal-Phalangeal Joint, Right Metatarsophalangeal (MTP) joint N Metatarsal-Phalangeal Joint, Left *See M Metatarsal-Phalangeal Joint, Right* P Toe Phalangeal Joint, Right Interphalangeal (IP) joint Q Toe Phalangeal Joint, Left *See P Toe Phalangeal Joint, Right*	Ø Open 3 Percutaneous 4 Percutaneous Endoscopic X External	Z No Device	Z No Qualifier

Non-OR ØSJ[Ø,2,3,4,5,6,7,8,9,B,C,D,F,G,H,J,K,L,M,N,P,Q][3,X]ZZ

Ø Medical and Surgical
S Lower Joints
N Release Definition: Freeing a body part from an abnormal physical constraint by cutting or by the use of force

Explanation: Some of the restraining tissue may be taken out but none of the body part is taken out

Body Part Character 4		Approach Character 5	Device Character 6	Qualifier Character 7
Ø Lumbar Vertebral Joint Lumbar facet joint 2 Lumbar Vertebral Disc 3 Lumbosacral Joint Lumbosacral facet joint 4 Lumbosacral Disc 5 Sacrococcygeal Joint Sacrococcygeal symphysis 6 Coccygeal Joint 7 Sacroiliac Joint, Right 8 Sacroiliac Joint, Left 9 Hip Joint, Right Acetabulofemoral joint B Hip Joint, Left *See 9 Hip Joint, Right* C Knee Joint, Right Femoropatellar joint Femorotibial joint Lateral meniscus Medial meniscus Patellofemoral joint Tibiofemoral joint D Knee Joint, Left *See C Knee Joint, Right* F Ankle Joint, Right Inferior tibiofibular joint Talocrural joint G Ankle Joint, Left *See F Ankle Joint, Right*	H Tarsal Joint, Right Calcaneocuboid joint Cuboideonavicular joint Cuneonavicular joint Intercuneiform joint Subtalar (talocalcaneal) joint Talocalcaneal (subtalar) joint Talocalcaneonavicular joint J Tarsal Joint, Left *See H Tarsal Joint, Right* K Tarsometatarsal Joint, Right L Tarsometatarsal Joint, Left M Metatarsal-Phalangeal Joint, Right Metatarsophalangeal (MTP) joint N Metatarsal-Phalangeal Joint, Left *See M Metatarsal-Phalangeal Joint, Right* P Toe Phalangeal Joint, Right Interphalangeal (IP) joint Q Toe Phalangeal Joint, Left *See P Toe Phalangeal Joint, Right*	Ø Open 3 Percutaneous 4 Percutaneous Endoscopic X External	Z No Device	Z No Qualifier

Non-OR ØSN[Ø,2,3,4,5,6,7,8,9,B,C,D,F,G,H,J,K,L,M,N,P,Q]XZZ

Ø Medical and Surgical
S Lower Joints
P Removal Definition: Taking out or off a device from a body part

Explanation: If a device is taken out and a similar device put in without cutting or puncturing the skin or mucous membrane, the procedure is coded to the root operation CHANGE. Otherwise, the procedure for taking out the device is coded to the root operation REMOVAL.

Body Part Character 4	Approach Character 5	Device Character 6	Qualifier Character 7
Ø Lumbar Vertebral Joint Lumbar facet joint 3 Lumbosacral Joint Lumbosacral facet joint	Ø Open 3 Percutaneous 4 Percutaneous Endoscopic	Ø Drainage Device 3 Infusion Device 4 Internal Fixation Device 7 Autologous Tissue Substitute 8 Spacer A Interbody Fusion Device J Synthetic Substitute K Nonautologous Tissue Substitute	Z No Qualifier
Ø Lumbar Vertebral Joint Lumbar facet joint 3 Lumbosacral Joint Lumbosacral facet joint	X External	Ø Drainage Device 3 Infusion Device 4 Internal Fixation Device	Z No Qualifier
2 Lumbar Vertebral Disc 4 Lumbosacral Disc	Ø Open 3 Percutaneous 4 Percutaneous Endoscopic	Ø Drainage Device 3 Infusion Device 7 Autologous Tissue Substitute J Synthetic Substitute K Nonautologous Tissue Substitute	Z No Qualifier
2 Lumbar Vertebral Disc 4 Lumbosacral Disc	X External	Ø Drainage Device 3 Infusion Device	Z No Qualifier
5 Sacrococcygeal Joint Sacrococcygeal symphysis 6 Coccygeal Joint 7 Sacroiliac Joint, Right 8 Sacroiliac Joint, Left	Ø Open 3 Percutaneous 4 Percutaneous Endoscopic	Ø Drainage Device 3 Infusion Device 4 Internal Fixation Device 7 Autologous Tissue Substitute 8 Spacer J Synthetic Substitute K Nonautologous Tissue Substitute	Z No Qualifier
5 Sacrococcygeal Joint Sacrococcygeal symphysis 6 Coccygeal Joint 7 Sacroiliac Joint, Right 8 Sacroiliac Joint, Left	X External	Ø Drainage Device 3 Infusion Device 4 Internal Fixation Device	Z No Qualifier
9 Hip Joint, Right ⊞ Acetabulofemoral joint B Hip Joint, Left ⊞ *See 9 Hip Joint, Right*	Ø Open	Ø Drainage Device 3 Infusion Device 4 Internal Fixation Device 5 External Fixation Device 7 Autologous Tissue Substitute 8 Spacer 9 Liner B Resurfacing Device E Articulating Spacer J Synthetic Substitute K Nonautologous Tissue Substitute	Z No Qualifier
9 Hip Joint, Right ⊞ Acetabulofemoral joint B Hip Joint, Left ⊞ *See 9 Hip Joint, Right*	3 Percutaneous 4 Percutaneous Endoscopic	Ø Drainage Device 3 Infusion Device 4 Internal Fixation Device 5 External Fixation Device 7 Autologous Tissue Substitute 8 Spacer J Synthetic Substitute K Nonautologous Tissue Substitute	Z No Qualifier
9 Hip Joint, Right Acetabulofemoral joint B Hip Joint, Left *See 9 Hip Joint, Right*	X External	Ø Drainage Device 3 Infusion Device 4 Internal Fixation Device 5 External Fixation Device	Z No Qualifier

Non-OR ØSP[Ø,3][Ø,3,4]8Z
Non-OR ØSP[Ø,3]3[Ø,3]Z
Non-OR ØSP[Ø,3]X[Ø,3,4]Z
Non-OR ØSP[2,4]3[Ø,3]Z
Non-OR ØSP[2,4]X[Ø,3]Z
Non-OR ØSP[5,6,7,8][Ø,3,4]8Z
Non-OR ØSP[5,6,7,8]3[Ø,3]Z
Non-OR ØSP[5,6,7,8]X[Ø,3,4]Z
Non-OR ØSP[9,B]3[Ø,3,8]Z
Non-OR ØSP[9,B]X[Ø,3,4,5]Z

See Appendix L for Procedure Combinations
Combo-only ØSP[9,B]48Z
⊞ ØSP[9,B]Ø[8,9,B,E,J]Z
⊞ ØSP[9,B]4JZ

ØSP Continued on next page

Ø Medical and Surgical
S Lower Joints
P Removal Definition: Taking out or off a device from a body part

Explanation: If a device is taken out and a similar device put in without cutting or puncturing the skin or mucous membrane, the procedure is coded to the root operation CHANGE. Otherwise, the procedure for taking out the device is coded to the root operation REMOVAL.

ØSP Continued

Body Part Character 4	Approach Character 5	Device Character 6	Qualifier Character 7
A Hip Joint, Acetabular Surface, Right ⊞ **E** Hip Joint, Acetabular Surface, Left ⊞ **R** Hip Joint, Femoral Surface, Right ⊞ **S** Hip Joint, Femoral Surface, Left ⊞ **T** Knee Joint, Femoral Surface, Right ⊞ Femoropatellar joint Patellofemoral joint **U** Knee Joint, Femoral Surface, Left ⊞ *See T Knee Joint, Femoral Surface, Right* **V** Knee Joint, Tibial Surface, Right ⊞ Femorotibial joint Tibiofemoral joint **W** Knee Joint, Tibial Surface, Left ⊞ *See V Knee Joint, Tibial Surface, Right*	**Ø** Open **3** Percutaneous **4** Percutaneous Endoscopic	**J** Synthetic Substitute	**Z** No Qualifier
C Knee Joint, Right ⊞ Femoropatellar joint Femorotibial joint Lateral meniscus Medial meniscus Patellofemoral joint Tibiofemoral joint **D** Knee Joint, Left ⊞ *See C Knee Joint, Right*	**Ø** Open	**Ø** Drainage Device **3** Infusion Device **4** Internal Fixation Device **5** External Fixation Device **7** Autologous Tissue Substitute **8** Spacer **9** Liner **E** Articulating Spacer **K** Nonautologous Tissue Substitute **L** Synthetic Substitute, Unicondylar Medial **M** Synthetic Substitute, Unicondylar Lateral **N** Synthetic Substitute, Patellofemoral	**Z** No Qualifier
C Knee Joint, Right ⊞ Femoropatellar joint Femorotibial joint Lateral meniscus Medial meniscus Patellofemoral joint Tibiofemoral joint **D** Knee Joint, Left ⊞ *See C Knee Joint, Right*	**Ø** Open	**J** Synthetic Substitute	**C** Patellar Surface **Z** No Qualifier
C Knee Joint, Right ⊞ Femoropatellar joint Femorotibial joint Lateral meniscus Medial meniscus Patellofemoral joint Tibiofemoral joint **D** Knee Joint, Left ⊞ *See C Knee Joint, Right*	**3** Percutaneous **4** Percutaneous Endoscopic	**Ø** Drainage Device **3** Infusion Device **4** Internal Fixation Device **5** External Fixation Device **7** Autologous Tissue Substitute **8** Spacer **K** Nonautologous Tissue Substitute **L** Synthetic Substitute, Unicondylar Medial **M** Synthetic Substitute, Unicondylar Lateral **N** Synthetic Substitute, Patellofemoral	**Z** No Qualifier
C Knee Joint, Right ⊞ Femoropatellar joint Femorotibial joint Lateral meniscus Medial meniscus Patellofemoral joint Tibiofemoral joint **D** Knee Joint, Left ⊞ *See C Knee Joint, Right*	**3** Percutaneous **4** Percutaneous Endoscopic	**J** Synthetic Substitute	**C** Patellar Surface **Z** No Qualifier

Non-OR ØSP[C,D]3[Ø,3]Z

See Appendix L for Procedure Combinations

Combo-only ØSP[C,D][3,4]8Z
⊞ ØSP[A,E,R,S,T,U,V,W][Ø,4]JZ
⊞ ØSP[C,D]Ø[8,9,E,L,M,N]Z
⊞ ØSP[C,D]Ø[C,Z]
⊞ ØSP[C,D]4[L,M,N]Z
⊞ ØSP[C,D]4J[C,Z]

ØSP Continued on next page

Ø Medical and Surgical
S Lower Joints
P Removal

ØSP Continued

Definition: Taking out or off a device from a body part

Explanation: If a device is taken out and a similar device put in without cutting or puncturing the skin or mucous membrane, the procedure is coded to the root operation CHANGE. Otherwise, the procedure for taking out the device is coded to the root operation REMOVAL.

Body Part Character 4	Approach Character 5	Device Character 6	Qualifier Character 7
C Knee Joint, Right Femoropatellar joint Femorotibial joint Lateral meniscus Medial meniscus Patellofemoral joint Tibiofemoral joint **D Knee Joint, Left** *See C Knee Joint, Right*	**X External**	**Ø Drainage Device** **3 Infusion Device** **4 Internal Fixation Device** **5 External Fixation Device**	**Z No Qualifier**
F Ankle Joint, Right Inferior tibiofibular joint Talocrural joint **G Ankle Joint, Left** *See F Ankle Joint, Right* **H Tarsal Joint, Right** Calcaneocuboid joint Cuboideonavicular joint Cuneonavicular joint Intercuneiform joint Subtalar (talocalcaneal) joint Talocalcaneal (subtalar) joint Talocalcaneonavicular joint **J Tarsal Joint, Left** *See H Tarsal Joint, Right* **K Tarsometatarsal Joint, Right** **L Tarsometatarsal Joint, Left** **M Metatarsal-Phalangeal Joint, Right** Metatarsophalangeal (MTP) joint **N Metatarsal-Phalangeal Joint, Left** *See M Metatarsal-Phalangeal Joint, Right* **P Toe Phalangeal Joint, Right** Interphalangeal (IP) joint **Q Toe Phalangeal Joint, Left** *See P Toe Phalangeal Joint, Right*	**Ø Open** **3 Percutaneous** **4 Percutaneous Endoscopic**	**Ø Drainage Device** **3 Infusion Device** **4 Internal Fixation Device** **5 External Fixation Device** **7 Autologous Tissue Substitute** **8 Spacer** **J Synthetic Substitute** **K Nonautologous Tissue Substitute**	**Z No Qualifier**
F Ankle Joint, Right Inferior tibiofibular joint Talocrural joint **G Ankle Joint, Left** *See F Ankle Joint, Right* **H Tarsal Joint, Right** Calcaneocuboid joint Cuboideonavicular joint Cuneonavicular joint Intercuneiform joint Subtalar (talocalcaneal) joint Talocalcaneal (subtalar) joint Talocalcaneonavicular joint **J Tarsal Joint, Left** *See H Tarsal Joint, Right* **K Tarsometatarsal Joint, Right** **L Tarsometatarsal Joint, Left** **M Metatarsal-Phalangeal Joint, Right** Metatarsophalangeal (MTP) joint **N Metatarsal-Phalangeal Joint, Left** *See M Metatarsal-Phalangeal Joint, Right* **P Toe Phalangeal Joint, Right** Interphalangeal (IP) joint **Q Toe Phalangeal Joint, Left** *See P Toe Phalangeal Joint, Right*	**X External**	**Ø Drainage Device** **3 Infusion Device** **4 Internal Fixation Device** **5 External Fixation Device**	**Z No Qualifier**

Non-OR ØSP[C,D]X[Ø,3,4,5]Z
Non-OR ØSP[F,G,H,J,K,L,M,N,P,Q]3[Ø,3,8]Z
Non-OR ØSP[F,G,H,J,K,L,M,N,P,Q][Ø,4]8Z
Non-OR ØSP[F,G,H,J,K,L,M,N,P,Q]X[Ø,3,4,5]Z

Ø Medical and Surgical
S Lower Joints
Q Repair Definition: Restoring, to the extent possible, a body part to its normal anatomic structure and function
Explanation: Used only when the method to accomplish the repair is not one of the other root operations

Body Part Character 4	Approach Character 5	Device Character 6	Qualifier Character 7
Ø Lumbar Vertebral Joint Lumbar facet joint **2 Lumbar Vertebral Disc** **3 Lumbosacral Joint** Lumbosacral facet joint **4 Lumbosacral Disc** **5 Sacrococcygeal Joint** Sacrococcygeal symphysis **6 Coccygeal Joint** **7 Sacroiliac Joint, Right** **8 Sacroiliac Joint, Left** **9 Hip Joint, Right** Acetabulofemoral joint **B Hip Joint, Left** *See 9 Hip Joint, Right* **C Knee Joint, Right** Femoropatellar joint Femorotibial joint Lateral meniscus Medial meniscus Patellofemoral joint Tibiofemoral joint **D Knee Joint, Left** *See C Knee Joint, Right* **F Ankle Joint, Right** Inferior tibiofibular joint Talocrural joint **G Ankle Joint, Left** *See F Ankle Joint, Right* **H Tarsal Joint, Right** Calcaneocuboid joint Cuboideonavicular joint Cuneonavicular joint Intercuneiform joint Subtalar (talocalcaneal) joint Talocalcaneal (subtalar) joint Talocalcaneonavicular joint **J Tarsal Joint, Left** *See H Tarsal Joint, Right* **K Tarsometatarsal Joint, Right** **L Tarsometatarsal Joint, Left** **M Metatarsal-Phalangeal Joint, Right** Metatarsophalangeal (MTP) joint **N Metatarsal-Phalangeal Joint, Left** *See M Metatarsal-Phalangeal Joint, Right* **P Toe Phalangeal Joint, Right** Interphalangeal (IP) joint **Q Toe Phalangeal Joint, Left** *See P Toe Phalangeal Joint, Right*	**Ø Open** **3 Percutaneous** **4 Percutaneous Endoscopic** **X External**	**Z No Device**	**Z No Qualifier**

Non-OR ØSQ[Ø,2,3,4,5,6,7,8,9,B,C,D,F,G,H,J,K,L,M,N,P,Q]XZZ

Ø Medical and Surgical
S Lower Joints
R Replacement Definition: Putting in or on biological or synthetic material that physically takes the place and/or function of all or a portion of a body part

Explanation: The body part may have been taken out or replaced, or may be taken out, physically eradicated, or rendered nonfunctional during the REPLACEMENT procedure. A REMOVAL procedure is coded for taking out the device used in a previous replacement procedure.

Body Part Character 4	Approach Character 5	Device Character 6	Qualifier Character 7
Ø Lumbar Vertebral Joint Lumbar facet joint **2 Lumbar Vertebral Disc** NC **3 Lumbosacral Joint** Lumbosacral facet joint **4 Lumbosacral Disc** NC **5 Sacrococcygeal Joint** Sacrococcygeal symphysis **6 Coccygeal Joint** **7 Sacroiliac Joint, Right** **8 Sacroiliac Joint, Left** **H Tarsal Joint, Right** Calcaneocuboid joint Cuboideonavicular joint Cuneonavicular joint Intercuneiform joint Subtalar (talocalcaneal) joint Talocalcaneal (subtalar) joint Talocalcaneonavicular joint **J Tarsal Joint, Left** *See H Tarsal Joint, Right* **K Tarsometatarsal Joint, Right** **L Tarsometatarsal Joint, Left** **M Metatarsal-Phalangeal Joint, Right** Metatarsophalangeal (MTP) joint **N Metatarsal-Phalangeal Joint, Left** *See M Metatarsal-Phalangeal Joint, Right* **P Toe Phalangeal Joint, Right** Interphalangeal (IP) joint **Q Toe Phalangeal Joint, Left** *See P Toe Phalangeal Joint, Right*	**Ø Open**	**7 Autologous Tissue Substitute** **J Synthetic Substitute** **K Nonautologous Tissue Substitute**	**Z No Qualifier**
9 Hip Joint, Right ⊞ Acetabulofemoral joint **B Hip Joint, Left** ⊞ *See 9 Hip Joint, Right*	**Ø Open**	**1 Synthetic Substitute, Metal** **2 Synthetic Substitute, Metal on Polyethylene** **3 Synthetic Substitute, Ceramic** **4 Synthetic Substitute, Ceramic on Polyethylene** **6 Synthetic Substitute, Oxidized Zirconium on Polyethylene** **J Synthetic Substitute**	**9 Cemented** **A Uncemented** **Z No Qualifier**
9 Hip Joint, Right ⊞ Acetabulofemoral joint **B Hip Joint, Left** ⊞ *See 9 Hip Joint, Right*	**Ø Open**	**7 Autologous Tissue Substitute** **E Articulating Spacer** **K Nonautologous Tissue Substitute**	**Z No Qualifier**
A Hip Joint, Acetabular Surface, Right ⊞ **E Hip Joint, Acetabular Surface, Left** ⊞	**Ø Open**	**Ø Synthetic Substitute, Polyethylene** **1 Synthetic Substitute, Metal** **3 Synthetic Substitute, Ceramic** **J Synthetic Substitute**	**9 Cemented** **A Uncemented** **Z No Qualifier**
A Hip Joint, Acetabular Surface, Right **E Hip Joint, Acetabular Surface, Left**	**Ø Open**	**7 Autologous Tissue Substitute** **K Nonautologous Tissue Substitute**	**Z No Qualifier**

HAC ØSR[9,B]Ø[1,2,3,4,6,J][9,A,Z] when reported with SDx of I26.Ø2-I26.Ø9, I26.92-I26.99, or I82.4Ø1-I82.4Z9

HAC ØSR[9,B]Ø[7,E,K]Z when reported with SDx of I26.Ø2-I26.Ø9, I26.92-I26.99, or I82.4Ø1-I82.4Z9

HAC ØSR[A,E]Ø[Ø,1,3,J][9,A,Z] when reported with SDx of I26.Ø2-I26.Ø9, I26.92-I26.99, or I82.4Ø1-I82.4Z9

HAC ØSR[A,E]Ø[7,K]Z when reported with SDx of I26.Ø2-I26.Ø9, I26.92-I26.99, or I82.4Ø1-I82.4Z9

NC ØSR[2,4]ØJZ when beneficiary age is over 6Ø

See Appendix L for Procedure Combinations

⊞ ØSR[9,B]Ø[1,2,3,4,6,J][9,A,Z]
⊞ ØSR[9,B]ØEZ
⊞ ØSR[A,E]Ø[Ø,1,3,J][9,A,Z]

ØSR Continued on next page

Ø Medical and Surgical
S Lower Joints
R Replacement Definition: Putting in or on biological or synthetic material that physically takes the place and/or function of all or a portion of a body part

Explanation: The body part may have been taken out or replaced, or may be taken out, physically eradicated, or rendered nonfunctional during the REPLACEMENT procedure. A REMOVAL procedure is coded for taking out the device used in a previous replacement procedure.

ØSR Continued

Body Part Character 4	Approach Character 5	Device Character 6	Qualifier Character 7
C Knee Joint, Right ⊞ Femoropatellar joint Femorotibial joint Lateral meniscus Medial meniscus Patellofemoral joint Tibiofemoral joint D Knee Joint, Left ⊞ *See C Knee Joint, Right*	Ø Open	6 Synthetic Substitute, Oxidized Zirconium on Polyethylene J Synthetic Substitute L Synthetic Substitute, Unicondylar Medial M Synthetic Substitute, Unicondylar Lateral N Synthetic Substitute, Patellofemoral	9 Cemented A Uncemented Z No Qualifier
C Knee Joint, Right ⊞ Femoropatellar joint Femorotibial joint Lateral meniscus Medial meniscus Patellofemoral joint Tibiofemoral joint D Knee Joint, Left ⊞ *See C Knee Joint, Right*	Ø Open	7 Autologous Tissue Substitute E Articulating Spacer K Nonautologous Tissue Substitute	Z No Qualifier
F Ankle Joint, Right Inferior tibiofibular joint Talocrural joint G Ankle Joint, Left *See F Ankle Joint, Right* T Knee Joint, Femoral Surface, Right Femoropatellar joint Patellofemoral joint U Knee Joint, Femoral Surface, Left *See T Knee Joint, Femoral Surface, Right* V Knee Joint, Tibial Surface, Right Femorotibial joint Tibiofemoral joint W Knee Joint, Tibial Surface, Left *See V Knee Joint, Tibial Surface, Right*	Ø Open	7 Autologous Tissue Substitute K Nonautologous Tissue Substitute	Z No Qualifier
F Ankle Joint, Right Inferior tibiofibular joint Talocrural joint G Ankle Joint, Left *See F Ankle Joint, Right* T Knee Joint, Femoral Surface, Right ⊞ Femoropatellar joint Patellofemoral joint U Knee Joint, Femoral Surface, Left ⊞ *See T Knee Joint, Femoral Surface, Right* V Knee Joint, Tibial Surface, Right ⊞ Femorotibial joint Tibiofemoral joint W Knee Joint, Tibial Surface, Left ⊞ *See V Knee Joint, Tibial Surface, Right*	Ø Open	J Synthetic Substitute	9 Cemented A Uncemented Z No Qualifier
R Hip Joint, Femoral Surface, Right ⊞ S Hip Joint, Femoral Surface, Left ⊞	Ø Open	1 Synthetic Substitute, Metal 3 Synthetic Substitute, Ceramic J Synthetic Substitute	9 Cemented A Uncemented Z No Qualifier
R Hip Joint, Femoral Surface, Right S Hip Joint, Femoral Surface, Left	Ø Open	7 Autologous Tissue Substitute K Nonautologous Tissue Substitute	Z No Qualifier

HAC ØSR[C,D]Ø[6,J,L,M,N][9,A,Z] when reported with SDx of I26.Ø2-I26.Ø9, I26.92-I26.99 or I82.4Ø1-I82.4Z9

HAC ØSR[C,D]Ø[7,E,K]Z when reported with SDx of I26.Ø2-I26.Ø9, I26.92-I26.99 or I82.4Ø1-I82.4Z9

HAC ØSR[T,U,V,W]Ø[7,K]Z when reported with SDx of I26.Ø2-I26.Ø9, I26.92-I26.99 or I82.4Ø1-I82.4Z9

HAC ØSR[T,U,V,W]ØJ[9,A,Z] when reported with SDx of I26.Ø2-I26.Ø9, I26.92-I26.99 or I82.4Ø1-I82.4Z9

HAC ØSR[R,S]Ø[1,3,J][9,A,Z] when reported with SDx of I26.Ø2-I26.Ø9, I26.92-I26.99, or I82.4Ø1-I82.4Z9

HAC ØSR[R,S]Ø[7,K]Z when reported with SDx of I26.Ø2-I26.Ø9, I26.92-I26.99, or I82.4Ø1-I82.4Z9

See Appendix L for Procedure Combinations

⊞ ØSR[C,D]Ø[6,J,L,M,N][9,A,Z]
⊞ ØSR[C,D]ØEZ
⊞ ØSR[T,U,V,W]ØJ[9,A,Z]
⊞ ØSR[R,S]Ø[1,3,J][9,A,Z]

Ø Medical and Surgical
S Lower Joints
S Reposition Definition: Moving to its normal location, or other suitable location, all or a portion of a body part

Explanation: The body part is moved to a new location from an abnormal location, or from a normal location where it is not functioning correctly. The body part may or may not be cut out or off to be moved to the new location.

Body Part Character 4		Approach Character 5	Device Character 6	Qualifier Character 7
Ø Lumbar Vertebral Joint Lumbar facet joint 3 Lumbosacral Joint Lumbosacral facet joint 5 Sacrococcygeal Joint Sacrococcygeal symphysis 6 Coccygeal Joint 7 Sacroiliac Joint, Right 8 Sacroiliac Joint, Left		Ø Open 3 Percutaneous 4 Percutaneous Endoscopic X External	4 Internal Fixation Device Z No Device	Z No Qualifier
9 Hip Joint, Right Acetabulofemoral joint B Hip Joint, Left *See 9 Hip Joint, Right* C Knee Joint, Right Femoropatellar joint Femorotibial joint Lateral meniscus Medial meniscus Patellofemoral joint Tibiofemoral joint D Knee Joint, Left *See C Knee Joint, Right* F Ankle Joint, Right Inferior tibiofibular joint Talocrural joint G Ankle Joint, Left *See F Ankle Joint, Right* H Tarsal Joint, Right Calcaneocuboid joint Cuboideonavicular joint Cuneonavicular joint Intercuneiform joint Subtalar (talocalcaneal) joint Talocalcaneal (subtalar) joint Talocalcaneonavicular joint	J Tarsal Joint, Left *See H Tarsal Joint, Right* K Tarsometatarsal Joint, Right L Tarsometatarsal Joint, Left M Metatarsal-Phalangeal Joint, Right Metatarsophalangeal (MTP) joint N Metatarsal-Phalangeal Joint, Left *See M Metatarsal-Phalangeal Joint, Right* P Toe Phalangeal Joint, Right Interphalangeal (IP) joint Q Toe Phalangeal Joint, Left *See P Toe Phalangeal Joint, Right*	Ø Open 3 Percutaneous 4 Percutaneous Endoscopic X External	4 Internal Fixation Device 5 External Fixation Device Z No Device	Z No Qualifier

Non-OR ØSS[Ø,3,5,6,7,8][3,4,X][4,Z]Z
Non-OR ØSS[9,B,C,D,F,G,H,J,K,L,M,N,P,Q][3,4,X][4,5,Z]Z

Ø Medical and Surgical
S Lower Joints
T Resection Definition: Cutting out or off, without replacement, all of a body part

Explanation: None

Body Part Character 4		Approach Character 5	Device Character 6	Qualifier Character 7
2 Lumbar Vertebral Disc 4 Lumbosacral Disc 5 Sacrococcygeal Joint Sacrococcygeal symphysis 6 Coccygeal Joint 7 Sacroiliac Joint, Right 8 Sacroiliac Joint, Left 9 Hip Joint, Right Acetabulofemoral joint B Hip Joint, Left *See 9 Hip Joint, Right* C Knee Joint, Right Femoropatellar joint Femorotibial joint Lateral meniscus Medial meniscus Patellofemoral joint Tibiofemoral joint D Knee Joint, Left *See C Knee Joint, Right* F Ankle Joint, Right Inferior tibiofibular joint Talocrural joint G Ankle Joint, Left *See F Ankle Joint, Right*	H Tarsal Joint, Right Calcaneocuboid joint Cuboideonavicular joint Cuneonavicular joint Intercuneiform joint Subtalar (talocalcaneal) joint Talocalcaneal (subtalar) joint Talocalcaneonavicular joint J Tarsal Joint, Left *See H Tarsal Joint, Right* K Tarsometatarsal Joint, Right L Tarsometatarsal Joint, Left M Metatarsal-Phalangeal Joint, Right Metatarsophalangeal (MTP) joint N Metatarsal-Phalangeal Joint, Left *See M Metatarsal-Phalangeal Joint, Right* P Toe Phalangeal Joint, Right Interphalangeal (IP) joint Q Toe Phalangeal Joint, Left *See P Toe Phalangeal Joint, Right*	Ø Open	Z No Device	Z No Qualifier

Ø Medical and Surgical
S Lower Joints
U Supplement Definition: Putting in or on biological or synthetic material that physically reinforces and/or augments the function of a portion of a body part

Explanation: The biological material is non-living, or is living and from the same individual. The body part may have been previously replaced, and the SUPPLEMENT procedure is performed to physically reinforce and/or augment the function of the replaced body part.

Body Part Character 4	Approach Character 5	Device Character 6	Qualifier Character 7
Ø Lumbar Vertebral Joint Lumbar facet joint **2 Lumbar Vertebral Disc** **3 Lumbosacral Joint** Lumbosacral facet joint **4 Lumbosacral Disc** **5 Sacrococcygeal Joint** Sacrococcygeal symphysis **6 Coccygeal Joint** **7 Sacroiliac Joint, Right** **8 Sacroiliac Joint, Left** **F Ankle Joint, Right** Inferior tibiofibular joint, Talocrural joint **G Ankle Joint, Left** *See F Ankle Joint, Right* **H Tarsal Joint, Right** Calcaneocuboid joint, Cuboideonavicular joint, Cuneonavicular joint, Intercuneiform joint, Subtalar (talocalcaneal) joint, Talocalcaneal (subtalar) joint, Talocalcaneonavicular joint **J Tarsal Joint, Left** *See H Tarsal Joint, Right* **K Tarsometatarsal Joint, Right** **L Tarsometatarsal Joint, Left** **M Metatarsal-Phalangeal Joint, Right** Metatarsophalangeal (MTP) joint **N Metatarsal-Phalangeal Joint, Left** *See M Metatarsal-Phalangeal Joint, Right* **P Toe Phalangeal Joint, Right** Interphalangeal (IP) joint **Q Toe Phalangeal Joint, Left** *See P Toe Phalangeal Joint, Right*	**Ø Open** **3 Percutaneous** **4 Percutaneous Endoscopic**	**7 Autologous Tissue Substitute** **J Synthetic Substitute** **K Nonautologous Tissue Substitute**	**Z No Qualifier**
9 Hip Joint, Right ⊞ Acetabulofemoral joint **B Hip Joint, Left** ⊞ *See 9 Hip Joint, Right*	**Ø Open**	**7 Autologous Tissue Substitute** **9 Liner** **B Resurfacing Device** **J Synthetic Substitute** **K Nonautologous Tissue Substitute**	**Z No Qualifier**
9 Hip Joint, Right Acetabulofemoral joint **B Hip Joint, Left** *See 9 Hip Joint, Right*	**3 Percutaneous** **4 Percutaneous Endoscopic**	**7 Autologous Tissue Substitute** **J Synthetic Substitute** **K Nonautologous Tissue Substitute**	**Z No Qualifier**
A Hip Joint, Acetabular Surface, Right ⊞ **E Hip Joint, Acetabular Surface, Left** ⊞ **R Hip Joint, Femoral Surface, Right** ⊞ **S Hip Joint, Femoral Surface, Left** ⊞	**Ø Open**	**9 Liner** **B Resurfacing Device**	**Z No Qualifier**
C Knee Joint, Right Femoropatellar joint, Femorotibial joint, Lateral meniscus, Medial meniscus, Patellofemoral joint, Tibiofemoral joint **D Knee Joint, Left** *See C Knee Joint, Right*	**Ø Open**	**7 Autologous Tissue Substitute** **J Synthetic Substitute** **K Nonautologous Tissue Substitute**	**Z No Qualifier**
C Knee Joint, Right Femoropatellar joint, Femorotibial joint, Lateral meniscus, Medial meniscus, Patellofemoral joint, Tibiofemoral joint **D Knee Joint, Left** *See C Knee Joint, Right*	**Ø Open**	**9 Liner**	**C Patellar Surface** **Z No Qualifier**

HAC ØSU[9,B]ØBZ when reported with SDx of I26.Ø2-I26.Ø9, I26.92-I26.99, or I82.4Ø1-I82.4Z9

HAC ØSU[A,E,R,S]ØBZ when reported with SDx of I26.Ø2-I26.Ø9, I26.92-I26.99, or I82.4Ø1-I82.4Z9

See Appendix L for Procedure Combinations
⊞ ØSU[9,B]Ø9Z
⊞ ØSU[A,E,R,S]Ø9Z

ØSU Continued on next page

ØSU Continued

Ø Medical and Surgical
S Lower Joints
U Supplement

Definition: Putting in or on biological or synthetic material that physically reinforces and/or augments the function of a portion of a body part

Explanation: The biological material is non-living, or is living and from the same individual. The body part may have been previously replaced, and the SUPPLEMENT procedure is performed to physically reinforce and/or augment the function of the replaced body part.

Body Part Character 4	Approach Character 5	Device Character 6	Qualifier Character 7
C Knee Joint, Right Femoropatellar joint Femorotibial joint Lateral meniscus Medial meniscus Patellofemoral joint Tibiofemoral joint **D Knee Joint, Left** *See C Knee Joint, Right*	**3 Percutaneous** **4 Percutaneous Endoscopic**	**7 Autologous Tissue Substitute** **J Synthetic Substitute** **K Nonautologous Tissue Substitute**	**Z No Qualifier**
T Knee Joint, Femoral Surface, Right Femoropatellar joint Patellofemoral joint **U Knee Joint, Femoral Surface, Left** *See T Knee Joint, Femoral Surface, Right* **V Knee Joint, Tibial Surface, Right** ⊞ Femorotibial joint Tibiofemoral joint **W Knee Joint, Tibial Surface, Left** ⊞ *See V Knee Joint, Tibial Surface, Right*	**Ø Open**	**9 Liner**	**Z No Qualifier**

See Appendix L for Procedure Combinations

⊞ ØSU[V,W]Ø9Z

Ø Medical and Surgical
S Lower Joints
W Revision Definition: Correcting, to the extent possible, a portion of a malfunctioning device or the position of a displaced device

Explanation: Revision can include correcting a malfunctioning or displaced device by taking out or putting in components of the device such as a screw or pin

Body Part Character 4	Approach Character 5	Device Character 6	Qualifier Character 7
Ø Lumbar Vertebral Joint Lumbar facet joint **3 Lumbosacral Joint** Lumbosacral facet joint	Ø Open 3 Percutaneous 4 Percutaneous Endoscopic X External	Ø Drainage Device 3 Infusion Device 4 Internal Fixation Device 7 Autologous Tissue Substitute 8 Spacer A Interbody Fusion Device J Synthetic Substitute K Nonautologous Tissue Substitute	Z No Qualifier
2 Lumbar Vertebral Disc **4 Lumbosacral Disc**	Ø Open 3 Percutaneous 4 Percutaneous Endoscopic X External	Ø Drainage Device 3 Infusion Device 7 Autologous Tissue Substitute J Synthetic Substitute K Nonautologous Tissue Substitute	Z No Qualifier
5 Sacrococcygeal Joint Sacrococcygeal symphysis **6 Coccygeal Joint** **7 Sacroiliac Joint, Right** **8 Sacroiliac Joint, Left**	Ø Open 3 Percutaneous 4 Percutaneous Endoscopic X External	Ø Drainage Device 3 Infusion Device 4 Internal Fixation Device 7 Autologous Tissue Substitute 8 Spacer J Synthetic Substitute K Nonautologous Tissue Substitute	Z No Qualifier
9 Hip Joint, Right Acetabulofemoral joint **B Hip Joint, Left** *See 9 Hip Joint, Right*	Ø Open	Ø Drainage Device 3 Infusion Device 4 Internal Fixation Device 5 External Fixation Device 7 Autologous Tissue Substitute 8 Spacer 9 Liner B Resurfacing Device J Synthetic Substitute K Nonautologous Tissue Substitute	Z No Qualifier
9 Hip Joint, Right Acetabulofemoral joint **B Hip Joint, Left** *See 9 Hip Joint, Right*	3 Percutaneous 4 Percutaneous Endoscopic X External	Ø Drainage Device 3 Infusion Device 4 Internal Fixation Device 5 External Fixation Device 7 Autologous Tissue Substitute 8 Spacer J Synthetic Substitute K Nonautologous Tissue Substitute	Z No Qualifier
A Hip Joint, Acetabular Surface, Right **E Hip Joint, Acetabular Surface, Left** **R Hip Joint, Femoral Surface, Right** **S Hip Joint, Femoral Surface, Left** **T Knee Joint, Femoral Surface, Right** Femoropatellar joint Patellofemoral joint **U Knee Joint, Femoral Surface, Left** *See T Knee Joint, Femoral Surface, Right* **V Knee Joint, Tibial Surface, Right** Femorotibial joint Tibiofemoral joint **W Knee Joint, Tibial Surface, Left** *See V Knee Joint, Tibial Surface, Right*	Ø Open 3 Percutaneous 4 Percutaneous Endoscopic X External	J Synthetic Substitute	Z No Qualifier
C Knee Joint, Right Femoropatellar joint Femorotibial joint Lateral meniscus Medial meniscus Patellofemoral joint Tibiofemoral joint **D Knee Joint, Left** *See C Knee Joint, Right*	Ø Open	Ø Drainage Device 3 Infusion Device 4 Internal Fixation Device 5 External Fixation Device 7 Autologous Tissue Substitute 8 Spacer 9 Liner K Nonautologous Tissue Substitute	Z No Qualifier

Non-OR ØSW[Ø,3]X[Ø,3,4,7,8,A,J,K]Z
Non-OR ØSW[2,4]X[Ø,3,7,J,K]Z
Non-OR ØSW[5,6,7,8]X[Ø,3,4,7,8,J,K]Z
Non-OR ØSW[9,B]X[Ø,3,4,5,7,8,J,K]Z
Non-OR ØSW[A,E,R,S,T,U,V,W]XJZ

ØSW Continued on next page

Ø Medical and Surgical
S Lower Joints
W Revision

ØSW Continued

Definition: Correcting, to the extent possible, a portion of a malfunctioning device or the position of a displaced device

Explanation: Revision can include correcting a malfunctioning or displaced device by taking out or putting in components of the device such as a screw or pin

Body Part Character 4	Approach Character 5	Device Character 6	Qualifier Character 7
C Knee Joint, Right Femoropatellar joint Femorotibial joint Lateral meniscus Medial meniscus Patellofemoral joint Tibiofemoral joint **D Knee Joint, Left** *See C Knee Joint, Right*	**Ø Open**	**J Synthetic Substitute**	**C Patellar Surface** **Z No Qualifier**
C Knee Joint, Right Femoropatellar joint Femorotibial joint Lateral meniscus Medial meniscus Patellofemoral joint Tibiofemoral joint **D Knee Joint, Left** *See C Knee Joint, Right*	**3 Percutaneous** **4 Percutaneous Endoscopic** **X External**	**Ø Drainage Device** **3 Infusion Device** **4 Internal Fixation Device** **5 External Fixation Device** **7 Autologous Tissue Substitute** **8 Spacer** **K Nonautologous Tissue Substitute**	**Z No Qualifier**
C Knee Joint, Right Femoropatellar joint Femorotibial joint Lateral meniscus Medial meniscus Patellofemoral joint Tibiofemoral joint **D Knee Joint, Left** *See C Knee Joint, Right*	**3 Percutaneous** **4 Percutaneous Endoscopic** **X External**	**J Synthetic Substitute**	**C Patellar Surface** **Z No Qualifier**
F Ankle Joint, Right Inferior tibiofibular joint Talocrural joint **G Ankle Joint, Left** *See F Ankle Joint, Right* **H Tarsal Joint, Right** Calcaneocuboid joint Cuboideonavicular joint Cuneonavicular joint Intercuneiform joint Subtalar (talocalcaneal) joint Talocalcaneal (subtalar) joint Talocalcaneonavicular joint **J Tarsal Joint, Left** *See H Tarsal Joint, Right* **K Tarsometatarsal Joint, Right** **L Tarsometatarsal Joint, Left** **M Metatarsal-Phalangeal Joint, Right** Metatarsophalangeal (MTP) joint **N Metatarsal-Phalangeal Joint, Left** *See M Metatarsal-Phalangeal Joint, Right* **P Toe Phalangeal Joint, Right** Interphalangeal (IP) joint **Q Toe Phalangeal Joint, Left** *See P Toe Phalangeal Joint, Right*	**Ø Open** **3 Percutaneous** **4 Percutaneous Endoscopic** **X External**	**Ø Drainage Device** **3 Infusion Device** **4 Internal Fixation Device** **5 External Fixation Device** **7 Autologous Tissue Substitute** **8 Spacer** **J Synthetic Substitute** **K Nonautologous Tissue Substitute**	**Z No Qualifier**

Non-OR ØSW[C,D]X[Ø,3,4,5,7,8,K]Z
Non-OR ØSW[C,D]XJ[C,Z]
Non-OR ØSW[F,G,H,J,K,L,M,N,P,Q]X[Ø,3,4,5,7,8,J,K]Z

Urinary System ØT1–ØTY

Character Meanings

This Character Meaning table is provided as a guide to assist the user in the identification of character members that may be found in this section of code tables. It **SHOULD NOT** be used to build a PCS code.

Operation–Character 3	Body Part–Character 4	Approach–Character 5	Device–Character 6	Qualifier–Character 7
1 Bypass	Ø Kidney, Right	Ø Open	Ø Drainage Device	Ø Allogeneic
2 Change	1 Kidney, Left	3 Percutaneous	1 Radioactive Element	1 Syngeneic
5 Destruction	2 Kidneys, Bilateral	4 Percutaneous Endoscopic	2 Monitoring Device	2 Zooplastic
7 Dilation	3 Kidney Pelvis, Right	7 Via Natural or Artificial Opening	3 Infusion Device	3 Kidney Pelvis, Right
8 Division	4 Kidney Pelvis, Left	8 Via Natural or Artificial Opening Endoscopic	7 Autologous Tissue Substitute	4 Kidney Pelvis, Left
9 Drainage	5 Kidney	X External	C Extraluminal Device	6 Ureter, Right
B Excision	6 Ureter, Right		D Intraluminal Device	7 Ureter, Left
C Extirpation	7 Ureter, Left		J Synthetic Substitute	8 Colon
D Extraction	8 Ureters, Bilateral		K Nonautologous Tissue Substitute	9 Colocutaneous
F Fragmentation	9 Ureter		L Artificial Sphincter	A Ileum
H Insertion	B Bladder		M Stimulator Lead	B Bladder
J Inspection	C Bladder Neck		Y Other Device	C Ileocutaneous
L Occlusion	D Urethra		Z No Device	D Cutaneous
M Reattachment				X Diagnostic
N Release				Z No Qualifier
P Removal				
Q Repair				
R Replacement				
S Reposition				
T Resection				
U Supplement				
V Restriction				
W Revision				
Y Transplantation				

AHA Coding Clinic for table ØT1
2017, 3Q, 20 Creation of Indiana pouch
2017, 3Q, 21 Augmentation cystoplasty with Indiana pouch and continent urinary diversion
2017, 1Q, 37 Perineal urethrostomy
2015, 3Q, 34 Redo urinary diversion surgery via left ureteral reimplantation

AHA Coding Clinic for table ØT7
2019, 2Q, 16 Reimplantation of ureters with insertion of tubes
2017, 4Q, 111 Exchange of ureteral stent
2016, 2Q, 27 Exchange of ureteral stents
2015, 2Q, 8 Urinary calculi fragmentation and evacuation
2013, 4Q, 123 Urolift® procedure

AHA Coding Clinic for table ØT9
2017, 3Q, 19 Ureteral stent placement for urinary leakage
2017, 3Q, 20 Creation of Indiana pouch
2017, 3Q, 21 Augmentation cystoplasty with Indiana pouch and continent urinary diversion

AHA Coding Clinic for table ØTB
2016, 1Q, 19 Biopsy of neobladder malignancy
2015, 3Q, 34 Excision of Mitrofanoff polyp
2014, 2Q, 8 Ileoscopy with excision of polyp of ileal loop urinary diversion

AHA Coding Clinic for table ØTC
2019, 3Q, 4 Evacuation of clots from bladder dome
2016, 3Q, 23 Ureteral stone migrating into bladder
2015, 2Q, 7 Urinary calculi fragmentation and evacuation
2015, 2Q, 8 Urinary calculi fragmentation and evacuation
2013, 4Q, 122 Laser lithotripsy with removal of fragments

AHA Coding Clinic for table ØTF
2015, 2Q, 7 Urinary calculi fragmentation and evacuation
2013, 4Q, 122 Extracorporeal shock wave lithotripsy
2013, 4Q, 122 Laser lithotripsy with removal of fragments

AHA Coding Clinic for table ØTH
2019, 2Q, 16 Reimplantation of ureters with insertion of tubes

AHA Coding Clinic for table ØTP
2017, 4Q, 111 Exchange of ureteral stent
2016, 2Q, 27 Exchange of ureteral stents

AHA Coding Clinic for table ØTQ
2018, 2Q, 27 Dismembered pyeloplasty
2017, 1Q, 37 Perineal urethrostomy

AHA Coding Clinic for table ØTR
2017, 3Q, 20 Creation of Indiana pouch

AHA Coding Clinic for table ØTS
2019, 1Q, 29 Young-Dees-Leadbetter bladder neck reconstruction
2018, 2Q, 27 Dismembered pyeloplasty
2017, 1Q, 36 Dismembered pyeloplasty
2016, 1Q, 15 Pubovaginal sling placement

AHA Coding Clinic for table ØTT
2014, 3Q, 16 Hand-assisted laparoscopy nephroureterectomy

AHA Coding Clinic for table ØTU
2019, 1Q, 29 Young-Dees-Leadbetter bladder neck reconstruction
2017, 3Q, 21 Augmentation cystoplasty with Indiana pouch and continent urinary diversion

AHA Coding Clinic for table ØTV
2015, 2Q, 11 Cystourethroscopic Deflux® injection

Urinary System

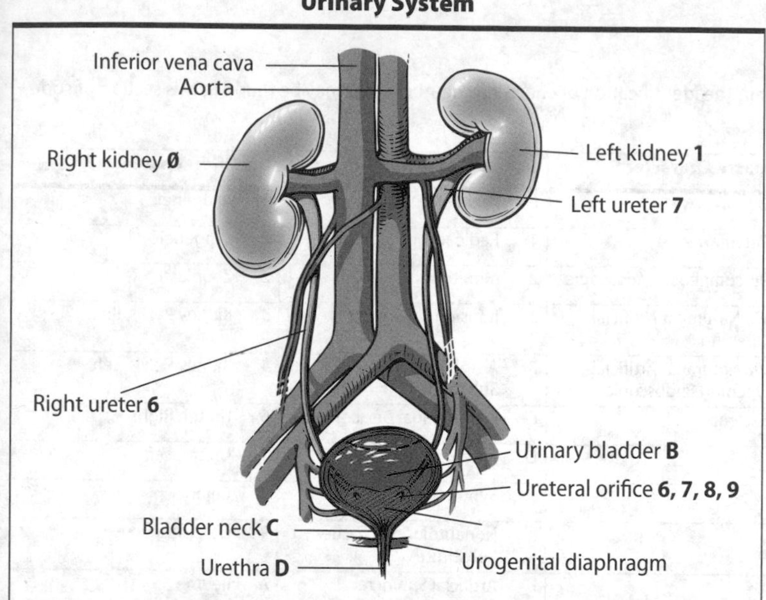

Kidney

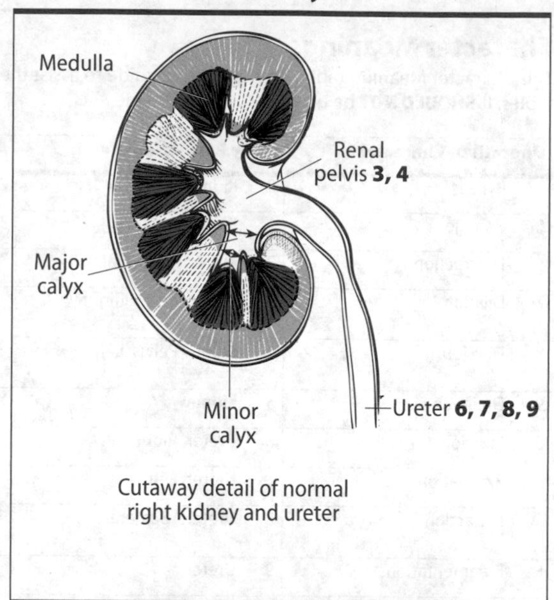

Cutaway detail of normal right kidney and ureter

Bladder

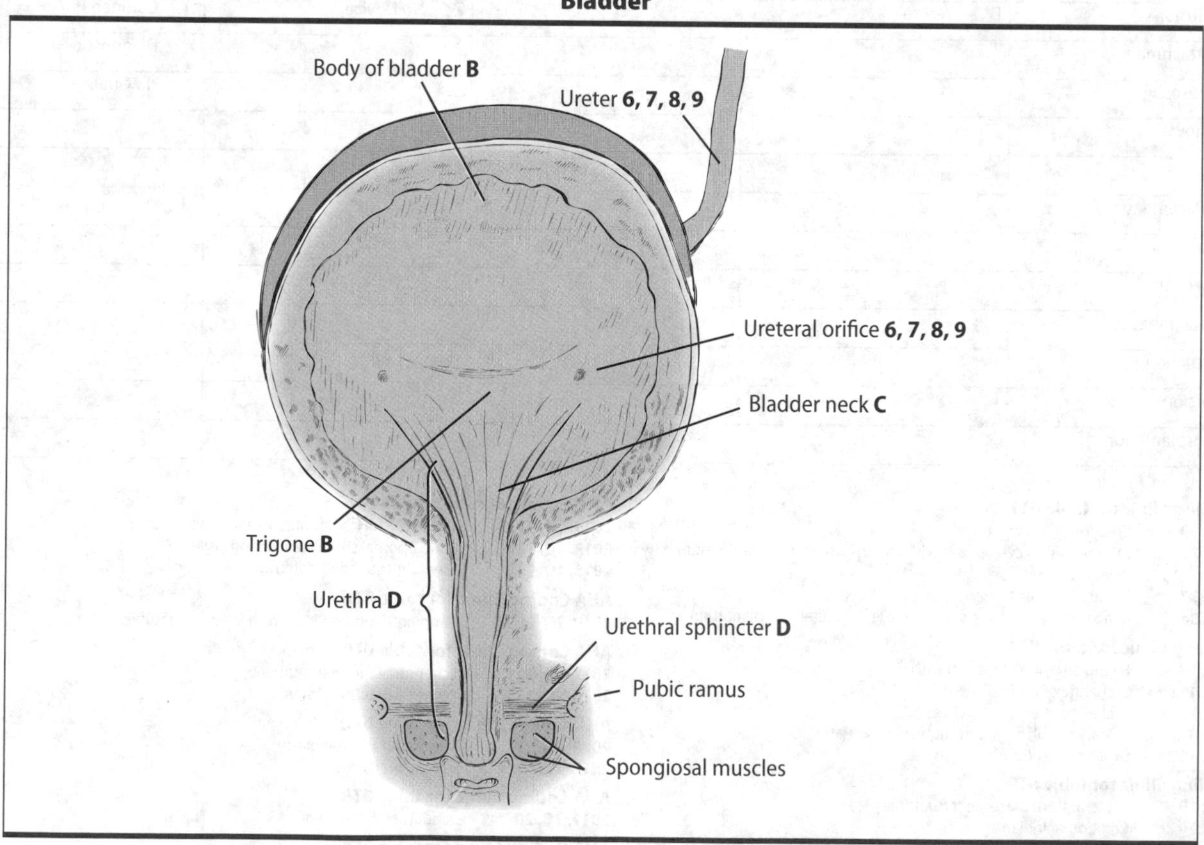

Ø Medical and Surgical
T Urinary System
1 Bypass Definition: Altering the route of passage of the contents of a tubular body part

Explanation: Rerouting contents of a body part to a downstream area of the normal route, to a similar route and body part, or to an abnormal route and dissimilar body part. Includes one or more anastomoses, with or without the use of a device.

Body Part Character 4	Approach Character 5	Device Character 6	Qualifier Character 7
3 Kidney Pelvis, Right Ureteropelvic junction (UPJ) **4 Kidney Pelvis, Left** *See 3 Kidney Pelvis, Right*	**Ø Open** **4 Percutaneous Endoscopic**	**7 Autologous Tissue Substitute** **J Synthetic Substitute** **K Nonautologous Tissue Substitute** **Z No Device**	**3 Kidney Pelvis, Right** **4 Kidney Pelvis, Left** **6 Ureter, Right** **7 Ureter, Left** **8 Colon** **9 Colocutaneous** **A Ileum** **B Bladder** **C Ileocutaneous** **D Cutaneous**
3 Kidney Pelvis, Right Ureteropelvic junction (UPJ) **4 Kidney Pelvis, Left** *See 3 Kidney Pelvis, Right*	**3 Percutaneous**	**J Synthetic Substitute**	**D Cutaneous**
6 Ureter, Right Ureteral orifice Ureterovesical orifice **7 Ureter, Left** *See 6 Ureter, Right* **8 Ureters, Bilateral** *See 6 Ureter, Right*	**Ø Open** **4 Percutaneous Endoscopic**	**7 Autologous Tissue Substitute** **J Synthetic Substitute** **K Nonautologous Tissue Substitute** **Z No Device**	**6 Ureter, Right** **7 Ureter, Left** **8 Colon** **9 Colocutaneous** **A Ileum** **B Bladder** **C Ileocutaneous** **D Cutaneous**
6 Ureter, Right Ureteral orifice Ureterovesical orifice **7 Ureter, Left** *See 6 Ureter, Right* **8 Ureters, Bilateral** *See 6 Ureter, Right*	**3 Percutaneous**	**J Synthetic Substitute**	**D Cutaneous**
B Bladder Trigone of bladder	**Ø Open** **4 Percutaneous Endoscopic**	**7 Autologous Tissue Substitute** **J Synthetic Substitute** **K Nonautologous Tissue Substitute** **Z No Device**	**9 Colocutaneous** **C Ileocutaneous** **D Cutaneous**
B Bladder Trigone of bladder	**3 Percutaneous**	**J Synthetic Substitute**	**D Cutaneous**

Ø Medical and Surgical
T Urinary System
2 Change Definition: Taking out or off a device from a body part and putting back an identical or similar device in or on the same body part without cutting or puncturing the skin or a mucous membrane

Explanation: All CHANGE procedures are coded using the approach EXTERNAL

Body Part Character 4	Approach Character 5	Device Character 6	Qualifier Character 7
5 Kidney Renal calyx Renal capsule Renal cortex Renal segment **9 Ureter** Ureteral orifice Ureterovesical orifice **B Bladder** Trigone of bladder **D Urethra** Bulbourethral (Cowper's) gland Cowper's (bulbourethral) gland External urethral sphincter Internal urethral sphincter Membranous urethra Penile urethra Prostatic urethra	**X External**	**Ø Drainage Device** **Y Other Device**	**Z No Qualifier**

Non-OR All body part, approach, device, and qualifier values

Ø Medical and Surgical
T Urinary System
5 Destruction Definition: Physical eradication of all or a portion of a body part by the direct use of energy, force, or a destructive agent
Explanation: None of the body part is physically taken out

Body Part Character 4	Approach Character 5	Device Character 6	Qualifier Character 7
Ø Kidney, Right Renal calyx Renal capsule Renal cortex Renal segment **1 Kidney, Left** *See Ø Kidney, Right* **3 Kidney Pelvis, Right** Ureteropelvic junction (UPJ) **4 Kidney Pelvis, Left** *See 3 Kidney Pelvis, Right* **6 Ureter, Right** Ureteral orifice Ureterovesical orifice **7 Ureter, Left** *See 6 Ureter, Right* **B Bladder** Trigone of bladder **C Bladder Neck**	**Ø Open** **3 Percutaneous** **4 Percutaneous Endoscopic** **7 Via Natural or Artificial Opening** **8 Via Natural or Artificial Opening Endoscopic**	**Z No Device**	**Z No Qualifier**
D Urethra Bulbourethral (Cowper's) gland Cowper's (bulbourethral) gland External urethral sphincter Internal urethral sphincter Membranous urethra Penile urethra Prostatic urethra	**Ø Open** **3 Percutaneous** **4 Percutaneous Endoscopic** **7 Via Natural or Artificial Opening** **8 Via Natural or Artificial Opening Endoscopic** **X External**	**Z No Device**	**Z No Qualifier**

Non-OR ØT5D[Ø,3,4,7,8,X]ZZ

Ø Medical and Surgical
T Urinary System
7 Dilation Definition: Expanding an orifice or the lumen of a tubular body part
Explanation: The orifice can be a natural orifice or an artificially created orifice. Accomplished by stretching a tubular body part using intraluminal pressure or by cutting part of the orifice or wall of the tubular body part.

Body Part Character 4	Approach Character 5	Device Character 6	Qualifier Character 7
3 Kidney Pelvis, Right Ureteropelvic junction (UPJ) **4 Kidney Pelvis, Left** *See 3 Kidney Pelvis, Right* **6 Ureter, Right** Ureteral orifice Ureterovesical orifice **7 Ureter, Left** *See 6 Ureter, Right* **8 Ureters, Bilateral** *See 6 Ureter, Right* **B Bladder** Trigone of bladder **C Bladder Neck** **D Urethra** Bulbourethral (Cowper's) gland Cowper's (bulbourethral) gland External urethral sphincter Internal urethral sphincter Membranous urethra Penile urethra Prostatic urethra	**Ø Open** **3 Percutaneous** **4 Percutaneous Endoscopic** **7 Via Natural or Artificial Opening** **8 Via Natural or Artificial Opening Endoscopic**	**D Intraluminal Device** **Z No Device**	**Z No Qualifier**

Non-OR ØT7[6,7,8][Ø,3,4,7]DZ
Non-OR ØT7[6,7,8]7ZZ
Non-OR ØT788ZZ
Non-OR ØT7B7[D,Z]Z
Non-OR ØT7C[Ø,3,4]ZZ
Non-OR ØT7[C,D][Ø,3,4]DZ
Non-OR ØT7[C,D][7,8][D,Z]Z

Ø Medical and Surgical
T Urinary System
8 Division Definition: Cutting into a body part, without draining fluids and/or gases from the body part, in order to separate or transect a body part
Explanation: All or a portion of the body part is separated into two or more portions

Body Part Character 4	Approach Character 5	Device Character 6	Qualifier Character 7
2 Kidneys, Bilateral Renal calyx Renal capsule Renal cortex Renal segment **C Bladder Neck**	**Ø Open** **3 Percutaneous** **4 Percutaneous Endoscopic**	**Z No Device**	**Z No Qualifier**

Ø Medical and Surgical
T Urinary System
9 Drainage Definition: Taking or letting out fluids and/or gases from a body part
Explanation: The qualifier DIAGNOSTIC is used to identify drainage procedures that are biopsies

Body Part Character 4	Approach Character 5	Device Character 6	Qualifier Character 7
Ø Kidney, Right Renal calyx Renal capsule Renal cortex Renal segment **1 Kidney, Left** *See Ø Kidney, Right* **3 Kidney Pelvis, Right** Ureteropelvic junction (UPJ) **4 Kidney Pelvis, Left** *See 3 Kidney Pelvis, Right* **6 Ureter, Right** Ureteral orifice Ureterovesical orifice **7 Ureter, Left** *See 6 Ureter, Right* **8 Ureters, Bilateral** *See 6 Ureter, Right* **B Bladder** Trigone of bladder **C Bladder Neck**	**Ø Open** **3 Percutaneous** **4 Percutaneous Endoscopic** **7 Via Natural or Artificial Opening** **8 Via Natural or Artificial Opening Endoscopic**	**Ø Drainage Device**	**Z No Qualifier**
Ø Kidney, Right Renal calyx Renal capsule Renal cortex Renal segment **1 Kidney, Left** *See Ø Kidney, Right* **3 Kidney Pelvis, Right** Ureteropelvic junction (UPJ) **4 Kidney Pelvis, Left** *See 3 Kidney Pelvis, Right* **6 Ureter, Right** Ureteral orifice Ureterovesical orifice **7 Ureter, Left** *See 6 Ureter, Right* **8 Ureters, Bilateral** *See 6 Ureter, Right* **B Bladder** Trigone of bladder **C Bladder Neck**	**Ø Open** **3 Percutaneous** **4 Percutaneous Endoscopic** **7 Via Natural or Artificial Opening** **8 Via Natural or Artificial Opening Endoscopic**	**Z No Device**	**X Diagnostic** **Z No Qualifier**
D Urethra Bulbourethral (Cowper's) gland Cowper's (bulbourethral) gland External urethral sphincter Internal urethral sphincter Membranous urethra Penile urethra Prostatic urethra	**Ø Open** **3 Percutaneous** **4 Percutaneous Endoscopic** **7 Via Natural or Artificial Opening** **8 Via Natural or Artificial Opening Endoscopic** **X External**	**Ø Drainage Device**	**Z No Qualifier**
D Urethra Bulbourethral (Cowper's) gland Cowper's (bulbourethral) gland External urethral sphincter Internal urethral sphincter Membranous urethra Penile urethra Prostatic urethra	**Ø Open** **3 Percutaneous** **4 Percutaneous Endoscopic** **7 Via Natural or Artificial Opening** **8 Via Natural or Artificial Opening Endoscopic** **X External**	**Z No Device**	**X Diagnostic** **Z No Qualifier**

Non-OR ØT9[Ø,1,3,4]3ØZ
Non-OR ØT9[6,7,8][Ø,3,4,7,8]ØZ
Non-OR ØT9[B,C][3,4,7,8]ØZ
Non-OR ØT9[Ø,1,3,4,6,7,8][3,4,7,8]ZX
Non-OR ØT9[Ø,1,3,4][3,4]ZZ
Non-OR ØT9[6,7,8]3ZZ
Non-OR ØT9[B,C][3,4,7,8]ZZ
Non-OR ØT9D3ØZ
Non-OR ØT9D[Ø,3,4,7,8,X]ZX
Non-OR ØT9D3ZZ

Ø Medical and Surgical
T Urinary System
B Excision Definition: Cutting out or off, without replacement, a portion of a body part
Explanation: The qualifier DIAGNOSTIC is used to identify excision procedures that are biopsies

Body Part Character 4	Approach Character 5	Device Character 6	Qualifier Character 7
Ø Kidney, Right Renal calyx Renal capsule Renal cortex Renal segment **1 Kidney, Left** *See Ø Kidney, Right* **3 Kidney Pelvis, Right** Ureteropelvic junction (UPJ) **4 Kidney Pelvis, Left** *See 3 Kidney Pelvis, Right* **6 Ureter, Right** Ureteral orifice Ureterovesical orifice **7 Ureter, Left** *See 6 Ureter, Right* **B Bladder** Trigone of bladder **C Bladder Neck**	**Ø Open** **3 Percutaneous** **4 Percutaneous Endoscopic** **7 Via Natural or Artificial Opening** **8 Via Natural or Artificial Opening Endoscopic**	**Z No Device**	**X Diagnostic** **Z No Qualifier**
D Urethra Bulbourethral (Cowper's) gland Cowper's (bulbourethral) gland External urethral sphincter Internal urethral sphincter Membranous urethra Penile urethra Prostatic urethra	**Ø Open** **3 Percutaneous** **4 Percutaneous Endoscopic** **7 Via Natural or Artificial Opening** **8 Via Natural or Artificial Opening Endoscopic** **X External**	**Z No Device**	**X Diagnostic** **Z No Qualifier**

Non-OR ØTB[Ø,1,3,4,6,7][3,4,7,8]ZX
Non-OR ØTBD[Ø,3,4,7,8,X]ZX

Ø Medical and Surgical
T Urinary System
C Extirpation Definition: Taking or cutting out solid matter from a body part
Explanation: The solid matter may be an abnormal byproduct of a biological function or a foreign body; it may be imbedded in a body part or in the lumen of a tubular body part. The solid matter may or may not have been previously broken into pieces.

Body Part Character 4	Approach Character 5	Device Character 6	Qualifier Character 7
Ø Kidney, Right Renal calyx Renal capsule Renal cortex Renal segment **1 Kidney, Left** *See Ø Kidney, Right* **3 Kidney Pelvis, Right** Ureteropelvic junction (UPJ) **4 Kidney Pelvis, Left** *See 3 Kidney Pelvis, Right* **6 Ureter, Right** Ureteral orifice Ureterovesical orifice **7 Ureter, Left** *See 6 Ureter, Right* **B Bladder** Trigone of bladder **C Bladder Neck**	**Ø Open** **3 Percutaneous** **4 Percutaneous Endoscopic** **7 Via Natural or Artificial Opening** **8 Via Natural or Artificial Opening Endoscopic**	**Z No Device**	**Z No Qualifier**
D Urethra Bulbourethral (Cowper's) gland Cowper's (bulbourethral) gland External urethral sphincter Internal urethral sphincter Membranous urethra Penile urethra Prostatic urethra	**Ø Open** **3 Percutaneous** **4 Percutaneous Endoscopic** **7 Via Natural or Artificial Opening** **8 Via Natural or Artificial Opening Endoscopic** **X External**	**Z No Device**	**Z No Qualifier**

Non-OR ØTC[B,C][7,8]ZZ
Non-OR ØTCD[7,8,X]ZZ

Ø Medical and Surgical
T Urinary System
D Extraction Definition: Pulling or stripping out or off all or a portion of a body part by the use of force

Explanation: The qualifier DIAGNOSTIC is used to identify extraction procedures that are biopsies

Body Part Character 4	Approach Character 5	Device Character 6	Qualifier Character 7
Ø Kidney, Right Renal calyx Renal capsule Renal cortex Renal segment **1 Kidney, Left** *See Ø Kidney, Right*	**Ø Open** **3 Percutaneous** **4 Percutaneous Endoscopic**	**Z No Device**	**Z No Qualifier**

Ø Medical and Surgical
T Urinary System
F Fragmentation Definition: Breaking solid matter in a body part into pieces

Explanation: Physical force (e.g., manual, ultrasonic) applied directly or indirectly is used to break the solid matter into pieces. The solid matter may be an abnormal byproduct of a biological function or a foreign body. The pieces of solid matter are not taken out.

Body Part Character 4	Approach Character 5	Device Character 6	Qualifier Character 7
3 Kidney Pelvis, Right Ureteropelvic junction (UPJ) **4 Kidney Pelvis, Left** *See 3 Kidney Pelvis, Right* **6 Ureter, Right** Ureteral orifice Ureterovesical orifice **7 Ureter, Left** *See 6 Ureter, Right* **B Bladder** Trigone of bladder **C Bladder Neck** **D Urethra** NC Bulbourethral (Cowper's) gland Cowper's (bulbourethral) gland External urethral sphincter Internal urethral sphincter Membranous urethra Penile urethra Prostatic urethra	**Ø Open** **3 Percutaneous** **4 Percutaneous Endoscopic** **7 Via Natural or Artificial Opening** **8 Via Natural or Artificial Opening Endoscopic** **X External**	**Z No Device**	**Z No Qualifier**

Non-OR ØTF[3,4][Ø,7,8]ZZ
Non-OR ØTF[6,7,B,C,D][Ø,3,4,7,8]ZZ
Non-OR ØTF[3,4,6,7,B,C,D]XZZ
NC ØTFDXZZ

Ø Medical and Surgical
T Urinary System
H Insertion Definition: Putting in a nonbiological appliance that monitors, assists, performs, or prevents a physiological function but does not physically take the place of a body part
Explanation: None

Body Part Character 4	Approach Character 5	Device Character 6	Qualifier Character 7
5 Kidney Renal calyx Renal capsule Renal cortex Renal segment	Ø Open 3 Percutaneous 4 Percutaneous Endoscopic 7 Via Natural or Artificial Opening 8 Via Natural or Artificial Opening Endoscopic	1 Radioactive Element 2 Monitoring Device 3 Infusion Device Y Other Device	Z No Qualifier
9 Ureter Ureteral orifice Ureterovesical orifice	Ø Open 3 Percutaneous 4 Percutaneous Endoscopic 7 Via Natural or Artificial Opening 8 Via Natural or Artificial Opening Endoscopic	1 Radioactive Element 2 Monitoring Device 3 Infusion Device M Stimulator Lead Y Other Device	Z No Qualifier
B Bladder NC Trigone of bladder	Ø Open 3 Percutaneous 4 Percutaneous Endoscopic 7 Via Natural or Artificial Opening 8 Via Natural or Artificial Opening Endoscopic	1 Radioactive Element 2 Monitoring Device 3 Infusion Device L Artificial Sphincter M Stimulator Lead Y Other Device	Z No Qualifier
C Bladder Neck	Ø Open 3 Percutaneous 4 Percutaneous Endoscopic 7 Via Natural or Artificial Opening 8 Via Natural or Artificial Opening Endoscopic	L Artificial Sphincter	Z No Qualifier
D Urethra Bulbourethral (Cowper's) gland Cowper's (bulbourethral) gland External urethral sphincter Internal urethral sphincter Membranous urethra Penile urethra Prostatic urethra	Ø Open 3 Percutaneous 4 Percutaneous Endoscopic 7 Via Natural or Artificial Opening 8 Via Natural or Artificial Opening Endoscopic	1 Radioactive Element 2 Monitoring Device 3 Infusion Device L Artificial Sphincter Y Other Device	Z No Qualifier
D Urethra Bulbourethral (Cowper's) gland Cowper's (bulbourethral) gland External urethral sphincter Internal urethral sphincter Membranous urethra Penile urethra Prostatic urethra	X External	2 Monitoring Device 3 Infusion Device L Artificial Sphincter	Z No Qualifier

Non-OR ØTH5Ø3Z
Non-OR ØTH5[3,4][3,Y]Z
Non-OR ØTH57[2,3,Y]Z
Non-OR ØTH58[2,3]Z
Non-OR ØTH9Ø3Z
Non-OR ØTH9[3,4][3,Y]Z
Non-OR ØTH97[2,3,Y]Z
Non-OR ØTH98[2,3]Z
Non-OR ØTHBØ3Z
Non-OR ØTHB[3,4][3,Y]Z
Non-OR ØTHB7[2,3,Y]Z
Non-OR ØTHB8[2,3]Z
Non-OR ØTHDØ3Z
Non-OR ØTHD[3,4][3,Y]Z
Non-OR ØTHD[7,8][2,3,Y]Z
Non-OR ØTHDX3Z
NC ØTHB[Ø,3,4,7,8]MZ

Ø Medical and Surgical
T Urinary System
J Inspection Definition: Visually and/or manually exploring a body part

Explanation: Visual exploration may be performed with or without optical instrumentation. Manual exploration may be performed directly or through intervening body layers.

Body Part Character 4	Approach Character 5	Device Character 6	Qualifier Character 7
5 Kidney Renal calyx Renal capsule Renal cortex Renal segment **9 Ureter** Ureteral orifice Ureterovesical orifice **B Bladder** Trigone of bladder **D Urethra** Bulbourethral (Cowper's) gland Cowper's (bulbourethral) gland External urethral sphincter Internal urethral sphincter Membranous urethra Penile urethra Prostatic urethra	**Ø Open** **3 Percutaneous** **4 Percutaneous Endoscopic** **7 Via Natural or Artificial Opening** **8 Via Natural or Artificial Opening Endoscopic** **X External**	**Z No Device**	**Z No Qualifier**

Non-OR ØTJ[5,9,D][3,4,7,8,X]ZZ
Non-OR ØTJB[3,7,8,X]ZZ

Ø Medical and Surgical
T Urinary System
L Occlusion Definition: Completely closing an orifice or the lumen of a tubular body part

Explanation: The orifice can be a natural orifice or an artificially created orifice

Body Part Character 4	Approach Character 5	Device Character 6	Qualifier Character 7
3 Kidney Pelvis, Right Ureteropelvic junction (UPJ) **4 Kidney Pelvis, Left** *See 3 Kidney Pelvis, Right* **6 Ureter, Right** Ureteral orifice Ureterovesical orifice **7 Ureter, Left** *See 6 Ureter, Right* **B Bladder** Trigone of bladder **C Bladder Neck**	**Ø Open** **3 Percutaneous** **4 Percutaneous Endoscopic**	**C Extraluminal Device** **D Intraluminal Device** **Z No Device**	**Z No Qualifier**
3 Kidney Pelvis, Right Ureteropelvic junction (UPJ) **4 Kidney Pelvis, Left** *See 3 Kidney Pelvis, Right* **6 Ureter, Right** Ureteral orifice Ureterovesical orifice **7 Ureter, Left** *See 6 Ureter, Right* **B Bladder** Trigone of bladder **C Bladder Neck**	**7 Via Natural or Artificial Opening** **8 Via Natural or Artificial Opening Endoscopic**	**D Intraluminal Device** **Z No Device**	**Z No Qualifier**
D Urethra Bulbourethral (Cowper's) gland Cowper's (bulbourethral) gland External urethral sphincter Internal urethral sphincter Membranous urethra Penile urethra Prostatic urethra	**Ø Open** **3 Percutaneous** **4 Percutaneous Endoscopic** **X External**	**C Extraluminal Device** **D Intraluminal Device** **Z No Device**	**Z No Qualifier**
D Urethra Bulbourethral (Cowper's) gland Cowper's (bulbourethral) gland External urethral sphincter Internal urethral sphincter Membranous urethra Penile urethra Prostatic urethra	**7 Via Natural or Artificial Opening** **8 Via Natural or Artificial Opening Endoscopic**	**D Intraluminal Device** **Z No Device**	**Z No Qualifier**

Ø Medical and Surgical
T Urinary System
M Reattachment Definition: Putting back in or on all or a portion of a separated body part to its normal location or other suitable location

Explanation: Vascular circulation and nervous pathways may or may not be reestablished

Body Part Character 4	Approach Character 5	Device Character 6	Qualifier Character 7
Ø Kidney, Right Renal calyx Renal capsule Renal cortex Renal segment **1 Kidney, Left** *See Ø Kidney, Right* **2 Kidneys, Bilateral** *See Ø Kidney, Right* **3 Kidney Pelvis, Right** Ureteropelvic junction (UPJ) **4 Kidney Pelvis, Left** *See 3 Kidney Pelvis, Right* **6 Ureter, Right** Ureteral orifice Ureterovesical orifice **7 Ureter, Left** *See 6 Ureter, Right* **8 Ureters, Bilateral** *See 6 Ureter, Right* **B Bladder** Trigone of bladder **C Bladder Neck** **D Urethra** Bulbourethral (Cowper's) gland Cowper's (bulbourethral) gland External urethral sphincter Internal urethral sphincter Membranous urethra Penile urethra Prostatic urethra	**Ø Open** **4 Percutaneous Endoscopic**	**Z No Device**	**Z No Qualifier**

Ø Medical and Surgical
T Urinary System
N Release Definition: Freeing a body part from an abnormal physical constraint by cutting or by the use of force

Explanation: Some of the restraining tissue may be taken out but none of the body part is taken out

Body Part Character 4	Approach Character 5	Device Character 6	Qualifier Character 7
Ø Kidney, Right Renal calyx Renal capsule Renal cortex Renal segment **1 Kidney, Left** *See Ø Kidney, Right* **3 Kidney Pelvis, Right** Ureteropelvic junction (UPJ) **4 Kidney Pelvis, Left** *See 3 Kidney Pelvis, Right* **6 Ureter, Right** Ureteral orifice Ureterovesical orifice **7 Ureter, Left** *See 6 Ureter, Right* **B Bladder** Trigone of bladder **C Bladder Neck**	**Ø Open** **3 Percutaneous** **4 Percutaneous Endoscopic** **7 Via Natural or Artificial Opening** **8 Via Natural or Artificial Opening Endoscopic**	**Z No Device**	**Z No Qualifier**
D Urethra Bulbourethral (Cowper's) gland Cowper's (bulbourethral) gland External urethral sphincter Internal urethral sphincter Membranous urethra Penile urethra Prostatic urethra	**Ø Open** **3 Percutaneous** **4 Percutaneous Endoscopic** **7 Via Natural or Artificial Opening** **8 Via Natural or Artificial Opening Endoscopic** **X External**	**Z No Device**	**Z No Qualifier**

Ø Medical and Surgical
T Urinary System
P Removal Definition: Taking out or off a device from a body part

Explanation: If a device is taken out and a similar device put in without cutting or puncturing the skin or mucous membrane, the procedure is coded to the root operation CHANGE. Otherwise, the procedure for taking out the device is coded to the root operation REMOVAL.

Body Part Character 4	Approach Character 5	Device Character 6	Qualifier Character 7
5 Kidney Renal calyx Renal capsule Renal cortex Renal segment	**Ø Open** **3 Percutaneous** **4 Percutaneous Endoscopic** **7 Via Natural or Artificial Opening** **8 Via Natural or Artificial Opening Endoscopic**	**Ø Drainage Device** **2 Monitoring Device** **3 Infusion Device** **7 Autologous Tissue Substitute** **C Extraluminal Device** **D Intraluminal Device** **J Synthetic Substitute** **K Nonautologous Tissue Substitute** **Y Other Device**	**Z No Qualifier**
5 Kidney Renal calyx Renal capsule Renal cortex Renal segment	**X External**	**Ø Drainage Device** **2 Monitoring Device** **3 Infusion Device** **D Intraluminal Device**	**Z No Qualifier**
9 Ureter Ureteral orifice Ureterovesical orifice	**Ø Open** **3 Percutaneous** **4 Percutaneous Endoscopic** **7 Via Natural or Artificial Opening** **8 Via Natural or Artificial Opening Endoscopic**	**Ø Drainage Device** **2 Monitoring Device** **3 Infusion Device** **7 Autologous Tissue Substitute** **C Extraluminal Device** **D Intraluminal Device** **J Synthetic Substitute** **K Nonautologous Tissue Substitute** **M Stimulator Lead** **Y Other Device**	**Z No Qualifier**
9 Ureter Ureteral orifice Ureterovesical orifice	**X External**	**Ø Drainage Device** **2 Monitoring Device** **3 Infusion Device** **D Intraluminal Device** **M Stimulator Lead**	**Z No Qualifier**
B Bladder NC Trigone of bladder	**Ø Open** **3 Percutaneous** **4 Percutaneous Endoscopic** **7 Via Natural or Artificial Opening** **8 Via Natural or Artificial Opening Endoscopic**	**Ø Drainage Device** **2 Monitoring Device** **3 Infusion Device** **7 Autologous Tissue Substitute** **C Extraluminal Device** **D Intraluminal Device** **J Synthetic Substitute** **K Nonautologous Tissue Substitute** **L Artificial Sphincter** **M Stimulator Lead** **Y Other Device**	**Z No Qualifier**
B Bladder Trigone of bladder	**X External**	**Ø Drainage Device** **2 Monitoring Device** **3 Infusion Device** **D Intraluminal Device** **L Artificial Sphincter** **M Stimulator Lead**	**Z No Qualifier**
D Urethra Bulbourethral (Cowper's) gland Cowper's (bulbourethral) gland External urethral sphincter Internal urethral sphincter Membranous urethra Penile urethra Prostatic urethra	**Ø Open** **3 Percutaneous** **4 Percutaneous Endoscopic** **7 Via Natural or Artificial Opening** **8 Via Natural or Artificial Opening Endoscopic**	**Ø Drainage Device** **2 Monitoring Device** **3 Infusion Device** **7 Autologous Tissue Substitute** **C Extraluminal Device** **D Intraluminal Device** **J Synthetic Substitute** **K Nonautologous Tissue Substitute** **L Artificial Sphincter** **Y Other Device**	**Z No Qualifier**
D Urethra Bulbourethral (Cowper's) gland Cowper's (bulbourethral) gland External urethral sphincter Internal urethral sphincter Membranous urethra Penile urethra Prostatic urethra	**X External**	**Ø Drainage Device** **2 Monitoring Device** **3 Infusion Device** **D Intraluminal Device** **L Artificial Sphincter**	**Z No Qualifier**

Non-OR ØTP5[3,4,7]YZ
Non-OR ØTP5[7,8][Ø,2,3,D]Z
Non-OR ØTP5X[Ø,2,3,D]Z
Non-OR ØTP9[3,4,7]YZ
Non-OR ØTP9[7,8][Ø,2,3,D]Z
Non-OR ØTP9X[Ø,2,3,D]Z
Non-OR ØTPB[3,4,7]YZ
Non-OR ØTPB[7,8][Ø,2,3,D]Z
Non-OR ØTPBX[Ø,2,3,D,L]Z
Non-OR ØTPD[3,4]YZ
Non-OR ØTPD[7,8][Ø,2,3,D,Y]Z
Non-OR ØTPDX[Ø,2,3,D]Z
NC ØTPB[Ø,3,4,7,8]MZ

Ø Medical and Surgical
T Urinary System
Q Repair Definition: Restoring, to the extent possible, a body part to its normal anatomic structure and function
Explanation: Used only when the method to accomplish the repair is not one of the other root operations

Body Part Character 4	Approach Character 5	Device Character 6	Qualifier Character 7
Ø Kidney, Right Renal calyx Renal capsule Renal cortex Renal segment **1 Kidney, Left** *See Ø Kidney, Right* **3 Kidney Pelvis, Right** Ureteropelvic junction (UPJ) **4 Kidney Pelvis, Left** *See 3 Kidney Pelvis, Right* **6 Ureter, Right** Ureteral orifice Ureterovesical orifice **7 Ureter, Left** *See 6 Ureter, Right* **B Bladder** ⊞ Trigone of bladder **C Bladder Neck**	**Ø Open** **3 Percutaneous** **4 Percutaneous Endoscopic** **7 Via Natural or Artificial Opening** **8 Via Natural or Artificial Opening Endoscopic**	**Z No Device**	**Z No Qualifier**
D Urethra Bulbourethral (Cowper's) gland Cowper's (bulbourethral) gland External urethral sphincter Internal urethral sphincter Membranous urethra Penile urethra Prostatic urethra	**Ø Open** **3 Percutaneous** **4 Percutaneous Endoscopic** **7 Via Natural or Artificial Opening** **8 Via Natural or Artificial Opening Endoscopic** **X External**	**Z No Device**	**Z No Qualifier**

See Appendix L for Procedure Combinations
⊞ ØTQB[Ø,3,4]ZZ

Ø Medical and Surgical
T Urinary System
R Replacement Definition: Putting in or on biological or synthetic material that physically takes the place and/or function of all or a portion of a body part
Explanation: The body part may have been taken out or replaced, or may be taken out, physically eradicated, or rendered nonfunctional during the REPLACEMENT procedure. A REMOVAL procedure is coded for taking out the device used in a previous replacement procedure.

Body Part Character 4	Approach Character 5	Device Character 6	Qualifier Character 7
3 Kidney Pelvis, Right Ureteropelvic junction (UPJ) **4 Kidney Pelvis, Left** *See 3 Kidney Pelvis, Right* **6 Ureter, Right** Ureteral orifice Ureterovesical orifice **7 Ureter, Left** *See 6 Ureter, Right* **B Bladder** Trigone of bladder **C Bladder Neck**	**Ø Open** **4 Percutaneous Endoscopic** **7 Via Natural or Artificial Opening** **8 Via Natural or Artificial Opening Endoscopic**	**7 Autologous Tissue Substitute** **J Synthetic Substitute** **K Nonautologous Tissue Substitute**	**Z No Qualifier**
D Urethra Bulbourethral (Cowper's) gland Cowper's (bulbourethral) gland External urethral sphincter Internal urethral sphincter Membranous urethra Penile urethra Prostatic urethra	**Ø Open** **4 Percutaneous Endoscopic** **7 Via Natural or Artificial Opening** **8 Via Natural or Artificial Opening Endoscopic** **X External**	**7 Autologous Tissue Substitute** **J Synthetic Substitute** **K Nonautologous Tissue Substitute**	**Z No Qualifier**

Ø Medical and Surgical
T Urinary System
S Reposition Definition: Moving to its normal location, or other suitable location, all or a portion of a body part

Explanation: The body part is moved to a new location from an abnormal location, or from a normal location where it is not functioning correctly. The body part may or may not be cut out or off to be moved to the new location.

Body Part Character 4	Approach Character 5	Device Character 6	Qualifier Character 7
Ø Kidney, Right Renal calyx Renal capsule Renal cortex Renal segment **1 Kidney, Left** *See Ø Kidney, Right* **2 Kidneys, Bilateral** *See Ø Kidney, Right* **3 Kidney Pelvis, Right** Ureteropelvic junction (UPJ) **4 Kidney Pelvis, Left** *See 3 Kidney Pelvis, Right* **6 Ureter, Right** Ureteral orifice Ureterovesical orifice **7 Ureter, Left** *See 6 Ureter, Right* **8 Ureters, Bilateral** *See 6 Ureter, Right* **B Bladder** Trigone of bladder **C Bladder Neck** **D Urethra** Bulbourethral (Cowper's) gland Cowper's (bulbourethral) gland External urethral sphincter Internal urethral sphincter Membranous urethra Penile urethra Prostatic urethra	**Ø Open** **4 Percutaneous Endoscopic**	**Z No Device**	**Z No Qualifier**

Ø Medical and Surgical
T Urinary System
T Resection Definition: Cutting out or off, without replacement, all of a body part

Explanation: None

Body Part Character 4	Approach Character 5	Device Character 6	Qualifier Character 7
Ø Kidney, Right Renal calyx Renal capsule Renal cortex Renal segment **1 Kidney, Left** *See Ø Kidney, Right* **2 Kidneys, Bilateral** *See Ø Kidney, Right*	**Ø Open** **4 Percutaneous Endoscopic**	**Z No Device**	**Z No Qualifier**
3 Kidney Pelvis, Right Ureteropelvic junction (UPJ) **4 Kidney Pelvis, Left** *See 3 Kidney Pelvis, Right* **6 Ureter, Right** Ureteral orifice Ureterovesical orifice **7 Ureter, Left** *See 6 Ureter, Right* **B Bladder** ⊞ Trigone of bladder **C Bladder Neck** **D Urethra** Bulbourethral (Cowper's) gland Cowper's (bulbourethral) gland External urethral sphincter Internal urethral sphincter Membranous urethra Penile urethra Prostatic urethra	**Ø Open** **4 Percutaneous Endoscopic** **7 Via Natural or Artificial Opening** **8 Via Natural or Artificial Opening Endoscopic**	**Z No Device**	**Z No Qualifier**

Non-OR ØTTD[4,7,8]ZZ

See Appendix L for Procedure Combinations

Combo-only ØTTDØZZ
⊞ ØTTBØZZ

Ø Medical and Surgical
T Urinary System
U Supplement Definition: Putting in or on biological or synthetic material that physically reinforces and/or augments the function of a portion of a body part

Explanation: The biological material is non-living, or is living and from the same individual. The body part may have been previously replaced, and the SUPPLEMENT procedure is performed to physically reinforce and/or augment the function of the replaced body part.

Body Part Character 4	Approach Character 5	Device Character 6	Qualifier Character 7
3 Kidney Pelvis, Right Ureteropelvic junction (UPJ) **4 Kidney Pelvis, Left** *See 3 Kidney Pelvis, Right* **6 Ureter, Right** Ureteral orifice Ureterovesical orifice **7 Ureter, Left** *See 6 Ureter, Right* **B Bladder** Trigone of bladder **C Bladder Neck**	**Ø Open** **4 Percutaneous Endoscopic** **7 Via Natural or Artificial Opening** **8 Via Natural or Artificial Opening Endoscopic**	**7 Autologous Tissue Substitute** **J Synthetic Substitute** **K Nonautologous Tissue Substitute**	**Z No Qualifier**
D Urethra Bulbourethral (Cowper's) gland Cowper's (bulbourethral) gland External urethral sphincter Internal urethral sphincter Membranous urethra Penile urethra Prostatic urethra	**Ø Open** **4 Percutaneous Endoscopic** **7 Via Natural or Artificial Opening** **8 Via Natural or Artificial Opening Endoscopic** **X External**	**7 Autologous Tissue Substitute** **J Synthetic Substitute** **K Nonautologous Tissue Substitute**	**Z No Qualifier**

Ø Medical and Surgical
T Urinary System
V Restriction Definition: Partially closing an orifice or the lumen of a tubular body part

Explanation: The orifice can be a natural orifice or an artificially created orifice

Body Part Character 4	Approach Character 5	Device Character 6	Qualifier Character 7
3 Kidney Pelvis, Right Ureteropelvic junction (UPJ) **4 Kidney Pelvis, Left** *See 3 Kidney Pelvis, Right* **6 Ureter, Right** Ureteral orifice Ureterovesical orifice **7 Ureter, Left** *See 6 Ureter, Right* **B Bladder** Trigone of bladder **C Bladder Neck**	**Ø Open** **3 Percutaneous** **4 Percutaneous Endoscopic**	**C Extraluminal Device** **D Intraluminal Device** **Z No Device**	**Z No Qualifier**
3 Kidney Pelvis, Right Ureteropelvic junction (UPJ) **4 Kidney Pelvis, Left** *See 3 Kidney Pelvis, Right* **6 Ureter, Right** Ureteral orifice Ureterovesical orifice **7 Ureter, Left** *See 6 Ureter, Right* **B Bladder** Trigone of bladder **C Bladder Neck**	**7 Via Natural or Artificial Opening** **8 Via Natural or Artificial Opening Endoscopic**	**D Intraluminal Device** **Z No Device**	**Z No Qualifier**
D Urethra Bulbourethral (Cowper's) gland Cowper's (bulbourethral) gland External urethral sphincter Internal urethral sphincter Membranous urethra Penile urethra Prostatic urethra	**Ø Open** **3 Percutaneous** **4 Percutaneous Endoscopic**	**C Extraluminal Device** **D Intraluminal Device** **Z No Device**	**Z No Qualifier**
D Urethra Bulbourethral (Cowper's) gland Cowper's (bulbourethral) gland External urethral sphincter Internal urethral sphincter Membranous urethra Penile urethra Prostatic urethra	**7 Via Natural or Artificial Opening** **8 Via Natural or Artificial Opening Endoscopic**	**D Intraluminal Device** **Z No Device**	**Z No Qualifier**
D Urethra Bulbourethral (Cowper's) gland Cowper's (bulbourethral) gland External urethral sphincter Internal urethral sphincter Membranous urethra Penile urethra Prostatic urethra	**X External**	**Z No Device**	**Z No Qualifier**

Ø Medical and Surgical
T Urinary System
W Revision Definition: Correcting, to the extent possible, a portion of a malfunctioning device or the position of a displaced device

Explanation: Revision can include correcting a malfunctioning or displaced device by taking out or putting in components of the device such as a screw or pin

Body Part Character 4	Approach Character 5	Device Character 6	Qualifier Character 7
5 Kidney Renal calyx Renal capsule Renal cortex Renal segment	**Ø Open** **3 Percutaneous** **4 Percutaneous Endoscopic** **7 Via Natural or Artificial Opening** **8 Via Natural or Artificial Opening Endoscopic**	**Ø Drainage Device** **2 Monitoring Device** **3 Infusion Device** **7 Autologous Tissue Substitute** **C Extraluminal Device** **D Intraluminal Device** **J Synthetic Substitute** **K Nonautologous Tissue Substitute** **Y Other Device**	**Z No Qualifier**
5 Kidney Renal calyx Renal capsule Renal cortex Renal segment	**X External**	**Ø Drainage Device** **2 Monitoring Device** **3 Infusion Device** **7 Autologous Tissue Substitute** **C Extraluminal Device** **D Intraluminal Device** **J Synthetic Substitute** **K Nonautologous Tissue Substitute**	**Z No Qualifier**
9 Ureter Ureteral orifice Ureterovesical orifice	**Ø Open** **3 Percutaneous** **4 Percutaneous Endoscopic** **7 Via Natural or Artificial Opening** **8 Via Natural or Artificial Opening Endoscopic**	**Ø Drainage Device** **2 Monitoring Device** **3 Infusion Device** **7 Autologous Tissue Substitute** **C Extraluminal Device** **D Intraluminal Device** **J Synthetic Substitute** **K Nonautologous Tissue Substitute** **M Stimulator Lead** **Y Other Device**	**Z No Qualifier**
9 Ureter Ureteral orifice Ureterovesical orifice	**X External**	**Ø Drainage Device** **2 Monitoring Device** **3 Infusion Device** **7 Autologous Tissue Substitute** **C Extraluminal Device** **D Intraluminal Device** **J Synthetic Substitute** **K Nonautologous Tissue Substitute** **M Stimulator Lead**	**Z No Qualifier**
B Bladder Trigone of bladder	**Ø Open** **3 Percutaneous** **4 Percutaneous Endoscopic** **7 Via Natural or Artificial Opening** **8 Via Natural or Artificial Opening Endoscopic**	**Ø Drainage Device** **2 Monitoring Device** **3 Infusion Device** **7 Autologous Tissue Substitute** **C Extraluminal Device** **D Intraluminal Device** **J Synthetic Substitute** **K Nonautologous Tissue Substitute** **L Artificial Sphincter** **M Stimulator Lead** **Y Other Device**	**Z No Qualifier**
B Bladder Trigone of bladder	**X External**	**Ø Drainage Device** **2 Monitoring Device** **3 Infusion Device** **7 Autologous Tissue Substitute** **C Extraluminal Device** **D Intraluminal Device** **J Synthetic Substitute** **K Nonautologous Tissue Substitute** **L Artificial Sphincter** **M Stimulator Lead**	**Z No Qualifier**

Non-OR ØTW5[3,4,7]YZ
Non-OR ØTW5X[Ø,2,3,7,C,D,J,K]Z
Non-OR ØTW9[3,4,7]YZ
Non-OR ØTW9X[Ø,2,3,7,C,D,J,K,M]Z
Non-OR ØTWB[3,4,7]YZ
Non-OR ØTWBX[Ø,2,3,7,C,D,J,K,L,M]Z

ØTW Continued on next page

Ø Medical and Surgical
T Urinary System
W Revision Definition: Correcting, to the extent possible, a portion of a malfunctioning device or the position of a displaced device

Explanation: Revision can include correcting a malfunctioning or displaced device by taking out or putting in components of the device such as a screw or pin

ØTW Continued

Body Part Character 4	Approach Character 5	Device Character 6	Qualifier Character 7
D Urethra Bulbourethral (Cowper's) gland Cowper's (bulbourethral) gland External urethral sphincter Internal urethral sphincter Membranous urethra Penile urethra Prostatic urethra	**Ø Open** **3 Percutaneous** **4 Percutaneous Endoscopic** **7 Via Natural or Artificial Opening** **8 Via Natural or Artificial Opening Endoscopic**	**Ø Drainage Device** **2 Monitoring Device** **3 Infusion Device** **7 Autologous Tissue Substitute** **C Extraluminal Device** **D Intraluminal Device** **J Synthetic Substitute** **K Nonautologous Tissue Substitute** **L Artificial Sphincter** **Y Other Device**	**Z No Qualifier**
D Urethra Bulbourethral (Cowper's) gland Cowper's (bulbourethral) gland External urethral sphincter Internal urethral sphincter Membranous urethra Penile urethra Prostatic urethra	**X External**	**Ø Drainage Device** **2 Monitoring Device** **3 Infusion Device** **7 Autologous Tissue Substitute** **C Extraluminal Device** **D Intraluminal Device** **J Synthetic Substitute** **K Nonautologous Tissue Substitute** **L Artificial Sphincter**	**Z No Qualifier**

Non-OR ØTWD[3,4,7,8]YZ
Non-OR ØTWDX[Ø,2,3,7,C,D,J,K,L]Z

Ø Medical and Surgical
T Urinary System
Y Transplantation Definition: Putting in or on all or a portion of a living body part taken from another individual or animal to physically take the place and/or function of all or a portion of a similar body part

Explanation: The native body part may or may not be taken out, and the transplanted body part may take over all or a portion of its function

Body Part Character 4	Approach Character 5	Device Character 6	Qualifier Character 7
Ø Kidney, Right LC ⊞ Renal calyx Renal capsule Renal cortex Renal segment **1 Kidney, Left** LC ⊞ *See Ø Kidney, Right*	**Ø Open**	**Z No Device**	**Ø Allogeneic** **1 Syngeneic** **2 Zooplastic**

LC ØTY[Ø,1]ØZ[Ø,1,2]

See Appendix L for Procedure Combinations
⊞ ØTY[Ø,1]ØZ[Ø,1,2]

Female Reproductive System ØU1–ØUY

Character Meanings

This Character Meaning table is provided as a guide to assist the user in the identification of character members that may be found in this section of code tables. It **SHOULD NOT** be used to build a PCS code.

Operation–Character 3	Body Part–Character 4	Approach–Character 5	Device–Character 6	Qualifier–Character 7
1 Bypass	Ø Ovary, Right	Ø Open	Ø Drainage Device	Ø Allogeneic
2 Change	1 Ovary, Left	3 Percutaneous	1 Radioactive Element	1 Syngeneic
5 Destruction	2 Ovaries, Bilateral	4 Percutaneous Endoscopic	3 Infusion Device	2 Zooplastic
7 Dilation	3 Ovary	7 Via Natural or Artificial Opening	7 Autologous Tissue Substitute	5 Fallopian Tube, Right
8 Division	4 Uterine Supporting Structure	8 Via Natural or Artificial Opening Endoscopic	C Extraluminal Device	6 Fallopian Tube, Left
9 Drainage	5 Fallopian Tube, Right	F Via Natural or Artificial Opening With Percutaneous Endoscopic Assistance	D Intraluminal Device	9 Uterus
B Excision	6 Fallopian Tube, Left	X External	G Intraluminal Device, Pessary	L Supracervical
C Extirpation	7 Fallopian Tubes, Bilateral		H Contraceptive Device	X Diagnostic
D Extraction	8 Fallopian Tube		J Synthetic Substitute	Z No Qualifier
F Fragmentation	9 Uterus		K Nonautologous Tissue Substitute	
H Insertion	B Endometrium		Y Other Device	
J Inspection	C Cervix		Z No Device	
L Occlusion	D Uterus and Cervix			
M Reattachment	F Cul-de-sac			
N Release	G Vagina			
P Removal	H Vagina and Cul-de-sac			
Q Repair	J Clitoris			
S Reposition	K Hymen			
T Resection	L Vestibular Gland			
U Supplement	M Vulva			
V Restriction	N Ova			
W Revision				
Y Transplantation				

AHA Coding Clinic for table ØU5
2015, 3Q, 31 Tubal ligation for sterilization

AHA Coding Clinic for table ØU7
2020, 2Q, 30 Duhrssen Cervical Incision

AHA Coding Clinic for table ØU9
2016, 4Q, 58 Longitudinal vaginal septum

AHA Coding Clinic for table ØUB
2018, 1Q, 23 Tubal ligation procedure
2015, 3Q, 31 Laparoscopic partial salpingectomy for ectopic pregnancy
2015, 3Q, 31 Tubal ligation for sterilization
2014, 4Q, 16 Excision of multiple uterine fibroids
2014, 3Q, 12 Excision of skin tag from labia majora

AHA Coding Clinic for table ØUC
2015, 3Q, 30 Removal of cervical cerclage
2013, 2Q, 38 Evacuation of clot post-partum

AHA Coding Clinic for table ØUH
2018, 1Q, 25 Intrauterine brachytherapy & placement of tandems & ovoids
2013, 2Q, 34 Placement of intrauterine device via open approach

AHA Coding Clinic for table ØUJ
2015, 1Q, 33 Robotic-assisted laparoscopic hysterectomy converted to open procedure

AHA Coding Clinic for table ØUL
2018, 1Q, 23 Tubal ligation procedure
2015, 3Q, 31 Tubal ligation for sterilization

AHA Coding Clinic for table ØUQ
2014, 4Q, 18 Obstetrical periurethral laceration
2013, 4Q, 120 Repair of clitoral obstetric laceration

AHA Coding Clinic for table ØUS
2016, 1Q, 9 Anteversion of retroverted pregnant uterus

AHA Coding Clinic for table ØUT
2017, 4Q, 68 New qualifier values - Supracervical hysterectomy
2015, 1Q, 33 Robotic-assisted laparoscopic hysterectomy converted to open procedure
2013, 3Q, 28 Total hysterectomy
2013, 1Q, 24 Excision versus Resection of remaining ovarian remnant following previous excision

AHA Coding Clinic for table ØUV
2015, 3Q, 30 Insertion of cervical cerclage

AHA Coding Clinic for table ØUY
2018, 4Q, 40 Uterus transplant

Female Reproductive System

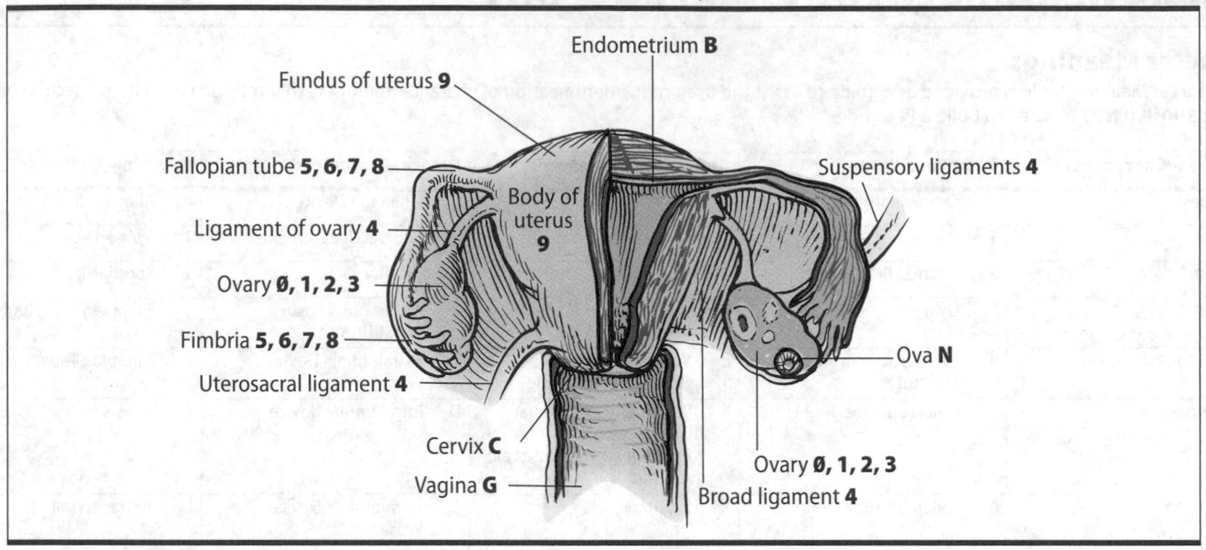

Female Internal/External Structures

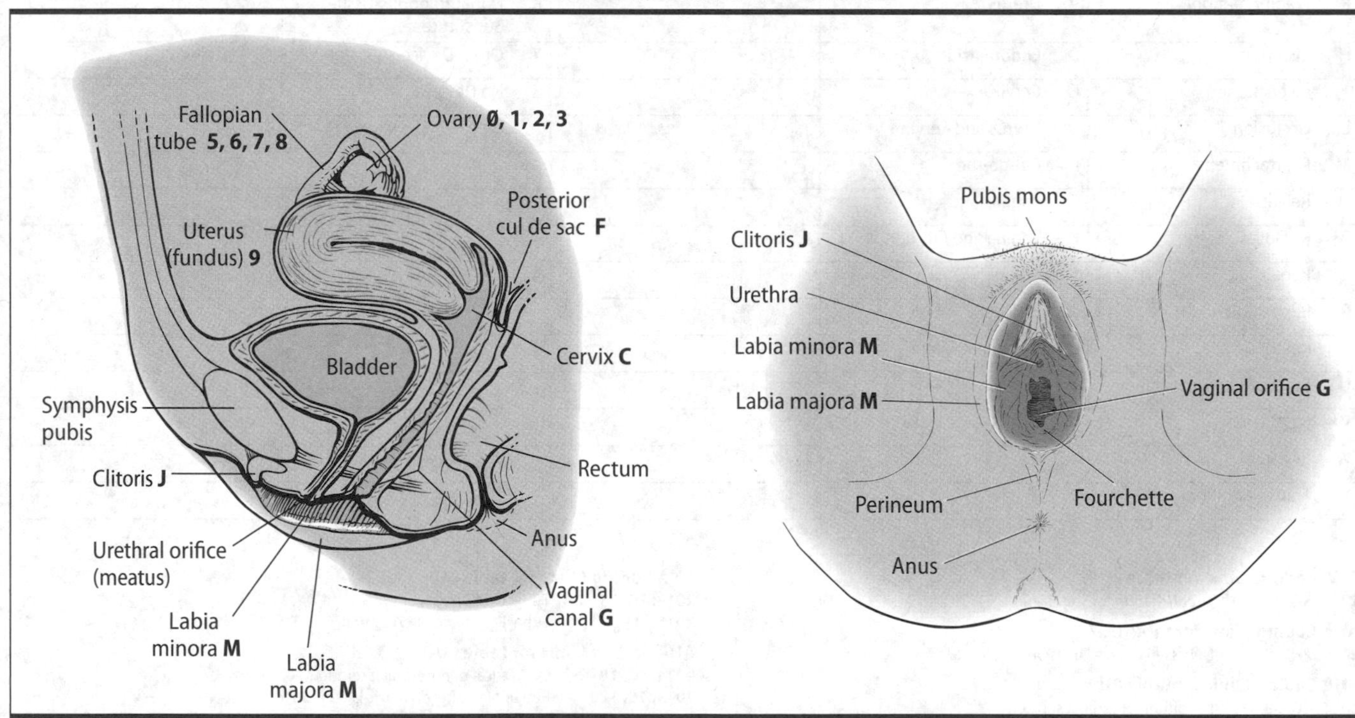

Ø Medical and Surgical
U Female Reproductive System
1 Bypass Definition: Altering the route of passage of the contents of a tubular body part

Explanation: Rerouting contents of a body part to a downstream area of the normal route, to a similar route and body part, or to an abnormal route and dissimilar body part. Includes one or more anastomoses, with or without the use of a device.

Body Part Character 4	Approach Character 5	Device Character 6	Qualifier Character 7
5 Fallopian Tube, Right ♀ Oviduct Salpinx Uterine tube **6 Fallopian Tube, Left** ♀ *See 5 Fallopian Tube, Right*	**Ø Open** **4 Percutaneous Endoscopic**	**7 Autologous Tissue Substitute** **J Synthetic Substitute** **K Nonautologous Tissue Substitute** **Z No Device**	**5 Fallopian Tube, Right** **6 Fallopian Tube, Left** **9 Uterus**

♀ All body part, approach, device, and qualifier values

Ø Medical and Surgical
U Female Reproductive System
2 Change Definition: Taking out or off a device from a body part and putting back an identical or similar device in or on the same body part without cutting or puncturing the skin or a mucous membrane

Explanation: All CHANGE procedures are coded using the approach EXTERNAL

Body Part Character 4	Approach Character 5	Device Character 6	Qualifier Character 7
3 Ovary ♀ **8 Fallopian Tube** ♀ **M Vulva** ♀ Labia majora Labia minora	**X External**	**Ø Drainage Device** **Y Other Device**	**Z No Qualifier**
D Uterus and Cervix ♀	**X External**	**Ø Drainage Device** **H Contraceptive Device** **Y Other Device**	**Z No Qualifier**
H Vagina and Cul-de-sac ♀	**X External**	**Ø Drainage Device** **G Intraluminal Device, Pessary** **Y Other Device**	**Z No Qualifier**

Non-OR All body part, approach, device, and qualifier values

♀ All body part, approach, device, and qualifier values

Ø Medical and Surgical
U Female Reproductive System
5 Destruction Definition: Physical eradication of all or a portion of a body part by the direct use of energy, force, or a destructive agent
Explanation: None of the body part is physically taken out

Body Part Character 4	Approach Character 5	Device Character 6	Qualifier Character 7
Ø Ovary, Right ♀ **1 Ovary, Left** ♀ **2 Ovaries, Bilateral** ♀ **4 Uterine Supporting Structure** ♀ Broad ligament Infundibulopelvic ligament Ovarian ligament Round ligament of uterus	**Ø Open** **3 Percutaneous** **4 Percutaneous Endoscopic** **8 Via Natural or Artificial Opening Endoscopic**	**Z No Device**	**Z No Qualifier**
5 Fallopian Tube, Right ♀ Oviduct Salpinx Uterine tube **6 Fallopian Tube, Left** ♀ *See 5 Fallopian Tube, Right* **7 Fallopian Tubes, Bilateral** NC ♀ **9 Uterus** ♀ Fundus uteri Myometrium Perimetrium Uterine cornu **B Endometrium** ♀ **C Cervix** ♀ **F Cul-de-sac** ♀	**Ø Open** **3 Percutaneous** **4 Percutaneous Endoscopic** **7 Via Natural or Artificial Opening** **8 Via Natural or Artificial Opening Endoscopic**	**Z No Device**	**Z No Qualifier**
G Vagina ♀ **K Hymen** ♀	**Ø Open** **3 Percutaneous** **4 Percutaneous Endoscopic** **7 Via Natural or Artificial Opening** **8 Via Natural or Artificial Opening Endoscopic** **X External**	**Z No Device**	**Z No Qualifier**
J Clitoris ♀ **L Vestibular Gland** ♀ Bartholin's (greater vestibular) gland Greater vestibular (Bartholin's) gland Paraurethral (Skene's) gland Skene's (paraurethral) gland **M Vulva** ♀ Labia majora Labia minora	**Ø Open** **X External**	**Z No Device**	**Z No Qualifier**

NC ØU57[Ø,3,4,7,8]ZZ with principal or secondary diagnosis of Z3Ø.2 ♀ All body part, approach, device, and qualifier values

Ø Medical and Surgical
U Female Reproductive System
7 Dilation Definition: Expanding an orifice or the lumen of a tubular body part

Explanation: The orifice can be a natural orifice or an artificially created orifice. Accomplished by stretching a tubular body part using intraluminal pressure or by cutting part of the orifice or wall of the tubular body part.

Body Part Character 4	Approach Character 5	Device Character 6	Qualifier Character 7
5 Fallopian Tube, Right ♀ Oviduct Salpinx Uterine tube **6 Fallopian Tube, Left** ♀ *See 5 Fallopian Tube, Right* **7 Fallopian Tubes, Bilateral** ♀ **9 Uterus** ♀ Fundus uteri Myometrium Perimetrium Uterine cornu **C Cervix** ♀ **G Vagina** ♀	**Ø Open** **3 Percutaneous** **4 Percutaneous Endoscopic** **7 Via Natural or Artificial Opening** **8 Via Natural or Artificial Opening Endoscopic**	**D Intraluminal Device** **Z No Device**	**Z No Qualifier**
K Hymen ♀	**Ø Open** **3 Percutaneous** **4 Percutaneous Endoscopic** **7 Via Natural or Artificial Opening** **8 Via Natural or Artificial Opening Endoscopic** **X External**	**D Intraluminal Device** **Z No Device**	**Z No Qualifier**

Non-OR ØU7C[Ø,3,4,7,8][D,Z]Z
Non-OR ØU7G[7,8][D,Z]Z

♀ All body part, approach, device, and qualifier values

Ø Medical and Surgical
U Female Reproductive System
8 Division Definition: Cutting into a body part, without draining fluids and/or gases from the body part, in order to separate or transect a body part

Explanation: All or a portion of the body part is separated into two or more portions

Body Part Character 4	Approach Character 5	Device Character 6	Qualifier Character 7
Ø Ovary, Right ♀ **1 Ovary, Left** ♀ **2 Ovaries, Bilateral** ♀ **4 Uterine Supporting Structure** ♀ Broad ligament Infundibulopelvic ligament Ovarian ligament Round ligament of uterus	**Ø Open** **3 Percutaneous** **4 Percutaneous Endoscopic**	**Z No Device**	**Z No Qualifier**
K Hymen ♀	**7 Via Natural or Artificial Opening** **8 Via Natural or Artificial Opening Endoscopic** **X External**	**Z No Device**	**Z No Qualifier**

Non-OR ØU8K[7,8,X]ZZ

♀ All body part, approach, device, and qualifier values

Ø Medical and Surgical
U Female Reproductive System
9 Drainage Definition: Taking or letting out fluids and/or gases from a body part
Explanation: The qualifier DIAGNOSTIC is used to identify drainage procedures that are biopsies

Body Part Character 4	Approach Character 5	Device Character 6	Qualifier Character 7
Ø Ovary, Right ♀ **1 Ovary, Left** ♀ **2 Ovaries, Bilateral** ♀	**Ø Open** **3 Percutaneous** **4 Percutaneous Endoscopic** **8 Via Natural or Artificial Opening Endoscopic**	**Ø Drainage Device**	**Z No Qualifier**
Ø Ovary, Right ♀ **1 Ovary, Left** ♀ **2 Ovaries, Bilateral** ♀	**Ø Open** **3 Percutaneous** **4 Percutaneous Endoscopic** **8 Via Natural or Artificial Opening Endoscopic**	**Z No Device**	**X Diagnostic** **Z No Qualifier**
Ø Ovary, Right ♀ **1 Ovary, Left** ♀ **2 Ovaries, Bilateral** ♀	**X External**	**Z No Device**	**Z No Qualifier**
4 Uterine Supporting Structure ♀ Broad ligament Infundibulopelvic ligament Ovarian ligament Round ligament of uterus	**Ø Open** **3 Percutaneous** **4 Percutaneous Endoscopic** **8 Via Natural or Artificial Opening Endoscopic**	**Ø Drainage Device**	**Z No Qualifier**
4 Uterine Supporting Structure ♀ Broad ligament Infundibulopelvic ligament Ovarian ligament Round ligament of uterus	**Ø Open** **3 Percutaneous** **4 Percutaneous Endoscopic** **8 Via Natural or Artificial Opening Endoscopic**	**Z No Device**	**X Diagnostic** **Z No Qualifier**
5 Fallopian Tube, Right ♀ Oviduct Salpinx Uterine tube **6 Fallopian Tube, Left** ♀ *See* 5 *Fallopian Tube, Right* **7 Fallopian Tubes, Bilateral** ♀ **9 Uterus** ♀ Fundus uteri Myometrium Perimetrium Uterine cornu **C Cervix** ♀ **F Cul-de-sac** ♀	**Ø Open** **3 Percutaneous** **4 Percutaneous Endoscopic** **7 Via Natural or Artificial Opening** **8 Via Natural or Artificial Opening Endoscopic**	**Ø Drainage Device**	**Z No Qualifier**
5 Fallopian Tube, Right ♀ Oviduct Salpinx Uterine tube **6 Fallopian Tube, Left** ♀ *See* 5 *Fallopian Tube, Right* **7 Fallopian Tubes, Bilateral** ♀ **9 Uterus** ♀ Fundus uteri Myometrium Perimetrium Uterine cornu **C Cervix** ♀ **F Cul-de-sac** ♀	**Ø Open** **3 Percutaneous** **4 Percutaneous Endoscopic** **7 Via Natural or Artificial Opening** **8 Via Natural or Artificial Opening Endoscopic**	**Z No Device**	**X Diagnostic** **Z No Qualifier**

Non-OR ØU9[Ø,1,2][3,8]ØZ
Non-OR ØU9[Ø,1,2][3,8]ZZ
Non-OR ØU9[Ø,1,2]8ZX
Non-OR ØU94[3,8]ØZ
Non-OR ØU94[3,8]ZZ
Non-OR ØU948ZX
Non-OR ØU9[5,6,7,9,C]3ØZ
Non-OR ØU9F[3,4]ØZ
Non-OR ØU9[5,6,7][3,4,7,8]ZZ
Non-OR ØU9[9,C]3ZZ
Non-OR ØU9F[3,4]ZZ
♀ All body part, approach, device, and qualifier values

ØU9 Continued on next page

ØU9 Continued

Ø Medical and Surgical
U Female Reproductive System
9 Drainage Definition: Taking or letting out fluids and/or gases from a body part

Explanation: The qualifier DIAGNOSTIC is used to identify drainage procedures that are biopsies

Body Part Character 4	Approach Character 5	Device Character 6	Qualifier Character 7
G Vagina ♀ K Hymen ♀	Ø Open 3 Percutaneous 4 Percutaneous Endoscopic 7 Via Natural or Artificial Opening 8 Via Natural or Artificial Opening Endoscopic X External	Ø Drainage Device	Z No Qualifier
G Vagina ♀ K Hymen ♀	Ø Open 3 Percutaneous 4 Percutaneous Endoscopic 7 Via Natural or Artificial Opening 8 Via Natural or Artificial Opening Endoscopic X External	Z No Device	X Diagnostic Z No Qualifier
J Clitoris ♀ L Vestibular Gland ♀ Bartholin's (greater vestibular) gland Greater vestibular (Bartholin's) gland Paraurethral (Skene's) gland Skene's (paraurethral) gland M Vulva ♀ Labia majora Labia minora	Ø Open X External	Ø Drainage Device	Z No Qualifier
J Clitoris ♀ L Vestibular Gland ♀ Bartholin's (greater vestibular) gland Greater vestibular (Bartholin's) gland Paraurethral (Skene's) gland Skene's (paraurethral) gland M Vulva ♀ Labia majora Labia minora	Ø Open X External	Z No Device	X Diagnostic Z No Qualifier

Non-OR ØU9G3ØZ
Non-OR ØU9K[Ø,3,4,7,8,X]ØZ
Non-OR ØU9G3ZZ
Non-OR ØU9K[Ø,3,4,7,8,X]ZZ
Non-OR ØU9L[Ø,X]ØZ
Non-OR ØU9L[Ø,X]ZZ
♀ All body part, approach, device, and qualifier values

Ø Medical and Surgical
U Female Reproductive System
B Excision Definition: Cutting out or off, without replacement, a portion of a body part
Explanation: The qualifier DIAGNOSTIC is used to identify excision procedures that are biopsies

Body Part Character 4	Approach Character 5	Device Character 6	Qualifier Character 7
Ø Ovary, Right ♀ **1 Ovary, Left** ♀ **2 Ovaries, Bilateral** ♀ **4 Uterine Supporting Structure** ♀ Broad ligament Infundibulopelvic ligament Ovarian ligament Round ligament of uterus **5 Fallopian Tube, Right** ♀ Oviduct Salpinx Uterine tube **6 Fallopian Tube, Left** ♀ *See 5 Fallopian Tube, Right* **7 Fallopian Tubes, Bilateral** ♀ **9 Uterus** ♀ Fundus uteri Myometrium Perimetrium Uterine cornu **C Cervix** ♀ **F Cul-de-sac** ♀	**Ø Open** **3 Percutaneous** **4 Percutaneous Endoscopic** **7 Via Natural or Artificial Opening** **8 Via Natural or Artificial Opening Endoscopic**	**Z No Device**	**X Diagnostic** **Z No Qualifier**
G Vagina ♀ **K Hymen** ♀	**Ø Open** **3 Percutaneous** **4 Percutaneous Endoscopic** **7 Via Natural or Artificial Opening** **8 Via Natural or Artificial Opening Endoscopic** **X External**	**Z No Device**	**X Diagnostic** **Z No Qualifier**
J Clitoris ♀ **L Vestibular Gland** ♀ Bartholin's (greater vestibular) gland Greater vestibular (Bartholin's) gland Paraurethral (Skene's) gland Skene's (paraurethral) gland **M Vulva** ♀ Labia majora Labia minora	**Ø Open** **X External**	**Z No Device**	**X Diagnostic** **Z No Qualifier**

♀ All body part, approach, device, and qualifier values

Ø Medical and Surgical
U Female Reproductive System
C Extirpation Definition: Taking or cutting out solid matter from a body part

Explanation: The solid matter may be an abnormal byproduct of a biological function or a foreign body; it may be imbedded in a body part or in the lumen of a tubular body part. The solid matter may or may not have been previously broken into pieces.

Body Part Character 4	Approach Character 5	Device Character 6	Qualifier Character 7
Ø Ovary, Right ♀ 1 Ovary, Left ♀ 2 Ovaries, Bilateral ♀ 4 Uterine Supporting Structure ♀ Broad ligament Infundibulopelvic ligament Ovarian ligament Round ligament of uterus	Ø Open 3 Percutaneous 4 Percutaneous Endoscopic 8 Via Natural or Artificial Opening Endoscopic	Z No Device	Z No Qualifier
5 Fallopian Tube, Right ♀ Oviduct Salpinx Uterine tube 6 Fallopian Tube, Left ♀ *See 5 Fallopian Tube, Right* 7 Fallopian Tubes, Bilateral ♀ 9 Uterus ♀ Fundus uteri Myometrium Perimetrium Uterine cornu B Endometrium ♀ C Cervix ♀ F Cul-de-sac ♀	Ø Open 3 Percutaneous 4 Percutaneous Endoscopic 7 Via Natural or Artificial Opening 8 Via Natural or Artificial Opening Endoscopic	Z No Device	Z No Qualifier
G Vagina ♀ K Hymen ♀	Ø Open 3 Percutaneous 4 Percutaneous Endoscopic 7 Via Natural or Artificial Opening 8 Via Natural or Artificial Opening Endoscopic X External	Z No Device	Z No Qualifier
J Clitoris ♀ L Vestibular Gland ♀ Bartholin's (greater vestibular) gland Greater vestibular (Bartholin's) gland Paraurethral (Skene's) gland Skene's (paraurethral) gland M Vulva ♀ Labia majora Labia minora	Ø Open X External	Z No Device	Z No Qualifier

Non-OR ØUC9[7,8]ZZ
Non-OR ØUCG[7,8,X]ZZ
Non-OR ØUCK[Ø,3,4,7,8,X]ZZ
Non-OR ØUCMXZZ
♀ All body part, approach, device, and qualifier values

Ø Medical and Surgical
U Female Reproductive System
D Extraction Definition: Pulling or stripping out or off all or a portion of a body part by the use of force

Explanation: The qualifier DIAGNOSTIC is used to identify extraction procedures that are biopsies

Body Part Character 4	Approach Character 5	Device Character 6	Qualifier Character 7
B Endometrium ♀	7 Via Natural or Artificial Opening 8 Via Natural or Artificial Opening Endoscopic	Z No Device	X Diagnostic Z No Qualifier
N Ova ♀	Ø Open 3 Percutaneous 4 Percutaneous Endoscopic	Z No Device	Z No Qualifier

♀ All body part, approach, device, and qualifier values

Ø Medical and Surgical
U Female Reproductive System
F Fragmentation Definition: Breaking solid matter in a body part into pieces

Explanation: Physical force (e.g., manual, ultrasonic) applied directly or indirectly is used to break the solid matter into pieces. The solid matter may be an abnormal byproduct of a biological function or a foreign body. The pieces of solid matter are not taken out.

Body Part Character 4	Approach Character 5	Device Character 6	Qualifier Character 7
5 Fallopian Tube, Right NC ♀ Oviduct Salpinx Uterine tube 6 Fallopian Tube, Left NC ♀ *See 5 Fallopian Tube, Right* 7 Fallopian Tubes, Bilateral NC ♀ 9 Uterus NC ♀ Fundus uteri Myometrium Perimetrium Uterine cornu	Ø Open 3 Percutaneous 4 Percutaneous Endoscopic 7 Via Natural or Artificial Opening 8 Via Natural or Artificial Opening Endoscopic X External	Z No Device	Z No Qualifier

Non-OR ØUF[5,6,7,9]XZZ
NC ØUF[5,6,7,9]XZZ
♀ All body part, approach, device, and qualifier values

Ø Medical and Surgical
U Female Reproductive System
H Insertion Definition: Putting in a nonbiological appliance that monitors, assists, performs, or prevents a physiological function but does not physically take the place of a body part

Explanation: None

Body Part Character 4	Approach Character 5	Device Character 6	Qualifier Character 7
3 Ovary ♀	Ø Open 3 Percutaneous 4 Percutaneous Endoscopic	1 Radioactive Element 3 Infusion Device Y Other Device	Z No Qualifier
3 Ovary ♀	7 Via Natural or Artificial Opening 8 Via Natural or Artificial Opening Endoscopic	1 Radioactive Element Y Other Device	Z No Qualifier
8 Fallopian Tube ♀ D Uterus and Cervix ♀ H Vagina and Cul-de-sac ♀	Ø Open 3 Percutaneous 4 Percutaneous Endoscopic 7 Via Natural or Artificial Opening 8 Via Natural or Artificial Opening Endoscopic	3 Infusion Device Y Other Device	Z No Qualifier
9 Uterus ♀ Fundus uteri Myometrium Perimetrium Uterine cornu	Ø Open 7 Via Natural or Artificial Opening 8 Via Natural or Artificial Opening Endoscopic	1 Radioactive Element H Contraceptive Device	Z No Qualifier
C Cervix ♀	Ø Open 3 Percutaneous 4 Percutaneous Endoscopic	1 Radioactive Element	Z No Qualifier
C Cervix ♀	7 Via Natural or Artificial Opening 8 Via Natural or Artificial Opening Endoscopic	1 Radioactive Element H Contraceptive Device	Z No Qualifier
F Cul-de-sac ♀	7 Via Natural or Artificial Opening 8 Via Natural or Artificial Opening Endoscopic	G Intraluminal Device, Pessary	Z No Qualifier
G Vagina ♀	Ø Open 3 Percutaneous 4 Percutaneous Endoscopic X External	1 Radioactive Element	Z No Qualifier
G Vagina ♀	7 Via Natural or Artificial Opening 8 Via Natural or Artificial Opening Endoscopic	1 Radioactive Element G Intraluminal Device, Pessary	Z No Qualifier

Non-OR ØUH3[Ø,3,4][3,Y]Z
Non-OR ØUH3[7,8]YZ
Non-OR ØUH[8,D][Ø,3,4,7,8][3,Y]Z
Non-OR ØUHH[3,4]YZ
Non-OR ØUHH[7,8][3,Y]Z
Non-OR ØUH9[Ø,7,8]HZ
Non-OR ØUHC[7,8]HZ
Non-OR ØUHF[7,8]GZ
Non-OR ØUHG[7,8]GZ
♀ All body part, approach, device, and qualifier values

Ø Medical and Surgical
U Female Reproductive System
J Inspection Definition: Visually and/or manually exploring a body part

Explanation: Visual exploration may be performed with or without optical instrumentation. Manual exploration may be performed directly or through intervening body layers.

Body Part Character 4	Approach Character 5	Device Character 6	Qualifier Character 7
3 Ovary ♀	**Ø Open** **3 Percutaneous** **4 Percutaneous Endoscopic** **8 Via Natural or Artificial Opening Endoscopic** **X External**	**Z No Device**	**Z No Qualifier**
8 Fallopian Tube ♀ **D Uterus and Cervix** ♀ **H Vagina and Cul-de-sac** ♀	**Ø Open** **3 Percutaneous** **4 Percutaneous Endoscopic** **7 Via Natural or Artificial Opening** **8 Via Natural or Artificial Opening Endoscopic** **X External**	**Z No Device**	**Z No Qualifier**
M Vulva ♀ Labia majora Labia minora	**Ø Open** **X External**	**Z No Device**	**Z No Qualifier**

Non-OR ØUJ3[3,8,X]ZZ
Non-OR ØUJ[8,D,H][3,7,8,X]ZZ
Non-OR ØUJMXZZ
♀ All body part, approach, device, and qualifier values

Ø Medical and Surgical
U Female Reproductive System
L Occlusion Definition: Completely closing an orifice or the lumen of a tubular body part

Explanation: The orifice can be a natural orifice or an artificially created orifice

Body Part Character 4	Approach Character 5	Device Character 6	Qualifier Character 7
5 Fallopian Tube, Right ♀ Oviduct Salpinx Uterine tube **6 Fallopian Tube, Left** ♀ *See 5 Fallopian Tube, Right* **7 Fallopian Tubes, Bilateral** NC ♀	**Ø Open** **3 Percutaneous** **4 Percutaneous Endoscopic**	**C Extraluminal Device** **D Intraluminal Device** **Z No Device**	**Z No Qualifier**
5 Fallopian Tube, Right ♀ Oviduct Salpinx Uterine tube **6 Fallopian Tube, Left** ♀ *See 5 Fallopian Tube, Right* **7 Fallopian Tubes, Bilateral** NC ♀	**7 Via Natural or Artificial Opening** **8 Via Natural or Artificial Opening Endoscopic**	**D Intraluminal Device** **Z No Device**	**Z No Qualifier**
F Cul-de-sac ♀ **G Vagina** ♀	**7 Via Natural or Artificial Opening** **8 Via Natural or Artificial Opening Endoscopic**	**D Intraluminal Device** **Z No Device**	**Z No Qualifier**

NC ØUL7[Ø,3,4][C,D,Z]Z with principal or secondary diagnosis of Z3Ø.2
NC ØUL7[7,8][D,Z]Z with principal or secondary diagnosis of Z3Ø.2
♀ All body part, approach, device, and qualifier values

Ø Medical and Surgical
U Female Reproductive System
M Reattachment Definition: Putting back in or on all or a portion of a separated body part to its normal location or other suitable location
Explanation: Vascular circulation and nervous pathways may or may not be reestablished

Body Part Character 4	Approach Character 5	Device Character 6	Qualifier Character 7
Ø Ovary, Right ♀ **1 Ovary, Left** ♀ **2 Ovaries, Bilateral** ♀ **4 Uterine Supporting Structure** ♀ Broad ligament Infundibulopelvic ligament Ovarian ligament Round ligament of uterus **5 Fallopian Tube, Right** ♀ Oviduct Salpinx Uterine tube **6 Fallopian Tube, Left** ♀ *See 5 Fallopian Tube, Right* **7 Fallopian Tubes, Bilateral** ♀ **9 Uterus** ♀ Fundus uteri Myometrium Perimetrium Uterine cornu **C Cervix** ♀ **F Cul-de-sac** ♀ **G Vagina** ♀	**Ø Open** **4 Percutaneous Endoscopic**	**Z No Device**	**Z No Qualifier**
J Clitoris ♀ **M Vulva** ♀ Labia majora Labia minora	**X External**	**Z No Device**	**Z No Qualifier**
K Hymen ♀	**Ø Open** **4 Percutaneous Endoscopic** **X External**	**Z No Device**	**Z No Qualifier**

♀ All body part, approach, device, and qualifier values

Ø Medical and Surgical
U Female Reproductive System
N Release Definition: Freeing a body part from an abnormal physical constraint by cutting or by the use of force
Explanation: Some of the restraining tissue may be taken out but none of the body part is taken out

Body Part Character 4	Approach Character 5	Device Character 6	Qualifier Character 7
Ø Ovary, Right ♀ **1 Ovary, Left** ♀ **2 Ovaries, Bilateral** ♀ **4 Uterine Supporting Structure** ♀ Broad ligament Infundibulopelvic ligament Ovarian ligament Round ligament of uterus	**Ø Open** **3 Percutaneous** **4 Percutaneous Endoscopic** **8 Via Natural or Artificial Opening Endoscopic**	**Z No Device**	**Z No Qualifier**
5 Fallopian Tube, Right ♀ Oviduct Salpinx Uterine tube **6 Fallopian Tube, Left** ♀ *See 5 Fallopian Tube, Right* **7 Fallopian Tubes, Bilateral** ♀ **9 Uterus** ♀ Fundus uteri Myometrium Perimetrium Uterine cornu **C Cervix** ♀ **F Cul-de-sac** ♀	**Ø Open** **3 Percutaneous** **4 Percutaneous Endoscopic** **7 Via Natural or Artificial Opening** **8 Via Natural or Artificial Opening Endoscopic**	**Z No Device**	**Z No Qualifier**
G Vagina ♀ **K Hymen** ♀	**Ø Open** **3 Percutaneous** **4 Percutaneous Endoscopic** **7 Via Natural or Artificial Opening** **8 Via Natural or Artificial Opening Endoscopic** **X External**	**Z No Device**	**Z No Qualifier**
J Clitoris ♀ **L Vestibular Gland** ♀ Bartholin's (greater vestibular) gland Greater vestibular (Bartholin's) gland Paraurethral (Skene's) gland Skene's (paraurethral) gland **M Vulva** ♀ Labia majora Labia minora	**Ø Open** **X External**	**Z No Device**	**Z No Qualifier**

♀ All body part, approach, device, and qualifier values

Ø Medical and Surgical
U Female Reproductive System
P Removal Definition: Taking out or off a device from a body part

Explanation: If a device is taken out and a similar device put in without cutting or puncturing the skin or mucous membrane, the procedure is coded to the root operation CHANGE. Otherwise, the procedure for taking out the device is coded to the root operation REMOVAL.

Body Part Character 4	Approach Character 5	Device Character 6	Qualifier Character 7
3 Ovary ♀	Ø Open 3 Percutaneous 4 Percutaneous Endoscopic	Ø Drainage Device 3 Infusion Device Y Other Device	Z No Qualifier
3 Ovary ♀	7 Via Natural or Artificial Opening 8 Via Natural or Artificial Opening Endoscopic	Y Other Device	Z No Qualifier
3 Ovary ♀	X External	Ø Drainage Device 3 Infusion Device	Z No Qualifier
8 Fallopian Tube ♀	Ø Open 3 Percutaneous 4 Percutaneous Endoscopic 7 Via Natural or Artificial Opening 8 Via Natural or Artificial Opening Endoscopic	Ø Drainage Device 3 Infusion Device 7 Autologous Tissue Substitute C Extraluminal Device D Intraluminal Device J Synthetic Substitute K Nonautologous Tissue Substitute Y Other Device	Z No Qualifier
8 Fallopian Tube ♀	X External	Ø Drainage Device 3 Infusion Device D Intraluminal Device	Z No Qualifier
D Uterus and Cervix ♀	Ø Open 3 Percutaneous 4 Percutaneous Endoscopic 7 Via Natural or Artificial Opening 8 Via Natural or Artificial Opening Endoscopic	Ø Drainage Device 1 Radioactive Element 3 Infusion Device 7 Autologous Tissue Substitute C Extraluminal Device D Intraluminal Device H Contraceptive Device J Synthetic Substitute K Nonautologous Tissue Substitute Y Other Device	Z No Qualifier
D Uterus and Cervix ♀	X External	Ø Drainage Device 3 Infusion Device D Intraluminal Device H Contraceptive Device	Z No Qualifier
H Vagina and Cul-de-sac ♀	Ø Open 3 Percutaneous 4 Percutaneous Endoscopic 7 Via Natural or Artificial Opening 8 Via Natural or Artificial Opening Endoscopic	Ø Drainage Device 1 Radioactive Element 3 Infusion Device 7 Autologous Tissue Substitute D Intraluminal Device J Synthetic Substitute K Nonautologous Tissue Substitute Y Other Device	Z No Qualifier
H Vagina and Cul-de-sac ♀	X External	Ø Drainage Device 1 Radioactive Element 3 Infusion Device D Intraluminal Device	Z No Qualifier
M Vulva Labia majora Labia minora ♀	Ø Open	Ø Drainage Device 7 Autologous Tissue Substitute J Synthetic Substitute K Nonautologous Tissue Substitute	Z No Qualifier
M Vulva Labia majora Labia minora ♀	X External	Ø Drainage Device	Z No Qualifier

Non-OR ØUP3[3,4]YZ
Non-OR ØUP3[7,8]YZ
Non-OR ØUP3X[Ø,3]Z
Non-OR ØUP8[3,4]YZ
Non-OR ØUP8[7,8][Ø,3,D,Y]Z
Non-OR ØUP8X[Ø,3,D]Z
Non-OR ØUPD[3,4][C,Y]Z
Non-OR ØUPD[7,8][Ø,3,C,D,H,Y]Z
Non-OR ØUPDX[Ø,3,D,H]Z
Non-OR ØUPH[3,4]YZ
Non-OR ØUPH[7,8][Ø,3,D,Y]Z
Non-OR ØUPHX[Ø,1,3,D]Z
Non-OR ØUPMXØZ
♀ All body part, approach, device, and qualifier values

Ø Medical and Surgical
U Female Reproductive System
Q Repair Definition: Restoring, to the extent possible, a body part to its normal anatomic structure and function
Explanation: Used only when the method to accomplish the repair is not one of the other root operations

Body Part Character 4	Approach Character 5	Device Character 6	Qualifier Character 7
Ø Ovary, Right ♀ **1 Ovary, Left** ♀ **2 Ovaries, Bilateral** ♀ **4 Uterine Supporting Structure** ♀ Broad ligament Infundibulopelvic ligament Ovarian ligament Round ligament of uterus	**Ø Open** **3 Percutaneous** **4 Percutaneous Endoscopic** **8 Via Natural or Artificial Opening Endoscopic**	**Z No Device**	**Z No Qualifier**
5 Fallopian Tube, Right ♀ Oviduct Salpinx Uterine tube **6 Fallopian Tube, Left** ♀ *See 5 Fallopian Tube, Right* **7 Fallopian Tubes, Bilateral** ♀ **9 Uterus** ♀ Fundus uteri Myometrium Perimetrium Uterine cornu **C Cervix** ♀ **F Cul-de-sac** ♀	**Ø Open** **3 Percutaneous** **4 Percutaneous Endoscopic** **7 Via Natural or Artificial Opening** **8 Via Natural or Artificial Opening Endoscopic**	**Z No Device**	**Z No Qualifier**
G Vagina ♀ **K Hymen** ♀	**Ø Open** **3 Percutaneous** **4 Percutaneous Endoscopic** **7 Via Natural or Artificial Opening** **8 Via Natural or Artificial Opening Endoscopic** **X External**	**Z No Device**	**Z No Qualifier**
J Clitoris ♀ **L Vestibular Gland** ♀ Bartholin's (greater vestibular) gland Greater vestibular (Bartholin's) gland Paraurethral (Skene's) gland Skene's (paraurethral) gland **M Vulva** ♀ Labia majora Labia minora	**Ø Open** **X External**	**Z No Device**	**Z No Qualifier**

Non-OR ØUQG[7,X]ZZ
Non-OR ØUQKXZZ
Non-OR ØUQMXZZ
♀ All body part, approach, device, and qualifier values

Ø Medical and Surgical
U Female Reproductive System
S Reposition Definition: Moving to its normal location, or other suitable location, all or a portion of a body part
Explanation: The body part is moved to a new location from an abnormal location, or from a normal location where it is not functioning correctly. The body part may or may not be cut out or off to be moved to the new location.

Body Part Character 4	Approach Character 5	Device Character 6	Qualifier Character 7
Ø Ovary, Right ♀ **1 Ovary, Left** ♀ **2 Ovaries, Bilateral** ♀ **4 Uterine Supporting Structure** ♀ Broad ligament Infundibulopelvic ligament Ovarian ligament Round ligament of uterus **5 Fallopian Tube, Right** ♀ Oviduct Salpinx Uterine tube **6 Fallopian Tube, Left** ♀ *See 5 Fallopian Tube, Right* **7 Fallopian Tubes, Bilateral** ♀ **C Cervix** ♀ **F Cul-de-sac** ♀	**Ø Open** **4 Percutaneous Endoscopic** **8 Via Natural or Artificial Opening Endoscopic**	**Z No Device**	**Z No Qualifier**
9 Uterus ♀ Fundus uteri Myometrium Perimetrium Uterine cornu **G Vagina** ♀	**Ø Open** **4 Percutaneous Endoscopic** **7 Via Natural or Artificial Opening** **8 Via Natural or Artificial Opening Endoscopic** **X External**	**Z No Device**	**Z No Qualifier**

Non-OR ØUS9XZZ
♀ All body part, approach, device, and qualifier values

Ø Medical and Surgical
U Female Reproductive System
T Resection Definition: Cutting out or off, without replacement, all of a body part
Explanation: None

Body Part Character 4	Approach Character 5	Device Character 6	Qualifier Character 7
Ø Ovary, Right ♀ **1 Ovary, Left** ♀ **2 Ovaries, Bilateral** ⊞♀ **5 Fallopian Tube, Right** ♀ Oviduct Salpinx Uterine tube **6 Fallopian Tube, Left** ♀ *See 5 Fallopian Tube, Right* **7 Fallopian Tubes, Bilateral** ⊞♀	**Ø Open** **4 Percutaneous Endoscopic** **7 Via Natural or Artificial Opening** **8 Via Natural or Artificial Opening Endoscopic** **F Via Natural or Artificial Opening With Percutaneous Endoscopic Assistance**	**Z No Device**	**Z No Qualifier**
4 Uterine Supporting Structure ⊞♀ Broad ligament Infundibulopelvic ligament Ovarian ligament Round ligament of uterus **C Cervix** ⊞♀ **F Cul-de-sac** ♀ **G Vagina** ⊞♀	**Ø Open** **4 Percutaneous Endoscopic** **7 Via Natural or Artificial Opening** **8 Via Natural or Artificial Opening Endoscopic**	**Z No Device**	**Z No Qualifier**
9 Uterus ⊞♀ Fundus uteri Myometrium Perimetrium Uterine cornu	**Ø Open** **4 Percutaneous Endoscopic** **7 Via Natural or Artificial Opening** **8 Via Natural or Artificial Opening Endoscopic** **F Via Natural or Artificial Opening With Percutaneous Endoscopic Assistance**	**Z No Device**	**L Supracervical** **Z No Qualifier**
J Clitoris ♀ **L Vestibular Gland** ♀ Bartholin's (greater vestibular) gland Greater vestibular (Bartholin's) gland Paraurethral (Skene's) gland Skene's (paraurethral) gland **M Vulva** ⊞♀ Labia majora Labia minora	**Ø Open** **X External**	**Z No Device**	**Z No Qualifier**
K Hymen ♀	**Ø Open** **4 Percutaneous Endoscopic** **7 Via Natural or Artificial Opening** **8 Via Natural or Artificial Opening Endoscopic** **X External**	**Z No Device**	**Z No Device**

♀ All body part, approach, device, and qualifier values

See Appendix L for Procedure Combinations
⊞ ØUT[2,7]ØZZ
⊞ ØUT[4,C][Ø,4,7,8]ZZ
⊞ ØUTGØZZ
⊞ ØUT9[Ø,4,7,8,F]ZZ
⊞ ØUTM[Ø,X]ZZ

Ø Medical and Surgical
U Female Reproductive System
U Supplement Definition: Putting in or on biological or synthetic material that physically reinforces and/or augments the function of a portion of a body part

Explanation: The biological material is non-living, or is living and from the same individual. The body part may have been previously replaced, and the SUPPLEMENT procedure is performed to physically reinforce and/or augment the function of the replaced body part.

Body Part Character 4	Approach Character 5	Device Character 6	Qualifier Character 7
4 Uterine Supporting Structure ♀ Broad ligament Infundibulopelvic ligament Ovarian ligament Round ligament of uterus	**Ø Open** **4 Percutaneous Endoscopic**	**7 Autologous Tissue Substitute** **J Synthetic Substitute** **K Nonautologous Tissue Substitute**	**Z No Qualifier**
5 Fallopian Tube, Right ♀ Oviduct Salpinx Uterine tube **6 Fallopian Tube, Left** ♀ *See 5 Fallopian Tube, Right* **7 Fallopian Tubes, Bilateral** ♀ **F Cul-de-sac** ♀	**Ø Open** **4 Percutaneous Endoscopic** **7 Via Natural or Artificial Opening** **8 Via Natural or Artificial Opening Endoscopic**	**7 Autologous Tissue Substitute** **J Synthetic Substitute** **K Nonautologous Tissue Substitute**	**Z No Qualifier**
G Vagina ♀ **K Hymen** ♀	**Ø Open** **4 Percutaneous Endoscopic** **7 Via Natural or Artificial Opening** **8 Via Natural or Artificial Opening Endoscopic** **X External**	**7 Autologous Tissue Substitute** **J Synthetic Substitute** **K Nonautologous Tissue Substitute**	**Z No Qualifier**
J Clitoris ♀ **M Vulva** ♀ Labia majora Labia minora	**Ø Open** **X External**	**7 Autologous Tissue Substitute** **J Synthetic Substitute** **K Nonautologous Tissue Substitute**	**Z No Qualifier**

♀ All body part, approach, device, and qualifier values

Ø Medical and Surgical
U Female Reproductive System
V Restriction Definition: Partially closing an orifice or the lumen of a tubular body part

Explanation: The orifice can be a natural orifice or an artificially created orifice

Body Part Character 4	Approach Character 5	Device Character 6	Qualifier Character 7
C Cervix ♀	**Ø Open** **3 Percutaneous** **4 Percutaneous Endoscopic**	**C Extraluminal Device** **D Intraluminal Device** **Z No Device**	**Z No Qualifier**
C Cervix ♀	**7 Via Natural or Artificial Opening** **8 Via Natural or Artificial Opening Endoscopic**	**D Intraluminal Device** **Z No Device**	**Z No Qualifier**

♀ All body part, approach, device, and qualifier values

Ø Medical and Surgical
U Female Reproductive System
W Revision Definition: Correcting, to the extent possible, a portion of a malfunctioning device or the position of a displaced device

Explanation: Revision can include correcting a malfunctioning or displaced device by taking out or putting in components of the device such as a screw or pin

Body Part Character 4	Approach Character 5	Device Character 6	Qualifier Character 7
3 Ovary ♀	**Ø Open** **3 Percutaneous** **4 Percutaneous Endoscopic**	**Ø Drainage Device** **3 Infusion Device** **Y Other Device**	**Z No Qualifier**
3 Ovary ♀	**7 Via Natural or Artificial Opening** **8 Via Natural or Artificial Opening Endoscopic**	**Y Other Device**	**Z No Qualifier**
3 Ovary ♀	**X External**	**Ø Drainage Device** **3 Infusion Device**	**Z No Qualifier**
8 Fallopian Tube ♀	**Ø Open** **3 Percutaneous** **4 Percutaneous Endoscopic** **7 Via Natural or Artificial Opening** **8 Via Natural or Artificial Opening Endoscopic**	**Ø Drainage Device** **3 Infusion Device** **7 Autologous Tissue Substitute** **C Extraluminal Device** **D Intraluminal Device** **J Synthetic Substitute** **K Nonautologous Tissue Substitute** **Y Other Device**	**Z No Qualifier**
8 Fallopian Tube ♀	**X External**	**Ø Drainage Device** **3 Infusion Device** **7 Autologous Tissue Substitute** **C Extraluminal Device** **D Intraluminal Device** **J Synthetic Substitute** **K Nonautologous Tissue Substitute**	**Z No Qualifier**
D Uterus and Cervix ♀	**Ø Open** **3 Percutaneous** **4 Percutaneous Endoscopic** **7 Via Natural or Artificial Opening** **8 Via Natural or Artificial Opening Endoscopic**	**Ø Drainage Device** **1 Radioactive Element** **3 Infusion Device** **7 Autologous Tissue Substitute** **C Extraluminal Device** **D Intraluminal Device** **H Contraceptive Device** **J Synthetic Substitute** **K Nonautologous Tissue Substitute** **Y Other Device**	**Z No Qualifier**
D Uterus and Cervix ♀	**X External**	**Ø Drainage Device** **3 Infusion Device** **7 Autologous Tissue Substitute** **C Extraluminal Device** **D Intraluminal Device** **H Contraceptive Device** **J Synthetic Substitute** **K Nonautologous Tissue Substitute**	**Z No Qualifier**
H Vagina and Cul-de-sac ♀	**Ø Open** **3 Percutaneous** **4 Percutaneous Endoscopic** **7 Via Natural or Artificial Opening** **8 Via Natural or Artificial Opening Endoscopic**	**Ø Drainage Device** **1 Radioactive Element** **3 Infusion Device** **7 Autologous Tissue Substitute** **D Intraluminal Device** **J Synthetic Substitute** **K Nonautologous Tissue Substitute** **Y Other Device**	**Z No Qualifier**
H Vagina and Cul-de-sac ♀	**X External**	**Ø Drainage Device** **3 Infusion Device** **7 Autologous Tissue Substitute** **D Intraluminal Device** **J Synthetic Substitute** **K Nonautologous Tissue Substitute**	**Z No Qualifier**
M Vulva ♀ Labia majora Labia minora	**Ø Open** **X External**	**Ø Drainage Device** **7 Autologous Tissue Substitute** **J Synthetic Substitute** **K Nonautologous Tissue Substitute**	**Z No Qualifier**

Non-OR ØUW3[3,4]YZ
Non-OR ØUW3[7,8]YZ
Non-OR ØUW3X[Ø,3]Z
Non-OR ØUW8[3,4,7,8]YZ
Non-OR ØUW8X[Ø,3,7,C,D,J,K]Z
Non-OR ØUWD[3,4,7,8]YZ
Non-OR ØUWDX[Ø,3,7,C,D,H,J,K]Z
Non-OR ØUWH[3,4,7,8]YZ
Non-OR ØUWHX[Ø,3,7,D,J,K]Z
Non-OR ØUWMX[Ø,7,J,K]Z
♀ All body part, approach, device, and qualifier values

Ø Medical and Surgical
U Female Reproductive System
Y Transplantation Definition: Putting in or on all or a portion of a living body part taken from another individual or animal to physically take the place and/or function of all or a portion of a similar body part

Explanation: The native body part may or may not be taken out, and the transplanted body part may take over all or a portion of its function

Body Part Character 4	Approach Character 5	Device Character 6	Qualifier Character 7
Ø Ovary, Right ♀ **1** Ovary, Left ♀ **9** Uterus ♀	**Ø** Open	**Z** No Device	**Ø** Allogeneic **1** Syngeneic **2** Zooplastic

♀ All body part, approach, device, and qualifier values

Male Reproductive System ØV1–ØVX

Character Meanings

This Character Meaning table is provided as a guide to assist the user in the identification of character members that may be found in this section of code tables. It **SHOULD NOT** be used to build a PCS code.

Operation–Character 3	Body Part–Character 4	Approach–Character 5	Device–Character 6	Qualifier–Character 7
1 Bypass	Ø Prostate	Ø Open	Ø Drainage Device	Ø Allogeneic
2 Change	1 Seminal Vesicle, Right	3 Percutaneous	1 Radioactive Element	1 Syngeneic
5 Destruction	2 Seminal Vesicle, Left	4 Percutaneous Endoscopic	3 Infusion Device	2 Zooplastic
7 Dilation	3 Seminal Vesicles, Bilateral	7 Via Natural or Artificial Opening	7 Autologous Tissue Substitute	D Urethra
9 Drainage	4 Prostate and Seminal Vesicles	8 Via Natural or Artificial Opening Endoscopic	C Extraluminal Device	J Epididymis, Right
B Excision	5 Scrotum	X External	D Intraluminal Device	K Epididymis, Left
C Extirpation	6 Tunica Vaginalis, Right		J Synthetic Substitute	N Vas Deferens, Right
H Insertion	7 Tunica Vaginalis, Left		K Nonautologous Tissue Substitute	P Vas Deferens, Left
J Inspection	8 Scrotum and Tunica Vaginalis		Y Other Device	S Penis
L Occlusion	9 Testis, Right		Z No Device	X Diagnostic
M Reattachment	B Testis, Left			Z No Qualifier
N Release	C Testes, Bilateral			
P Removal	D Testis			
Q Repair	F Spermatic Cord, Right			
R Replacement	G Spermatic Cord, Left			
S Reposition	H Spermatic Cords, Bilateral			
T Resection	J Epididymis, Right			
U Supplement	K Epididymis, Left			
W Revision	L Epididymis, Bilateral			
X Transfer	M Epididymis and Spermatic Cord			
Y Transplantation	N Vas Deferens, Right			
	P Vas Deferens, Left			
	Q Vas Deferens, Bilateral			
	R Vas Deferens			
	S Penis			
	T Prepuce			

AHA Coding Clinic for table ØV1
2018, 3Q, 12 Al-Ghorab distal penile shunt surgery

AHA Coding Clinic for table ØV9
2018, 3Q, 12 Al-Ghorab distal penile shunt surgery

AHA Coding Clinic for table ØVB
2020, 1Q, 31 Repair of buried penis
2019, 3Q, 18 Radical prostatectomy and lymph node dissection with biopsy of neurovascular bundle
2016, 1Q, 23 Transurethral resection of ejaculatory ducts
2014, 4Q, 33 Radical prostatectomy

AHA Coding Clinic for table ØVP
2016, 2Q, 28 Removal of multi-component inflatable penile prosthesis with placement of new malleable device

AHA Coding Clinic for table ØVQ
2018, 3Q, 12 Al-Ghorab distal penile shunt surgery

AHA Coding Clinic for table ØVT
2019, 3Q, 18 Radical prostatectomy and lymph node dissection with biopsy of neurovascular bundle
2014, 4Q, 33 Radical prostatectomy

AHA Coding Clinic for table ØVU
2020, 1Q, 31 Repair of buried penis
2016, 2Q, 28 Removal of multi-component inflatable penile prosthesis with placement of new malleable device
2015, 3Q, 25 Placement of inflatable penile prosthesis

AHA Coding Clinic for table ØVX
2018, 4Q, 40 Transfer of prepuce

Male Reproductive System

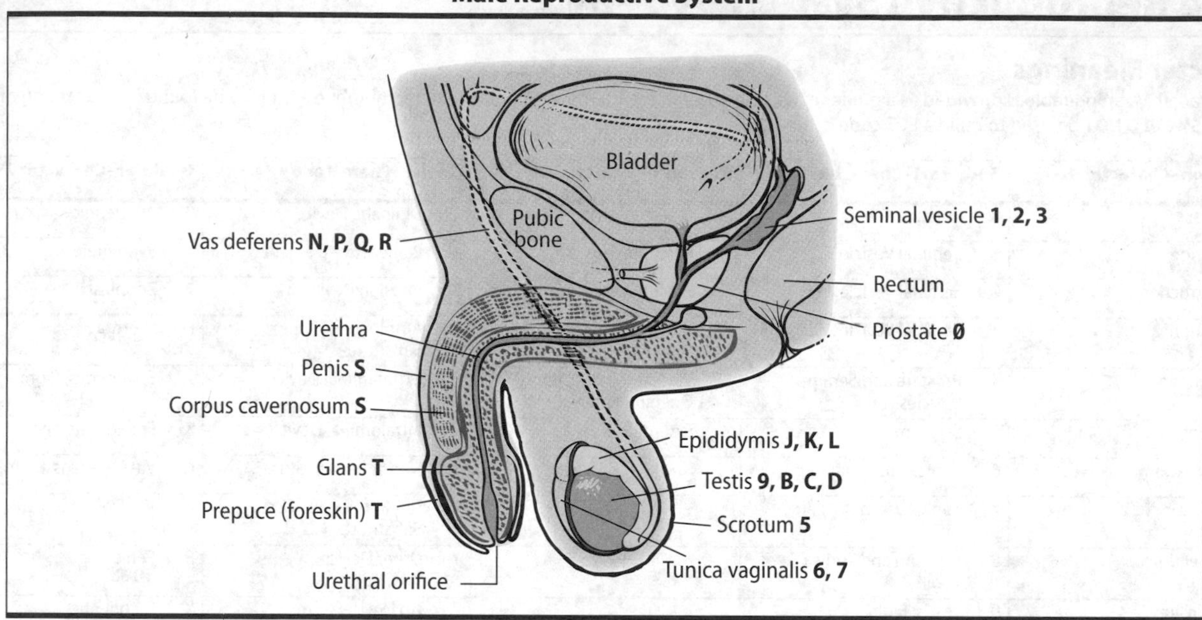

Penis

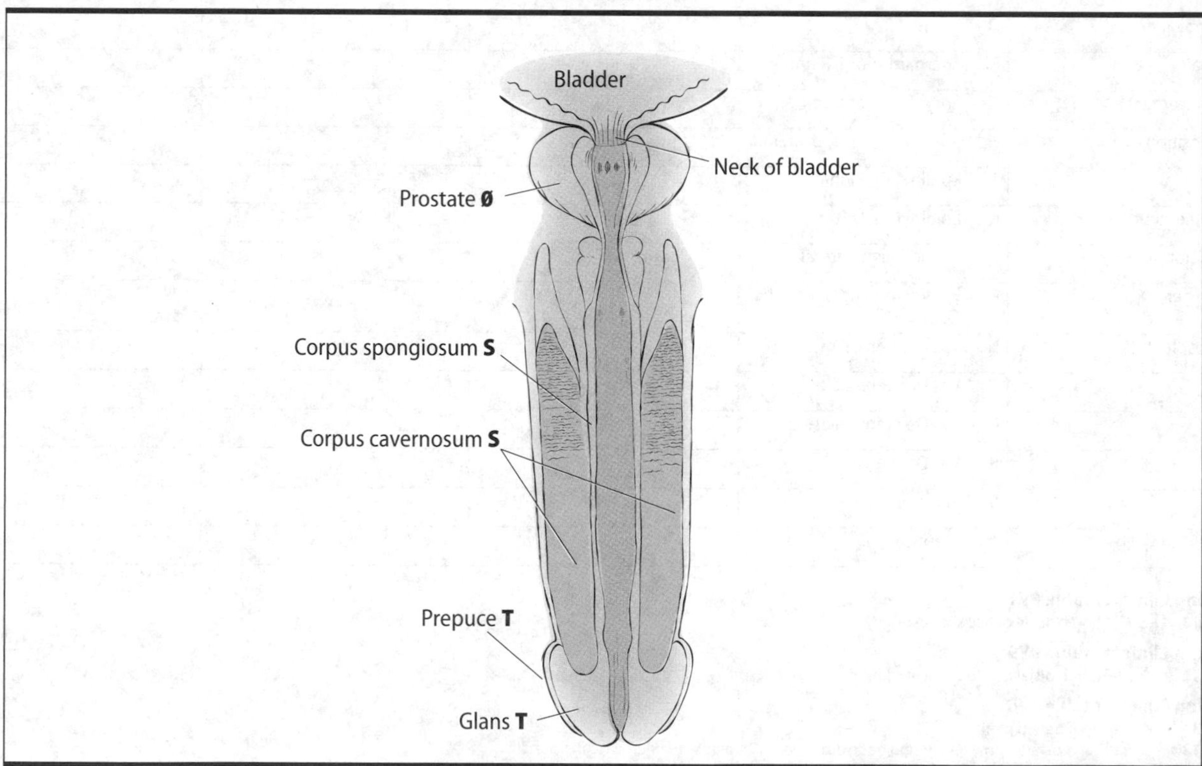

Ø Medical and Surgical
V Male Reproductive System
1 Bypass Definition: Altering the route of passage of the contents of a tubular body part

Explanation: Rerouting contents of a body part to a downstream area of the normal route, to a similar route and body part, or to an abnormal route and dissimilar body part. Includes one or more anastomoses, with or without the use of a device.

Body Part Character 4	Approach Character 5	Device Character 6	Qualifier Character 7
N Vas Deferens, Right ♂ Ductus deferens Ejaculatory duct P Vas Deferens, Left ♂ *See N Vas Deferens, Right* Q Vas Deferens, Bilateral ♂ *See N Vas Deferens, Right*	Ø Open 4 Percutaneous Endoscopic	7 Autologous Tissue Substitute J Synthetic Substitute K Nonautologous Tissue Substitute Z No Device	J Epididymis, Right K Epididymis, Left N Vas Deferens, Right P Vas Deferens, Left

♂ All body part, approach, device, and qualifier values

Ø Medical and Surgical
V Male Reproductive System
2 Change Definition: Taking out or off a device from a body part and putting back an identical or similar device in or on the same body part without cutting or puncturing the skin or a mucous membrane

Explanation: All CHANGE procedures are coded using the approach EXTERNAL

Body Part Character 4	Approach Character 5	Device Character 6	Qualifier Character 7
4 Prostate and Seminal Vesicles ♂ 8 Scrotum and Tunica Vaginalis ♂ D Testis ♂ M Epididymis and Spermatic Cord ♂ R Vas Deferens ♂ Ductus deferens Ejaculatory duct S Penis ♂ Corpus cavernosum Corpus spongiosum	X External	Ø Drainage Device Y Other Device	Z No Qualifier

Non-OR All body part, approach, device, and qualifier values
♂ All body part, approach, device, and qualifier values

Ø Medical and Surgical
V Male Reproductive System
5 Destruction Definition: Physical eradication of all or a portion of a body part by the direct use of energy, force, or a destructive agent

Explanation: None of the body part is physically taken out

Body Part Character 4	Approach Character 5	Device Character 6	Qualifier Character 7
Ø Prostate ♂	Ø Open 3 Percutaneous 4 Percutaneous Endoscopic 7 Via Natural or Artificial Opening 8 Via Natural or Artificial Opening Endoscopic	Z No Device	Z No Qualifier
1 Seminal Vesicle, Right ♂ 2 Seminal Vesicle, Left ♂ 3 Seminal Vesicles, Bilateral ♂ 6 Tunica Vaginalis, Right ♂ 7 Tunica Vaginalis, Left ♂ 9 Testis, Right ♂ B Testis, Left ♂ C Testes, Bilateral ♂	Ø Open 3 Percutaneous 4 Percutaneous Endoscopic	Z No Device	Z No Qualifier
5 Scrotum ♂ S Penis ♂ Corpus cavernosum Corpus spongiosum T Prepuce ♂ Foreskin Glans penis	Ø Open 3 Percutaneous 4 Percutaneous Endoscopic X External	Z No Device	Z No Qualifier
F Spermatic Cord, Right ♂ G Spermatic Cord, Left ♂ H Spermatic Cords, Bilateral ♂ J Epididymis, Right ♂ K Epididymis, Left ♂ L Epididymis, Bilateral ♂ N Vas Deferens, Right NC ♂ Ductus deferens Ejaculatory duct P Vas Deferens, Left NC ♂ *See N Vas Deferens, Right* Q Vas Deferens, Bilateral NC ♂ *See N Vas Deferens, Right*	Ø Open 3 Percutaneous 4 Percutaneous Endoscopic 8 Via Natural or Artificial Opening Endoscopic	Z No Device	Z No Qualifier

Non-OR ØV55[Ø,3,4,X]ZZ
Non-OR ØV5[N,P,Q][Ø,3,4,8]ZZ
NC ØV5[N,P,Q][Ø,3,4]ZZ with principal or secondary diagnosis of Z3Ø.2
♂ All body part, approach, device, and qualifier values

Ø Medical and Surgical
V Male Reproductive System
7 Dilation Definition: Expanding an orifice or the lumen of a tubular body part

Explanation: The orifice can be a natural orifice or an artificially created orifice. Accomplished by stretching a tubular body part using intraluminal pressure or by cutting part of the orifice or wall of the tubular body part.

Body Part Character 4	Approach Character 5	Device Character 6	Qualifier Character 7
N Vas Deferens, Right ♂ Ductus deferens Ejaculatory duct P Vas Deferens, Left ♂ *See* N Vas Deferens, Right Q Vas Deferens, Bilateral ♂ *See* N Vas Deferens, Right	Ø Open 3 Percutaneous 4 Percutaneous Endoscopic	D Intraluminal Device Z No Device	Z No Qualifier

♂ All body part, approach, device, and qualifier values

Ø Medical and Surgical
V Male Reproductive System
9 Drainage Definition: Taking or letting out fluids and/or gases from a body part

Explanation: The qualifier DIAGNOSTIC is used to identify drainage procedures that are biopsies

Body Part Character 4	Approach Character 5	Device Character 6	Qualifier Character 7
Ø Prostate ♂	Ø Open 3 Percutaneous 4 Percutaneous Endoscopic 7 Via Natural or Artificial Opening 8 Via Natural or Artificial Opening Endoscopic	Ø Drainage Device	Z No Qualifier
Ø Prostate ♂	Ø Open 3 Percutaneous 4 Percutaneous Endoscopic 7 Via Natural or Artificial Opening 8 Via Natural or Artificial Opening Endoscopic	Z No Device	X Diagnostic Z No Qualifier
1 Seminal Vesicle, Right ♂ 2 Seminal Vesicle, Left ♂ 3 Seminal Vesicles, Bilateral ♂ 6 Tunica Vaginalis, Right ♂ 7 Tunica Vaginalis, Left ♂ 9 Testis, Right ♂ B Testis, Left ♂ C Testes, Bilateral ♂ F Spermatic Cord, Right ♂ G Spermatic Cord, Left ♂ H Spermatic Cords, Bilateral ♂ J Epididymis, Right ♂ K Epididymis, Left ♂ L Epididymis, Bilateral ♂ N Vas Deferens, Right ♂ Ductus deferens Ejaculatory duct P Vas Deferens, Left ♂ *See* N Vas Deferens, Right Q Vas Deferens, Bilateral ♂ *See* N Vas Deferens, Right	Ø Open 3 Percutaneous 4 Percutaneous Endoscopic	Ø Drainage Device	Z No Qualifier

Non-OR ØV9Ø[3,4]ØZ
Non-OR ØV9Ø[3,4]Z[X,Z]
Non-OR ØV9Ø[7,8]ZX
Non-OR ØV9[1,2,3,9,B,C][3,4]ØZ
Non-OR ØV9[6,7,F,G,H,N,P,Q][Ø,3,4]ØZ
Non-OR ØV9[J,K,L]3ØZ
♂ All body part, approach, device, and qualifier values

ØV9 Continued on next page

ØV9 Continued

Ø Medical and Surgical
V Male Reproductive System
9 Drainage Definition: Taking or letting out fluids and/or gases from a body part
Explanation: The qualifier DIAGNOSTIC is used to identify drainage procedures that are biopsies

Body Part Character 4	Approach Character 5	Device Character 6	Qualifier Character 7
1 Seminal Vesicle, Right ♂ 2 Seminal Vesicle, Left ♂ 3 Seminal Vesicles, Bilateral ♂ 6 Tunica Vaginalis, Right ♂ 7 Tunica Vaginalis, Left ♂ 9 Testis, Right ♂ B Testis, Left ♂ C Testes, Bilateral ♂ F Spermatic Cord, Right ♂ G Spermatic Cord, Left ♂ H Spermatic Cords, Bilateral ♂ J Epididymis, Right ♂ K Epididymis, Left ♂ L Epididymis, Bilateral ♂ N Vas Deferens, Right ♂ Ductus deferens Ejaculatory duct P Vas Deferens, Left ♂ *See N Vas Deferens, Right* Q Vas Deferens, Bilateral ♂ *See N Vas Deferens, Right*	Ø Open 3 Percutaneous 4 Percutaneous Endoscopic	Z No Device	X Diagnostic Z No Qualifier
5 Scrotum ♂ S Penis ♂ Corpus cavernosum Corpus spongiosum T Prepuce ♂ Foreskin Glans penis	Ø Open 3 Percutaneous 4 Percutaneous Endoscopic X External	Ø Drainage Device	Z No Qualifier
5 Scrotum ♂ S Penis ♂ Corpus cavernosum Corpus spongiosum T Prepuce ♂ Foreskin Glans penis	Ø Open 3 Percutaneous 4 Percutaneous Endoscopic X External	Z No Device	X Diagnostic Z No Qualifier

Non-OR ØV9[1,2,3,9,B,C][3,4]Z[X,Z]
Non-OR ØV9[6,7,F,G,H,J,K,L,N,P,Q][Ø,3,4]ZX
Non-OR ØV9[6,7,F,G,H,N,P,Q][Ø,3,4]ZZ
Non-OR ØV9[J,K,L]3ZZ
Non-OR ØV95[Ø,3,4,X]ØZ
Non-OR ØV9[S,T]3ØZ
Non-OR ØV95ØZX
Non-OR ØV95[3,4,X]Z[X,Z]
Non-OR ØV9[S,T]3ZZ
♂ All body part, approach, device, and qualifier values

Ø Medical and Surgical
V Male Reproductive System
B Excision Definition: Cutting out or off, without replacement, a portion of a body part
Explanation: The qualifier DIAGNOSTIC is used to identify excision procedures that are biopsies

Body Part Character 4	Approach Character 5	Device Character 6	Qualifier Character 7
Ø Prostate ♂	**Ø Open** **3 Percutaneous** **4 Percutaneous Endoscopic** **7 Via Natural or Artificial Opening** **8 Via Natural or Artificial Opening Endoscopic**	**Z No Device**	**X Diagnostic** **Z No Qualifier**
1 Seminal Vesicle, Right ♂ **2 Seminal Vesicle, Left** ♂ **3 Seminal Vesicles, Bilateral** ♂ **6 Tunica Vaginalis, Right** ♂ **7 Tunica Vaginalis, Left** ♂ **9 Testis, Right** ♂ **B Testis, Left** ♂ **C Testes, Bilateral** ♂	**Ø Open** **3 Percutaneous** **4 Percutaneous Endoscopic**	**Z No Device**	**X Diagnostic** **Z No Qualifier**
5 Scrotum ♂ **S Penis** ♂ Corpus cavernosum Corpus spongiosum **T Prepuce** ♂ Foreskin Glans penis	**Ø Open** **3 Percutaneous** **4 Percutaneous Endoscopic** **X External**	**Z No Device**	**X Diagnostic** **Z No Qualifier**
F Spermatic Cord, Right ♂ **G Spermatic Cord, Left** ♂ **H Spermatic Cords, Bilateral** ♂ **J Epididymis, Right** ♂ **K Epididymis, Left** ♂ **L Epididymis, Bilateral** ♂ **N Vas Deferens, Right** NC ♂ Ductus deferens Ejaculatory duct **P Vas Deferens, Left** NC ♂ *See* *N Vas Deferens, Right* **Q Vas Deferens, Bilateral** NC ♂ *See* *N Vas Deferens, Right*	**Ø Open** **3 Percutaneous** **4 Percutaneous Endoscopic** **8 Via Natural or Artificial Opening Endoscopic**	**Z No Device**	**X Diagnostic** **Z No Qualifier**

Non-OR ØVBØ[3,4,7,8]ZX
Non-OR ØVB[1,2,3,9,B,C][3,4]ZX
Non-OR ØVB[6,7][Ø,3,4]ZX
Non-OR ØVB5ØZX
Non-OR ØVB5[3,4,X]Z[X,Z]
Non-OR ØVB[F,G,H,J,K,L][Ø,3,4,8]ZX
Non-OR ØVB[N,P,Q][Ø,3,4,8]Z[X,Z]
NC ØVB[N,P,Q][Ø,3,4]ZZ with principal or secondary diagnosis of Z3Ø.2
♂ All body part, approach, device, and qualifier values

Ø Medical and Surgical
V Male Reproductive System
C Extirpation Definition: Taking or cutting out solid matter from a body part

Explanation: The solid matter may be an abnormal byproduct of a biological function or a foreign body; it may be imbedded in a body part or in the lumen of a tubular body part. The solid matter may or may not have been previously broken into pieces.

Body Part Character 4	Approach Character 5	Device Character 6	Qualifier Character 7
Ø Prostate ♂	Ø Open 3 Percutaneous 4 Percutaneous Endoscopic 7 Via Natural or Artificial Opening 8 Via Natural or Artificial Opening Endoscopic	Z No Device	Z No Qualifier
1 Seminal Vesicle, Right ♂ 2 Seminal Vesicle, Left ♂ 3 Seminal Vesicles, Bilateral ♂ 6 Tunica Vaginalis, Right ♂ 7 Tunica Vaginalis, Left ♂ 9 Testis, Right ♂ B Testis, Left ♂ C Testes, Bilateral ♂ F Spermatic Cord, Right ♂ G Spermatic Cord, Left ♂ H Spermatic Cords, Bilateral ♂ J Epididymis, Right ♂ K Epididymis, Left ♂ L Epididymis, Bilateral ♂ N Vas Deferens, Right ♂ Ductus deferens Ejaculatory duct P Vas Deferens, Left ♂ *See N Vas Deferens, Right* Q Vas Deferens, Bilateral ♂ *See N Vas Deferens, Right*	Ø Open 3 Percutaneous 4 Percutaneous Endoscopic	Z No Device	Z No Qualifier
5 Scrotum ♂ S Penis ♂ Corpus cavernosum Corpus spongiosum T Prepuce ♂ Foreskin Glans penis	Ø Open 3 Percutaneous 4 Percutaneous Endoscopic X External	Z No Device	Z No Qualifier

Non-OR ØVC[6,7,N,P,Q][Ø,3,4]ZZ
Non-OR ØVC5[3,4,X]ZZ
Non-OR ØVCSXZZ
♂ All body part, approach, device, and qualifier values

Ø Medical and Surgical
V Male Reproductive System
H Insertion Definition: Putting in a nonbiological appliance that monitors, assists, performs, or prevents a physiological function but does not physically take the place of a body part

Explanation: None

Body Part Character 4	Approach Character 5	Device Character 6	Qualifier Character 7
Ø Prostate ♂	Ø Open 3 Percutaneous 4 Percutaneous Endoscopic 7 Via Natural or Artificial Opening 8 Via Natural or Artificial Opening Endoscopic	1 Radioactive Element	Z No Qualifier
4 Prostate and Seminal Vesicles ♂ 8 Scrotum and Tunica Vaginalis ♂ M Epididymis and Spermatic Cord ♂ R Vas Deferens ♂ Ductus deferens Ejaculatory duct	Ø Open 3 Percutaneous 4 Percutaneous Endoscopic 7 Via Natural or Artificial Opening 8 Via Natural or Artificial Opening Endoscopic	3 Infusion Device Y Other Device	Z No Qualifier
D Testis ♂	Ø Open 3 Percutaneous 4 Percutaneous Endoscopic 7 Via Natural or Artificial Opening 8 Via Natural or Artificial Opening Endoscopic	1 Radioactive Element 3 Infusion Device Y Other Device	Z No Qualifier
S Penis ♂ Corpus cavernosum Corpus spongiosum	Ø Open 3 Percutaneous 4 Percutaneous Endoscopic	3 Infusion Device Y Other Device	Z No Qualifier
S Penis ♂ Corpus cavernosum Corpus spongiosum	7 Via Natural or Artificial Opening 8 Via Natural or Artificial Opening Endoscopic	Y Other Device	Z No Qualifier
S Penis ♂ Corpus cavernosum Corpus spongiosum	X External	3 Infusion Device	Z No Qualifier

Non-OR ØVH[4,8,M,R][Ø,3,4,7,8][3,Y]Z
Non-OR ØVHD[Ø,3,4,7,8][3,Y]Z
Non-OR ØVHS[Ø,3,4][3,Y]Z
Non-OR ØVHS[7,8]YZ
Non-OR ØVHSX3Z
♂ All body part, approach, device, and qualifier values

Ø Medical and Surgical
V Male Reproductive System
J Inspection Definition: Visually and/or manually exploring a body part

Explanation: Visual exploration may be performed with or without optical instrumentation. Manual exploration may be performed directly or through intervening body layers.

Body Part Character 4	Approach Character 5	Device Character 6	Qualifier Character 7
4 Prostate and Seminal Vesicles ♂ 8 Scrotum and Tunica Vaginalis ♂ D Testis ♂ M Epididymis and Spermatic Cord ♂ R Vas Deferens ♂ Ductus deferens Ejaculatory duct S Penis ♂ Corpus cavernosum Corpus spongiosum	Ø Open 3 Percutaneous 4 Percutaneous Endoscopic X External	Z No Device	Z No Qualifier

Non-OR ØVJ[4,D,M,R][3,X]ZZ
Non-OR ØVJ8[Ø,3,4,X]ZZ
Non-OR ØVJS[3,4,X]ZZ
♂ All body part, approach, device, and qualifier values

Ø Medical and Surgical
V Male Reproductive System
L Occlusion Definition: Completely closing an orifice or the lumen of a tubular body part
Explanation: The orifice can be a natural orifice or an artificially created orifice

Body Part Character 4	Approach Character 5	Device Character 6	Qualifier Character 7
F Spermatic Cord, Right NC ♂ **G** Spermatic Cord, Left NC ♂ **H** Spermatic Cords, Bilateral NC ♂ **N** Vas Deferens, Right NC ♂ Ductus deferens Ejaculatory duct **P** Vas Deferens, Left NC ♂ *See N Vas Deferens, Right* **Q** Vas Deferens, Bilateral NC ♂ *See N Vas Deferens, Right*	**Ø** Open **3** Percutaneous **4** Percutaneous Endoscopic **8** Via Natural or Artificial Opening Endoscopic	**C** Extraluminal Device **D** Intraluminal Device **Z** No Device	**Z** No Qualifier

Non-OR ØVL[F,G,H][Ø,3,4,8][C,D,Z]Z
Non-OR ØVL[N,P,Q][Ø,3,4,8][C,Z]Z

NC ØVL[F,G,H][Ø,3,4][C,D,Z]Z with principal or secondary diagnosis of Z3Ø.2
NC ØVL[N,P,Q][Ø,3,4][C,Z]Z with principal or secondary diagnosis of Z3Ø.2
♂ All body part, approach, device, and qualifier values

Ø Medical and Surgical
V Male Reproductive System
M Reattachment Definition: Putting back in or on all or a portion of a separated body part to its normal location or other suitable location
Explanation: Vascular circulation and nervous pathways may or may not be reestablished

Body Part Character 4	Approach Character 5	Device Character 6	Qualifier Character 7
5 Scrotum ♂ **S** Penis ♂ Corpus cavernosum Corpus spongiosum	**X** External	**Z** No Device	**Z** No Qualifier
6 Tunica Vaginalis, Right ♂ **7** Tunica Vaginalis, Left ♂ **9** Testis, Right ♂ **B** Testis, Left ♂ **C** Testes, Bilateral ♂ **F** Spermatic Cord, Right ♂ **G** Spermatic Cord, Left ♂ **H** Spermatic Cords, Bilateral ♂	**Ø** Open **4** Percutaneous Endoscopic	**Z** No Device	**Z** No Qualifier

♂ All body part, approach, device, and qualifier values

Ø Medical and Surgical
V Male Reproductive System
N Release Definition: Freeing a body part from an abnormal physical constraint by cutting or by the use of force
Explanation: Some of the restraining tissue may be taken out but none of the body part is taken out

Body Part Character 4	Approach Character 5	Device Character 6	Qualifier Character 7
Ø Prostate ♂	**Ø Open** **3 Percutaneous** **4 Percutaneous Endoscopic** **7 Via Natural or Artificial Opening** **8 Via Natural or Artificial Opening Endoscopic**	**Z No Device**	**Z No Qualifier**
1 Seminal Vesicle, Right ♂ **2 Seminal Vesicle, Left** ♂ **3 Seminal Vesicles, Bilateral** ♂ **6 Tunica Vaginalis, Right** ♂ **7 Tunica Vaginalis, Left** ♂ **9 Testis, Right** ♂ **B Testis, Left** ♂ **C Testes, Bilateral** ♂	**Ø Open** **3 Percutaneous** **4 Percutaneous Endoscopic**	**Z No Device**	**Z No Qualifier**
5 Scrotum ♂ **S Penis** ♂ Corpus cavernosum Corpus spongiosum **T Prepuce** ♂ Foreskin Glans penis	**Ø Open** **3 Percutaneous** **4 Percutaneous Endoscopic** **X External**	**Z No Device**	**Z No Qualifier**
F Spermatic Cord, Right ♂ **G Spermatic Cord, Left** ♂ **H Spermatic Cords, Bilateral** ♂ **J Epididymis, Right** ♂ **K Epididymis, Left** ♂ **L Epididymis, Bilateral** ♂ **N Vas Deferens, Right** ♂ Ductus deferens Ejaculatory duct **P Vas Deferens, Left** ♂ *See N Vas Deferens, Right* **Q Vas Deferens, Bilateral** ♂ *See N Vas Deferens, Right*	**Ø Open** **3 Percutaneous** **4 Percutaneous Endoscopic** **8 Via Natural or Artificial Opening Endoscopic**	**Z No Device**	**Z No Qualifier**

Non-OR ØVN[9,B,C][Ø,3,4]ZZ
Non-OR ØVNT[Ø,3,4,X]ZZ

♂ All body part, approach, device, and qualifier values

Ø Medical and Surgical
V Male Reproductive System
P Removal Definition: Taking out or off a device from a body part

Explanation: If a device is taken out and a similar device put in without cutting or puncturing the skin or mucous membrane, the procedure is coded to the root operation CHANGE. Otherwise, the procedure for taking out the device is coded to the root operation REMOVAL.

Body Part Character 4	Approach Character 5	Device Character 6	Qualifier Character 7
4 Prostate and Seminal Vesicles ♂	Ø Open 3 Percutaneous 4 Percutaneous Endoscopic 7 Via Natural or Artificial Opening 8 Via Natural or Artificial Opening Endoscopic	Ø Drainage Device 1 Radioactive Element 3 Infusion Device 7 Autologous Tissue Substitute J Synthetic Substitute K Nonautologous Tissue Substitute Y Other Device	Z No Qualifier
4 Prostate and Seminal Vesicles ♂	X External	Ø Drainage Device 1 Radioactive Element 3 Infusion Device	Z No Qualifier
8 Scrotum and Tunica Vaginalis ♂ D Testis ♂ S Penis ♂ Corpus cavernosum Corpus spongiosum	Ø Open 3 Percutaneous 4 Percutaneous Endoscopic 7 Via Natural or Artificial Opening 8 Via Natural or Artificial Opening Endoscopic	Ø Drainage Device 3 Infusion Device 7 Autologous Tissue Substitute J Synthetic Substitute K Nonautologous Tissue Substitute Y Other Device	Z No Qualifier
8 Scrotum and Tunica Vaginalis ♂ D Testis ♂ S Penis ♂ Corpus cavernosum Corpus spongiosum	X External	Ø Drainage Device 3 Infusion Device	Z No Qualifier
M Epididymis and Spermatic Cord ♂	Ø Open 3 Percutaneous 4 Percutaneous Endoscopic 7 Via Natural or Artificial Opening 8 Via Natural or Artificial Opening Endoscopic	Ø Drainage Device 3 Infusion Device 7 Autologous Tissue Substitute C Extraluminal Device J Synthetic Substitute K Nonautologous Tissue Substitute Y Other Device	Z No Qualifier
M Epididymis and Spermatic Cord ♂	X External	Ø Drainage Device 3 Infusion Device	Z No Qualifier
R Vas Deferens ♂ Ductus deferens Ejaculatory duct	Ø Open 3 Percutaneous 4 Percutaneous Endoscopic 7 Via Natural or Artificial Opening 8 Via Natural or Artificial Opening Endoscopic	Ø Drainage Device 3 Infusion Device 7 Autologous Tissue Substitute C Extraluminal Device D Intraluminal Device J Synthetic Substitute K Nonautologous Tissue Substitute Y Other Device	Z No Qualifier
R Vas Deferens ♂ Ductus deferens Ejaculatory duct	X External	Ø Drainage Device 3 Infusion Device D Intraluminal Device	Z No Qualifier

Non-OR ØVP4[3,4]YZ
Non-OR ØVP4[7,8][Ø,3,Y]Z
Non-OR ØVP4X[Ø,1,3]Z
Non-OR ØVP8[Ø,3,4,7,8][Ø,3,7,J,K,Y]Z
Non-OR ØVP[D,S][3,4]YZ
Non-OR ØVP[D,S][7,8][Ø,3,Y]Z
Non-OR ØVP[8,D,S]X[Ø,3]Z
Non-OR ØVPM[3,4]YZ
Non-OR ØVPM[7,8][Ø,3,Y]Z
Non-OR ØVPMX[Ø,3]Z
Non-OR ØVPR[Ø,3,4][Ø,3,7,C,J,K,Y]Z
Non-OR ØVPR[7,8][Ø,3,7,C,D,J,K,Y]Z
Non-OR ØVPRX[Ø,3,D]Z
♂ All body part, approach, device, and qualifier values

Ø Medical and Surgical
V Male Reproductive System
Q Repair Definition: Restoring, to the extent possible, a body part to its normal anatomic structure and function

Explanation: Used only when the method to accomplish the repair is not one of the other root operations

Body Part Character 4	Approach Character 5	Device Character 6	Qualifier Character 7
Ø Prostate ♂	Ø Open 3 Percutaneous 4 Percutaneous Endoscopic 7 Via Natural or Artificial Opening 8 Via Natural or Artificial Opening Endoscopic	Z No Device	Z No Qualifier
1 Seminal Vesicle, Right ♂ 2 Seminal Vesicle, Left ♂ 3 Seminal Vesicles, Bilateral ♂ 6 Tunica Vaginalis, Right ♂ 7 Tunica Vaginalis, Left ♂ 9 Testis, Right ♂ B Testis, Left ♂ C Testes, Bilateral ♂	Ø Open 3 Percutaneous 4 Percutaneous Endoscopic	Z No Device	Z No Qualifier
5 Scrotum ♂ S Penis ♂ Corpus cavernosum Corpus spongiosum T Prepuce ♂ Foreskin Glans penis	Ø Open 3 Percutaneous 4 Percutaneous Endoscopic X External	Z No Device	Z No Qualifier
F Spermatic Cord, Right ♂ G Spermatic Cord, Left ♂ H Spermatic Cords, Bilateral ♂ J Epididymis, Right ♂ K Epididymis, Left ♂ L Epididymis, Bilateral ♂ N Vas Deferens, Right ♂ Ductus deferens Ejaculatory duct P Vas Deferens, Left ♂ *See N Vas Deferens, Right* Q Vas Deferens, Bilateral ♂ *See N Vas Deferens, Right*	Ø Open 3 Percutaneous 4 Percutaneous Endoscopic 8 Via Natural or Artificial Opening Endoscopic	Z No Device	Z No Qualifier

Non-OR ØVQ[6,7][Ø,3,4]ZZ
Non-OR ØVQ5[Ø,3,4,X]ZZ

♂ All body part, approach, device, and qualifier values

Ø Medical and Surgical
V Male Reproductive System
R Replacement Definition: Putting in or on biological or synthetic material that physically takes the place and/or function of all or a portion of a body part

Explanation: The body part may have been taken out or replaced, or may be taken out, physically eradicated, or rendered nonfunctional during the REPLACEMENT procedure. A REMOVAL procedure is coded for taking out the device used in a previous replacement procedure.

Body Part Character 4	Approach Character 5	Device Character 6	Qualifier Character 7
9 Testis, Right ♂ B Testis, Left ♂ C Testes, Bilateral ♂	Ø Open	J Synthetic Substitute	Z No Qualifier

♂ All body part, approach, device, and qualifier values

Ø Medical and Surgical
V Male Reproductive System
S Reposition Definition: Moving to its normal location, or other suitable location, all or a portion of a body part

Explanation: The body part is moved to a new location from an abnormal location, or from a normal location where it is not functioning correctly. The body part may or may not be cut out or off to be moved to the new location.

Body Part Character 4	Approach Character 5	Device Character 6	Qualifier Character 7
9 Testis, Right ♂ B Testis, Left ♂ C Testes, Bilateral ♂ F Spermatic Cord, Right ♂ G Spermatic Cord, Left ♂ H Spermatic Cords, Bilateral ♂	Ø Open 3 Percutaneous 4 Percutaneous Endoscopic 8 Via Natural or Artificial Opening Endoscopic	Z No Device	Z No Qualifier

♂ All body part, approach, device, and qualifier values

Ø Medical and Surgical
V Male Reproductive System
T Resection Definition: Cutting out or off, without replacement, all of a body part
Explanation: None

Body Part Character 4	Approach Character 5	Device Character 6	Qualifier Character 7
Ø Prostate ⊞♂	**Ø Open** **4 Percutaneous Endoscopic** **7 Via Natural or Artificial Opening** **8 Via Natural or Artificial Opening Endoscopic**	**Z No Device**	**Z No Qualifier**
1 Seminal Vesicle, Right ♂ **2 Seminal Vesicle, Left** ♂ **3 Seminal Vesicles, Bilateral** ⊞♂ **6 Tunica Vaginalis, Right** ♂ **7 Tunica Vaginalis, Left** ♂ **9 Testis, Right** ♂ **B Testis, Left** ♂ **C Testes, Bilateral** ♂ **F Spermatic Cord, Right** ♂ **G Spermatic Cord, Left** ♂ **H Spermatic Cords, Bilateral** ♂ **J Epididymis, Right** ♂ **K Epididymis, Left** ♂ **L Epididymis, Bilateral** ♂ **N Vas Deferens, Right** NC♂ Ductus deferens Ejaculatory duct **P Vas Deferens, Left** NC♂ *See N Vas Deferens, Right* **Q Vas Deferens, Bilateral** NC♂ *See N Vas Deferens, Right*	**Ø Open** **4 Percutaneous Endoscopic**	**Z No Device**	**Z No Qualifier**
5 Scrotum ♂ **S Penis** ♂ Corpus cavernosum Corpus spongiosum **T Prepuce** ♂ Foreskin Glans penis	**Ø Open** **4 Percutaneous Endoscopic** **X External**	**Z No Device**	**Z No Qualifier**

Non-OR ØVT[N,P,Q][Ø,4]ZZ
Non-OR ØVT[5,T][Ø,4,X]ZZ
NC ØVT[N,P,Q][Ø,4]ZZ with principal or secondary diagnosis of Z3Ø.2
♂ All body part, approach, device, and qualifier values

See Appendix L for Procedure Combinations
⊞ ØVTØ[Ø,4,7,8]ZZ
⊞ ØVT3[Ø,4]ZZ

Ø Medical and Surgical
V Male Reproductive System
U Supplement Definition: Putting in or on biological or synthetic material that physically reinforces and/or augments the function of a portion of a body part

Explanation: The biological material is non-living, or is living and from the same individual. The body part may have been previously replaced, and the SUPPLEMENT procedure is performed to physically reinforce and/or augment the function of the replaced body part.

Body Part Character 4	Approach Character 5	Device Character 6	Qualifier Character 7
1 Seminal Vesicle, Right ♂ **2 Seminal Vesicle, Left** ♂ **3 Seminal Vesicles, Bilateral** ♂ **6 Tunica Vaginalis, Right** ♂ **7 Tunica Vaginalis, Left** ♂ **F Spermatic Cord, Right** ♂ **G Spermatic Cord, Left** ♂ **H Spermatic Cords, Bilateral** ♂ **J Epididymis, Right** ♂ **K Epididymis, Left** ♂ **L Epididymis, Bilateral** ♂ **N Vas Deferens, Right** ♂ Ductus deferens Ejaculatory duct **P Vas Deferens, Left** ♂ *See N Vas Deferens, Right* **Q Vas Deferens, Bilateral** ♂ *See N Vas Deferens, Right*	**Ø Open** **4 Percutaneous Endoscopic** **8 Via Natural or Artificial Opening Endoscopic**	**7 Autologous Tissue Substitute** **J Synthetic Substitute** **K Nonautologous Tissue Substitute**	**Z No Qualifier**
5 Scrotum ♂ **S Penis** ♂ Corpus cavernosum Corpus spongiosum **T Prepuce** ♂ Foreskin Glans penis	**Ø Open** **4 Percutaneous Endoscopic** **X External**	**7 Autologous Tissue Substitute** **J Synthetic Substitute** **K Nonautologous Tissue Substitute**	**Z No Qualifier**
9 Testis, Right ♂ **B Testis, Left** ♂ **C Testes, Bilateral** ♂	**Ø Open**	**7 Autologous Tissue Substitute** **J Synthetic Substitute** **K Nonautologous Tissue Substitute**	**Z No Qualifier**

Non-OR ØVUSX[7,J,K]Z

♂ All body part, approach, device, and qualifier values

Ø Medical and Surgical
V Male Reproductive System
W Revision Definition: Correcting, to the extent possible, a portion of a malfunctioning device or the position of a displaced device

Explanation: Revision can include correcting a malfunctioning or displaced device by taking out or putting in components of the device such as a screw or pin

Body Part Character 4	Approach Character 5	Device Character 6	Qualifier Character 7
4 Prostate and Seminal Vesicles ♂ **8** Scrotum and Tunica Vaginalis ♂ **D** Testis ♂ **S** Penis ♂ Corpus cavernosum Corpus spongiosum	**Ø** Open **3** Percutaneous **4** Percutaneous Endoscopic **7** Via Natural or Artificial Opening **8** Via Natural or Artificial Opening Endoscopic	**Ø** Drainage Device **3** Infusion Device **7** Autologous Tissue Substitute **J** Synthetic Substitute **K** Nonautologous Tissue Substitute **Y** Other Device	**Z** No Qualifier
4 Prostate and Seminal Vesicles ♂ **8** Scrotum and Tunica Vaginalis ♂ **D** Testis ♂ **S** Penis ♂ Corpus cavernosum Corpus spongiosum	**X** External	**Ø** Drainage Device **3** Infusion Device **7** Autologous Tissue Substitute **J** Synthetic Substitute **K** Nonautologous Tissue Substitute	**Z** No Qualifier
M Epididymis and Spermatic Cord ♂	**Ø** Open **3** Percutaneous **4** Percutaneous Endoscopic **7** Via Natural or Artificial Opening **8** Via Natural or Artificial Opening Endoscopic	**Ø** Drainage Device **3** Infusion Device **7** Autologous Tissue Substitute **C** Extraluminal Device **J** Synthetic Substitute **K** Nonautologous Tissue Substitute **Y** Other Device	**Z** No Qualifier
M Epididymis and Spermatic Cord ♂	**X** External	**Ø** Drainage Device **3** Infusion Device **7** Autologous Tissue Substitute **C** Extraluminal Device **J** Synthetic Substitute **K** Nonautologous Tissue Substitute	**Z** No Qualifier
R Vas Deferens ♂ Ductus deferens Ejaculatory duct	**Ø** Open **3** Percutaneous **4** Percutaneous Endoscopic **7** Via Natural or Artificial Opening **8** Via Natural or Artificial Opening Endoscopic	**Ø** Drainage Device **3** Infusion Device **7** Autologous Tissue Substitute **C** Extraluminal Device **D** Intraluminal Device **J** Synthetic Substitute **K** Nonautologous Tissue Substitute **Y** Other Device	**Z** No Qualifier
R Vas Deferens ♂ Ductus deferens Ejaculatory duct	**X** External	**Ø** Drainage Device **3** Infusion Device **7** Autologous Tissue Substitute **C** Extraluminal Device **D** Intraluminal Device **J** Synthetic Substitute **K** Nonautologous Tissue Substitute	**Z** No Qualifier

Non-OR ØVW[4,D,S][3,4,7,8]YZ
Non-OR ØVW8[Ø,3,4,7,8][Ø,3,7,J,K,Y]Z
Non-OR ØVW[4,8,D,S]X[Ø,3,7,J,K]Z
Non-OR ØVWM[3,4,7,8]YZ
Non-OR ØVWMX[Ø,3,7,C,J,K]Z
Non-OR ØVWR[Ø,3,4,7,8][Ø,3,7,C,D,J,K,Y]Z
Non-OR ØVWRX[Ø,3,7,C,D,J,K]Z
♂ All body part, approach, device, and qualifier values

Ø Medical and Surgical
V Male Reproductive System
X Transfer Definition: Moving, without taking out, all or a portion of a body part to another location to take over the function of all or a portion of a body part

Explanation: The body part transferred remains connected to its vascular and nervous supply

Body Part Character 4	Approach Character 5	Device Character 6	Qualifier Character 7
T Prepuce Foreskin Glans penis	**Ø** Open **X** External	**Z** No Device	**D** Urethra **S** Penis

Ø Medical and Surgical
V Male Reproductive System
Y Transplantation Definition: Putting in or on all or a portion of a living body part taken from another individual or animal to physically take the place and/or function of all or a portion of a similar body part

Explanation: The native body part may or may not be taken out, and the transplanted body part may take over all or a portion of its function

Body Part Character 4	Approach Character 5	Device Character 6	Qualifier Character 7
5 Scrotum ♂ **S Penis** ♂ Corpus cavernosum Corpus spongiosum	**Ø Open**	**Z No Device**	**Ø Allogeneic** **1 Syngeneic** **2 Zooplastic**

♂ All body part, approach, device, and qualifier values

Anatomical Regions, General ØWØ–ØWY

Character Meanings

This Character Meaning table is provided as a guide to assist the user in the identification of character members that may be found in this section of code tables. It **SHOULD NOT** be used to build a PCS code.

Operation–Character 3		Body Region–Character 4		Approach–Character 5		Device–Character 6		Qualifier–Character 7	
Ø	Alteration	Ø	Head	Ø	Open	Ø	Drainage Device	Ø	Vagina OR Allogeneic
1	Bypass	1	Cranial Cavity	3	Percutaneous	1	Radioactive Element	1	Penis OR Syngeneic
2	Change	2	Face	4	Percutaneous Endoscopic	3	Infusion Device	2	Stoma
3	Control	3	Oral Cavity and Throat	7	Via Natural or Artificial Opening	7	Autologous Tissue Substitute	4	Cutaneous
4	Creation	4	Upper Jaw	8	Via Natural or Artificial Opening Endoscopic	J	Synthetic Substitute	6	Bladder
8	Division	5	Lower Jaw	X	External	K	Nonautologous Tissue Substitute	9	Pleural Cavity, Right
9	Drainage	6	Neck			Y	Other Device	B	Pleural Cavity, Left
B	Excision	8	Chest Wall			Z	No Device	G	Peritoneal Cavity
C	Extirpation	9	Pleural Cavity, Right					J	Pelvic Cavity
F	Fragmentation	B	Pleural Cavity, Left					W	Upper Vein
H	Insertion	C	Mediastinum					X	Diagnostic
J	Inspection	D	Pericardial Cavity					Y	Lower Vein
M	Reattachment	F	Abdominal Wall					Z	No Qualifier
P	Removal	G	Peritoneal Cavity						
Q	Repair	H	Retroperitoneum						
U	Supplement	J	Pelvic Cavity						
W	Revision	K	Upper Back						
Y	Transplantation	L	Lower Back						
		M	Perineum, Male						
		N	Perineum, Female						
		P	Gastrointestinal Tract						
		Q	Respiratory Tract						
		R	Genitourinary Tract						

AHA Coding Clinic for table ØWØ
2015, 1Q, 31 Bilateral browpexy

AHA Coding Clinic for table ØW1
2018, 4Q, 41-42 Anatomical regions bypass qualifiers
2015, 2Q, 36 Insertion of infusion device into peritoneal cavity
2013, 4Q, 126-127 Creation of percutaneous cutaneoperitoneal fistula

AHA Coding Clinic for table ØW3
2019, 3Q, 4 Evacuation of subdural hematoma and control of bleeding artery
2018, 4Q, 38 Control of epistaxis
2018, 1Q, 19 Argon plasma coagulation of duodenal arteriovenous malformation
2018, 1Q, 19 Control of epistaxis via silver nitrate cauterization
2017, 4Q, 57-58 Added approach values - Transorifice esophageal vein banding
2017, 4Q, 105 Control of gastrointestinal bleeding
2017, 4Q, 106 Control of bleeding of external naris using suture
2017, 4Q, 106 Nasal packing for epistaxis
2016, 4Q, 99-100 Root operation Control
2014, 4Q, 44 Bakri balloon for control of postpartum hemorrhage
2013, 3Q, 23 Control of intraoperative bleeding

AHA Coding Clinic for table ØW4
2019, 4Q, 30 Transfer large intestine to vagina
2016, 4Q, 101 Root operation Creation

AHA Coding Clinic for table ØW9
2017, 3Q, 12 Therapeutic and diagnostic paracentesis
2017, 2Q, 16 Incision and drainage of floor of mouth

AHA Coding Clinic for table ØWB
2019, 1Q, 27 Excision of pelvic sidewall mass
2017, 2Q, 16 Excision of floor of mouth
2016, 1Q, 21 Excision of urachal mass
2013, 4Q, 119 Excision of inclusion cyst of perineum

AHA Coding Clinic for table ØWC
2019, 4Q, 35 Extirpation of jaw
2017, 2Q, 16 Excision of floor of mouth

AHA Coding Clinic for table ØWH
2019, 4Q, 43 Unidirectional source brachytherapy
2018, 1Q, 25 Intrauterine brachytherapy & placement of tandems & ovoids
2017, 4Q, 104 Intrauterine brachytherapy & placement of tandems & ovoids
2016, 2Q, 14 Insertion of peritoneal totally implantable venous access device
2015, 2Q, 36 Insertion of infusion device into peritoneal cavity

AHA Coding Clinic for table ØWJ
2019, 1Q, 3-8 Whipple procedure
2019, 1Q, 25 Laparoscopic appendectomy converted to open procedure
2018, 3Q, 29 Decommissioning of left ventricular assist device with exploration of mediastinum
2016, 4Q, 58 Longitudinal vaginal septum
2013, 2Q, 36 Insertion of ventriculoperitoneal shunt with laparoscopic assistance

AHA Coding Clinic for table ØWQ
2017, 4Q, 106 Control of bleeding of external naris using suture
2017, 3Q, 8 Removal of silo and closure of gastroschisis
2016, 3Q, 3-7 Stoma creation & takedown procedures
2014, 4Q, 38 Abdominoplasty and abdominal wall plication for hernia repair
2014, 3Q, 28 Ileostomy takedown and parastomal hernia repair

AHA Coding Clinic for table ØWU
2017, 3Q, 8 First stage of gastroschisis repair with silo placement
2016, 3Q, 40 Omentoplasty
2015, 2Q, 29 Placement of Ioban™ antimicrobial drape over surgical wound
2014, 4Q, 39 Abdominal component release with placement of mesh for hernia repair
2012, 4Q, 101 Rib resection with reconstruction of anterior chest wall

AHA Coding Clinic for table ØWW
2015, 2Q, 9 Revision of ventriculoperitoneal (VP) shunt

AHA Coding Clinic for table ØWY
2016, 4Q, 112-113 Transplantation

Ø Medical and Surgical
W Anatomical Regions, General
Ø Alteration Definition: Modifying the anatomic structure of a body part without affecting the function of the body part
Explanation: Principal purpose is to improve appearance

Body Part Character 4	Approach Character 5	Device Character 6	Qualifier Character 7
Ø Head **2** Face **4** Upper Jaw **5** Lower Jaw **6** Neck **8** Chest Wall **F** Abdominal Wall **K** Upper Back **L** Lower Back **M** Perineum, Male ♂ **N** Perineum, Female ♀	**Ø** Open **3** Percutaneous **4** Percutaneous Endoscopic	**7** Autologous Tissue Substitute **J** Synthetic Substitute **K** Nonautologous Tissue Substitute **Z** No Device	**Z** No Qualifier

♂ ØWØM[Ø,3,4][7,J,K,Z]Z
♀ ØWØN[Ø,3,4][7,J,K,Z]Z

Ø Medical and Surgical
W Anatomical Regions, General
1 Bypass Definition: Altering the route of passage of the contents of a tubular body part
Explanation: Rerouting contents of a body part to a downstream area of the normal route, to a similar route and body part, or to an abnormal route and dissimilar body part. Includes one or more anastomoses, with or without the use of a device.

Body Part Character 4	Approach Character 5	Device Character 6	Qualifier Character 7
1 Cranial Cavity	**Ø** Open	**J** Synthetic Substitute	**9** Pleural Cavity, Right **B** Pleural Cavity, Left **G** Peritoneal Cavity **J** Pelvic Cavity
9 Pleural Cavity, Right **B** Pleural Cavity, Left **J** Pelvic Cavity Retropubic space	**Ø** Open **3** Percutaneous **4** Percutaneous Endoscopic	**J** Synthetic Substitute	**4** Cutaneous **9** Pleural Cavity, Right **B** Pleural Cavity, Left **G** Peritoneal Cavity **J** Pelvic Cavity **W** Upper Vein **Y** Lower Vein
G Peritoneal Cavity	**Ø** Open **3** Percutaneous **4** Percutaneous Endoscopic	**J** Synthetic Substitute	**4** Cutaneous **6** Bladder **9** Pleural Cavity, Right **B** Pleural Cavity, Left **G** Peritoneal Cavity **J** Pelvic Cavity **W** Upper Vein **Y** Lower Vein

Non-OR ØW1[9,B][Ø,3,4]J[4,G,W,Y]
Non-OR ØW1J[Ø,3,4]J[4,W,Y]
Non-OR ØW1G[Ø,3,4]J[9,B,G,J]

Ø Medical and Surgical
W Anatomical Regions, General
2 Change Definition: Taking out or off a device from a body part and putting back an identical or similar device in or on the same body part without cutting or puncturing the skin or a mucous membrane

Explanation: All CHANGE procedures are coded using the approach EXTERNAL

Body Part Character 4	Approach Character 5	Device Character 6	Qualifier Character 7
Ø Head 1 Cranial Cavity 2 Face 4 Upper Jaw 5 Lower Jaw 6 Neck 8 Chest Wall 9 Pleural Cavity, Right B Pleural Cavity, Left C Mediastinum Mediastinal cavity Mediastinal space D Pericardial Cavity F Abdominal Wall G Peritoneal Cavity H Retroperitoneum Retroperitoneal cavity Retroperitoneal space J Pelvic Cavity Retropubic space K Upper Back L Lower Back M Perineum, Male ♂ N Perineum, Female ♀	X External	Ø Drainage Device Y Other Device	Z No Qualifier

Non-OR All body part, approach, device, and qualifier values
♂ ØW2MX[Ø,Y]Z
♀ ØW2NX[Ø,Y]Z

Ø Medical and Surgical
W Anatomical Regions, General
3 Control Definition: Stopping, or attempting to stop, postprocedural or other acute bleeding
Explanation: None

Body Part Character 4	Approach Character 5	Device Character 6	Qualifier Character 7
Ø Head 1 Cranial Cavity 2 Face 4 Upper Jaw 5 Lower Jaw 6 Neck 8 Chest Wall 9 Pleural Cavity, Right B Pleural Cavity, Left C Mediastinum Mediastinal cavity Mediastinal space D Pericardial Cavity F Abdominal Wall G Peritoneal Cavity H Retroperitoneum Retroperitoneal cavity Retroperitoneal space J Pelvic Cavity Retropubic space K Upper Back L Lower Back M Perineum, Male ♂ N Perineum, Female ♀	Ø Open 3 Percutaneous 4 Percutaneous Endoscopic	Z No Device	Z No Qualifier
3 Oral Cavity and Throat	Ø Open 3 Percutaneous 4 Percutaneous Endoscopic 7 Via Natural or Artificial Opening 8 Via Natural or Artificial Opening Endoscopic X External	Z No Device	Z No Qualifier
P Gastrointestinal Tract Q Respiratory Tract R Genitourinary Tract	Ø Open 3 Percutaneous 4 Percutaneous Endoscopic 7 Via Natural or Artificial Opening 8 Via Natural or Artificial Opening Endoscopic	Z No Device	Z No Qualifier

Non-OR ØW3P8ZZ

♂ ØW3M[Ø,3,4]ZZ
♀ ØW3N[Ø,3,4]ZZ

Ø Medical and Surgical
W Anatomical Regions, General
4 Creation Definition: Putting in or on biological or synthetic material to form a new body part that to the extent possible replicates the anatomic structure or function of an absent body part
Explanation: Used for gender reassignment surgery and corrective procedures in individuals with congenital anomalies

Body Part Character 4	Approach Character 5	Device Character 6	Qualifier Character 7
M Perineum, Male ♂	Ø Open	7 Autologous Tissue Substitute J Synthetic Substitute K Nonautologous Tissue Substitute	Ø Vagina
N Perineum, Female ♀	Ø Open	7 Autologous Tissue Substitute J Synthetic Substitute K Nonautologous Tissue Substitute	1 Penis

♂ ØW4MØ[7,J,K]Ø
♀ ØW4NØ[7,J,K]1

Ø Medical and Surgical
W Anatomical Regions, General
8 Division Definition: Cutting into a body part, without draining fluids and/or gases from the body part, in order to separate or transect a body part
Explanation: All or a portion of the body part is separated into two or more portions

Body Part Character 4	Approach Character 5	Device Character 6	Qualifier Character 7
N Perineum, Female ♀	X External	Z No Device	Z No Qualifier

Non-OR ØW8NXZZ

♀ ØW8NXZZ

Ø Medical and Surgical
W Anatomical Regions, General
9 Drainage Definition: Taking or letting out fluids and/or gases from a body part
Explanation: The qualifier DIAGNOSTIC is used to identify drainage procedures that are biopsies

Body Part Character 4	Approach Character 5	Device Character 6	Qualifier Character 7
Ø Head 1 Cranial Cavity 2 Face 3 Oral Cavity and Throat 4 Upper Jaw 5 Lower Jaw 6 Neck 8 Chest Wall 9 Pleural Cavity, Right B Pleural Cavity, Left C Mediastinum Mediastinal cavity Mediastinal space D Pericardial Cavity F Abdominal Wall G Peritoneal Cavity H Retroperitoneum Retroperitoneal cavity Retroperitoneal space K Upper Back L Lower Back M Perineum, Male ♂ N Perineum, Female ♀	Ø Open 3 Percutaneous 4 Percutaneous Endoscopic	Ø Drainage Device	Z No Qualifier
Ø Head 1 Cranial Cavity 2 Face 3 Oral Cavity and Throat 4 Upper Jaw 5 Lower Jaw 6 Neck 8 Chest Wall 9 Pleural Cavity, Right B Pleural Cavity, Left C Mediastinum Mediastinal cavity Mediastinal space D Pericardial Cavity F Abdominal Wall G Peritoneal Cavity H Retroperitoneum Retroperitoneal cavity Retroperitoneal space K Upper Back L Lower Back M Perineum, Male ♂ N Perineum, Female ♀	Ø Open 3 Percutaneous 4 Percutaneous Endoscopic	Z No Device	X Diagnostic Z No Qualifier
J Pelvic Cavity Retropubic space	Ø Open 3 Percutaneous 4 Percutaneous Endoscopic 7 Via Natural or Artificial Opening 8 Via Natural or Artificial Opening Endoscopic	Ø Drainage Device	Z No Qualifier
J Pelvic Cavity Retropubic space	Ø Open 3 Percutaneous 4 Percutaneous Endoscopic 7 Via Natural or Artificial Opening 8 Via Natural or Artificial Opening Endoscopic	Z No Device	X Diagnostic Z No Qualifier

Non-OR ØW9[Ø,8,9,B,K,L,M]ØØZ
Non-OR ØW9[Ø,1,2,3,4,5,6,8,9,B,C,D,F,G,H,K,L,M,N]3ØZ
Non-OR ØW9[Ø,1,8,F,K,L,M]4ØZ
Non-OR ØW9[Ø,2,3,4,5,6,8,9,B,K,L,M,N]ØZX
Non-OR ØW9[Ø,1,2,3,4,5,6,8,9,B,C,D,G,K,L,M,N]3ZX
Non-OR ØW9[Ø,1,2,3,4,5,6,8,C,K,L,M,N]4ZX
Non-OR ØW9[Ø,8,9,B,K,L,M]ØZZ
Non-OR ØW9[Ø,1,2,3,4,5,6,8,9,B,C,D,F,G,H,K,L,M,N]3ZZ
Non-OR ØW9[Ø,1,8,F,K,L,M]4ZZ
Non-OR ØW9J[3,7,8]ØZ
Non-OR ØW9J[3,7,8]Z[X,Z]

♂ ØW9M[Ø,3,4]ØZ
♂ ØW9M[Ø,3,4]Z[X,Z]
♀ ØW9N[Ø,3,4]ØZ
♀ ØW9N[Ø,3]Z[X,Z]
♀ ØW9N4ZZ

Ø Medical and Surgical
W Anatomical Regions, General
B Excision Definition: Cutting out or off, without replacement, a portion of a body part
Explanation: The qualifier DIAGNOSTIC is used to identify excision procedures that are biopsies

Body Part Character 4	Approach Character 5	Device Character 6	Qualifier Character 7
Ø Head 2 Face 3 Oral Cavity and Throat 4 Upper Jaw 5 Lower Jaw 8 Chest Wall K Upper Back L Lower Back M Perineum, Male ♂ N Perineum, Female ♀	Ø Open 3 Percutaneous 4 Percutaneous Endoscopic X External	Z No Device	X Diagnostic Z No Qualifier
6 Neck F Abdominal Wall	Ø Open 3 Percutaneous 4 Percutaneous Endoscopic	Z No Device	X Diagnostic Z No Qualifier
6 Neck F Abdominal Wall	X External	Z No Device	2 Stoma X Diagnostic Z No Qualifier
C Mediastinum Mediastinal cavity Mediastinal space H Retroperitoneum Retroperitoneal cavity Retroperitoneal space	Ø Open 3 Percutaneous 4 Percutaneous Endoscopic	Z No Device	X Diagnostic Z No Qualifier

Non-OR ØWB[Ø,2,4,5,8,K,L,M][Ø,3,4,X]ZX
Non-OR ØWB6[Ø,3,4]ZX
Non-OR ØWB6XZX
Non-OR ØWBH[3,4]ZX

♂ ØWBM[Ø,3,4,X]Z[X,Z]
♀ ØWBN[Ø,3,4,X]Z[X,Z]

Ø Medical and Surgical
W Anatomical Regions, General
C Extirpation Definition: Taking or cutting out solid matter from a body part
Explanation: The solid matter may be an abnormal byproduct of a biological function or a foreign body; it may be imbedded in a body part or in the lumen of a tubular body part. The solid matter may or may not have been previously broken into pieces.

Body Part Character 4	Approach Character 5	Device Character 6	Qualifier Character 7
1 Cranial Cavity 3 Oral Cavity and Throat 9 Pleural Cavity, Right B Pleural Cavity, Left C Mediastinum Mediastinal cavity Mediastinal space D Pericardial Cavity G Peritoneal Cavity H Retroperitoneum Retroperitoneal cavity Retroperitoneal space J Pelvic Cavity Retropubic space	Ø Open 3 Percutaneous 4 Percutaneous Endoscopic X External	Z No Device	Z No Qualifier
4 Upper Jaw 5 Lower Jaw	Ø Open 3 Percutaneous 4 Percutaneous Endoscopic	Z No Device	Z No Qualifier
P Gastrointestinal Tract Q Respiratory Tract R Genitourinary Tract	Ø Open 3 Percutaneous 4 Percutaneous Endoscopic 7 Via Natural or Artificial Opening 8 Via Natural or Artificial Opening Endoscopic X External	Z No Device	Z No Qualifier

Non-OR ØWC[1,3]XZZ
Non-OR ØWC[9,B][Ø,3,4,X]ZZ
Non-OR ØWC[C,D,G,H,J]XZZ
Non-OR ØWC[4,5][Ø,3,4]ZZ
Non-OR ØWC[P,R][7,8,X]ZZ
Non-OR ØWCQ[Ø,3,4,X]ZZ

Ø Medical and Surgical
W Anatomical Regions, General
F Fragmentation Definition: Breaking solid matter in a body part into pieces

Explanation: Physical force (e.g., manual, ultrasonic) applied directly or indirectly is used to break the solid matter into pieces. The solid matter may be an abnormal byproduct of a biological function or a foreign body. The pieces of solid matter are not taken out.

Body Part Character 4	Approach Character 5	Device Character 6	Qualifier Character 7
1 Cranial Cavity NC 3 Oral Cavity and Throat NC 9 Pleural Cavity, Right NC B Pleural Cavity, Left NC C Mediastinum NC Mediastinal cavity Mediastinal space D Pericardial Cavity G Peritoneal Cavity NC J Pelvic Cavity NC Retropubic space	Ø Open 3 Percutaneous 4 Percutaneous Endoscopic X External	Z No Device	Z No Qualifier
P Gastrointestinal Tract NC Q Respiratory Tract NC R Genitourinary Tract	Ø Open 3 Percutaneous 4 Percutaneous Endoscopic 7 Via Natural or Artificial Opening 8 Via Natural or Artificial Opening Endoscopic X External	Z No Device	Z No Qualifier

Non-OR ØWF[1,3,9,B,C,G]XZZ
Non-OR ØWFJ[Ø,3,4,X]ZZ
Non-OR ØWFP[Ø,3,4,7,8,X]ZZ
Non-OR ØWFQXZZ
Non-OR ØWFR[Ø,3,4,7,8,X]ZZ
NC ØWF[1,3,9,B,C,G,J]XZZ
NC ØWF[P,Q]XZZ

Ø Medical and Surgical
W Anatomical Regions, General
H Insertion Definition: Putting in a nonbiological appliance that monitors, assists, performs, or prevents a physiological function but does not physically take the place of a body part

Explanation: None

Body Part Character 4	Approach Character 5	Device Character 6	Qualifier Character 7
Ø Head 1 Cranial Cavity 2 Face 3 Oral Cavity and Throat 4 Upper Jaw 5 Lower Jaw 6 Neck 8 Chest Wall 9 Pleural Cavity, Right B Pleural Cavity, Left C Mediastinum Mediastinal cavity Mediastinal space D Pericardial Cavity F Abdominal Wall G Peritoneal Cavity H Retroperitoneum Retroperitoneal cavity Retroperitoneal space J Pelvic Cavity Retropubic space K Upper Back L Lower Back M Perineum, Male N Perineum, Female ♀	Ø Open 3 Percutaneous 4 Percutaneous Endoscopic	1 Radioactive Element 3 Infusion Device Y Other Device	Z No Qualifier
P Gastrointestinal Tract Q Respiratory Tract R Genitourinary Tract	Ø Open 3 Percutaneous 4 Percutaneous Endoscopic 7 Via Natural or Artificial Opening 8 Via Natural or Artificial Opening Endoscopic	1 Radioactive Element 3 Infusion Device Y Other Device	Z No Qualifier

DRG Non-OR ØWH[Ø,2,4,5,6,K,L,M][Ø,3,4][3,Y]Z
Non-OR ØWH1[Ø,3,4]3Z
Non-OR ØWH[8,9,B][Ø,3,4][3,Y]Z
Non-OR ØWHPØYZ
Non-OR ØWHP[3,4,7,8][3,Y]Z
Non-OR ØWHQ[Ø,7,8][3,Y]Z
Non-OR ØWHR[Ø,3,4,7,8][3,Y]Z
♀ ØWHN[Ø,3,4][3,Y]Z

Ø Medical and Surgical
W Anatomical Regions, General
J Inspection Definition: Visually and/or manually exploring a body part

Explanation: Visual exploration may be performed with or without optical instrumentation. Manual exploration may be performed directly or through intervening body layers.

Body Part Character 4	Approach Character 5	Device Character 6	Qualifier Character 7
Ø Head **2** Face **3** Oral Cavity and Throat **4** Upper Jaw **5** Lower Jaw **6** Neck **8** Chest Wall **F** Abdominal Wall **K** Upper Back **L** Lower Back **M** Perineum, Male ♂ **N** Perineum, Female ♀	**Ø** Open **3** Percutaneous **4** Percutaneous Endoscopic **X** External	**Z** No Device	**Z** No Qualifier
1 Cranial Cavity **9** Pleural Cavity, Right **B** Pleural Cavity, Left **C** Mediastinum Mediastinal cavity Mediastinal space **D** Pericardial Cavity **G** Peritoneal Cavity **H** Retroperitoneum Retroperitoneal cavity Retroperitoneal space **J** Pelvic Cavity Retropubic space	**Ø** Open **3** Percutaneous **4** Percutaneous Endoscopic	**Z** No Device	**Z** No Qualifier
P Gastrointestinal Tract **Q** Respiratory Tract **R** Genitourinary Tract	**Ø** Open **3** Percutaneous **4** Percutaneous Endoscopic **7** Via Natural or Artificial Opening **8** Via Natural or Artificial Opening Endoscopic	**Z** No Device	**Z** No Qualifier

DRG Non-OR ØWJ[Ø,2,4,5,K,L]ØZZ
DRG Non-OR ØWJM[Ø,4]ZZ
Non-OR ØWJ3ØZZ
Non-OR ØWJ[Ø,2,3,4,5,6,8,F,K,L,M,N][3,X]ZZ
Non-OR ØWJ[Ø,2,3,4,5,K,L]4ZZ
Non-OR ØWJDØZZ
Non-OR ØWJ[1,9,B,C,D,G,H,J]3ZZ
Non-OR ØWJ[P,Q,R][3,7,8]ZZ

♂ ØWJM[Ø,3,4,X]ZZ
♀ ØWJN[Ø,3,4,X]ZZ

Ø Medical and Surgical
W Anatomical Regions, General
M Reattachment Definition: Putting back in or on all or a portion of a separated body part to its normal location or other suitable location

Explanation: Vascular circulation and nervous pathways may or may not be reestablished

Body Part Character 4	Approach Character 5	Device Character 6	Qualifier Character 7
2 Face **4** Upper Jaw **5** Lower Jaw **6** Neck **8** Chest Wall **F** Abdominal Wall **K** Upper Back **L** Lower Back **M** Perineum, Male ♂ **N** Perineum, Female ♀	**Ø** Open	**Z** No Device	**Z** No Qualifier

♂ ØWMMØZZ
♀ ØWMNØZZ

Ø Medical and Surgical
W Anatomical Regions, General
P Removal Definition: Taking out or off a device from a body part

Explanation: If a device is taken out and a similar device put in without cutting or puncturing the skin or mucous membrane, the procedure is coded to the root operation CHANGE. Otherwise, the procedure for taking out the device is coded to the root operation REMOVAL.

Body Part Character 4	Approach Character 5	Device Character 6	Qualifier Character 7
Ø Head 2 Face 4 Upper Jaw 5 Lower Jaw 6 Neck 8 Chest Wall C Mediastinum Mediastinal cavity Mediastinal space F Abdominal Wall K Upper Back L Lower Back M Perineum, Male ♂ N Perineum, Female ♀	Ø Open 3 Percutaneous 4 Percutaneous Endoscopic X External	Ø Drainage Device 1 Radioactive Element 3 Infusion Device 7 Autologous Tissue Substitute J Synthetic Substitute K Nonautologous Tissue Substitute Y Other Device	Z No Qualifier
1 Cranial Cavity 9 Pleural Cavity, Right B Pleural Cavity, Left G Peritoneal Cavity J Pelvic Cavity Retropubic space	Ø Open 3 Percutaneous 4 Percutaneous Endoscopic	Ø Drainage Device 1 Radioactive Element 3 Infusion Device J Synthetic Substitute Y Other Device	Z No Qualifier
1 Cranial Cavity 9 Pleural Cavity, Right B Pleural Cavity, Left G Peritoneal Cavity J Pelvic Cavity Retropubic space	X External	Ø Drainage Device 1 Radioactive Element 3 Infusion Device	Z No Qualifier
D Pericardial Cavity H Retroperitoneum Retroperitoneal cavity Retroperitoneal space	Ø Open 3 Percutaneous 4 Percutaneous Endoscopic	Ø Drainage Device 1 Radioactive Element 3 Infusion Device Y Other Device	Z No Qualifier
D Pericardial Cavity H Retroperitoneum Retroperitoneal cavity Retroperitoneal space	X External	Ø Drainage Device 1 Radioactive Element 3 Infusion Device	Z No Qualifier
P Gastrointestinal Tract Q Respiratory Tract R Genitourinary Tract	Ø Open 3 Percutaneous 4 Percutaneous Endoscopic 7 Via Natural or Artificial Opening 8 Via Natural or Artificial Opening Endoscopic X External	1 Radioactive Element 3 Infusion Device Y Other Device	Z No Qualifier

Non-OR ØWP[Ø,2,4,5,6,8][Ø,3,4,X][Ø,1,3,7,J,K,Y]Z
Non-OR ØWP[C,F]X[Ø,1,3,7,J,K,Y]Z
Non-OR ØWP[K,L][Ø,3,4,X][Ø,1,3,7,J,K,Y]Z
Non-OR ØWPM[Ø,3,4][Ø,1,3,J,Y]Z
Non-OR ØWPMX[Ø,1,3,Y]Z
Non-OR ØWPNX[Ø,1,3,7,J,K,Y]Z
Non-OR ØWP1[Ø,3,4]3Z
Non-OR ØWP[9,B,J][Ø,3,4][Ø,1,3,J,Y]Z
Non-OR ØWP[1,9,B,G,J]X[Ø,1,3]Z
Non-OR ØWP[D,H]X[Ø,1,3]Z
Non-OR ØWPP[3,4,7,8,X][1,3,Y]Z
Non-OR ØWPQ73Z
Non-OR ØWPQ8[3,Y]Z
Non-OR ØWPQ[Ø,X][1,3,Y]Z
Non-OR ØWPR[Ø,3,4,7,8,X][1,3,Y]Z

♂ ØWPM[Ø,3,4,X][Ø,1,3,7,J,K,Y]Z
♀ ØWPN[Ø,3,4,X][Ø,1,3,7,J,K,Y]Z

Ø Medical and Surgical
W Anatomical Regions, General
Q Repair Definition: Restoring, to the extent possible, a body part to its normal anatomic structure and function
Explanation: Used only when the method to accomplish the repair is not one of the other root operations

Body Part Character 4	Approach Character 5	Device Character 6	Qualifier Character 7
Ø Head **2** Face **3** Oral Cavity and Throat **4** Upper Jaw **5** Lower Jaw **8** Chest Wall **K** Upper Back **L** Lower Back **M** Perineum, Male ♂ **N** Perineum, Female ♀	**Ø** Open **3** Percutaneous **4** Percutaneous Endoscopic **X** External	**Z** No Device	**Z** No Qualifier
6 Neck **F** Abdominal Wall	**Ø** Open **3** Percutaneous **4** Percutaneous Endoscopic	**Z** No Device	**Z** No Qualifier
6 Neck **F** Abdominal Wall ⊞	**X** External	**Z** No Device	**2** Stoma **Z** No Qualifier
C Mediastinum Mediastinal cavity Mediastinal space	**Ø** Open **3** Percutaneous **4** Percutaneous Endoscopic	**Z** No Device	**Z** No Qualifier

Non-OR ØWQNXZZ
♂ ØWQM[Ø,3,4,X]ZZ
♀ ØWQN[Ø,3,4,X]ZZ

See Appendix L for Procedure Combinations
⊞ ØWQFXZ[2,Z]

Ø Medical and Surgical
W Anatomical Regions, General
U Supplement Definition: Putting in or on biological or synthetic material that physically reinforces and/or augments the function of a portion of a body part
Explanation: The biological material is non-living, or is living and from the same individual. The body part may have been previously replaced, and the SUPPLEMENT procedure is performed to physically reinforce and/or augment the function of the replaced body part.

Body Part Character 4	Approach Character 5	Device Character 6	Qualifier Character 7
Ø Head **2** Face **4** Upper Jaw **5** Lower Jaw **6** Neck **8** Chest Wall **C** Mediastinum Mediastinal cavity Mediastinal space **F** Abdominal Wall **K** Upper Back **L** Lower Back **M** Perineum, Male ♂ **N** Perineum, Female ♀	**Ø** Open **4** Percutaneous Endoscopic	**7** Autologous Tissue Substitute **J** Synthetic Substitute **K** Nonautologous Tissue Substitute	**Z** No Qualifier

♂ ØWUM[Ø,4][7,J,K]Z
♀ ØWUN[Ø,4][7,J,K]Z

Ø Medical and Surgical
W Anatomical Regions, General
W Revision Definition: Correcting, to the extent possible, a portion of a malfunctioning device or the position of a displaced device

Explanation: Revision can include correcting a malfunctioning or displaced device by taking out or putting in components of the device such as a screw or pin

Body Part Character 4	Approach Character 5	Device Character 6	Qualifier Character 7
Ø Head **2** Face **4** Upper Jaw **5** Lower Jaw **6** Neck **8** Chest Wall **C** Mediastinum Mediastinal cavity Mediastinal space **F** Abdominal Wall **K** Upper Back **L** Lower Back **M** Perineum, Male ♂ **N** Perineum, Female ♀	**Ø** Open **3** Percutaneous **4** Percutaneous Endoscopic **X** External	**Ø** Drainage Device **1** Radioactive Element **3** Infusion Device **7** Autologous Tissue Substitute **J** Synthetic Substitute **K** Nonautologous Tissue Substitute **Y** Other Device	**Z** No Qualifier
1 Cranial Cavity **9** Pleural Cavity, Right **B** Pleural Cavity, Left **G** Peritoneal Cavity **J** Pelvic Cavity Retropubic space	**Ø** Open **3** Percutaneous **4** Percutaneous Endoscopic **X** External	**Ø** Drainage Device **1** Radioactive Element **3** Infusion Device **J** Synthetic Substitute **Y** Other Device	**Z** No Qualifier
D Pericardial Cavity **H** Retroperitoneum Retroperitoneal cavity Retroperitoneal space	**Ø** Open **3** Percutaneous **4** Percutaneous Endoscopic **X** External	**Ø** Drainage Device **1** Radioactive Element **3** Infusion Device **Y** Other Device	**Z** No Qualifier
P Gastrointestinal Tract **Q** Respiratory Tract **R** Genitourinary Tract	**Ø** Open **3** Percutaneous **4** Percutaneous Endoscopic **7** Via Natural or Artificial Opening **8** Via Natural or Artificial Opening Endoscopic **X** External	**1** Radioactive Element **3** Infusion Device **Y** Other Device	**Z** No Qualifier

DRG Non-OR ØWW[Ø,2,4,5,6,K,L][Ø,3,4][Ø,1,3,7,J,K,Y]Z
DRG Non-OR ØWWM[Ø,3,4][Ø,1,3,J,Y]Z
Non-OR ØWW[Ø,2,4,5,6,C,F,K,L,M,N]X[Ø,1,3,7,J,K,Y]Z
Non-OR ØWW8[Ø,3,4,X][Ø,1,3,7,J,K,Y]Z
Non-OR ØWW[1,G,J]X[Ø,1,3,J,Y]Z
Non-OR ØWW[9,B][Ø,3,4,X][Ø,1,3,J,Y]Z
Non-OR ØWW[D,H]X[Ø,1,3,Y]Z
Non-OR ØWWP[3,4,7,8,X][1,3,Y]Z
Non-OR ØWWQ[Ø,X][1,3,Y]Z
Non-OR ØWWR[Ø,3,4,7,8,X][1,3,Y]Z

♂ ØWWM[Ø,3,4,X][Ø,1,3,7,K,Y]Z
♀ ØWWN[Ø,3,4,X][Ø,1,3,7,K,Y]Z

Ø Medical and Surgical
W Anatomical Regions, General
Y Transplantation Definition: Putting in or on all or a portion of a living body part taken from another individual or animal to physically take the place and/or function of all or a portion of a similar body part

Explanation: The native body part may or may not be taken out, and the transplanted body part may take over all or a portion of its function

Body Part Character 4	Approach Character 5	Device Character 6	Qualifier Character 7
2 Face	**Ø** Open	**Z** No Device	**Ø** Allogeneic **1** Syngeneic

Anatomical Regions, Upper Extremities ØXØ–ØXY

Character Meanings

This Character Meaning table is provided as a guide to assist the user in the identification of character members that may be found in this section of code tables. It **SHOULD NOT** be used to build a PCS code.

Operation–Character 3	Body Part–Character 4	Approach–Character 5	Device–Character 6	Qualifier–Character 7
Ø Alteration	Ø Forequarter, Right	Ø Open	Ø Drainage Device	Ø Allogeneic OR Complete
2 Change	1 Forequarter, Left	3 Percutaneous	1 Radioactive Element	1 High OR Syngeneic
3 Control	2 Shoulder Region, Right	4 Percutaneous Endoscopic	3 Infusion Device	2 Mid
6 Detachment	3 Shoulder Region, Left	X External	7 Autologous Tissue Substitute	3 Low
9 Drainage	4 Axilla, Right		J Synthetic Substitute	4 Complete 1st Ray
B Excision	5 Axilla, Left		K Nonautologous Tissue Substitute	5 Complete 2nd Ray
H Insertion	6 Upper Extremity, Right		Y Other Device	6 Complete 3rd Ray
J Inspection	7 Upper Extremity, Left		Z No Device	7 Complete 4th Ray
M Reattachment	8 Upper Arm, Right			8 Complete 5th Ray
P Removal	9 Upper Arm, Left			9 Partial 1st Ray
Q Repair	B Elbow Region, Right			B Partial 2nd Ray
R Replacement	C Elbow Region, Left			C Partial 3rd Ray
U Supplement	D Lower Arm, Right			D Partial 4th Ray
W Revision	F Lower Arm, Left			F Partial 5th Ray
X Transfer	G Wrist Region, Right			L Thumb, Right
Y Transplantation	H Wrist Region, Left			M Thumb, Left
	J Hand, Right			N Toe, Right
	K Hand, Left			P Toe, Left
	L Thumb, Right			X Diagnostic
	M Thumb, Left			Z No Qualifier
	N Index Finger, Right			
	P Index Finger, Left			
	Q Middle Finger, Right			
	R Middle Finger, Left			
	S Ring Finger, Right			
	T Ring Finger, Left			
	V Little Finger, Right			
	W Little Finger, Left			

AHA Coding Clinic for table ØX3

2016, 4Q, 99 Root operation Control
2015, 1Q, 35 Evacuation of hematoma for control of postprocedural bleeding
2013, 3Q, 23 Control of intraoperative bleeding

AHA Coding Clinic for table ØX6

2017, 2Q, 3-4 Qualifiers for the root operation detachment
2017, 2Q, 18 Removal of polydactyl digits
2017, 1Q, 52 Further distal phalangeal amputation
2016, 3Q, 33 Traumatic amputation of fingers with further revision amputation

AHA Coding Clinic for table ØXH

2017, 2Q, 20 Exchange of intramedullary antibiotic impregnated spacer

AHA Coding Clinic for table ØXP

2017, 2Q, 20 Exchange of intramedullary antibiotic impregnated spacer

AHA Coding Clinic for table ØXY

2016, 4Q, 112-113 Transplantation

Detachment Qualifier Descriptions

Qualifier Definition	Upper Arm	Lower Arm
1 **High:** Amputation at the proximal portion of the shaft of the:	Humerus	Radius/Ulna
2 **Mid:** Amputation at the middle portion of the shaft of the:	Humerus	Radius/Ulna
3 **Low:** Amputation at the distal portion of the shaft of the:	Humerus	Radius/Ulna

Qualifier Definition	Hand
Ø Complete 1st through 5th Rays Ray: digit of hand or foot with corresponding metacarpus or metatarsus	Through carpo-metacarpal joint, **Wrist**
4 Complete 1st Ray	Through carpo-metacarpal joint, **Thumb**
5 Complete 2nd Ray	Through carpo-metacarpal joint, **Index Finger**
6 Complete 3rd Ray	Through carpo-metacarpal joint, **Middle Finger**
7 Complete 4th Ray	Through carpo-metacarpal joint, **Ring Finger**
8 Complete 5th Ray	Through carpo-metacarpal joint, **Little Finger**
9 Partial 1st Ray	Anywhere along shaft or head of metacarpal bone, **Thumb**
B Partial 2nd Ray	Anywhere along shaft or head of metacarpal bone, **Index Finger**
C Partial 3rd Ray	Anywhere along shaft or head of metacarpal bone, **Middle Finger**
D Partial 4th Ray	Anywhere along shaft or head of metacarpal bone, **Ring Finger**
F Partial 5th Ray	Anywhere along shaft or head of metacarpal bone, **Little Finger**

Qualifier Definition	Thumb/Finger
Ø Complete	At the metacarpophalangeal joint
1 High	Anywhere along the proximal phalanx
2 Mid	Through the proximal interphalangeal joint or anywhere along the middle phalanx
3 Low	Through the distal interphalangeal joint or anywhere along the distal phalanx

Ø Medical and Surgical
X Anatomical Regions, Upper Extremities
Ø Alteration Definition: Modifying the anatomic structure of a body part without affecting the function of the body part
Explanation: Principal purpose is to improve appearance

Body Part Character 4	Approach Character 5	Device Character 6	Qualifier Character 7
2 Shoulder Region, Right 3 Shoulder Region, Left 4 Axilla, Right 5 Axilla, Left 6 Upper Extremity, Right 7 Upper Extremity, Left 8 Upper Arm, Right 9 Upper Arm, Left B Elbow Region, Right C Elbow Region, Left D Lower Arm, Right F Lower Arm, Left G Wrist Region, Right H Wrist Region, Left	Ø Open 3 Percutaneous 4 Percutaneous Endoscopic	7 Autologous Tissue Substitute J Synthetic Substitute K Nonautologous Tissue Substitute Z No Device	Z No Qualifier

Ø Medical and Surgical
X Anatomical Regions, Upper Extremities
2 Change Definition: Taking out or off a device from a body part and putting back an identical or similar device in or on the same body part without cutting or puncturing the skin or a mucous membrane
Explanation: All CHANGE procedures are coded using the approach EXTERNAL

Body Part Character 4	Approach Character 5	Device Character 6	Qualifier Character 7
6 Upper Extremity, Right 7 Upper Extremity, Left	X External	Ø Drainage Device Y Other Device	Z No Qualifier

Non-OR All body part, approach, device, and qualifier values

Ø Medical and Surgical
X Anatomical Regions, Upper Extremities
3 Control Definition: Stopping, or attempting to stop, postprocedural or other acute bleeding
Explanation: None

Body Part Character 4	Approach Character 5	Device Character 6	Qualifier Character 7
2 Shoulder Region, Right 3 Shoulder Region, Left 4 Axilla, Right 5 Axilla, Left 6 Upper Extremity, Right 7 Upper Extremity, Left 8 Upper Arm, Right 9 Upper Arm, Left B Elbow Region, Right C Elbow Region, Left D Lower Arm, Right F Lower Arm, Left G Wrist Region, Right H Wrist Region, Left J Hand, Right K Hand, Left	Ø Open 3 Percutaneous 4 Percutaneous Endoscopic	Z No Device	Z No Qualifier

Ø Medical and Surgical
X Anatomical Regions, Upper Extremities
6 Detachment Definition: Cutting off all or a portion of the upper or lower extremities

Explanation: The body part value is the site of the detachment, with a qualifier if applicable to further specify the level where the extremity was detached

Body Part Character 4	Approach Character 5	Device Character 6	Qualifier Character 7
Ø Forequarter, Right 1 Forequarter, Left 2 Shoulder Region, Right 3 Shoulder Region, Left B Elbow Region, Right C Elbow Region, Left	Ø Open	Z No Device	Z No Qualifier
8 Upper Arm, Right 9 Upper Arm, Left D Lower Arm, Right F Lower Arm, Left	Ø Open	Z No Device	1 High 2 Mid 3 Low
J Hand, Right K Hand, Left	Ø Open	Z No Device	Ø Complete 4 Complete 1st Ray 5 Complete 2nd Ray 6 Complete 3rd Ray 7 Complete 4th Ray 8 Complete 5th Ray 9 Partial 1st Ray B Partial 2nd Ray C Partial 3rd Ray D Partial 4th Ray F Partial 5th Ray
L Thumb, Right M Thumb, Left N Index Finger, Right P Index Finger, Left Q Middle Finger, Right R Middle Finger, Left S Ring Finger, Right T Ring Finger, Left V Little Finger, Right W Little Finger, Left	Ø Open	Z No Device	Ø Complete 1 High 2 Mid 3 Low

Ø Medical and Surgical
X Anatomical Regions, Upper Extremities
9 Drainage Definition: Taking or letting out fluids and/or gases from a body part
Explanation: The qualifier DIAGNOSTIC is used to identify drainage procedures that are biopsies

Body Part Character 4	Approach Character 5	Device Character 6	Qualifier Character 7
2 Shoulder Region, Right 3 Shoulder Region, Left 4 Axilla, Right 5 Axilla, Left 6 Upper Extremity, Right 7 Upper Extremity, Left 8 Upper Arm, Right 9 Upper Arm, Left B Elbow Region, Right C Elbow Region, Left D Lower Arm, Right F Lower Arm, Left G Wrist Region, Right H Wrist Region, Left J Hand, Right K Hand, Left	Ø Open 3 Percutaneous 4 Percutaneous Endoscopic	Ø Drainage Device	Z No Qualifier
2 Shoulder Region, Right 3 Shoulder Region, Left 4 Axilla, Right 5 Axilla, Left 6 Upper Extremity, Right 7 Upper Extremity, Left 8 Upper Arm, Right 9 Upper Arm, Left B Elbow Region, Right C Elbow Region, Left D Lower Arm, Right F Lower Arm, Left G Wrist Region, Right H Wrist Region, Left J Hand, Right K Hand, Left	Ø Open 3 Percutaneous 4 Percutaneous Endoscopic	Z No Device	X Diagnostic Z No Qualifier

Non-OR All body part, approach, device, and qualifier values

Ø Medical and Surgical
X Anatomical Regions, Upper Extremities
B Excision Definition: Cutting out or off, without replacement, a portion of a body part
Explanation: The qualifier DIAGNOSTIC is used to identify excision procedures that are biopsies

Body Part Character 4	Approach Character 5	Device Character 6	Qualifier Character 7
2 Shoulder Region, Right 3 Shoulder Region, Left 4 Axilla, Right 5 Axilla, Left 6 Upper Extremity, Right 7 Upper Extremity, Left 8 Upper Arm, Right 9 Upper Arm, Left B Elbow Region, Right C Elbow Region, Left D Lower Arm, Right F Lower Arm, Left G Wrist Region, Right H Wrist Region, Left J Hand, Right K Hand, Left	Ø Open 3 Percutaneous 4 Percutaneous Endoscopic	Z No Device	X Diagnostic Z No Qualifier

Non-OR ØXB[2,3,4,5,6,7,8,9,B,C,D,F,G,H,J,K][Ø,3,4]ZX

Ø Medical and Surgical
X Anatomical Regions, Upper Extremities
H Insertion Definition: Putting in a nonbiological appliance that monitors, assists, performs, or prevents a physiological function but does not physically take the place of a body part

Explanation: None

Body Part Character 4	Approach Character 5	Device Character 6	Qualifier Character 7
2 Shoulder Region, Right 3 Shoulder Region, Left 4 Axilla, Right 5 Axilla, Left 6 Upper Extremity, Right 7 Upper Extremity, Left 8 Upper Arm, Right 9 Upper Arm, Left B Elbow Region, Right C Elbow Region, Left D Lower Arm, Right F Lower Arm, Left G Wrist Region, Right H Wrist Region, Left J Hand, Right K Hand, Left	Ø Open 3 Percutaneous 4 Percutaneous Endoscopic	1 Radioactive Element 3 Infusion Device Y Other Device	Z No Qualifier

DRG Non-OR ØXH[2,3,4,5,6,7,8,9,B,C,D,F,G,H,J,K][Ø,3,4][3,Y]Z

Ø Medical and Surgical
X Anatomical Regions, Upper Extremities
J Inspection Definition: Visually and/or manually exploring a body part

Explanation: Visual exploration may be performed with or without optical instrumentation. Manual exploration may be performed directly or through intervening body layers.

Body Part Character 4	Approach Character 5	Device Character 6	Qualifier Character 7
2 Shoulder Region, Right 3 Shoulder Region, Left 4 Axilla, Right 5 Axilla, Left 6 Upper Extremity, Right 7 Upper Extremity, Left 8 Upper Arm, Right 9 Upper Arm, Left B Elbow Region, Right C Elbow Region, Left D Lower Arm, Right F Lower Arm, Left G Wrist Region, Right H Wrist Region, Left J Hand, Right K Hand, Left	Ø Open 3 Percutaneous 4 Percutaneous Endoscopic X External	Z No Device	Z No Qualifier

DRG Non-OR ØXJ[2,3,4,5,6,7,8,9,B,C,D,F,G,H,J,K]ØZZ
Non-OR ØXJ[2,3,4,5,6,7,8,9,B,C,D,F,G,H][3,4,X]ZZ
Non-OR ØXJ[J,K][3,X]ZZ

Ø Medical and Surgical
X Anatomical Regions, Upper Extremities
M Reattachment Definition: Putting back in or on all or a portion of a separated body part to its normal location or other suitable location

Explanation: Vascular circulation and nervous pathways may or may not be reestablished

Body Part Character 4	Approach Character 5	Device Character 6	Qualifier Character 7
Ø Forequarter, Right 1 Forequarter, Left 2 Shoulder Region, Right 3 Shoulder Region, Left 4 Axilla, Right 5 Axilla, Left 6 Upper Extremity, Right 7 Upper Extremity, Left 8 Upper Arm, Right 9 Upper Arm, Left B Elbow Region, Right C Elbow Region, Left D Lower Arm, Right F Lower Arm, Left G Wrist Region, Right H Wrist Region, Left J Hand, Right K Hand, Left L Thumb, Right M Thumb, Left N Index Finger, Right P Index Finger, Left Q Middle Finger, Right R Middle Finger, Left S Ring Finger, Right T Ring Finger, Left V Little Finger, Right W Little Finger, Left	Ø Open	Z No Device	Z No Qualifier

Ø Medical and Surgical
X Anatomical Regions, Upper Extremities
P Removal Definition: Taking out or off a device from a body part

Explanation: If a device is taken out and a similar device put in without cutting or puncturing the skin or mucous membrane, the procedure is coded to the root operation CHANGE. Otherwise, the procedure for taking out the device is coded to the root operation REMOVAL.

Body Part Character 4	Approach Character 5	Device Character 6	Qualifier Character 7
6 Upper Extremity, Right 7 Upper Extremity, Left	Ø Open 3 Percutaneous 4 Percutaneous Endoscopic X External	Ø Drainage Device 1 Radioactive Element 3 Infusion Device 7 Autologous Tissue Substitute J Synthetic Substitute K Nonautologous Tissue Substitute Y Other Device	Z No Qualifier

Non-OR All body part, approach, device, and qualifier values

Ø Medical and Surgical
X Anatomical Regions, Upper Extremities
Q Repair Definition: Restoring, to the extent possible, a body part to its normal anatomic structure and function

Explanation: Used only when the method to accomplish the repair is not one of the other root operations

Body Part Character 4	Approach Character 5	Device Character 6	Qualifier Character 7
2 Shoulder Region, Right 3 Shoulder Region, Left 4 Axilla, Right 5 Axilla, Left 6 Upper Extremity, Right 7 Upper Extremity, Left 8 Upper Arm, Right 9 Upper Arm, Left B Elbow Region, Right C Elbow Region, Left D Lower Arm, Right F Lower Arm, Left G Wrist Region, Right H Wrist Region, Left J Hand, Right K Hand, Left L Thumb, Right M Thumb, Left N Index Finger, Right P Index Finger, Left Q Middle Finger, Right R Middle Finger, Left S Ring Finger, Right T Ring Finger, Left V Little Finger, Right W Little Finger, Left	Ø Open 3 Percutaneous 4 Percutaneous Endoscopic X External	Z No Device	Z No Qualifier

Ø Medical and Surgical
X Anatomical Regions, Upper Extremities
R Replacement Definition: Putting in or on biological or synthetic material that physically takes the place and/or function of all or a portion of a body part

Explanation: The body part may have been taken out or replaced, or may be taken out, physically eradicated, or rendered nonfunctional during the REPLACEMENT procedure. A REMOVAL procedure is coded for taking out the device used in a previous replacement procedure.

Body Part Character 4	Approach Character 5	Device Character 6	Qualifier Character 7
L Thumb, Right M Thumb, Left	Ø Open 4 Percutaneous Endoscopic	7 Autologous Tissue Substitute	N Toe, Right P Toe, Left

Ø Medical and Surgical
X Anatomical Regions, Upper Extremities
U Supplement Definition: Putting in or on biological or synthetic material that physically reinforces and/or augments the function of a portion of a body part

Explanation: The biological material is non-living, or is living and from the same individual. The body part may have been previously replaced, and the SUPPLEMENT procedure is performed to physically reinforce and/or augment the function of the replaced body part.

Body Part Character 4	Approach Character 5	Device Character 6	Qualifier Character 7
2 Shoulder Region, Right 3 Shoulder Region, Left 4 Axilla, Right 5 Axilla, Left 6 Upper Extremity, Right 7 Upper Extremity, Left 8 Upper Arm, Right 9 Upper Arm, Left B Elbow Region, Right C Elbow Region, Left D Lower Arm, Right F Lower Arm, Left G Wrist Region, Right H Wrist Region, Left J Hand, Right K Hand, Left L Thumb, Right M Thumb, Left N Index Finger, Right P Index Finger, Left Q Middle Finger, Right R Middle Finger, Left S Ring Finger, Right T Ring Finger, Left V Little Finger, Right W Little Finger, Left	Ø Open 4 Percutaneous Endoscopic	7 Autologous Tissue Substitute J Synthetic Substitute K Nonautologous Tissue Substitute	Z No Qualifier

Ø Medical and Surgical
X Anatomical Regions, Upper Extremities
W Revision Definition: Correcting, to the extent possible, a portion of a malfunctioning device or the position of a displaced device

Explanation: Revision can include correcting a malfunctioning or displaced device by taking out or putting in components of the device such as a screw or pin

Body Part Character 4	Approach Character 5	Device Character 6	Qualifier Character 7
6 Upper Extremity, Right 7 Upper Extremity, Left	Ø Open 3 Percutaneous 4 Percutaneous Endoscopic X External	Ø Drainage Device 3 Infusion Device 7 Autologous Tissue Substitute J Synthetic Substitute K Nonautologous Tissue Substitute Y Other Device	Z No Qualifier

DRG Non-OR ØXW[6,7][Ø,3,4][Ø,3,7,J,K,Y]Z
Non-OR ØXW[6,7]X[Ø,3,7,J,K,Y]Z

Ø Medical and Surgical
X Anatomical Regions, Upper Extremities
X Transfer Definition: Moving, without taking out, all or a portion of a body part to another location to take over the function of all or a portion of a body part

Explanation: The body part transferred remains connected to its vascular and nervous supply

Body Part Character 4	Approach Character 5	Device Character 6	Qualifier Character 7
N Index Finger, Right	Ø Open	Z No Device	L Thumb, Right
P Index Finger, Left	Ø Open	Z No Device	M Thumb, Left

Ø Medical and Surgical
X Anatomical Regions, Upper Extremities
Y Transplantation Definition: Putting in or on all or a portion of a living body part taken from another individual or animal to physically take the place and/or function of all or a portion of a similar body part

Explanation: The native body part may or may not be taken out, and the transplanted body part may take over all or a portion of its function

Body Part Character 4	Approach Character 5	Device Character 6	Qualifier Character 7
J Hand, Right K Hand, Left	Ø Open	Z No Device	Ø Allogeneic 1 Syngeneic

Anatomical Regions, Lower Extremities ØYØ–ØYW

Character Meanings

This Character Meaning table is provided as a guide to assist the user in the identification of character members that may be found in this section of code tables. It **SHOULD NOT** be used to build a PCS code.

Operation–Character 3	Body Part–Character 4	Approach–Character 5	Device–Character 6	Qualifier–Character 7
Ø Alteration	Ø Buttock, Right	Ø Open	Ø Drainage Device	Ø Complete
2 Change	1 Buttock, Left	3 Percutaneous	1 Radioactive Element	1 High
3 Control	2 Hindquarter, Right	4 Percutaneous Endoscopic	3 Infusion Device	2 Mid
6 Detachment	3 Hindquarter, Left	X External	7 Autologous Tissue Substitute	3 Low
9 Drainage	4 Hindquarter, Bilateral		J Synthetic Substitute	4 Complete 1st Ray
B Excision	5 Inguinal Region, Right		K Nonautologous Tissue Substitute	5 Complete 2nd Ray
H Insertion	6 Inguinal Region, Left		Y Other Device	6 Complete 3rd Ray
J Inspection	7 Femoral Region, Right		Z No Device	7 Complete 4th Ray
M Reattachment	8 Femoral Region, Left			8 Complete 5th Ray
P Removal	9 Lower Extremity, Right			9 Partial 1st Ray
Q Repair	A Inguinal Region, Bilateral			B Partial 2nd Ray
U Supplement	B Lower Extremity, Left			C Partial 3rd Ray
W Revision	C Upper Leg, Right			D Partial 4th Ray
	D Upper Leg, Left			F Partial 5th Ray
	E Femoral Region, Bilateral			X Diagnostic
	F Knee Region, Right			Z No Qualifier
	G Knee Region, Left			
	H Lower Leg, Right			
	J Lower Leg, Left			
	K Ankle Region, Right			
	L Ankle Region, Left			
	M Foot, Right			
	N Foot, Left			
	P 1st Toe, Right			
	Q 1st Toe, Left			
	R 2nd Toe, Right			
	S 2nd Toe, Left			
	T 3rd Toe, Right			
	U 3rd Toe, Left			
	V 4th Toe, Right			
	W 4th Toe, Left			
	X 5th Toe, Right			
	Y 5th Toe, Left			

AHA Coding Clinic for table ØY3

2016, 4Q, 99 Root operation Control
2013, 3Q, 23 Control of intraoperative bleeding

AHA Coding Clinic for table ØY6

2019, 2Q, 17 Cryoamputation of lower leg
2017, 2Q, 3-4 Qualifiers for the root operation detachment
2017, 1Q, 22 Chopart amputation of foot
2015, 2Q, 28 Partial amputation of hallux at interphalangeal Joint
2015, 1Q, 28 Mid-foot amputation

AHA Coding Clinic for table ØY9

2015, 1Q, 22 Incision and drainage of abscess of femoropopliteal bypass site
2015, 1Q, 22 Incision and drainage of groin abscess

Detachment Qualifier Descriptions

Qualifier Definition	Upper Leg	Lower Leg
1 **High:** Amputation at the proximal portion of the shaft of the:	Femur	Tibia/Fibula
2 **Mid:** Amputation at the middle portion of the shaft of the:	Femur	Tibia/Fibula
3 **Low:** Amputation at the distal portion of the shaft of the:	Femur	Tibia/Fibula

Qualifier Definition	Foot
Ø Complete 1st through 5th Rays Ray: digit of hand or foot with corresponding metacarpus or metatarsus	Through tarso-metatarsal Joint, **Ankle**
4 Complete 1st Ray	Through tarso-metatarsal joint, **Great Toe**
5 Complete 2nd Ray	Through tarso-metatarsal joint, **2nd Toe**
6 Complete 3rd Ray	Through tarso-metatarsal joint, **3rd Toe**
7 Complete 4th Ray	Through tarso-metatarsal joint, **4th Toe**
8 Complete 5th Ray	Through tarso-metatarsal joint, **Little Toe**
9 Partial 1st Ray	Anywhere along shaft or head of metatarsal bone, **Great Toe**
B Partial 2nd Ray	Anywhere along shaft or head of metatarsal bone, **2nd Toe**
C Partial 3rd Ray	Anywhere along shaft or head of metatarsal bone, **3rd Toe**
D Partial 4th Ray	Anywhere along shaft or head of metatarsal bone, **4th Toe**
F Partial 5th Ray	Anywhere along shaft or head of metatarsal bone, **Little Toe**

Qualifier Definition	Toe
Ø Complete	At the metatarsal-phalangeal joint
1 High	Anywhere along the proximal phalanx
2 Mid	Through the proximal interphalangeal joint or anywhere along the middle phalanx
3 Low	Through the distal interphalangeal joint or anywhere along the distal phalanx

Ø Medical and Surgical
Y Anatomical Regions, Lower Extremities
Ø Alteration Definition: Modifying the anatomic structure of a body part without affecting the function of the body part
Explanation: Principal purpose is to improve appearance

Body Part Character 4	Approach Character 5	Device Character 6	Qualifier Character 7
Ø Buttock, Right 1 Buttock, Left 9 Lower Extremity, Right B Lower Extremity, Left C Upper Leg, Right D Upper Leg, Left F Knee Region, Right G Knee Region, Left H Lower Leg, Right J Lower Leg, Left K Ankle Region, Right L Ankle Region, Left	Ø Open 3 Percutaneous 4 Percutaneous Endoscopic	7 Autologous Tissue Substitute J Synthetic Substitute K Nonautologous Tissue Substitute Z No Device	Z No Qualifier

Ø Medical and Surgical
Y Anatomical Regions, Lower Extremities
2 Change Definition: Taking out or off a device from a body part and putting back an identical or similar device in or on the same body part without cutting or puncturing the skin or a mucous membrane
Explanation: All CHANGE procedures are coded using the approach EXTERNAL

Body Part Character 4	Approach Character 5	Device Character 6	Qualifier Character 7
9 Lower Extremity, Right B Lower Extremity, Left	X External	Ø Drainage Device Y Other Device	Z No Qualifier

Non-OR All body part, approach, device, and qualifier values

Ø Medical and Surgical
Y Anatomical Regions, Lower Extremities
3 Control Definition: Stopping, or attempting to stop, postprocedural or other acute bleeding
Explanation: None

Body Part Character 4	Approach Character 5	Device Character 6	Qualifier Character 7
Ø Buttock, Right 1 Buttock, Left 5 Inguinal Region, Right Inguinal canal Inguinal triangle 6 Inguinal Region, Left *See 5 Inguinal Region, Right* 7 Femoral Region, Right 8 Femoral Region, Left 9 Lower Extremity, Right B Lower Extremity, Left C Upper Leg, Right D Upper Leg, Left F Knee Region, Right G Knee Region, Left H Lower Leg, Right J Lower Leg, Left K Ankle Region, Right L Ankle Region, Left M Foot, Right N Foot, Left	Ø Open 3 Percutaneous 4 Percutaneous Endoscopic	Z No Device	Z No Qualifier

Ø Medical and Surgical
Y Anatomical Regions, Lower Extremities
6 Detachment Definition: Cutting off all or a portion of the upper or lower extremities

Explanation: The body part value is the site of the detachment, with a qualifier if applicable to further specify the level where the extremity was detached

Body Part Character 4	Approach Character 5	Device Character 6	Qualifier Character 7
2 Hindquarter, Right **3** Hindquarter, Left **4** Hindquarter, Bilateral **7** Femoral Region, Right **8** Femoral Region, Left **F** Knee Region, Right **G** Knee Region, Left	**Ø** Open	**Z** No Device	**Z** No Qualifier
C Upper Leg, Right **D** Upper Leg, Left **H** Lower Leg, Right **J** Lower Leg, Left	**Ø** Open	**Z** No Device	**1** High **2** Mid **3** Low
M Foot, Right **N** Foot, Left	**Ø** Open	**Z** No Device	**Ø** Complete **4** Complete 1st Ray **5** Complete 2nd Ray **6** Complete 3rd Ray **7** Complete 4th Ray **8** Complete 5th Ray **9** Partial 1st Ray **B** Partial 2nd Ray **C** Partial 3rd Ray **D** Partial 4th Ray **F** Partial 5th Ray
P 1st Toe, Right Hallux **Q** 1st Toe, Left *See 1st Toe, Right* **R** 2nd Toe, Right **S** 2nd Toe, Left **T** 3rd Toe, Right **U** 3rd Toe, Left **V** 4th Toe, Right **W** 4th Toe, Left **X** 5th Toe, Right **Y** 5th Toe, Left	**Ø** Open	**Z** No Device	**Ø** Complete **1** High **2** Mid **3** Low

Ø Medical and Surgical
Y Anatomical Regions, Lower Extremities
9 Drainage Definition: Taking or letting out fluids and/or gases from a body part
Explanation: The qualifier DIAGNOSTIC is used to identify drainage procedures that are biopsies

Body Part Character 4	Approach Character 5	Device Character 6	Qualifier Character 7
Ø Buttock, Right **1 Buttock, Left** **5 Inguinal Region, Right** Inguinal canal Inguinal triangle **6 Inguinal Region, Left** *See 5 Inguinal Region, Right* **7 Femoral Region, Right** **8 Femoral Region, Left** **9 Lower Extremity, Right** **B Lower Extremity, Left** **C Upper Leg, Right** **D Upper Leg, Left** **F Knee Region, Right** **G Knee Region, Left** **H Lower Leg, Right** **J Lower Leg, Left** **K Ankle Region, Right** **L Ankle Region, Left** **M Foot, Right** **N Foot, Left**	**Ø Open** **3 Percutaneous** **4 Percutaneous Endoscopic**	**Ø Drainage Device**	**Z No Qualifier**
Ø Buttock, Right **1 Buttock, Left** **5 Inguinal Region, Right** Inguinal canal Inguinal triangle **6 Inguinal Region, Left** *See 5 Inguinal Region, Right* **7 Femoral Region, Right** **8 Femoral Region, Left** **9 Lower Extremity, Right** **B Lower Extremity, Left** **C Upper Leg, Right** **D Upper Leg, Left** **F Knee Region, Right** **G Knee Region, Left** **H Lower Leg, Right** **J Lower Leg, Left** **K Ankle Region, Right** **L Ankle Region, Left** **M Foot, Right** **N Foot, Left**	**Ø Open** **3 Percutaneous** **4 Percutaneous Endoscopic**	**Z No Device**	**X Diagnostic** **Z No Qualifier**

Non-OR ØY9[Ø,1,7,8,9,B,C,D,F,G,H,J,K,L,M,N][Ø,3,4]ØZ
Non-OR ØY9[5,6]3ØZ
Non-OR ØY9[Ø,1,7,8,9,B,C,D,F,G,H,J,K,L,M,N][Ø,3,4]Z[X,Z]
Non-OR ØY9[5,6]3ZZ

Ø Medical and Surgical
Y Anatomical Regions, Lower Extremities
B Excision Definition: Cutting out or off, without replacement, a portion of a body part
Explanation: The qualifier DIAGNOSTIC is used to identify excision procedures that are biopsies

Body Part Character 4	Approach Character 5	Device Character 6	Qualifier Character 7
Ø Buttock, Right 1 Buttock, Left 5 Inguinal Region, Right Inguinal canal Inguinal triangle 6 Inguinal Region, Left *See 5 Inguinal Region, Right* 7 Femoral Region, Right 8 Femoral Region, Left 9 Lower Extremity, Right B Lower Extremity, Left C Upper Leg, Right D Upper Leg, Left F Knee Region, Right G Knee Region, Left H Lower Leg, Right J Lower Leg, Left K Ankle Region, Right L Ankle Region, Left M Foot, Right N Foot, Left	Ø Open 3 Percutaneous 4 Percutaneous Endoscopic	Z No Device	X Diagnostic Z No Qualifier

Non-OR ØYB[Ø,1,9,B,C,D,F,G,H,J,K,L,M,N][Ø,3,4]ZX

Ø Medical and Surgical
Y Anatomical Regions, Lower Extremities
H Insertion Definition: Putting in a nonbiological appliance that monitors, assists, performs, or prevents a physiological function but does not physically take the place of a body part
Explanation: None

Body Part Character 4	Approach Character 5	Device Character 6	Qualifier Character 7
Ø Buttock, Right 1 Buttock, Left 5 Inguinal Region, Right Inguinal canal Inguinal triangle 6 Inguinal Region, Left *See 5 Inguinal Region, Right* 7 Femoral Region, Right 8 Femoral Region, Left 9 Lower Extremity, Right B Lower Extremity, Left C Upper Leg, Right D Upper Leg, Left F Knee Region, Right G Knee Region, Left H Lower Leg, Right J Lower Leg, Left K Ankle Region, Right L Ankle Region, Left M Foot, Right N Foot, Left	Ø Open 3 Percutaneous 4 Percutaneous Endoscopic	1 Radioactive Element 3 Infusion Device Y Other Device	Z No Qualifier

DRG Non-OR ØYH[Ø,1,5,6,7,8,9,B,C,D,F,G,H,J,K,L,M,N][Ø,3,4][3,Y]Z

Ø Medical and Surgical
Y Anatomical Regions, Lower Extremities
J Inspection Definition: Visually and/or manually exploring a body part

Explanation: Visual exploration may be performed with or without optical instrumentation. Manual exploration may be performed directly or through intervening body layers.

Body Part Character 4	Approach Character 5	Device Character 6	Qualifier Character 7
Ø Buttock, Right **1 Buttock, Left** **5 Inguinal Region, Right** Inguinal canal Inguinal triangle **6 Inguinal Region, Left** *See 5 Inguinal Region, Right* **7 Femoral Region, Right** **8 Femoral Region, Left** **9 Lower Extremity, Right** **A Inguinal Region, Bilateral** *See 5 Inguinal Region, Right* **B Lower Extremity, Left** **C Upper Leg, Right** **D Upper Leg, Left** **E Femoral Region, Bilateral** **F Knee Region, Right** **G Knee Region, Left** **H Lower Leg, Right** **J Lower Leg, Left** **K Ankle Region, Right** **L Ankle Region, Left** **M Foot, Right** **N Foot, Left**	**Ø Open** **3 Percutaneous** **4 Percutaneous Endoscopic** **X External**	**Z No Device**	**Z No Qualifier**

DRG Non-OR ØYJ[Ø,1,8,9,B,C,D,E,F,G,H,J,K,L,M,N]ØZZ
Non-OR ØYJ[Ø,1,9,B,C,D,F,G,H,J,K,L,M,N][3,4,X]ZZ
Non-OR ØYJ[5,6,7,8,A,E][3,X]ZZ

Ø Medical and Surgical
Y Anatomical Regions, Lower Extremities
M Reattachment Definition: Putting back in or on all or a portion of a separated body part to its normal location or other suitable location

Explanation: Vascular circulation and nervous pathways may or may not be reestablished

Body Part Character 4	Approach Character 5	Device Character 6	Qualifier Character 7
Ø Buttock, Right 1 Buttock, Left 2 Hindquarter, Right 3 Hindquarter, Left 4 Hindquarter, Bilateral 5 Inguinal Region, Right Inguinal canal Inguinal triangle 6 Inguinal Region, Left *See 5 Inguinal Region, Right* 7 Femoral Region, Right 8 Femoral Region, Left 9 Lower Extremity, Right B Lower Extremity, Left C Upper Leg, Right D Upper Leg, Left F Knee Region, Right G Knee Region, Left H Lower Leg, Right J Lower Leg, Left K Ankle Region, Right L Ankle Region, Left M Foot, Right N Foot, Left P 1st Toe, Right Hallux Q 1st Toe, Left *See 1st Toe, Right* R 2nd Toe, Right S 2nd Toe, Left T 3rd Toe, Right U 3rd Toe, Left V 4th Toe, Right W 4th Toe, Left X 5th Toe, Right Y 5th Toe, Left	Ø Open	Z No Device	Z No Qualifier

Ø Medical and Surgical
Y Anatomical Regions, Lower Extremities
P Removal Definition: Taking out or off a device from a body part

Explanation: If a device is taken out and a similar device put in without cutting or puncturing the skin or mucous membrane, the procedure is coded to the root operation CHANGE. Otherwise, the procedure for taking out the device is coded to the root operation REMOVAL.

Body Part Character 4	Approach Character 5	Device Character 6	Qualifier Character 7
9 Lower Extremity, Right B Lower Extremity, Left	Ø Open 3 Percutaneous 4 Percutaneous Endoscopic X External	Ø Drainage Device 1 Radioactive Element 3 Infusion Device 7 Autologous Tissue Substitute J Synthetic Substitute K Nonautologous Tissue Substitute Y Other Device	Z No Qualifier

Non-OR All body part, approach, device, and qualifier values

Ø Medical and Surgical
Y Anatomical Regions, Lower Extremities
Q Repair Definition: Restoring, to the extent possible, a body part to its normal anatomic structure and function
Explanation: Used only when the method to accomplish the repair is not one of the other root operations

Body Part Character 4	Approach Character 5	Device Character 6	Qualifier Character 7
Ø Buttock, Right **1** Buttock, Left **5** Inguinal Region, Right Inguinal canal Inguinal triangle **6** Inguinal Region, Left *See 5 Inguinal Region, Right* **7** Femoral Region, Right **8** Femoral Region, Left **9** Lower Extremity, Right **A** Inguinal Region, Bilateral *See 5 Inguinal Region, Right* **B** Lower Extremity, Left **C** Upper Leg, Right **D** Upper Leg, Left **E** Femoral Region, Bilateral **F** Knee Region, Right **G** Knee Region, Left **H** Lower Leg, Right **J** Lower Leg, Left **K** Ankle Region, Right **L** Ankle Region, Left **M** Foot, Right **N** Foot, Left **P** 1st Toe, Right Hallux **Q** 1st Toe, Left *See 1st Toe, Right* **R** 2nd Toe, Right **S** 2nd Toe, Left **T** 3rd Toe, Right **U** 3rd Toe, Left **V** 4th Toe, Right **W** 4th Toe, Left **X** 5th Toe, Right **Y** 5th Toe, Left	**Ø** Open **3** Percutaneous **4** Percutaneous Endoscopic **X** External	**Z** No Device	**Z** No Qualifier

Non-OR ØYQ[5,6,7,8,A,E]XZZ

Ø Medical and Surgical
Y Anatomical Regions, Lower Extremities
U Supplement Definition: Putting in or on biological or synthetic material that physically reinforces and/or augments the function of a portion of a body part

Explanation: The biological material is non-living, or is living and from the same individual. The body part may have been previously replaced, and the SUPPLEMENT procedure is performed to physically reinforce and/or augment the function of the replaced body part.

Body Part Character 4	Approach Character 5	Device Character 6	Qualifier Character 7
Ø Buttock, Right 1 Buttock, Left 5 Inguinal Region, Right Inguinal canal Inguinal triangle 6 Inguinal Region, Left *See 5 Inguinal Region, Right* 7 Femoral Region, Right 8 Femoral Region, Left 9 Lower Extremity, Right A Inguinal Region, Bilateral *See 5 Inguinal Region, Right* B Lower Extremity, Left C Upper Leg, Right D Upper Leg, Left E Femoral Region, Bilateral F Knee Region, Right G Knee Region, Left H Lower Leg, Right J Lower Leg, Left K Ankle Region, Right L Ankle Region, Left M Foot, Right N Foot, Left P 1st Toe, Right Hallux Q 1st Toe, Left *See 1st Toe, Right* R 2nd Toe, Right S 2nd Toe, Left T 3rd Toe, Right U 3rd Toe, Left V 4th Toe, Right W 4th Toe, Left X 5th Toe, Right Y 5th Toe, Left	Ø Open 4 Percutaneous Endoscopic	7 Autologous Tissue Substitute J Synthetic Substitute K Nonautologous Tissue Substitute	Z No Qualifier

Ø Medical and Surgical
Y Anatomical Regions, Lower Extremities
W Revision Definition: Correcting, to the extent possible, a portion of a malfunctioning device or the position of a displaced device

Explanation: Revision can include correcting a malfunctioning or displaced device by taking out or putting in components of the device such as a screw or pin

Body Part Character 4	Approach Character 5	Device Character 6	Qualifier Character 7
9 Lower Extremity, Right B Lower Extremity, Left	Ø Open 3 Percutaneous 4 Percutaneous Endoscopic X External	Ø Drainage Device 3 Infusion Device 7 Autologous Tissue Substitute J Synthetic Substitute K Nonautologous Tissue Substitute Y Other Device	Z No Qualifier

DRG Non-OR ØYW[9,B][Ø,3,4][Ø,3,7,J,K,Y]Z
Non-OR ØYW[9,B]X[Ø,3,7,J,K,Y]Z

Obstetrics 1Ø2–1ØY

Character Meanings

This Character Meaning table is provided as a guide to assist the user in the identification of character members that may be found in this section of code tables. It **SHOULD NOT** be used to build a PCS code.

Ø: Pregnancy

Operation–Character 3	Body Part–Character 4	Approach–Character 5	Device–Character 6	Qualifier–Character 7
2 Change	Ø Products of Conception	Ø Open	3 Monitoring Electrode	Ø High
9 Drainage	1 Products of Conception, Retained	3 Percutaneous	Y Other Device	1 Low
A Abortion	2 Products of Conception, Ectopic	4 Percutaneous Endoscopic	Z No Device	2 Extraperitoneal
D Extraction		7 Via Natural or Artificial Opening		3 Low Forceps
E Delivery		8 Via Natural or Artificial Opening Endoscopic		4 Mid Forceps
H Insertion		X External		5 High Forceps
J Inspection				6 Vacuum
P Removal				7 Internal Version
Q Repair				8 Other
S Reposition				9 Fetal Blood OR Manual
T Resection				A Fetal Cerebrospinal Fluid
Y Transplantation				B Fetal Fluid, Other
				C Amniotic Fluid, Therapeutic
				D Fluid, Other
				E Nervous System
				F Cardiovascular System
				G Lymphatics & Hemic
				H Eye
				J Ear, Nose & Sinus
				K Respiratory System
				L Mouth & Throat
				M Gastrointestinal System
				N Hepatobiliary & Pancreas
				P Endocrine System
				Q Skin
				R Musculoskeletal System
				S Urinary System
				T Female Reproductive System
				U Amniotic Fluid, Diagnostic
				V Male Reproductive System
				W Laminaria
				X Abortifacient
				Y Other Body System
				Z No Qualifier

AHA Coding Clinic for table 1Ø9
2014, 3Q, 12 Fetoscopic laser photocoagulation and laser microseptostomy for twin-twin transfusion syndrome
2014, 2Q, 9 Pitocin administration to augment labor

AHA Coding Clinic for table 1ØD
2018, 4Q, 49-51 Revised qualifier values for root operation "extraction" (cesarean delivery)
2018, 2Q, 17 High transverse cesarean section
2016, 1Q, 9 Vaginal delivery assisted by vacuum and low forceps extraction
2014, 4Q, 43 Cesarean delivery assisted by vacuum extraction
2014, 4Q, 43 Vacuum dilation and curettage for blighted ovum

AHA Coding Clinic for table 1ØE
2017, 3Q, 5 Delivery of placenta
2016, 2Q, 34 Assisted vaginal delivery
2014, 4Q, 17 RH (D) alloimmunization (sensitization)
2014, 2Q, 9 Pitocin administration to augment labor

AHA Coding Clinic for table 1ØH
2013, 2Q, 36 Intrauterine pressure monitor

AHA Coding Clinic for table 1ØQ
2014, 3Q, 12 Fetoscopic laser photocoagulation and laser microseptostomy for twin-twin transfusion syndrome

AHA Coding Clinic for table 1ØT
2015, 3Q, 31 Laparoscopic partial salpingectomy for ectopic pregnancy

1 Obstetrics
Ø Pregnancy
2 Change

Definition: Taking out or off a device from a body part and putting back an identical or similar device in or on the same body part without cutting or puncturing the skin or a mucous membrane

Explanation: None

Body Part Character 4	Approach Character 5	Device Character 6	Qualifier Character 7
Ø Products of Conception ♀	7 Via Natural or Artificial Opening	3 Monitoring Electrode Y Other Device	Z No Qualifier

Non-OR All body part, approach, device, and qualifier values
♀ All body part, approach, device, and qualifier values

1 Obstetrics
Ø Pregnancy
9 Drainage

Definition: Taking or letting out fluids and/or gases from a body part

Explanation: None

Body Part Character 4	Approach Character 5	Device Character 6	Qualifier Character 7
Ø Products of Conception ♀	Ø Open 3 Percutaneous 4 Percutaneous Endoscopic 7 Via Natural or Artificial Opening 8 Via Natural or Artificial Opening Endoscopic	Z No Device	9 Fetal Blood A Fetal Cerebrospinal Fluid B Fetal Fluid, Other C Amniotic Fluid, Therapeutic D Fluid, Other U Amniotic Fluid, Diagnostic

Non-OR All body part, approach, device, and qualifier values
♀ All body part, approach, device, and qualifier values

1 Obstetrics
Ø Pregnancy
A Abortion

Definition: Artificially terminating a pregnancy

Explanation: None

Body Part Character 4	Approach Character 5	Device Character 6	Qualifier Character 7
Ø Products of Conception ♀	Ø Open 3 Percutaneous 4 Percutaneous Endoscopic 8 Via Natural or Artificial Opening Endoscopic	Z No Device	Z No Qualifier
Ø Products of Conception ♀	7 Via Natural or Artificial Opening	Z No Device	6 Vacuum W Laminaria X Abortifacient Z No Qualifier

Non-OR 1ØAØ7Z[6,W,X]
♀ All body part, approach, device, and qualifier values

1 Obstetrics
Ø Pregnancy
D Extraction

Definition: Pulling or stripping out or off all or a portion of a body part by the use of force

Explanation: None

Body Part Character 4	Approach Character 5	Device Character 6	Qualifier Character 7
Ø Products of Conception QA ♀	Ø Open	Z No Device	Ø High 1 Low 2 Extraperitoneal
Ø Products of Conception QA ♀	7 Via Natural or Artificial Opening	Z No Device	3 Low Forceps 4 Mid Forceps 5 High Forceps 6 Vacuum 7 Internal Version 8 Other
1 Products of Conception, Retained ♀	7 Via Natural or Artificial Opening 8 Via Natural or Artificial Opening Endoscopic	Z No Device	9 Manual Z No Qualifier
2 Products of Conception, Ectopic ♀	Ø Open 4 Percutaneous Endoscopic 7 Via Natural or Artificial Opening 8 Via Natural or Artificial Opening Endoscopic	Z No Device	Z No Qualifier

DRG Non-OR 1ØDØ7Z[3,4,5,6,7,8]
QA 1ØDØØZ[Ø,1,2] except when a corresponding SDX of Z37.Ø-Z37.9 is also reported
QA 1ØDØ7Z[3,4,5,7] except when a corresponding SDX of Z37.Ø-Z37.9 is also reported
♀ All body part, approach, device, and qualifier values

1 Obstetrics
Ø Pregnancy
E Delivery Definition: Assisting the passage of the products of conception from the genital canal
Explanation: None

Body Part Character 4	Approach Character 5	Device Character 6	Qualifier Character 7
Ø Products of Conception QA ♀	X External	Z No Device	Z No Qualifier

DRG Non-OR 1ØEØXZZ
QA 1ØEØXZZ except when a corresponding SDX of Z37.Ø-Z37.9 is also reported
♀ All body part, approach, device, and qualifier values

1 Obstetrics
Ø Pregnancy
H Insertion Definition: Putting in a nonbiological appliance that monitors, assists, performs, or prevents a physiological function but does not physically take the place of a body part
Explanation: None

Body Part Character 4	Approach Character 5	Device Character 6	Qualifier Character 7
Ø Products of Conception ♀	Ø Open 7 Via Natural or Artificial Opening	3 Monitoring Electrode Y Other Device	Z No Qualifier

Non-OR All body part, approach, device, and qualifier values
♀ All body part, approach, device, and qualifier values

1 Obstetrics
Ø Pregnancy
J Inspection Definition: Visually and/or manually exploring a body part
Explanation: Visual exploration may be performed with or without optical instrumentation. Manual exploration may be performed directly or through intervening body layers.

Body Part Character 4	Approach Character 5	Device Character 6	Qualifier Character 7
Ø Products of Conception ♀ 1 Products of Conception, Retained ♀ 2 Products of Conception, Ectopic ♀	Ø Open 3 Percutaneous 4 Percutaneous Endoscopic 7 Via Natural or Artificial Opening 8 Via Natural or Artificial Opening Endoscopic X External	Z No Device	Z No Qualifier

Non-OR All body part, approach, device, and qualifier values
♀ All body part, approach, device, and qualifier values

1 Obstetrics
Ø Pregnancy
P Removal Definition: Taking out or off a device from a body part, region or orifice
Explanation: If a device is taken out and a similar device put in without cutting or puncturing the skin or mucous membrane, the procedure is coded to the root operation CHANGE. Otherwise, the procedure for taking out a device is coded to the root operation REMOVAL.

Body Part Character 4	Approach Character 5	Device Character 6	Qualifier Character 7
Ø Products of Conception ♀	Ø Open 7 Via Natural or Artificial Opening	3 Monitoring Electrode Y Other Device	Z No Qualifier

Non-OR All body part, approach, device, and qualifier values
♀ All body part, approach, device, and qualifier values

1 Obstetrics
Ø Pregnancy
Q Repair Definition: Restoring, to the extent possible, a body part to its normal anatomic structure and function
Explanation: Used only when the method to accomplish the repair is not one of the other root operations

Body Part Character 4	Approach Character 5	Device Character 6	Qualifier Character 7
Ø Products of Conception ♀	Ø Open 3 Percutaneous 4 Percutaneous Endoscopic 7 Via Natural or Artificial Opening 8 Via Natural or Artificial Opening Endoscopic	Y Other Device Z No Device	E Nervous System F Cardiovascular System G Lymphatics and Hemic H Eye J Ear, Nose and Sinus K Respiratory System L Mouth and Throat M Gastrointestinal System N Hepatobiliary and Pancreas P Endocrine System Q Skin R Musculoskeletal System S Urinary System T Female Reproductive System V Male Reproductive System Y Other Body System

Non-OR All body part, approach, device, and qualifier values
♀ All body part, approach, device, and qualifier values

1 Obstetrics
Ø Pregnancy
S Reposition

Definition: Moving to its normal location, or other suitable location, all or a portion of a body part

Explanation: The body part is moved to a new location from an abnormal location, or from a normal location where it is not functioning correctly. The body part may or may not be cut out or off to be moved to the new location.

Body Part Character 4	Approach Character 5	Device Character 6	Qualifier Character 7
Ø Products of Conception ♀	7 Via Natural or Artificial Opening X External	Z No Device	Z No Qualifier
2 Products of Conception, Ectopic ♀	Ø Open 3 Percutaneous 4 Percutaneous Endoscopic 7 Via Natural or Artificial Opening 8 Via Natural or Artificial Opening Endoscopic	Z No Device	Z No Qualifier

Non-OR 1ØSØ[7,X]ZZ

♀ All body part, approach, device, and qualifier values

1 Obstetrics
Ø Pregnancy
T Resection

Definition: Cutting out or off, without replacement, all of a body part

Explanation: None

Body Part Character 4	Approach Character 5	Device Character 6	Qualifier Character 7
2 Products of Conception, Ectopic ♀	Ø Open 3 Percutaneous 4 Percutaneous Endoscopic 7 Via Natural or Artificial Opening 8 Via Natural or Artificial Opening Endoscopic	Z No Device	Z No Qualifier

♀ All body part, approach, device, and qualifier values

1 Obstetrics
Ø Pregnancy
Y Transplantation

Definition: Putting in or on all or a portion of a living body part taken from another individual or animal to physically take the place and/or function of all or a portion of a similar body part

Explanation: The native body part may or may not be taken out, and the transplanted body part may take over all or a portion of its function

Body Part Character 4	Approach Character 5	Device Character 6	Qualifier Character 7
Ø Products of Conception ♀	3 Percutaneous 4 Percutaneous Endoscopic 7 Via Natural or Artificial Opening	Z No Device	E Nervous System F Cardiovascular System G Lymphatics and Hemic H Eye J Ear, Nose and Sinus K Respiratory System L Mouth and Throat M Gastrointestinal System N Hepatobiliary and Pancreas P Endocrine System Q Skin R Musculoskeletal System S Urinary System T Female Reproductive System V Male Reproductive System Y Other Body System

Non-OR All body part, approach, device, and qualifier values

♀ All body part, approach, device, and qualifier values

Placement 2WØ–2Y5

AHA Coding Clinic for table 2W6
2015, 2Q, 35 Application of tongs to reduce and stabilize cervical fracture
2013, 2Q, 39 Application of cervical tongs for reduction of cervical fracture

AHA Coding Clinic for table 2Y4
2018, 4Q, 38 Control of epistaxis
2017, 4Q, 106 Nasal packing for epistaxis

2 Placement
W Anatomical Regions
Ø Change Definition: Taking out or off a device from a body part and putting back an identical or similar device in or on the same body part without cutting or puncturing the skin or a mucous membrane

Body Region Character 4	Approach Character 5	Device Character 6	Qualifier Character 7
Ø Head 2 Neck 3 Abdominal Wall 4 Chest Wall 5 Back 6 Inguinal Region, Right 7 Inguinal Region, Left 8 Upper Extremity, Right 9 Upper Extremity, Left A Upper Arm, Right B Upper Arm, Left C Lower Arm, Right D Lower Arm, Left E Hand, Right F Hand, Left G Thumb, Right H Thumb, Left J Finger, Right K Finger, Left L Lower Extremity, Right M Lower Extremity, Left N Upper Leg, Right P Upper Leg, Left Q Lower Leg, Right R Lower Leg, Left S Foot, Right T Foot, Left U Toe, Right V Toe, Left	X External	Ø Traction Apparatus 1 Splint 2 Cast 3 Brace 4 Bandage 5 Packing Material 6 Pressure Dressing 7 Intermittent Pressure Device Y Other Device	Z No Qualifier
1 Face	X External	Ø Traction Apparatus 1 Splint 2 Cast 3 Brace 4 Bandage 5 Packing Material 6 Pressure Dressing 7 Intermittent Pressure Device 9 Wire Y Other Device	Z No Qualifier

2 Placement
W Anatomical Regions
1 Compression Definition: Putting pressure on a body region

Body Region Character 4	Approach Character 5	Device Character 6	Qualifier Character 7
Ø Head 1 Face 2 Neck 3 Abdominal Wall 4 Chest Wall 5 Back 6 Inguinal Region, Right 7 Inguinal Region, Left 8 Upper Extremity, Right 9 Upper Extremity, Left A Upper Arm, Right B Upper Arm, Left C Lower Arm, Right D Lower Arm, Left E Hand, Right F Hand, Left G Thumb, Right H Thumb, Left J Finger, Right K Finger, Left L Lower Extremity, Right M Lower Extremity, Left N Upper Leg, Right P Upper Leg, Left Q Lower Leg, Right R Lower Leg, Left S Foot, Right T Foot, Left U Toe, Right V Toe, Left	X External	6 Pressure Dressing 7 Intermittent Pressure Device	Z No Qualifier

2 Placement
W Anatomical Regions
2 Dressing Definition: Putting material on a body region for protection

Body Region Character 4	Approach Character 5	Device Character 6	Qualifier Character 7
Ø Head 1 Face 2 Neck 3 Abdominal Wall 4 Chest Wall 5 Back 6 Inguinal Region, Right 7 Inguinal Region, Left 8 Upper Extremity, Right 9 Upper Extremity, Left A Upper Arm, Right B Upper Arm, Left C Lower Arm, Right D Lower Arm, Left E Hand, Right F Hand, Left G Thumb, Right H Thumb, Left J Finger, Right K Finger, Left L Lower Extremity, Right M Lower Extremity, Left N Upper Leg, Right P Upper Leg, Left Q Lower Leg, Right R Lower Leg, Left S Foot, Right T Foot, Left U Toe, Right V Toe, Left	X External	4 Bandage	Z No Qualifier

2 Placement
W Anatomical Regions
3 Immobilization Definition: Limiting or preventing motion of a body region

Body Region Character 4	Approach Character 5	Device Character 6	Qualifier Character 7
Ø Head **2** Neck **3** Abdominal Wall **4** Chest Wall **5** Back **6** Inguinal Region, Right **7** Inguinal Region, Left **8** Upper Extremity, Right **9** Upper Extremity, Left **A** Upper Arm, Right **B** Upper Arm, Left **C** Lower Arm, Right **D** Lower Arm, Left **E** Hand, Right **F** Hand, Left **G** Thumb, Right **H** Thumb, Left **J** Finger, Right **K** Finger, Left **L** Lower Extremity, Right **M** Lower Extremity, Left **N** Upper Leg, Right **P** Upper Leg, Left **Q** Lower Leg, Right **R** Lower Leg, Left **S** Foot, Right **T** Foot, Left **U** Toe, Right **V** Toe, Left	**X** External	**1** Splint **2** Cast **3** Brace **Y** Other Device	**Z** No Qualifier
1 Face	**X** External	**1** Splint **2** Cast **3** Brace **9** Wire **Y** Other Device	**Z** No Qualifier

2 Placement
W Anatomical Regions
4 Packing Definition: Putting material in a body region or orifice

Body Region Character 4	Approach Character 5	Device Character 6	Qualifier Character 7
Ø Head **1** Face **2** Neck **3** Abdominal Wall **4** Chest Wall **5** Back **6** Inguinal Region, Right **7** Inguinal Region, Left **8** Upper Extremity, Right **9** Upper Extremity, Left **A** Upper Arm, Right **B** Upper Arm, Left **C** Lower Arm, Right **D** Lower Arm, Left **E** Hand, Right **F** Hand, Left **G** Thumb, Right **H** Thumb, Left **J** Finger, Right **K** Finger, Left **L** Lower Extremity, Right **M** Lower Extremity, Left **N** Upper Leg, Right **P** Upper Leg, Left **Q** Lower Leg, Right **R** Lower Leg, Left **S** Foot, Right **T** Foot, Left **U** Toe, Right **V** Toe, Left	**X** External	**5** Packing Material	**Z** No Qualifier

2 Placement
W Anatomical Regions
5 Removal Definition: Taking out or off a device from a body part

Body Region Character 4	Approach Character 5	Device Character 6	Qualifier Character 7
Ø Head 2 Neck 3 Abdominal Wall 4 Chest Wall 5 Back 6 Inguinal Region, Right 7 Inguinal Region, Left 8 Upper Extremity, Right 9 Upper Extremity, Left A Upper Arm, Right B Upper Arm, Left C Lower Arm, Right D Lower Arm, Left E Hand, Right F Hand, Left G Thumb, Right H Thumb, Left J Finger, Right K Finger, Left L Lower Extremity, Right M Lower Extremity, Left N Upper Leg, Right P Upper Leg, Left Q Lower Leg, Right R Lower Leg, Left S Foot, Right T Foot, Left U Toe, Right V Toe, Left	X External	Ø Traction Apparatus 1 Splint 2 Cast 3 Brace 4 Bandage 5 Packing Material 6 Pressure Dressing 7 Intermittent Pressure Device Y Other Device	Z No Qualifier
1 Face	X External	Ø Traction Apparatus 1 Splint 2 Cast 3 Brace 4 Bandage 5 Packing Material 6 Pressure Dressing 7 Intermittent Pressure Device 9 Wire Y Other Device	Z No Qualifier

2 Placement
W Anatomical Regions
6 Traction Definition: Exerting a pulling force on a body region in a distal direction

Body Region Character 4	Approach Character 5	Device Character 6	Qualifier Character 7
Ø Head 1 Face 2 Neck 3 Abdominal Wall 4 Chest Wall 5 Back 6 Inguinal Region, Right 7 Inguinal Region, Left 8 Upper Extremity, Right 9 Upper Extremity, Left A Upper Arm, Right B Upper Arm, Left C Lower Arm, Right D Lower Arm, Left E Hand, Right F Hand, Left G Thumb, Right H Thumb, Left J Finger, Right K Finger, Left L Lower Extremity, Right M Lower Extremity, Left N Upper Leg, Right P Upper Leg, Left Q Lower Leg, Right R Lower Leg, Left S Foot, Right T Foot, Left U Toe, Right V Toe, Left	X External	Ø Traction Apparatus Z No Device	Z No Qualifier

2 Placement
Y Anatomical Orifices
Ø Change Definition: Taking out or off a device from a body part and putting back an identical or similar device in or on the same body part without cutting or puncturing the skin or a mucous membrane

Body Region Character 4	Approach Character 5	Device Character 6	Qualifier Character 7
Ø Mouth and Pharynx 1 Nasal 2 Ear 3 Anorectal 4 Female Genital Tract ♀ 5 Urethra	X External	5 Packing Material	Z No Qualifier

♀ 2YØ4X5Z

2 Placement
Y Anatomical Orifices
4 Packing Definition: Putting material in a body region or orifice

Body Region Character 4	Approach Character 5	Device Character 6	Qualifier Character 7
Ø Mouth and Pharynx 1 Nasal 2 Ear 3 Anorectal 4 Female Genital Tract ♀ 5 Urethra	X External	5 Packing Material	Z No Qualifier

♀ 2Y44X5Z

2 Placement
Y Anatomical Orifices
5 Removal Definition: Taking out or off a device from a body part

Body Region Character 4	Approach Character 5	Device Character 6	Qualifier Character 7
Ø Mouth and Pharynx 1 Nasal 2 Ear 3 Anorectal 4 Female Genital Tract ♀ 5 Urethra	X External	5 Packing Material	Z No Qualifier

♀ 2Y54X5Z

Administration 3Ø2–3E1

AHA Coding Clinic for table 3Ø2

2019, 4Q, 35 Transfusion of blood products
2019, 4Q, 36 T-cell depleted hematopoietic stem cells for transplantation
2016, 4Q, 113 Bone marrow and stem cell transfusion (Transplantation)

AHA Coding Clinic for table 3EØ

2019, 4Q, 36-37 Hyperthermic antineoplastic chemotherapy
2018, 3Q, 7 Coronary brachytherapy with angioplasty
2018, 1Q, 8 Placement of bone morphogenetic protein & spinal fusion surgery
2017, 2Q, 14 Infusion of tPA into pleural cavity
2017, 1Q, 37 Injection of glue into enteric fistula tract
2016, 4Q, 113-114 Substances applied to cranial cavity and brain
2016, 3Q, 29 Closure of bilateral alveolar clefts
2016, 1Q, 20 Metatarsophalangeal joint resection arthroplasty
2015, 3Q, 24 Esophagogastroduodenoscopy with epinephrine injection for control of bleeding
2015, 3Q, 29 Placement of adhesion barrier
2015, 2Q, 29 Insertion of nasogastric tube for drainage and feeding
2015, 2Q, 31 Thoracoscopic talc pleurodesis

AHA Coding Clinic for table 3EØ (Continued)

2015, 1Q, 31 Intrathecal chemotherapy
2015, 1Q, 38 Chemoembolization of the hepatic artery
2014, 4Q, 16 Administration of RH (D) immunoglobulin
2014, 4Q, 17 RH (D) alloimmunization (sensitization)
2014, 4Q, 19 Ultrasound accelerated thrombolysis
2014, 4Q, 34 Resection of brain malignancy with implantation of chemotherapeutic wafer
2014, 4Q, 38 Placement of saline and seprafilm solution into abdominal cavity
2014, 3Q, 26 Coil embolization of gastroduodenal artery with chemoembolization of hepatic artery
2014, 2Q, 8 Medical induction of labor with Cervidil tampon insertion
2014, 2Q, 10 Prophylactic Neulasta injection for infection prevention
2013, 4Q, 124 Administration of tPA for stroke treatment prior to transfer
2013, 1Q, 27 Injection of sclerosing agent into an esophageal varix

AHA Coding Clinic for table 3E1

2019, 4Q, 38 Irrigation of joint using irrigating substance
2017, 3Q, 14 Bronchoscopy with suctioning and washings for removal of mucus plug

3 Administration
Ø Circulatory
2 Transfusion Definition: Putting in blood or blood products

Body System/Region Character 4	Approach Character 5	Substance Character 6	Qualifier Character 7
3 Peripheral Vein NC 4 Central Vein NC	Ø Open 3 Percutaneous	A Stem Cells, Embryonic	Z No Qualifier
3 Peripheral Vein 4 Central Vein	Ø Open 3 Percutaneous	C Hematopoietic Stem/Progenitor Cells, Genetically Modified	Ø Autologous
3 Peripheral Vein NC 4 Central Vein NC	Ø Open 3 Percutaneous	G Bone Marrow X Stem Cells, Cord Blood Y Stem Cells, Hematopoietic	Ø Autologous 2 Allogeneic, Related 3 Allogeneic, Unrelated 4 Allogeneic, Unspecified
3 Peripheral Vein 4 Central Vein	Ø Open 3 Percutaneous	H Whole Blood J Serum Albumin K Frozen Plasma L Fresh Plasma M Plasma Cryoprecipitate N Red Blood Cells P Frozen Red Cells Q White Cells R Platelets S Globulin T Fibrinogen V Antihemophilic Factors W Factor IX	Ø Autologous 1 Nonautologous
3 Peripheral Vein 4 Central Vein	Ø Open 3 Percutaneous	U Stem Cells, T-cell Depleted Hematopoietic	2 Allogeneic, Related 3 Allogeneic, Unrelated 4 Allogeneic, Unspecified
7 Products of Conception, Circulatory ♀	3 Percutaneous 7 Via Natural or Artificial Opening	H Whole Blood J Serum Albumin K Frozen Plasma L Fresh Plasma M Plasma Cryoprecipitate N Red Blood Cells P Frozen Red Cells Q White Cells R Platelets S Globulin T Fibrinogen V Antihemophilic Factors W Factor IX	1 Nonautologous
8 Vein	Ø Open 3 Percutaneous	B 4-Factor Prothrombin Complex Concentrate	1 Nonautologous

DRG-Non-OR 3Ø2[3,4][Ø,3]AZ
DRG-Non-OR 3Ø2[3,4][Ø,3][G,X,Y][Ø,2,3,4]
DRG-Non-OR 3Ø2[3,4][Ø,3]U[2,3,4]

NC 3Ø2[3,4][Ø,3]AZ Only when reported with PDx or SDx of C91.ØØ, C92.ØØ, C92.1Ø, C92.11, C92.4Ø, C92.5Ø, C92.6Ø, C92.AØ, C93.ØØ, C94.ØØ, C95.ØØ
NC 3Ø2[3,4][Ø,3][G,Y]Ø Only when reported with PDx or SDx of C91.ØØ, C92.ØØ, C92.1Ø, C92.11, C92.4Ø, C92.5Ø, C92.6Ø, C92.AØ, C93.ØØ, C94.ØØ, C95.ØØ
NC 3Ø2[3,4][Ø,3][G,Y][2,3,4]
♀ 3Ø27[3,7][H,J,K,L,M,N,P,Q,R,S,T,V,W]1

3 Administration
C Indwelling Device
1 Irrigation Definition: Putting in or on a cleansing substance

Body System/Region Character 4	Approach Character 5	Substance Character 6	Qualifier Character 7
Z None	X External	8 Irrigating Substance	Z No Qualifier

3 Administration
E Physiological Systems and Anatomical Regions
Ø Introduction Definition: Putting in or on a therapeutic, diagnostic, nutritional, physiological, or prophylactic substance except blood or blood products

Body System/Region Character 4	Approach Character 5	Substance Character 6	Qualifier Character 7
Ø Skin and Mucous Membranes	X External	Ø Antineoplastic	5 Other Antineoplastic M Monoclonal Antibody
Ø Skin and Mucous Membranes	X External	2 Anti-infective	8 Oxazolidinones 9 Other Anti-infective
Ø Skin and Mucous Membranes	X External	3 Anti-inflammatory 4 Serum, Toxoid and Vaccine B Anesthetic Agent K Other Diagnostic Substance M Pigment N Analgesics, Hypnotics, Sedatives T Destructive Agent	Z No Qualifier
Ø Skin and Mucous Membranes	X External	G Other Therapeutic Substance	C Other Substance
1 Subcutaneous Tissue	Ø Open	2 Anti-infective	A Anti-Infective Envelope
1 Subcutaneous Tissue	3 Percutaneous	Ø Antineoplastic	5 Other Antineoplastic M Monoclonal Antibody
1 Subcutaneous Tissue	3 Percutaneous	2 Anti-infective	8 Oxazolidinones 9 Other Anti-infective A Anti-Infective Envelope
1 Subcutaneous Tissue	3 Percutaneous	3 Anti-inflammatory 6 Nutritional Substance 7 Electrolytic and Water Balance Substance B Anesthetic Agent H Radioactive Substance K Other Diagnostic Substance N Analgesics, Hypnotics, Sedatives T Destructive Agent	Z No Qualifier
1 Subcutaneous Tissue	3 Percutaneous	4 Serum, Toxoid and Vaccine	Ø Influenza Vaccine Z No Qualifier
1 Subcutaneous Tissue	3 Percutaneous	G Other Therapeutic Substance	C Other Substance
1 Subcutaneous Tissue	3 Percutaneous	V Hormone	G Insulin J Other Hormone
2 Muscle	3 Percutaneous	Ø Antineoplastic	5 Other Antineoplastic M Monoclonal Antibody
2 Muscle	3 Percutaneous	2 Anti-infective	8 Oxazolidinones 9 Other Anti-infective
2 Muscle	3 Percutaneous	3 Anti-inflammatory 6 Nutritional Substance 7 Electrolytic and Water Balance Substance B Anesthetic Agent H Radioactive Substance K Other Diagnostic Substance N Analgesics, Hypnotics, Sedatives T Destructive Agent	Z No Qualifier
2 Muscle	3 Percutaneous	4 Serum, Toxoid and Vaccine	Ø Influenza Vaccine Z No Qualifier
2 Muscle	3 Percutaneous	G Other Therapeutic Substance	C Other Substance
3 Peripheral Vein	Ø Open	Ø Antineoplastic	2 High-dose Interleukin-2 3 Low-dose Interleukin-2 5 Other Antineoplastic M Monoclonal Antibody P Clofarabine
3 Peripheral Vein	Ø Open	1 Thrombolytic	6 Recombinant Human- activated Protein C 7 Other Thrombolytic
3 Peripheral Vein	Ø Open	2 Anti-infective	8 Oxazolidinones 9 Other Anti-infective

DRG Non-OR 3EØ3ØØ2
DRG Non-OR 3EØ3Ø17

3EØ Continued on next page

3EØ Continued

3 Administration
E Physiological Systems and Anatomical Regions
Ø Introduction Definition: Putting in or on a therapeutic, diagnostic, nutritional, physiological, or prophylactic substance except blood or blood products

Body System/Region Character 4	Approach Character 5	Substance Character 6	Qualifier Character 7
3 Peripheral Vein	Ø Open	3 Anti-inflammatory 4 Serum, Toxoid and Vaccine 6 Nutritional Substance 7 Electrolytic and Water Balance Substance F Intracirculatory Anesthetic H Radioactive Substance K Other Diagnostic Substance N Analgesics, Hypnotics, Sedatives P Platelet Inhibitor R Antiarrhythmic T Destructive Agent X Vasopressor	Z No Qualifier
3 Peripheral Vein	Ø Open	G Other Therapeutic Substance	C Other Substance N Blood Brain Barrier Disruption
3 Peripheral Vein	Ø Open	U Pancreatic Islet Cells	Ø Autologous 1 Nonautologous
3 Peripheral Vein	Ø Open	V Hormone	G Insulin H Human B-type Natriuretic Peptide J Other Hormone
3 Peripheral Vein	Ø Open	W Immunotherapeutic	K Immunostimulator L Immunosuppressive
3 Peripheral Vein	3 Percutaneous	Ø Antineoplastic	2 High-dose Interleukin-2 3 Low-dose Interleukin-2 5 Other Antineoplastic M Monoclonal Antibody P Clofarabine
3 Peripheral Vein	3 Percutaneous	1 Thrombolytic	6 Recombinant Human- activated Protein C 7 Other Thrombolytic
3 Peripheral Vein	3 Percutaneous	2 Anti-infective	8 Oxazolidinones 9 Other Anti-infective
3 Peripheral Vein	3 Percutaneous	3 Anti-inflammatory 4 Serum, Toxoid and Vaccine 6 Nutritional Substance 7 Electrolytic and Water Balance Substance F Intracirculatory Anesthetic H Radioactive Substance K Other Diagnostic Substance N Analgesics, Hypnotics, Sedatives P Platelet Inhibitor R Antiarrhythmic T Destructive Agent X Vasopressor	Z No Qualifier
3 Peripheral Vein	3 Percutaneous	G Other Therapeutic Substance	C Other Substance N Blood Brain Barrier Disruption Q Glucarpidase
3 Peripheral Vein	3 Percutaneous	U Pancreatic Islet Cells	Ø Autologous 1 Nonautologous
3 Peripheral Vein	3 Percutaneous	V Hormone	G Insulin H Human B-type Natriuretic Peptide J Other Hormone
3 Peripheral Vein	3 Percutaneous	W Immunotherapeutic	K Immunostimulator L Immunosuppressive
4 Central Vein	Ø Open	Ø Antineoplastic	2 High-dose Interleukin-2 3 Low-dose Interleukin-2 5 Other Antineoplastic M Monoclonal Antibody P Clofarabine
4 Central Vein	Ø Open	1 Thrombolytic	6 Recombinant Human- activated Protein C 7 Other Thrombolytic

Valid OR 3EØ3ØTZ
DRG Non-OR 3EØ3ØU[Ø,1]
DRG Non-OR 3EØ33Ø2
DRG Non-OR 3EØ3317
DRG Non-OR 3EØ33U[Ø,1]
DRG Non-OR 3EØ4ØØ2
DRG Non-OR 3EØ4Ø17

3EØ Continued on next page

3EØ Continued

3 Administration
E Physiological Systems and Anatomical Regions
Ø Introduction Definition: Putting in or on a therapeutic, diagnostic, nutritional, physiological, or prophylactic substance except blood or blood products

Body System/Region Character 4	Approach Character 5	Substance Character 6	Qualifier Character 7
4 Central Vein	Ø Open	2 Anti-infective	8 Oxazolidinones 9 Other Anti-infective
4 Central Vein	Ø Open	3 Anti-inflammatory 4 Serum, Toxoid and Vaccine 6 Nutritional Substance 7 Electrolytic and Water Balance Substance F Intracirculatory Anesthetic H Radioactive Substance K Other Diagnostic Substance N Analgesics, Hypnotics, Sedatives P Platelet Inhibitor R Antiarrhythmic T Destructive Agent X Vasopressor	Z No Qualifier
4 Central Vein	Ø Open	G Other Therapeutic Substance	C Other Substance N Blood Brain Barrier Disruption
4 Central Vein	Ø Open	V Hormone	G Insulin H Human B-type Natriuretic Peptide J Other Hormone
4 Central Vein	Ø Open	W Immunotherapeutic	K Immunostimulator L Immunosuppressive
4 Central Vein	3 Percutaneous	Ø Antineoplastic	2 High-dose Interleukin-2 3 Low-dose Interleukin-2 5 Other Antineoplastic M Monoclonal Antibody P Clofarabine
4 Central Vein	3 Percutaneous	1 Thrombolytic	6 Recombinant Human-activated Protein C 7 Other Thrombolytic
4 Central Vein	3 Percutaneous	2 Anti-infective	8 Oxazolidinones 9 Other Anti-infective
4 Central Vein	3 Percutaneous	3 Anti-inflammatory 4 Serum, Toxoid and Vaccine 6 Nutritional Substance 7 Electrolytic and Water Balance Substance F Intracirculatory Anesthetic H Radioactive Substance K Other Diagnostic Substance N Analgesics, Hypnotics, Sedatives P Platelet Inhibitor R Antiarrhythmic T Destructive Agent X Vasopressor	Z No Qualifier
4 Central Vein	3 Percutaneous	G Other Therapeutic Substance	C Other Substance N Blood Brain Barrier Disruption Q Glucarpidase
4 Central Vein	3 Percutaneous	V Hormone	G Insulin H Human B-type Natriuretic Peptide J Other Hormone
4 Central Vein	3 Percutaneous	W Immunotherapeutic	K Immunostimulator L Immunosuppressive
5 Peripheral Artery 6 Central Artery	Ø Open 3 Percutaneous	Ø Antineoplastic	2 High-dose Interleukin-2 3 Low-dose Interleukin-2 5 Other Antineoplastic M Monoclonal Antibody P Clofarabine
5 Peripheral Artery 6 Central Artery	Ø Open 3 Percutaneous	1 Thrombolytic	6 Recombinant Human-activated Protein C 7 Other Thrombolytic
5 Peripheral Artery 6 Central Artery	Ø Open 3 Percutaneous	2 Anti-infective	8 Oxazolidinones 9 Other Anti-infective

Valid OR 3E04ØTZ
DRG Non-OR 3E043Ø2
DRG Non-OR 3E04317
DRG Non-OR 3EØ[5,6][Ø,3]Ø2
DRG Non-OR 3EØ[5,6][Ø,3]17

3EØ Continued on next page

3EØ Continued

3 Administration
E Physiological Systems and Anatomical Regions
Ø Introduction Definition: Putting in or on a therapeutic, diagnostic, nutritional, physiological, or prophylactic substance except blood or blood products

Body System/Region Character 4	Approach Character 5	Substance Character 6	Qualifier Character 7
5 Peripheral Artery 6 Central Artery	Ø Open 3 Percutaneous	3 Anti-inflammatory 4 Serum, Toxoid and Vaccine 6 Nutritional Substance 7 Electrolytic and Water Balance Substance F Intracirculatory Anesthetic H Radioactive Substance K Other Diagnostic Substance N Analgesics, Hypnotics, Sedatives P Platelet Inhibitor R Antiarrhythmic T Destructive Agent X Vasopressor	Z No Qualifier
5 Peripheral Artery 6 Central Artery	Ø Open 3 Percutaneous	G Other Therapeutic Substance	C Other Substance N Blood Brain Barrier Disruption
5 Peripheral Artery 6 Central Artery	Ø Open 3 Percutaneous	V Hormone	G Insulin H Human B-type Natriuretic Peptide J Other Hormone
5 Peripheral Artery 6 Central Artery	Ø Open 3 Percutaneous	W Immunotherapeutic	K Immunostimulator L Immunosuppressive
7 Coronary Artery 8 Heart	Ø Open 3 Percutaneous	1 Thrombolytic	6 Recombinant Human-activated Protein C 7 Other Thrombolytic
7 Coronary Artery 8 Heart	Ø Open 3 Percutaneous	G Other Therapeutic Substance	C Other Substance
7 Coronary Artery 8 Heart	Ø Open 3 Percutaneous	K Other Diagnostic Substance P Platelet Inhibitor	Z No Qualifier
7 Coronary Artery 8 Heart	4 Percutaneous Endoscopic	G Other Therapeutic Substance	C Other Substance
9 Nose	3 Percutaneous 7 Via Natural or Artificial Opening X External	Ø Antineoplastic	5 Other Antineoplastic M Monoclonal Antibody
9 Nose	3 Percutaneous 7 Via Natural or Artificial Opening X External	2 Anti-infective	8 Oxazolidinones 9 Other Anti-infective
9 Nose	3 Percutaneous 7 Via Natural or Artificial Opening X External	3 Anti-inflammatory 4 Serum, Toxoid and Vaccine B Anesthetic Agent H Radioactive Substance K Other Diagnostic Substance N Analgesics, Hypnotics, Sedatives T Destructive Agent	Z No Qualifier
9 Nose	3 Percutaneous 7 Via Natural or Artificial Opening X External	G Other Therapeutic Substance	C Other Substance
A Bone Marrow	3 Percutaneous	Ø Antineoplastic	5 Other Antineoplastic M Monoclonal Antibody
A Bone Marrow	3 Percutaneous	G Other Therapeutic Substance	C Other Substance
B Ear	3 Percutaneous 7 Via Natural or Artificial Opening X External	Ø Antineoplastic	4 Liquid Brachytherapy Radioisotope 5 Other Antineoplastic M Monoclonal Antibody
B Ear	3 Percutaneous 7 Via Natural or Artificial Opening X External	2 Anti-infective	8 Oxazolidinones 9 Other Anti-infective
B Ear	3 Percutaneous 7 Via Natural or Artificial Opening X External	3 Anti-inflammatory B Anesthetic Agent H Radioactive Substance K Other Diagnostic Substance N Analgesics, Hypnotics, Sedatives T Destructive Agent	Z No Qualifier
B Ear	3 Percutaneous 7 Via Natural or Artificial Opening X External	G Other Therapeutic Substance	C Other Substance

DRG Non-OR 3EØ8[Ø,3]17

3EØ Continued on next page

3 Administration
E Physiological Systems and Anatomical Regions
Ø Introduction Definition: Putting in or on a therapeutic, diagnostic, nutritional, physiological, or prophylactic substance except blood or blood products

3EØ Continued

Body System/Region Character 4	Approach Character 5	Substance Character 6	Qualifier Character 7
C Eye	**3** Percutaneous **7** Via Natural or Artificial Opening **X** External	**Ø** Antineoplastic	**4** Liquid Brachytherapy Radioisotope **5** Other Antineoplastic **M** Monoclonal Antibody
C Eye	**3** Percutaneous **7** Via Natural or Artificial Opening **X** External	**2** Anti-infective	**8** Oxazolidinones **9** Other Anti-infective
C Eye	**3** Percutaneous **7** Via Natural or Artificial Opening **X** External	**3** Anti-inflammatory **B** Anesthetic Agent **H** Radioactive Substance **K** Other Diagnostic Substance **M** Pigment **N** Analgesics, Hypnotics, Sedatives **T** Destructive Agent	**Z** No Qualifier
C Eye	**3** Percutaneous **7** Via Natural or Artificial Opening **X** External	**G** Other Therapeutic Substance	**C** Other Substance
C Eye	**3** Percutaneous **7** Via Natural or Artificial Opening **X** External	**S** Gas	**F** Other Gas
D Mouth and Pharynx	**3** Percutaneous **7** Via Natural or Artificial Opening **X** External	**Ø** Antineoplastic	**4** Liquid Brachytherapy Radioisotope **5** Other Antineoplastic **M** Monoclonal Antibody
D Mouth and Pharynx	**3** Percutaneous **7** Via Natural or Artificial Opening **X** External	**2** Anti-infective	**8** Oxazolidinones **9** Other Anti-infective
D Mouth and Pharynx	**3** Percutaneous **7** Via Natural or Artificial Opening **X** External	**3** Anti-inflammatory **4** Serum, Toxoid and Vaccine **6** Nutritional Substance **7** Electrolytic and Water Balance Substance **B** Anesthetic Agent **H** Radioactive Substance **K** Other Diagnostic Substance **N** Analgesics, Hypnotics, Sedatives **R** Antiarrhythmic **T** Destructive Agent	**Z** No Qualifier
D Mouth and Pharynx	**3** Percutaneous **7** Via Natural or Artificial Opening **X** External	**G** Other Therapeutic Substance	**C** Other Substance
E Products of Conception ♀ **G** Upper GI **H** Lower GI **K** Genitourinary Tract **N** Male Reproductive ♂	**3** Percutaneous **7** Via Natural or Artificial Opening **8** Via Natural or Artificial Opening Endoscopic	**Ø** Antineoplastic	**4** Liquid Brachytherapy Radioisotope **5** Other Antineoplastic **M** Monoclonal Antibody
E Products of Conception ♀ **G** Upper GI **H** Lower GI **K** Genitourinary Tract **N** Male Reproductive ♂	**3** Percutaneous **7** Via Natural or Artificial Opening **8** Via Natural or Artificial Opening Endoscopic	**2** Anti-infective	**8** Oxazolidinones **9** Other Anti-infective
E Products of Conception ♀ **G** Upper GI **H** Lower GI **K** Genitourinary Tract **N** Male Reproductive ♂	**3** Percutaneous **7** Via Natural or Artificial Opening **8** Via Natural or Artificial Opening Endoscopic	**3** Anti-inflammatory **6** Nutritional Substance **7** Electrolytic and Water Balance Substance **B** Anesthetic Agent **H** Radioactive Substance **K** Other Diagnostic Substance **N** Analgesics, Hypnotics, Sedatives **T** Destructive Agent	**Z** No Qualifier
E Products of Conception ♀ **G** Upper GI **H** Lower GI **K** Genitourinary Tract **N** Male Reproductive ♂	**3** Percutaneous **7** Via Natural or Artificial Opening **8** Via Natural or Artificial Opening Endoscopic	**G** Other Therapeutic Substance	**C** Other Substance

♂ All approach, substance, and qualifier values for body system/region (character 4) with this icon
♀ All approach, substance, and qualifier values for body system/region (character 4) with this icon

3EØ Continued on next page

3EØ Continued

3 Administration
E Physiological Systems and Anatomical Regions
Ø Introduction Definition: Putting in or on a therapeutic, diagnostic, nutritional, physiological, or prophylactic substance except blood or blood products

Body System/Region Character 4	Approach Character 5	Substance Character 6	Qualifier Character 7
E Products of Conception ♀ G Upper GI H Lower GI K Genitourinary Tract N Male Reproductive ♂	3 Percutaneous 7 Via Natural or Artificial Opening 8 Via Natural or Artificial Opening Endoscopic	S Gas	F Other Gas
E Products of Conception ♀ G Upper GI H Lower GI K Genitourinary Tract N Male Reproductive ♂	4 Percutaneous Endoscopic	G Other Therapeutic Substance	C Other Substance
F Respiratory Tract	3 Percutaneous 7 Via Natural or Artificial Opening 8 Via Natural or Artificial Opening Endoscopic	Ø Antineoplastic	4 Liquid Brachytherapy Radioisotope 5 Other Antineoplastic M Monoclonal Antibody
F Respiratory Tract	3 Percutaneous 7 Via Natural or Artificial Opening 8 Via Natural or Artificial Opening Endoscopic	2 Anti-infective	8 Oxazolidinones 9 Other Anti-infective
F Respiratory Tract	3 Percutaneous 7 Via Natural or Artificial Opening 8 Via Natural or Artificial Opening Endoscopic	3 Anti-inflammatory 6 Nutritional Substance 7 Electrolytic and Water Balance Substance B Anesthetic Agent H Radioactive Substance K Other Diagnostic Substance N Analgesics, Hypnotics, Sedatives T Destructive Agent	Z No Qualifier
F Respiratory Tract	3 Percutaneous 7 Via Natural or Artificial Opening 8 Via Natural or Artificial Opening Endoscopic	G Other Therapeutic Substance	C Other Substance
F Respiratory Tract	3 Percutaneous 7 Via Natural or Artificial Opening 8 Via Natural or Artificial Opening Endoscopic	S Gas	D Nitric Oxide F Other Gas
F Respiratory Tract	4 Percutaneous Endoscopic	G Other Therapeutic Substance	C Other Substance
J Biliary and Pancreatic Tract	3 Percutaneous 7 Via Natural or Artificial Opening 8 Via Natural or Artificial Opening Endoscopic	Ø Antineoplastic	4 Liquid Brachytherapy Radioisotope 5 Other Antineoplastic M Monoclonal Antibody
J Biliary and Pancreatic Tract	3 Percutaneous 7 Via Natural or Artificial Opening 8 Via Natural or Artificial Opening Endoscopic	2 Anti-infective	8 Oxazolidinones 9 Other Anti-infective
J Biliary and Pancreatic Tract	3 Percutaneous 7 Via Natural or Artificial Opening 8 Via Natural or Artificial Opening Endoscopic	3 Anti-inflammatory 6 Nutritional Substance 7 Electrolytic and Water Balance Substance B Anesthetic Agent H Radioactive Substance K Other Diagnostic Substance N Analgesics, Hypnotics, Sedatives T Destructive Agent	Z No Qualifier
J Biliary and Pancreatic Tract	3 Percutaneous 7 Via Natural or Artificial Opening 8 Via Natural or Artificial Opening Endoscopic	G Other Therapeutic Substance	C Other Substance
J Biliary and Pancreatic Tract	3 Percutaneous 7 Via Natural or Artificial Opening 8 Via Natural or Artificial Opening Endoscopic	S Gas	F Other Gas

♂ All approach, substance, and qualifier values for body system/region (character 4) with this icon
♀ All approach, substance, and qualifier values for body system/region (character 4) with this icon

3EØ Continued on next page

3 Administration
E Physiological Systems and Anatomical Regions
0 Introduction Definition: Putting in or on a therapeutic, diagnostic, nutritional, physiological, or prophylactic substance except blood or blood products

3E0 Continued

Body System/Region Character 4	Approach Character 5	Substance Character 6	Qualifier Character 7
J Biliary and Pancreatic Tract	3 Percutaneous 7 Via Natural or Artificial Opening 8 Via Natural or Artificial Opening Endoscopic	U Pancreatic Islet Cells	0 Autologous 1 Nonautologous
J Biliary and Pancreatic Tract	4 Percutaneous Endoscopic	G Other Therapeutic Substance	C Other Substance
L Pleural Cavity	0 Open	5 Adhesion Barrier	Z No Qualifier
L Pleural Cavity	3 Percutaneous	0 Antineoplastic	4 Liquid Brachytherapy Radioisotope 5 Other Antineoplastic M Monoclonal Antibody
L Pleural Cavity	3 Percutaneous	2 Anti-infective	8 Oxazolidinones 9 Other Anti-infective
L Pleural Cavity	3 Percutaneous	3 Anti-inflammatory 5 Adhesion Barrier 6 Nutritional Substance 7 Electrolytic and Water Balance Substance B Anesthetic Agent H Radioactive Substance K Other Diagnostic Substance N Analgesics, Hypnotics, Sedatives T Destructive Agent	Z No Qualifier
L Pleural Cavity	3 Percutaneous	G Other Therapeutic Substance	C Other Substance
L Pleural Cavity	3 Percutaneous	S Gas	F Other Gas
L Pleural Cavity	4 Percutaneous Endoscopic	5 Adhesion Barrier	Z No Qualifier
L Pleural Cavity	4 Percutaneous Endoscopic	G Other Therapeutic Substance	C Other Substance
L Pleural Cavity	7 Via Natural or Artificial Opening	0 Antineoplastic	4 Liquid Brachytherapy Radioisotope 5 Other Antineoplastic M Monoclonal Antibody
L Pleural Cavity	7 Via Natural or Artificial Opening	S Gas	F Other Gas
M Peritoneal Cavity	0 Open	5 Adhesion Barrier	Z No Qualifier
M Peritoneal Cavity	3 Percutaneous	0 Antineoplastic	4 Liquid Brachytherapy Radioisotope 5 Other Antineoplastic M Monoclonal Antibody Y Hyperthermic
M Peritoneal Cavity	3 Percutaneous	2 Anti-infective	8 Oxazolidinones 9 Other Anti-infective
M Peritoneal Cavity	3 Percutaneous	3 Anti-inflammatory 5 Adhesion Barrier 6 Nutritional Substance 7 Electrolytic and Water Balance Substance B Anesthetic Agent H Radioactive Substance K Other Diagnostic Substance N Analgesics, Hypnotics, Sedatives T Destructive Agent	Z No Qualifier
M Peritoneal Cavity	3 Percutaneous	G Other Therapeutic Substance	C Other Substance
M Peritoneal Cavity	3 Percutaneous	S Gas	F Other Gas
M Peritoneal Cavity	4 Percutaneous Endoscopic	5 Adhesion Barrier	Z No Qualifier
M Peritoneal Cavity	4 Percutaneous Endoscopic	G Other Therapeutic Substance	C Other Substance
M Peritoneal Cavity	7 Via Natural or Artificial Opening	0 Antineoplastic	4 Liquid Brachytherapy Radioisotope 5 Other Antineoplastic M Monoclonal Antibody
M Peritoneal Cavity	7 Via Natural or Artificial Opening	S Gas	F Other Gas
P Female Reproductive ♀	0 Open	5 Adhesion Barrier	Z No Qualifier
P Female Reproductive ♀	3 Percutaneous	0 Antineoplastic	4 Liquid Brachytherapy Radioisotope 5 Other Antineoplastic M Monoclonal Antibody
P Female Reproductive ♀	3 Percutaneous	2 Anti-infective	8 Oxazolidinones 9 Other Anti-infective

Valid OR 3E0L4GC
DRG Non-OR 3E0J[3,7,8]U[0,1]
♀ All approach, substance, and qualifier values for body system/region (character 4) with this icon

3E0 Continued on next page

3 Administration
E Physiological Systems and Anatomical Regions
Ø Introduction Definition: Putting in or on a therapeutic, diagnostic, nutritional, physiological, or prophylactic substance except blood or blood products

3EØ Continued

Body System/Region Character 4	Approach Character 5	Substance Character 6	Qualifier Character 7
P Female Reproductive ♀	**3** Percutaneous	**3** Anti-inflammatory **5** Adhesion Barrier **6** Nutritional Substance **7** Electrolytic and Water Balance Substance **B** Anesthetic Agent **H** Radioactive Substance **K** Other Diagnostic Substance **L** Sperm **N** Analgesics, Hypnotics, Sedatives **T** Destructive Agent **V** Hormone	**Z** No Qualifier
P Female Reproductive ♀	**3** Percutaneous	**G** Other Therapeutic Substance	**C** Other Substance
P Female Reproductive ♀	**3** Percutaneous	**Q** Fertilized Ovum	**Ø** Autologous **1** Nonautologous
P Female Reproductive ♀	**3** Percutaneous	**S** Gas	**F** Other Gas
P Female Reproductive ♀	**4** Percutaneous Endoscopic	**5** Adhesion Barrier	**Z** No Qualifier
P Female Reproductive ♀	**4** Percutaneous Endoscopic	**G** Other Therapeutic Substance	**C** Other Substance
P Female Reproductive ♀	**7** Via Natural or Artificial Opening	**Ø** Antineoplastic	**4** Liquid Brachytherapy Radioisotope **5** Other Antineoplastic **M** Monoclonal Antibody
P Female Reproductive ♀	**7** Via Natural or Artificial Opening	**2** Anti-infective	**8** Oxazolidinones **9** Other Anti-infective
P Female Reproductive ♀	**7** Via Natural or Artificial Opening	**3** Anti-inflammatory **6** Nutritional Substance **7** Electrolytic and Water Balance Substance **B** Anesthetic Agent **H** Radioactive Substance **K** Other Diagnostic Substance **L** Sperm **N** Analgesics, Hypnotics, Sedatives **T** Destructive Agent **V** Hormone	**Z** No Qualifier
P Female Reproductive ♀	**7** Via Natural or Artificial Opening	**G** Other Therapeutic Substance	**C** Other Substance
P Female Reproductive ♀	**7** Via Natural or Artificial Opening	**Q** Fertilized Ovum	**Ø** Autologous **1** Nonautologous
P Female Reproductive ♀	**7** Via Natural or Artificial Opening	**S** Gas	**F** Other Gas
P Female Reproductive ♀	**8** Via Natural or Artificial Opening Endoscopic	**Ø** Antineoplastic	**4** Liquid Brachytherapy Radioisotope **5** Other Antineoplastic **M** Monoclonal Antibody
P Female Reproductive ♀	**8** Via Natural or Artificial Opening Endoscopic	**2** Anti-infective	**8** Oxazolidinones **9** Other Anit-infection
P Female Reproductive ♀	**8** Via Natural or Artificial Opening Endoscopic	**3** Anti-inflammatory **6** Nutritional Substance **7** Electrolytic and Water Balance Substance **B** Anesthetic Agent **H** Radioactive Substance **K** Other Diagnostic Substance **N** Analgesics, Hypnotics, Sedative **T** Destructive Agent	**Z** No Qualifier
P Female Reproductive ♀	**8** Via Natural or Artificial Opening Endoscopic	**G** Other Therapeutic Substance	**C** Other Substance
P Female Reproductive ♀	**8** Via Natural or Artificial Opening Endoscopic	**S** Gas	**F** Other Gas
Q Cranial Cavity and Brain	**Ø** Open **3** Percutaneous	**Ø** Antineoplastic	**4** Liquid Brachytherapy Radioisotope **5** Other Antineoplastic **M** Monoclonal Antibody
Q Cranial Cavity and Brain	**Ø** Open **3** Percutaneous	**2** Anti-infective	**8** Oxazolidinones **9** Other Anti-infective

Valid OR 3EØP3Q[Ø,1]
Valid OR 3EØP7Q[Ø,1]
DRG Non-OR 3EØQ[Ø,3]Ø5
♀ All approach, substance, and qualifier values for body system/region (character 4) with this icon

3EØ Continued on next page

3 Administration
E Physiological Systems and Anatomical Regions
Ø Introduction Definition: Putting in or on a therapeutic, diagnostic, nutritional, physiological, or prophylactic substance except blood or blood products

3EØ Continued

Body System/Region Character 4	Approach Character 5	Substance Character 6	Qualifier Character 7
Q Cranial Cavity and Brain	Ø Open 3 Percutaneous	3 Anti-inflammatory 6 Nutritional Substance 7 Electrolytic and Water Balance Substance A Stem Cells, Embryonic B Anesthetic Agent H Radioactive Substance K Other Diagnostic Substance N Analgesics, Hypnotics, Sedatives T Destructive Agent	Z No Qualifier
Q Cranial Cavity and Brain	Ø Open 3 Percutaneous	E Stem Cells, Somatic	Ø Autologous 1 Nonautologous
Q Cranial Cavity and Brain	Ø Open 3 Percutaneous	G Other Therapeutic Substance	C Other Substance
Q Cranial Cavity and Brain	Ø Open 3 Percutaneous	S Gas	F Other Gas
Q Cranial Cavity and Brain	7 Via Natural or Artificial Opening	Ø Antineoplastic	4 Liquid Brachytherapy Radioisotope 5 Other Antineoplastic M Monoclonal Antibody
Q Cranial Cavity and Brain	7 Via Natural or Artificial Opening	S Gas	F Other Gas
R Spinal Canal	Ø Open	A Stem Cells, Embryonic	Z No Qualifier
R Spinal Canal	Ø Open	E Stem Cells, Somatic	Ø Autologous 1 Nonautologous
R Spinal Canal	3 Percutaneous	Ø Antineoplastic	2 High-dose Interleukin-2 3 Low-dose Interleukin-2 4 Liquid Brachytherapy Radioisotope 5 Other Antineoplastic M Monoclonal Antibody
R Spinal Canal	3 Percutaneous	2 Anti-infective	8 Oxazolidinones 9 Other Anti-infective
R Spinal Canal	3 Percutaneous	3 Anti-inflammatory 6 Nutritional Substance 7 Electrolytic and Water Balance Substance A Stem Cells, Embryonic B Anesthetic Agent H Radioactive Substance K Other Diagnostic Substance N Analgesics, Hypnotics, Sedatives T Destructive Agent	Z No Qualifier
R Spinal Canal	3 Percutaneous	E Stem Cells, Somatic	Ø Autologous 1 Nonautologous
R Spinal Canal	3 Percutaneous	G Other Therapeutic Substance	C Other Substance
R Spinal Canal	3 Percutaneous	S Gas	F Other Gas
R Spinal Canal	7 Via Natural or Artificial Opening	S Gas	F Other Gas
S Epidural Space	3 Percutaneous	Ø Antineoplastic	2 High-dose Interleukin-2 3 Low-dose Interleukin-2 4 Liquid Brachytherapy Radioisotope 5 Other Antineoplastic M Monoclonal Antibody
S Epidural Space	3 Percutaneous	2 Anti-infective	8 Oxazolidinones 9 Other Anti-infective
S Epidural Space	3 Percutaneous	3 Anti-inflammatory 6 Nutritional Substance 7 Electrolytic and Water Balance Substance B Anesthetic Agent H Radioactive Substance K Other Diagnostic Substance N Analgesics, Hypnotics, Sedatives T Destructive Agent	Z No Qualifier

DRG Non-OR 3EØQ7Ø5
DRG Non-OR 3EØR3Ø2
DRG Non-OR 3EØS3Ø2

3EØ Continued on next page

3EØ Continued

3 Administration
E Physiological Systems and Anatomical Regions
Ø Introduction Definition: Putting in or on a therapeutic, diagnostic, nutritional, physiological, or prophylactic substance except blood or blood products

Body System/Region Character 4	Approach Character 5	Substance Character 6	Qualifier Character 7
S Epidural Space	3 Percutaneous	G Other Therapeutic Substance	C Other Substance
S Epidural Space	3 Percutaneous	S Gas	F Other Gas
S Epidural Space	7 Via Natural or Artificial Opening	S Gas	F Other Gas
T Peripheral Nerves and Plexi X Cranial Nerves	3 Percutaneous	3 Anti-inflammatory B Anesthetic Agent T Destructive Agent	Z No Qualifier
T Peripheral Nerves and Plexi X Cranial Nerves	3 Percutaneous	G Other Therapeutic Substance	C Other Substance
U Joints	Ø Open	2 Anti-infective	8 Oxazolidinones 9 Other Anti-infective
U Joints	Ø Open	G Other Therapeutic Substance	B Recombinant Bone Morphogenetic Protein
U Joints	3 Percutaneous	Ø Antineoplastic	4 Liquid Brachytherapy Radioisotope 5 Other Antineoplastic M Monoclonal Antibody
U Joints	3 Percutaneous	2 Anti-infective	8 Oxazolidinones 9 Other Anti-infective
U Joints	3 Percutaneous	3 Anti-inflammatory 6 Nutritional Substance 7 Electrolytic and Water Balance Substance B Anesthetic Agent H Radioactive Substance K Other Diagnostic Substance N Analgesics, Hypnotics, Sedatives T Destructive Agent	Z No Qualifier
U Joints	3 Percutaneous	G Other Therapeutic Substance	B Recombinant Bone Morphogenetic Protein C Other Substance
U Joints	3 Percutaneous	S Gas	F Other Gas
U Joints	4 Percutaneous Endoscopic	G Other Therapeutic Substance	C Other Substance
V Bones	Ø Open	G Other Therapeutic Substance	B Recombinant Bone Morphogenetic Protein
V Bones	3 Percutaneous	Ø Antineoplastic	5 Other Antineoplastic M Monoclonal Antibody
V Bones	3 Percutaneous	2 Anti-infective	8 Oxazolidinones 9 Other Anti-infective
V Bones	3 Percutaneous	3 Anti-inflammatory 6 Nutritional Substance 7 Electrolytic and Water Balance Substance B Anesthetic Agent H Radioactive Substance K Other Diagnostic Substance N Analgesics, Hypnotics, Sedatives T Destructive Agent	Z No Qualifier
V Bones	3 Percutaneous	G Other Therapeutic Substance	B Recombinant Bone Morphogenetic Protein C Other Substance
W Lymphatics	3 Percutaneous	Ø Antineoplastic	5 Other Antineoplastic M Monoclonal Antibody
W Lymphatics	3 Percutaneous	2 Anti-infective	8 Oxazolidinones 9 Other Anti-infective
W Lymphatics	3 Percutaneous	3 Anti-inflammatory 6 Nutritional Substance 7 Electrolytic and Water Balance Substance B Anesthetic Agent H Radioactive Substance K Other Diagnostic Substance N Analgesics, Hypnotics, Sedatives T Destructive Agent	Z No Qualifier
W Lymphatics	3 Percutaneous	G Other Therapeutic Substance	C Other Substance

3EØ Continued on next page

3 Administration
E Physiological Systems and Anatomical Regions
Ø Introduction Definition: Putting in or on a therapeutic, diagnostic, nutritional, physiological, or prophylactic substance except blood or blood products

3EØ Continued

Body System/Region Character 4	Approach Character 5	Substance Character 6	Qualifier Character 7
Y Pericardial Cavity	3 Percutaneous	Ø Antineoplastic	4 Liquid Brachytherapy Radioisotope 5 Other Antineoplastic M Monoclonal Antibody
Y Pericardial Cavity	3 Percutaneous	2 Anti-infective	8 Oxazolidinones 9 Other Anti-infective
Y Pericardial Cavity	3 Percutaneous	3 Anti-inflammatory 6 Nutritional Substance 7 Electrolytic and Water Balance Substance B Anesthetic Agent H Radioactive Substance K Other Diagnostic Substance N Analgesics, Hypnotics, Sedatives T Destructive Agent	Z No Qualifier
Y Pericardial Cavity	3 Percutaneous	G Other Therapeutic Substance	C Other Substance
Y Pericardial Cavity	3 Percutaneous	S Gas	F Other Gas
Y Pericardial Cavity	4 Percutaneous Endoscopic	G Other Therapeutic Substance	C Other Substance
Y Pericardial Cavity	7 Via Natural or Artificial Opening	Ø Antineoplastic	4 Liquid Brachytherapy Radioisotope 5 Other Antineoplastic M Monoclonal Antibody
Y Pericardial Cavity	7 Via Natural or Artificial Opening	S Gas	F Other Gas

3 Administration
E Physiological Systems and Anatomical Regions
1 Irrigation Definition: Putting in or on a cleansing substance

Body System/Region Character 4	Approach Character 5	Substance Character 6	Qualifier Character 7
Ø Skin and Mucous Membranes C Eye	3 Percutaneous X External	8 Irrigating Substance	X Diagnostic Z No Qualifier
9 Nose B Ear F Respiratory Tract G Upper GI H Lower GI J Biliary and Pancreatic Tract K Genitourinary Tract N Male Reproductive ♂ P Female Reproductive ♀	3 Percutaneous 7 Via Natural or Artificial Opening 8 Via Natural or Artificial Opening Endoscopic	8 Irrigating Substance	X Diagnostic Z No Qualifier
L Pleural Cavity Q Cranial Cavity and Brain R Spinal Canal S Epidural Space Y Pericardial Cavity	3 Percutaneous	8 Irrigating Substance	X Diagnostic Z No Qualifier
M Peritoneal Cavity	3 Percutaneous	8 Irrigating Substance	X Diagnostic Z No Qualifier
M Peritoneal Cavity	3 Percutaneous	9 Dialysate	Z No Qualifier
U Joints	3 Percutaneous 4 Percutaneous Endoscopic	8 Irrigating Substance	X Diagnostic Z No Qualifier

♂ 3E1N[3,7,8]8[X,Z]
♀ 3E1P[3,7,8]8[X,Z]

Measurement and Monitoring 4AØ–4BØ

AHA Coding Clinic for table 4AØ

2019, 3Q, 32	Endomyocardial biopsy and right heart catheterization
2018, 1Q, 12	Percutaneous balloon valvuloplasty & cardiac catheterization with ventriculogram
2016, 3Q, 37	Fractional flow reserve
2015, 3Q, 29	Approach value for esophageal electrophysiology study

AHA Coding Clinic for table 4A1

2019, 4Q, 38-39	Intraoperative fluorescence lymphatic mapping using Indocyanine green dye
2016, 4Q, 114	Fluorescence vascular angiography
2016, 2Q, 29	Decompressive craniectomy with cryopreservation and storage of bone flap
2016, 2Q, 33	Monitoring of arterial pressure & pulse
2015, 3Q, 35	Swan Ganz catheterization
2015, 2Q, 14	Intraoperative EMG monitoring via endotracheal tube
2015, 1Q, 26	Intraoperative monitoring using Sentio MMG®
2014, 4Q, 28	Removal and replacement of displaced growing rods

4 Measurement and Monitoring
A Physiological Systems
Ø Measurement Definition: Determining the level of a physiological or physical function at a point in time

Body System Character 4	Approach Character 5	Function/Device Character 6	Qualifier Character 7
Ø Central Nervous	**Ø** Open	**2** Conductivity **4** Electrical Activity **B** Pressure	**Z** No Qualifier
Ø Central Nervous	**3** Percutaneous **7** Via Natural or Artificial Opening **8** Via Natural or Artificial Opening Endoscopic	**4** Electrical Activity	**Z** No Qualifier
Ø Central Nervous	**3** Percutaneous **7** Via Natural or Artificial Opening **8** Via Natural or Artificial Opening Endoscopic	**B** Pressure **K** Temperature **R** Saturation	**D** Intracranial
Ø Central Nervous	**X** External	**2** Conductivity **4** Electrical Activity	**Z** No Qualifier
1 Peripheral Nervous	**Ø** Open **3** Percutaneous **7** Via Natural or Artificial Opening **8** Via Natural or Artificial Opening Endoscopic **X** External	**2** Conductivity	**9** Sensory **B** Motor
1 Peripheral Nervous	**Ø** Open **3** Percutaneous **7** Via Natural or Artificial Opening **8** Via Natural or Artificial Opening Endoscopic **X** External	**4** Electrical Activity	**Z** No Qualifier
2 Cardiac	**Ø** Open **3** Percutaneous **7** Via Natural or Artificial Opening **8** Via Natural or Artificial Opening Endoscopic	**4** Electrical Activity **9** Output **C** Rate **F** Rhythm **H** Sound **P** Action Currents	**Z** No Qualifier
2 Cardiac	**Ø** Open **3** Percutaneous **7** Via Natural or Artificial Opening **8** Via Natural or Artificial Opening Endoscopic	**N** Sampling and Pressure	**6** Right Heart **7** Left Heart **8** Bilateral
2 Cardiac	**X** External	**4** Electrical Activity	**A** Guidance **Z** No Qualifier
2 Cardiac	**X** External	**9** Output **C** Rate **F** Rhythm **H** Sound **P** Action Currents	**Z** No Qualifier
2 Cardiac	**X** External	**M** Total Activity	**4** Stress
3 Arterial	**Ø** Open **3** Percutaneous	**5** Flow **J** Pulse	**1** Peripheral **3** Pulmonary **C** Coronary
3 Arterial	**Ø** Open **3** Percutaneous	**B** Pressure	**1** Peripheral **3** Pulmonary **C** Coronary **F** Other Thoracic

DRG Non-OR 4AØ2[3,7,8]FZ
DRG Non-OR 4AØ2[Ø,3,7,8]N[6,7,8]

4AØ Continued on next page

4AØ Continued

4 Measurement and Monitoring
A Physiological Systems
Ø Measurement Definition: Determining the level of a physiological or physical function at a point in time

Body System Character 4	Approach Character 5	Function/Device Character 6	Qualifier Character 7
3 Arterial	Ø Open 3 Percutaneous	H Sound R Saturation	1 Peripheral
3 Arterial	X External	5 Flow	1 Peripheral D Intracranial
3 Arterial	X External	B Pressure H Sound J Pulse R Saturation	1 Peripheral
4 Venous	Ø Open 3 Percutaneous	5 Flow B Pressure J Pulse	Ø Central 1 Peripheral 2 Portal 3 Pulmonary
4 Venous	Ø Open 3 Percutaneous	R Saturation	1 Peripheral
4 Venous	4 Percutaneous Endoscopic	B Pressure	2 Portal
4 Venous	X External	5 Flow B Pressure J Pulse R Saturation	1 Peripheral
5 Circulatory	X External	L Volume	Z No Qualifier
6 Lymphatic	Ø Open 3 Percutaneous 7 Via Natural or Artificial Opening 8 Via Natural or Artificial Opening Endoscopic	5 Flow B Pressure	Z No Qualifier
7 Visual	X External	Ø Acuity 7 Mobility B Pressure	Z No Qualifier
8 Olfactory	X External	Ø Acuity	Z No Qualifier
9 Respiratory	7 Via Natural or Artificial Opening 8 Via Natural or Artificial Opening Endoscopic X External	1 Capacity 5 Flow C Rate D Resistance L Volume M Total Activity	Z No Qualifier
B Gastrointestinal	7 Via Natural or Artificial Opening 8 Via Natural or Artificial Opening Endoscopic	8 Motility B Pressure G Secretion	Z No Qualifier
C Biliary	3 Percutaneous 4 Percutaneous Endoscopic 7 Via Natural or Artificial Opening 8 Via Natural or Artificial Opening Endoscopic	5 Flow B Pressure	Z No Qualifier
D Urinary	7 Via Natural or Artificial Opening 8 Via Natural or Artificial Opening Endoscopic	3 Contractility 5 Flow B Pressure D Resistance L Volume	Z No Qualifier
F Musculoskeletal	3 Percutaneous	3 Contractility	Z No Qualifier
F Musculoskeletal	3 Percutaneous	B Pressure	E Compartment
F Musculoskeletal	X External	3 Contractility	Z No Qualifier
H Products of Conception, Cardiac ♀	7 Via Natural or Artificial Opening 8 Via Natural or Artificial Opening Endoscopic X External	4 Electrical Activity C Rate F Rhythm H Sound	Z No Qualifier
J Products of Conception, Nervous ♀	7 Via Natural or Artificial Opening 8 Via Natural or Artificial Opening Endoscopic X External	2 Conductivity 4 Electrical Activity B Pressure	Z No Qualifier
Z None	7 Via Natural or Artificial Opening	6 Metabolism K Temperature	Z No Qualifier
Z None	X External	6 Metabolism K Temperature Q Sleep	Z No Qualifier

Valid OR 4AØ6Ø[5,B]Z
Valid OR 4AØC4[5,B]Z
♀ 4AØH[7,8,X][4,C,F,H]Z
♀ 4AØJ[7,8,X][2,4,B]Z

4 Measurement and Monitoring
A Physiological Systems
1 Monitoring Definition: Determining the level of a physiological or physical function repetitively over a period of time

Body System Character 4	Approach Character 5	Function/Device Character 6	Qualifier Character 7
Ø Central Nervous	Ø Open	2 Conductivity B Pressure	Z No Qualifier
Ø Central Nervous	Ø Open	4 Electrical Activity	G Intraoperative Z No Qualifier
Ø Central Nervous	3 Percutaneous 7 Via Natural or Artificial Opening 8 Via Natural or Artificial Opening Endoscopic	4 Electrical Activity	G Intraoperative Z No Qualifier
Ø Central Nervous	3 Percutaneous 7 Via Natural or Artificial Opening 8 Via Natural or Artificial Opening Endoscopic	B Pressure K Temperature R Saturation	D Intracranial
Ø Central Nervous	X External	2 Conductivity	Z No Qualifier
Ø Central Nervous	X External	4 Electrical Activity	G Intraoperative Z No Qualifier
1 Peripheral Nervous	Ø Open 3 Percutaneous 7 Via Natural or Artificial Opening 8 Via Natural or Artificial Opening Endoscopic X External	2 Conductivity	9 Sensory B Motor
1 Peripheral Nervous	Ø Open 3 Percutaneous 7 Via Natural or Artificial Opening 8 Via Natural or Artificial Opening Endoscopic X External	4 Electrical Activity	G Intraoperative Z No Qualifier
2 Cardiac	Ø Open 3 Percutaneous 7 Via Natural or Artificial Opening 8 Via Natural or Artificial Opening Endoscopic	4 Electrical Activity 9 Output C Rate F Rhythm H Sound	Z No Qualifier
2 Cardiac	X External	4 Electrical Activity	5 Ambulatory Z No Qualifier
2 Cardiac	X External	9 Output C Rate F Rhythm H Sound	Z No Qualifier
2 Cardiac	X External	M Total Activity	4 Stress
2 Cardiac	X External	S Vascular Perfusion	H Indocyanine Green Dye
3 Arterial	Ø Open 3 Percutaneous	5 Flow B Pressure J Pulse	1 Peripheral 3 Pulmonary C Coronary
3 Arterial	Ø Open 3 Percutaneous	H Sound R Saturation	1 Peripheral
3 Arterial	X External	5 Flow B Pressure H Sound J Pulse R Saturation	1 Peripheral
4 Venous	Ø Open 3 Percutaneous	5 Flow B Pressure J Pulse	Ø Central 1 Peripheral 2 Portal 3 Pulmonary
4 Venous	Ø Open 3 Percutaneous	R Saturation	Ø Central 2 Portal 3 Pulmonary
4 Venous	X External	5 Flow B Pressure J Pulse	1 Peripheral
6 Lymphatic	Ø Open 3 Percutaneous 7 Via Natural or Artificial Opening 8 Via Natural or Artificial Opening Endoscopic	5 Flow	H Indocyanine Green Dye Z No Qualifier

Valid OR 4A16Ø5Z

4A1 Continued on next page

4 Measurement and Monitoring
A Physiological Systems
1 Monitoring Definition: Determining the level of a physiological or physical function repetitively over a period of time

4A1 Continued

Body System Character 4	Approach Character 5	Function/Device Character 6	Qualifier Character 7
6 Lymphatic	**Ø** Open **3** Percutaneous **7** Via Natural or Artificial Opening **8** Via Natural or Artificial Opening Endoscopic	**B** Pressure	**Z** No Qualifier
9 Respiratory	**7** Via Natural or Artificial Opening **X** External	**1** Capacity **5** Flow **C** Rate **D** Resistance **L** Volume	**Z** No Qualifier
B Gastrointestinal	**7** Via Natural or Artificial Opening **8** Via Natural or Artificial Opening Endoscopic	**8** Motility **B** Pressure **G** Secretion	**Z** No Qualifier
B Gastrointestinal	**X** External	**S** Vascular Perfusion	**H** Indocyanine Green Dye
D Urinary	**7** Via Natural or Artificial Opening **8** Via Natural or Artificial Opening Endoscopic	**3** Contractility **5** Flow **B** Pressure **D** Resistance **L** Volume	**Z** No Qualifier
G Skin and Breast	**X** External	**S** Vascular Perfusion	**H** Indocyanine Green Dye
H Products of Conception, Cardiac ♀	**7** Via Natural or Artificial Opening **8** Via Natural or Artificial Opening Endoscopic **X** External	**4** Electrical Activity **C** Rate **F** Rhythm **H** Sound	**Z** No Qualifier
J Products of Conception, Nervous ♀	**7** Via Natural or Artificial Opening **8** Via Natural or Artificial Opening Endoscopic **X** External	**2** Conductivity **4** Electrical Activity **B** Pressure	**Z** No Qualifier
Z None	**7** Via Natural or Artificial Opening	**K** Temperature	**Z** No Qualifier
Z None	**X** External	**K** Temperature **Q** Sleep	**Z** No Qualifier

Valid OR 4A16ØBZ
♀ 4A1H[7,8,X][4,C,F,H]Z
♀ 4A1J[7,8,X][2,4,B]Z

4 Measurement and Monitoring
B Physiological Devices
Ø Measurement Definition: Determining the level of a physiological or physical function at a point in time

Body System Character 4	Approach Character 5	Function/Device Character 6	Qualifier Character 7
Ø Central Nervous **1** Peripheral Nervous **F** Musculoskeletal	**X** External	**V** Stimulator	**Z** No Qualifier
2 Cardiac	**X** External	**S** Pacemaker **T** Defibrillator	**Z** No Qualifier
9 Respiratory	**X** External	**S** Pacemaker	**Z** No Qualifier

Extracorporeal or Systemic Assistance and Performance 5AØ–5A2

AHA Coding Clinic for table 5AØ

2020, 1Q, 10	Intermittent use of continuous positive airway pressure
2018, 2Q, 3-5	Intra-aortic balloon pump
2017, 4Q, 43-44	Insertion of external heart assist devices
2017, 3Q, 18	Intra-aortic balloon pump removal
2017, 1Q, 10-11	External heart assist device
2017, 1Q, 29	Newborn resuscitation using positive pressure ventilation
2017, 1Q, 29	Newborn noninvasive ventilation
2016, 4Q, 137-139	Heart assist device systems
2014, 4Q, 9	Mechanical ventilation
2014, 3Q, 19	Ablation of ventricular tachycardia with Impella® support
2013, 3Q, 18	Heart transplant surgery

AHA Coding Clinic for table 5A1

2019, 4Q, 39-41	Intraoperative extracorporeal membrane oxygenation
2019, 3Q, 19	Insertion of left ventricular catheter
2019, 3Q, 20	Removal and revision of ECMO component
2019, 3Q, 21	Exchange of extracorporeal membrane oxygenation component (oxygenator)
2019, 2Q, 36	Veno-arterial extracorporeal membrane oxygenation via sternotomy

AHA Coding Clinic for table 5A1 (Continued)

2019, 3Q, 22	Extracorporeal membrane oxygenation and Centrimag™ pump
2019, 3Q, 22	Extracorporeal membrane oxygenation transfers
2018, 4Q, 52-54	Percutaneous extracorporeal membrane oxygenation
2018, 1Q, 13	Mechanical ventilation using patient's equipment
2017, 4Q, 71-73	Hemodialysis and renal replacement therapy
2017, 3Q, 7	Senning procedure (arterial switch)
2017, 1Q, 19	Norwood Sano procedure
2016, 1Q, 27	Aortocoronary bypass graft utilizing Y-graft
2016, 1Q, 28	Extracorporeal liver assist device
2016, 1Q, 29	Duration of hemodialysis
2015, 4Q, 22-24	Congenital heart corrective procedures
2014, 4Q, 3-10	Mechanical ventilation
2014, 4Q, 11-15	Sequencing of mechanical ventilation with other procedures
2014, 3Q, 16	Repair of Tetralogy of Fallot
2014, 3Q, 20	MAZE procedure performed with coronary artery bypass graft
2014, 1Q, 10	Repair of thoracic aortic aneurysm & coronary artery bypass graft
2013, 3Q, 18	Heart transplant surgery

5 Extracorporeal or Systemic Assistance and Performance
A Physiological Systems
Ø Assistance Definition: Taking over a portion of a physiological function by extracorporeal means

Body System Character 4	Duration Character 5	Function Character 6	Qualifier Character 7
2 Cardiac	1 Intermittent 2 Continuous	1 Output	Ø Balloon Pump 5 Pulsatile Compression 6 Other Pump D Impeller Pump
5 Circulatory	1 Intermittent 2 Continuous	2 Oxygenation	1 Hyperbaric C Supersaturated
9 Respiratory	2 Continuous	Ø Filtration	Z No Qualifier
9 Respiratory	3 Less than 24 Consecutive Hours 4 24-96 Consecutive Hours 5 Greater than 96 Consecutive Hours	5 Ventilation	7 Continuous Positive Airway Pressure 8 Intermittent Positive Airway Pressure 9 Continuous Negative Airway Pressure A High Nasal Flow/Velocity B Intermittent Negative Airway Pressure Z No Qualifier

Valid OR 5AØ2[1,2]1[Ø,6,D]

5 Extracorporeal or Systemic Assistance and Performance
A Physiological Systems
1 Performance Definition: Completely taking over a physiological function by extracorporeal means

Body System Character 4	Duration Character 5	Function Character 6	Qualifier Character 7
2 Cardiac	Ø Single	1 Output	2 Manual
2 Cardiac	1 Intermittent	3 Pacing	Z No Qualifier
2 Cardiac	2 Continuous	1 Output 3 Pacing	Z No Qualifier
5 Circulatory	2 Continuous A Intraoperative	2 Oxygenation	F Membrane, Central G Membrane, Peripheral Veno-arterial H Membrane, Peripheral Veno-venous
9 Respiratory	Ø Single	5 Ventilation	4 Nonmechanical
9 Respiratory	3 Less than 24 Consecutive Hours 4 24-96 Consecutive Hours 5 Greater than 96 Consecutive Hours	5 Ventilation	Z No Qualifier
C Biliary	Ø Single 6 Multiple	Ø Filtration	Z No Qualifier
D Urinary	7 Intermittent, Less than 6 Hours per day 8 Prolonged Intermittent, 6-18 Hours per day 9 Continuous, Greater than 18 Hours per day	Ø Filtration	Z No Qualifier

Valid OR 5A1522F
DRG Non-OR 5A1522[G,H]
DRG Non-OR 5A19[3,4]5Z
DRG Non-OR 5A1955Z Length of stay must be > 4 consecutive days.
DRG Non-OR 5A1D[7,8,9]ØZ

5 Extracorporeal or Systemic Assistance and Performance
A Physiological Systems
2 Restoration Definition: Returning, or attempting to return, a physiological function to its original state by extracorporeal means.

Body System Character 4	Duration Character 5	Function Character 6	Qualifier Character 7
2 Cardiac	Ø Single	4 Rhythm	Z No Qualifier

Extracorporeal or Systemic Therapies 6AØ–6AB

AHA Coding Clinic for table 6A4
2019, 2Q, 17 Cryoamputation of lower leg

AHA Coding Clinic for table 6A7
2014, 4Q, 19 Ultrasound accelerated thrombolysis

AHA Coding Clinic for table 6AB
2016, 4Q, 115 Donor organ perfusion

6 Extracorporeal or Systemic Therapies
A Physiological Systems
Ø Atmospheric Control Definition: Extracorporeal control of atmospheric pressure and composition

Body System Character 4	Duration Character 5	Qualifier Character 6	Qualifier Character 7
Z None	Ø Single 1 Multiple	Z No Qualifier	Z No Qualifier

6 Extracorporeal or Systemic Therapies
A Physiological Systems
1 Decompression Definition: Extracorporeal elimination of undissolved gas from body fluids

Body System Character 4	Duration Character 5	Qualifier Character 6	Qualifier Character 7
5 Circulatory	Ø Single 1 Multiple	Z No Qualifier	Z No Qualifier

6 Extracorporeal or Systemic Therapies
A Physiological Systems
2 Electromagnetic Therapy Definition: Extracorporeal treatment by electromagnetic rays

Body System Character 4	Duration Character 5	Qualifier Character 6	Qualifier Character 7
1 Urinary 2 Central Nervous	Ø Single 1 Multiple	Z No Qualifier	Z No Qualifier

6 Extracorporeal or Systemic Therapies
A Physiological Systems
3 Hyperthermia Definition: Extracorporeal raising of body temperature

Body System Character 4	Duration Character 5	Qualifier Character 6	Qualifier Character 7
Z None	Ø Single 1 Multiple	Z No Qualifier	Z No Qualifier

6 Extracorporeal or Systemic Therapies
A Physiological Systems
4 Hypothermia Definition: Extracorporeal lowering of body temperature

Body System Character 4	Duration Character 5	Qualifier Character 6	Qualifier Character 7
Z None	Ø Single 1 Multiple	Z No Qualifier	Z No Qualifier

6 Extracorporeal or Systemic Therapies
A Physiological Systems
5 Pheresis Definition: Extracorporeal separation of blood products

Body System Character 4	Duration Character 5	Qualifier Character 6	Qualifier Character 7
5 Circulatory	Ø Single 1 Multiple	Z No Qualifier	Ø Erythrocytes 1 Leukocytes 2 Platelets 3 Plasma T Stem Cells, Cord Blood V Stem Cells, Hematopoietic

6 Extracorporeal or Systemic Therapies
A Physiological Systems
6 Phototherapy Definition: Extracorporeal treatment by light rays

Body System Character 4	Duration Character 5	Qualifier Character 6	Qualifier Character 7
Ø Skin 5 Circulatory	Ø Single 1 Multiple	Z No Qualifier	Z No Qualifier

Extracorporeal or Systemic Therapies

6 Extracorporeal or Systemic Therapies
A Physiological Systems
7 Ultrasound Therapy Definition: Extracorporeal treatment by ultrasound

Body System Character 4	Duration Character 5	Qualifier Character 6	Qualifier Character 7
5 Circulatory	Ø Single 1 Multiple	Z No Qualifier	4 Head and Neck Vessels 5 Heart 6 Peripheral Vessels 7 Other Vessels Z No Qualifier

6 Extracorporeal or Systemic Therapies
A Physiological Systems
8 Ultraviolet Light Therapy Definition: Extracorporeal treatment by ultraviolet light

Body System Character 4	Duration Character 5	Qualifier Character 6	Qualifier Character 7
Ø Skin	Ø Single 1 Multiple	Z No Qualifier	Z No Qualifier

6 Extracorporeal or Systemic Therapies
A Physiological Systems
9 Shock Wave Therapy Definition: Extracorporeal treatment by shock waves

Body System Character 4	Duration Character 5	Qualifier Character 6	Qualifier Character 7
3 Musculoskeletal	Ø Single 1 Multiple	Z No Qualifier	Z No Qualifier

6 Extracorporeal or Systemic Therapies
A Physiological Systems
B Perfusion Definition: Extracorporeal treatment by diffusion of therapeutic fluid

Body System Character 4	Duration Character 5	Qualifier Character 6	Qualifier Character 7
5 Circulatory B Respiratory System F Hepatobiliary System and Pancreas T Urinary System	Ø Single	B Donor Organ	Z No Qualifier

Osteopathic 7WØ

7 Osteopathic
W Anatomical Regions
Ø Treatment Definition: Manual treatment to eliminate or alleviate somatic dysfunction and related disorders

Body Region Character 4	Approach Character 5	Method Character 6	Qualifier Character 7
Ø Head 1 Cervical 2 Thoracic 3 Lumbar 4 Sacrum 5 Pelvis 6 Lower Extremities 7 Upper Extremities 8 Rib Cage 9 Abdomen	X External	Ø Articulatory-Raising 1 Fascial Release 2 General Mobilization 3 High Velocity-Low Amplitude 4 Indirect 5 Low Velocity-High Amplitude 6 Lymphatic Pump 7 Muscle Energy-Isometric 8 Muscle Energy-Isotonic 9 Other Method	Z None

Other Procedures 8CØ–8EØ

AHA Coding Clinic for table 8EØ
2019, 4Q, 41-42 Intraoperative fluorescence guidance
2019, 1Q, 30 Laparoscopic-assisted rectopexy with manual reduction of prolapse
2015, 1Q, 33 Robotic-assisted laparoscopic hysterectomy converted to open procedure
2014, 4Q, 33 Radical prostatectomy

8 Other Procedures
C Indwelling Device
Ø Other Procedures Definition: Methodologies which attempt to remediate or cure a disorder or disease

Body Region Character 4	Approach Character 5	Method Character 6	Qualifier Character 7
1 Nervous System	X External	6 Collection	J Cerebrospinal Fluid L Other Fluid
2 Circulatory System	X External	6 Collection	K Blood L Other Fluid

8 Other Procedures
E Physiological Systems and Anatomical Regions
Ø Other Procedures Definition: Methodologies which attempt to remediate or cure a disorder or disease

Body Region Character 4	Approach Character 5	Method Character 6	Qualifier Character 7
1 Nervous System U Female Reproductive System ♀	X External	Y Other Method	7 Examination
2 Circulatory System	3 Percutaneous X External	D Near Infrared Spectroscopy	Z No Qualifier
9 Head and Neck Region	Ø Open	C Robotic Assisted Procedure	Z No Qualifier
9 Head and Neck Region	Ø Open	E Fluorescence Guided Procedure	M Aminolevulinic Acid Z No Qualifier
9 Head and Neck Region	3 Percutaneous 4 Percutaneous Endoscopic 7 Via Natural or Artificial Opening 8 Via Natural or Artificial Opening Endoscopic	C Robotic Assisted Procedure E Fluorescence Guided Procedure	Z No Qualifier
9 Head and Neck Region	X External	B Computer Assisted Procedure	F With Fluoroscopy G With Computerized Tomography H With Magnetic Resonance Imaging Z No Qualifier
9 Head and Neck Region	X External	C Robotic Assisted Procedure	Z No Qualifier
9 Head and Neck Region	X External	Y Other Method	8 Suture Removal
H Integumentary System and Breast	3 Percutaneous	Ø Acupuncture	Ø Anesthesia Z No Qualifier
H Integumentary System and Breast ♀	X External	6 Collection	2 Breast Milk
H Integumentary System and Breast	X External	Y Other Method	9 Piercing
K Musculoskeletal System	X External	1 Therapeutic Massage	Z No Qualifier
K Musculoskeletal System	X External	Y Other Method	7 Examination
V Male Reproductive System ♂	X External	1 Therapeutic Massage	C Prostate D Rectum
V Male Reproductive System ♂	X External	6 Collection	3 Sperm
W Trunk Region	Ø Open 3 Percutaneous 4 Percutaneous Endoscopic 7 Via Natural or Artificial Opening 8 Via Natural or Artificial Opening Endoscopic	C Robotic Assisted Procedure E Fluorescence Guided Procedure	Z No Qualifier
W Trunk Region	X External	B Computer Assisted Procedure	F With Fluoroscopy G With Computerized Tomography H With Magnetic Resonance Imaging Z No Qualifier
W Trunk Region	X External	C Robotic Assisted Procedure	Z No Qualifier
W Trunk Region	X External	Y Other Method	8 Suture Removal
X Upper Extremity Y Lower Extremity	Ø Open 3 Percutaneous 4 Percutaneous Endoscopic	C Robotic Assisted Procedure E Fluorescence Guided Procedure	Z No Qualifier

♂ 8EØVX1C
♂ 8EØVX63
♀ 8EØUXY7
♀ 8EØHX62

8EØ Continued on next page

8 Other Procedures
E Physiological Systems and Anatomical Regions
Ø Other Procedures Definition: Methodologies which attempt to remediate or cure a disorder or disease

8EØ Continued

Body Region Character 4	Approach Character 5	Method Character 6	Qualifier Character 7
X Upper Extremity Y Lower Extremity	X External	B Computer Assisted Procedure	F With Fluoroscopy G With Computerized Tomography H With Magnetic Resonance Imaging Z No Qualifier
X Upper Extremity Y Lower Extremity	X External	C Robotic Assisted Procedure	Z No Qualifier
X Upper Extremity Y Lower Extremity	X External	Y Other Method	8 Suture Removal
Z None	X External	Y Other Method	1 In Vitro Fertilization 4 Yoga Therapy 5 Meditation 6 Isolation

Chiropractic 9WB

9 Chiropractic
W Anatomical Regions
B Manipulation Definition: Manual procedure that involves a directed thrust to move a joint past the physiological range of motion, without exceeding the anatomical limit

Body Region Character 4	Approach Character 5	Method Character 6	Qualifier Character 7
Ø Head 1 Cervical 2 Thoracic 3 Lumbar 4 Sacrum 5 Pelvis 6 Lower Extremities 7 Upper Extremities 8 Rib Cage 9 Abdomen	X External	B Non-Manual C Indirect Visceral D Extra-Articular F Direct Visceral G Long Lever Specific Contact H Short Lever Specific Contact J Long and Short Lever Specific Contact K Mechanically Assisted L Other Method	Z None

Imaging BØØ–BY4

AHA Coding Clinic for table B21
2018, 1Q, 12 Percutaneous balloon valvuloplasty & cardiac catheterization with ventriculogram
2016, 3Q, 36 Type of contrast medium for angiography (high osmolar, low osmolar, and other)

AHA Coding Clinic for table B41
2015, 3Q, 9 Aborted endovascular stenting of superficial femoral artery

AHA Coding Clinic for table B51
2015, 4Q, 30 Vascular access devices

AHA Coding Clinic for table BF4
2014, 3Q, 15 Drainage of pancreatic pseudocyst

B Imaging
Ø Central Nervous System
Ø Plain Radiography Definition: Planar display of an image developed from the capture of external ionizing radiation on photographic or photoconductive plate

Body Part Character 4	Contrast Character 5	Qualifier Character 6	Qualifier Character 7
B Spinal Cord	Ø High Osmolar 1 Low Osmolar Y Other Contrast Z None	Z None	Z None

B Imaging
Ø Central Nervous System
1 Fluoroscopy Definition: Single plane or bi-plane real time display of an image developed from the capture of external ionizing radioation on a fluorescent screen. The image may also be stored by either digital or analog means.

Body Part Character 4	Contrast Character 5	Qualifier Character 6	Qualifier Character 7
B Spinal Cord	Ø High Osmolar 1 Low Osmolar Y Other Contrast Z None	Z None	Z None

B Imaging
Ø Central Nervous System
2 Computerized Tomography (CT Scan) Definition: Computer reformatted digital display of multiplanar images developed from the capture of multiple exposures of external ionizing radiation

Body Part Character 4	Contrast Character 5	Qualifier Character 6	Qualifier Character 7
Ø Brain 7 Cisterna 8 Cerebral Ventricle(s) 9 Sella Turcica/Pituitary Gland B Spinal Cord	Ø High Osmolar 1 Low Osmolar Y Other Contrast	Ø Unenhanced and Enhanced Z None	Z None
Ø Brain 7 Cisterna 8 Cerebral Ventricle(s) 9 Sella Turcica/Pituitary Gland B Spinal Cord	Z None	Z None	Z None

B Imaging
Ø Central Nervous System
3 Magnetic Resonance Imaging (MRI) Definition: Computer reformatted digital display of multiplanar images developed from the capture of radio-frequency signals emitted by nuclei in a body site excited within a magnetic field

Body Part Character 4	Contrast Character 5	Qualifier Character 6	Qualifier Character 7
Ø Brain 9 Sella Turcica/Pituitary Gland B Spinal Cord C Acoustic Nerves	Y Other Contrast	Ø Unenhanced and Enhanced Z None	Z None
Ø Brain 9 Sella Turcica/Pituitary Gland B Spinal Cord C Acoustic Nerves	Z None	Z None	Z None

B Imaging
Ø Central Nervous System
4 Ultrasonography Definition: Real time display of images of anatomy or flow information developed from the capture of relected and attenuated high frequency sound waves

Body Part Character 4	Contrast Character 5	Qualifier Character 6	Qualifier Character 7
Ø Brain B Spinal Cord	Z None	Z None	Z None

B Imaging
2 Heart
Ø Plain Radiography Definition: Planar display of an image developed from the capture of external ionizing radiation on photographic or photoconductive plate

Body Part Character 4	Contrast Character 5	Qualifier Character 6	Qualifier Character 7
Ø Coronary Artery, Single 1 Coronary Arteries, Multiple 2 Coronary Artery Bypass Graft, Single 3 Coronary Artery Bypass Grafts, Multiple 4 Heart, Right 5 Heart, Left 6 Heart, Right and Left 7 Internal Mammary Bypass Graft, Right 8 Internal Mammary Bypass Graft, Left F Bypass Graft, Other	Ø High Osmolar 1 Low Osmolar Y Other Contrast	Z None	Z None

DRG Non-OR All body part, contrast, and qualifier values

B Imaging
2 Heart
1 Fluoroscopy Definition: Single plane or bi-plane real time display of an image developed from the capture of external ionizing radioation on a fluorescent screen. The image may also be stored by either digital or analog means.

Body Part Character 4	Contrast Character 5	Qualifier Character 6	Qualifier Character 7
Ø Coronary Artery, Single 1 Coronary Arteries, Multiple 2 Coronary Artery Bypass Graft, Single 3 Coronary Artery Bypass Grafts, Multiple	Ø High Osmolar 1 Low Osmolar Y Other Contrast	1 Laser	Ø Intraoperative
Ø Coronary Artery, Single 1 Coronary Arteries, Multiple 2 Coronary Artery Bypass Graft, Single 3 Coronary Artery Bypass Grafts, Multiple	Ø High Osmolar 1 Low Osmolar Y Other Contrast	Z None	Z None
4 Heart, Right 5 Heart, Left 6 Heart, Right and Left 7 Internal Mammary Bypass Graft, Right 8 Internal Mammary Bypass Graft, Left F Bypass Graft, Other	Ø High Osmolar 1 Low Osmolar Y Other Contrast	Z None	Z None

DRG Non-OR All body part, contrast, and qualifier values

B Imaging
2 Heart
2 Computerized Tomography (CT Scan) Definition: Computer reformatted digital display of multiplanar images developed from the capture of multiple exposures of external ionizing radiation

Body Part Character 4	Contrast Character 5	Qualifier Character 6	Qualifier Character 7
1 Coronary Arteries, Multiple 3 Coronary Artery Bypass Grafts, Multiple 6 Heart, Right and Left	Ø High Osmolar 1 Low Osmolar Y Other Contrast	Ø Unenhanced and Enhanced Z None	Z None
1 Coronary Arteries, Multiple 3 Coronary Artery Bypass Grafts, Multiple 6 Heart, Right and Left	Z None	2 Intravascular Optical Coherence Z None	Z None

B Imaging
2 Heart
3 Magnetic Resonance Imaging (MRI) Definition: Computer reformatted digital display of multiplanar images developed from the capture of radio-frequency signals emitted by nuclei in a body site excited within a magnetic field

Body Part Character 4	Contrast Character 5	Qualifier Character 6	Qualifier Character 7
1 Coronary Arteries, Multiple 3 Coronary Artery Bypass Grafts, Multiple 6 Heart, Right and Left	Y Other Contrast	Ø Unenhanced and Enhanced Z None	Z None
1 Coronary Arteries, Multiple 3 Coronary Artery Bypass Grafts, Multiple 6 Heart, Right and Left	Z None	Z None	Z None

B Imaging
2 Heart
4 Ultrasonography Definition: Real time display of images of anatomy or flow information developed from the capture of relected and attenuated high frequency sound waves

Body Part Character 4	Contrast Character 5	Qualifier Character 6	Qualifier Character 7
Ø Coronary Artery, Single 1 Coronary Arteries, Multiple 4 Heart, Right 5 Heart, Left 6 Heart, Right and Left B Heart with Aorta C Pericardium D Pediatric Heart	Y Other Contrast	Z None	Z None
Ø Coronary Artery, Single 1 Coronary Arteries, Multiple 4 Heart, Right 5 Heart, Left 6 Heart, Right and Left B Heart with Aorta C Pericardium D Pediatric Heart	Z None	Z None	3 Intravascular 4 Transesophageal Z None

B Imaging
3 Upper Arteries
Ø Plain Radiography Definition: Planar display of an image developed from the capture of external ionizing radiation on photographic or photoconductive plate

Body Part Character 4	Contrast Character 5	Qualifier Character 6	Qualifier Character 7
Ø Thoracic Aorta 1 Brachiocephalic-Subclavian Artery, Right 2 Subclavian Artery, Left 3 Common Carotid Artery, Right 4 Common Carotid Artery, Left 5 Common Carotid Arteries, Bilateral 6 Internal Carotid Artery, Right 7 Internal Carotid Artery, Left 8 Internal Carotid Arteries, Bilateral 9 External Carotid Artery, Right B External Carotid Artery, Left C External Carotid Arteries, Bilateral D Vertebral Artery, Right F Vertebral Artery, Left G Vertebral Arteries, Bilateral H Upper Extremity Arteries, Right J Upper Extremity Arteries, Left K Upper Extremity Arteries, Bilateral L Intercostal and Bronchial Arteries M Spinal Arteries N Upper Arteries, Other P Thoraco-Abdominal Aorta Q Cervico-Cerebral Arch R Intracranial Arteries S Pulmonary Artery, Right T Pulmonary Artery, Left	Ø High Osmolar 1 Low Osmolar Y Other Contrast Z None	Z None	Z None

B Imaging
3 Upper Arteries
1 Fluoroscopy Definition: Single plane or bi-plane real time display of an image developed from the capture of external ionizing radiation on a fluorescent screen. The image may also be stored by either digital or analog means.

Body Part Character 4	Contrast Character 5	Qualifier Character 6	Qualifier Character 7
Ø Thoracic Aorta 1 Brachiocephalic-Subclavian Artery, Right 2 Subclavian Artery, Left 3 Common Carotid Artery, Right 4 Common Carotid Artery, Left 5 Common Carotid Arteries, Bilateral 6 Internal Carotid Artery, Right 7 Internal Carotid Artery, Left 8 Internal Carotid Arteries, Bilateral 9 External Carotid Artery, Right B External Carotid Artery, Left C External Carotid Arteries, Bilateral D Vertebral Artery, Right F Vertebral Artery, Left G Vertebral Arteries, Bilateral H Upper Extremity Arteries, Right J Upper Extremity Arteries, Left K Upper Extremity Arteries, Bilateral L Intercostal and Bronchial Arteries M Spinal Arteries N Upper Arteries, Other P Thoraco-Abdominal Aorta Q Cervico-Cerebral Arch R Intracranial Arteries S Pulmonary Artery, Right T Pulmonary Artery, Left U Pulmonary Trunk	Ø High Osmolar 1 Low Osmolar Y Other Contrast	1 Laser	Ø Intraoperative
Ø Thoracic Aorta 1 Brachiocephalic-Subclavian Artery, Right 2 Subclavian Artery, Left 3 Common Carotid Artery, Right 4 Common Carotid Artery, Left 5 Common Carotid Arteries, Bilateral 6 Internal Carotid Artery, Right 7 Internal Carotid Artery, Left 8 Internal Carotid Arteries, Bilateral 9 External Carotid Artery, Right B External Carotid Artery, Left C External Carotid Arteries, Bilateral D Vertebral Artery, Right F Vertebral Artery, Left G Vertebral Arteries, Bilateral H Upper Extremity Arteries, Right J Upper Extremity Arteries, Left K Upper Extremity Arteries, Bilateral L Intercostal and Bronchial Arteries M Spinal Arteries N Upper Arteries, Other P Thoraco-Abdominal Aorta Q Cervico-Cerebral Arch R Intracranial Arteries S Pulmonary Artery, Right T Pulmonary Artery, Left U Pulmonary Trunk	Ø High Osmolar 1 Low Osmolar Y Other Contrast	Z None	Z None

B31 Continued on next page

B31 Continued

B Imaging
3 Upper Arteries
1 Fluoroscopy Definition: Single plane or bi-plane real time display of an image developed from the capture of external ionizing radiation on a fluorescent screen. The image may also be stored by either digital or analog means.

Body Part Character 4	Contrast Character 5	Qualifier Character 6	Qualifier Character 7
Ø Thoracic Aorta 1 Brachiocephalic-Subclavian Artery, Right 2 Subclavian Artery, Left 3 Common Carotid Artery, Right 4 Common Carotid Artery, Left 5 Common Carotid Arteries, Bilateral 6 Internal Carotid Artery, Right 7 Internal Carotid Artery, Left 8 Internal Carotid Arteries, Bilateral 9 External Carotid Artery, Right B External Carotid Artery, Left C External Carotid Arteries, Bilateral D Vertebral Artery, Right F Vertebral Artery, Left G Vertebral Arteries, Bilateral H Upper Extremity Arteries, Right J Upper Extremity Arteries, Left K Upper Extremity Arteries, Bilateral L Intercostal and Bronchial Arteries M Spinal Arteries N Upper Arteries, Other P Thoraco-Abdominal Aorta Q Cervico-Cerebral Arch R Intracranial Arteries S Pulmonary Artery, Right T Pulmonary Artery, Left U Pulmonary Trunk	Z None	Z None	Z None

B Imaging
3 Upper Arteries
2 Computerized Tomography (CT Scan) Definition: Computer reformatted digital display of multiplanar images developed from the capture of multiple exposures of external ionizing radiation

Body Part Character 4	Contrast Character 5	Qualifier Character 6	Qualifier Character 7
Ø Thoracic Aorta 5 Common Carotid Arteries, Bilateral 8 Internal Carotid Arteries, Bilateral G Vertebral Arteries, Bilateral R Intracranial Arteries S Pulmonary Artery, Right T Pulmonary Artery, Left	Ø High Osmolar 1 Low Osmolar Y Other Contrast	Z None	Z None
Ø Thoracic Aorta 5 Common Carotid Arteries, Bilateral 8 Internal Carotid Arteries, Bilateral G Vertebral Arteries, Bilateral R Intracranial Arteries S Pulmonary Artery, Right T Pulmonary Artery, Left	Z None	2 Intravascular Optical Coherence Z None	Z None

B Imaging
3 Upper Arteries
3 Magnetic Resonance Imaging (MRI) Definition: Computer reformatted digital display of multiplanar images developed from the capture of radio-frequency signals emitted by nuclei in a body site excited within a magnetic field

Body Part Character 4	Contrast Character 5	Qualifier Character 6	Qualifier Character 7
Ø Thoracic Aorta 5 Common Carotid Arteries, Bilateral 8 Internal Carotid Arteries, Bilateral G Vertebral Arteries, Bilateral H Upper Extremity Arteries, Right J Upper Extremity Arteries, Left K Upper Extremity Arteries, Bilateral M Spinal Arteries Q Cervico-Cerebral Arch R Intracranial Arteries	Y Other Contrast	Ø Unenhanced and Enhanced Z None	Z None
Ø Thoracic Aorta 5 Common Carotid Arteries, Bilateral 8 Internal Carotid Arteries, Bilateral G Vertebral Arteries, Bilateral H Upper Extremity Arteries, Right J Upper Extremity Arteries, Left K Upper Extremity Arteries, Bilateral M Spinal Arteries Q Cervico-Cerebral Arch R Intracranial Arteries	Z None	Z None	Z None

B Imaging
3 Upper Arteries
4 Ultrasonography Definition: Real time display of images of anatomy or flow information developed from the capture of relected and attenuated high frequency sound waves

Body Part Character 4	Contrast Character 5	Qualifier Character 6	Qualifier Character 7
Ø Thoracic Aorta 1 Brachiocephalic-Subclavian Artery, Right 2 Subclavian Artery, Left 3 Common Carotid Artery, Right 4 Common Carotid Artery, Left 5 Common Carotid Arteries, Bilateral 6 Internal Carotid Artery, Right 7 Internal Carotid Artery, Left 8 Internal Carotid Arteries, Bilateral H Upper Extremity Arteries, Right J Upper Extremity Arteries, Left K Upper Extremity Arteries, Bilateral R Intracranial Arteries S Pulmonary Artery, Right T Pulmonary Artery, Left V Ophthalmic Arteries	Z None	Z None	3 Intravascular Z None

B Imaging
4 Lower Arteries
Ø Plain Radiography Definition: Planar display of an image developed from the capture of external ionizing radiation on photographic or photoconductive plate

Body Part Character 4	Contrast Character 5	Qualifier Character 6	Qualifier Character 7
Ø Abdominal Aorta 2 Hepatic Artery 3 Splenic Arteries 4 Superior Mesenteric Artery 5 Inferior Mesenteric Artery 6 Renal Artery, Right 7 Renal Artery, Left 8 Renal Arteries, Bilateral 9 Lumbar Arteries B Intra-Abdominal Arteries, Other C Pelvic Arteries D Aorta and Bilateral Lower Extremity Arteries F Lower Extremity Arteries, Right G Lower Extremity Arteries, Left J Lower Arteries, Other M Renal Artery Transplant	Ø High Osmolar 1 Low Osmolar Y Other Contrast	Z None	Z None

B Imaging
4 Lower Arteries
1 Fluoroscopy Definition: Single plane or bi-plane real time display of an image developed from the capture of external ionizing radiation on a fluorescent screen. The image may also be stored by either digital or analog means.

Body Part Character 4	Contrast Character 5	Qualifier Character 6	Qualifier Character 7
Ø Abdominal Aorta 2 Hepatic Artery 3 Splenic Arteries 4 Superior Mesenteric Artery 5 Inferior Mesenteric Artery 6 Renal Artery, Right 7 Renal Artery, Left 8 Renal Arteries, Bilateral 9 Lumbar Arteries B Intra-Abdominal Arteries, Other C Pelvic Arteries D Aorta and Bilateral Lower Extremity Arteries F Lower Extremity Arteries, Right G Lower Extremity Arteries, Left J Lower Arteries, Other	Ø High Osmolar 1 Low Osmolar Y Other Contrast	1 Laser	Ø Intraoperative
Ø Abdominal Aorta 2 Hepatic Artery 3 Splenic Arteries 4 Superior Mesenteric Artery 5 Inferior Mesenteric Artery 6 Renal Artery, Right 7 Renal Artery, Left 8 Renal Arteries, Bilateral 9 Lumbar Arteries B Intra-Abdominal Arteries, Other C Pelvic Arteries D Aorta and Bilateral Lower Extremity Arteries F Lower Extremity Arteries, Right G Lower Extremity Arteries, Left J Lower Arteries, Other	Ø High Osmolar 1 Low Osmolar Y Other Contrast	Z None	Z None
Ø Abdominal Aorta 2 Hepatic Artery 3 Splenic Arteries 4 Superior Mesenteric Artery 5 Inferior Mesenteric Artery 6 Renal Artery, Right 7 Renal Artery, Left 8 Renal Arteries, Bilateral 9 Lumbar Arteries B Intra-Abdominal Arteries, Other C Pelvic Arteries D Aorta and Bilateral Lower Extremity Arteries F Lower Extremity Arteries, Right G Lower Extremity Arteries, Left J Lower Arteries, Other	Z None	Z None	Z None

B Imaging
4 Lower Arteries
2 Computerized Tomography (CT Scan) Definition: Computer reformatted digital display of multiplanar images developed from the capture of multiple exposures of external ionizing radiation

Body Part Character 4	Contrast Character 5	Qualifier Character 6	Qualifier Character 7
Ø Abdominal Aorta 1 Celiac Artery 4 Superior Mesenteric Artery 8 Renal Arteries, Bilateral C Pelvic Arteries F Lower Extremity Arteries, Right G Lower Extremity Arteries, Left H Lower Extremity Arteries, Bilateral M Renal Artery Transplant	Ø High Osmolar 1 Low Osmolar Y Other Contrast	Z None	Z None
Ø Abdominal Aorta 1 Celiac Artery 4 Superior Mesenteric Artery 8 Renal Arteries, Bilateral C Pelvic Arteries F Lower Extremity Arteries, Right G Lower Extremity Arteries, Left H Lower Extremity Arteries, Bilateral M Renal Artery Transplant	Z None	2 Intravascular Optical Coherence Z None	Z None

B Imaging
4 Lower Arteries
3 Magnetic Resonance Imaging (MRI) Definition: Computer reformatted digital display of multiplanar images developed from the capture of radio-frequency signals emitted by nuclei in a body site excited within a magnetic field

Body Part Character 4	Contrast Character 5	Qualifier Character 6	Qualifier Character 7
Ø Abdominal Aorta 1 Celiac Artery 4 Superior Mesenteric Artery 8 Renal Arteries, Bilateral C Pelvic Arteries F Lower Extremity Arteries, Right G Lower Extremity Arteries, Left H Lower Extremity Arteries, Bilateral	Y Other Contrast	Ø Unenhanced and Enhanced Z None	Z None
Ø Abdominal Aorta 1 Celiac Artery 4 Superior Mesenteric Artery 8 Renal Arteries, Bilateral C Pelvic Arteries F Lower Extremity Arteries, Right G Lower Extremity Arteries, Left H Lower Extremity Arteries, Bilateral	Z None	Z None	Z None

B Imaging
4 Lower Arteries
4 Ultrasonography Definition: Real time display of images of anatomy or flow information developed from the capture of relected and attenuated high frequency sound waves

Body Part Character 4	Contrast Character 5	Qualifier Character 6	Qualifier Character 7
Ø Abdominal Aorta 4 Superior Mesenteric Artery 5 Inferior Mesenteric Artery 6 Renal Artery, Right 7 Renal Artery, Left 8 Renal Arteries, Bilateral B Intra-Abdominal Arteries, Other F Lower Extremity Arteries, Right G Lower Extremity Arteries, Left H Lower Extremity Arteries, Bilateral K Celiac and Mesenteric Arteries L Femoral Artery N Penile Arteries	Z None	Z None	3 Intravascular Z None

B Imaging
5 Veins
Ø Plain Radiography Definition: Planar display of an image developed from the capture of external ionizing radiation on photographic or photoconductive plate

Body Part Character 4	Contrast Character 5	Qualifier Character 6	Qualifier Character 7
Ø Epidural Veins 1 Cerebral and Cerebellar Veins 2 Intracranial Sinuses 3 Jugular Veins, Right 4 Jugular Veins, Left 5 Jugular Veins, Bilateral 6 Subclavian Vein, Right 7 Subclavian Vein, Left 8 Superior Vena Cava 9 Inferior Vena Cava B Lower Extremity Veins, Right C Lower Extremity Veins, Left D Lower Extremity Veins, Bilateral F Pelvic (Iliac) Veins, Right G Pelvic (Iliac) Veins, Left H Pelvic (Iliac) Veins, Bilateral J Renal Vein, Right K Renal Vein, Left L Renal Veins, Bilateral M Upper Extremity Veins, Right N Upper Extremity Veins, Left P Upper Extremity Veins, Bilateral Q Pulmonary Vein, Right R Pulmonary Vein, Left S Pulmonary Veins, Bilateral T Portal and Splanchnic Veins V Veins, Other W Dialysis Shunt/Fistula	Ø High Osmolar 1 Low Osmolar Y Other Contrast	Z None	Z None

B Imaging
5 Veins
1 Fluoroscopy Definition: Single plane or bi-plane real time display of an image developed from the capture of external ionizing radioation on a fluorescent screen. The image may also be stored by either digital or analog means.

Body Part Character 4	Contrast Character 5	Qualifier Character 6	Qualifier Character 7
Ø Epidural Veins 1 Cerebral and Cerebellar Veins 2 Intracranial Sinuses 3 Jugular Veins, Right 4 Jugular Veins, Left 5 Jugular Veins, Bilateral 6 Subclavian Vein, Right 7 Subclavian Vein, Left 8 Superior Vena Cava 9 Inferior Vena Cava B Lower Extremity Veins, Right C Lower Extremity Veins, Left D Lower Extremity Veins, Bilateral F Pelvic (Iliac) Veins, Right G Pelvic (Iliac) Veins, Left H Pelvic (Iliac) Veins, Bilateral J Renal Vein, Right K Renal Vein, Left L Renal Veins, Bilateral M Upper Extremity Veins, Right N Upper Extremity Veins, Left P Upper Extremity Veins, Bilateral Q Pulmonary Vein, Right R Pulmonary Vein, Left S Pulmonary Veins, Bilateral T Portal and Splanchnic Veins V Veins, Other W Dialysis Shunt/Fistula	Ø High Osmolar 1 Low Osmolar Y Other Contrast Z None	Z None	A Guidance Z None

B Imaging
5 Veins
2 Computerized Tomography (CT Scan) Definition: Computer reformatted digital display of multiplanar images developed from the capture of multiple exposures of external ionizing radiation

Body Part Character 4	Contrast Character 5	Qualifier Character 6	Qualifier Character 7
2 Intracranial Sinuses 8 Superior Vena Cava 9 Inferior Vena Cava F Pelvic (Iliac) Veins, Right G Pelvic (Iliac) Veins, Left H Pelvic (Iliac) Veins, Bilateral J Renal Vein, Right K Renal Vein, Left L Renal Veins, Bilateral Q Pulmonary Vein, Right R Pulmonary Vein, Left S Pulmonary Veins, Bilateral T Portal and Splanchnic Veins	Ø High Osmolar 1 Low Osmolar Y Other Contrast	Ø Unenhanced and Enhanced Z None	Z None
2 Intracranial Sinuses 8 Superior Vena Cava 9 Inferior Vena Cava F Pelvic (Iliac) Veins, Right G Pelvic (Iliac) Veins, Left H Pelvic (Iliac) Veins, Bilateral J Renal Vein, Right K Renal Vein, Left L Renal Veins, Bilateral Q Pulmonary Vein, Right R Pulmonary Vein, Left S Pulmonary Veins, Bilateral T Portal and Splanchnic Veins	Z None	2 Intravascular Optical Coherence Z None	Z None

B Imaging
5 Veins
3 Magnetic Resonance Imaging (MRI) Definition: Computer reformatted digital display of multiplanar images developed from the capture of radio-frequency signals emitted by nuclei in a body site excited within a magnetic field

Body Part Character 4	Contrast Character 5	Qualifier Character 6	Qualifier Character 7
1 Cerebral and Cerebellar Veins 2 Intracranial Sinuses 5 Jugular Veins, Bilateral 8 Superior Vena Cava 9 Inferior Vena Cava B Lower Extremity Veins, Right C Lower Extremity Veins, Left D Lower Extremity Veins, Bilateral H Pelvic (Iliac) Veins, Bilateral L Renal Veins, Bilateral M Upper Extremity Veins, Right N Upper Extremity Veins, Left P Upper Extremity Veins, Bilateral S Pulmonary Veins, Bilateral T Portal and Splanchnic Veins V Veins, Other	Y Other Contrast	Ø Unenhanced and Enhanced Z None	Z None
1 Cerebral and Cerebellar Veins 2 Intracranial Sinuses 5 Jugular Veins, Bilateral 8 Superior Vena Cava 9 Inferior Vena Cava B Lower Extremity Veins, Right C Lower Extremity Veins, Left D Lower Extremity Veins, Bilateral H Pelvic (Iliac) Veins, Bilateral L Renal Veins, Bilateral M Upper Extremity Veins, Right N Upper Extremity Veins, Left P Upper Extremity Veins, Bilateral S Pulmonary Veins, Bilateral T Portal and Splanchnic Veins V Veins, Other	Z None	Z None	Z None

B Imaging
5 Veins
4 Ultrasonography Definition: Real time display of images of anatomy or flow information developed from the capture of relected and attenuated high frequency sound waves

Body Part Character 4	Contrast Character 5	Qualifier Character 6	Qualifier Character 7
3 Jugular Veins, Right **4** Jugular Veins, Left **6** Subclavian Vein, Right **7** Subclavian Vein, Left **8** Superior Vena Cava **9** Inferior Vena Cava **B** Lower Extremity Veins, Right **C** Lower Extremity Veins, Left **D** Lower Extremity Veins, Bilateral **J** Renal Vein, Right **K** Renal Vein, Left **L** Renal Veins, Bilateral **M** Upper Extremity Veins, Right **N** Upper Extremity Veins, Left **P** Upper Extremity Veins, Bilateral **T** Portal and Splanchnic Veins	**Z** None	**Z** None	**3** Intravascular **A** Guidance **Z** None

B Imaging
7 Lymphatic System
Ø Plain Radiography Definition: Planar display of an image developed from the capture of external ionizing radiation on photographic or photoconductive plate

Body Part Character 4	Contrast Character 5	Qualifier Character 6	Qualifier Character 7
Ø Abdominal/Retroperitoneal Lymphatics, Unilateral **1** Abdominal/Retroperitoneal Lymphatics, Bilateral **4** Lymphatics, Head and Neck **5** Upper Extremity Lymphatics, Right **6** Upper Extremity Lymphatics, Left **7** Upper Extremity Lymphatics, Bilateral **8** Lower Extremity Lymphatics, Right **9** Lower Extremity Lymphatics, Left **B** Lower Extremity Lymphatics, Bilateral **C** Lymphatics, Pelvic	**Ø** High Osmolar **1** Low Osmolar **Y** Other Contrast	**Z** None	**Z** None

B Imaging
8 Eye
Ø Plain Radiography Definition: Planar display of an image developed from the capture of external ionizing radiation on photographic or photoconductive plate

Body Part Character 4	Contrast Character 5	Qualifier Character 6	Qualifier Character 7
Ø Lacrimal Duct, Right **1** Lacrimal Duct, Left **2** Lacrimal Ducts, Bilateral	**Ø** High Osmolar **1** Low Osmolar **Y** Other Contrast	**Z** None	**Z** None
3 Optic Foramina, Right **4** Optic Foramina, Left **5** Eye, Right **6** Eye, Left **7** Eyes, Bilateral	**Z** None	**Z** None	**Z** None

B Imaging
8 Eye
2 Computerized Tomography (CT Scan) Definition: Computer reformatted digital display of multiplanar images developed from the capture of multiple exposures of external ionizing radiation

Body Part Character 4	Contrast Character 5	Qualifier Character 6	Qualifier Character 7
5 Eye, Right **6** Eye, Left **7** Eyes, Bilateral	**Ø** High Osmolar **1** Low Osmolar **Y** Other Contrast	**Ø** Unenhanced and Enhanced **Z** None	**Z** None
5 Eye, Right **6** Eye, Left **7** Eyes, Bilateral	**Z** None	**Z** None	**Z** None

B Imaging
8 Eye
3 Magnetic Resonance Imaging (MRI) Definition: Computer reformatted digital display of multiplanar images developed from the capture of radio-frequency signals emitted by nuclei in a body site excited within a magnetic field

Body Part Character 4	Contrast Character 5	Qualifier Character 6	Qualifier Character 7
5 Eye, Right 6 Eye, Left 7 Eyes, Bilateral	Y Other Contrast	Ø Unenhanced and Enhanced Z None	Z None
5 Eye, Right 6 Eye, Left 7 Eyes, Bilateral	Z None	Z None	Z None

B Imaging
8 Eye
4 Ultrasonography Definition: Real time display of images of anatomy or flow information developed from the capture of relected and attenuated high frequency sound waves

Body Part Character 4	Contrast Character 5	Qualifier Character 6	Qualifier Character 7
5 Eye, Right 6 Eye, Left 7 Eyes, Bilateral	Z None	Z None	Z None

B Imaging
9 Ear, Nose, Mouth and Throat
Ø Plain Radiography Definition: Planar display of an image developed from the capture of external ionizing radiation on photographic or photoconductive plate

Body Part Character 4	Contrast Character 5	Qualifier Character 6	Qualifier Character 7
2 Paranasal Sinuses F Nasopharynx/Oropharynx H Mastoids	Z None	Z None	Z None
4 Parotid Gland, Right 5 Parotid Gland, Left 6 Parotid Glands, Bilateral 7 Submandibular Gland, Right 8 Submandibular Gland, Left 9 Submandibular Glands, Bilateral B Salivary Gland, Right C Salivary Gland, Left D Salivary Glands, Bilateral	Ø High Osmolar 1 Low Osmolar Y Other Contrast	Z None	Z None

B Imaging
9 Ear, Nose, Mouth and Throat
1 Fluoroscopy Definition: Single plane or bi-plane real time display of an image developed from the capture of external ionizing radioation on a fluorescent screen. The image may also be stored by either digital or analog means.

Body Part Character 4	Contrast Character 5	Qualifier Character 6	Qualifier Character 7
G Pharynx and Epiglottis J Larynx	Y Other Contrast Z None	Z None	Z None

B Imaging
9 Ear, Nose, Mouth and Throat
2 Computerized Tomography (CT Scan) Definition: Computer reformatted digital display of multiplanar images developed from the capture of multiple exposures of external ionizing radiation

Body Part Character 4	Contrast Character 5	Qualifier Character 6	Qualifier Character 7
Ø Ear 2 Paranasal Sinuses 6 Parotid Glands, Bilateral 9 Submandibular Glands, Bilateral D Salivary Glands, Bilateral F Nasopharynx/Oropharynx J Larynx	Ø High Osmolar 1 Low Osmolar Y Other Contrast	Ø Unenhanced and Enhanced Z None	Z None
Ø Ear 2 Paranasal Sinuses 6 Parotid Glands, Bilateral 9 Submandibular Glands, Bilateral D Salivary Glands, Bilateral F Nasopharynx/Oropharynx J Larynx	Z None	Z None	Z None

B Imaging
9 Ear, Nose, Mouth and Throat
3 Magnetic Resonance Imaging (MRI) Definition: Computer reformatted digital display of multiplanar images developed from the capture of radio-frequency signals emitted by nuclei in a body site excited within a magnetic field

Body Part Character 4	Contrast Character 5	Qualifier Character 6	Qualifier Character 7
Ø Ear 2 Paranasal Sinuses 6 Parotid Glands, Bilateral 9 Submandibular Glands, Bilateral D Salivary Glands, Bilateral F Nasopharynx/Oropharynx J Larynx	Y Other Contrast	Ø Unenhanced and Enhanced Z None	Z None
Ø Ear 2 Paranasal Sinuses 6 Parotid Glands, Bilateral 9 Submandibular Glands, Bilateral D Salivary Glands, Bilateral F Nasopharynx/Oropharynx J Larynx	Z None	Z None	Z None

B Imaging
B Respiratory System
Ø Plain Radiography Definition: Planar display of an image developed from the capture of external ionizing radiation on photographic or photoconductive plate

Body Part Character 4	Contrast Character 5	Qualifier Character 6	Qualifier Character 7
7 Tracheobronchial Tree, Right 8 Tracheobronchial Tree, Left 9 Tracheobronchial Trees, Bilateral	Y Other Contrast	Z None	Z None
D Upper Airways	Z None	Z None	Z None

B Imaging
B Respiratory System
1 Fluoroscopy Definition: Single plane or bi-plane real time display of an image developed from the capture of external ionizing radioation on a fluorescent screen. The image may also be stored by either digital or analog means.

Body Part Character 4	Contrast Character 5	Qualifier Character 6	Qualifier Character 7
2 Lung, Right 3 Lung, Left 4 Lungs, Bilateral 6 Diaphragm C Mediastinum D Upper Airways	Z None	Z None	Z None
7 Tracheobronchial Tree, Right 8 Tracheobronchial Tree, Left 9 Tracheobronchial Trees, Bilateral	Y Other Contrast	Z None	Z None

B Imaging
B Respiratory System
2 Computerized Tomography (CT Scan) Definition: Computer reformatted digital display of multiplanar images developed from the capture of multiple exposures of external ionizing radiation

Body Part Character 4	Contrast Character 5	Qualifier Character 6	Qualifier Character 7
4 Lungs, Bilateral 7 Tracheobronchial Tree, Right 8 Tracheobronchial Tree, Left 9 Tracheobronchial Trees, Bilateral F Trachea/Airways	Ø High Osmolar 1 Low Osmolar Y Other Contrast	Ø Unenhanced and Enhanced Z None	Z None
4 Lungs, Bilateral 7 Tracheobronchial Tree, Right 8 Tracheobronchial Tree, Left 9 Tracheobronchial Trees, Bilateral F Trachea/Airways	Z None	Z None	Z None

B Imaging
B Respiratory System
3 Magnetic Resonance Imaging (MRI) Definition: Computer reformatted digital display of multiplanar images developed from the capture of radio-frequency signals emitted by nuclei in a body site excited within a magnetic field

Body Part Character 4	Contrast Character 5	Qualifier Character 6	Qualifier Character 7
G Lung Apices	Y Other Contrast	Ø Unenhanced and Enhanced Z None	Z None
G Lung Apices	Z None	Z None	Z None

B Imaging
B Respiratory System
4 Ultrasonography Definition: Real time display of images of anatomy or flow information developed from the capture of relected and attenuated high frequency sound waves

Body Part Character 4	Contrast Character 5	Qualifier Character 6	Qualifier Character 7
B Pleura C Mediastinum	Z None	Z None	Z None

B Imaging
D Gastrointestinal System
1 Fluoroscopy Definition: Single plane or bi-plane real time display of an image developed from the capture of external ionizing radioation on a fluorescent screen. The image may also be stored by either digital or analog means.

Body Part Character 4	Contrast Character 5	Qualifier Character 6	Qualifier Character 7
1 Esophagus 2 Stomach 3 Small Bowel 4 Colon 5 Upper GI 6 Upper GI and Small Bowel 9 Duodenum B Mouth/Oropharynx	Y Other Contrast Z None	Z None	Z None

B Imaging
D Gastrointestinal System
2 Computerized Tomography (CT Scan) Definition: Computer reformatted digital display of multiplanar images developed from the capture of multiple exposures of external ionizing radiation

Body Part Character 4	Contrast Character 5	Qualifier Character 6	Qualifier Character 7
4 Colon	Ø High Osmolar 1 Low Osmolar Y Other Contrast	Ø Unenhanced and Enhanced Z None	Z None
4 Colon	Z None	Z None	Z None

B Imaging
D Gastrointestinal System
4 Ultrasonography Definition: Real time display of images of anatomy or flow information developed from the capture of relected and attenuated high frequency sound waves

Body Part Character 4	Contrast Character 5	Qualifier Character 6	Qualifier Character 7
1 Esophagus 2 Stomach 7 Gastrointestinal Tract 8 Appendix 9 Duodenum C Rectum	Z None	Z None	Z None

B Imaging
F Hepatobiliary System and Pancreas
Ø Plain Radiography Definition: Planar display of an image developed from the capture of external ionizing radiation on photographic or photoconductive plate

Body Part Character 4	Contrast Character 5	Qualifier Character 6	Qualifier Character 7
Ø Bile Ducts 3 Gallbladder and Bile Ducts C Hepatobiliary System, All	Ø High Osmolar 1 Low Osmolar Y Other Contrast	Z None	Z None

B Imaging
F Hepatobiliary System and Pancreas
1 Fluoroscopy Definition: Single plane or bi-plane real time display of an image developed from the capture of external ionizing radioation on a fluorescent screen. The image may also be stored by either digital or analog means.

Body Part Character 4	Contrast Character 5	Qualifier Character 6	Qualifier Character 7
Ø Bile Ducts 1 Biliary and Pancreatic Ducts 2 Gallbladder 3 Gallbladder and Bile Ducts 4 Gallbladder, Bile Ducts and Pancreatic Ducts 8 Pancreatic Ducts	Ø High Osmolar 1 Low Osmolar Y Other Contrast	Z None	Z None

B Imaging
F Hepatobiliary System and Pancreas
2 Computerized Tomography (CT Scan) Definition: Computer reformatted digital display of multiplanar images developed from the capture of multiple exposures of external ionizing radiation

Body Part Character 4	Contrast Character 5	Qualifier Character 6	Qualifier Character 7
5 Liver 6 Liver and Spleen 7 Pancreas C Hepatobiliary System, All	Ø High Osmolar 1 Low Osmolar Y Other Contrast	Ø Unenhanced and Enhanced Z None	Z None
5 Liver 6 Liver and Spleen 7 Pancreas C Hepatobiliary System, All	Z None	Z None	Z None

B Imaging
F Hepatobiliary System and Pancreas
3 Magnetic Resonance Imaging (MRI) Definition: Computer reformatted digital display of multiplanar images developed from the capture of radio-frequency signals emitted by nuclei in a body site excited within a magnetic field

Body Part Character 4	Contrast Character 5	Qualifier Character 6	Qualifier Character 7
5 Liver 6 Liver and Spleen 7 Pancreas	Y Other Contrast	Ø Unenhanced and Enhanced Z None	Z None
5 Liver 6 Liver and Spleen 7 Pancreas	Z None	Z None	Z None

B Imaging
F Hepatobiliary System and Pancreas
4 Ultrasonography Definition: Real time display of images of anatomy or flow information developed from the capture of relected and attenuated high frequency sound waves

Body Part Character 4	Contrast Character 5	Qualifier Character 6	Qualifier Character 7
Ø Bile Ducts 2 Gallbladder 3 Gallbladder and Bile Ducts 5 Liver 6 Liver and Spleen 7 Pancreas C Hepatobiliary System, All	Z None	Z None	Z None

B Imaging
F Hepatobiliary System and Pancreas
5 Other Imaging Definition: Other specified modality for visualizing a body part

Body Part Character 4	Contrast Character 5	Qualifier Character 6	Qualifier Character 7
Ø Bile Ducts 2 Gallbladder 3 Gallbladder and Bile Ducts 5 Liver 6 Liver and Spleen 7 Pancreas C Hepatobiliary System, All	2 Fluorescing Agent	Ø Indocyanine Green Dye Z None	Ø Intraoperative Z None

B Imaging
G Endocrine System
2 Computerized Tomography (CT Scan) Definition: Computer reformatted digital display of multiplanar images developed from the capture of multiple exposures of external ionizing radiation

Body Part Character 4	Contrast Character 5	Qualifier Character 6	Qualifier Character 7
2 Adrenal Glands, Bilateral 3 Parathyroid Glands 4 Thyroid Gland	Ø High Osmolar 1 Low Osmolar Y Other Contrast	Ø Unenhanced and Enhanced Z None	Z None
2 Adrenal Glands, Bilateral 3 Parathyroid Glands 4 Thyroid Gland	Z None	Z None	Z None

B Imaging
G Endocrine System
3 Magnetic Resonance Imaging (MRI) Definition: Computer reformatted digital display of multiplanar images developed from the capture of radio-frequency signals emitted by nuclei in a body site excited within a magnetic field

Body Part Character 4	Contrast Character 5	Qualifier Character 6	Qualifier Character 7
2 Adrenal Glands, Bilateral 3 Parathyroid Glands 4 Thyroid Gland	Y Other Contrast	Ø Unenhanced and Enhanced Z None	Z None
2 Adrenal Glands, Bilateral 3 Parathyroid Glands 4 Thyroid Gland	Z None	Z None	Z None

B Imaging
G Endocrine System
4 Ultrasonography Definition: Real time display of images of anatomy or flow information developed from the capture of relected and attenuated high frequency sound waves

Body Part Character 4	Contrast Character 5	Qualifier Character 6	Qualifier Character 7
Ø Adrenal Gland, Right 1 Adrenal Gland, Left 2 Adrenal Glands, Bilateral 3 Parathyroid Glands 4 Thyroid Gland	Z None	Z None	Z None

B Imaging
H Skin, Subcutaneous Tissue and Breast
Ø Plain Radiography Definition: Planar display of an image developed from the capture of external ionizing radiation on photographic or photoconductive plate

Body Part Character 4	Contrast Character 5	Qualifier Character 6	Qualifier Character 7
Ø Breast, Right 1 Breast, Left 2 Breasts, Bilateral	Z None	Z None	Z None
3 Single Mammary Duct, Right 4 Single Mammary Duct, Left 5 Multiple Mammary Ducts, Right 6 Multiple Mammary Ducts, Left	Ø High Osmolar 1 Low Osmolar Y Other Contrast Z None	Z None	Z None

B Imaging
H Skin, Subcutaneous Tissue and Breast
3 Magnetic Resonance Imaging (MRI) Definition: Computer reformatted digital display of multiplanar images developed from the capture of radio-frequency signals emitted by nuclei in a body site excited within a magnetic field

Body Part Character 4	Contrast Character 5	Qualifier Character 6	Qualifier Character 7
Ø Breast, Right 1 Breast, Left 2 Breasts, Bilateral D Subcutaneous Tissue, Head/Neck F Subcutaneous Tissue, Upper Extremity G Subcutaneous Tissue, Thorax H Subcutaneous Tissue, Abdomen and Pelvis J Subcutaneous Tissue, Lower Extremity	Y Other Contrast	Ø Unenhanced and Enhanced Z None	Z None
Ø Breast, Right 1 Breast, Left 2 Breasts, Bilateral D Subcutaneous Tissue, Head/Neck F Subcutaneous Tissue, Upper Extremity G Subcutaneous Tissue, Thorax H Subcutaneous Tissue, Abdomen and Pelvis J Subcutaneous Tissue, Lower Extremity	Z None	Z None	Z None

B Imaging
H Skin, Subcutaneous Tissue and Breast
4 Ultrasonography Definition: Real time display of images of anatomy or flow information developed from the capture of relected and attenuated high frequency sound waves

Body Part Character 4	Contrast Character 5	Qualifier Character 6	Qualifier Character 7
Ø Breast, Right 1 Breast, Left 2 Breasts, Bilateral 7 Extremity, Upper 8 Extremity, Lower 9 Abdominal Wall B Chest Wall C Head and Neck	Z None	Z None	Z None

B Imaging
L Connective Tissue
3 Magnetic Resonance Imaging (MRI) Definition: Computer reformatted digital display of multiplanar images developed from the capture of radio-frequency signals emitted by nuclei in a body site excited within a magnetic field

Body Part Character 4	Contrast Character 5	Qualifier Character 6	Qualifier Character 7
Ø Connective Tissue, Upper Extremity 1 Connective Tissue, Lower Extremity 2 Tendons, Upper Extremity 3 Tendons, Lower Extremity	Y Other Contrast	Ø Unenhanced and Enhanced Z None	Z None
Ø Connective Tissue, Upper Extremity 1 Connective Tissue, Lower Extremity 2 Tendons, Upper Extremity 3 Tendons, Lower Extremity	Z None	Z None	Z None

B Imaging
L Connective Tissue
4 Ultrasonography Definition: Real time display of images of anatomy or flow information developed from the capture of relected and attenuated high frequency sound waves

Body Part Character 4	Contrast Character 5	Qualifier Character 6	Qualifier Character 7
Ø Connective Tissue, Upper Extremity 1 Connective Tissue, Lower Extremity 2 Tendons, Upper Extremity 3 Tendons, Lower Extremity	Z None	Z None	Z None

B Imaging
N Skull and Facial Bones
Ø Plain Radiography **Definition:** Planar display of an image developed from the capture of external ionizing radiation on photographic or photoconductive plate

Body Part Character 4	Contrast Character 5	Qualifier Character 6	Qualifier Character 7
Ø Skull 1 Orbit, Right 2 Orbit, Left 3 Orbits, Bilateral 4 Nasal Bones 5 Facial Bones 6 Mandible B Zygomatic Arch, Right C Zygomatic Arch, Left D Zygomatic Arches, Bilateral G Tooth, Single H Teeth, Multiple J Teeth, All	Z None	Z None	Z None
7 Temporomandibular Joint, Right 8 Temporomandibular Joint, Left 9 Temporomandibular Joints, Bilateral	Ø High Osmolar 1 Low Osmolar Y Other Contrast Z None	Z None	Z None

B Imaging
N Skull and Facial Bones
1 Fluoroscopy **Definition:** Single plane or bi-plane real time display of an image developed from the capture of external ionizing radioation on a fluorescent screen. The image may also be stored by either digital or analog means.

Body Part Character 4	Contrast Character 5	Qualifier Character 6	Qualifier Character 7
7 Temporomandibular Joint, Right 8 Temporomandibular Joint, Left 9 Temporomandibular Joints, Bilateral	Ø High Osmolar 1 Low Osmolar Y Other Contrast Z None	Z None	Z None

B Imaging
N Skull and Facial Bones
2 Computerized Tomography (CT Scan) **Definition:** Computer reformatted digital display of multiplanar images developed from the capture of multiple exposures of external ionizing radiation

Body Part Character 4	Contrast Character 5	Qualifier Character 6	Qualifier Character 7
Ø Skull 3 Orbits, Bilateral 5 Facial Bones 6 Mandible 9 Temporomandibular Joints, Bilateral F Temporal Bones	Ø High Osmolar 1 Low Osmolar Y Other Contrast Z None	Z None	Z None

B Imaging
N Skull and Facial Bones
3 Magnetic Resonance Imaging (MRI) **Definition:** Computer reformatted digital display of multiplanar images developed from the capture of radio-frequency signals emitted by nuclei in a body site excited within a magnetic field

Body Part Character 4	Contrast Character 5	Qualifier Character 6	Qualifier Character 7
9 Temporomandibular Joints, Bilateral	Y Other Contrast Z None	Z None	Z None

B Imaging
P Non-Axial Upper Bones
Ø Plain Radiography Definition: Planar display of an image developed from the capture of external ionizing radiation on photographic or photoconductive plate

Body Part Character 4	Contrast Character 5	Qualifier Character 6	Qualifier Character 7
Ø Sternoclavicular Joint, Right 1 Sternoclavicular Joint, Left 2 Sternoclavicular Joints, Bilateral 3 Acromioclavicular Joints, Bilateral 4 Clavicle, Right 5 Clavicle, Left 6 Scapula, Right 7 Scapula, Left A Humerus, Right B Humerus, Left E Upper Arm, Right F Upper Arm, Left J Forearm, Right K Forearm, Left N Hand, Right P Hand, Left R Finger(s), Right S Finger(s), Left X Ribs, Right Y Ribs, Left	Z None	Z None	Z None
8 Shoulder, Right 9 Shoulder, Left C Hand/Finger Joint, Right D Hand/Finger Joint, Left G Elbow, Right H Elbow, Left L Wrist, Right M Wrist, Left	Ø High Osmolar 1 Low Osmolar Y Other Contrast Z None	Z None	Z None

B Imaging
P Non-Axial Upper Bones
1 Fluoroscopy Definition: Single plane or bi-plane real time display of an image developed from the capture of external ionizing radioation on a fluorescent screen. The image may also be stored by either digital or analog means.

Body Part Character 4	Contrast Character 5	Qualifier Character 6	Qualifier Character 7
Ø Sternoclavicular Joint, Right 1 Sternoclavicular Joint, Left 2 Sternoclavicular Joints, Bilateral 3 Acromioclavicular Joints, Bilateral 4 Clavicle, Right 5 Clavicle, Left 6 Scapula, Right 7 Scapula, Left A Humerus, Right B Humerus, Left E Upper Arm, Right F Upper Arm, Left J Forearm, Right K Forearm, Left N Hand, Right P Hand, Left R Finger(s), Right S Finger(s), Left X Ribs, Right Y Ribs, Left	Z None	Z None	Z None
8 Shoulder, Right 9 Shoulder, Left L Wrist, Right M Wrist, Left	Ø High Osmolar 1 Low Osmolar Y Other Contrast Z None	Z None	Z None
C Hand/Finger Joint, Right D Hand/Finger Joint, Left G Elbow, Right H Elbow, Left	Ø High Osmolar 1 Low Osmolar Y Other Contrast	Z None	Z None

B Imaging
P Non-Axial Upper Bones
2 Computerized Tomography (CT Scan) Definition: Computer reformatted digital display of multiplanar images developed from the capture of multiple exposures of external ionizing radiation

Body Part Character 4	Contrast Character 5	Qualifier Character 6	Qualifier Character 7
Ø Sternoclavicular Joint, Right 1 Sternoclavicular Joint, Left W Thorax	Ø High Osmolar 1 Low Osmolar Y Other Contrast	Z None	Z None
2 Sternoclavicular Joints, Bilateral 3 Acromioclavicular Joints, Bilateral 4 Clavicle, Right 5 Clavicle, Left 6 Scapula, Right 7 Scapula, Left 8 Shoulder, Right 9 Shoulder, Left A Humerus, Right B Humerus, Left E Upper Arm, Right F Upper Arm, Left G Elbow, Right H Elbow, Left J Forearm, Right K Forearm, Left L Wrist, Right M Wrist, Left N Hand, Right P Hand, Left Q Hands and Wrists, Bilateral R Finger(s), Right S Finger(s), Left T Upper Extremity, Right U Upper Extremity, Left V Upper Extremities, Bilateral X Ribs, Right Y Ribs, Left	Ø High Osmolar 1 Low Osmolar Y Other Contrast Z None	Z None	Z None
C Hand/Finger Joint, Right D Hand/Finger Joint, Left	Z None	Z None	Z None

B Imaging
P Non-Axial Upper Bones
3 Magnetic Resonance Imaging (MRI) Definition: Computer reformatted digital display of multiplanar images developed from the capture of radio-frequency signals emitted by nuclei in a body site excited within a magnetic field

Body Part Character 4	Contrast Character 5	Qualifier Character 6	Qualifier Character 7
8 Shoulder, Right 9 Shoulder, Left C Hand/Finger Joint, Right D Hand/Finger Joint, Left E Upper Arm, Right F Upper Arm, Left G Elbow, Right H Elbow, Left J Forearm, Right K Forearm, Left L Wrist, Right M Wrist, Left	Y Other Contrast	Ø Unenhanced and Enhanced Z None	Z None
8 Shoulder, Right 9 Shoulder, Left C Hand/Finger Joint, Right D Hand/Finger Joint, Left E Upper Arm, Right F Upper Arm, Left G Elbow, Right H Elbow, Left J Forearm, Right K Forearm, Left L Wrist, Right M Wrist, Left	Z None	Z None	Z None

B Imaging
P Non-Axial Upper Bones
4 Ultrasonography Definition: Real time display of images of anatomy or flow information developed from the capture of relected and attenuated high frequency sound waves

Body Part Character 4	Contrast Character 5	Qualifier Character 6	Qualifier Character 7
8 Shoulder, Right 9 Shoulder, Left G Elbow, Right H Elbow, Left L Wrist, Right M Wrist, Left N Hand, Right P Hand, Left	Z None	Z None	1 Densitometry Z None

B Imaging
Q Non-Axial Lower Bones
Ø Plain Radiography Definition: Planar display of an image developed from the capture of external ionizing radiation on photographic or photoconductive plate

Body Part Character 4	Contrast Character 5	Qualifier Character 6	Qualifier Character 7
Ø Hip, Right 1 Hip, Left	Ø High Osmolar 1 Low Osmolar Y Other Contrast	Z None	Z None
Ø Hip, Right 1 Hip, Left	Z None	Z None	1 Densitometry Z None
3 Femur, Right 4 Femur, Left	Z None	Z None	1 Densitometry Z None
7 Knee, Right 8 Knee, Left G Ankle, Right H Ankle, Left	Ø High Osmolar 1 Low Osmolar Y Other Contrast Z None	Z None	Z None
D Lower Leg, Right F Lower Leg, Left J Calcaneus, Right K Calcaneus, Left L Foot, Right M Foot, Left P Toe(s), Right Q Toe(s), Left V Patella, Right W Patella, Left	Z None	Z None	Z None
X Foot/Toe Joint, Right Y Foot/Toe Joint, Left	Ø High Osmolar 1 Low Osmolar Y Other Contrast	Z None	Z None

B Imaging
Q Non-Axial Lower Bones
1 Fluoroscopy Definition: Single plane or bi-plane real time display of an image developed from the capture of external ionizing radioation on a fluorescent screen. The image may also be stored by either digital or analog means.

Body Part Character 4	Contrast Character 5	Qualifier Character 6	Qualifier Character 7
Ø Hip, Right 1 Hip, Left 7 Knee, Right 8 Knee, Left G Ankle, Right H Ankle, Left X Foot/Toe Joint, Right Y Foot/Toe Joint, Left	Ø High Osmolar 1 Low Osmolar Y Other Contrast Z None	Z None	Z None
3 Femur, Right 4 Femur, Left D Lower Leg, Right F Lower Leg, Left J Calcaneus, Right K Calcaneus, Left L Foot, Right M Foot, Left P Toe(s), Right Q Toe(s), Left V Patella, Right W Patella, Left	Z None	Z None	Z None

B Imaging
Q Non-Axial Lower Bones
2 Computerized Tomography (CT Scan) Definition: Computer reformatted digital display of multiplanar images developed from the capture of multiple exposures of external ionizing radiation

Body Part Character 4	Contrast Character 5	Qualifier Character 6	Qualifier Character 7
Ø Hip, Right 1 Hip, Left 3 Femur, Right 4 Femur, Left 7 Knee, Right 8 Knee, Left D Lower Leg, Right F Lower Leg, Left G Ankle, Right H Ankle, Left J Calcaneus, Right K Calcaneus, Left L Foot, Right M Foot, Left P Toe(s), Right Q Toe(s), Left R Lower Extremity, Right S Lower Extremity, Left V Patella, Right W Patella, Left X Foot/Toe Joint, Right Y Foot/Toe Joint, Left	Ø High Osmolar 1 Low Osmolar Y Other Contrast Z None	Z None	Z None
B Tibia/Fibula, Right C Tibia/Fibula, Left	Ø High Osmolar 1 Low Osmolar Y Other Contrast	Z None	Z None

B Imaging
Q Non-Axial Lower Bones
3 Magnetic Resonance Imaging (MRI) Definition: Computer reformatted digital display of multiplanar images developed from the capture of radio-frequency signals emitted by nuclei in a body site excited within a magnetic field

Body Part Character 4	Contrast Character 5	Qualifier Character 6	Qualifier Character 7
Ø Hip, Right 1 Hip, Left 3 Femur, Right 4 Femur, Left 7 Knee, Right 8 Knee, Left D Lower Leg, Right F Lower Leg, Left G Ankle, Right H Ankle, Left J Calcaneus, Right K Calcaneus, Left L Foot, Right M Foot, Left P Toe(s), Right Q Toe(s), Left V Patella, Right W Patella, Left	Y Other Contrast	Ø Unenhanced and Enhanced Z None	Z None
Ø Hip, Right 1 Hip, Left 3 Femur, Right 4 Femur, Left 7 Knee, Right 8 Knee, Left D Lower Leg, Right F Lower Leg, Left G Ankle, Right H Ankle, Left J Calcaneus, Right K Calcaneus, Left L Foot, Right M Foot, Left P Toe(s), Right Q Toe(s), Left V Patella, Right W Patella, Left	Z None	Z None	Z None

B Imaging
Q Non-Axial Lower Bones
4 Ultrasonography Definition: Real time display of images of anatomy or flow information developed from the capture of relected and attenuated high frequency sound waves

Body Part Character 4	Contrast Character 5	Qualifier Character 6	Qualifier Character 7
Ø Hip, Right 1 Hip, Left 2 Hips, Bilateral 7 Knee, Right 8 Knee, Left 9 Knees, Bilateral	Z None	Z None	Z None

B Imaging
R Axial Skeleton, Except Skull and Facial Bones
Ø Plain Radiography Definition: Planar display of an image developed from the capture of external ionizing radiation on photographic or photoconductive plate

Body Part Character 4	Contrast Character 5	Qualifier Character 6	Qualifier Character 7
Ø Cervical Spine 7 Thoracic Spine 9 Lumbar Spine G Whole Spine	Z None	Z None	1 Densitometry Z None
1 Cervical Disc(s) 2 Thoracic Disc(s) 3 Lumbar Disc(s) 4 Cervical Facet Joint(s) 5 Thoracic Facet Joint(s) 6 Lumbar Facet Joint(s) D Sacroiliac Joints	Ø High Osmolar 1 Low Osmolar Y Other Contrast Z None	Z None	Z None
8 Thoracolumbar Joint B Lumbosacral Joint C Pelvis F Sacrum and Coccyx H Sternum	Z None	Z None	Z None

B Imaging
R Axial Skeleton, Except Skull and Facial Bones
1 Fluoroscopy Definition: Single plane or bi-plane real time display of an image developed from the capture of external ionizing radioation on a fluorescent screen. The image may also be stored by either digital or analog means.

Body Part Character 4	Contrast Character 5	Qualifier Character 6	Qualifier Character 7
Ø Cervical Spine 1 Cervical Disc(s) 2 Thoracic Disc(s) 3 Lumbar Disc(s) 4 Cervical Facet Joint(s) 5 Thoracic Facet Joint(s) 6 Lumbar Facet Joint(s) 7 Thoracic Spine 8 Thoracolumbar Joint 9 Lumbar Spine B Lumbosacral Joint C Pelvis D Sacroiliac Joints F Sacrum and Coccyx G Whole Spine H Sternum	Ø High Osmolar 1 Low Osmolar Y Other Contrast Z None	Z None	Z None

B Imaging
R Axial Skeleton, Except Skull and Facial Bones
2 Computerized Tomography (CT Scan) Definition: Computer reformatted digital display of multiplanar images developed from the capture of multiple exposures of external ionizing radiation

Body Part Character 4	Contrast Character 5	Qualifier Character 6	Qualifier Character 7
Ø Cervical Spine 7 Thoracic Spine 9 Lumbar Spine C Pelvis D Sacroiliac Joints F Sacrum and Coccyx	Ø High Osmolar 1 Low Osmolar Y Other Contrast Z None	Z None	Z None

B Imaging
R Axial Skeleton, Except Skull and Facial Bones
3 Magnetic Resonance Imaging (MRI) Definition: Computer reformatted digital display of multiplanar images developed from the capture of radio-frequency signals emitted by nuclei in a body site excited within a magnetic field

Body Part Character 4	Contrast Character 5	Qualifier Character 6	Qualifier Character 7
Ø Cervical Spine 1 Cervical Disc(s) 2 Thoracic Disc(s) 3 Lumbar Disc(s) 7 Thoracic Spine 9 Lumbar Spine C Pelvis F Sacrum and Coccyx	Y Other Contrast	Ø Unenhanced and Enhanced Z None	Z None
Ø Cervical Spine 1 Cervical Disc(s) 2 Thoracic Disc(s) 3 Lumbar Disc(s) 7 Thoracic Spine 9 Lumbar Spine C Pelvis F Sacrum and Coccyx	Z None	Z None	Z None

B Imaging
R Axial Skeleton, Except Skull and Facial Bones
4 Ultrasonography Definition: Real time display of images of anatomy or flow information developed from the capture of relected and attenuated high frequency sound waves

Body Part Character 4	Contrast Character 5	Qualifier Character 6	Qualifier Character 7
Ø Cervical Spine 7 Thoracic Spine 9 Lumbar Spine F Sacrum and Coccyx	Z None	Z None	Z None

B Imaging
T Urinary System
Ø Plain Radiography Definition: Planar display of an image developed from the capture of external ionizing radiation on photographic or photoconductive plate

Body Part Character 4	Contrast Character 5	Qualifier Character 6	Qualifier Character 7
Ø Bladder 1 Kidney, Right 2 Kidney, Left 3 Kidneys, Bilateral 4 Kidneys, Ureters and Bladder 5 Urethra 6 Ureter, Right 7 Ureter, Left 8 Ureters, Bilateral B Bladder and Urethra C Ileal Diversion Loop	Ø High Osmolar 1 Low Osmolar Y Other Contrast Z None	Z None	Z None

B Imaging
T Urinary System
1 Fluoroscopy Definition: Single plane or bi-plane real time display of an image developed from the capture of external ionizing radioation on a fluorescent screen. The image may also be stored by either digital or analog means.

Body Part Character 4	Contrast Character 5	Qualifier Character 6	Qualifier Character 7
Ø Bladder 1 Kidney, Right 2 Kidney, Left 3 Kidneys, Bilateral 4 Kidneys, Ureters and Bladder 5 Urethra 6 Ureter, Right 7 Ureter, Left B Bladder and Urethra C Ileal Diversion Loop D Kidney, Ureter and Bladder, Right F Kidney, Ureter and Bladder, Left G Ileal Loop, Ureters and Kidneys	Ø High Osmolar 1 Low Osmolar Y Other Contrast Z None	Z None	Z None

B Imaging
T Urinary System
2 Computerized Tomography (CT Scan) Definition: Computer reformatted digital display of multiplanar images developed from the capture of multiple exposures of external ionizing radiation

Body Part Character 4	Contrast Character 5	Qualifier Character 6	Qualifier Character 7
Ø Bladder 1 Kidney, Right 2 Kidney, Left 3 Kidneys, Bilateral 9 Kidney Transplant	Ø High Osmolar 1 Low Osmolar Y Other Contrast	Ø Unenhanced and Enhanced Z None	Z None
Ø Bladder 1 Kidney, Right 2 Kidney, Left 3 Kidneys, Bilateral 9 Kidney Transplant	Z None	Z None	Z None

B Imaging
T Urinary System
3 Magnetic Resonance Imaging (MRI) Definition: Computer reformatted digital display of multiplanar images developed from the capture of radio-frequency signals emitted by nuclei in a body site excited within a magnetic field

Body Part Character 4	Contrast Character 5	Qualifier Character 6	Qualifier Character 7
Ø Bladder 1 Kidney, Right 2 Kidney, Left 3 Kidneys, Bilateral 9 Kidney Transplant	Y Other Contrast	Ø Unenhanced and Enhanced Z None	Z None
Ø Bladder 1 Kidney, Right 2 Kidney, Left 3 Kidneys, Bilateral 9 Kidney Transplant	Z None	Z None	Z None

B Imaging
T Urinary System
4 Ultrasonography Definition: Real time display of images of anatomy or flow information developed from the capture of relected and attenuated high frequency sound waves

Body Part Character 4	Contrast Character 5	Qualifier Character 6	Qualifier Character 7
Ø Bladder 1 Kidney, Right 2 Kidney, Left 3 Kidneys, Bilateral 5 Urethra 6 Ureter, Right 7 Ureter, Left 8 Ureters, Bilateral 9 Kidney Transplant J Kidneys and Bladder	Z None	Z None	Z None

B Imaging
U Female Reproductive System
Ø Plain Radiography Definition: Planar display of an image developed from the capture of external ionizing radiation on photographic or photoconductive plate

Body Part Character 4	Contrast Character 5	Qualifier Character 6	Qualifier Character 7
Ø Fallopian Tube, Right ♀ 1 Fallopian Tube, Left ♀ 2 Fallopian Tubes, Bilateral ♀ 6 Uterus ♀ 8 Uterus and Fallopian Tubes ♀ 9 Vagina ♀	Ø High Osmolar 1 Low Osmolar Y Other Contrast	Z None	Z None

♀ All body part, contrast, and qualifier values

B Imaging
U Female Reproductive System
1 Fluoroscopy Definition: Single plane or bi-plane real time display of an image developed from the capture of external ionizing radioation on a fluorescent screen. The image may also be stored by either digital or analog means.

Body Part Character 4	Contrast Character 5	Qualifier Character 6	Qualifier Character 7
Ø Fallopian Tube, Right ♀ 1 Fallopian Tube, Left ♀ 2 Fallopian Tubes, Bilateral ♀ 6 Uterus ♀ 8 Uterus and Fallopian Tubes ♀ 9 Vagina ♀	Ø High Osmolar 1 Low Osmolar Y Other Contrast Z None	Z None	Z None

♀ All body part, contrast, and qualifier values

B Imaging
U Female Reproductive System
3 Magnetic Resonance Imaging (MRI) Definition: Computer reformatted digital display of multiplanar images developed from the capture of radio-frequency signals emitted by nuclei in a body site excited within a magnetic field

Body Part Character 4	Contrast Character 5	Qualifier Character 6	Qualifier Character 7
3 Ovary, Right ♀ 4 Ovary, Left ♀ 5 Ovaries, Bilateral ♀ 6 Uterus ♀ 9 Vagina ♀ B Pregnant Uterus ♀ C Uterus and Ovaries ♀	Y Other Contrast	Ø Unenhanced and Enhanced Z None	Z None
3 Ovary, Right ♀ 4 Ovary, Left ♀ 5 Ovaries, Bilateral ♀ 6 Uterus ♀ 9 Vagina ♀ B Pregnant Uterus ♀ C Uterus and Ovaries ♀	Z None	Z None	Z None

♀ All body part, contrast, and qualifier values

B Imaging
U Female Reproductive System
4 Ultrasonography Definition: Real time display of images of anatomy or flow information developed from the capture of relected and attenuated high frequency sound waves

Body Part Character 4	Contrast Character 5	Qualifier Character 6	Qualifier Character 7
Ø Fallopian Tube, Right ♀ 1 Fallopian Tube, Left ♀ 2 Fallopian Tubes, Bilateral ♀ 3 Ovary, Right ♀ 4 Ovary, Left ♀ 5 Ovaries, Bilateral ♀ 6 Uterus ♀ C Uterus and Ovaries ♀	Y Other Contrast Z None	Z None	Z None

♀ All body part, contrast, and qualifier values

B Imaging
V Male Reproductive System
Ø Plain Radiography Definition: Planar display of an image developed from the capture of external ionizing radiation on photographic or photoconductive plate

Body Part Character 4	Contrast Character 5	Qualifier Character 6	Qualifier Character 7
Ø Corpora Cavernosa ♂ 1 Epididymis, Right ♂ 2 Epididymis, Left ♂ 3 Prostate ♂ 5 Testicle, Right ♂ 6 Testicle, Left ♂ 8 Vasa Vasorum ♂	Ø High Osmolar 1 Low Osmolar Y Other Contrast	Z None	Z None

♂ All body part, contrast, and qualifier values

B Imaging
V Male Reproductive System
1 Fluoroscopy Definition: Single plane or bi-plane real time display of an image developed from the capture of external ionizing radioation on a fluorescent screen. The image may also be stored by either digital or analog means.

Body Part Character 4	Contrast Character 5	Qualifier Character 6	Qualifier Character 7
Ø Corpora Cavernosa ♂ 8 Vasa Vasorum ♂	Ø High Osmolar 1 Low Osmolar Y Other Contrast Z None	Z None	Z None

♂ All body part, contrast, and qualifier values

B Imaging
V Male Reproductive System
2 Computerized Tomography (CT Scan) Definition: Computer reformatted digital display of multiplanar images developed from the capture of multiple exposures of external ionizing radiation

Body Part Character 4	Contrast Character 5	Qualifier Character 6	Qualifier Character 7
3 Prostate ♂	Ø High Osmolar 1 Low Osmolar Y Other Contrast	Ø Unenhanced and Enhanced Z None	Z None
3 Prostate ♂	Z None	Z None	Z None

♂ BV23[Ø,Y][Ø,Z]Z
♂ BV231ØZ
♂ BV23ZZZ

B Imaging
V Male Reproductive System
3 Magnetic Resonance Imaging (MRI) Definition: Computer reformatted digital display of multiplanar images developed from the capture of radio-frequency signals emitted by nuclei in a body site excited within a magnetic field

Body Part Character 4	Contrast Character 5	Qualifier Character 6	Qualifier Character 7
Ø Corpora Cavernosa ♂ 3 Prostate ♂ 4 Scrotum ♂ 5 Testicle, Right ♂ 6 Testicle, Left ♂ 7 Testicles, Bilateral ♂	Y Other Contrast	Ø Unenhanced and Enhanced Z None	Z None
Ø Corpora Cavernosa ♂ 3 Prostate ♂ 4 Scrotum ♂ 5 Testicle, Right ♂ 6 Testicle, Left ♂ 7 Testicles, Bilateral ♂	Z None	Z None	Z None

♂ All body part, contrast, and qualifier values

B Imaging
V Male Reproductive System
4 Ultrasonography Definition: Real time display of images of anatomy or flow information developed from the capture of relected and attenuated high frequency sound waves

Body Part Character 4	Contrast Character 5	Qualifier Character 6	Qualifier Character 7
4 Scrotum ♂ 9 Prostate and Seminal Vesicles ♂ B Penis ♂	Z None	Z None	Z None

♂ All body part, contrast, and qualifier values

B Imaging
W Anatomical Regions
Ø Plain Radiography Definition: Planar display of an image developed from the capture of external ionizing radiation on photographic or photoconductive plate

Body Part Character 4	Contrast Character 5	Qualifier Character 6	Qualifier Character 7
Ø Abdomen 1 Abdomen and Pelvis 3 Chest B Long Bones, All C Lower Extremity J Upper Extremity K Whole Body L Whole Skeleton M Whole Body, Infant	Z None	Z None	Z None

B Imaging
W Anatomical Regions
1 Fluoroscopy Definition: Single plane or bi-plane real time display of an image developed from the capture of external ionizing radioation on a fluorescent screen. The image may also be stored by either digital or analog means.

Body Part Character 4	Contrast Character 5	Qualifier Character 6	Qualifier Character 7
1 Abdomen and Pelvis 9 Head and Neck C Lower Extremity J Upper Extremity	Ø High Osmolar 1 Low Osmolar Y Other Contrast Z None	Z None	Z None

B Imaging
W Anatomical Regions
2 Computerized Tomography (CT Scan) Definition: Computer reformatted digital display of multiplanar images developed from the capture of multiple exposures of external ionizing radiation

Body Part Character 4	Contrast Character 5	Qualifier Character 6	Qualifier Character 7
Ø Abdomen 1 Abdomen and Pelvis 4 Chest and Abdomen 5 Chest, Abdomen and Pelvis 8 Head 9 Head and Neck F Neck G Pelvic Region	Ø High Osmolar 1 Low Osmolar Y Other Contrast	Ø Unenhanced and Enhanced Z None	Z None
Ø Abdomen 1 Abdomen and Pelvis 4 Chest and Abdomen 5 Chest, Abdomen and Pelvis 8 Head 9 Head and Neck F Neck G Pelvic Region	Z None	Z None	Z None

B Imaging
W Anatomical Regions
3 Magnetic Resonance Imaging (MRI) Definition: Computer reformatted digital display of multiplanar images developed from the capture of radio-frequency signals emitted by nuclei in a body site excited within a magnetic field

Body Part Character 4	Contrast Character 5	Qualifier Character 6	Qualifier Character 7
Ø Abdomen 8 Head F Neck G Pelvic Region H Retroperitoneum P Brachial Plexus	Y Other Contrast	Ø Unenhanced and Enhanced Z None	Z None
Ø Abdomen 8 Head F Neck G Pelvic Region H Retroperitoneum P Brachial Plexus	Z None	Z None	Z None
3 Chest	Y Other Contrast	Ø Unenhanced and Enhanced Z None	Z None

B Imaging
W Anatomical Regions
4 Ultrasonography Definition: Real time display of images of anatomy or flow information developed from the capture of relected and attenuated high frequency sound waves

Body Part Character 4	Contrast Character 5	Qualifier Character 6	Qualifier Character 7
Ø Abdomen 1 Abdomen and Pelvis F Neck G Pelvic Region	Z None	Z None	Z None

B Imaging
W Anatomical Regions
5 Other Imaging Definition: Other specified modality for visualizing a body part

Body Part Character 4	Contrast Character 5	Qualifier Character 6	Qualifier Character 7
2 Trunk 9 Head and Neck C Lower Extremity J Upper Extremity	Z None	1 Bacterial Autofluorescence	Z None

B Imaging
Y Fetus and Obstetrical
3 Magnetic Resonance Imaging (MRI) Definition: Computer reformatted digital display of multiplanar images developed from the capture of radio-frequency signals emitted by nuclei in a body site excited within a magnetic field

Body Part Character 4	Contrast Character 5	Qualifier Character 6	Qualifier Character 7
Ø Fetal Head ♀ 1 Fetal Heart ♀ 2 Fetal Thorax ♀ 3 Fetal Abdomen ♀ 4 Fetal Spine ♀ 5 Fetal Extremities ♀ 6 Whole Fetus ♀	Y Other Contrast	Ø Unenhanced and Enhanced Z None	Z None
Ø Fetal Head ♀ 1 Fetal Heart ♀ 2 Fetal Thorax ♀ 3 Fetal Abdomen ♀ 4 Fetal Spine ♀ 5 Fetal Extremities ♀ 6 Whole Fetus ♀	Z None	Z None	Z None

♀ BY3[Ø,1,2,3,5,6]Y[Ø,Z]Z
♀ BY34YZZ
♀ BY3[Ø,1,2,3,4,5,6]ZZZ

B Imaging
Y Fetus and Obstetrical
4 Ultrasonography Definition: Real time display of images of anatomy or flow information developed from the capture of relected and attenuated high frequency sound waves

Body Part Character 4	Contrast Character 5	Qualifier Character 6	Qualifier Character 7
7 Fetal Umbilical Cord ♀ 8 Placenta ♀ 9 First Trimester, Single Fetus ♀ B First Trimester, Multiple Gestation ♀ C Second Trimester, Single Fetus ♀ D Second Trimester, Multiple Gestation ♀ F Third Trimester, Single Fetus ♀ G Third Trimester, Multiple Gestation ♀	Z None	Z None	Z None

♀ All body part, contrast, and qualifier values

Nuclear Medicine CØ1–CW7

C Nuclear Medicine
Ø Central Nervous System
1 Planar Nuclear Medicine Imaging Definition: Introduction of radioactive materials into the body for single plane display of images developed from the capture of radioactive emissions

Body Part Character 4	Radionuclide Character 5	Qualifier Character 6	Qualifier Character 7
Ø Brain	**1** Technetium 99m (Tc-99m) **Y** Other Radionuclide	**Z** None	**Z** None
5 Cerebrospinal Fluid	**D** Indium 111 (In-111) **Y** Other Radionuclide	**Z** None	**Z** None
Y Central Nervous System	**Y** Other Radionuclide	**Z** None	**Z** None

C Nuclear Medicine
Ø Central Nervous System
2 Tomographic (Tomo) Nuclear Medicine Imaging Definition: Introduction of radioactive materials into the body for three dimensional display of images developed from the capture of radioactive emissions

Body Part Character 4	Radionuclide Character 5	Qualifier Character 6	Qualifier Character 7
Ø Brain	**1** Technetium 99m (Tc-99m) **F** Iodine 123 (I-123) **S** Thallium 201 (Tl-201) **Y** Other Radionuclide	**Z** None	**Z** None
5 Cerebrospinal Fluid	**D** Indium 111 (In-111) **Y** Other Radionuclide	**Z** None	**Z** None
Y Central Nervous System	**Y** Other Radionuclide	**Z** None	**Z** None

C Nuclear Medicine
Ø Central Nervous System
3 Positron Emission Tomographic (PET) Imaging Definition: Introduction of radioactive materials into the body for three dimensional display of images developed from the simultaneous capture, 180 degrees apart, of radioactive emissions

Body Part Character 4	Radionuclide Character 5	Qualifier Character 6	Qualifier Character 7
Ø Brain	**B** Carbon 11 (C-11) **K** Fluorine 18 (F-18) **M** Oxygen 15 (O-15) **Y** Other Radionuclide	**Z** None	**Z** None
Y Central Nervous System	**Y** Other Radionuclide	**Z** None	**Z** None

C Nuclear Medicine
Ø Central Nervous System
5 Nonimaging Nuclear Medicine Probe Definition: Introduction of radioactive materials into the body for the study of distribution and fate of certain substances by the detection of radioactive emissions; or, alternatively, measurement of absorption of radioactive emissions from an external source

Body Part Character 4	Radionuclide Character 5	Qualifier Character 6	Qualifier Character 7
Ø Brain	**V** Xenon 133 (Xe-133) **Y** Other Radionuclide	**Z** None	**Z** None
Y Central Nervous System	**Y** Other Radionuclide	**Z** None	**Z** None

C Nuclear Medicine
2 Heart
1 Planar Nuclear Medicine Imaging Definition: Introduction of radioactive materials into the body for single plane display of images developed from the capture of radioactive emissions

Body Part Character 4	Radionuclide Character 5	Qualifier Character 6	Qualifier Character 7
6 Heart, Right and Left	**1** Technetium 99m (Tc-99m) **Y** Other Radionuclide	**Z** None	**Z** None
G Myocardium	**1** Technetium 99m (Tc-99m) **D** Indium 111 (In-111) **S** Thallium 201 (Tl-201) **Y** Other Radionuclide **Z** None	**Z** None	**Z** None
Y Heart	**Y** Other Radionuclide	**Z** None	**Z** None

C Nuclear Medicine
2 Heart
2 Tomographic (Tomo) Nuclear Medicine Imaging Definition: Introduction of radioactive materials into the body for three dimensional display of images developed from the capture of radioactive emissions

Body Part Character 4	Radionuclide Character 5	Qualifier Character 6	Qualifier Character 7
6 Heart, Right and Left	1 Technetium 99m (Tc-99m) Y Other Radionuclide	Z None	Z None
G Myocardium	1 Technetium 99m (Tc-99m) D Indium 111 (In-111) K Fluorine 18 (F-18) S Thallium 201 (Tl-201) Y Other Radionuclide Z None	Z None	Z None
Y Heart	Y Other Radionuclide	Z None	Z None

C Nuclear Medicine
2 Heart
3 Positron Emission Tomographic (PET) Imaging Definition: Introduction of radioactive materials into the body for three dimensional display of images developed from the simultaneous capture, 180 degrees apart, of radioactive emissions

Body Part Character 4	Radionuclide Character 5	Qualifier Character 6	Qualifier Character 7
G Myocardium	K Fluorine 18 (F-18) M Oxygen 15 (O-15) Q Rubidium 82 (Rb-82) R Nitrogen 13 (N-13) Y Other Radionuclide	Z None	Z None
Y Heart	Y Other Radionuclide	Z None	Z None

C Nuclear Medicine
2 Heart
5 Nonimaging Nuclear Medicine Probe Definition: Introduction of radioactive materials into the body for the study of distribution and fate of certain substances by the detection of radioactive emissions; or, alternatively, measurement of absorption of radioactive emissions from an external source

Body Part Character 4	Radionuclide Character 5	Qualifier Character 6	Qualifier Character 7
6 Heart, Right and Left	1 Technetium 99m (Tc-99m) Y Other Radionuclide	Z None	Z None
Y Heart	Y Other Radionuclide	Z None	Z None

C Nuclear Medicine
5 Veins
1 Planar Nuclear Medicine Imaging Definition: Introduction of radioactive materials into the body for single plane display of images developed from the capture of radioactive emissions

Body Part Character 4	Radionuclide Character 5	Qualifier Character 6	Qualifier Character 7
B Lower Extremity Veins, Right C Lower Extremity Veins, Left D Lower Extremity Veins, Bilateral N Upper Extremity Veins, Right P Upper Extremity Veins, Left Q Upper Extremity Veins, Bilateral R Central Veins	1 Technetium 99m (Tc-99m) Y Other Radionuclide	Z None	Z None
Y Veins	Y Other Radionuclide	Z None	Z None

C Nuclear Medicine
7 Lymphatic and Hematologic System
1 Planar Nuclear Medicine Imaging Definition: Introduction of radioactive materials into the body for single plane display of images developed from the capture of radioactive emissions

Body Part Character 4	Radionuclide Character 5	Qualifier Character 6	Qualifier Character 7
Ø Bone Marrow	1 Technetium 99m (Tc-99m) D Indium 111 (In-111) Y Other Radionuclide	Z None	Z None
2 Spleen 5 Lymphatics, Head and Neck D Lymphatics, Pelvic J Lymphatics, Head K Lymphatics, Neck L Lymphatics, Upper Chest M Lymphatics, Trunk N Lymphatics, Upper Extremity P Lymphatics, Lower Extremity	1 Technetium 99m (Tc-99m) Y Other Radionuclide	Z None	Z None
3 Blood	D Indium 111 (In-111) Y Other Radionuclide	Z None	Z None
Y Lymphatic and Hematologic System	Y Other Radionuclide	Z None	Z None

C Nuclear Medicine
7 Lymphatic and Hematologic System
2 Tomographic (Tomo) Nuclear Medicine Imaging Definition: Introduction of radioactive materials into the body for three dimensional display of images developed from the capture of radioactive emissions

Body Part Character 4	Radionuclide Character 5	Qualifier Character 6	Qualifier Character 7
2 Spleen	1 Technetium 99m (Tc-99m) Y Other Radionuclide	Z None	Z None
Y Lymphatic and Hematologic System	Y Other Radionuclide	Z None	Z None

C Nuclear Medicine
7 Lymphatic and Hematologic System
5 Nonimaging Nuclear Medicine Probe Definition: Introduction of radioactive materials into the body for the study of distribution and fate of certain substances by the detection of radioactive emissions; or, alternatively, measurement of absorption of radioactive emissions from an external source

Body Part Character 4	Radionuclide Character 5	Qualifier Character 6	Qualifier Character 7
5 Lymphatics, Head and Neck D Lymphatics, Pelvic J Lymphatics, Head K Lymphatics, Neck L Lymphatics, Upper Chest M Lymphatics, Trunk N Lymphatics, Upper Extremity P Lymphatics, Lower Extremity	1 Technetium 99m (Tc-99m) Y Other Radionuclide	Z None	Z None
Y Lymphatic and Hematologic System	Y Other Radionuclide	Z None	Z None

C Nuclear Medicine
7 Lymphatic and Hematologic System
6 Nonimaging Nuclear Medicine Assay Definition: Introduction of radioactive materials into the body for the study of body fluids and blood elements, by the detection of radioactive emissions

Body Part Character 4	Radionuclide Character 5	Qualifier Character 6	Qualifier Character 7
3 Blood	1 Technetium 99m (Tc-99m) 7 Cobalt 58 (Co-58) C Cobalt 57 (Co-57) D Indium 111 (In-111) H Iodine 125 (I-125) W Chromium (Cr-51) Y Other Radionuclide	Z None	Z None
Y Lymphatic and Hematologic System	Y Other Radionuclide	Z None	Z None

C Nuclear Medicine
8 Eye
1 Planar Nuclear Medicine Imaging Definition: Introduction of radioactive materials into the body for single plane display of images developed from the capture of radioactive emissions

Body Part Character 4	Radionuclide Character 5	Qualifier Character 6	Qualifier Character 7
9 Lacrimal Ducts, Bilateral	1 Technetium 99m (Tc-99m) Y Other Radionuclide	Z None	Z None
Y Eye	Y Other Radionuclide	Z None	Z None

C Nuclear Medicine
9 Ear, Nose, Mouth and Throat
1 Planar Nuclear Medicine Imaging Definition: Introduction of radioactive materials into the body for single plane display of images developed from the capture of radioactive emissions

Body Part Character 4	Radionuclide Character 5	Qualifier Character 6	Qualifier Character 7
B Salivary Glands, Bilateral	1 Technetium 99m (Tc-99m) Y Other Radionuclide	Z None	Z None
Y Ear, Nose, Mouth and Throat	Y Other Radionuclide	Z None	Z None

C Nuclear Medicine
B Respiratory System
1 Planar Nuclear Medicine Imaging Definition: Introduction of radioactive materials into the body for single plane display of images developed from the capture of radioactive emissions

Body Part Character 4	Radionuclide Character 5	Qualifier Character 6	Qualifier Character 7
2 Lungs and Bronchi	1 Technetium 99m (Tc-99m) 9 Krypton (Kr-81m) T Xenon 127 (Xe-127) V Xenon 133 (Xe-133) Y Other Radionuclide	Z None	Z None
Y Respiratory System	Y Other Radionuclide	Z None	Z None

C Nuclear Medicine
B Respiratory System
2 Tomographic (Tomo) Nuclear Medicine Imaging Definition: Introduction of radioactive materials into the body for three dimensional display of images developed from the capture of radioactive emissions

Body Part Character 4	Radionuclide Character 5	Qualifier Character 6	Qualifier Character 7
2 Lungs and Bronchi	1 Technetium 99m (Tc-99m) 9 Krypton (Kr-81m) Y Other Radionuclide	Z None	Z None
Y Respiratory System	Y Other Radionuclide	Z None	Z None

C Nuclear Medicine
B Respiratory System
3 Positron Emission Tomographic (PET) Imaging Definition: Introduction of radioactive materials into the body for three dimensional display of images developed from the simultaneous capture, 180 degrees apart, of radioactive emissions

Body Part Character 4	Radionuclide Character 5	Qualifier Character 6	Qualifier Character 7
2 Lungs and Bronchi	K Fluorine 18 (F-18) Y Other Radionuclide	Z None	Z None
Y Respiratory System	Y Other Radionuclide	Z None	Z None

C Nuclear Medicine
D Gastrointestinal System
1 Planar Nuclear Medicine Imaging Definition: Introduction of radioactive materials into the body for single plane display of images developed from the capture of radioactive emissions

Body Part Character 4	Radionuclide Character 5	Qualifier Character 6	Qualifier Character 7
5 Upper Gastrointestinal Tract 7 Gastrointestinal Tract	1 Technetium 99m (Tc-99m) D Indium 111 (In-111) Y Other Radionuclide	Z None	Z None
Y Digestive System	Y Other Radionuclide	Z None	Z None

C Nuclear Medicine
D Gastrointestinal System
2 Tomographic (Tomo) Nuclear Medicine Imaging Definition: Introduction of radioactive materials into the body for three dimensional display of images developed from the capture of radioactive emissions

Body Part Character 4	Radionuclide Character 5	Qualifier Character 6	Qualifier Character 7
7 Gastrointestinal Tract	1 Technetium 99m (Tc-99m) D Indium 111 (In-111) Y Other Radionuclide	Z None	Z None
Y Digestive System	Y Other Radionuclide	Z None	Z None

C Nuclear Medicine
F Hepatobiliary System and Pancreas
1 Planar Nuclear Medicine Imaging Definition: Introduction of radioactive materials into the body for single plane display of images developed from the capture of radioactive emissions

Body Part Character 4	Radionuclide Character 5	Qualifier Character 6	Qualifier Character 7
4 Gallbladder 5 Liver 6 Liver and Spleen C Hepatobiliary System, All	1 Technetium 99m (Tc-99m) Y Other Radionuclide	Z None	Z None
Y Hepatobiliary System and Pancreas	Y Other Radionuclide	Z None	Z None

C Nuclear Medicine
F Hepatobiliary System and Pancreas
2 Tomographic (Tomo) Nuclear Medicine Imaging Definition: Introduction of radioactive materials into the body for three dimensional display of images developed from the capture of radioactive emissions

Body Part Character 4	Radionuclide Character 5	Qualifier Character 6	Qualifier Character 7
4 Gallbladder 5 Liver 6 Liver and Spleen	1 Technetium 99m (Tc-99m) Y Other Radionuclide	Z None	Z None
Y Hepatobiliary System and Pancreas	Y Other Radionuclide	Z None	Z None

C Nuclear Medicine
G Endocrine System
1 Planar Nuclear Medicine Imaging Definition: Introduction of radioactive materials into the body for single plane display of images developed from the capture of radioactive emissions

Body Part Character 4	Radionuclide Character 5	Qualifier Character 6	Qualifier Character 7
1 Parathyroid Glands	1 Technetium 99m (Tc-99m) S Thallium 201 (Tl-201) Y Other Radionuclide	Z None	Z None
2 Thyroid Gland	1 Technetium 99m (Tc-99m) F Iodine 123 (I-123) G Iodine 131 (I-131) Y Other Radionuclide	Z None	Z None
4 Adrenal Glands, Bilateral	G Iodine 131 (I-131) Y Other Radionuclide	Z None	Z None
Y Endocrine System	Y Other Radionuclide	Z None	Z None

C Nuclear Medicine
G Endocrine System
2 Tomographic (Tomo) Nuclear Medicine Imaging Definition: Introduction of radioactive materials into the body for three dimensional display of images developed from the capture of radioactive emissions

Body Part Character 4	Radionuclide Character 5	Qualifier Character 6	Qualifier Character 7
1 Parathyroid Glands	1 Technetium 99m (Tc-99m) S Thallium 201 (Tl-201) Y Other Radionuclide	Z None	Z None
Y Endocrine System	Y Other Radionuclide	Z None	Z None

C Nuclear Medicine
G Endocrine System
4 Nonimaging Nuclear Medicine Uptake

Definition: Introduction of radioactive materials into the body for measurements of organ function, from the detection of radioactive emmissions

Body Part Character 4	Radionuclide Character 5	Qualifier Character 6	Qualifier Character 7
2 Thyroid Gland	1 Technetium 99m (Tc-99m) F Iodine 123 (I-123) G Iodine 131 (I-131) Y Other Radionuclide	Z None	Z None
Y Endocrine System	Y Other Radionuclide	Z None	Z None

C Nuclear Medicine
H Skin, Subcutaneous Tissue and Breast
1 Planar Nuclear Medicine Imaging

Definition: Introduction of radioactive materials into the body for single plane display of images developed from the capture of radioactive emissions

Body Part Character 4	Radionuclide Character 5	Qualifier Character 6	Qualifier Character 7
Ø Breast, Right 1 Breast, Left 2 Breasts, Bilateral	1 Technetium 99m (Tc-99m) S Thallium 201 (Tl-201) Y Other Radionuclide	Z None	Z None
Y Skin, Subcutaneous Tissue and Breast	Y Other Radionuclide	Z None	Z None

C Nuclear Medicine
H Skin, Subcutaneous Tissue and Breast
2 Tomographic (Tomo) Nuclear Medicine Imaging

Definition: Introduction of radioactive materials into the body for three dimensional display of images developed from the capture of radioactive emissions

Body Part Character 4	Radionuclide Character 5	Qualifier Character 6	Qualifier Character 7
Ø Breast, Right 1 Breast, Left 2 Breasts, Bilateral	1 Technetium 99m (Tc-99m) S Thallium 201 (Tl-201) Y Other Radionuclide	Z None	Z None
Y Skin, Subcutaneous Tissue and Breast	Y Other Radionuclide	Z None	Z None

C Nuclear Medicine
P Musculoskeletal System
1 Planar Nuclear Medicine Imaging

Definition: Introduction of radioactive materials into the body for single plane display of images developed from the capture of radioactive emissions

Body Part Character 4	Radionuclide Character 5	Qualifier Character 6	Qualifier Character 7
1 Skull 4 Thorax 5 Spine 6 Pelvis 7 Spine and Pelvis 8 Upper Extremity, Right 9 Upper Extremity, Left B Upper Extremities, Bilateral C Lower Extremity, Right D Lower Extremity, Left F Lower Extremities, Bilateral Z Musculoskeletal System, All	1 Technetium 99m (Tc-99m) Y Other Radionuclide	Z None	Z None
Y Musculoskeletal System, Other	Y Other Radionuclide	Z None	Z None

C Nuclear Medicine
P Musculoskeletal System
2 Tomographic (Tomo) Nuclear Medicine Imaging Definition: Introduction of radioactive materials into the body for three dimensional display of images developed from the capture of radioactive emissions

Body Part Character 4	Radionuclide Character 5	Qualifier Character 6	Qualifier Character 7
1 Skull 2 Cervical Spine 3 Skull and Cervical Spine 4 Thorax 6 Pelvis 7 Spine and Pelvis 8 Upper Extremity, Right 9 Upper Extremity, Left B Upper Extremities, Bilateral C Lower Extremity, Right D Lower Extremity, Left F Lower Extremities, Bilateral G Thoracic Spine H Lumbar Spine J Thoracolumbar Spine	1 Technetium 99m (Tc-99m) Y Other Radionuclide	Z None	Z None
Y Musculoskeletal System, Other	Y Other Radionuclide	Z None	Z None

C Nuclear Medicine
P Musculoskeletal System
5 Nonimaging Nuclear Medicine Probe Definition: Introduction of radioactive materials into the body for the study of distribution and fate of certain substances by the detection of radioactive emissions; or, alternatively, measurement of absorption of radioactive emissions from an external source

Body Part Character 4	Radionuclide Character 5	Qualifier Character 6	Qualifier Character 7
5 Spine N Upper Extremities P Lower Extremities	Z None	Z None	Z None
Y Musculoskeletal System, Other	Y Other Radionuclide	Z None	Z None

C Nuclear Medicine
T Urinary System
1 Planar Nuclear Medicine Imaging Definition: Introduction of radioactive materials into the body for single plane display of images developed from the capture of radioactive emissions

Body Part Character 4	Radionuclide Character 5	Qualifier Character 6	Qualifier Character 7
3 Kidneys, Ureters and Bladder	1 Technetium 99m (Tc-99m) F Iodine 123 (I-123) G Iodine 131 (I-131) Y Other Radionuclide	Z None	Z None
H Bladder and Ureters	1 Technetium 99m (Tc-99m) Y Other Radionuclide	Z None	Z None
Y Urinary System	Y Other Radionuclide	Z None	Z None

C Nuclear Medicine
T Urinary System
2 Tomographic (Tomo) Nuclear Medicine Imaging Definition: Introduction of radioactive materials into the body for three dimensional display of images developed from the capture of radioactive emissions

Body Part Character 4	Radionuclide Character 5	Qualifier Character 6	Qualifier Character 7
3 Kidneys, Ureters and Bladder	1 Technetium 99m (Tc-99m) Y Other Radionuclide	Z None	Z None
Y Urinary System	Y Other Radionuclide	Z None	Z None

C Nuclear Medicine
T Urinary System
6 Nonimaging Nuclear Medicine Assay Definition: Introduction of radioactive materials into the body for the study of body fluids and blood elements, by the detection of radioactive emissions

Body Part Character 4	Radionuclide Character 5	Qualifier Character 6	Qualifier Character 7
3 Kidneys, Ureters and Bladder	1 Technetium 99m (Tc-99m) F Iodine 123 (I-123) G Iodine 131 (I-131) H Iodine 125 (I-125) Y Other Radionuclide	Z None	Z None
Y Urinary System	Y Other Radionuclide	Z None	Z None

C Nuclear Medicine
V Male Reproductive System
1 Planar Nuclear Medicine Imaging

Definition: Introduction of radioactive materials into the body for single plane display of images developed from the capture of radioactive emissions

Body Part Character 4	Radionuclide Character 5	Qualifier Character 6	Qualifier Character 7
9 Testicles, Bilateral ♂	**1** Technetium 99m (Tc-99m) **Y** Other Radionuclide	**Z** None	**Z** None
Y Male Reproductive System ♂	**Y** Other Radionuclide	**Z** None	**Z** None

♂ All body part, radionuclide, and qualifier values

C Nuclear Medicine
W Anatomical Regions
1 Planar Nuclear Medicine Imaging

Definition: Introduction of radioactive materials into the body for single plane display of images developed from the capture of radioactive emissions

Body Part Character 4	Radionuclide Character 5	Qualifier Character 6	Qualifier Character 7
Ø Abdomen **1** Abdomen and Pelvis **4** Chest and Abdomen **6** Chest and Neck **B** Head and Neck **D** Lower Extremity **J** Pelvic Region **M** Upper Extremity **N** Whole Body	**1** Technetium 99m (Tc-99m) **D** Indium 111 (In-111) **F** Iodine 123 (I-123) **G** Iodine 131 (I-131) **L** Gallium 67 (Ga-67) **S** Thallium 201 (Tl-201) **Y** Other Radionuclide	**Z** None	**Z** None
3 Chest	**1** Technetium 99m (Tc-99m) **D** Indium 111 (In-111) **F** Iodine 123 (I-123) **G** Iodine 131 (I-131) **K** Fluorine 18 (F-18) **L** Gallium 67 (Ga-67) **S** Thallium 201 (Tl-201) **Y** Other Radionuclide	**Z** None	**Z** None
Y Anatomical Regions, Multiple	**Y** Other Radionuclide	**Z** None	**Z** None
Z Anatomical Region, Other	**Z** None	**Z** None	**Z** None

C Nuclear Medicine
W Anatomical Regions
2 Tomographic (Tomo) Nuclear Medicine Imaging

Definition: Introduction of radioactive materials into the body for three dimensional display of images developed from the capture of radioactive emissions

Body Part Character 4	Radionuclide Character 5	Qualifier Character 6	Qualifier Character 7
Ø Abdomen **1** Abdomen and Pelvis **3** Chest **4** Chest and Abdomen **6** Chest and Neck **B** Head and Neck **D** Lower Extremity **J** Pelvic Region **M** Upper Extremity	**1** Technetium 99m (Tc-99m) **D** Indium 111 (In-111) **F** Iodine 123 (I-123) **G** Iodine 131 (I-131) **K** Fluorine 18 (F-18) **L** Gallium 67 (Ga-67) **S** Thallium 201 (Tl-201) **Y** Other Radionuclide	**Z** None	**Z** None
Y Anatomical Regions, Multiple	**Y** Other Radionuclide	**Z** None	**Z** None

C Nuclear Medicine
W Anatomical Regions
3 Positron Emission Tomographic (PET) Imaging

Definition: Introduction of radioactive materials into the body for three dimensional display of images developed from the simultaneous capture, 180 degrees apart, of radioactive emissions

Body Part Character 4	Radionuclide Character 5	Qualifier Character 6	Qualifier Character 7
N Whole Body	**Y** Other Radionuclide	**Z** None	**Z** None

C Nuclear Medicine
W Anatomical Regions
5 Nonimaging Nuclear Medicine Probe Definition: Introduction of radioactive materials into the body for the study of distribution and fate of certain substances by the detection of radioactive emissions; or, alternatively, measurement of absorption of radioactive emissions from an external source

Body Part Character 4	Radionuclide Character 5	Qualifier Character 6	Qualifier Character 7
Ø Abdomen **1** Abdomen and Pelvis **3** Chest **4** Chest and Abdomen **6** Chest and Neck **B** Head and Neck **D** Lower Extremity **J** Pelvic Region **M** Upper Extremity	**1** Technetium 99m (Tc-99m) **D** Indium 111 (In-111) **Y** Other Radionuclide	**Z** None	**Z** None

C Nuclear Medicine
W Anatomical Regions
7 Systemic Nuclear Medicine Therapy Definition: Introduction of unsealed radioactive materials into the body for treatment

Body Part Character 4	Radionuclide Character 5	Qualifier Character 6	Qualifier Character 7
Ø Abdomen **3** Chest	**N** Phosphorus 32 (P-32) **Y** Other Radionuclide	**Z** None	**Z** None
G Thyroid	**G** Iodine 131 (I-131) **Y** Other Radionuclide	**Z** None	**Z** None
N Whole Body	**8** Samarium 153 (Sm-153) **G** Iodine 131 (I-131) **N** Phosphorus 32 (P-32) **P** Strontium 89 (Sr-89) **Y** Other Radionuclide	**Z** None	**Z** None
Y Anatomical Regions, Multiple	**Y** Other Radionuclide	**Z** None	**Z** None

Radiation Therapy DØØ–DWY

AHA Coding Clinic for table DØ1
2019, 4Q, 42-44 Unidirectional source brachytherapy

AHA Coding Clinic for table D71
2019, 4Q, 42-44 Unidirectional source brachytherapy

AHA Coding Clinic for table D81
2019, 4Q, 42-44 Unidirectional source brachytherapy

AHA Coding Clinic for table D91
2019, 4Q, 42-44 Unidirectional source brachytherapy

AHA Coding Clinic for table DB1
2019, 4Q, 42-44 Unidirectional source brachytherapy

AHA Coding Clinic for table DD1
2019, 4Q, 42-44 Unidirectional source brachytherapy

AHA Coding Clinic for table DF1
2019, 4Q, 42-44 Unidirectional source brachytherapy

AHA Coding Clinic for table DG1
2019, 4Q, 42-44 Unidirectional source brachytherapy

AHA Coding Clinic for table DM1
2019, 4Q, 42-44 Unidirectional source brachytherapy

AHA Coding Clinic for table DT1
2019, 4Q, 42-44 Unidirectional source brachytherapy

AHA Coding Clinic for table DU1
2019, 4Q, 42-44 Unidirectional source brachytherapy
2017, 4Q, 104 Intrauterine brachytherapy & placement of tandems & ovoids

AHA Coding Clinic for table DV1
2019, 4Q, 42-44 Unidirectional source brachytherapy

AHA Coding Clinic for table DW1
2019, 4Q, 42-44 Unidirectional source brachytherapy

AHA Coding Clinic for table DWY
2019, 4Q, 37 Hyperthermic antineoplastic chemotherapy

D Radiation Therapy
Ø Central and Peripheral Nervous System
Ø Beam Radiation

Treatment Site Character 4	Modality Qualifier Character 5	Isotope Character 6	Qualifier Character 7
Ø Brain 1 Brain Stem 6 Spinal Cord 7 Peripheral Nerve	Ø Photons <1 MeV 1 Photons 1- 10 MeV 2 Photons >10 MeV 4 Heavy Particles (Protons, Ions) 5 Neutrons 6 Neutron Capture	Z None	Z None
Ø Brain 1 Brain Stem 6 Spinal Cord 7 Peripheral Nerve	3 Electrons	Z None	Ø Intraoperative Z None

D Radiation Therapy
Ø Central and Peripheral Nervous System
1 Brachytherapy

Treatment Site Character 4	Modality Qualifier Character 5	Isotope Character 6	Qualifier Character 7
Ø Brain 1 Brain Stem 6 Spinal Cord 7 Peripheral Nerve	9 High Dose Rate (HDR)	7 Cesium 137 (Cs-137) 8 Iridium 192 (Ir-192) 9 Iodine 125 (I-125) B Palladium 103 (Pd-103) C Californium 252 (Cf-252) Y Other Isotope	Z None
Ø Brain 1 Brain Stem 6 Spinal Cord 7 Peripheral Nerve	B Low Dose Rate (LDR)	6 Cesium 131 (Cs-131) 7 Cesium 137 (Cs-137) 8 Iridium 192 (Ir-192) 9 Iodine 125 (I-125) C Californium 252 (Cf-252) Y Other Isotope	Z None
Ø Brain 1 Brain Stem 6 Spinal Cord 7 Peripheral Nerve	B Low Dose Rate (LDR)	B Palladium 103 (Pd-103)	1 Unidirectional Source Z None

D Radiation Therapy
Ø Central and Peripheral Nervous System
2 Stereotactic Radiosurgery

Treatment Site Character 4	Modality Qualifier Character 5	Isotope Character 6	Qualifier Character 7
Ø Brain 1 Brain Stem 6 Spinal Cord 7 Peripheral Nerve	D Stereotactic Other Photon Radiosurgery H Stereotactic Particulate Radiosurgery J Stereotactic Gamma Beam Radiosurgery	Z None	Z None

DRG Non-OR All treatment site, modality, isotope, and qualifier values

D Radiation Therapy
Ø Central and Peripheral Nervous System
Y Other Radiation

Treatment Site Character 4	Modality Qualifier Character 5	Isotope Character 6	Qualifier Character 7
Ø Brain 1 Brain Stem 6 Spinal Cord 7 Peripheral Nerve	7 Contact Radiation 8 Hyperthermia C Intraoperative Radiation Therapy (IORT) F Plaque Radiation K Laser Interstitial Thermal Therapy	Z None	Z None

Valid OR DØY[Ø,1,6,7]KZZ

D Radiation Therapy
7 Lymphatic and Hematologic System
Ø Beam Radiation

Treatment Site Character 4	Modality Qualifier Character 5	Isotope Character 6	Qualifier Character 7
Ø Bone Marrow 1 Thymus 2 Spleen 3 Lymphatics, Neck 4 Lymphatics, Axillary 5 Lymphatics, Thorax 6 Lymphatics, Abdomen 7 Lymphatics, Pelvis 8 Lymphatics, Inguinal	Ø Photons <1 MeV 1 Photons 1 - 10 MeV 2 Photons >10 MeV 4 Heavy Particles (Protons, Ions) 5 Neutrons 6 Neutron Capture	Z None	Z None
Ø Bone Marrow 1 Thymus 2 Spleen 3 Lymphatics, Neck 4 Lymphatics, Axillary 5 Lymphatics, Thorax 6 Lymphatics, Abdomen 7 Lymphatics, Pelvis 8 Lymphatics, Inguinal	3 Electrons	Z None	Ø Intraoperative Z None

D Radiation Therapy
7 Lymphatic and Hematologic System
1 Brachytherapy

Treatment Site Character 4	Modality Qualifier Character 5	Isotope Character 6	Qualifier Character 7
Ø Bone Marrow 1 Thymus 2 Spleen 3 Lymphatics, Neck 4 Lymphatics, Axillary 5 Lymphatics, Thorax 6 Lymphatics, Abdomen 7 Lymphatics, Pelvis 8 Lymphatics, Inguinal	9 High Dose Rate (HDR)	7 Cesium 137 (Cs-137) 8 Iridium 192 (Ir-192) 9 Iodine 125 (I-125) B Palladium 103 (Pd-103) C Californium 252 (Cf-252) Y Other Isotope	Z None
Ø Bone Marrow 1 Thymus 2 Spleen 3 Lymphatics, Neck 4 Lymphatics, Axillary 5 Lymphatics, Thorax 6 Lymphatics, Abdomen 7 Lymphatics, Pelvis 8 Lymphatics, Inguinal	B Low Dose Rate (LDR)	6 Cesium 131 (Cs-131) 7 Cesium 137 (Cs-137) 8 Iridium 192 (Ir-192) 9 Iodine 125 (I-125) C Californium 252 (Cf-252) Y Other Isotope	Z None
Ø Bone Marrow 1 Thymus 2 Spleen 3 Lymphatics, Neck 4 Lymphatics, Axillary 5 Lymphatics, Thorax 6 Lymphatics, Abdomen 7 Lymphatics, Pelvis 8 Lymphatics, Inguinal	B Low Dose Rate (LDR)	B Palladium 103 (Pd-103)	1 Unidirectional Source Z None

D Radiation Therapy
7 Lymphatic and Hematologic System
2 Stereotactic Radiosurgery

Treatment Site Character 4	Modality Qualifier Character 5	Isotope Character 6	Qualifier Character 7
Ø Bone Marrow **1** Thymus **2** Spleen **3** Lymphatics, Neck **4** Lymphatics, Axillary **5** Lymphatics, Thorax **6** Lymphatics, Abdomen **7** Lymphatics, Pelvis **8** Lymphatics, Inguinal	**D** Stereotactic Other Photon Radiosurgery **H** Stereotactic Particulate Radiosurgery **J** Stereotactic Gamma Beam Radiosurgery	**Z** None	**Z** None

DRG Non-OR All treatment site, modality, isotope, and qualifier values

D Radiation Therapy
7 Lymphatic and Hematologic System
Y Other Radiation

Treatment Site Character 4	Modality Qualifier Character 5	Isotope Character 6	Qualifier Character 7
Ø Bone Marrow **1** Thymus **2** Spleen **3** Lymphatics, Neck **4** Lymphatics, Axillary **5** Lymphatics, Thorax **6** Lymphatics, Abdomen **7** Lymphatics, Pelvis **8** Lymphatics, Inguinal	**8** Hyperthermia **F** Plaque Radiation	**Z** None	**Z** None

D Radiation Therapy
8 Eye
Ø Beam Radiation

Treatment Site Character 4	Modality Qualifier Character 5	Isotope Character 6	Qualifier Character 7
Ø Eye	**Ø** Photons <1 MeV **1** Photons 1- 10 MeV **2** Photons >10 MeV **4** Heavy Particles (Protons, Ions) **5** Neutrons **6** Neutron Capture	**Z** None	**Z** None
Ø Eye	**3** Electrons	**Z** None	**Ø** Intraoperative **Z** None

D Radiation Therapy
8 Eye
1 Brachytherapy

Treatment Site Character 4	Modality Qualifier Character 5	Isotope Character 6	Qualifier Character 7
Ø Eye	**9** High Dose Rate (HDR)	**7** Cesium 137 (Cs-137) **8** Iridium 192 (Ir-192) **9** Iodine 125 (I-125) **B** Palladium 103 (Pd-103) **C** Californium 252 (Cf-252) **Y** Other Isotope	**Z** None
Ø Eye	**B** Low Dose Rate (LDR)	**6** Cesium 131 (Cs-131) **7** Cesium 137 (Cs-137) **8** Iridium 192 (Ir-192) **9** Iodine 125 (I-125) **C** Californium 252 (Cf-252) **Y** Other Isotope	**Z** None
Ø Eye	**B** Low Dose Rate (LDR)	**B** Palladium 103 (Pd-103)	**1** Unidirectional Source **Z** None

D Radiation Therapy
8 Eye
2 Stereotactic Radiosurgery

Treatment Site Character 4	Modality Qualifier Character 5	Isotope Character 6	Qualifier Character 7
Ø Eye	D Stereotactic Other Photon Radiosurgery H Stereotactic Particulate Radiosurgery J Stereotactic Gamma Beam Radiosurgery	Z None	Z None

DRG Non-OR All treatment site, modality, isotope, and qualifier values

D Radiation Therapy
8 Eye
Y Other Radiation

Treatment Site Character 4	Modality Qualifier Character 5	Isotope Character 6	Qualifier Character 7
Ø Eye	7 Contact Radiation 8 Hyperthermia F Plaque Radiation	Z None	Z None

D Radiation Therapy
9 Ear, Nose, Mouth and Throat
Ø Beam Radiation

Treatment Site Character 4	Modality Qualifier Character 5	Isotope Character 6	Qualifier Character 7
Ø Ear 1 Nose 3 Hypopharynx 4 Mouth 5 Tongue 6 Salivary Glands 7 Sinuses 8 Hard Palate 9 Soft Palate B Larynx D Nasopharynx F Oropharynx	Ø Photons <1 MeV 1 Photons 1- 10 MeV 2 Photons >10 MeV 4 Heavy Particles (Protons, Ions) 5 Neutrons 6 Neutron Capture	Z None	Z None
Ø Ear 1 Nose 3 Hypopharynx 4 Mouth 5 Tongue 6 Salivary Glands 7 Sinuses 8 Hard Palate 9 Soft Palate B Larynx D Nasopharynx F Oropharynx	3 Electrons	Z None	Ø Intraoperative Z None

D Radiation Therapy
9 Ear, Nose, Mouth and Throat
1 Brachytherapy

Treatment Site Character 4	Modality Qualifier Character 5	Isotope Character 6	Qualifier Character 7
Ø Ear 1 Nose 3 Hypopharynx 4 Mouth 5 Tongue 6 Salivary Glands 7 Sinuses 8 Hard Palate 9 Soft Palate B Larynx D Nasopharynx F Oropharynx	9 High Dose Rate (HDR)	7 Cesium 137 (Cs-137) 8 Iridium 192 (Ir-192) 9 Iodine 125 (I-125) B Palladium 103 (Pd-103) C Californium 252 (Cf-252) Y Other Isotope	Z None
Ø Ear 1 Nose 3 Hypopharynx 4 Mouth 5 Tongue 6 Salivary Glands 7 Sinuses 8 Hard Palate 9 Soft Palate B Larynx D Nasopharynx F Oropharynx	B Low Dose Rate (LDR)	6 Cesium 131 (Cs-131) 7 Cesium 137 (Cs-137) 8 Iridium 192 (Ir-192) 9 Iodine 125 (I-125) C Californium 252 (Cf-252) Y Other Isotope	Z None
Ø Ear 1 Nose 3 Hypopharynx 4 Mouth 5 Tongue 6 Salivary Glands 7 Sinuses 8 Hard Palate 9 Soft Palate B Larynx D Nasopharynx F Oropharynx	B Low Dose Rate (LDR)	B Palladium 103 (Pd-103)	1 Unidirectional Source Z None

D Radiation Therapy
9 Ear, Nose, Mouth and Throat
2 Stereotactic Radiosurgery

Treatment Site Character 4	Modality Qualifier Character 5	Isotope Character 6	Qualifier Character 7
Ø Ear 1 Nose 4 Mouth 5 Tongue 6 Salivary Glands 7 Sinuses 8 Hard Palate 9 Soft Palate B Larynx C Pharynx D Nasopharynx	D Stereotactic Other Photon Radiosurgery H Stereotactic Particulate Radiosurgery J Stereotactic Gamma Beam Radiosurgery	Z None	Z None

DRG Non-OR All treatment site, modality, isotope, and qualifier values

D Radiation Therapy
9 Ear, Nose, Mouth and Throat
Y Other Radiation

Treatment Site Character 4	Modality Qualifier Character 5	Isotope Character 6	Qualifier Character 7
Ø Ear 1 Nose 5 Tongue 6 Salivary Glands 7 Sinuses 8 Hard Palate 9 Soft Palate	7 Contact Radiation 8 Hyperthermia F Plaque Radiation	Z None	Z None
3 Hypopharynx F Oropharynx	7 Contact Radiation 8 Hyperthermia	Z None	Z None
4 Mouth B Larynx D Nasopharynx	7 Contact Radiation 8 Hyperthermia C Intraoperative Radiation Therapy (IORT) F Plaque Radiation	Z None	Z None
C Pharynx	C Intraoperative Radiation Therapy (IORT) F Plaque Radiation	Z None	Z None

D Radiation Therapy
B Respiratory System
Ø Beam Radiation

Treatment Site Character 4	Modality Qualifier Character 5	Isotope Character 6	Qualifier Character 7
Ø Trachea 1 Bronchus 2 Lung 5 Pleura 6 Mediastinum 7 Chest Wall 8 Diaphragm	Ø Photons <1 MeV 1 Photons 1- 10 MeV 2 Photons >10 MeV 4 Heavy Particles (Protons, Ions) 5 Neutrons 6 Neutron Capture	Z None	Z None
Ø Trachea 1 Bronchus 2 Lung 5 Pleura 6 Mediastinum 7 Chest Wall 8 Diaphragm	3 Electrons	Z None	Ø Intraoperative Z None

D Radiation Therapy
B Respiratory System
1 Brachytherapy

Treatment Site Character 4	Modality Qualifier Character 5	Isotope Character 6	Qualifier Character 7
Ø Trachea 1 Bronchus 2 Lung 5 Pleura 6 Mediastinum 7 Chest Wall 8 Diaphragm	9 High Dose Rate (HDR)	7 Cesium 137 (Cs-137) 8 Iridium 192 (Ir-192) 9 Iodine 125 (I-125) B Palladium 103 (Pd-103) C Californium 252 (Cf-252) Y Other Isotope	Z None
Ø Trachea 1 Bronchus 2 Lung 5 Pleura 6 Mediastinum 7 Chest Wall 8 Diaphragm	B Low Dose Rate (LDR)	6 Cesium 131 (Cs-131) 7 Cesium 137 (Cs-137) 8 Iridium 192 (Ir-192) 9 Iodine 125 (I-125) C Californium 252 (Cf-252) Y Other Isotope	Z None
Ø Trachea 1 Bronchus 2 Lung 5 Pleura 6 Mediastinum 7 Chest Wall 8 Diaphragm	B Low Dose Rate (LDR)	B Palladium 103 (Pd-103)	1 Unidirectional Source Z None

D Radiation Therapy
B Respiratory System
2 Stereotactic Radiosurgery

Treatment Site Character 4	Modality Qualifier Character 5	Isotope Character 6	Qualifier Character 7
Ø Trachea 1 Bronchus 2 Lung 5 Pleura 6 Mediastinum 7 Chest Wall 8 Diaphragm	D Stereotactic Other Photon Radiosurgery H Stereotactic Particulate Radiosurgery J Stereotactic Gamma Beam Radiosurgery	Z None	Z None

DRG Non-OR All treatment site, modality, isotope, and qualifier values

D Radiation Therapy
B Respiratory System
Y Other Radiation

Treatment Site Character 4	Modality Qualifier Character 5	Isotope Character 6	Qualifier Character 7
Ø Trachea 1 Bronchus 2 Lung 5 Pleura 6 Mediastinum 7 Chest Wall 8 Diaphragm	7 Contact Radiation 8 Hyperthermia F Plaque Radiation K Laser Interstitial Thermal Therapy	Z None	Z None

Valid OR DBY[Ø,1,2,5,6,7,8]KZZ

D Radiation Therapy
D Gastrointestinal System
Ø Beam Radiation

Treatment Site Character 4	Modality Qualifier Character 5	Isotope Character 6	Qualifier Character 7
Ø Esophagus 1 Stomach 2 Duodenum 3 Jejunum 4 Ileum 5 Colon 7 Rectum	Ø Photons <1 MeV 1 Photons 1- 10 MeV 2 Photons >10 MeV 4 Heavy Particles (Protons, Ions) 5 Neutrons 6 Neutron Capture	Z None	Z None
Ø Esophagus 1 Stomach 2 Duodenum 3 Jejunum 4 Ileum 5 Colon 7 Rectum	3 Electrons	Z None	Ø Intraoperative Z None

D Radiation Therapy
D Gastrointestinal System
1 Brachytherapy

Treatment Site Character 4	Modality Qualifier Character 5	Isotope Character 6	Qualifier Character 7
Ø Esophagus 1 Stomach 2 Duodenum 3 Jejunum 4 Ileum 5 Colon 7 Rectum	9 High Dose Rate (HDR)	7 Cesium 137 (Cs-137) 8 Iridium 192 (Ir-192) 9 Iodine 125 (I-125) B Palladium 103 (Pd-103) C Californium 252 (Cf-252) Y Other Isotope	Z None
Ø Esophagus 1 Stomach 2 Duodenum 3 Jejunum 4 Ileum 5 Colon 7 Rectum	B Low Dose Rate (LDR)	6 Cesium 131 (Cs-131) 7 Cesium 137 (Cs-137) 8 Iridium 192 (Ir-192) 9 Iodine 125 (I-125) C Californium 252 (Cf-252) Y Other Isotope	Z None
Ø Esophagus 1 Stomach 2 Duodenum 3 Jejunum 4 Ileum 5 Colon 7 Rectum	B Low Dose Rate (LDR)	B Palladium 103 (Pd-103)	1 Unidirectional Source Z None

D Radiation Therapy
D Gastrointestinal System
2 Stereotactic Radiosurgery

Treatment Site Character 4	Modality Qualifier Character 5	Isotope Character 6	Qualifier Character 7
Ø Esophagus 1 Stomach 2 Duodenum 3 Jejunum 4 Ileum 5 Colon 7 Rectum	D Stereotactic Other Photon Radiosurgery H Stereotactic Particulate Radiosurgery J Stereotactic Gamma Beam Radiosurgery	Z None	Z None

DRG Non-OR All treatment site, modality, isotope, and qualifier values

D Radiation therapy
D Gastrointestinal System
Y Other Radiation

Treatment Site Character 4	Modality Qualifier Character 5	Isotope Character 6	Qualifier Character 7
Ø Esophagus	7 Contact Radiation 8 Hyperthermia F Plaque Radiation K Laser Interstitial Thermal Therapy	Z None	Z None
1 Stomach 2 Duodenum 3 Jejunum 4 Ileum 5 Colon 7 Rectum	7 Contact Radiation 8 Hyperthermia C Intraoperative Radiation Therapy (IORT) F Plaque Radiation K Laser Interstitial Thermal Therapy	Z None	Z None
8 Anus	C Intraoperative Radiation Therapy (IORT) F Plaque Radiation K Laser Interstitial Thermal Therapy	Z None	Z None

Valid OR DDYØKZZ
Valid OR DDY[1,2,3,4,5,7]KZZ
Valid OR DDY8KZZ

D Radiation Therapy
F Hepatobiliary System and Pancreas
Ø Beam Radiation

Treatment Site Character 4	Modality Qualifier Character 5	Isotope Character 6	Qualifier Character 7
Ø Liver 1 Gallbladder 2 Bile Ducts 3 Pancreas	Ø Photons <1 MeV 1 Photons 1- 10 MeV 2 Photons >10 MeV 4 Heavy Particles (Protons, Ions) 5 Neutrons 6 Neutron Capture	Z None	Z None
Ø Liver 1 Gallbladder 2 Bile Ducts 3 Pancreas	3 Electrons	Z None	Ø Intraoperative Z None

D Radiation Therapy
F Hepatobiliary System and Pancreas
1 Brachytherapy

Treatment Site Character 4	Modality Qualifier Character 5	Isotope Character 6	Qualifier Character 7
Ø Liver 1 Gallbladder 2 Bile Ducts 3 Pancreas	9 High Dose Rate (HDR)	7 Cesium 137 (Cs-137) 8 Iridium 192 (Ir-192) 9 Iodine 125 (I-125) B Palladium 103 (Pd-103) C Californium 252 (Cf-252) Y Other Isotope	Z None
Ø Liver 1 Gallbladder 2 Bile Ducts 3 Pancreas	B Low Dose Rate (LDR)	6 Cesium 131 (Cs-131) 7 Cesium 137 (Cs-137) 8 Iridium 192 (Ir-192) 9 Iodine 125 (I-125) C Californium 252 (Cf-252) Y Other Isotope	Z None
Ø Liver 1 Gallbladder 2 Bile Ducts 3 Pancreas	B Low Dose Rate (LDR)	B Palladium 103 (Pd-103)	1 Unidirectional Source Z None

D Radiation Therapy
F Hepatobiliary System and Pancreas
2 Stereotactic Radiosurgery

Treatment Site Character 4	Modality Qualifier Character 5	Isotope Character 6	Qualifier Character 7
Ø Liver 1 Gallbladder 2 Bile Ducts 3 Pancreas	D Stereotactic Other Photon Radiosurgery H Stereotactic Particulate Radiosurgery J Stereotactic Gamma Beam Radiosurgery	Z None	Z None

DRG Non-OR All treatment site, modality, isotope, and qualifier values

D Radiation Therapy
F Hepatobiliary System and Pancreas
Y Other Radiation

Treatment Site Character 4	Modality Qualifier Character 5	Isotope Character 6	Qualifier Character 7
Ø Liver 1 Gallbladder 2 Bile Ducts 3 Pancreas	7 Contact Radiation 8 Hyperthermia C Intraoperative Radiation Therapy (IORT) F Plaque Radiation K Laser Interstitial Thermal Therapy	Z None	Z None

Valid OR DFY[Ø,1,2,3]KZZ

D Radiation Therapy
G Endocrine System
Ø Beam Radiation

Treatment Site Character 4	Modality Qualifier Character 5	Isotope Character 6	Qualifier Character 7
Ø Pituitary Gland **1** Pineal Body **2** Adrenal Glands **4** Parathyroid Glands **5** Thyroid	**Ø** Photons <1 MeV **1** Photons 1- 10 MeV **2** Photons >10 MeV **5** Neutrons **6** Neutron Capture	**Z** None	**Z** None
Ø Pituitary Gland **1** Pineal Body **2** Adrenal Glands **4** Parathyroid Glands **5** Thyroid	**3** Electrons	**Z** None	**Ø** Intraoperative **Z** None

D Radiation Therapy
G Endocrine System
1 Brachytherapy

Treatment Site Character 4	Modality Qualifier Character 5	Isotope Character 6	Qualifier Character 7
Ø Pituitary Gland **1** Pineal Body **2** Adrenal Glands **4** Parathyroid Glands **5** Thyroid	**9** High Dose Rate (HDR)	**7** Cesium 137 (Cs-137) **8** Iridium 192 (Ir-192) **9** Iodine 125 (I-125) **B** Palladium 103 (Pd-103) **C** Californium 252 (Cf-252) **Y** Other Isotope	**Z** None
Ø Pituitary Gland **1** Pineal Body **2** Adrenal Glands **4** Parathyroid Glands **5** Thyroid	**B** Low Dose Rate (LDR)	**6** Cesium 131 (Cs-131) **7** Cesium 137 (Cs-137) **8** Iridium 192 (Ir-192) **9** Iodine 125 (I-125) **C** Californium 252 (Cf-252) **Y** Other Isotope	**Z** None
Ø Pituitary Gland **1** Pineal Body **2** Adrenal Glands **4** Parathyroid Glands **5** Thyroid	**B** Low Dose Rate (LDR)	**B** Palladium 103 (Pd-103)	**1** Unidirectional Source **Z** None

D Radiation Therapy
G Endocrine System
2 Stereotactic Radiosurgery

Treatment Site Character 4	Modality Qualifier Character 5	Isotope Character 6	Qualifier Character 7
Ø Pituitary Gland **1** Pineal Body **2** Adrenal Glands **4** Parathyroid Glands **5** Thyroid	**D** Stereotactic Other Photon Radiosurgery **H** Stereotactic Particulate Radiosurgery **J** Stereotactic Gamma Beam Radiosurgery	**Z** None	**Z** None

DRG Non-OR All treatment site, modality, isotope, and qualifier values

D Radiation therapy
G Endocrine System
Y Other Radiation

Treatment Site Character 4	Modality Qualifier Character 5	Isotope Character 6	Qualifier Character 7
Ø Pituitary Gland **1** Pineal Body **2** Adrenal Glands **4** Parathyroid Glands **5** Thyroid	**7** Contact Radiation **8** Hyperthermia **F** Plaque Radiation **K** Laser Interstitial Thermal Therapy	**Z** None	**Z** None

Valid OR DGY[Ø,1,2,4,5]KZZ

D Radiation Therapy
H Skin
Ø Beam Radiation

Treatment Site Character 4	Modality Qualifier Character 5	Isotope Character 6	Qualifier Character 7
2 Skin, Face 3 Skin, Neck 4 Skin, Arm 6 Skin, Chest 7 Skin, Back 8 Skin, Abdomen 9 Skin, Buttock B Skin, Leg	Ø Photons <1 MeV 1 Photons 1- 10 MeV 2 Photons >10 MeV 4 Heavy Particles (Protons, Ions) 5 Neutrons 6 Neutron Capture	Z None	Z None
2 Skin, Face 3 Skin, Neck 4 Skin, Arm 6 Skin, Chest 7 Skin, Back 8 Skin, Abdomen 9 Skin, Buttock B Skin, Leg	3 Electrons	Z None	Ø Intraoperative Z None

D Radiation Therapy
H Skin
Y Other Radiation

Treatment Site Character 4	Modality Qualifier Character 5	Isotope Character 6	Qualifier Character 7
2 Skin, Face 3 Skin, Neck 4 Skin, Arm 6 Skin, Chest 7 Skin, Back 8 Skin, Abdomen 9 Skin, Buttock B Skin, Leg	7 Contact Radiation 8 Hyperthermia F Plaque Radiation	Z None	Z None
5 Skin, Hand C Skin, Foot	F Plaque Radiation	Z None	Z None

D Radiation Therapy
M Breast
Ø Beam Radiation

Treatment Site Character 4	Modality Qualifier Character 5	Isotope Character 6	Qualifier Character 7
Ø Breast, Left 1 Breast, Right	Ø Photons <1 MeV 1 Photons 1- 10 MeV 2 Photons >10 MeV 4 Heavy Particles (Protons, Ions) 5 Neutrons 6 Neutron Capture	Z None	Z None
Ø Breast, Left 1 Breast, Right	3 Electrons	Z None	Ø Intraoperative Z None

D Radiation Therapy
M Breast
1 Brachytherapy

Treatment Site Character 4	Modality Qualifier Character 5	Isotope Character 6	Qualifier Character 7
Ø Breast, Left 1 Breast, Right	9 High Dose Rate (HDR)	7 Cesium 137 (Cs-137) 8 Iridium 192 (Ir-192) 9 Iodine 125 (I-125) B Palladium 103 (Pd-103) C Californium 252 (Cf-252) Y Other Isotope	Z None
Ø Breast, Left 1 Breast, Right	B Low Dose Rate (LDR)	6 Cesium 131 (Cs-131) 7 Cesium 137 (Cs-137) 8 Iridium 192 (Ir-192) 9 Iodine 125 (I-125) C Californium 252 (Cf-252) Y Other Isotope	Z None
Ø Breast, Left 1 Breast, Right	B Low Dose Rate (LDR)	B Palladium 103 (Pd-103)	1 Unidirectional Source Z None

D Radiation Therapy
M Breast
2 Stereotactic Radiosurgery

Treatment Site Character 4	Modality Qualifier Character 5	Isotope Character 6	Qualifier Character 7
Ø Breast, Left 1 Breast, Right	D Stereotactic Other Photon Radiosurgery H Stereotactic Particulate Radiosurgery J Stereotactic Gamma Beam Radiosurgery	Z None	Z None

DRG Non-OR All treatment site, modality, isotope, and qualifier values

D Radiation Therapy
M Breast
Y Other Radiation

Treatment Site Character 4	Modality Qualifier Character 5	Isotope Character 6	Qualifier Character 7
Ø Breast, Left 1 Breast, Right	7 Contact Radiation 8 Hyperthermia F Plaque Radiation K Laser Interstitial Thermal Therapy	Z None	Z None

Valid OR DMY[Ø,1]KZZ

D Radiation Therapy
P Musculoskeletal System
Ø Beam Radiation

Treatment Site Character 4	Modality Qualifier Character 5	Isotope Character 6	Qualifier Character 7
Ø Skull 2 Maxilla 3 Mandible 4 Sternum 5 Rib(s) 6 Humerus 7 Radius/Ulna 8 Pelvic Bones 9 Femur B Tibia/Fibula C Other Bone	Ø Photons <1 MeV 1 Photons 1- 10 MeV 2 Photons >10 MeV 4 Heavy Particles (Protons, Ions) 5 Neutrons 6 Neutron Capture	Z None	Z None
Ø Skull 2 Maxilla 3 Mandible 4 Sternum 5 Rib(s) 6 Humerus 7 Radius/Ulna 8 Pelvic Bones 9 Femur B Tibia/Fibula C Other Bone	3 Electrons	Z None	Ø Intraoperative Z None

D Radiation Therapy
P Musculoskeletal System
Y Other Radiation

Treatment Site Character 4	Modality Qualifier Character 5	Isotope Character 6	Qualifier Character 7
Ø Skull 2 Maxilla 3 Mandible 4 Sternum 5 Rib(s) 6 Humerus 7 Radius/Ulna 8 Pelvic Bones 9 Femur B Tibia/Fibula C Other Bone	7 Contact Radiation 8 Hyperthermia F Plaque Radiation	Z None	Z None

D Radiation Therapy
T Urinary System
Ø Beam Radiation

Treatment Site Character 4	Modality Qualifier Character 5	Isotope Character 6	Qualifier Character 7
Ø Kidney **1** Ureter **2** Bladder **3** Urethra	**Ø** Photons <1 MeV **1** Photons 1- 10 MeV **2** Photons >10 MeV **4** Heavy Particles (Protons, Ions) **5** Neutrons **6** Neutron Capture	**Z** None	**Z** None
Ø Kidney **1** Ureter **2** Bladder **3** Urethra	**3** Electrons	**Z** None	**Ø** Intraoperative **Z** None

D Radiation Therapy
T Urinary System
1 Brachytherapy

Treatment Site Character 4	Modality Qualifier Character 5	Isotope Character 6	Qualifier Character 7
Ø Kidney **1** Ureter **2** Bladder **3** Urethra	**9** High Dose Rate (HDR)	**7** Cesium 137 (Cs-137) **8** Iridium 192 (Ir-192) **9** Iodine 125 (I-125) **B** Palladium 103 (Pd-103) **C** Californium 252 (Cf-252) **Y** Other Isotope	**Z** None
Ø Kidney **1** Ureter **2** Bladder **3** Urethra	**B** Low Dose Rate (LDR)	**6** Cesium 131 (Cs-131) **7** Cesium 137 (Cs-137) **8** Iridium 192 (Ir-192) **9** Iodine 125 (I-125) **C** Californium 252 (Cf-252) **Y** Other Isotope	**Z** None
Ø Kidney **1** Ureter **2** Bladder **3** Urethra	**B** Low Dose Rate (LDR)	**B** Palladium 103 (Pd-103)	**1** Unidirectional Source **Z** None

D Radiation Therapy
T Urinary System
2 Stereotactic Radiosurgery

Treatment Site Character 4	Modality Qualifier Character 5	Isotope Character 6	Qualifier Character 7
Ø Kidney **1** Ureter **2** Bladder **3** Urethra	**D** Stereotactic Other Photon Radiosurgery **H** Stereotactic Particulate Radiosurgery **J** Stereotactic Gamma Beam Radiosurgery	**Z** None	**Z** None

DRG Non-OR All treatment site, modality, isotope, and qualifier values

D Radiation Therapy
T Urinary System
Y Other Radiation

Treatment Site Character 4	Modality Qualifier Character 5	Isotope Character 6	Qualifier Character 7
Ø Kidney **1** Ureter **2** Bladder **3** Urethra	**7** Contact Radiation **8** Hyperthermia **C** Intraoperative Radiation Therapy (IORT) **F** Plaque Radiation	**Z** None	**Z** None

D Radiation Therapy
U Female Reproductive System
Ø Beam Radiation

Treatment Site Character 4	Modality Qualifier Character 5	Isotope Character 6	Qualifier Character 7
Ø Ovary ♀ 1 Cervix ♀ 2 Uterus ♀	Ø Photons <1 MeV 1 Photons 1- 10 MeV 2 Photons >10 MeV 4 Heavy Particles (Protons, Ions) 5 Neutrons 6 Neutron Capture	Z None	Z None
Ø Ovary ♀ 1 Cervix ♀ 2 Uterus ♀	3 Electrons	Z None	Ø Intraoperative Z None

♀ All treatment site, modality, isotope, and qualifier values

D Radiation Therapy
U Female Reproductive System
1 Brachytherapy

Treatment Site Character 4	Modality Qualifier Character 5	Isotope Character 6	Qualifier Character 7
Ø Ovary ♀ 1 Cervix ♀ 2 Uterus ♀	9 High Dose Rate (HDR)	7 Cesium 137 (Cs-137) 8 Iridium 192 (Ir-192) 9 Iodine 125 (I-125) B Palladium 103 (Pd-103) C Californium 252 (Cf-252) Y Other Isotope	Z None
Ø Ovary ♀ 1 Cervix ♀ 2 Uterus ♀	B Low Dose Rate (LDR)	6 Cesium 131 (Cs-131) 7 Cesium 137 (Cs-137) 8 Iridium 192 (Ir-192) 9 Iodine 125 (I-125) C Californium 252 (Cf-252) Y Other Isotope	Z None
Ø Ovary ♀ 1 Cervix ♀ 2 Uterus ♀	B Low Dose Rate (LDR)	B Palladium 103 (Pd-103)	1 Unidirectional Source Z None

♀ All treatment site, modality, isotope, and qualifier values

D Radiation Therapy
U Female Reproductive System
2 Stereotactic Radiosurgery

Treatment Site Character 4	Modality Qualifier Character 5	Isotope Character 6	Qualifier Character 7
Ø Ovary ♀ 1 Cervix ♀ 2 Uterus ♀	D Stereotactic Other Photon Radiosurgery H Stereotactic Particulate Radiosurgery J Stereotactic Gamma Beam Radiosurgery	Z None	Z None

DRG Non-OR All treatment site, modality, isotope, and qualifier values
♀ All treatment site, modality, isotope, and qualifier values

D Radiation Therapy
U Female Reproductive System
Y Other Radiation

Treatment Site Character 4	Modality Qualifier Character 5	Isotope Character 6	Qualifier Character 7
Ø Ovary ♀ 1 Cervix ♀ 2 Uterus ♀	7 Contact Radiation 8 Hyperthermia C Intraoperative Radiation Therapy (IORT) F Plaque Radiation	Z None	Z None

♀ All treatment site, modality, isotope, and qualifier values

D Radiation Therapy
V Male Reproductive System
Ø Beam Radiation

Treatment Site Character 4	Modality Qualifier Character 5	Isotope Character 6	Qualifier Character 7
Ø Prostate ♂ 1 Testis ♂	Ø Photons <1 MeV 1 Photons 1- 10 MeV 2 Photons >10 MeV 4 Heavy Particles (Protons, Ions) 5 Neutrons 6 Neutron Capture	Z None	Z None
Ø Prostate ♂ 1 Testis ♂	3 Electrons	Z None	Ø Intraoperative Z None

♂ All treatment site, modality, isotope, and qualifier values

D Radiation Therapy
V Male Reproductive System
1 Brachytherapy

Treatment Site Character 4	Modality Qualifier Character 5	Isotope Character 6	Qualifier Character 7
Ø Prostate ♂ 1 Testis ♂	9 High Dose Rate (HDR)	7 Cesium 137 (Cs-137) 8 Iridium 192 (Ir-192) 9 Iodine 125 (I-125) B Palladium 103 (Pd-103) C Californium 252 (Cf-252) Y Other Isotope	Z None
Ø Prostate ♂ 1 Testis ♂	B Low Dose Rate (LDR)	6 Cesium 131 (Cs-131) 7 Cesium 137 (Cs-137) 8 Iridium 192 (Ir-192) 9 Iodine 125 (I-125) C Californium 252 (Cf-252) Y Other Isotope	Z None
Ø Prostate ♂ 1 Testis ♂	B Low Dose Rate (LDR)	B Palladium 103 (Pd-103)	1 Unidirectional Source Z None

♂ All treatment site, modality, isotope, and qualifier values

D Radiation Therapy
V Male Reproductive System
2 Stereotactic Radiosurgery

Treatment Site Character 4	Modality Qualifier Character 5	Isotope Character 6	Qualifier Character 7
Ø Prostate ♂ 1 Testis ♂	D Stereotactic Other Photon Radiosurgery H Stereotactic Particulate Radiosurgery J Stereotactic Gamma Beam Radiosurgery	Z None	Z None

DRG Non-OR All treatment site, modality, isotope, and qualifier values
♂ All treatment site, modality, isotope, and qualifier values

D Radiation Therapy
V Male Reproductive System
Y Other Radiation

Treatment Site Character 4	Modality Qualifier Character 5	Isotope Character 6	Qualifier Character 7
Ø Prostate ♂	7 Contact Radiation 8 Hyperthermia C Intraoperative Radiation Therapy (IORT) F Plaque Radiation K Laser Interstitial Thermal Therapy	Z None	Z None
1 Testis ♂	7 Contact Radiation 8 Hyperthermia F Plaque Radiation	Z None	Z None

Valid OR DVYØKZZ
♂ All treatment site, modality, isotope, and qualifier values

D Radiation Therapy
W Anatomical Regions
Ø Beam Radiation

Treatment Site Character 4	Modality Qualifier Character 5	Isotope Character 6	Qualifier Character 7
1 Head and Neck 2 Chest 3 Abdomen 4 Hemibody 5 Whole Body 6 Pelvic Region	Ø Photons <1 MeV 1 Photons 1- 10 MeV 2 Photons >10 MeV 4 Heavy Particles (Protons, Ions) 5 Neutrons 6 Neutron Capture	Z None	Z None
1 Head and Neck 2 Chest 3 Abdomen 4 Hemibody 5 Whole Body 6 Pelvic Region	3 Electrons	Z None	Ø Intraoperative Z None

D Radiation Therapy
W Anatomical Regions
1 Brachytherapy

Treatment Site Character 4	Modality Qualifier Character 5	Isotope Character 6	Qualifier Character 7
Ø Cranial Cavity K Upper Back L Lower Back P Gastrointestinal Tract Q Respiratory Tract R Genitourinary Tract X Upper Extremity Y Lower Extremity	B Low Dose Rate (LDR)	B Palladium 103 (Pd-103)	1 Unidirectional Source Z None
1 Head and Neck 2 Chest 3 Abdomen 6 Pelvic Region	9 High Dose Rate (HDR)	7 Cesium 137 (Cs-137) 8 Iridium 192 (Ir-192) 9 Iodine 125 (I-125) B Palladium 103 (Pd-103) C Californium 252 (Cf-252) Y Other Isotope	Z None
1 Head and Neck 2 Chest 3 Abdomen 6 Pelvic Region	B Low Dose Rate (LDR)	6 Cesium 131 (Cs-131) 7 Cesium 137 (Cs-137) 8 Iridium 192 (Ir-192) 9 Iodine 125 (I-125) C Californium 252 (Cf-252) Y Other Isotope	Z None
1 Head and Neck 2 Chest 3 Abdomen 6 Pelvic Region	B Low Dose Rate (LDR)	B Palladium 103 (Pd-103)	1 Unidirectional Source Z None

D Radiation Therapy
W Anatomical Regions
2 Stereotactic Radiosurgery

Treatment Site Character 4	Modality Qualifier Character 5	Isotope Character 6	Qualifier Character 7
1 Head and Neck 2 Chest 3 Abdomen 6 Pelvic Region	D Stereotactic Other Photon Radiosurgery H Stereotactic Particulate Radiosurgery J Stereotactic Gamma Beam Radiosurgery	Z None	Z None

DRG Non-OR All treatment site, modality, isotope, and qualifier values

D Radiation Therapy
W Anatomical Regions
Y Other Radiation

Treatment Site Character 4	Modality Qualifier Character 5	Isotope Character 6	Qualifier Character 7
1 Head and Neck 2 Chest 3 Abdomen 4 Hemibody 6 Pelvic Region	7 Contact Radiation 8 Hyperthermia F Plaque Radiation	Z None	Z None
5 Whole Body	7 Contact Radiation 8 Hyperthermia F Plaque Radiation	Z None	Z None
5 Whole Body	G Isotope Administration	D Iodine 131 (I-131) F Phosphorus 32 (P-32) G Strontium 89 (Sr-89) H Strontium 90 (Sr-90) Y Other Isotope	Z None

Physical Rehabilitation and Diagnostic Audiology FØØ–F15

F Physical Rehabilitation and Diagnostic Audiology
Ø Rehabilitation
Ø Speech Assessment Definition: Measurement of speech and related functions

Body System/Region Character 4	Type Qualifier Character 5	Equipment Character 6	Qualifier Character 7
3 Neurological System - Whole Body	G Communicative/Cognitive Integration Skills	K Audiovisual M Augmentative / Alternative Communication P Computer Y Other Equipment Z None	Z None
Z None	Ø Filtered Speech 3 Staggered Spondaic Word Q Performance Intensity Phonetically Balanced Speech Discrimination R Brief Tone Stimuli S Distorted Speech T Dichotic Stimuli V Temporal Ordering of Stimuli W Masking Patterns	1 Audiometer 2 Sound Field / Booth K Audiovisual Z None	Z None
Z None	1 Speech Threshold 2 Speech/Word Recognition	1 Audiometer 2 Sound Field / Booth 9 Cochlear Implant K Audiovisual Z None	Z None
Z None	4 Sensorineural Acuity Level	1 Audiometer 2 Sound Field / Booth Z None	Z None
Z None	5 Synthetic Sentence Identification	1 Audiometer 2 Sound Field / Booth 9 Cochlear Implant K Audiovisual	Z None
Z None	6 Speech and/or Language Screening 7 Nonspoken Language 8 Receptive/Expressive Language C Aphasia G Communicative/Cognitive Integration Skills L Augmentative/Alternative Communication System	K Audiovisual M Augmentative / Alternative Communication P Computer Y Other Equipment Z None	Z None
Z None	9 Articulation/Phonology	K Audiovisual P Computer Q Speech Analysis Y Other Equipment Z None	Z None
Z None	B Motor Speech	K Audiovisual N Biosensory Feedback P Computer Q Speech Analysis T Aerodynamic Function Y Other Equipment Z None	Z None
Z None	D Fluency	K Audiovisual N Biosensory Feedback P Computer Q Speech Analysis S Voice Analysis T Aerodynamic Function Y Other Equipment Z None	Z None
Z None	F Voice	K Audiovisual N Biosensory Feedback P Computer S Voice Analysis T Aerodynamic Function Y Other Equipment Z None	Z None

DRG Non-OR All body system/region, type qualifier, equipment, and qualifier values

FØØ Continued on next page

F Physical Rehabilitation and Diagnostic Audiology
0 Rehabilitation
0 Speech Assessment Definition: Measurement of speech and related functions

F00 Continued

Body System/Region Character 4	Type Qualifier Character 5	Equipment Character 6	Qualifier Character 7
Z None	**H** Bedside Swallowing and Oral Function **P** Oral Peripheral Mechanism	**Y** Other Equipment **Z** None	**Z** None
Z None	**J** Instrumental Swallowing and Oral Function	**T** Aerodynamic Function **W** Swallowing **Y** Other Equipment	**Z** None
Z None	**K** Orofacial Myofunctional	**K** Audiovisual **P** Computer **Y** Other Equipment **Z** None	**Z** None
Z None	**M** Voice Prosthetic	**K** Audiovisual **P** Computer **S** Voice Analysis **V** Speech Prosthesis **Y** Other Equipment **Z** None	**Z** None
Z None	**N** Non-invasive Instrumental Status	**N** Biosensory Feedback **P** Computer **Q** Speech Analysis **S** Voice Analysis **T** Aerodynamic Function **Y** Other Equipment	**Z** None
Z None	**X** Other Specified Central Auditory Processing	**Z** None	**Z** None

DRG Non-OR All body system/region, type qualifier, equipment, and qualifier values

F Physical Rehabilitation and Diagnostic Audiology
0 Rehabilitation
1 Motor and/or Nerve Function Assessment Definition: Measurement of motor, nerve, and related functions

Body System/Region Character 4	Type Qualifier Character 5	Equipment Character 6	Qualifier Character 7
0 Neurological System - Head and Neck **1** Neurological System - Upper Back/ Upper Extremity **2** Neurological System - Lower Back/ Lower Extremity **3** Neurological System - Whole Body	**0** Muscle Performance	**E** Orthosis **F** Assistive, Adaptive, Supportive or Protective **U** Prosthesis **Y** Other Equipment **Z** None	**Z** None
0 Neurological System - Head and Neck **1** Neurological System - Upper Back/ Upper Extremity **2** Neurological System - Lower Back/ Lower Extremity **3** Neurological System - Whole Body	**1** Integumentary Integrity **3** Coordination/Dexterity **4** Motor Function **G** Reflex Integrity	**Z** None	**Z** None
0 Neurological System - Head and Neck **1** Neurological System - Upper Back/ Upper Extremity **2** Neurological System - Lower Back/ Lower Extremity **3** Neurological System - Whole Body	**5** Range of Motion and Joint Integrity **6** Sensory Awareness/Processing/ Integrity	**Y** Other Equipment **Z** None	**Z** None
D Integumentary System - Head and Neck **F** Integumentary System - Upper Back/ Upper Extremity **G** Integumentary System - Lower Back/ Lower Extremity **H** Integumentary System - Whole Body **J** Musculoskeletal System - Head and Neck **K** Musculoskeletal System - Upper Back/ Upper Extremity **L** Musculoskeletal System - Lower Back/ Lower Extremity **M** Musculoskeletal System - Whole Body	**0** Muscle Performance	**E** Orthosis **F** Assistive, Adaptive, Supportive or Protective **U** Prosthesis **Y** Other Equipment **Z** None	**Z** None

DRG Non-OR All body system/region, type qualifier, equipment, and qualifier values

F01 Continued on next page

F01 Continued

F Physical Rehabilitation and Diagnostic Audiology
0 Rehabilitation
1 Motor and/or Nerve Function Assessment Definition: Measurement of motor, nerve, and related functions

Body System/Region Character 4	Type Qualifier Character 5	Equipment Character 6	Qualifier Character 7
D Integumentary System - Head and Neck F Integumentary System - Upper Back/ Upper Extremity G Integumentary System - Lower Back/ Lower Extremity H Integumentary System - Whole Body J Musculoskeletal System - Head and Neck K Musculoskeletal System - Upper Back/ Upper Extremity L Musculoskeletal System - Lower Back/ Lower Extremity M Musculoskeletal System - Whole Body	1 Integumentary Integrity	Z None	Z None
D Integumentary System - Head and Neck F Integumentary System - Upper Back/ Upper Extremity G Integumentary System - Lower Back/ Lower Extremity H Integumentary System - Whole Body J Musculoskeletal System - Head and Neck K Musculoskeletal System - Upper Back/ Upper Extremity L Musculoskeletal System - Lower Back/ Lower Extremity M Musculoskeletal System - Whole Body	5 Range of Motion and Joint Integrity 6 Sensory Awareness/Processing/ Integrity	Y Other Equipment Z None	Z None
N Genitourinary System	0 Muscle Performance	E Orthosis F Assistive, Adaptive, Supportive or Protective U Prosthesis Y Other Equipment Z None	Z None
Z None	2 Visual Motor Integration	K Audiovisual M Augmentative / Alternative Communication N Biosensory Feedback P Computer Q Speech Analysis S Voice Analysis Y Other Equipment Z None	Z None
Z None	7 Facial Nerve Function	7 Electrophysiologic	Z None
Z None	9 Somatosensory Evoked Potentials	J Somatosensory	Z None
Z None	B Bed Mobility C Transfer F Wheelchair Mobility	E Orthosis F Assistive, Adaptive, Supportive or Protective U Prosthesis Z None	Z None
Z None	D Gait and/or Balance	E Orthosis F Assistive, Adaptive, Supportive or Protective U Prosthesis Y Other Equipment Z None	Z None

DRG Non-OR All body system/region, type qualifier, equipment, and qualifier values

F Physical Rehabilitation and Diagnostic Audiology
Ø Rehabilitation
2 Activities of Daily Living Assessment Definition: Measurement of functional level for activities of daily living

Body System/Region Character 4	Type Qualifier Character 5	Equipment Character 6	Qualifier Character 7
Ø Neurological System - Head and Neck	9 Cranial Nerve Integrity D Neuromotor Development	Y Other Equipment Z None	Z None
1 Neurological System - Upper Back/ Upper Extremity 2 Neurological System - Lower Back/ Lower Extremity 3 Neurological System - Whole Body	D Neuromotor Development	Y Other Equipment Z None	Z None
4 Circulatory System - Head and Neck 5 Circulatory System - Upper Back/ Upper Extremity 6 Circulatory System - Lower Back/ Lower Extremity 8 Respiratory System - Head and Neck 9 Respiratory System - Upper Back/ Upper Extremity B Respiratory System - Lower Back/ Lower Extremity	G Ventilation, Respiration and Circulation	C Mechanical G Aerobic Endurance and Conditioning Y Other Equipment Z None	Z None
7 Circulatory System - Whole Body C Respiratory System - Whole Body	7 Aerobic Capacity and Endurance	E Orthosis G Aerobic Endurance and Conditioning U Prosthesis Y Other Equipment Z None	Z None
7 Circulatory System - Whole Body C Respiratory System - Whole Body	G Ventilation, Respiration and Circulation	C Mechanical G Aerobic Endurance and Conditioning Y Other Equipment Z None	Z None
Z None	Ø Bathing/Showering 1 Dressing 3 Grooming/Personal Hygiene 4 Home Management	E Orthosis F Assistive, Adaptive, Supportive or Protective U Prosthesis Z None	Z None
Z None	2 Feeding/Eating 8 Anthropometric Characteristics F Pain	Y Other Equipment Z None	Z None
Z None	5 Perceptual Processing	K Audiovisual M Augmentative / Alternative Communication N Biosensory Feedback P Computer Q Speech Analysis S Voice Analysis Y Other Equipment Z None	Z None
Z None	6 Psychosocial Skills	Z None	Z None
Z None	B Environmental, Home and Work Barriers C Ergonomics and Body Mechanics	E Orthosis F Assistive, Adaptive, Supportive or Protective U Prosthesis Y Other Equipment Z None	Z None
Z None	H Vocational Activities and Functional Community or Work Reintegration Skills	E Orthosis F Assistive, Adaptive, Supportive or Protective G Aerobic Endurance and Conditioning U Prosthesis Y Other Equipment Z None	Z None

DRG Non-OR All body system/region, type qualifier, equipment, and qualifier values

F Physical Rehabilitation and Diagnostic Audiology
Ø Rehabilitation
6 Speech Treatment Definition: Application of techniques to improve, augment, or compensate for speech and related functional impairment

Body System/Region Character 4	Type Qualifier Character 5	Equipment Character 6	Qualifier Character 7
3 Neurological System - Whole Body	6 Communicative/Cognitive Integration Skills	K Audiovisual M Augmentative / Alternative Communication P Computer Y Other Equipment Z None	Z None
Z None	Ø Nonspoken Language 3 Aphasia 6 Communicative/Cognitive Integration Skills	K Audiovisual M Augmentative / Alternative Communication P Computer Y Other Equipment Z None	Z None
Z None	1 Speech-Language Pathology and Related Disorders Counseling 2 Speech-Language Pathology and Related Disorders Prevention	K Audiovisual Z None	Z None
Z None	4 Articulation/Phonology	K Audiovisual P Computer Q Speech Analysis T Aerodynamic Function Y Other Equipment Z None	Z None
Z None	5 Aural Rehabilitation	K Audiovisual L Assistive Listening M Augmentative / Alternative Communication N Biosensory Feedback P Computer Q Speech Analysis S Voice Analysis Y Other Equipment Z None	Z None
Z None	7 Fluency	4 Electroacoustic Immitance / Acoustic Reflex K Audiovisual N Biosensory Feedback Q Speech Analysis S Voice Analysis T Aerodynamic Function Y Other Equipment Z None	Z None
Z None	8 Motor Speech	K Audiovisual N Biosensory Feedback P Computer Q Speech Analysis S Voice Analysis T Aerodynamic Function Y Other Equipment Z None	Z None
Z None	9 Orofacial Myofunctional	K Audiovisual P Computer Y Other Equipment Z None	Z None
Z None	B Receptive/Expressive Language	K Audiovisual L Assistive Listening M Augmentative / Alternative Communication P Computer Y Other Equipment Z None	Z None

DRG Non-OR All body system/region, type qualifier, equipment, and qualifier values

FØ6 Continued on next page

F Physical Rehabilitation and Diagnostic Audiology
Ø Rehabilitation
6 Speech Treatment Definition: Application of techniques to improve, augment, or compensate for speech and related functional impairment

FØ6 Continued

Body System/Region Character 4	Type Qualifier Character 5	Equipment Character 6	Qualifier Character 7
Z None	C Voice	K Audiovisual N Biosensory Feedback P Computer S Voice Analysis T Aerodynamic Function V Speech Prosthesis Y Other Equipment Z None	Z None
Z None	D Swallowing Dysfunction	M Augmentative / Alternative Communication T Aerodynamic Function V Speech Prosthesis Y Other Equipment Z None	Z None

DRG Non-OR All body system/region, type qualifier, equipment, and qualifier values

F Physical Rehabilitation and Diagnostic Audiology
Ø Rehabilitation
7 Motor Treatment Definition: Exercise or activities to increase or facilitate motor function

Body System/Region Character 4	Type Qualifier Character 5	Equipment Character 6	Qualifier Character 7
Ø Neurological System - Head and Neck 1 Neurological System - Upper Back/ Upper Extremity 2 Neurological System - Lower Back/ Lower Extremity 3 Neurological System - Whole Body D Integumentary System - Head and Neck F Integumentary System - Upper Back/Upper Extremity G Integumentary System - Lower Back/Lower Extremity H Integumentary System - Whole Body J Musculoskeletal System - Head and Neck K Musculoskeletal System - Upper Back/Upper Extremity L Musculoskeletal System - Lower Back/Lower Extremity M Musculoskeletal System - Whole Body	Ø Range of Motion and Joint Mobility 1 Muscle Performance 2 Coordination/Dexterity 3 Motor Function	E Orthosis F Assistive, Adaptive, Supportive or Protective U Prosthesis Y Other Equipment Z None	Z None
Ø Neurological System - Head and Neck 1 Neurological System - Upper Back/ Upper Extremity 2 Neurological System - Lower Back/ Lower Extremity 3 Neurological System - Whole Body D Integumentary System - Head and Neck F Integumentary System - Upper Back/Upper Extremity G Integumentary System - Lower Back/Lower Extremity H Integumentary System - Whole Body J Musculoskeletal System - Head and Neck K Musculoskeletal System - Upper Back/Upper Extremity L Musculoskeletal System - Lower Back/Lower Extremity M Musculoskeletal System - Whole Body	6 Therapeutic Exercise	B Physical Agents C Mechanical D Electrotherapeutic E Orthosis F Assistive, Adaptive, Supportive or Protective G Aerobic Endurance and Conditioning H Mechanical or Electromechanical U Prosthesis Y Other Equipment Z None	Z None

DRG Non-OR All body system/region, type qualifier, equipment, and qualifier values

FØ7 Continued on next page

F07 Continued

F Physical Rehabilitation and Diagnostic Audiology
0 Rehabilitation
7 Motor Treatment Definition: Exercise or activities to increase or facilitate motor function

Body System/Region Character 4	Type Qualifier Character 5	Equipment Character 6	Qualifier Character 7
0 Neurological System - Head and Neck 1 Neurological System - Upper Back/Upper Extremity 2 Neurological System - Lower Back/Lower Extremity 3 Neurological System - Whole Body D Integumentary System - Head and Neck F Integumentary System - Upper Back/Upper Extremity G Integumentary System - Lower Back/Lower Extremity H Integumentary System - Whole Body J Musculoskeletal System - Head and Neck K Musculoskeletal System - Upper Back/Upper Extremity L Musculoskeletal System - Lower Back/Lower Extremity M Musculoskeletal System - Whole Body	7 Manual Therapy Techniques	Z None	Z None
4 Circulatory System - Head and Neck 5 Circulatory System - Upper Back / Upper Extremity 6 Circulatory System - Lower Back / Lower Extremity 7 Circulatory System - Whole Body 8 Respiratory System - Head and Neck 9 Respiratory System - Upper Back / Upper Extremity B Respiratory System -Lower Back / Lower Extremity C Respiratory System -Whole Body	6 Therapeutic Exercise	B Physical Agents C Mechanical D Electrotherapeutic E Orthosis F Assistive, Adaptive, Supportive or Protective G Aerobic Endurance and Conditioning H Mechanical or Electromechanical U Prosthesis Y Other Equipment Z None	Z None
N Genitourinary System	1 Muscle Performance	E Orthosis F Assistive, Adaptive, Supportive or Protective U Prosthesis Y Other Equipment Z None	Z None
N Genitourinary System	6 Therapeutic Exercise	B Physical Agents C Mechanical D Electrotherapeutic E Orthosis F Assistive, Adaptive, Supportive or Protective G Aerobic Endurance and Conditioning H Mechanical or Electromechanical U Prosthesis Y Other Equipment Z None	Z None
Z None	4 Wheelchair Mobility	D Electrotherapeutic E Orthosis F Assistive, Adaptive, Supportive or Protective U Prosthesis Y Other Equipment Z None	Z None
Z None	5 Bed Mobility	C Mechanical E Orthosis F Assistive, Adaptive, Supportive or Protective U Prosthesis Y Other Equipment Z None	Z None

DRG Non-OR All body system/region, type qualifier, equipment, and qualifier values

F Physical Rehabilitation and Diagnostic Audiology
Ø Rehabilitation
8 Activities of Daily Living Treatment Definition: Exercise or activities to facilitate functional competence for activities of daily living

Body System/Region Character 4	Type Qualifier Character 5	Equipment Character 6	Qualifier Character 7
Z None	8 Transfer Training	C Mechanical D Electrotherapeutic E Orthosis F Assistive, Adaptive, Supportive or Protective U Prosthesis Y Other Equipment Z None	Z None
Z None	9 Gait Training/Functional Ambulation	C Mechanical D Electrotherapeutic E Orthosis F Assistive, Adaptive, Supportive or Protective G Aerobic Endurance and Conditioning U Prosthesis Y Other Equipment Z None	Z None
D Integumentary System - Head and Neck F Integumentary System - Upper Back/Upper Extremity G Integumentary System - Lower Back/Lower Extremity H Integumentary System - Whole Body J Musculoskeletal System - Head and Neck K Musculoskeletal System - Upper Back/Upper Extremity L Musculoskeletal System - Lower Back/Lower Extremity M Musculoskeletal System - Whole Body	5 Wound Management	B Physical Agents C Mechanical D Electrotherapeutic E Orthosis F Assistive, Adaptive, Supportive or Protective U Prosthesis Y Other Equipment Z None	Z None
Z None	Ø Bathing/Showering Techniques 1 Dressing Techniques 2 Grooming/Personal Hygiene	E Orthosis F Assistive, Adaptive, Supportive or Protective U Prosthesis Y Other Equipment Z None	Z None
Z None	3 Feeding/Eating	C Mechanical D Electrotherapeutic E Orthosis F Assistive, Adaptive, Supportive or Protective U Prosthesis Y Other Equipment Z None	Z None
Z None	4 Home Management	D Electrotherapeutic E Orthosis F Assistive, Adaptive, Supportive or Protective U Prosthesis Y Other Equipment Z None	Z None
Z None	6 Psychosocial Skills	Z None	Z None
Z None	7 Vocational Activities and Functional Community or Work Reintegration Skills	B Physical Agents C Mechanical D Electrotherapeutic E Orthosis F Assistive, Adaptive, Supportive or Protective G Aerobic Endurance and Conditioning U Prosthesis Y Other Equipment Z None	Z None

DRG Non-OR All body system/region, type qualifier, equipment, and qualifier values

F Physical Rehabilitation and Diagnostic Audiology
Ø Rehabilitation
9 Hearing Treatment Definition: Application of techniques to improve, augment, or compensate for hearing and related functional impairment

Body System/Region Character 4	Type Qualifier Character 5	Equipment Character 6	Qualifier Character 7
Z None	Ø Hearing and Related Disorders Counseling 1 Hearing and Related Disorders Prevention	K Audiovisual Z None	Z None
Z None	2 Auditory Processing	K Audiovisual L Assistive Listening P Computer Y Other Equipment Z None	Z None
Z None	3 Cerumen Management	X Cerumen Management Z None	Z None

DRG Non-OR All body system/region, type qualifier, equipment, and qualifier values

F Physical Rehabilitation and Diagnostic Audiology
Ø Rehabilitation
B Cochlear Implant Treatment Definition: Application of techniques to improve the communication abilities of individuals with cochlear implant

Body System/Region Character 4	Type Qualifier Character 5	Equipment Character 6	Qualifier Character 7
Z None	Ø Cochlear Implant Rehabilitation	1 Audiometer 2 Sound Field / Booth 9 Cochlear Implant K Audiovisual P Computer Y Other Equipment	Z None

DRG Non-OR All body system/region, type qualifier, equipment, and qualifier values

F Physical Rehabilitation and Diagnostic Audiology
Ø Rehabilitation
C Vestibular Treatment Definition: Application of techniques to improve, augment, or compensate for vestibular and related functional impairment

Body System/Region Character 4	Type Qualifier Character 5	Equipment Character 6	Qualifier Character 7
3 Neurological System - Whole Body H Integumentary System - Whole Body M Musculoskeletal System - Whole Body	3 Postural Control	E Orthosis F Assistive, Adaptive, Supportive or Protective U Prosthesis Y Other Equipment Z None	Z None
Z None	Ø Vestibular	8 Vestibular / Balance Z None	Z None
Z None	1 Perceptual Processing 2 Visual Motor Integration	K Audiovisual L Assistive Listening N Biosensory Feedback P Computer Q Speech Analysis S Voice Analysis T Aerodynamic Function Y Other Equipment Z None	Z None

DRG Non-OR All body system/region, type qualifier, equipment, and qualifier values

F Physical Rehabilitation and Diagnostic Audiology
Ø Rehabilitation
D Device Fitting Definition: Fitting of a device designed to facilitate or support achievement of a higher level of function

Body System/Region Character 4	Type Qualifier Character 5	Equipment Character 6	Qualifier Character 7
Z None	Ø Tinnitus Masker	5 Hearing Aid Selection / Fitting / Test Z None	Z None
Z None	1 Monaural Hearing Aid 2 Binaural Hearing Aid 5 Assistive Listening Device	1 Audiometer 2 Sound Field / Booth 5 Hearing Aid Selection / Fitting / Test K Audiovisual L Assistive Listening Z None	Z None
Z None	3 Augmentative/Alternative Communication System	M Augmentative / Alternative Communication	Z None
Z None	4 Voice Prosthetic	S Voice Analysis V Speech Prosthesis	Z None
Z None	6 Dynamic Orthosis 7 Static Orthosis 8 Prosthesis 9 Assistive, Adaptive,Supportive or Protective Devices	E Orthosis F Assistive, Adaptive, Supportive or Protective U Prosthesis Z None	Z None

DRG Non-OR FØDZØ[5,Z]Z
DRG Non-OR FØDZ[1, 2,5][1,2,5, K,L,Z]Z
DRG Non-OR FØDZ3MZ
DRG Non-OR FØDZ4[S,V]Z
DRG Non-OR FØDZ[6,7][E,F,U,Z]Z
DRG Non-OR FØDZ8[E,F,U]Z

F Physical Rehabilitation and Diagnostic Audiology
Ø Rehabilitation
F Caregiver Training Definition: Training in activities to support patient's optimal level of function

Body System/Region Character 4	Type Qualifier Character 5	Equipment Character 6	Qualifier Character 7
Z None	Ø Bathing/Showering Technique 1 Dressing 2 Feeding and Eating 3 Grooming/Personal Hygiene 4 Bed Mobility 5 Transfer 6 Wheelchair Mobility 7 Therapeutic Exercise 8 Airway Clearance Techniques 9 Wound Management B Vocational Activities and Functional Community or Work Reintegration Skills C Gait Training/Functional Ambulation D Application, Proper Use and Care of Devices F Application, Proper Use and Care of Orthoses G Application, Proper Use and Care of Prosthesis H Home Management	E Orthosis F Assistive, Adaptive, Supportive or Protective U Prosthesis Z None	Z None
Z None	J Communication Skills	K Audiovisual L Assistive Listening M Augmentative / Alternative Communication P Computer Z None	Z None

DRG Non-OR All body system/region, type qualifier, equipment, and qualifier values

F Physical Rehabilitation and Diagnostic Audiology
1 Diagnostic Audiology
3 Hearing Assessment Definition: Measurement of hearing and related functions

Body System/Region Character 4	Type Qualifier Character 5	Equipment Character 6	Qualifier Character 7
Z None	Ø Hearing Screening	Ø Occupational Hearing 1 Audiometer 2 Sound Field / Booth 3 Tympanometer 8 Vestibular / Balance 9 Cochlear Implant Z None	Z None
Z None	1 Pure Tone Audiometry, Air 2 Pure Tone Audiometry, Air and Bone	Ø Occupational Hearing 1 Audiometer 2 Sound Field / Booth Z None	Z None
Z None	3 Bekesy Audiometry 6 Visual Reinforcement Audiometry 9 Short Increment Sensitivity Index B Stenger C Pure Tone Stenger	1 Audiometer 2 Sound Field / Booth Z None	Z None
Z None	4 Conditioned Play Audiometry 5 Select Picture Audiometry	1 Audiometer 2 Sound Field / Booth K Audiovisual Z None	Z None
Z None	7 Alternate Binaural or Monaural Loudness Balance	1 Audiometer K Audiovisual Z None	Z None
Z None	8 Tone Decay D Tympanometry F Eustachian Tube Function G Acoustic Reflex Patterns H Acoustic Reflex Threshold J Acoustic Reflex Decay	3 Tympanometer 4 Electroacoustic Immitance / Acoustic Reflex Z None	Z None
Z None	K Electrocochleography L Auditory Evoked Potentials	7 Electrophysiologic Z None	Z None
Z None	M Evoked Otoacoustic Emissions, Screening N Evoked Otoacoustic Emissions, Diagnostic	6 Otoacoustic Emission (OAE) Z None	Z None
Z None	P Aural Rehabilitation Status	1 Audiometer 2 Sound Field / Booth 4 Electroacoustic Immitance / Acoustic Reflex 9 Cochlear Implant K Audiovisual L Assistive Listening P Computer Z None	Z None
Z None	Q Auditory Processing	K Audiovisual P Computer Y Other Equipment Z None	Z None

F Physical Rehabilitation and Diagnostic Audiology
1 Diagnostic Audiology
4 Hearing Aid Assessment Definition: Measurement of the appropriateness and/or effectiveness of a hearing device

Body System/Region Character 4	Type Qualifier Character 5	Equipment Character 6	Qualifier Character 7
Z None	Ø Cochlear Implant	1 Audiometer 2 Sound Field / Booth 3 Tympanometer 4 Electroacoustic Immitance / Acoustic Reflex 5 Hearing Aid Selection / Fitting / Test 7 Electrophysiologic 9 Cochlear Implant K Audiovisual L Assistive Listening P Computer Y Other Equipment Z None	Z None
Z None	1 Ear Canal Probe Microphone 6 Binaural Electroacoustic Hearing Aid Check 8 Monaural Electroacoustic Hearing Aid Check	5 Hearing Aid Selection / Fitting / Test Z None	Z None
Z None	2 Monaural Hearing Aid 3 Binaural Hearing Aid	1 Audiometer 2 Sound Field / Booth 3 Tympanometer 4 Electroacoustic Immitance / Acoustic Reflex 5 Hearing Aid Selection / Fitting / Test K Audiovisual L Assistive Listening P Computer Z None	Z None
Z None	4 Assistive Listening System/Device Selection	1 Audiometer 2 Sound Field / Booth 3 Tympanometer 4 Electroacoustic Immitance / Acoustic Reflex K Audiovisual L Assistive Listening Z None	Z None
Z None	5 Sensory Aids	1 Audiometer 2 Sound Field / Booth 3 Tympanometer 4 Electroacoustic Immitance / Acoustic Reflex 5 Hearing Aid Selection / Fitting / Test K Audiovisual L Assistive Listening Z None	Z None
Z None	7 Ear Protector Attentuation	Ø Occupational Hearing Z None	Z None

F Physical Rehabilitation and Diagnostic Audiology
1 Diagnostic Audiology
5 Vestibular Assessment Definition: Measurement of the vestibular system and related functions

Body System/Region Character 4	Type Qualifier Character 5	Equipment Character 6	Qualifier Character 7
Z None	Ø Bithermal, Binaural Caloric Irrigation 1 Bithermal, Monaural Caloric Irrigation 2 Unithermal Binaural Screen 3 Oscillating Tracking 4 Sinusoidal Vertical Axis Rotational 5 Dix-Hallpike Dynamic 6 Computerized Dynamic Posturography	8 Vestibular / Balance Z None	Z None
Z None	7 Tinnitus Masker	5 Hearing Aid Selection / Fitting / Test Z None	Z None

Mental Health GZ1–GZJ

G Mental Health
Z None
1 Psychological Tests Definition: The administration and interpretation of standardized psychological tests and measurement instruments for the assessment of psychological function

Qualifier Character 4	Qualifier Character 5	Qualifier Character 6	Qualifier Character 7
Ø Developmental 1 Personality and Behavioral 2 Intellectual and Psychoeducational 3 Neuropsychological 4 Neurobehavioral and Cognitive Status	Z None	Z None	Z None

G Mental Health
Z None
2 Crisis Intervention Definition: Treatment of a traumatized, acutely disturbed or distressed individual for the purpose of short-term stabilization

Qualifier Character 4	Qualifier Character 5	Qualifier Character 6	Qualifier Character 7
Z None	Z None	Z None	Z None

G Mental Health
Z None
3 Medication Management Definition: Monitoring and adjusting the use of medications for the treatment of a mental health disorder

Qualifier Character 4	Qualifier Character 5	Qualifier Character 6	Qualifier Character 7
Z None	Z None	Z None	Z None

G Mental Health
Z None
5 Individual Psychotherapy Definition: Treatment of an individual with a mental health disorder by behavioral, cognitive, psychoanalytic, psychodynamic or psychophysiological means to improve functioning or well-being

Qualifier Character 4	Qualifier Character 5	Qualifier Character 6	Qualifier Character 7
Ø Interactive 1 Behavioral 2 Cognitive 3 Interpersonal 4 Psychoanalysis 5 Psychodynamic 6 Supportive 8 Cognitive-Behavioral 9 Psychophysiological	Z None	Z None	Z None

G Mental Health
Z None
6 Counseling Definition: The application of psychological methods to treat an individual with normal developmental issues and psychological problems in order to increase function, improve well-being, alleviate distress, maladjustment or resolve crises

Qualifier Character 4	Qualifier Character 5	Qualifier Character 6	Qualifier Character 7
Ø Educational 1 Vocational 3 Other Counseling	Z None	Z None	Z None

G Mental Health
Z None
7 Family Psychotherapy Definition: Treatment that includes one or more family members of an individual with a mental health disorder by behavioral, cognitive, psychoanalytic, psychodynamic or psychophysiological means to improve functioning or well-being
Explanation: Remediation of emotional or behavioral problems presented by one or more family members in cases where psychotherapy with more than one family member is indicated

Qualifier Character 4	Qualifier Character 5	Qualifier Character 6	Qualifier Character 7
2 Other Family Psychotherapy	Z None	Z None	Z None

G Mental Health
Z None
B Electroconvulsive Therapy Definition: The application of controlled electrical voltages to treat a mental health disorder

Qualifier Character 4	Qualifier Character 5	Qualifier Character 6	Qualifier Character 7
Ø Unilateral-Single Seizure 1 Unilateral-Multiple Seizure 2 Bilateral-Single Seizure 3 Bilateral-Multiple Seizure 4 Other Electroconvulsive Therapy	Z None	Z None	Z None

G Mental Health
Z None
C Biofeedback Definition: Provision of information from the monitoring and regulating of physiological processes in conjunction with cognitive-behavioral techniques to improve patient functioning or well-being

Qualifier Character 4	Qualifier Character 5	Qualifier Character 6	Qualifier Character 7
9 Other Biofeedback	Z None	Z None	Z None

G Mental Health
Z None
F Hypnosis Definition: Induction of a state of heightened suggestibility by auditory, visual and tactile techniques to elicit an emotional or behavioral response

Qualifier Character 4	Qualifier Character 5	Qualifier Character 6	Qualifier Character 7
Z None	Z None	Z None	Z None

G Mental Health
Z None
G Narcosynthesis Definition: Administration of intravenous barbiturates in order to release suppressed or repressed thoughts

Qualifier Character 4	Qualifier Character 5	Qualifier Character 6	Qualifier Character 7
Z None	Z None	Z None	Z None

G Mental Health
Z None
H Group Psychotherapy Definition: Treatment of two or more individuals with a mental health disorder by behavioral, cognitive, psychoanalytic, psychodynamic or psychophysiological means to improve functioning or well-being

Qualifier Character 4	Qualifier Character 5	Qualifier Character 6	Qualifier Character 7
Z None	Z None	Z None	Z None

G Mental Health
Z None
J Light Therapy Definition: Application of specialized light treatments to improve functioning or well-being

Qualifier Character 4	Qualifier Character 5	Qualifier Character 6	Qualifier Character 7
Z None	Z None	Z None	Z None

Substance Abuse Treatment HZ2–HZ9

AHA Coding Clinic for table HZ2
2020, 1Q, 21 Inpatient detoxification services

AHA Coding Clinic for table HZ9
2020, 1Q, 21 Inpatient detoxification services

H Substance Abuse Treatment
Z None
2 Detoxification Services

Definition: Detoxification from alcohol and/or drugs
Explanation: Not a treatment modality, but helps the patient stabilize physically and psychologically until the body becomes free of drugs and the effects of alcohol

Qualifier Character 4	Qualifier Character 5	Qualifier Character 6	Qualifier Character 7
Z None	Z None	Z None	Z None

H Substance Abuse Treatment
Z None
3 Individual Counseling

Definition: The application of psychological methods to treat an individual with addictive behavior
Explanation: Comprised of several different techniques, which apply various strategies to address drug addiction

Qualifier Character 4	Qualifier Character 5	Qualifier Character 6	Qualifier Character 7
Ø Cognitive 1 Behavioral 2 Cognitive-Behavioral 3 12-Step 4 Interpersonal 5 Vocational 6 Psychoeducation 7 Motivational Enhancement 8 Confrontational 9 Continuing Care B Spiritual C Pre/Post-Test Infectious Disease	Z None	Z None	Z None

DRG Non-OR HZ3[Ø,1,2,3,4,5,6,7,8,9,B]ZZZ

H Substance Abuse Treatment
Z None
4 Group Counseling

Definition: The application of psychological methods to treat two or more individuals with addictive behavior
Explanation: Provides structured group counseling sessions and healing power through the connection with others

Qualifier Character 4	Qualifier Character 5	Qualifier Character 6	Qualifier Character 7
Ø Cognitive 1 Behavioral 2 Cognitive-Behavioral 3 12-Step 4 Interpersonal 5 Vocational 6 Psychoeducation 7 Motivational Enhancement 8 Confrontational 9 Continuing Care B Spiritual C Pre/Post-Test Infectious Disease	Z None	Z None	Z None

DRG Non-OR HZ4[Ø,1,2,3,4,5,6,7,8,9,B]ZZZ

H Substance Abuse Treatment
Z None
5 Individual Psychotherapy Definition: Treatment of an individual with addictive behavior by behavioral, cognitive, psychoanalytic, psychodynamic or psychophysiological means

Qualifier Character 4	Qualifier Character 5	Qualifier Character 6	Qualifier Character 7
Ø Cognitive 1 Behavioral 2 Cognitive-Behavioral 3 12-Step 4 Interpersonal 5 Interactive 6 Psychoeducation 7 Motivational Enhancement 8 Confrontational 9 Supportive B Psychoanalysis C Psychodynamic D Psychophysiological	Z None	Z None	Z None

DRG Non-OR For all qualifier values

H Substance Abuse Treatment
Z None
6 Family Counseling Definition: The application of psychological methods that includes one or more family members to treat an individual with addictive behavior

Explanation: Provides support and education for family members of addicted individuals. Family member participation is seen as a critical area of substance abuse treatment

Qualifier Character 4	Qualifier Character 5	Qualifier Character 6	Qualifier Character 7
3 Other Family Counseling	Z None	Z None	Z None

H Substance Abuse Treatment
Z None
8 Medication Management Definition: Monitoring or adjusting the use of replacement medications for the treatment of addiction

Qualifier Character 4	Qualifier Character 5	Qualifier Character 6	Qualifier Character 7
Ø Nicotine Replacement 1 Methadone Maintenance 2 Levo-alpha-acetyl-methadol (LAAM) 3 Antabuse 4 Naltrexone 5 Naloxone 6 Clonidine 7 Bupropion 8 Psychiatric Medication 9 Other Replacement Medication	Z None	Z None	Z None

H Substance Abuse Treatment
Z None
9 Pharmacotherapy Definition: The use of replacement medications for the treatment of addiction

Qualifier Character 4	Qualifier Character 5	Qualifier Character 6	Qualifier Character 7
Ø Nicotine Replacement 1 Methadone Maintenance 2 Levo-alpha-acetyl-methadol (LAAM) 3 Antabuse 4 Naltrexone 5 Naloxone 6 Clonidine 7 Bupropion 8 Psychiatric Medication 9 Other Replacement Medication	Z None	Z None	Z None

New Technology X27–XYØ

AHA Coding Clinic for all tables in the New Technology Section
2015, 4Q, 8-11 New Section X codes - New Technology procedures

AHA Coding Clinic for table X27
2019, 4Q, 45-46 Sustained released drug-eluting stent

AHA Coding Clinic for table X2A
2019, 4Q, 46 Cerebral embolic filtration
2016, 4Q, 115-116 Cerebral embolic filtration

AHA Coding Clinic for table X2C
2016, 4Q, 82-83 Coronary artery, number of arteries
2015, 4Q, 8-14 New Section X codes—New Technology procedures

AHA Coding Clinic for table X2R
2016, 4Q, 116 Aortic valve rapid deployment
2015, 4Q, 8-12 New Section X codes—New Technology procedures

AHA Coding Clinic for table XHR
2016, 4Q, 116 Application of wound matrix

AHA Coding Clinic for table XKØ
2017, 4Q, 74 Intramuscular autologous bone marrow cell therapy

AHA Coding Clinic for table XNS
2017, 4Q, 74-75 Magnetic growth rods
2016, 4Q, 117 Placement of magnetic growth rods

AHA Coding Clinic for table XRG
2017, 4Q, 76 Radiolucent porous interbody fusion device

AHA Coding Clinic for table XT2
2019, 4Q, 46-47 Renal function monitoring

AHA Coding Clinic for table XV5
2018, 4Q, 55 Robotic waterjet ablation

AHA Coding Clinic for table XWØ
2019, 4Q, 47-50 New therapeutic substances
2018, 4Q, 56 New therapeutic substances
2015, 4Q, 8-15 New Section X codes—New Technology procedures

AHA Coding Clinic for table XXE
2019, 4Q, 50-51 Whole blood nucleic acid-base microbial detection

AHA Coding Clinic for table XYØ
2017, 4Q, 78 Intraoperative treatment of vascular grafts

X New Technology
2 Cardiovascular System
7 Dilation **Definition: Expanding an orifice or the lumen of a tubular body part**
Explanation: The orifice can be a natural orifice or an artificially created orifice. Accomplished by stretching a tubular body part using intraluminal pressure or by cutting part of the orifice or wall of the tubular body part.

Body Part Character 4	Approach Character 5	Device/Substance/Technology Character 6	Qualifier Character 7
H Femoral Artery, Right J Femoral Artery, Left K Popliteal Artery, Proximal Right L Popliteal Artery, Proximal Left M Popliteal Artery, Distal Right N Popliteal Artery, Distal Left P Anterior Tibial Artery, Right Q Anterior Tibial Artery, Left R Posterior Tibial Artery, Right S Posterior Tibial Artery, Left T Peroneal Artery, Right U Peroneal Artery, Left	3 Percutaneous	8 Intraluminal Device, Sustained Release Drug-eluting 9 Intraluminal Device, Sustained Release Drug-eluting, Two B Intraluminal Device, Sustained Release Drug-eluting, Three C Intraluminal Device, Sustained Release Drug-eluting, Four or More	5 New Technology Group 5

Valid OR All body part, approach, device/substance/technology, and qualifier values

X New Technology
2 Cardiovascular System
A Assistance **Definition: Taking over a portion of a physiological function by extracorporeal means**
Explanation: None

Body Part Character 4	Approach Character 5	Device/Substance/Technology Character 6	Qualifier Character 7
5 Innominate Artery and Left Common Carotid Artery	3 Percutaneous	1 Cerebral Embolic Filtration, Dual Filter	2 New Technology Group 2
6 Aortic Arch	3 Percutaneous	2 Cerebral Embolic Filtration, Single Deflection Filter	5 New Technology Group 5
H Common Carotid Artery, Right J Common Carotid Artery, Left	3 Percutaneous	3 Cerebral Embolic Filtration, Extracorporeal Flow Reversal Circuit	6 New Technology Group 6

X New Technology
2 Cardiovascular System
C Extirpation **Definition: Taking or cutting out solid matter from a body part**
Explanation: The solid matter may be an abnormal byproduct of a biological function or a foreign body; it may be imbedded in a body part or in the lumen of a tubular body part. The solid matter may or may not have been previously broken into pieces.

Body Part Character 4	Approach Character 5	Device/Substance/Technology Character 6	Qualifier Character 7
Ø Coronary Artery, One Artery 1 Coronary Artery, Two Arteries 2 Coronary Artery, Three Arteries 3 Coronary Artery, Four or More Arteries	3 Percutaneous	6 Orbital Atherectomy Technology	1 New Technology Group 1

Valid OR All body part, approach, device/substance/technology, and qualifier values

X New Technology
2 Cardiovascular System
R Replacement Definition: Putting in or on biological or synthetic material that physically takes the place and/or function of all or a portion of a body part

Explanation: The body part may have been taken out or replaced, or may be taken out, physically eradicated, or rendered nonfunctional during the REPLACEMENT procedure. A REMOVAL procedure is coded for taking out the device used in a previous replacement procedure

Body Part Character 4	Approach Character 5	Device/Substance/Technology Character 6	Qualifier Character 7
F Aortic Valve	Ø Open 3 Percutaneous 4 Percutaneous Endoscopic	3 Zooplastic Tissue, Rapid Deployment Technique	2 New Technology Group 2

Valid OR All body part, approach, device/substance/technology, and qualifier values

X New Technology
H Skin, Subcutaneous Tissue, Fascia and Breast
R Replacement Definition: Putting in or on biological or synthetic material that physically takes the place and/or function of all or a portion of a body part

Explanation: The body part may have been taken out or replaced, or may be taken out, physically eradicated, or rendered nonfunctional during the REPLACEMENT procedure. A REMOVAL procedure is coded for taking out the device used in a previous replacement procedure

Body Part Character 4	Approach Character 5	Device/Substance/Technology Character 6	Qualifier Character 7
P Skin	X External	L Skin Substitute, Porcine Liver Derived	2 New Technology Group 2

Valid OR All body part, approach, device/substance/technology, and qualifier values

X New Technology
K Muscles, Tendons, Bursae and Ligaments
Ø Introduction Definition: Putting in or on a therapeutic, diagnostic, nutritional, physiological, or prophylactic substance except blood or blood products

Explanation: None

Body Part Character 4	Approach Character 5	Device/Substance/Technology Character 6	Qualifier Character 7
2 Muscle	3 Percutaneous	Ø Concentrated Bone Marrow Aspirate	3 New Technology Group 3

X New Technology
N Bones
S Reposition Definition: Moving to its normal location, or other suitable location, all or a portion of a body part

Explanation: The body part is moved to a new location from an abnormal location, or from a normal location where it is not functioning correctly. The body part may or may not be cut out or off to be moved to the new location.

Body Part Character 4	Approach Character 5	Device/Substance/Technology Character 6	Qualifier Character 7
Ø Lumbar Vertebra 3 Cervical Vertebra 4 Thoracic Vertebra	Ø Open 3 Percutaneous	3 Magnetically Controlled Growth Rod(s)	2 New Technology Group 2

Valid OR All body part, approach, device/substance/technology, and qualifier values

X New Technology
N Bones
U Supplement Definition: Putting in or on biological or synthetic material that physically reinforces and/or augments the function of a portion of a body part

Explanation: None

Body Part Character 4	Approach Character 5	Device/Substance/Technology Character 6	Qualifier Character 7
Ø Lumbar Vertebra 4 Thoracic Vertebra	3 Percutaneous	5 Synthetic Substitute, Mechanically Expandable (Paired)	6 New Technology Group 6

X New Technology
R Joints
2 Monitoring Definition: Determining the level of a physiological or physical function repetitively over a period of time

Explanation: None

Body Part Character 4	Approach Character 5	Device/Substance/Technology Character 6	Qualifier Character 7
G Knee Joint, Right H Knee Joint, Left	Ø Open	2 Intraoperative Knee Replacement Sensor	1 New Technology Group 1

Valid OR All body part, approach, device/substance/technology, and qualifier values

X New Technology
R Joints
G Fusion Definition: Joining together portions of an articular body part rendering the articular body part immobile
Explanation: The body part is joined together by fixation device, bone graft, or other means

Body Part Character 4	Approach Character 5	Device/Substance/Technology Character 6	Qualifier Character 7
Ø Occipital-cervical Joint	Ø Open	9 Interbody Fusion Device, Nanotextured Surface	2 New Technology Group 2
Ø Occipital-cervical Joint	Ø Open	F Interbody Fusion Device, Radiolucent Porous	3 New Technology Group 3
1 Cervical Vertebral Joint	Ø Open	9 Interbody Fusion Device, Nanotextured Surface	2 New Technology Group 2
1 Cervical Vertebral Joint	Ø Open	F Interbody Fusion Device, Radiolucent Porous	3 New Technology Group 3
2 Cervical Vertebral Joints, 2 or more	Ø Open	9 Interbody Fusion Device, Nanotextured Surface	2 New Technology Group 2
2 Cervical Vertebral Joints, 2 or more	Ø Open	F Interbody Fusion Device, Radiolucent Porous	3 New Technology Group 3
4 Cervicothoracic Vertebral Joint	Ø Open	9 Interbody Fusion Device, Nanotextured Surface	2 New Technology Group 2
4 Cervicothoracic Vertebral Joint	Ø Open	F Interbody Fusion Device, Radiolucent Porous	3 New Technology Group 3
6 Thoracic Vertebral Joint	Ø Open	9 Interbody Fusion Device, Nanotextured Surface	2 New Technology Group 2
6 Thoracic Vertebral Joint	Ø Open	F Interbody Fusion Device, Radiolucent Porous	3 New Technology Group 3
7 Thoracic Vertebral Joints, 2 to 7 ⊞	Ø Open	9 Interbody Fusion Device, Nanotextured Surface	2 New Technology Group 2
7 Thoracic Vertebral Joints, 2 to 7 ⊞	Ø Open	F Interbody Fusion Device, Radiolucent Porous	3 New Technology Group 3
8 Thoracic Vertebral Joints, 8 or more	Ø Open	9 Interbody Fusion Device, Nanotextured Surface	2 New Technology Group 2
8 Thoracic Vertebral Joints, 8 or more	Ø Open	F Interbody Fusion Device, Radiolucent Porous	3 New Technology Group 3
A Thoracolumbar Vertebral Joint	Ø Open	9 Interbody Fusion Device, Nanotextured Surface	2 New Technology Group 2
A Thoracolumbar Vertebral Joint	Ø Open	F Interbody Fusion Device, Radiolucent Porous	3 New Technology Group 3
B Lumbar Vertebral Joint	Ø Open	9 Interbody Fusion Device, Nanotextured Surface	2 New Technology Group 2
B Lumbar Vertebral Joint	Ø Open	F Interbody Fusion Device, Radiolucent Porous	3 New Technology Group 3
C Lumbar Vertebral Joints, 2 or more ⊞	Ø Open	9 Interbody Fusion Device, Nanotextured Surface	2 New Technology Group 2
C Lumbar Vertebral Joints,2 or more ⊞	Ø Open	F Interbody Fusion Device, Radiolucent Porous	3 New Technology Group 3
D Lumbosacral Joint	Ø Open	9 Interbody Fusion Device, Nanotextured Surface	2 New Technology Group 2
D Lumbosacral Joint	Ø Open	F Interbody Fusion Device, Radiolucent Porous	3 New Technology Group 3

Valid OR All body part, approach, device/substance/technology, and qualifier values
HAC XRG[Ø,1,2,4,6,7,8,A,B,C,D]Ø92 when reported with SDx K68.11 or T81.4Ø–T81.49, T84.6Ø-T84.619, T84.63-T84.7 with 7th character A
HAC XRG[Ø,1,2,4,6,7,8,A,B,C,D]ØF3 when reported with SDx K68.11 or T81.4Ø–T81.49, T84.6Ø-T84.619, T84.63-T84.7 with 7th character A

See Appendix L for Procedure Combinations
⊞ XRG7Ø92
⊞ XRG7ØF3
⊞ XRGCØ92
⊞ XRGCØF3

X New Technology
T Urinary System
2 Monitoring Definition: Determining the level of a physiological or physical function repetitively over a period of time
Explanation: None

Body Part Character 4	Approach Character 5	Device/Substance/Technology Character 6	Qualifier Character 7
5 Kidney	X External	E Fluorescent Pyrazine	5 New Technology Group 5

X New Technology
V Male Reproductive System
5 Destruction Definition: Physical eradication of all or a portion of a body part by the direct use of energy, force, or a destructive agent
Explanation: None of the body part is physically taken out

Body Part Character 4	Approach Character 5	Device/Substance/Technology Character 6	Qualifier Character 7
Ø Prostate	8 Via Natural or Artificial Opening Endoscopic	A Robotic Waterjet Ablation	4 New Technology Group 4

Valid OR All body part, approach, device/substance/technology, and qualifier values

X New Technology
W Anatomical Regions
Ø Introduction Definition: Putting in or on a therapeutic, diagnostic, nutritional, physiological, or prophylactic substance except blood or blood products
Explanation: None

Body Part Character 4	Approach Character 5	Device/Substance/Technology Character 6	Qualifier Character 7
1 Subcutaneous Tissue	3 Percutaneous	W Caplacizumab	5 New Technology Group 5
3 Peripheral Vein	3 Percutaneous	Ø Brexanolone	6 New Technology Group 6
3 Peripheral Vein	3 Percutaneous	2 Ceftazidime-Avibactam Anti-infective	1 New Technology Group 1
3 Peripheral Vein	3 Percutaneous	2 Nerinitide	6 New Technology Group 6
3 Peripheral Vein	3 Percutaneous	3 Idarucizumab, Dabigatran Reversal Agent	1 New Technology Group 1
3 Peripheral Vein	3 Percutaneous	3 Durvalumab Antineoplastic	6 New Technology Group 6
3 Peripheral Vein	3 Percutaneous	4 Isavuconazole Anti-infective 5 Blinatumomab Antineoplastic Immunotherapy	1 New Technology Group 1
3 Peripheral Vein	3 Percutaneous	6 Lefamulin Anti-infective	6 New Technology Group 6
3 Peripheral Vein	3 Percutaneous	7 Coagulation Factor Xa, Inactivated 9 Defibrotide Sodium Anticoagulant	2 New Technology Group 2
3 Peripheral Vein	3 Percutaneous	9 Ceftolozane/Tazobacatam Anti-infective	6 New Technology Group 6
3 Peripheral Vein	3 Percutaneous	A Bezlotoxumab Monoclonal Antibody	3 New Technology Group 3
3 Peripheral Vein	3 Percutaneous	A Cefiderocol Anti-infective	6 New Technology Group 6
3 Peripheral Vein	3 Percutaneous	B Cytarabine and Daunorubicin Liposome Antineoplastic	3 New Technology Group 3
3 Peripheral Vein	3 Percutaneous	B Omadacycline Anti-infective	6 New Technology Group 6
3 Peripheral Vein	3 Percutaneous	C Engineered Autologous Chimeric Antigen Receptor T-cell Immunotherapy	3 New Technology Group 3
3 Peripheral Vein	3 Percutaneous	C Eculizumab D Atezolizumab Antineoplastic	6 New Technology Group 6
3 Peripheral Vein	3 Percutaneous	F Other New Technology Therapeutic Substance	3 New Technology Group 3
3 Peripheral Vein	3 Percutaneous	G Plazomicin Anti-infective H Synthetic Human Angiotensin II	4 New Technology Group 4
3 Peripheral Vein	3 Percutaneous	K Fosfomycin Anti-infective N Meropenem-vaborbactam Anti-infective Q Tagraxofusp-erzs Antineoplastic S Iobenguane I-131 Antineoplastic U Imipenem-cilastatin-relebactam Anti-infective W Caplacizumab	5 New Technology Group 5
4 Central Vein	3 Percutaneous	Ø Brexanolone	6 New Technology Group 6
4 Central Vein	3 Percutaneous	2 Ceftazidime-Avibactam Anti-infective	1 New Technology Group 1
4 Central Vein	3 Percutaneous	2 Nerinitide	6 New Technology Group 6
4 Central Vein	3 Percutaneous	3 Idarucizumab, Dabigatran Reversal Agent	1 New Technology Group 1
4 Central Vein	3 Percutaneous	3 Durvalumab Antineoplastic	6 New Technology Group 6
4 Central Vein	3 Percutaneous	4 Isavuconazole Anti-infective 5 Blinatumomab Antineoplastic Immunotherapy	1 New Technology Group 1
4 Central Vein	3 Percutaneous	6 Lefamulin Anti-infective	6 New Technology Group 6
4 Central Vein	3 Percutaneous	7 Coagulation Factor Xa, Inactivated 9 Defibrotide Sodium Anticoagulant	2 New Technology Group 2
4 Central Vein	3 Percutaneous	9 Ceftolozane/Tazobacatam Anti-infective	6 New Technology Group 6
4 Central Vein	3 Percutaneous	A Bezlotoxumab Monoclonal Antibody	3 New Technology Group 3
4 Central Vein	3 Percutaneous	A Cefiderocol Anti-infective	6 New Technology Group 6
4 Central Vein	3 Percutaneous	B Cytarabine and Daunorubicin Liposome Antineoplastic	3 New Technology Group 3
4 Central Vein	3 Percutaneous	B Omadacycline Anti-infective	6 New Technology Group 6

DRG Non-OR XWØ33C3

XWØ Continued on next page

XWØ Continued

X New Technology
W Anatomical Regions
Ø Introduction Definition: Putting in or on a therapeutic, diagnostic, nutritional, physiological, or prophylactic substance except blood or blood products
Explanation: None

Body Part Character 4	Approach Character 5	Device/Substance/Technology Character 6	Qualifier Character 7
4 Central Vein	3 Percutaneous	C Engineered Autologous Chimeric Antigen Receptor T-cell Immunotherapy	3 New Technology Group 3
4 Central Vein	3 Percutaneous	C Eculizumab D Atezolizumab Antineoplastic	6 New Technology Group 6
4 Central Vein	3 Percutaneous	F Other New Technology Therapeutic Substance	3 New Technology Group 3
4 Central Vein	3 Percutaneous	G Plazomicin Anti-infective H Synthetic Human Angiotensin II	4 New Technology Group 4
4 Central Vein	3 Percutaneous	K Fosfomycin Anti-infective N Meropenem-vaborbactam Anti-infective Q Tagraxofusp-erzs Antineoplastic S Iobenguane I-131 Antineoplastic U Imipenem-cilastatin-relebactam Anti-infective W Caplacizumab	5 New Technology Group 5
9 Nose	7 Via Natural or Artificial Opening	M Esketamine Hydrochloride	5 New Technology Group 5
D Mouth and Pharynx	X External	6 Lefamulin Anti-infective	6 New Technology Group 6
D Mouth and Pharynx	X External	8 Uridine Triacetate	2 New Technology Group 2
D Mouth and Pharynx	X External	J Apalutamide Antineoplastic L Erdafitinib Antineoplastic R Venetoclax Antineoplastic T Ruxolitinib V Gilteritinib Antineoplastic	5 New Technology Group 5
G Upper GI H Lower GI	8 Via Natural or Artificial Opening Endoscopic	8 Mineral-based Topical Hemostatic Agent	6 New Technology Group 6
Q Cranial Cavity and Brain	3 Percutaneous	1 Eladocagene exuparvovec	6 New Technology Group 6

DRG Non-OR XWØ43C3

X New Technology
W Anatomical Regions
2 Transfusion Definition: Putting in blood or blood products
Explanation: None

Body Part Character 4	Approach Character 5	Device/Substance/Technology Character 6	Qualifier Character 7
3 Peripheral Vein 4 Central Vein	3 Percutaneous	4 Brexucabtagene Autoleucel Immunotherapy 7 Lisocabtagene Maraleucel Immunotherapy	6 New Technology Group 6

X New Technology
X Physiological Systems
E Measurement Definition: Determining the level of a physiological or physical function at a point in time
Explanation: None

Body Part Character 4	Approach Character 5	Device/Substance/Technology Character 6	Qualifier Character 7
5 Circulatory	X External	M Infection, Whole Blood Nucleic Acid-base Microbial Detection	5 New Technology Group 5
5 Circulatory	X External	N Infection, Positive Blood Culture Fluorescence Hybridization for Organism Identification, Concentration and Susceptibility	6 New Technology Group 6
B Respiratory	X External	Q Infection, Lower Respiratory Fluid Nucleic Acid-base Microbial Detection	6 New Technology Group 6

X New Technology
Y Extracorporeal
Ø Introduction Definition: Putting in or on a therapeutic, diagnostic, nutritional, physiological, or prophylactic substance except blood or blood products
Explanation: None

Body Part Character 4	Approach Character 5	Device/Substance/Technology Character 6	Qualifier Character 7
V Vein Graft	X External	8 Endothelial Damage Inhibitor	3 New Technology Group 3

Appendixes

Appendix A: Components of the Medical and Surgical Approach Definitions

ICD-10-PCS Value	Definition	Access Location	Method	Type of Instrumentation	Example
Open (Ø)	Cutting through the skin or mucous membrane and any other body layers necessary to expose the site of the procedure	Skin or mucous membrane, any other body layers	Cutting	None	Abdominal hysterectomy
Percutaneous (3)	Entry, by puncture or minor incision, of instrumentation through the skin or mucous membrane and any other body layers necessary to reach the site of the procedure	Skin or mucous membrane, any other body layers	Puncture or minor incision	Without visualization	Needle biopsy of liver, Liposuction
Percutaneous endoscopic (4)	Entry, by puncture or minor incision, of instrumentation through the skin or mucous membrane and any other body layers necessary to reach and visualize the site of the procedure	Skin or mucous membrane, any other body layers	Puncture or minor incision	With visualization	Arthroscopy, Laparoscopic cholecystectomy
Via natural or artificial opening (7)	Entry of instrumentation through a natural or artificial external opening to reach the site of the procedure	Natural or artificial external opening	Direct entry	Without visualization	Endotracheal tube insertion, Foley catheter placement
Via natural or artificial opening endoscopic (8)	Entry of instrumentation through a natural or artificial external opening to reach and visualize the site of the procedure	Natural or artificial external opening	Direct entry	With visualization	Sigmoidoscopy, EGD, ERCP
Via natural or artificial opening with percutaneous endoscopic assistance (F)	Entry of instrumentation through a natural or artificial external opening and entry, by puncture or minor incision, of instrumentation through the skin or mucous membrane and any other body layers necessary to aid in the performance of the procedure	Skin or mucous membrane, any other body layers	Direct entry with puncture or minor incision for instrumentation only	With visualization	Laparoscopic-assisted vaginal hysterectomy
External (X)	Procedures performed directly on the skin or mucous membrane and procedures performed indirectly by the application of external force through the skin or mucous membrane	Skin or mucous membrane	Direct or indirect application	None	Closed fracture reduction, Resection of tonsils

Open (Ø)

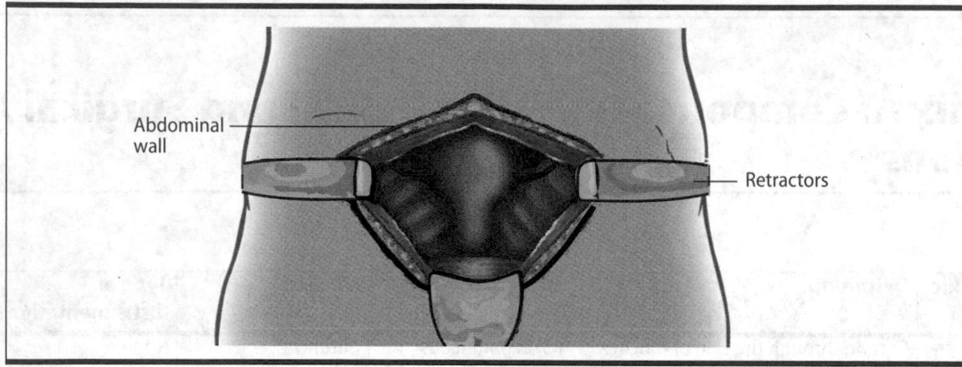

Percutaneous (3)

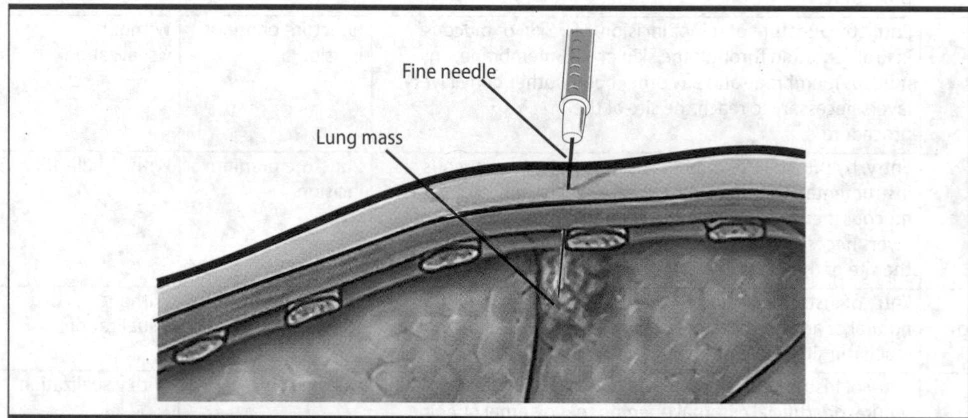

Percutaneous Endoscopic (4)

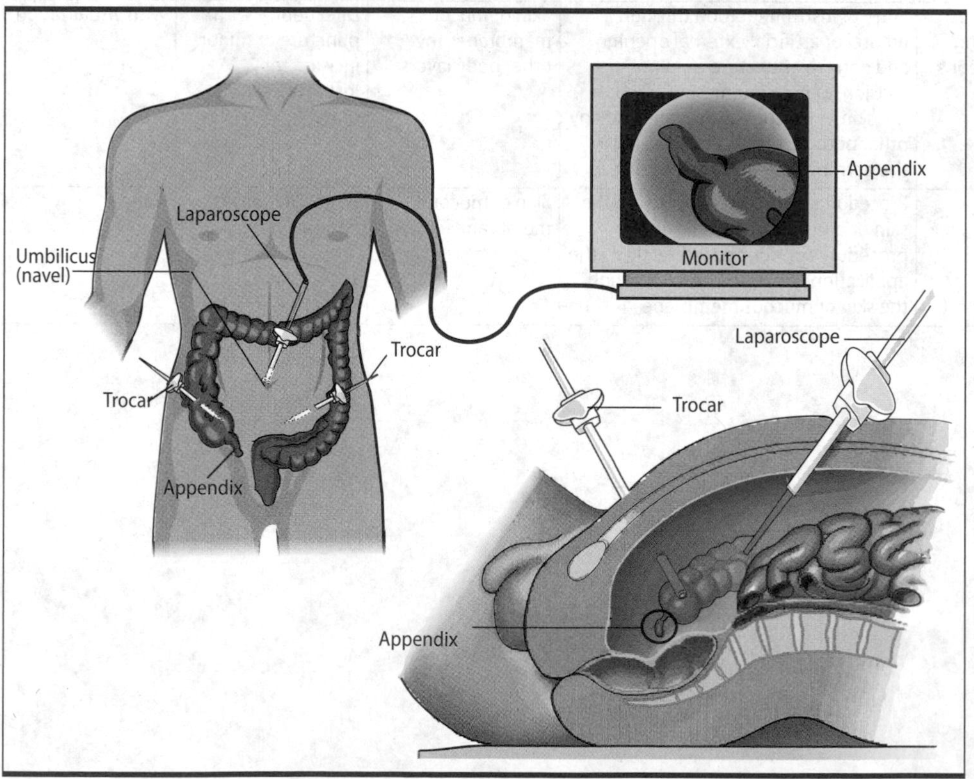

Via Natural or Artificial Opening (7)

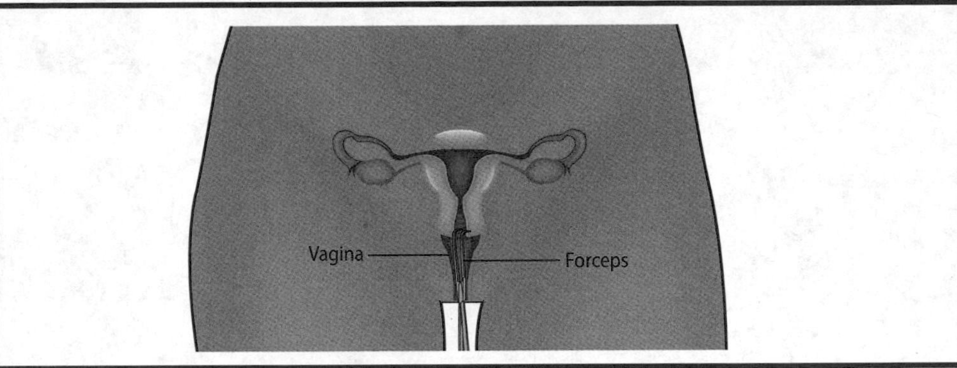

Via Natural or Artificial Opening, Endoscopic (8)

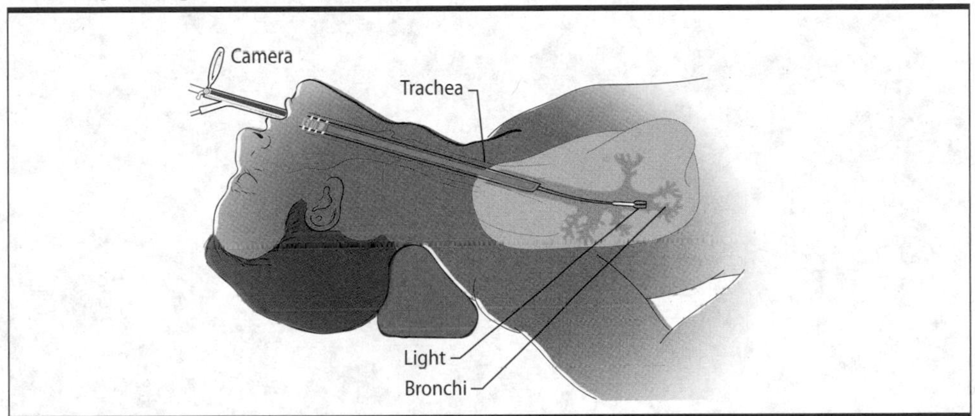

Via Natural or Artificial Opening with Percutaneous Endoscopic Assistance (F)

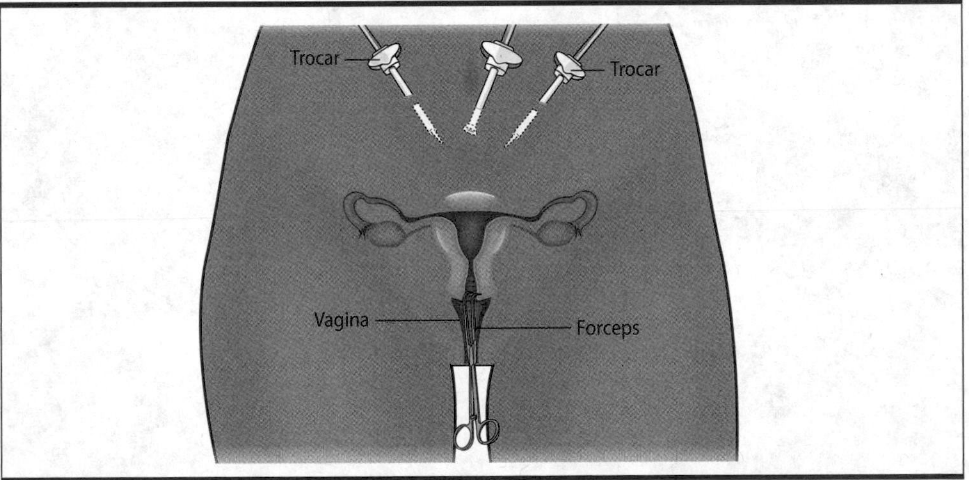

External (X)

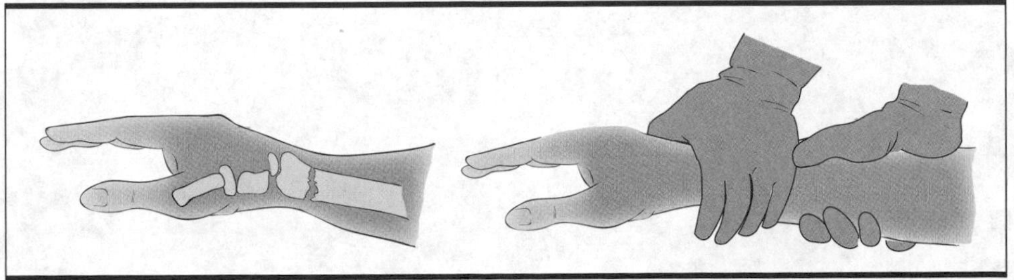

Appendix B: Root Operation Definitions

The character 3 value in the Medical and Surgical section (Ø) and the Medical and Surgical-related sections (1-9) represents the root operation. This resource provides each root operation (character 3) value, found in sections Ø-9, as well as their associated definition, explanation, and examples, where applicable. The Ancillary sections (B-H) do not include root operations; instead the character 3 value represents the type of procedure performed with additional detail provided by the character 4 or 5 value, when applicable. For the character 3, character 4, and character 5 values used in the Ancillary sections of B-H, along with their definitions, see appendix J.

Ø	Medical and Surgical		
ICD-10-PCS Value		**Definition**	
Ø	Alteration	Definition:	Modifying the anatomic structure of a body part without affecting the function of the body part
		Explanation:	Principal purpose is to improve appearance
		Examples:	Face lift, breast augmentation
1	Bypass	Definition:	Altering the route of passage of the contents of a tubular body part
		Explanation:	Rerouting contents of a body part to a downstream area of the normal route, to a similar route and body part, or to an abnormal route and dissimilar body part. Includes one or more anastomoses, with or without the use of a device.
		Examples:	Coronary artery bypass, colostomy formation
2	Change	Definition:	Taking out or off a device from a body part and putting back an identical or similar device in or on the same body part without cutting or puncturing the skin or a mucous membrane
		Explanation:	All CHANGE procedures are coded using the approach EXTERNAL
		Example:	Urinary catheter change, gastrostomy tube change
3	Control	Definition:	Stopping, or attempting to stop, postprocedural or other acute bleeding
		Explanation:	None
		Examples:	Control of post-prostatectomy hemorrhage, control of intracranial subdural hemorrhage, control of bleeding duodenal ulcer, control of retroperitoneal hemorrhage
4	Creation	Definition:	Putting in or on biological or synthetic material to form a new body part that to the extent possible replicates the anatomic structure or function of an absent body part
		Explanation:	Used for gender reassignment surgery and corrective procedures in individuals with congenital anomalies
		Examples:	Creation of vagina in a male, creation of right and left atrioventricular valve from common atrioventricular valve
5	Destruction	Definition:	Physical eradication of all or a portion of a body part by the direct use of energy, force, or a destructive agent
		Explanation:	None of the body part is physically taken out
		Examples:	Fulguration of rectal polyp, cautery of skin lesion
6	Detachment	Definition:	Cutting off all or a portion of the upper or lower extremities
		Explanation:	The body part value is the site of the detachment, with a qualifier if applicable to further specify the level where the extremity was detached
		Examples:	Below knee amputation, disarticulation of shoulder
7	Dilation	Definition:	Expanding an orifice or the lumen of a tubular body part
		Explanation:	The orifice can be a natural orifice or an artificially created orifice. Accomplished by stretching a tubular body part using intraluminal pressure or by cutting part of the orifice or wall of the tubular body part.
		Examples:	Percutaneous transluminal angioplasty, internal urethrotomy
8	Division	Definition:	Cutting into a body part, without draining fluids and/or gases from the body part, in order to separate or transect a body part
		Explanation:	All or a portion of the body part is separated into two or more portions
		Examples:	Spinal cordotomy, osteotomy
9	Drainage	Definition:	Taking or letting out fluids and/or gases from a body part
		Explanation:	The qualifier DIAGNOSTIC is used to identify drainage procedures that are biopsies
		Examples:	Thoracentesis, incision and drainage
B	Excision	Definition:	Cutting out or off, without replacement, a portion of a body part
		Explanation:	The qualifier DIAGNOSTIC is used to identify excision procedures that are biopsies
		Examples:	Partial nephrectomy, liver biopsy

Continued on next page

Ø Medical and Surgical

Continued from previous page

ICD-10-PCS Value		Definition	
C	Extirpation	Definition:	Taking or cutting out solid matter from a body part
		Explanation:	The solid matter may be an abnormal byproduct of a biological function or a foreign body; it may be imbedded in a body part or in the lumen of a tubular body part. The solid matter may or may not have been previously broken into pieces.
		Examples:	Thrombectomy, choledocholithotomy
D	Extraction	Definition:	Pulling or stripping out or off all or a portion of a body part by the use of force
		Explanation:	The qualifier DIAGNOSTIC is used to identify extractions that are biopsies
		Examples:	Dilation and curettage, vein stripping
F	Fragmentation	Definition:	Breaking solid matter in a body part into pieces
		Explanation:	Physical force (e.g., manual, ultrasonic) applied directly or indirectly is used to break the solid matter into pieces. The solid matter may be an abnormal byproduct of a biological function or a foreign body. The pieces of solid matter are not taken out.
		Examples:	Extracorporeal shockwave lithotripsy, transurethral lithotripsy
G	Fusion	Definition:	Joining together portions of an articular body part rendering the articular body part immobile
		Explanation:	The body part is joined together by fixation device, bone graft, or other means
		Examples:	Spinal fusion, ankle arthrodesis
H	Insertion	Definition:	Putting in a nonbiological appliance that monitors, assists, performs, or prevents a physiological function but does not physically take the place of a body part
		Explanation:	None
		Examples:	Insertion of radioactive implant, insertion of central venous catheter
J	Inspection	Definition:	Visually and/or manually exploring a body part
		Explanation:	Visual exploration may be performed with or without optical instrumentation. Manual exploration may be performed directly or through intervening body layers.
		Examples:	Diagnostic arthroscopy, exploratory laparotomy
K	Map	Definition:	Locating the route of passage of electrical impulses and/or locating functional areas in a body part
		Explanation:	Applicable only to the cardiac conduction mechanism and the central nervous system
		Examples:	Cardiac mapping, cortical mapping
L	Occlusion	Definition:	Completely closing an orifice or lumen of a tubular body part
		Explanation:	The orifice can be a natural orifice or an artificially created orifice
		Examples:	Fallopian tube ligation, ligation of inferior vena cava
M	Reattachment	Definition:	Putting back in or on all or a portion of a separated body part to its normal location or other suitable location
		Explanation:	Vascular circulation and nervous pathways may or may not be reestablished
		Examples:	Reattachment of hand, reattachment of avulsed kidney
N	Release	Definition:	Freeing a body part from an abnormal physical constraint by cutting or by use of force
		Explanation:	Some of the restraining tissue may be taken out but none of the body part is taken out
		Examples:	Adhesiolysis, carpal tunnel release
P	Removal	Definition:	Taking out or off a device from a body part
		Explanation:	If a device is taken out and a similar device put in without cutting or puncturing the skin or mucous membrane, the procedure is coded to the root operation CHANGE. Otherwise, the procedure for taking out a device is coded to the root operation REMOVAL.
		Examples:	Drainage tube removal, cardiac pacemaker removal
Q	Repair	Definition:	Restoring, to the extent possible, a body part to its normal anatomic structure and function
		Explanation:	Used only when the method to accomplish the repair is not one of the other root operations
		Examples:	Colostomy takedown, suture of laceration
R	Replacement	Definition:	Putting in or on biological or synthetic material that physically takes the place and/or function of all or a portion of a body part
		Explanation:	The body part may have been taken out or replaced, or may be taken out, physically eradicated, or rendered nonfunctional during the REPLACEMENT procedure. A REMOVAL procedure is coded for taking out the device used in a previous replacement procedure.
		Examples:	Total hip replacement, bone graft, free skin graft

Continued on next page

Ø Medical and Surgical

Continued from previous page

ICD-10-PCS Value		Definition	
S	Reposition	Definition:	Moving to its normal location, or other suitable location, all or a portion of a body part
		Explanation:	The body part is moved to a new location from an abnormal location, or from a normal location where it is not functioning correctly. The body part may or may not be cut out or off to be moved to the new location.
		Examples:	Reposition of undescended testicle, fracture reduction
T	Resection	Definition:	Cutting out or off, without replacement, all of a body part
		Explanation:	None
		Examples:	Total nephrectomy, total lobectomy of lung
V	Restriction	Definition:	Partially closing an orifice or the lumen of a tubular body part
		Explanation:	The orifice can be a natural orifice or an artificially created orifice
		Examples:	Esophagogastric fundoplication, cervical cerclage
W	Revision	Definition:	Correcting, to the extent possible, a portion of a malfunctioning device or the position of a displaced device
		Explanation:	Revision can include correcting a malfunctioning or displaced device by taking out or putting in components of the device such as a screw or pin
		Examples:	Adjustment of position of pacemaker lead, recementing of hip prosthesis
U	Supplement	Definition:	Putting in or on biological or synthetic material that physically reinforces and/or augments the function of a portion of a body part
		Explanation:	The biological material is non-living, or is living and from the same individual. The body part may have been previously replaced, and the SUPPLEMENT procedure is performed to physically reinforce and/or augment the function of the replaced body part.
		Examples:	Herniorrhaphy using mesh, mitral valve ring annuloplasty, put a new acetabular liner in a previous hip replacement
X	Transfer	Definition:	Moving, without taking out, all or a portion of a body part to another location to take over the function of all or a portion of a body part
		Explanation:	The body part transferred remains connected to its vascular and nervous supply
		Examples:	Tendon transfer, skin pedicle flap transfer
Y	Transplantation	Definition:	Putting in or on all or a portion of a living body part taken from another individual or animal to physically take the place and/or function of all or a portion of a similar body part
		Explanation:	The native body part may or may not be taken out, and the transplanted body part may take over all or a portion of its function
		Examples:	Kidney transplant, heart transplant

Root Operation Definitions for Other Sections

1 Obstetrics

ICD-10-PCS Value		Definition	
2	Change	Definition:	Taking out or off a device from a body part and putting back an identical or similar device in or on the same body part without cutting or puncturing the skin or a mucous membrane
		Explanation:	None
		Examples:	Replacement of fetal scalp electrode
9	Drainage	Definition:	Taking or letting out fluids and/or gases from a body part
		Explanation:	None
		Examples:	Biopsy of amniotic fluid
A	Abortion	Definition:	Artificially terminating a pregnancy
		Explanation:	None
		Examples:	Transvaginal abortion using vacuum aspiration technique
D	Extraction	Definition:	Pulling or stripping out or off all or a portion of a body part by the use of force
		Explanation:	None
		Examples:	Low-transverse C-section
E	Delivery	Definition:	Assisting the passage of the products of conception from the genital canal
		Explanation:	None
		Examples:	Manually-assisted delivery

Continued on next page

1 Obstetrics

Continued from previous page

ICD-10-PCS Value		Definition	
H	Insertion	Definition:	Putting in a nonbiological appliance that monitors, assists, performs, or prevents a physiological function but does not physically take the place of a body part
		Explanation:	None
		Examples:	Placement of fetal scalp electrode
J	Inspection	Definition:	Visually and/or manually exploring a body part
		Explanation:	Visual exploration may be performed with or without optical instrumentation. Manual exploration may be performed directly or through intervening body layers.
		Examples:	Bimanual pregnancy exam
P	Removal	Definition:	Taking out or off a device from a body part, region or orifice
		Explanation:	If a device is taken out and a similar device put in without cutting or puncturing the skin or mucous membrane, the procedure is coded to the root operation CHANGE. Otherwise, the procedure for taking out a device is coded to the root operation REMOVAL.
		Examples:	Removal of fetal monitoring electrode
Q	Repair	Definition:	Restoring, to the extent possible, a body part to its normal anatomic structure and function
		Explanation:	Used only when the method to accomplish the repair is not one of the other root operations
		Examples:	In utero repair of congenital diaphragmatic hernia
S	Reposition	Definition:	Moving to its normal location, or other suitable location, all or a portion of a body part
		Explanation:	The body part is moved to a new location from an abnormal location, or from a normal location where it is not functioning correctly. The body part may or may not be cut out or off to be moved to the new location.
		Examples:	External version of fetus
T	Resection	Definition:	Cutting out or off, without replacement, all of a body part
		Explanation:	None
		Examples:	Total excision of tubal pregnancy
Y	Transplantation	Definition:	Putting in or on all or a portion of a living body part taken from another individual or animal to physically take the place and/or function of all or a portion of a similar body part
		Explanation:	The native body part may or may not be taken out, and the transplanted body part may take over all or a portion of its function
		Examples:	In utero fetal kidney transplant

2 Placement

ICD-10-PCS Value		Definition	
Ø	Change	Definition:	Taking out or off a device from a body part and putting back an identical or similar device in or on the same body part without cutting or puncturing the skin or a mucous membrane
		Examples:	Change of vaginal packing
1	Compression	Definition:	Putting pressure on a body region
		Examples:	Placement of pressure dressing on abdominal wall
2	Dressing	Definition:	Putting material on a body region for protection
		Examples:	Application of sterile dressing to head wound
3	Immobilization	Definition:	Limiting or preventing motion of a body region
		Examples:	Placement of splint on left finger
4	Packing	Definition:	Putting material in a body region or orifice
		Examples:	Placement of nasal packing
5	Removal	Definition:	Taking out or off a device from a body part
		Examples:	Removal of stereotactic head frame
6	Traction	Definition:	Exerting a pulling force on a body region in a distal direction
		Examples:	Lumbar traction using motorized split-traction table

3 Administration

ICD-10-PCS Value		Definition	
Ø	Introduction	Definition:	Putting in or on a therapeutic, diagnostic, nutritional, physiological, or prophylactic substance except blood or blood products
		Examples:	Nerve block injection to median nerve
1	Irrigation	Definition:	Putting in or on a cleansing substance
		Examples:	Flushing of eye
2	Transfusion	Definition:	Putting in blood or blood products
		Examples:	Transfusion of cell saver red cells into central venous line

4 Measurement and Monitoring

ICD-10-PCS Value		Definition	
Ø	Measurement	Definition:	Determining the level of a physiological or physical function at a point in time
		Examples:	External electrocardiogram(EKG), single reading
1	Monitoring	Definition:	Determining the level of a physiological or physical function repetitively over a period of time
		Examples:	Urinary pressure monitoring

5 Extracorporeal or Systemic Assistance and Performance

ICD-10-PCS Value		Definition	
Ø	Assistance	Definition:	Taking over a portion of a physiological function by extracorporeal means
		Examples:	Hyperbaric oxygenation of wound
1	Performance	Definition:	Completely taking over a physiological function by extracorporeal means
		Examples:	Cardiopulmonary bypass in conjunction with CABG
2	Restoration	Definition:	Returning, or attempting to return, a physiological function to its original state by extracorporeal means
		Examples:	Attempted cardiac defibrillation, unsuccessful

6 Extracorporeal or Systemic Therapies

ICD-10-PCS Value		Definition	
Ø	Atmospheric Control	Definition:	Extracorporeal control of atmospheric pressure and composition
		Examples:	Antigen-free air conditioning, series treatment
1	Decompression	Definition:	Extracorporeal elimination of undissolved gas from body fluids
		Examples:	Hyperbaric decompression treatment, single
2	Electromagnetic Therapy	Definition:	Extracorporeal treatment by electromagnetic rays
		Examples:	TMS (transcranial magnetic stimulation), series treatment
3	Hyperthermia	Definition:	Extracorporeal raising of body temperature
		Examples:	None
4	Hypothermia	Definition:	Extracorporeal lowering of body temperature
		Examples:	Whole body hypothermia treatment for temperature imbalances, series
5	Pheresis	Definition:	Extracorporeal separation of blood products
		Examples:	Therapeutic leukopheresis, single treatment
6	Phototherapy	Definition:	Extracorporeal treatment by light rays
		Examples:	Phototherapy of circulatory system, series treatment
7	Ultrasound Therapy	Definition:	Extracorporeal treatment by ultrasound
		Examples:	Therapeutic ultrasound of peripheral vessels, single treatment
8	Ultraviolet Light Therapy	Definition:	Extracorporeal treatment by ultraviolet light
		Examples:	Ultraviolet light phototherapy, series treatment
9	Shock Wave Therapy	Definition:	Extracorporeal treatment by shock waves
		Examples:	Shockwave therapy of plantar fascia, single treatment
B	Perfusion	Definition:	Extracorporeal treatment by diffusion of therapeutic fluid
		Examples:	Perfusion of donor liver while preparing transplant patient

7 Osteopathic

ICD-10-PCS Value			Definition
Ø	Treatment	Definition:	Manual treatment to eliminate or alleviate somatic dysfunction and related disorders
		Examples:	Fascial release of abdomen, osteopathic treatment

8 Other Procedures

ICD-10-PCS Value			Definition
Ø	Other Procedures	Definition:	Methodologies which attempt to remediate or cure a disorder or disease
		Examples:	Acupuncture, yoga therapy

9 Chiropractic

ICD-10-PCS Value			Definition
B	Manipulation	Definition:	Manual procedure that involves a directed thrust to move a joint past the physiological range of motion, without exceeding the anatomical limit
		Examples:	Chiropractic treatment of cervical spine, short lever specific contact

Appendix C: Comparison of Medical and Surgical Root Operations

Note: the character associated with each operation appears in parentheses after its title.

Procedures That Take Out Some or All of a Body Part

Root Operation	Objective of Procedure	Site of Procedure	Example
Destruction (5)	Eradicating without taking out or replacement	Some/all of a body part	Fulguration of endometrium
Detachment (6)	Cutting out/off without replacement	Extremity only, any level	Amputation above elbow
Excision (B)	Cutting out/off without replacement	Some of a body part	Breast lumpectomy
Extraction (D)	Pulling out or off without replacement	Some/all of a body part	Suction D&C
Resection (T)	Cutting out/off without replacement	All of a body part	Total mastectomy

Procedures That Put in/Put Back or Move Some/All of a Body Part

Root Operation	Objective of Procedure	Site of Procedure	Example
Reattachment (M)	Putting back a detached body part	Some/all of a body part	Reattach finger
Reposition (S)	Moving a body part to normal or other suitable location	Some/all of a body part	Move undescended testicle
Transfer (X)	Moving a body part to function for a similar body part	Some/all of a body part	Skin pedicle transfer flap
Transplantation (Y)	Putting in a living body part from a person/animal	Some/all of a body part	Kidney transplant

Procedures That Take Out or Eliminate Solid Matter, Fluids, or Gases From a Body Part

Root Operation	Objective of Procedure	Site of Procedure	Example
Drainage (9)	Taking or letting out	Fluids and/or gases from a body part	Incision and drainage
Extirpation (C)	Taking or cutting out	Solid matter in a body part	Thrombectomy
Fragmentation (F)	Breaking into pieces	Solid matter within a body part	Lithotripsy

Procedures That Involve Only Examination of Body Parts and Regions

Root Operation	Objective of Procedure	Site of Procedure	Example
Inspection (J)	Visual/manual exploration	Some/all of a body part	Diagnostic cystoscopy Exploratory laparoscopy
Map (K)	Locating electrical impulse route/functional areas	Brain/cardiac conduction mechanism	Cardiac mapping

Procedures That Alter the Diameter/Route of a Tubular Body Part

Root Operation	Objective of Procedure	Site of Procedure	Example
Bypass (1)	Altering route of passage of contents	Tubular body part	Coronary artery bypass graft (CABG)
Dilation (7)	Expanding natural or artificially created orifice/lumen	Tubular body part	Percutaneous transluminal coronary angioplasty (PTCA)
Occlusion (L)	Completely closing natural or artificially created orifice/lumen	Tubular body part	Fallopian tube ligation
Restriction (V)	Partially closing natural or artificially created orifice/lumen	Tubular body part	Gastroesophageal fundoplication

Procedures That Always Involve Devices

Root Operation	Objective of Procedure	Site of Procedure	Example
Change (2) DVC	Exchanging device w/out cutting/puncturing	In/on a body part	Gastrostomy tube change
Insertion (H) DVC	Putting in nonbiological device	In/on a body part	Central line insertion
Removal (P) DVC	Taking out device	In/on a body part	Central line removal
Replacement (R) DVC	Putting in device that replaces a body part	Some/all of a body part	Total hip replacement
Revision (W) DVC	Correcting a malfunctioning/displaced device	In/on a body part	Revision of pacemaker
Supplement (U) DVC	Putting in device that reinforces or augments a body part	In/on a body part	Abdominal wall herniorrhaphy using mesh

DVC = Device involved in root operation

Procedures Involving Cutting or Separation Only

Root Operation	Objective of Procedure	Site of Procedure	Example
Division (8)	Cutting into/separating	A body part	Neurotomy
Release (N)	Freeing a body part from constraint	Around a body part	Adhesiolysis

Procedures That Define Other Repairs

Root Operation	Objective of Procedure	Site of Procedure	Example
Control (3)	Stopping/attempting to stop postprocedural or other acute bleeding	Anatomical region or nasal mucosa/soft tissue	Post-prostatectomy bleeding control, control subdural hemorrhage, bleeding ulcer, retroperitoneal hemorrhage
Repair (Q)	Restoring body part to its normal structure/function	Some/all of a body part	Suture laceration

Procedures That Define Other Objectives

Root Operation	Objective of Procedure	Site of Procedure	Example
Alteration (Ø)	Modifying body part for cosmetic purposes without affecting function	Some/all of a body part	Face lift
Creation (4)	Using biological or synthetic material to form a new body part that replicates the anatomic structure or function of a missing body part	Perineum, valve	Sex change/artificial vagina/penis, atrioventricular valve creation
Fusion (G)	Unification or immobilization	Joint or articular body part	Spinal fusion

Appendix D: Body Part Key

Term	ICD-10-PCS Value
Abdominal aortic plexus	Abdominal Sympathetic Nerve
Abdominal esophagus	Esophagus, Lower
Abductor hallucis muscle	Foot Muscle, Right
	Foot Muscle, Left
Accessory cephalic vein	Cephalic Vein, Right
	Cephalic Vein, Left
Accessory obturator nerve	Lumbar Plexus
Accessory phrenic nerve	Phrenic nerve
Accessory spleen	Spleen
Acetabulofemoral joint	Hip Joint, Right
	Hip Joint, Left
Achilles tendon	Lower Leg Tendon, Right
	Lower Leg Tendon, Left
Acromioclavicular ligament	Shoulder Bursa and Ligament, Right
	Shoulder Bursa and Ligament, Left
Acromion (process)	Scapula, Right
	Scapula, Left
Adductor brevis muscle	Upper Leg Muscle, Right
	Upper Leg Muscle, Left
Adductor hallucis muscle	Foot Muscle, Right
	Foot Muscle, Left
Adductor longus muscle	Upper Leg Muscle, Right
	Upper Leg Muscle, Left
Adductor magnus muscle	Upper Leg Muscle, Right
	Upper Leg Muscle, Left
Adenohypophysis	Pituitary Gland
Alar ligament of axis	Head and Neck Bursa and Ligament
Alveolar process of mandible	Mandible, Right
	Mandible, Left
Alveolar process of maxilla	Maxilla
Anal orifice	Anus
Anatomical snuffbox	Lower Arm and Wrist Muscle, Right
	Lower Arm and Wrist Muscle, Left
Angular artery	Face Artery
Angular vein	Face Vein, Right
	Face Vein, Left
Annular ligament	Elbow Bursa and Ligament, Right
	Elbow Bursa and Ligament, Left
Anorectal junction	Rectum
Ansa cervicalis	Cervical Plexus
Antebrachial fascia	Subcutaneous Tissue and Fascia, Right Lower Arm
	Subcutaneous Tissue and Fascia, Left Lower Arm
Anterior (pectoral) lymph node	Lymphatic, Right Axillary
	Lymphatic, Left Axillary
Anterior cerebral artery	Intracranial Artery
Anterior cerebral vein	Intracranial Vein
Anterior choroidal artery	Intracranial Artery
Anterior circumflex humeral artery	Axillary Artery, Right
	Axillary Artery, Left
Anterior communicating artery	Intracranial Artery

Term	ICD-10-PCS Value
Anterior cruciate ligament (ACL)	Knee Bursa and Ligament, Right
	Knee Bursa and Ligament, Left
Anterior crural nerve	Femoral Nerve
Anterior facial vein	Face Vein, Right
	Face Vein, Left
Anterior intercostal artery	Internal Mammary Artery, Right
	Internal Mammary Artery, Left
Anterior interosseous nerve	Median Nerve
Anterior lateral malleolar artery	Anterior Tibial Artery, Right
	Anterior Tibial Artery, Left
Anterior lingual gland	Minor Salivary Gland
Anterior medial malleolar artery	Anterior Tibial Artery, Right
	Anterior Tibial Artery, Left
Anterior spinal artery	Vertebral Artery, Right
	Vertebral Artery, Left
Anterior tibial recurrent artery	Anterior Tibial Artery, Right
	Anterior Tibial Artery, Left
Anterior ulnar recurrent artery	Ulnar Artery, Right
	Ulnar Artery, Left
Anterior vagal trunk	Vagus Nerve
Anterior vertebral muscle	Neck Muscle, Right
	Neck Muscle, Left
Antihelix	External Ear, Right
	External Ear, Left
	External Ear, Bilateral
Antitragus	External Ear, Right
	External Ear, Left
	External Ear, Bilateral
Antrum of Highmore	Maxillary Sinus, Right
	Maxillary Sinus, Left
Aortic annulus	Aortic Valve
Aortic arch	Thoracic Aorta, Ascending/Arch
Aortic intercostal artery	Upper Artery
Apical (subclavicular) lymph node	Lymphatic, Right Axillary
	Lymphatic, Left Axillary
Apneustic center	Pons
Aqueduct of Sylvius	Cerebral Ventricle
Aqueous humour	Anterior Chamber, Right
	Anterior Chamber, Left
Arachnoid mater, intracranial	Cerebral Meninges
Arachnoid mater, spinal	Spinal Meninges
Arcuate artery	Foot Artery, Right
	Foot Artery, Left
Areola	Nipple, Right
	Nipple, Left
Arterial canal (duct)	Pulmonary Artery, Left
Aryepiglottic fold	Larynx
Arytenoid cartilage	Larynx
Arytenoid muscle	Neck Muscle, Right
	Neck Muscle, Left
Ascending aorta	Thoracic Aorta, Ascending/Arch
Ascending palatine artery	Face Artery

Term	ICD-10-PCS Value
Ascending pharyngeal artery	External Carotid Artery, Right
	External Carotid Artery, Left
Atlantoaxial joint	Cervical Vertebral Joint
Atrioventricular node	Conduction Mechanism
Atrium dextrum cordis	Atrium, Right
Atrium pulmonale	Atrium, Left
Auditory tube	Eustachian Tube, Right
	Eustachian Tube, Left
Auerbach's (myenteric)plexus	Abdominal Sympathetic Nerve
Auricle	External Ear, Right
	External Ear, Left
	External Ear, Bilateral
Auricularis muscle	Head Muscle
Axillary fascia	Subcutaneous Tissue and Fascia, Right Upper Arm
	Subcutaneous Tissue and Fascia, Left Upper Arm
Axillary nerve	Brachial Plexus
Bartholin's (greater vestibular) gland	Vestibular Gland
Basal (internal) cerebral vein	Intracranial Vein
Basal nuclei	Basal Ganglia
Base of tongue	Pharynx
Basilar artery	Intracranial Artery
Basis pontis	Pons
Biceps brachii muscle	Upper Arm Muscle, Right
	Upper Arm Muscle, Left
Biceps femoris muscle	Upper Leg Muscle, Right
	Upper Leg Muscle, Left
Bicipital aponeurosis	Subcutaneous Tissue and Fascia, Right Lower Arm
	Subcutaneous Tissue and Fascia, Left Lower Arm
Bicuspid valve	Mitral Valve
Body of femur	Femoral Shaft, Right
	Femoral Shaft, Left
Body of fibula	Fibula, Right
	Fibula, Left
Bony labyrinth	Inner Ear, Right
	Inner Ear, Left
Bony orbit	Orbit, Right
	Orbit, Left
Bony vestibule	Inner Ear, Right
	Inner Ear, Left
Botallo's duct	Pulmonary Artery, Left
Brachial (lateral) lymph node	Lymphatic, Right Axillary
	Lymphatic, Left Axillary
Brachialis muscle	Upper Arm Muscle, Right
	Upper Arm Muscle, Left
Brachiocephalic artery	Innominate Artery
Brachiocephalic trunk	Innominate Artery
Brachiocephalic vein	Innominate Vein, Right
	Innominate Vein, Left
Brachioradialis muscle	Lower Arm and Wrist Muscle, Right
	Lower Arm and Wrist Muscle, Left

Term	ICD-10-PCS Value
Breast procedures, skin only	Skin, Chest
Broad ligament	Uterine Supporting Structure
Bronchial artery	Upper Artery
Bronchus intermedius	Main Bronchus, Right
Buccal gland	Buccal Mucosa
Buccinator lymph node	Lymphatic, Head
Buccinator muscle	Facial Muscle
Bulbospongiosus muscle	Perineum Muscle
Bulbourethral (Cowper's) gland	Urethra
Bundle of His	Conduction Mechanism
Bundle of Kent	Conduction Mechanism
Calcaneocuboid joint	Tarsal Joint, Right
	Tarsal Joint, Left
Calcaneocuboid ligament	Foot Bursa and Ligament, Right
	Foot Bursa and Ligament, Left
Calcaneofibular ligament	Ankle Bursa and Ligament, Right
	Ankle Bursa and Ligament, Left
Calcaneus	Tarsal, Right
	Tarsal, Left
Capitate bone	Carpal, Right
	Carpal, Left
Cardia	Esophagogastric Junction
Cardiac plexus	Thoracic Sympathetic Nerve
Cardioesophageal junction	Esophagogastric Junction
Caroticotympanic artery	Internal Carotid Artery, Right
	Internal Carotid Artery, Left
Carotid glomus	Carotid Body, Right
	Carotid Body, Left
	Carotid Bodies, Bilateral
Carotid sinus	Internal Carotid Artery, Right
	Internal Carotid Artery, Left
Carotid sinus nerve	Glossopharyngeal Nerve
Carpometacarpal ligament	Hand Bursa and Ligament, Right
	Hand Bursa and Ligament, Left
Cauda equina	Lumbar Spinal Cord
Cavernous plexus	Head and Neck Sympathetic Nerve
Celiac ganglion	Abdominal Sympathetic Nerve
Celiac (solar) plexus	Abdominal Sympathetic Nerve
Celiac lymph node	Lymphatic, Aortic
Celiac trunk	Celiac Artery
Central axillary lymph node	Lymphatic, Right Axillary
	Lymphatic, Left Axillary
Cerebral aqueduct (Sylvius)	Cerebral Ventricle
Cerebrum	Brain
Cervical esophagus	Esophagus, Upper
Cervical facet joint	Cervical Vertebral Joint
	Cervical Vertebral Joints, 2 or more
Cervical ganglion	Head and Neck Sympathetic Nerve
Cervical interspinous ligament	Head and Neck Bursa and Ligament
Cervical intertransverse ligament	Head and Neck Bursa and Ligament
Cervical ligamentum flavum	Head and Neck Bursa and Ligament

Term	ICD-10-PCS Value
Cervical lymph node	Lymphatic, Right Neck
	Lymphatic, Left Neck
Cervicothoracic facet joint	Cervicothoracic Vertebral Joint
Choana	Nasopharynx
Chondroglossus muscle	Tongue, Palate, Pharynx Muscle
Chorda tympani	Facial Nerve
Choroid plexus	Cerebral Ventricle
Ciliary body	Eye, Right
	Eye, Left
Ciliary ganglion	Head and Neck Sympathetic Nerve
Circle of Willis	Intracranial Artery
Circumflex illiac artery	Femoral Artery, Right
	Femoral Artery, Left
Claustrum	Basal Ganglia
Coccygeal body	Coccygeal Glomus
Coccygeus muscle	Trunk Muscle, Right
	Trunk Muscle, Left
Cochlea	Inner Ear, Right
	Inner Ear, Left
Cochlear nerve	Acoustic Nerve
Columella	Nasal Mucosa and Soft Tissue
Common digital vein	Foot Vein, Right
	Foot Vein, Left
Common facial vein	Face Vein, Right
	Face Vein, Left
Common fibular nerve	Peroneal Nerve
Common hepatic artery	Hepatic Artery
Common iliac (subaortic) lymph node	Lymphatic, Pelvis
Common interosseous artery	Ulnar Artery, Right
	Ulnar Artery, Left
Common peroneal nerve	Peroneal Nerve
Condyloid process	Mandible, Right
	Mandible, Left
Conus arteriosus	Ventricle, Right
Conus medullaris	Lumbar Spinal Cord
Coracoacromial ligament	Shoulder Bursa and Ligament, Right
	Shoulder Bursa and Ligament, Left
Coracobrachialis muscle	Upper Arm Muscle, Right
	Upper Arm Muscle, Left
Coracoclavicular ligament	Shoulder Bursa and Ligament, Right
	Shoulder Bursa and Ligament, Left
Coracohumeral ligament	Shoulder Bursa and Ligament, Right
	Shoulder Bursa and Ligament, Left
Coracoid process	Scapula, Right
	Scapula, Left
Corniculate cartilage	Larynx
Corpus callosum	Brain
Corpus cavernosum	Penis
Corpus spongiosum	Penis
Corpus striatum	Basal Ganglia
Corrugator supercilii muscle	Facial Muscle
Costocervical trunk	Subclavian Artery, Right
	Subclavian Artery, Left

Term	ICD-10-PCS Value
Costoclavicular ligament	Shoulder Bursa and Ligament, Right
	Shoulder Bursa and Ligament, Left
Costotransverse joint	Thoracic Vertebral Joint
Costotransverse ligament	Rib(s) Bursa and Ligament
Costovertebral joint	Thoracic Vertebral Joint
Costoxiphoid ligament	Sternum Bursa and Ligament
Cowper's (bulbourethral) gland	Urethra
Cremaster muscle	Perineum Muscle
Cribriform plate	Ethmoid Bone, Right
	Ethmoid Bone, Left
Cricoid cartilage	Trachea
Cricothyroid artery	Thyroid Artery, Right
	Thyroid Artery, Left
Cricothyroid muscle	Neck Muscle, Right
	Neck Muscle, Left
Crural fascia	Subcutaneous Tissue and Fascia, Right Upper Leg
	Subcutaneous Tissue and Fascia, Left Upper Leg
Cubital lymph node	Lymphatic, Right Upper Extremity
	Lymphatic, Left Upper Extremity
Cubital nerve	Ulnar Nerve
Cuboid bone	Tarsal, Right
	Tarsal, Left
Cuboideonavicular joint	Tarsal Joint, Right
	Tarsal Joint, Left
Culmen	Cerebellum
Cuneiform cartilage	Larynx
Cuneonavicular joint	Tarsal Joint, Right
	Tarsal Joint, Left
Cuneonavicular ligament	Foot Bursa and Ligament, Right
	Foot Bursa and Ligament, Left
Cutaneous (transverse) cervical nerve	Cervical Plexus
Deep cervical fascia	Subcutaneous Tissue and Fascia, Right Neck
	Subcutaneous Tissue and Fascia, Left Neck
Deep cervical vein	Vertebral Vein, Right
	Vertebral Vein, Left
Deep circumflex iliac artery	External Iliac Artery, Right
	External Iliac Artery, Left
Deep facial vein	Face Vein, Right
	Face Vein, Left
Deep femoral artery	Femoral Artery, Right
	Femoral Artery, Left
Deep femoral (profunda femoris) vein	Femoral Vein, Right
	Femoral Vein, Left
Deep palmar arch	Hand Artery, Right
	Hand Artery, Left
Deep transverse perineal muscle	Perineum Muscle
Deferential artery	Internal Iliac Artery, Right
	Internal Iliac Artery, Left

Term	ICD-10-PCS Value
Deltoid fascia	Subcutaneous Tissue and Fascia, Right Upper Arm
	Subcutaneous Tissue and Fascia, Left Upper Arm
Deltoid ligament	Ankle Bursa and Ligament, Right
	Ankle Bursa and Ligament, Left
Deltoid muscle	Shoulder Muscle, Right
	Shoulder Muscle, Left
Deltopectoral (infraclavicular) lymph node	Lymphatic, Right Upper Extremity
	Lymphatic, Left Upper Extremity
Dens	Cervical Vertebra
Denticulate (dentate) ligament	Spinal Meninges
Depressor anguli oris muscle	Facial Muscle
Depressor labii inferioris muscle	Facial Muscle
Depressor septi nasi muscle	Facial Muscle
Depressor supercilii muscle	Facial Muscle
Dermis	Skin
Descending genicular artery	Femoral Artery, Right
	Femoral Artery, Left
Diaphragma sellae	Dura Mater
Distal humerus	Humeral Shaft, Right
	Humeral Shaft, Left
Distal humerus, involving joint	Elbow Joint, Right
	Elbow Joint, Left
Distal radioulnar joint	Wrist Joint, Right
	Wrist Joint, Left
Dorsal digital nerve	Radial Nerve
Dorsal metacarpal vein	Hand Vein, Right
	Hand Vein, Left
Dorsal metatarsal artery	Foot Artery, Right
	Foot Artery, Left
Dorsal metatarsal vein	Foot Vein, Right
	Foot Vein, Left
Dorsal scapular artery	Subclavian Artery, Right
	Subclavian Artery, Left
Dorsal scapular nerve	Brachial Plexus
Dorsal venous arch	Foot Vein, Right
	Foot Vein, Left
Dorsalis pedis artery	Anterior Tibial Artery, Right
	Anterior Tibial Artery, Left
Duct of Santorini	Pancreatic Duct, Accessory
Duct of Wirsung	Pancreatic Duct
Ductus deferens	Vas Deferens, Right
	Vas Deferens, Left
	Vas Deferens, Bilateral
	Vas Deferens
Duodenal ampulla	Ampulla of Vater
Duodenojejunal flexure	Jejunum
Dura mater, intracranial	Dura Mater
Dura mater, spinal	Spinal Meninges
Dural venous sinus	Intracranial Vein
Earlobe	External Ear, Right
	External Ear, Left
	External Ear, Bilateral
Eighth cranial nerve	Acoustic Nerve
Ejaculatory duct	Vas Deferens, Right
	Vas Deferens, Left
	Vas Deferens, Bilateral
	Vas Deferens
Eleventh cranial nerve	Accessory Nerve
Encephalon	Brain
Ependyma	Cerebral Ventricle
Epidermis	Skin
Epidural space, spinal	Spinal Canal
Epiploic foramen	Peritoneum
Epithalamus	Thalamus
Epitroclear lymph node	Lymphatic, Right Upper Extremity
	Lymphatic, Left Upper Extremity
Erector spinae muscle	Trunk Muscle, Right
	Trunk Muscle, Left
Esophageal artery	Upper Artery
Esophageal plexus	Thoracic Sympathetic Nerve
Ethmoidal air cell	Ethmoid Sinus, Right
	Ethmoid Sinus, Left
Extensor carpi radialis muscle	Lower Arm and Wrist Muscle, Right
	Lower Arm and Wrist Muscle, Left
Extensor carpi ulnaris muscle	Lower Arm and Wrist Muscle, Right
	Lower Arm and Wrist Muscle, Left
Extensor digitorum brevis muscle	Foot Muscle, Right
	Foot Muscle, Left
Extensor digitorum longus muscle	Lower Leg Muscle, Right
	Lower Leg Muscle, Left
Extensor hallucis brevis muscle	Foot Muscle, Right
	Foot Muscle, Left
Extensor hallucis longus muscle	Lower Leg Muscle, Right
	Lower Leg Muscle, Left
External anal sphincter	Anal Sphincter
External auditory meatus	External Auditory Canal, Right
	External Auditory Canal, Left
External maxillary artery	Face Artery
External naris	Nasal Mucosa and Soft Tissue
External oblique aponeurosis	Subcutaneous Tissue and Fascia, Trunk
External oblique muscle	Abdomen Muscle, Right
	Abdomen Muscle, Left
External popliteal nerve	Peroneal Nerve
External pudendal artery	Femoral Artery, Right
	Femoral Artery, Left
External pudendal vein	Saphenous Vein, Right
	Saphenous Vein, Left
External urethral sphincter	Urethra
Extradural space, intracranial	Epidural Space, Intracranial
Extradural space, spinal	Spinal Canal
Facial artery	Face Artery
False vocal cord	Larynx
Falx cerebri	Dura Mater

Term	ICD-10-PCS Value
Fascia lata	Subcutaneous Tissue and Fascia, Right Upper Leg
	Subcutaneous Tissue and Fascia, Left Upper Leg
Femoral head	Upper Femur, Right
	Upper Femur, Left
Femoral lymph node	Lymphatic, Right Lower Extremity
	Lymphatic, Left Lower Extremity
Femoropatellar joint	Knee Joint, Right
	Knee Joint, Left
	Knee Joint, Femoral Surface, Right
	Knee Joint, Femoral Surface, Left
Femorotibial joint	Knee Joint, Right
	Knee Joint, Left
	Knee Joint, Tibial Surface, Right
	Knee Joint, Tibial Surface, Left
Fibular artery	Peroneal Artery, Right
	Peroneal Artery, Left
Fibularis brevis muscle	Lower Leg Muscle, Right
	Lower Leg Muscle, Left
Fibularis longus muscle	Lower Leg Muscle, Right
	Lower Leg Muscle, Left
Fifth cranial nerve	Trigeminal Nerve
Filum terminale	Spinal Meninges
First cranial nerve	Olfactory Nerve
First intercostal nerve	Brachial Plexus
Flexor carpi radialis muscle	Lower Arm and Wrist Muscle, Right
	Lower Arm and Wrist Muscle, Left
Flexor carpi ulnaris muscle	Lower Arm and Wrist Muscle, Right
	Lower Arm and Wrist Muscle, Left
Flexor digitorum brevis muscle	Foot Muscle, Right
	Foot Muscle, Left
Flexor digitorum longus muscle	Lower Leg Muscle, Right
	Lower Leg Muscle, Left
Flexor hallucis brevis muscle	Foot Muscle, Right
	Foot Muscle, Left
Flexor hallucis longus muscle	Lower Leg Muscle, Right
	Lower Leg Muscle, Left
Flexor pollicis longus muscle	Lower Arm and Wrist Muscle, Right
	Lower Arm and Wrist Muscle, Left
Foramen magnum	Occipital Bone
Foramen of Monro (intraventricular)	Cerebral Ventricle
Foreskin	Prepuce
Fossa of Rosenmuller	Nasopharynx
Fourth cranial nerve	Trochlear Nerve
Fourth ventricle	Cerebral Ventricle
Fovea	Retina, Right
	Retina, Left
Frenulum labii inferioris	Lower Lip
Frenulum labii superioris	Upper Lip
Frenulum linguae	Tongue
Frontal lobe	Cerebral Hemisphere
Frontal vein	Face Vein, Right
	Face Vein, Left
Fundus uteri	Uterus

Term	ICD-10-PCS Value
Galea aponeurotica	Subcutaneous Tissue and Fascia, Scalp
Ganglion impar (ganglion of Walther)	Sacral Sympathetic Nerve
Gasserian ganglion	Trigeminal Nerve
Gastric lymph node	Lymphatic, Aortic
Gastric plexus	Abdominal Sympathetic Nerve
Gastrocnemius muscle	Lower Leg Muscle, Right
	Lower Leg Muscle, Left
Gastrocolic ligament	Omentum
Gastrocolic omentum	Omentum
Gastroduodenal artery	Hepatic Artery
Gastroesophageal (GE) junction	Esophagogastric Junction
Gastrohepatic omentum	Omentum
Gastrophrenic ligament	Omentum
Gastrosplenic ligament	Omentum
Gemellus muscle	Hip Muscle, Right
	Hip Muscle, Left
Geniculate ganglion	Facial Nerve
Geniculate nucleus	Thalamus
Genioglossus muscle	Tongue, Palate, Pharynx Muscle
Genitofemoral nerve	Lumbar Plexus
Glans penis	Prepuce
Glenohumeral joint	Shoulder Joint, Right
	Shoulder Joint, Left
Glenohumeral ligament	Shoulder Bursa and Ligament, Right
	Shoulder Bursa and Ligament, Left
Glenoid fossa (of scapula)	Glenoid Cavity, Right
	Glenoid Cavity, Left
Glenoid ligament (labrum)	Shoulder Joint, Right
	Shoulder Joint, Left
Globus pallidus	Basal Ganglia
Glossoepiglottic fold	Epiglottis
Glottis	Larynx
Gluteal lymph node	Lymphatic, Pelvis
Gluteal vein	Hypogastric Vein, Right
	Hypogastric Vein, Left
Gluteus maximus muscle	Hip Muscle, Right
	Hip Muscle, Left
Gluteus medius muscle	Hip Muscle, Right
	Hip Muscle, Left
Gluteus minimus muscle	Hip Muscle, Right
	Hip Muscle, Left
Gracilis muscle	Upper Leg Muscle, Right
	Upper Leg Muscle, Left
Great auricular nerve	Cervical Plexus
Great cerebral vein	Intracranial Vein
Great(er) saphenous vein	Saphenous Vein, Right
	Saphenous Vein, Left
Greater alar cartilage	Nasal Mucosa and Soft Tissue
Greater occipital nerve	Cervical Nerve
Greater omentum	Omentum
Greater splanchnic nerve	Thoracic Sympathetic Nerve
Greater superficial petrosal nerve	Facial Nerve

Term	ICD-10-PCS Value
Greater trochanter	Upper Femur, Right
	Upper Femur, Left
Greater tuberosity	Humeral Head, Right
	Humeral Head, Left
Greater vestibular (Bartholin's) gland	Vestibular Gland
Greater wing	Sphenoid Bone
Hallux	1st Toe, Right
	1st Toe, Left
Hamate bone	Carpal, Right
	Carpal, Left
Head of fibula	Fibula, Right
	Fibula, Left
Helix	External Ear, Right
	External Ear, Left
	External Ear, Bilateral
Hepatic artery proper	Hepatic Artery
Hepatic flexure	Transverse Colon
Hepatic lymph node	Lymphatic, Aortic
Hepatic plexus	Abdominal Sympathetic Nerve
Hepatic portal vein	Portal Vein
Hepatogastric ligament	Omentum
Hepatopancreatic ampulla	Ampulla of Vater
Humeroradial joint	Elbow Joint, Right
	Elbow Joint, Left
Humeroulnar joint	Elbow Joint, Right
	Elbow Joint, Left
Humerus, distal	Humeral Shaft, Right
	Humeral Shaft, Left
Hyoglossus muscle	Tongue, Palate, Pharynx Muscle
Hyoid artery	Thyroid Artery, Right
	Thyroid Artery, Left
Hypogastric artery	Internal Iliac Artery, Right
	Internal Iliac Artery, Left
Hypopharynx	Pharynx
Hypophysis	Pituitary Gland
Hypothenar muscle	Hand Muscle, Right
	Hand Muscle, Left
Ileal artery	Superior Mesenteric Artery
Ileocolic artery	Superior Mesenteric Artery
Ileocolic vein	Colic Vein
Iliac crest	Pelvic Bone, Right
	Pelvic Bone, Left
Iliac fascia	Subcutaneous Tissue and Fascia, Right Upper Leg
	Subcutaneous Tissue and Fascia, Left Upper Leg
Iliac lymph node	Lymphatic, Pelvis
Iliacus muscle	Hip Muscle, Right
	Hip Muscle, Left
Iliofemoral ligament	Hip Bursa and Ligament, Right
	Hip Bursa and Ligament, Left
Iliohypogastric nerve	Lumbar Plexus
Ilioinguinal nerve	Lumbar Plexus
Iliolumbar artery	Internal Iliac Artery, Right
	Internal Iliac Artery, Left
Iliolumbar ligament	Lower Spine Bursa and Ligament
Iliotibial tract (band)	Subcutaneous Tissue and Fascia, Right Upper Leg
	Subcutaneous Tissue and Fascia, Left Upper Leg
Ilium	Pelvic Bone, Right
	Pelvic Bone, Left
Incus	Auditory Ossicle, Right
	Auditory Ossicle, Left
Inferior cardiac nerve	Thoracic Sympathetic Nerve
Inferior cerebellar vein	Intracranial Vein
Inferior cerebral vein	Intracranial Vein
Inferior epigastric artery	External Iliac Artery, Right
	External Iliac Artery, Left
Inferior epigastric lymph node	Lymphatic, Pelvis
Inferior genicular artery	Popliteal Artery, Right
	Popliteal Artery, Left
Inferior gluteal artery	Internal Iliac Artery, Right
	Internal Iliac Artery, Left
Inferior gluteal nerve	Sacral Plexus
Inferior hypogastric plexus	Abdominal Sympathetic Nerve
Inferior labial artery	Face Artery
Inferior longitudinal muscle	Tongue, Palate, Pharynx Muscle
Inferior mesenteric ganglion	Abdominal Sympathetic Nerve
Inferior mesenteric lymph node	Lymphatic, Mesenteric
Inferior mesenteric plexus	Abdominal Sympathetic Nerve
Inferior oblique muscle	Extraocular Muscle, Right
	Extraocular Muscle, Left
Inferior pancreaticoduodenal artery	Superior Mesenteric Artery
Inferior phrenic artery	Abdominal Aorta
Inferior rectus muscle	Extraocular Muscle, Right
	Extraocular Muscle, Left
Inferior suprarenal artery	Renal Artery, Right
	Renal Artery, Left
Inferior tarsal plate	Lower Eyelid, Right
	Lower Eyelid, Left
Inferior thyroid vein	Innominate Vein, Right
	Innominate Vein, Left
Inferior tibiofibular joint	Ankle Joint, Right
	Ankle Joint, Left
Inferior turbinate	Nasal Turbinate
Inferior ulnar collateral artery	Brachial Artery, Right
	Brachial Artery, Left
Inferior vesical artery	Internal Iliac Artery, Right
	Internal Iliac Artery, Left
Infraauricular lymph node	Lymphatic, Head
Infraclavicular (deltopectoral) lymph node	Lymphatic, Right Upper Extremity
	Lymphatic, Left Upper Extremity
Infrahyoid muscle	Neck Muscle, Right
	Neck Muscle, Left
Infraparotid lymph node	Lymphatic, Head

Term	ICD-10-PCS Value
Infraspinatus fascia	Subcutaneous Tissue and Fascia, Right Upper Arm
	Subcutaneous Tissue and Fascia, Left Upper Arm
Infraspinatus muscle	Shoulder Muscle, Right
	Shoulder Muscle, Left
Infundibulopelvic ligament	Uterine Supporting Structure
Inguinal canal	Inguinal Region, Right
	Inguinal Region, Left
	Inguinal Region, Bilateral
Inguinal triangle	Inguinal Region, Right
	Inguinal Region, Left
	Inguinal Region, Bilateral
Interatrial septum	Atrial Septum
Intercarpal joint	Carpal Joint, Right
	Carpal Joint, Left
Intercarpal ligament	Hand Bursa and Ligament, Right
	Hand Bursa and Ligament, Left
Interclavicular ligament	Shoulder Bursa and Ligament, Right
	Shoulder Bursa and Ligament, Left
Intercostal lymph node	Lymphatic, Thorax
Intercostal muscle	Thorax Muscle, Right
	Thorax Muscle, Left
Intercostal nerve	Thoracic Nerve
Intercostobrachial nerve	Thoracic Nerve
Intercuneiform joint	Tarsal Joint, Right
	Tarsal Joint, Left
Intercuneiform ligament	Foot Bursa and Ligament, Right
	Foot Bursa and Ligament, Left
Intermediate bronchus	Main Bronchus, Right
Intermediate cuneiform bone	Tarsal, Right
	Tarsal, Left
Internal anal sphincter	Anal Sphincter
Internal (basal) cerebral vein	Intracranial Vein
Internal carotid artery, intracranial portion	Intracranial Artery
Internal carotid plexus	Head and Neck Sympathetic Nerve
Internal iliac vein	Hypogastric Vein, Right
	Hypogastric Vein, Left
Internal maxillary artery	External Carotid Artery, Right
	External Carotid Artery, Left
Internal naris	Nasal Mucosa and Soft Tissue
Internal oblique muscle	Abdomen Muscle, Right
	Abdomen Muscle, Left
Internal pudendal artery	Internal Iliac Artery, Right
	Internal Iliac Artery, Left
Internal pudendal vein	Hypogastric Vein, Right
	Hypogastric Vein, Left
Internal thoracic artery	Internal Mammary Artery, Right
	Internal Mammary Artery, Left
	Subclavian Artery, Right
	Subclavian Artery, Left
Internal urethral sphincter	Urethra

Term	ICD-10-PCS Value
Interphalangeal (IP) joint	Finger Phalangeal Joint, Right
	Finger Phalangeal Joint, Left
	Toe Phalangeal Joint, Right
	Toe Phalangeal Joint, Left
Interphalangeal ligament	Foot Bursa and Ligament, Right
	Foot Bursa and Ligament, Left
	Hand Bursa and Ligament, Right
	Hand Bursa and Ligament, Left
Interspinalis muscle	Trunk Muscle, Right
	Trunk Muscle, Left
Interspinous ligament, cervical	Head and Neck Bursa and Ligament
Interspinous ligament, lumbar	Lower Spine Bursa and Ligament
Interspinous ligament, thoracic	Upper Spine Bursa and Ligament
Intertransversarius muscle	Trunk Muscle, Right
	Trunk Muscle, Left
Intertransverse ligament, cervical	Head and Neck Bursa and Ligament
Intertransverse ligament, lumbar	Lower Spine Bursa and Ligament
Intertransverse ligament, thoracic	Upper Spine Bursa and Ligament
Interventricular foramen (Monro)	Cerebral Ventricle
Interventricular septum	Ventricular Septum
Intestinal lymphatic trunk	Cisterna Chyli
Ischiatic nerve	Sciatic Nerve
Ischiocavernosus muscle	Perineum Muscle
Ischiofemoral ligament	Hip Bursa and Ligament, Right
	Hip Bursa and Ligament, Left
Ischium	Pelvic Bone, Right
	Pelvic Bone, Left
Jejunal artery	Superior Mesenteric Artery
Jugular body	Glomus Jugulare
Jugular lymph node	Lymphatic, Right Neck
	Lymphatic, Left Neck
Labia majora	Vulva
Labia minora	Vulva
Labial gland	Upper Lip
	Lower Lip
Lacrimal canaliculus	Lacrimal Duct, Right
	Lacrimal Duct, Left
Lacrimal punctum	Lacrimal Duct, Right
	Lacrimal Duct, Left
Lacrimal sac	Lacrimal Duct, Right
	Lacrimal Duct, Left
Laryngopharynx	Pharynx
Lateral (brachial) lymph node	Lymphatic, Right Axillary
	Lymphatic, Left Axillary
Lateral canthus	Upper Eyelid, Right
	Upper Eyelid, Left
Lateral collateral ligament (LCL)	Knee Bursa and Ligament, Right
	Knee Bursa and Ligament, Left
Lateral condyle of femur	Lower Femur, Right
	Lower Femur, Left

Term	ICD-10-PCS Value
Lateral condyle of tibia	Tibia, Right
	Tibia, Left
Lateral cuneiform bone	Tarsal, Right
	Tarsal, Left
Lateral epicondyle of femur	Lower Femur, Right
	Lower Femur, Left
Lateral epicondyle of humerus	Humeral Shaft, Right
	Humeral Shaft, Left
Lateral femoral cutaneous nerve	Lumbar Plexus
Lateral malleolus	Fibula, Right
	Fibula, Left
Lateral meniscus	Knee Joint, Right
	Knee Joint, Left
Lateral nasal cartilage	Nasal Mucosa and Soft Tissue
Lateral plantar artery	Foot Artery, Right
	Foot Artery, Left
Lateral plantar nerve	Tibial Nerve
Lateral rectus muscle	Extraocular Muscle, Right
	Extraocular Muscle, Left
Lateral sacral artery	Internal Iliac Artery, Right
	Internal Iliac Artery, Left
Lateral sacral vein	Hypogastric Vein, Right
	Hypogastric Vein, Left
Lateral sural cutaneous nerve	Peroneal Nerve
Lateral tarsal artery	Foot Artery, Right
	Foot Artery, Left
Lateral temporomandibular ligament	Head and Neck Bursa and Ligament
Lateral thoracic artery	Axillary Artery, Right
	Axillary Artery, Left
Latissimus dorsi muscle	Trunk Muscle, Right
	Trunk Muscle, Left
Least splanchnic nerve	Thoracic Sympathetic Nerve
Left ascending lumbar vein	Hemiazygos Vein
Left atrioventricular valve	Mitral Valve
Left auricular appendix	Atrium, Left
Left colic vein	Colic Vein
Left coronary sulcus	Heart, Left
Left gastric artery	Gastric Artery
Left gastroepiploic artery	Splenic Artery
Left gastroepiploic vein	Splenic Vein
Left inferior phrenic vein	Renal Vein, Left
Left inferior pulmonary vein	Pulmonary Vein, Left
Left jugular trunk	Thoracic Duct
Left lateral ventricle	Cerebral Ventricle
Left ovarian vein	Renal Vein, Left
Left second lumbar vein	Renal Vein, Left
Left subclavian trunk	Thoracic Duct
Left subcostal vein	Hemiazygos Vein
Left superior pulmonary vein	Pulmonary Vein, Left
Left suprarenal vein	Renal Vein, Left
Left testicular vein	Renal Vein, Left

Term	ICD-10-PCS Value
Leptomeninges, intracranial	Cerebral Meninges
Leptomeninges, spinal	Spinal Meninges
Lesser alar cartilage	Nasal Mucosa and Soft Tissue
Lesser occipital nerve	Cervical Plexus
Lesser omentum	Omentum
Lesser saphenous vein	Saphenous Vein, Right
	Saphenous Vein, Left
Lesser splanchnic nerve	Thoracic Sympathetic Nerve
Lesser trochanter	Upper Femur, Right
	Upper Femur, Left
Lesser tuberosity	Humeral Head, Right
	Humeral Head, Left
Lesser wing	Sphenoid Bone
Levator anguli oris muscle	Facial Muscle
Levator ani muscle	Perineum Muscle
Levator labii superioris alaeque nasi muscle	Facial Muscle
Levator labii superioris muscle	Facial Muscle
Levator palpebrae superioris muscle	Upper Eyelid, Right
	Upper Eyelid, Left
Levator scapulae muscle	Neck Muscle, Right
	Neck Muscle, Left
Levator veli palatini muscle	Tongue, Palate, Pharynx Muscle
Levatores costarum muscle	Thorax Muscle, Right
	Thorax Muscle, Left
Ligament of head of fibula	Knee Bursa and Ligament, Right
	Knee Bursa and Ligament, Left
Ligament of the lateral malleolus	Ankle Bursa and Ligament, Right
	Ankle Bursa and Ligament, Left
Ligamentum flavum, cervical	Head and Neck Bursa and Ligament
Ligamentum flavum, lumbar	Lower Spine Bursa and Ligament
Ligamentum flavum, thoracic	Upper Spine Bursa and Ligament
Lingual artery	External Carotid Artery, Right
	External Carotid Artery, Left
Lingual tonsil	Pharynx
Locus ceruleus	Pons
Long thoracic nerve	Brachial Plexus
Lumbar artery	Abdominal Aorta
Lumbar facet joint	Lumbar Vertebral Joint
Lumbar ganglion	Lumbar Sympathetic Nerve
Lumbar lymph node	Lymphatic, Aortic
Lumbar lymphatic trunk	Cisterna Chyli
Lumbar splanchnic nerve	Lumbar Sympathetic Nerve
Lumbosacral facet joint	Lumbosacral Joint
Lumbosacral trunk	Lumbar Nerve
Lunate bone	Carpal, Right
	Carpal, Left
Lunotriquetral ligament	Hand Bursa and Ligament, Right
	Hand Bursa and Ligament, Left
Macula	Retina, Right
	Retina, Left

Term	ICD-10-PCS Value
Malleus	Auditory Ossicle, Right
	Auditory Ossicle, Left
Mammary duct	Breast, Right
	Breast, Left
	Breast, Bilateral
Mammary gland	Breast, Right
	Breast, Left
	Breast, Bilateral
Mammillary body	Hypothalamus
Mandibular nerve	Trigeminal Nerve
Mandibular notch	Mandible, Right
	Mandible, Left
Manubrium	Sternum
Masseter muscle	Head Muscle
Masseteric fascia	Subcutaneous Tissue and Fascia, Face
Mastoid (postauricular) lymph node	Lymphatic, Right Neck
	Lymphatic, Left Neck
Mastoid air cells	Mastoid Sinus, Right
	Mastoid Sinus, Left
Mastoid process	Temporal Bone, Right
	Temporal Bone, Left
Maxillary artery	External Carotid Artery, Right
	External Carotid Artery, Left
Maxillary nerve	Trigeminal Nerve
Medial canthus	Lower Eyelid, Right
	Lower Eyelid, Left
Medial collateral ligament (MCL)	Knee Bursa and Ligament, Right
	Knee Bursa and Ligament, Left
Medial condyle of femur	Lower Femur, Right
	Lower Femur, Left
Medial condyle of tibia	Tibia, Right
	Tibia, Left
Medial cuneiform bone	Tarsal, Right
	Tarsal, Left
Medial epicondyle of femur	Lower Femur, Right
	Lower Femur, Left
Medial epicondyle of humerus	Humeral Shaft, Right
	Humeral Shaft, Left
Medial malleolus	Tibia, Right
	Tibia, Left
Medial meniscus	Knee Joint, Right
	Knee Joint, Left
Medial plantar artery	Foot Artery, Right
	Foot Artery, Left
Medial plantar nerve	Tibial Nerve
Medial popliteal nerve	Tibial Nerve
Medial rectus muscle	Extraocular Muscle, Right
	Extraocular Muscle, Left
Medial sural cutaneous nerve	Tibial Nerve
Median antebrachial vein	Basilic Vein, Right
	Basilic Vein, Left
Median cubital vein	Basilic Vein, Right
	Basilic Vein, Left
Median sacral artery	Abdominal Aorta

Term	ICD-10-PCS Value
Mediastinal cavity	Mediastinum
Mediastinal lymph node	Lymphatic, Thorax
Mediastinal space	Mediastinum
Meissner's (submucous) plexus	Abdominal Sympathetic Nerve
Membranous urethra	Urethra
Mental foramen	Mandible, Right
	Mandible, Left
Mentalis muscle	Facial Muscle
Mesoappendix	Mesentery
Mesocolon	Mesentery
Metacarpal ligament	Hand Bursa and Ligament, Right
	Hand Bursa and Ligament, Left
Metacarpophalangeal ligament	Hand Bursa and Ligament, Right
	Hand Bursa and Ligament, Left
Metatarsal ligament	Foot Bursa and Ligament, Right
	Foot Bursa and Ligament, Left
Metatarsophalangeal ligament	Foot Bursa and Ligament, Right
	Foot Bursa and Ligament, Left
Metatarsophalangeal (MTP) joint	Metatarsal-Phalangeal Joint, Right
	Metatarsal-Phalangeal Joint, Left
Metathalamus	Thalamus
Midcarpal joint	Carpal Joint, Right
	Carpal Joint, Left
Middle cardiac nerve	Thoracic Sympathetic Nerve
Middle cerebral artery	Intracranial Artery
Middle cerebral vein	Intracranial Vein
Middle colic vein	Colic Vein
Middle genicular artery	Popliteal Artery, Right
	Popliteal Artery, Left
Middle hemorrhoidal vein	Hypogastric Vein, Right
	Hypogastric Vein, Left
Middle rectal artery	Internal Iliac Artery, Right
	Internal Iliac Artery, Left
Middle suprarenal artery	Abdominal Aorta
Middle temporal artery	Temporal Artery, Right
	Temporal Artery, Left
Middle turbinate	Nasal Turbinate
Mitral annulus	Mitral Valve
Molar gland	Buccal Mucosa
Musculocutaneous nerve	Brachial Plexus
Musculophrenic artery	Internal Mammary Artery, Right
	Internal Mammary Artery, Left
Musculospiral nerve	Radial Nerve
Myelencephalon	Medulla Oblongata
Myenteric (Auerbach's) plexus	Abdominal Sympathetic Nerve
Myometrium	Uterus
Nail bed	Finger Nail
	Toe Nail
Nail plate	Finger Nail
	Toe Nail
Nasal cavity	Nasal Mucosa and Soft Tissue
Nasal concha	Nasal Turbinate
Nasalis muscle	Facial Muscle

Term	ICD-10-PCS Value
Nasolacrimal duct	Lacrimal Duct, Right
	Lacrimal Duct, Left
Navicular bone	Tarsal, Right
	Tarsal, Left
Neck of femur	Upper Femur, Right
	Upper Femur, Left
Neck of humerus (anatomical) (surgical)	Humeral Head, Right
	Humeral Head, Left
Nerve to the stapedius	Facial Nerve
Neurohypophysis	Pituitary Gland
Ninth cranial nerve	Glossopharyngeal Nerve
Nostril	Nasal Mucosa and Soft Tissue
Obturator artery	Internal Iliac Artery, Right
	Internal Iliac Artery, Left
Obturator lymph node	Lymphatic, Pelvis
Obturator muscle	Hip Muscle, Right
	Hip Muscle, Left
Obturator nerve	Lumbar Plexus
Obturator vein	Hypogastric Vein, Right
	Hypogastric Vein, Left
Obtuse margin	Heart, Left
Occipital artery	External Carotid Artery, Right
	External Carotid Artery, Left
Occipital lobe	Cerebral Hemisphere
Occipital lymph node	Lymphatic, Right Neck
	Lymphatic, Left Neck
Occipitofrontalis muscle	Facial Muscle
Odontoid process	Cervical Vertebra
Olecranon bursa	Elbow Bursa and Ligament, Right
	Elbow Bursa and Ligament, Left
Olecranon process	Ulna, Right
	Ulna, Left
Olfactory bulb	Olfactory Nerve
Ophthalmic artery	Intracranial Artery
Ophthalmic nerve	Trigeminal Nerve
Ophthalmic vein	Intracranial Vein
Optic chiasma	Optic Nerve
Optic disc	Retina, Right
	Retina, Left
Optic foramen	Sphenoid Bone
Orbicularis oculi muscle	Upper Eyelid, Right
	Upper Eyelid, Left
Orbicularis oris muscle	Facial Muscle
Orbital fascia	Subcutaneous Tissue and Fascia, Face
Orbital portion of ethmoid bone	Orbit, Right
	Orbit, Left
Orbital portion of frontal bone	Orbit, Right
	Orbit, Left
Orbital portion of lacrimal bone	Orbit, Right
	Orbit, Left
Orbital portion of maxilla	Orbit, Right
	Orbit, Left
Orbital portion of palatine bone	Orbit, Right
	Orbit, Left

Term	ICD-10-PCS Value
Orbital portion of sphenoid bone	Orbit, Right
	Orbit, Left
Orbital portion of zygomatic bone	Orbit, Right
	Orbit, Left
Oropharynx	Pharynx
Otic ganglion	Head and Neck Sympathetic Nerve
Oval window	Middle Ear, Right
	Middle Ear, Left
Ovarian artery	Abdominal Aorta
Ovarian ligament	Uterine Supporting Structure
Oviduct	Fallopian Tube, Right
	Fallopian Tube, Left
Palatine gland	Buccal Mucosa
Palatine tonsil	Tonsils
Palatine uvula	Uvula
Palatoglossal muscle	Tongue, Palate, Pharynx Muscle
Palatopharyngeal muscle	Tongue, Palate, Pharynx Muscle
Palmar (volar) digital vein	Hand Vein, Right
	Hand Vein, Left
Palmar (volar) metacarpal vein	Hand Vein, Right
	Hand Vein, Left
Palmar cutaneous nerve	Median Nerve
	Radial Nerve
Palmar fascia (aponeurosis)	Subcutaneous Tissue and Fascia, Right Hand
	Subcutaneous Tissue and Fascia, Left Hand
Palmar interosseous muscle	Hand Muscle, Right
	Hand Muscle, Left
Palmar ulnocarpal ligament	Wrist Bursa and Ligament, Right
	Wrist Bursa and Ligament, Left
Palmaris longus muscle	Lower Arm and Wrist Muscle, Right
	Lower Arm and Wrist Muscle, Left
Pancreatic artery	Splenic Artery
Pancreatic plexus	Abdominal Sympathetic Nerve
Pancreatic vein	Splenic Vein
Pancreaticosplenic lymph node	Lymphatic, Aortic
Paraaortic lymph node	Lymphatic, Aortic
Pararectal lymph node	Lymphatic, Mesenteric
Parasternal lymph node	Lymphatic, Thorax
Paratracheal lymph node	Lymphatic, Thorax
Paraurethral (Skene's) gland	Vestibular Gland
Parietal lobe	Cerebral Hemisphere
Parotid lymph node	Lymphatic, Head
Parotid plexus	Facial Nerve
Pars flaccida	Tympanic Membrane, Right
	Tympanic Membrane, Left
Patellar ligament	Knee Bursa and Ligament, Right
	Knee Bursa and Ligament, Left
Patellar tendon	Knee Tendon, Right
	Knee Tendon, Left
Patellofemoral joint	Knee Joint, Right
	Knee Joint, Left
	Knee Joint, Femoral Surface, Right
	Knee Joint, Femoral Surface, Left

Term	ICD-10-PCS Value
Pectineus muscle	Upper Leg Muscle, Right
	Upper Leg Muscle, Left
Pectoral (anterior) lymph node	Lymphatic, Right Axillary
	Lymphatic, Left Axillary
Pectoral fascia	Subcutaneous Tissue and Fascia, Chest
Pectoralis major muscle	Thorax Muscle, Right
	Thorax Muscle, Left
Pectoralis minor muscle	Thorax Muscle, Right
	Thorax Muscle, Left
Pelvic splanchnic nerve	Abdominal Sympathetic Nerve
	Sacral Sympathetic Nerve
Penile urethra	Urethra
Pericardiophrenic artery	Internal Mammary Artery, Right
	Internal Mammary Artery, Left
Perimetrium	Uterus
Peroneus brevis muscle	Lower Leg Muscle, Right
	Lower Leg Muscle, Left
Peroneus longus muscle	Lower Leg Muscle, Right
	Lower Leg Muscle, Left
Petrous part of temporal bone	Temporal Bone, Right
	Temporal Bone, Left
Pharyngeal constrictor muscle	Tongue, Palate, Pharynx Muscle
Pharyngeal plexus	Vagus Nerve
Pharyngeal recess	Nasopharynx
Pharyngeal tonsil	Adenoids
Pharyngotympanic tube	Eustachian Tube, Right
	Eustachian Tube, Left
Pia mater, intracranial	Cerebral Meninges
Pia mater, spinal	Spinal Meninges
Pinna	External Ear, Right
	External Ear, Left
	External Ear, Bilateral
Piriform recess (sinus)	Pharynx
Piriformis muscle	Hip Muscle, Right
	Hip Muscle, Left
Pisiform bone	Carpal, Right
	Carpal, Left
Pisohamate ligament	Hand Bursa and Ligament, Right
	Hand Bursa and Ligament, Left
Pisometacarpal ligament	Hand Bursa and Ligament, Right
	Hand Bursa and Ligament, Left
Plantar digital vein	Foot Vein, Right
	Foot Vein, Left
Plantar fascia (aponeurosis)	Subcutaneous Tissue and Fascia, Right Foot
	Subcutaneous Tissue and Fascia, Left Foot
Plantar metatarsal vein	Foot Vein, Right
	Foot Vein, Left
Plantar venous arch	Foot Vein, Right
	Foot Vein, Left
Platysma muscle	Neck Muscle, Right
	Neck Muscle, Left
Plica semilunaris	Conjunctiva, Right
	Conjunctiva, Left
Pneumogastric nerve	Vagus Nerve

Term	ICD-10-PCS Value
Pneumotaxic center	Pons
Pontine tegmentum	Pons
Popliteal ligament	Knee Bursa and Ligament, Right
	Knee Bursa and Ligament, Left
Popliteallymph node	Lymphatic, Left Lower Extremity
	Lymphatic, Right Lower Extremity
Popliteal vein	Femoral Vein, Right
	Femoral Vein, Left
Popliteus muscle	Lower Leg Muscle, Right
	Lower Leg Muscle, Left
Postauricular (mastoid) lymph node	Lymphatic, Right Neck
	Lymphatic, Left Neck
Postcava	Inferior Vena Cava
Posterior (subscapular) lymph node	Lymphatic, Right Axillary
	Lymphatic, Left Axillary
Posterior auricular artery	External Carotid Artery, Right
	External Carotid Artery, Left
Posterior auricular nerve	Facial Nerve
Posterior auricular vein	External Jugular Vein, Right
	External Jugular Vein, Left
Posterior cerebral artery	Intracranial Artery
Posterior chamber	Eye, Right
	Eye, Left
Posterior circumflex humeral artery	Axillary Artery, Right
	Axillary Artery, Left
Posterior communicating artery	Intracranial Artery
Posterior cruciate ligament (PCL)	Knee Bursa and Ligament, Right
	Knee Bursa and Ligament, Left
Posterior facial (retromandibular) vein	Face Vein, Right
	Face Vein, Left
Posterior femoral cutaneous nerve	Sacral Plexus
Posterior inferior cerebellar artery (PICA)	Intracranial Artery
Posterior interosseous nerve	Radial Nerve
Posterior labial nerve	Pudendal Nerve
Posterior scrotal nerve	Pudendal Nerve
Posterior spinal artery	Vertebral Artery, Right
	Vertebral Artery, Left
Posterior tibial recurrent artery	Anterior Tibial Artery, Right
	Anterior Tibial Artery, Left
Posterior ulnar recurrent artery	Ulnar Artery, Right
	Ulnar Artery, Left
Posterior vagal trunk	Vagus Nerve
Preauricular lymph node	Lymphatic, Head
Precava	Superior Vena Cava
Prepatellar bursa	Knee Bursa and Ligament, Right
	Knee Bursa and Ligament, Left
Pretracheal fascia	Subcutaneous Tissue and Fascia, Right Neck
	Subcutaneous Tissue and Fascia, Left Neck
Prevertebral fascia	Subcutaneous Tissue and Fascia, Right Neck
	Subcutaneous Tissue and Fascia, Left Neck

Term	ICD-10-PCS Value
Princeps pollicis artery	Hand Artery, Right
	Hand Artery, Left
Procerus muscle	Facial Muscle
Profunda brachii	Brachial Artery, Right
	Brachial Artery, Left
Profunda femoris (deep femoral) vein	Femoral Vein, Right
	Femoral Vein, Left
Pronator quadratus muscle	Lower Arm and Wrist Muscle, Right
	Lower Arm and Wrist Muscle, Left
Pronator teres muscle	Lower Arm and Wrist Muscle, Right
	Lower Arm and Wrist Muscle, Left
Prostatic urethra	Urethra
Proximal radioulnar joint	Elbow Joint, Right
	Elbow Joint, Left
Psoas muscle	Hip Muscle, Right
	Hip Muscle, Left
Pterygoid muscle	Head Muscle
Pterygoid process	Sphenoid Bone
Pterygopalatine (sphenopalatine) ganglion	Head and Neck Sympathetic Nerve
Pubis	Pelvic Bone, Right
	Pelvic Bone, Left
Pubofemoral ligament	Hip Bursa and Ligament, Right
	Hip Bursa and Ligament, Left
Pudendal nerve	Sacral Plexus
Pulmoaortic canal	Pulmonary Artery, Left
Pulmonary annulus	Pulmonary Valve
Pulmonary plexus	Thoracic Sympathetic Nerve
	Vagus Nerve
Pulmonic valve	Pulmonary Valve
Pulvinar	Thalamus
Pyloric antrum	Stomach, Pylorus
Pyloric canal	Stomach, Pylorus
Pyloric sphincter	Stomach, Pylorus
Pyramidalis muscle	Abdomen Muscle, Right
	Abdomen Muscle, Left
Quadrangular cartilage	Nasal Septum
Quadrate lobe	Liver
Quadratus femoris muscle	Hip Muscle, Right
	Hip Muscle, Left
Quadratus lumborum muscle	Trunk Muscle, Right
	Trunk Muscle, Left
Quadratus plantae muscle	Foot Muscle, Right
	Foot Muscle, Left
Quadriceps (femoris)	Upper Leg Muscle, Right
	Upper Leg Muscle, Left
Radial collateral carpal ligament	Wrist Bursa and Ligament, Right
	Wrist Bursa and Ligament, Left
Radial collateral ligament	Elbow Bursa and Ligament, Right
	Elbow Bursa and Ligament, Left
Radial notch	Ulna, Right
	Ulna, Left
Radial recurrent artery	Radial Artery, Right
	Radial Artery, Left
Radial vein	Brachial Vein, Right
	Brachial Vein, Left
Radialis indicis	Hand Artery, Right
	Hand Artery, Left
Radiocarpal joint	Wrist Joint, Right
	Wrist Joint, Left
Radiocarpal ligament	Wrist Bursa and Ligament, Right
	Wrist Bursa and Ligament, Left
Radioulnar ligament	Wrist Bursa and Ligament, Right
	Wrist Bursa and Ligament, Left
Rectosigmoid junction	Sigmoid Colon
Rectus abdominis muscle	Abdomen Muscle, Right
	Abdomen Muscle, Left
Rectus femoris muscle	Upper Leg Muscle, Right
	Upper Leg Muscle, Left
Recurrent laryngeal nerve	Vagus Nerve
Renal calyx	Kidney, Right
	Kidney, Left
	Kidneys, Bilateral
	Kidney
Renal capsule	Kidney, Right
	Kidney, Left
	Kidneys, Bilateral
	Kidney
Renal cortex	Kidney, Right
	Kidney, Left
	Kidneys, Bilateral
	Kidney
Renal nerve	Abdominal sympathetic Nerve
Renal plexus	Abdominal Sympathetic Nerve
Renal segment	Kidney, Right
	Kidney, Left
	Kidneys, Bilateral
	Kidney
Renal segmental artery	Renal Artery, Right
	Renal Artery, Left
Retroperitoneal cavity	Retroperitoneum
Retroperitoneal lymph node	Lymphatic, Aortic
Retroperitoneal space	Retroperitoneum
Retropharyngeal lymph node	Lymphatic, Right Neck
	Lymphatic, Left Neck
Retropubic space	Pelvic Cavity
Rhinopharynx	Nasopharynx
Rhomboid major muscle	Trunk Muscle, Right
	Trunk Muscle, Left
Rhomboid minor muscle	Trunk Muscle, Right
	Trunk Muscle, Left
Right ascending lumbar vein	Azygos Vein
Right atrioventricular valve	Tricuspid Valve
Right auricular appendix	Atrium, Right
Right colic vein	Colic Vein
Right coronary sulcus	Heart, Right
Right gastric artery	Gastric Artery

Term	ICD-10-PCS Value
Right gastroepiploic vein	Superior Mesenteric Vein
Right inferior phrenic vein	Inferior Vena Cava
Right inferior pulmonary vein	Pulmonary Vein, Right
Right jugular trunk	Lymphatic, Right Neck
Right lateral ventricle	Cerebral Ventricle
Right lymphatic duct	Lymphatic, Right Neck
Right ovarian vein	Inferior Vena Cava
Right second lumbar vein	Inferior Vena Cava
Right subclavian trunk	Lymphatic, Right Neck
Right subcostal vein	Azygos Vein
Right superior pulmonary vein	Pulmonary Vein, Right
Right suprarenal vein	Inferior Vena Cava
Right testicular vein	Inferior Vena Cava
Rima glottidis	Larynx
Risorius muscle	Facial Muscle
Round ligament of uterus	Uterine Supporting Structure
Round window	Inner Ear, Right
	Inner Ear, Left
Sacral ganglion	Sacral Sympathetic Nerve
Sacral lymph node	Lymphatic, Pelvis
Sacral splanchnic nerve	Sacral Sympathetic Nerve
Sacrococcygeal ligament	Lower Spine Bursa and Ligament
Sacrococcygeal symphysis	Sacrococcygeal Joint
Sacroiliac ligament	Lower Spine Bursa and Ligament
Sacrospinous ligament	Lower Spine Bursa and Ligament
Sacrotuberous ligament	Lower Spine Bursa and Ligament
Salpingopharyngeus muscle	Tongue, Palate, Pharynx Muscle
Salpinx	Fallopian Tube, Right
	Fallopian Tube, Left
Saphenous nerve	Femoral Nerve
Sartorius muscle	Upper Leg Muscle, Right
	Upper Leg Muscle, Left
Scalene muscle	Neck Muscle, Right
	Neck Muscle, Left
Scaphoid bone	Carpal, Right
	Carpal, Left
Scapholunate ligament	Wrist Bursa and Ligament, Right
	Wrist Bursa and Ligament, Left
Scaphotrapezium ligament	Hand Bursa and Ligament, Right
	Hand Bursa and Ligament, Left
Scarpa's (vestibular) ganglion	Acoustic Nerve
Sebaceous gland	Skin
Second cranial nerve	Optic Nerve
Sella turcica	Sphenoid Bone
Semicircular canal	Inner Ear, Right
	Inner Ear, Left
Semimembranosus muscle	Upper Leg Muscle, Right
	Upper Leg Muscle, Left
Semitendinosus muscle	Upper Leg Muscle, Right
	Upper Leg Muscle, Left
Septal cartilage	Nasal Septum

Term	ICD-10-PCS Value
Serratus anterior muscle	Thorax Muscle, Right
	Thorax Muscle, Left
Serratus posterior muscle	Trunk Muscle, Right
	Trunk Muscle, Left
Seventh cranial nerve	Facial Nerve
Short gastric artery	Splenic Artery
Sigmoid artery	Inferior Mesenteric Artery
Sigmoid flexure	Sigmoid Colon
Sigmoid vein	Inferior Mesenteric Vein
Sinoatrial node	Conduction Mechanism
Sinus venosus	Atrium, Right
Sixth cranial nerve	Abducens Nerve
Skene's (paraurethral) gland	Vestibular Gland
Small saphenous vein	Saphenous Vein, Right
	Saphenous Vein, Left
Solar (celiac) plexus	Abdominal Sympathetic Nerve
Soleus muscle	Lower Leg Muscle, Right
	Lower Leg Muscle, Left
Sphenomandibular ligament	Head and Neck Bursa and Ligament
Sphenopalatine (pterygopalatine) ganglion	Head and Neck Sympathetic Nerve
Spinal nerve, cervical	Cervical Nerve
Spinal nerve, lumbar	Lumbar Nerve
Spinal nerve, sacral	Sacral Nerve
Spinal nerve, thoracic	Thoracic Nerve
Spinous process	Cervical Vertebra
	Lumbar Vertebra
	Thoracic Vertebra
Spiral ganglion	Acoustic Nerve
Splenic flexure	Transverse Colon
Splenic plexus	Abdominal Sympathetic Nerve
Splenius capitis muscle	Head Muscle
Splenius cervicis muscle	Neck Muscle, Right
	Neck Muscle, Left
Stapes	Auditory Ossicle, Right
	Auditory Ossicle, Left
Stellate ganglion	Head and Neck Sympathetic Nerve
Stensen's duct	Parotid Duct, Right
	Parotid Duct, Left
Sternoclavicular ligament	Shoulder Bursa and Ligament, Right
	Shoulder Bursa and Ligament, Left
Sternocleidomastoid artery	Thyroid Artery, Right
	Thyroid Artery, Left
Sternocleidomastoid muscle	Neck Muscle, Right
	Neck Muscle, Left
Sternocostal ligament	Sternum Bursa and Ligament
Styloglossus muscle	Tongue, Palate, Pharynx Muscle
Stylomandibular ligament	Head and Neck Bursa and Ligament
Stylopharyngeus muscle	Tongue, Palate, Pharynx Muscle
Subacromial bursa	Shoulder Bursa and Ligament, Right
	Shoulder Bursa and Ligament, Left
Subaortic (common iliac) lymph node	Lymphatic, Pelvis
Subarachnoid space, spinal	Spinal Canal

Term	ICD-10-PCS Value
Subclavicular (apical) lymph node	Lymphatic, Right Axillary
	Lymphatic, Left Axillary
Subclavius muscle	Thorax Muscle, Right
	Thorax Muscle, Left
Subclavius nerve	Brachial Plexus
Subcostal artery	Upper Artery
Subcostal muscle	Thorax Muscle, Right
	Thorax Muscle, Left
Subcostal nerve	Thoracic Nerve
Subdural space, spinal	Spinal Canal
Submandibular ganglion	Facial Nerve
	Head and Neck Sympathetic Nerve
Submandibular gland	Submaxillary Gland, Right
	Submaxillary Gland, Left
Submandibular lymph node	Lymphatic, Head
Submandibular space	Subcutaneous Tissue and Fascia, Face
Submaxillary ganglion	Head and Neck Sympathetic Nerve
Submaxillary lymph node	Lymphatic, Head
Submental artery	Face Artery
Submental lymph node	Lymphatic, Head
Submucous (Meissner's) plexus	Abdominal Sympathetic Nerve
Suboccipital nerve	Cervical Nerve
Suboccipital venous plexus	Vertebral Vein, Right
	Vertebral Vein, Left
Subparotid lymph node	Lymphatic, Head
Subscapular aponeurosis	Subcutaneous Tissue and Fascia, Right Upper Arm
	Subcutaneous Tissue and Fascia, Left Upper Arm
Subscapular artery	Axillary Artery, Right
	Axillary Artery, Left
Subscapular (posterior) lymph node	Lymphatic, Right Axillary
	Lymphatic, Left Axillary
Subscapularis muscle	Shoulder Muscle, Right
	Shoulder Muscle, Left
Substantia nigra	Basal Ganglia
Subtalar (talocalcaneal) joint	Tarsal Joint, Right
	Tarsal Joint, Left
Subtalar ligament	Foot Bursa and Ligament, Right
	Foot Bursa and Ligament, Left
Subthalamic nucleus	Basal Ganglia
Superficial circumflex iliac vein	Saphenous Vein, Right
	Saphenous Vein, Left
Superficial epigastric artery	Femoral Artery, Right
	Femoral Artery, Left
Superficial epigastric vein	Saphenous Vein, Right
	Saphenous Vein, Left
Superficial palmar arch	Hand Artery, Right
	Hand Artery, Left
Superficial palmar venous arch	Hand Vein, Right
	Hand Vein, Left
Superficial temporal artery	Temporal Artery, Right
	Temporal Artery, Left
Superficial transverse perineal muscle	Perineum Muscle
Superior cardiac nerve	Thoracic Sympathetic Nerve
Superior cerebellar vein	Intracranial Vein
Superior cerebral vein	Intracranial Vein
Superior clunic (cluneal) nerve	Lumbar Nerve
Superior epigastric artery	Internal Mammary Artery, Right
	Internal Mammary Artery, Left
Superior genicular artery	Popliteal Artery, Right
	Popliteal Artery, Left
Superior gluteal artery	Internal Iliac Artery, Right
	Internal Iliac Artery, Left
Superior gluteal nerve	Lumbar Plexus
Superior hypogastric plexus	Abdominal Sympathetic Nerve
Superior labial artery	Face Artery
Superior laryngeal artery	Thyroid Artery, Right
	Thyroid Artery, Left
Superior laryngeal nerve	Vagus Nerve
Superior longitudinal muscle	Tongue, Palate, Pharynx Muscle
Superior mesenteric ganglion	Abdominal Sympathetic Nerve
Superior mesenteric lymph node	Lymphatic, Mesenteric
Superior mesenteric plexus	Abdominal Sympathetic Nerve
Superior oblique muscle	Extraocular Muscle, Right
	Extraocular Muscle, Left
Superior olivary nucleus	Pons
Superior rectal artery	Inferior Mesenteric Artery
Superior rectal vein	Inferior Mesenteric Vein
Superior rectus muscle	Extraocular Muscle, Right
	Extraocular Muscle, Left
Superior tarsal plate	Upper Eyelid, Right
	Upper Eyelid, Left
Superior thoracic artery	Axillary Artery, Right
	Axillary Artery, Left
Superior thyroid artery	External Carotid Artery, Right
	External Carotid Artery, Left
	Thyroid Artery, Right
	Thyroid Artery, Left
Superior turbinate	Nasal Turbinate
Superior ulnar collateral artery	Brachial Artery, Right
	Brachial Artery, Left
Supraclavicular nerve	Cervical Plexus
Supraclavicular (Virchow's) lymph node	Lymphatic, Right Neck
	Lymphatic, Left Neck
Suprahyoid lymph node	Lymphatic, Head
Suprahyoid muscle	Neck Muscle, Right
	Neck Muscle, Left
Suprainguinal lymph node	Lymphatic, Pelvis
Supraorbital vein	Face Vein, Right
	Face Vein, Left

Term	ICD-10-PCS Value
Suprarenal gland	Adrenal Gland, Right
	Adrenal Gland, Left
	Adrenal Glands, Bilateral
	Adrenal Gland
Suprarenal plexus	Abdominal Sympathetic Nerve
Suprascapular nerve	Brachial Plexus
Supraspinatus fascia	Subcutaneous Tissue and Fascia, Right Upper Arm
	Subcutaneous Tissue and Fascia, Left Upper Arm
Supraspinatus muscle	Shoulder Muscle, Right
	Shoulder Muscle, Left
Supraspinous ligament	Upper Spine Bursa and Ligament
	Lower Spine Bursa and Ligament
Suprasternal notch	Sternum
Supratrochlear lymph node	Lymphatic, Right Upper Extremity
	Lymphatic, Left Upper Extremity
Sural artery	Popliteal Artery, Right
	Popliteal Artery, Left
Sweat gland	Skin
Talocalcaneal ligament	Foot Bursa and Ligament, Right
	Foot Bursa and Ligament, Left
Talocalcaneal (subtalar) joint	Tarsal Joint, Right
	Tarsal Joint, Left
Talocalcaneonavicular joint	Tarsal Joint, Right
	Tarsal Joint, Left
Talocalcaneonavicular ligament	Foot Bursa and Ligament, Right
	Foot Bursa and Ligament, Left
Talocrural joint	Ankle Joint, Right
	Ankle Joint, Left
Talofibular ligament	Ankle Bursa and Ligament, Right
	Ankle Bursa and Ligament, Left
Talus bone	Tarsal, Right
	Tarsal, Left
Tarsometatarsal ligament	Foot Bursa and Ligament, Right
	Foot Bursa and Ligament, Left
Temporal lobe	Cerebral Hemisphere
Temporalis muscle	Head Muscle
Temporoparietalis muscle	Head Muscle
Tensor fasciae latae muscle	Hip Muscle, Right
	Hip Muscle, Left
Tensor veli palatini muscle	Tongue, Palate, Pharynx Muscle
Tenth cranial nerve	Vagus Nerve
Tentorium cerebelli	Dura Mater
Teres major muscle	Shoulder Muscle, Right
	Shoulder Muscle, Left
Teres minor muscle	Shoulder Muscle, Right
	Shoulder Muscle, Left
Testicular artery	Abdominal Aorta
Thenar muscle	Hand Muscle, Right
	Hand Muscle, Left
Third cranial nerve	Oculomotor Nerve
Third occipital nerve	Cervical Nerve
Third ventricle	Cerebral Ventricle
Thoracic aortic plexus	Thoracic Sympathetic Nerve

Term	ICD-10-PCS Value
Thoracic esophagus	Esophagus, Middle
Thoracic facet joint	Thoracic Vertebral Joint
Thoracic ganglion	Thoracic Sympathetic Nerve
Thoracoacromial artery	Axillary Artery, Right
	Axillary Artery, Left
Thoracolumbar facet joint	Thoracolumbar Vertebral Joint
Thymus gland	Thymus
Thyroarytenoid muscle	Neck Muscle, Right
	Neck Muscle, Left
Thyrocervical trunk	Thyroid Artery, Right
	Thyroid Artery, Left
Thyroid cartilage	Larynx
Tibialis anterior muscle	Lower Leg Muscle, Right
	Lower Leg Muscle, Left
Tibialis posterior muscle	Lower Leg Muscle, Right
	Lower Leg Muscle, Left
Tibiofemoral joint	Knee Joint, Right
	Knee Joint, Left
	Knee Joint, Tibial Surface, Right
	Knee Joint, Tibial Surface, Left
Tibioperoneal trunk	Popliteal Artery, Right
	Popliteal Artery, Left
Tongue, base of	Pharynx
Tracheobronchial lymph node	Lymphatic, Thorax
Tragus	External Ear, Right
	External Ear, Left
	External Ear, Bilateral
Transversalis fascia	Subcutaneous Tissue and Fascia, Trunk
Transverse acetabular ligament	Hip Bursa and Ligament, Right
	Hip Bursa and Ligament, Left
Transverse (cutaneous) cervical nerve	Cervical Plexus
Transverse facial artery	Temporal Artery, Right
	Temporal Artery, Left
Transverse foramen	Cervical Vertebra
Transverse humeral ligament	Shoulder Bursa and Ligament, Right
	Shoulder Bursa and Ligament, Left
Transverse ligament of atlas	Head and Neck Bursa and Ligament
Transverse process	Cervical Vertebra
	Thoracic Vertebra
	Lumbar Vertebra
Transverse scapular ligament	Shoulder Bursa and Ligament, Right
	Shoulder Bursa and Ligament, Left
Transverse thoracis muscle	Thorax Muscle, Right
	Thorax Muscle, Left
Transversospinalis muscle	Trunk Muscle, Right
	Trunk Muscle, Left
Transversus abdominis muscle	Abdomen Muscle, Right
	Abdomen Muscle, Left
Trapezium bone	Carpal, Right
	Carpal, Left
Trapezius muscle	Trunk Muscle, Right
	Trunk Muscle, Left

Term	ICD-10-PCS Value
Trapezoid bone	Carpal, Right
	Carpal, Left
Triceps brachii muscle	Upper Arm Muscle, Right
	Upper Arm Muscle, Left
Tricuspid annulus	Tricuspid Valve
Trifacial nerve	Trigeminal Nerve
Trigone of bladder	Bladder
Triquetral bone	Carpal, Right
	Carpal, Left
Trochantericbursa	Hip Bursa and Ligament, Right
	Hip Bursa and Ligament, Left
Twelfth cranial nerve	Hypoglossal Nerve
Tympanic cavity	Middle Ear, Right
	Middle Ear, Left
Tympanic nerve	Glossopharyngeal Nerve
Tympanic part of temoporal bone	Temporal Bone, Right
	Temporal Bone, Left
Ulnar collateral carpal ligament	Wrist Bursa and Ligament, Right
	Wrist Bursa and Ligament, Left
Ulnar collateral ligament	Elbow Bursa and Ligament, Right
	Elbow Bursa and Ligament, Left
Ulnar notch	Radius, Right
	Radius, Left
Ulnar vein	Brachial Vein, Right
	Brachial Vein, Left
Umbilical artery	Internal Iliac Artery, Right
	Internal Iliac Artery, Left
	Lower Artery
Ureteral orifice	Ureter, Right
	Ureter, Left
	Ureters, Bilateral
	Ureter
Ureteropelvic junction (UPJ)	Kidney Pelvis, Right
	Kidney Pelvis, Left
Ureterovesical orifice	Ureter, Right
	Ureter, Left
	Ureters, Bilateral
	Ureter
Uterine artery	Internal Iliac Artery, Right
	Internal Iliac Artery, Left
Uterine cornu	Uterus
Uterine tube	Fallopian Tube, Right
	Fallopian Tube, Left
Uterine vein	Hypogastric Vein, Right
	Hypogastric Vein, Left
Vaginal artery	Internal Iliac Artery, Right
	Internal Iliac Artery, Left
Vaginal vein	Hypogastric Vein, Right
	Hypogastric Vein, Left
Vastus intermedius muscle	Upper Leg Muscle, Right
	Upper Leg Muscle, Left
Vastus lateralis muscle	Upper Leg Muscle, Right
	Upper Leg Muscle, Left
Vastus medialis muscle	Upper Leg Muscle, Right
	Upper Leg Muscle, Left

Term	ICD-10-PCS Value
Ventricular fold	Larynx
Vermiform appendix	Appendix
Vermilion border	Upper Lip
	Lower Lip
Vertebral arch	Cervical Vertebra
	Lumbar Vertebra
	Thoracic Vertebra
Vertebral body	Cervical Vertebra
	Lumbar Vertebra
	Thoracic Vertebra
Vertebral canal	Spinal Canal
Vertebral foramen	Cervical Vertebra
	Lumbar Vertebra
	Thoracic Vertebra
Vertebral lamina	Cervical Vertebra
	Lumbar Vertebra
	Thoracic Vertebra
Vertebral pedicle	Cervical Vertebra
	Lumbar Vertebra
	Thoracic Vertebra
Vesical vein	Hypogastric Vein, Right
	Hypogastric Vein, Left
Vestibular (Scarpa's) ganglion	Acoustic Nerve
Vestibular nerve	Acoustic Nerve
Vestibulocochlear nerve	Acoustic Nerve
Virchow's (supraclavicular) lymph node	Lymphatic, Right Neck
	Lymphatic, Left Neck
Vitreous body	Vitreous, Right
	Vitreous, Left
Vocal fold	Vocal Cord, Right
	Vocal Cord, Left
Volar (palmar) digital vein	Hand Vein, Right
	Hand Vein, Left
Volar (palmar) metacarpal vein	Hand Vein, Right
	Hand Vein, Left
Vomer bone	Nasal Septum
Vomer of nasal septum	Nasal Bone
Xiphoid process	Sternum
Zonule of Zinn	Lens, Right
	Lens, Left
Zygomatic process of frontal bone	Frontal Bone
Zygomatic process of temporal bone	Temporal Bone, Right
	Temporal Bone, Left
Zygomaticus muscle	Facial Muscle

Appendix E: Body Part Definitions

ICD-10-PCS Value	Definition
1st Toe, Left **1st Toe, Right**	**Includes:** Hallux
Abdomen Muscle, Left **Abdomen Muscle, Right**	**Includes:** External oblique muscle Internal oblique muscle Pyramidalis muscle Rectus abdominis muscle Transversus abdominis muscle
Abdominal Aorta	**Includes:** Inferior phrenic artery Lumbar artery Median sacral artery Middle suprarenal artery Ovarian artery Testicular artery
Abdominal Sympathetic Nerve	**Includes:** Abdominal aortic plexus Auerbach's (myenteric) plexus Celiac (solar) plexus Celiac ganglion Gastric plexus Hepatic plexus Inferior hypogastric plexus Inferior mesenteric ganglion Inferior mesenteric plexus Meissner's (submucous) plexus Myenteric (Auerbach's) plexus Pancreatic plexus Pelvic splanchnic nerve Renal nerve Renal plexus Solar (celiac) plexus Splenic plexus Submucous (Meissner's) plexus Superior hypogastric plexus Superior mesenteric ganglion Superior mesenteric plexus Suprarenal plexus
Abducens Nerve	**Includes:** Sixth cranial nerve
Accessory Nerve	**Includes:** Eleventh cranial nerve
Acoustic Nerve	**Includes:** Cochlear nerve Eighth cranial nerve Scarpa's (vestibular) ganglion Spiral ganglion Vestibular (Scarpa's) ganglion Vestibular nerve Vestibulocochlear nerve
Adenoids	**Includes:** Pharyngeal tonsil
Adrenal Gland **Adrenal Gland, Left** **Adrenal Gland, Right** **Adrenal Glands, Bilateral**	**Includes:** Suprarenal gland
Ampulla of Vater	**Includes:** Duodenal ampulla Hepatopancreatic ampulla
Anal Sphincter	**Includes:** External anal sphincter Internal anal sphincter

ICD-10-PCS Value	Definition
Ankle Bursa and Ligament, Left **Ankle Bursa and Ligament, Right**	**Includes:** Calcaneofibular ligament Deltoid ligament Ligament of the lateral malleolus Talofibular ligament
Ankle Joint, Left **Ankle Joint, Right**	**Includes:** Inferior tibiofibular joint Talocrural joint
Anterior Chamber, Left **Anterior Chamber, Right**	**Includes:** Aqueous humour
Anterior Tibial Artery, Left **Anterior Tibial Artery, Right**	**Includes:** Anterior lateral malleolar artery Anterior medial malleolar artery Anterior tibial recurrent artery Dorsalis pedis artery Posterior tibial recurrent artery
Anus	**Includes:** Anal orifice
Aortic Valve	**Includes:** Aortic annulus
Appendix	**Includes:** Vermiform appendix
Atrial Septum	**Includes:** Interatrial septum
Atrium, Left	**Includes:** Atrium pulmonale Left auricular appendix
Atrium, Right	**Includes:** Atrium dextrum cordis Right auricular appendix Sinus venosus
Auditory Ossicle, Left **Auditory Ossicle, Right**	**Includes:** Incus Malleus Stapes
Axillary Artery, Left **Axillary Artery, Right**	**Includes:** Anterior circumflex humeral artery Lateral thoracic artery Posterior circumflex humeral artery Subscapular artery Superior thoracic artery Thoracoacromial artery
Azygos Vein	**Includes:** Right ascending lumbar vein Right subcostal vein
Basal Ganglia	**Includes:** Basal nuclei Claustrum Corpus striatum Globus pallidus Substantia nigra Subthalamic nucleus
Basilic Vein, Left **Basilic Vein, Right**	**Includes:** Median antebrachial vein Median cubital vein
Bladder	**Includes:** Trigone of bladder
Brachial Artery, Left **Brachial Artery, Right**	**Includes:** Inferior ulnar collateral artery Profunda brachii Superior ulnar collateral artery

ICD-10-PCS Value	Definition
Brachial Plexus	Includes: Axillary nerve Dorsal scapular nerve First intercostal nerve Long thoracic nerve Musculocutaneous nerve Subclavius nerve Suprascapular nerve
Brachial Vein, Left Brachial Vein, Right	Includes: Radial vein Ulnar vein
Brain	Includes: Cerebrum Corpus callosum Encephalon
Breast, Bilateral Breast, Left Breast, Right	Includes: Mammary duct Mammary gland
Buccal Mucosa	Includes: Buccal gland Molar gland Palatine gland
Carotid Bodies, Bilateral Carotid Body, Left Carotid Body, Right	Includes: Carotid glomus
Carpal Joint, Left Carpal Joint, Right	Includes: Intercarpal joint Midcarpal joint
Carpal, Left Carpal, Right	Includes: Capitate bone Hamate bone Lunate bone Pisiform bone Scaphoid bone Trapezium bone Trapezoid bone Triquetral bone
Celiac Artery	Includes: Celiac trunk
Cephalic Vein, Left Cephalic Vein, Right	Includes: Accessory cephalic vein
Cerebellum	Includes: Culmen
Cerebral Hemisphere	Includes: Frontal lobe Occipital lobe Parietal lobe Temporal lobe
Cerebral Meninges	Includes: Arachnoid mater, intracranial Leptomeninges, intracranial Pia mater, intracranial
Cerebral Ventricle	Includes: Aqueduct of Sylvius Cerebral aqueduct (Sylvius) Choroid plexus Ependyma Foramen of Monro (intraventricular) Fourth ventricle Interventricular foramen (Monro) Left lateral ventricle Right lateral ventricle Third ventricle

ICD-10-PCS Value	Definition
Cervical Nerve	Includes: Greater occipital nerve Spinal nerve, cervical Suboccipital nerve Third occipital nerve
Cervical Plexus	Includes: Ansa cervicalis Cutaneous (transverse) cervical nerve Great auricular nerve Lesser occipital nerve Supraclavicular nerve Transverse (cutaneous) cervical nerve
Cervical Vertebra	Includes: Dens Odontoid process Spinous process Transverse foramen Transverse process Vertebral arch Vertebral body Vertebral foramen Vertebral lamina Vertebral pedicle
Cervical Vertebral Joint	Includes: Atlantoaxial joint Cervical facet joint
Cervical Vertebral Joints, 2 or more	Includes: Cervical facet joint
Cervicothoracic Vertebral Joint	Includes: Cervicothoracic facet joint
Cisterna Chyli	Includes: Intestinal lymphatic trunk Lumbar lymphatic trunk
Coccygeal Glomus	Includes: Coccygeal body
Colic Vein	Includes: Ileocolic vein Left colic vein Middle colic vein Right colic vein
Conduction Mechanism	Includes: Atrioventricular node Bundle of His Bundle of Kent Sinoatrial node
Conjunctiva, Left Conjunctiva, Right	Includes: Plica semilunaris
Dura Mater	Includes: Diaphragma sellae Dura mater, intracranial Falx cerebri Tentorium cerebelli
Elbow Bursa and Ligament, Left Elbow Bursa and Ligament, Right	Includes: Annular ligament Olecranon bursa Radial collateral ligament Ulnar collateral ligament
Elbow Joint, Left Elbow Joint, Right	Includes: Distal humerus, involving joint Humeroradial joint Humeroulnar joint Proximal radioulnar joint
Epidural Space, Intracranial	Includes: Extradural space, intracranial

ICD-10-PCS Value	Definition
Epiglottis	**Includes:** Glossoepiglottic fold
Esophagogastric Junction	**Includes:** Cardia Cardioesophageal junction Gastroesophageal (GE) junction
Esophagus, Lower	**Includes:** Abdominal esophagus
Esophagus, Middle	**Includes:** Thoracic esophagus
Esophagus, Upper	**Includes:** Cervical esophagus
Ethmoid Bone, Left **Ethmoid Bone, Right**	**Includes:** Cribriform plate
Ethmoid Sinus, Left **Ethmoid Sinus, Right**	**Includes:** Ethmoidal air cell
Eustachian Tube, Left **Eustachian Tube, Right**	**Includes:** Auditory tube Pharyngotympanic tube
External Auditory Canal, Left **External Auditory Canal, Right**	**Includes:** External auditory meatus
External Carotid Artery, Left **External Carotid Artery, Right**	**Includes:** Ascending pharyngeal artery Internal maxillary artery Lingual artery Maxillary artery Occipital artery Posterior auricular artery Superior thyroid artery
External Ear, Bilateral **External Ear, Left** **External Ear, Right**	**Includes:** Antihelix Antitragus Auricle Earlobe Helix Pinna Tragus
External Iliac Artery, Left **External Iliac Artery, Right**	**Includes:** Deep circumflex iliac artery Inferior epigastric artery
External Jugular Vein, Left **External Jugular Vein, Right**	**Includes:** Posterior auricular vein
Extraocular Muscle, Left **Extraocular Muscle, Right**	**Includes:** Inferior oblique muscle Inferior rectus muscle Lateral rectus muscle Medial rectus muscle Superior oblique muscle Superior rectus muscle
Eye, Left **Eye, Right**	**Includes:** Ciliary body Posterior chamber
Face Artery	**Includes:** Angular artery Ascending palatine artery External maxillary artery Facial artery Inferior labial artery Submental artery Superior labial artery
Face Vein, Left **Face Vein, Right**	**Includes:** Angular vein Anterior facial vein Common facial vein Deep facial vein Frontal vein Posterior facial (retromandibular) vein Supraorbital vein
Facial Muscle	**Includes:** Buccinator muscle Corrugator supercilii muscle Depressor anguli oris muscle Depressor labii inferioris muscle Depressor septi nasi muscle Depressor supercilii muscle Levator anguli oris muscle Levator labii superioris alaeque nasi muscle Levator labii superioris muscle Mentalis muscle Nasalis muscle Occipitofrontalis muscle Orbicularis oris muscle Procerus muscle Risorius muscle Zygomaticus muscle
Facial Nerve	**Includes:** Chorda tympani Geniculate ganglion Greater superficial petrosal nerve Nerve to the stapedius Parotid plexus Posterior auricular nerve Seventh cranial nerve Submandibular ganglion
Fallopian Tube, Left **Fallopian Tube, Right**	**Includes:** Oviduct Salpinx Uterine tube
Femoral Artery, Left **Femoral Artery, Right**	**Includes:** Circumflex iliac artery Deep femoral artery Descending genicular artery External pudendal artery Superficial epigastric artery
Femoral Nerve	**Includes:** Anterior crural nerve Saphenous nerve
Femoral Shaft, Left **Femoral Shaft, Right**	**Includes:** Body of femur
Femoral Vein, Left **Femoral Vein, Right**	**Includes:** Deep femoral (profunda femoris) vein Popliteal vein Profunda femoris (deep femoral) vein
Fibula, Left **Fibula, Right**	**Includes:** Body of fibula Head of fibula Lateral malleolus
Finger Nail	**Includes:** Nail bed Nail plate

ICD-10-PCS Value	Definition
Finger Phalangeal Joint, Left **Finger Phalangeal Joint, Right**	**Includes:** Interphalangeal (IP) joint
Foot Artery, Left **Foot Artery, Right**	**Includes:** Arcuate artery Dorsal metatarsal artery Lateral plantar artery Lateral tarsal artery Medial plantar artery
Foot Bursa and Ligament, Left **Foot Bursa and Ligament, Right**	**Includes:** Calcaneocuboid ligament Cuneonavicular ligament Intercuneiform ligament Interphalangeal ligament Metatarsal ligament Metatarsophalangeal ligament Subtalar ligament Talocalcaneal ligament Talocalcaneonavicular ligament Tarsometatarsal ligament
Foot Muscle, Left **Foot Muscle, Right**	**Includes:** Abductor hallucis muscle Adductor hallucis muscle Extensor digitorum brevis muscle Extensor hallucis brevis muscle Flexor digitorum brevis muscle Flexor hallucis brevis muscle Quadratus plantae muscle
Foot Vein, Left **Foot Vein, Right**	**Includes:** Common digital vein Dorsal metatarsal vein Dorsal venous arch Plantar digital vein Plantar metatarsal vein Plantar venous arch
Frontal Bone	**Includes:** Zygomatic process of frontal bone
Gastric Artery	**Includes:** Left gastric artery Right gastric artery
Glenoid Cavity, Left **Glenoid Cavity, Right**	**Includes:** Glenoid fossa (of scapula)
Glomus Jugulare	**Includes:** Jugular body
Glossopharyngeal Nerve	**Includes:** Carotid sinus nerve Ninth cranial nerve Tympanic nerve
Hand Artery, Left **Hand Artery, Right**	**Includes:** Deep palmar arch Princeps pollicis artery Radialis indicis Superficial palmar arch
Hand Bursa and Ligament, Left **Hand Bursa and Ligament, Right**	**Includes:** Carpometacarpal ligament Intercarpal ligament Interphalangeal ligament Lunotriquetral ligament Metacarpal ligament Metacarpophalangeal ligament Pisohamate ligament Pisometacarpal ligament Scaphotrapezium ligament
Hand Muscle, Left **Hand Muscle, Right**	**Includes:** Hypothenar muscle Palmar interosseous muscle Thenar muscle
Hand Vein, Left **Hand Vein, Right**	**Includes:** Dorsal metacarpal vein Palmar (volar) digital vein Palmar (volar) metacarpal vein Superficial palmar venous arch Volar (palmar) digital vein Volar (palmar) metacarpal vein
Head and Neck Bursa and Ligament	**Includes:** Alar ligament of axis Cervical interspinous ligament Cervical intertransverse ligament Cervical ligamentum flavum Interspinous ligament, cervical Intertransverse ligament, cervical Lateral temporomandibular ligament Ligamentum flavum, cervical Sphenomandibular ligament Stylomandibular ligament Transverse ligament of atlas
Head and Neck Sympathetic Nerve	**Includes:** Cavernous plexus Cervical ganglion Ciliary ganglion Internal carotid plexus Otic ganglion Pterygopalatine (sphenopalatine) ganglion Sphenopalatine (pterygopalatine) ganglion Stellate ganglion Submandibular ganglion Submaxillary ganglion
Head Muscle	**Includes:** Auricularis muscle Masseter muscle Pterygoid muscle Splenius capitis muscle Temporalis muscle Temporoparietalis muscle
Heart, Left	**Includes:** Left coronary sulcus Obtuse margin
Heart, Right	**Includes:** Right coronary sulcus
Hemiazygos Vein	**Includes:** Left ascending lumbar vein Left subcostal vein
Hepatic Artery	**Includes:** Common hepatic artery Gastroduodenal artery Hepatic artery proper
Hip Bursa and Ligament, Left **Hip Bursa and Ligament, Right**	**Includes:** Iliofemoral ligament Ischiofemoral ligament Pubofemoral ligament Transverse acetabular ligament Trochanteric bursa
Hip Joint, Left **Hip Joint, Right**	**Includes:** Acetabulofemoral joint

ICD-10-PCS Value	Definition
Hip Muscle, Left **Hip Muscle, Right**	**Includes:** Gemellus muscle Gluteus maximus muscle Gluteus medius muscle Gluteus minimus muscle Iliacus muscle Obturator muscle Piriformis muscle Psoas muscle Quadratus femoris muscle Tensor fasciae latae muscle
Humeral Head, Left **Humeral Head, Right**	**Includes:** Greater tuberosity Lesser tuberosity Neck of humerus (anatomical)(surgical)
Humeral Shaft, Left **Humeral Shaft, Right**	**Includes:** Distal humerus Humerus, distal Lateral epicondyle of humerus Medial epicondyle of humerus
Hypogastric Vein, Left **Hypogastric Vein, Right**	**Includes:** Gluteal vein Internal iliac vein Internal pudendal vein Lateral sacral vein Middle hemorrhoidal vein Obturator vein Uterine vein Vaginal vein Vesical vein
Hypoglossal Nerve	**Includes:** Twelfth cranial nerve
Hypothalamus	**Includes:** Mammillary body
Inferior Mesenteric Artery	**Includes:** Sigmoid artery Superior rectal artery
Inferior Mesenteric Vein	**Includes:** Sigmoid vein Superior rectal vein
Inferior Vena Cava	**Includes:** Postcava Right inferior phrenic vein Right ovarian vein Right second lumbar vein Right suprarenal vein Right testicular vein
Inguinal Region, Bilateral **Inguinal Region, Left** **Inguinal Region, Right**	**Includes:** Inguinal canal Inguinal triangle
Inner Ear, Left **Inner Ear, Right**	**Includes:** Bony labyrinth Bony vestibule Cochlea Round window Semicircular canal
Innominate Artery	**Includes:** Brachiocephalic artery Brachiocephalic trunk
Innominate Vein, Left **Innominate Vein, Right**	**Includes:** Brachiocephalic vein Inferior thyroid vein
Internal Carotid Artery, Left **Internal Carotid Artery, Right**	**Includes:** Caroticotympanic artery Carotid sinus
Internal Iliac Artery, Left **Internal Iliac Artery, Right**	**Includes:** Deferential artery Hypogastric artery Iliolumbar artery Inferior gluteal artery Inferior vesical artery Internal pudendal artery Lateral sacral artery Middle rectal artery Obturator artery Superior gluteal artery Umbilical artery Uterine artery Vaginal artery
Internal Mammary Artery, Left **Internal Mammary Artery, Right**	**Includes:** Anterior intercostal artery Internal thoracic artery Musculophrenic artery Pericardiophrenic artery Superior epigastric artery
Intracranial Artery	**Includes:** Anterior cerebral artery Anterior choroidal artery Anterior communicating artery Basilar artery Circle of Willis Internal carotid artery, intracranial portion Middle cerebral artery Ophthalmic artery Posterior cerebral artery Posterior communicating artery Posterior inferior cerebellar artery (PICA)
Intracranial Vein	**Includes:** Anterior cerebral vein Basal (internal) cerebral vein Dural venous sinus Great cerebral vein Inferior cerebellar vein Inferior cerebral vein Internal (basal) cerebral vein Middle cerebral vein Ophthalmic vein Superior cerebellar vein Superior cerebral vein
Jejunum	**Includes:** Duodenojejunal flexure
Kidney	**Includes:** Renal calyx Renal capsule Renal cortex Renal segment
Kidney Pelvis, Left **Kidney Pelvis, Right**	**Includes:** Ureteropelvic junction (UPJ)
Kidney, Left **Kidney, Right** **Kidneys, Bilateral**	**Includes:** Renal calyx Renal capsule Renal cortex Renal segment

ICD-10-PCS Value	Definition
Knee Bursa and Ligament, Left Knee Bursa and Ligament, Right	Includes: Anterior cruciate ligament (ACL) Lateral collateral ligament (LCL) Ligament of head of fibula Medial collateral ligament (MCL) Patellar ligament Popliteal ligament Posterior cruciate ligament (PCL) Prepatellar bursa
Knee Joint, Femoral Surface, Left Knee Joint, Femoral Surface, Right	Includes: Femoropatellar joint Patellofemoral joint
Knee Joint, Left Knee Joint, Right	Includes: Femoropatellar joint Femorotibial joint Lateral meniscus Medial meniscus Patellofemoral joint Tibiofemoral joint
Knee Joint, Tibial Surface, Left Knee Joint, Tibial Surface, Right	Includes: Femorotibial joint Tibiofemoral joint
Knee Tendon, Left Knee Tendon, Right	Includes: Patellar tendon
Lacrimal Duct, Left Lacrimal Duct, Right	Includes: Lacrimal canaliculus Lacrimal punctum Lacrimal sac Nasolacrimal duct
Larynx	Includes: Aryepiglottic fold Arytenoid cartilage Corniculate cartilage Cuneiform cartilage False vocal cord Glottis Rima glottidis Thyroid cartilage Ventricular fold
Lens, Left Lens, Right	Includes: Zonule of Zinn
Liver	Includes: Quadrate lobe
Lower Arm and Wrist Muscle, Left Lower Arm and Wrist Muscle, Right	Includes: Anatomical snuffbox Brachioradialis muscle Extensor carpi radialis muscle Extensor carpi ulnaris muscle Flexor carpi radialis muscle Flexor carpi ulnaris muscle Flexor pollicis longus muscle Palmaris longus muscle Pronator quadratus muscle Pronator teres muscle
Lower Artery	Includes: Umbilical artery
Lower Eyelid, Left Lower Eyelid, Right	Includes: Inferior tarsal plate Medial canthus
Lower Femur, Left Lower Femur, Right	Includes: Lateral condyle of femur Lateral epicondyle of femur Medial condyle of femur Medial epicondyle of femur

ICD-10-PCS Value	Definition
Lower Leg Muscle, Left Lower Leg Muscle, Right	Includes: Extensor digitorum longus muscle Extensor hallucis longus muscle Fibularis brevis muscle Fibularis longus muscle Flexor digitorum longus muscle Flexor hallucis longus muscle Gastrocnemius muscle Peroneus brevis muscle Peroneus longus muscle Popliteus muscle Soleus muscle Tibialis anterior muscle Tibialis posterior muscle
Lower Leg Tendon, Left Lower Leg Tendon, Right	Includes: Achilles tendon
Lower Lip	Includes: Frenulum labii inferioris Labial gland Vermilion border
Lower Spine Bursa and Ligament	Includes: Iliolumbar ligament Interspinous ligament, lumbar Intertransverse ligament, lumbar Ligamentum flavum, lumbar Sacrococcygeal ligament Sacroiliac ligament Sacrospinous ligament Sacrotuberous ligament Supraspinous ligament
Lumbar Nerve	Includes: Lumbosacral trunk Spinal nerve, lumbar Superior clunic (cluneal) nerve
Lumbar Plexus	Includes: Accessory obturator nerve Genitofemoral nerve Iliohypogastric nerve Ilioinguinal nerve Lateral femoral cutaneous nerve Obturator nerve Superior gluteal nerve
Lumbar Spinal Cord	Includes: Cauda equina Conus medullaris
Lumbar Sympathetic Nerve	Includes: Lumbar ganglion Lumbar splanchnic nerve
Lumbar Vertebra	Includes: Spinous process Transverse process Vertebral arch Vertebral body Vertebral foramen Vertebral lamina Vertebral pedicle
Lumbar Vertebral Joint	Includes: Lumbar facet joint
Lumbosacral Joint	Includes: Lumbosacral facet joint

ICD-10-PCS Value	Definition
Lymphatic, Aortic	**Includes:** Celiac lymph node Gastric lymph node Hepatic lymph node Lumbar lymph node Pancreaticosplenic lymph node Paraaortic lymph node Retroperitoneal lymph node
Lymphatic, Head	**Includes:** Buccinator lymph node Infraauricular lymph node Infraparotid lymph node Parotid lymph node Preauricular lymph node Submandibular lymph node Submaxillary lymph node Submental lymph node Subparotid lymph node Suprahyoid lymph node
Lymphatic, Left Axillary	**Includes:** Anterior (pectoral) lymph node Apical (subclavicular) lymph node Brachial (lateral) lymph node Central axillary lymph node Lateral (brachial) lymph node Pectoral (anterior) lymph node Posterior (subscapular) lymph node Subclavicular (apical) lymph node Subscapular (posterior) lymph node
Lymphatic, Left Lower Extremity	**Includes:** Femoral lymph node Popliteal lymph node
Lymphatic, Left Neck	**Includes:** Cervical lymph node Jugular lymph node Mastoid (postauricular) lymph node Occipital lymph node Postauricular (mastoid) lymph node Retropharyngeal lymph node Supraclavicular (Virchow's) lymph node Virchow's (supraclavicular) lymph node
Lymphatic, Left Upper Extremity	**Includes:** Cubital lymph node Deltopectoral (infraclavicular) lymph node Epitrochlear lymph node Infraclavicular (deltopectoral) lymph node Supratrochlear lymph node
Lymphatic, Mesenteric	**Includes:** Inferior mesenteric lymph node Pararectal lymph node Superior mesenteric lymph node
Lymphatic, Pelvis	**Includes:** Common iliac (subaortic) lymph node Gluteal lymph node Iliac lymph node Inferior epigastric lymph node Obturator lymph node Sacral lymph node Subaortic (common iliac) lymph node Suprainguinal lymph node
Lymphatic, Right Axillary	**Includes:** Anterior (pectoral) lymph node Apical (subclavicular) lymph node Brachial (lateral) lymph node Central axillary lymph node Lateral (brachial) lymph node Pectoral (anterior) lymph node Posterior (subscapular) lymph node Subclavicular (apical) lymph node Subscapular (posterior) lymph node
Lymphatic, Right Lower Extremity	**Includes:** Femoral lymph node Popliteal lymph node
Lymphatic, Right Neck	**Includes:** Cervical lymph node Jugular lymph node Mastoid (postauricular) lymph node Occipital lymph node Postauricular (mastoid) lymph node Retropharyngeal lymph node Right jugular trunk Right lymphatic duct Right subclavian trunk Supraclavicular (Virchow's) lymph node Virchow's (supraclavicular) lymph node
Lymphatic, Right Upper Extremity	**Includes:** Cubital lymph node Deltopectoral (infraclavicular) lymph node Epitrochlear lymph node Infraclavicular (deltopectoral) lymph node Supratrochlear lymph node
Lymphatic, Thorax	**Includes:** Intercostal lymph node Mediastinal lymph node Parasternal lymph node Paratracheal lymph node Tracheobronchial lymph node
Main Bronchus, Right	**Includes:** Bronchus intermedius Intermediate bronchus
Mandible, Left **Mandible, Right**	**Includes:** Alveolar process of mandible Condyloid process Mandibular notch Mental foramen
Mastoid Sinus, Left **Mastoid Sinus, Right**	**Includes:** Mastoid air cells
Maxilla	**Includes:** Alveolar process of maxilla
Maxillary Sinus, Left **Maxillary Sinus, Right**	**Includes:** Antrum of Highmore
Median Nerve	**Includes:** Anterior interosseous nerve Palmar cutaneous nerve
Mediastinum	**Includes:** Mediastinal cavity Mediastinal space
Medulla Oblongata	**Includes:** Myelencephalon
Mesentery	**Includes:** Mesoappendix Mesocolon

ICD-10-PCS Value	Definition
Metatarsal-Phalangeal Joint, Left **Metatarsal-Phalangeal Joint, Right**	**Includes:** Metatarsophalangeal (MTP) joint
Middle Ear, Left **Middle Ear, Right**	**Includes:** Oval window Tympanic cavity
Minor Salivary Gland	**Includes:** Anterior lingual gland
Mitral Valve	**Includes:** Bicuspid valve Left atrioventricular valve Mitral annulus
Nasal Bone	**Includes:** Vomer of nasal septum
Nasal Mucosa and Soft Tissue	**Includes:** Columella External naris Greater alar cartilage Internal naris Lateral nasal cartilage Lesser alar cartilage Nasal cavity Nostril
Nasal Septum	**Includes:** Quadrangular cartilage Septal cartilage Vomer bone
Nasal Turbinate	**Includes:** Inferior turbinate Middle turbinate Nasal concha Superior turbinate
Nasopharynx	**Includes:** Choana Fossa of Rosenmuller Pharyngeal recess Rhinopharynx
Neck Muscle, Left **Neck Muscle, Right**	**Includes:** Anterior vertebral muscle Arytenoid muscle Cricothyroid muscle Infrahyoid muscle Levator scapulae muscle Platysma muscle Scalene muscle Splenius cervicis muscle Sternocleidomastoid muscle Suprahyoid muscle Thyroarytenoid muscle
Nipple, Left **Nipple, Right**	**Includes:** Areola
Occipital Bone	**Includes:** Foramen magnum
Oculomotor Nerve	**Includes:** Third cranial nerve
Olfactory Nerve	**Includes:** First cranial nerve Olfactory bulb

ICD-10-PCS Value	Definition
Omentum	**Includes:** Gastrocolic ligament Gastrocolic omentum Gastrohepatic omentum Gastrophrenic ligament Gastrosplenic ligament Greater Omentum Hepatogastric ligament Lesser Omentum
Optic Nerve	**Includes:** Optic chiasma Second cranial nerve
Orbit, Left **Orbit, Right**	**Includes:** Bony orbit Orbital portion of ethmoid bone Orbital portion of frontal bone Orbital portion of lacrimal bone Orbital portion of maxilla Orbital portion of palatine bone Orbital portion of sphenoid bone Orbital portion of zygomatic bone
Pancreatic Duct	**Includes:** Duct of Wirsung
Pancreatic Duct, Accessory	**Includes:** Duct of Santorini
Parotid Duct, Left **Parotid Duct, Right**	**Includes:** Stensen's duct
Pelvic Bone, Left **Pelvic Bone, Right**	**Includes:** Iliac crest Ilium Ischium Pubis
Pelvic Cavity	**Includes:** Retropubic space
Penis	**Includes:** Corpus cavernosum Corpus spongiosum
Perineum Muscle	**Includes:** Bulbospongiosus muscle Cremaster muscle Deep transverse perineal muscle Ischiocavernosus muscle Levator ani muscle Superficial transverse perineal muscle
Peritoneum	**Includes:** Epiploic foramen
Peroneal Artery, Left **Peroneal Artery, Right**	**Includes:** Fibular artery
Peroneal Nerve	**Includes:** Common fibular nerve Common peroneal nerve External popliteal nerve Lateral sural cutaneous nerve
Pharynx	**Includes:** Base of Tongue Hypopharynx Laryngopharynx Lingual tonsil Oropharynx Piriform recess (sinus) Tongue, base of
Phrenic Nerve	**Includes:** Accessory phrenic nerve

ICD-10-PCS Value	Definition
Pituitary Gland	**Includes:** Adenohypophysis Hypophysis Neurohypophysis
Pons	**Includes:** Apneustic center Basis pontis Locus ceruleus Pneumotaxic center Pontine tegmentum Superior olivary nucleus
Popliteal Artery, Left **Popliteal Artery, Right**	**Includes:** Inferior genicular artery Middle genicular artery Superior genicular artery Sural artery Tibioperoneal trunk
Portal Vein	**Includes:** Hepatic portal vein
Prepuce	**Includes:** Foreskin Glans penis
Pudendal Nerve	**Includes:** Posterior labial nerve Posterior scrotal nerve
Pulmonary Artery, Left	**Includes:** Arterial canal (duct) Botallo's duct Pulmoaortic canal
Pulmonary Valve	**Includes:** Pulmonary annulus Pulmonic valve
Pulmonary Vein, Left	**Includes:** Left inferior pulmonary vein Left superior pulmonary vein
Pulmonary Vein, Right	**Includes:** Right inferior pulmonary vein Right superior pulmonary vein
Radial Artery, Left **Radial Artery, Right**	**Includes:** Radial recurrent artery
Radial Nerve	**Includes:** Dorsal digital nerve Musculospiral nerve Palmar cutaneous nerve Posterior interosseous nerve
Radius, Left **Radius, Right**	**Includes:** Ulnar notch
Rectum	**Includes:** Anorectal junction
Renal Artery, Left **Renal Artery, Right**	**Includes:** Inferior suprarenal artery Renal segmental artery
Renal Vein, Left	**Includes:** Left inferior phrenic vein Left ovarian vein Left second lumbar vein Left suprarenal vein Left testicular vein
Retina, Left **Retina, Right**	**Includes:** Fovea Macula Optic disc
Retroperitoneum	**Includes:** Retroperitoneal cavity Retroperitoneal space

ICD-10-PCS Value	Definition
Rib(s) Bursa and Ligament	**Includes:** Costotransverse ligament
Sacral Nerve	**Includes:** Spinal nerve, sacral
Sacral Plexus	**Includes:** Inferior gluteal nerve Posterior femoral cutaneous nerve Pudendal nerve
Sacral Sympathetic Nerve	**Includes:** Ganglion impar (ganglion of Walther) Pelvic splanchnic nerve Sacral ganglion Sacral splanchnic nerve
Sacrococcygeal Joint	**Includes:** Sacrococcygeal symphysis
Saphenous Vein, Left **Saphenous Vein, Right**	**Includes:** External pudendal vein Great(er) saphenous vein Lesser saphenous vein Small saphenous vein Superficial circumflex iliac vein Superficial epigastric vein
Scapula, Left **Scapula, Right**	**Includes:** Acromion (process) Coracoid process
Sciatic Nerve	**Includes:** Ischiatic nerve
Shoulder Bursa and Ligament, Left **Shoulder Bursa and Ligament, Right**	**Includes:** Acromioclavicular ligament Coracoacromial ligament Coracoclavicular ligament Coracohumeral ligament Costoclavicular ligament Glenohumeral ligament Interclavicular ligament Sternoclavicular ligament Subacromial bursa Transverse humeral ligament Transverse scapular ligament
Shoulder Joint, Left **Shoulder Joint, Right**	**Includes:** Glenohumeral joint Glenoid ligament (labrum)
Shoulder Muscle, Left **Shoulder Muscle, Right**	**Includes:** Deltoid muscle Infraspinatus muscle Subscapularis muscle Supraspinatus muscle Teres major muscle Teres minor muscle
Sigmoid Colon	**Includes:** Rectosigmoid junction Sigmoid flexure
Skin	**Includes:** Dermis Epidermis Sebaceous gland Sweat gland
Skin, Chest	**Includes:** Breast procedures, skin only
Sphenoid Bone	**Includes:** Greater wing Lesser wing Optic foramen Pterygoid process Sella turcica

ICD-10-PCS Value	Definition
Spinal Canal	**Includes:** Epidural space, spinal Extradural space, spinal Subarachnoid space, spinal Subdural space, spinal Vertebral canal
Spinal Meninges	**Includes:** Arachnoid mater, spinal Denticulate (dentate) ligament Dura mater, spinal Filum terminale Leptomeninges, spinal Pia mater, spinal
Spleen	**Includes:** Accessory spleen
Splenic Artery	**Includes:** Left gastroepiploic artery Pancreatic artery Short gastric artery
Splenic Vein	**Includes:** Left gastroepiploic vein Pancreatic vein
Sternum	**Includes:** Manubrium Suprasternal notch Xiphoid process
Sternum Bursa and Ligament	**Includes:** Costoxiphoid ligament Sternocostal ligament
Stomach, Pylorus	**Includes:** Pyloric antrum Pyloric canal Pyloric sphincter
Subclavian Artery, Left **Subclavian Artery, Right**	**Includes:** Costocervical trunk Dorsal scapular artery Internal thoracic artery
Subcutaneous Tissue and Fascia, Chest	**Includes:** Pectoral fascia
Subcutaneous Tissue and Fascia, Face	**Includes:** Masseteric fascia Orbital fascia Submandibular space
Subcutaneous Tissue and Fascia, Left Foot	**Includes:** Plantar fascia (aponeurosis)
Subcutaneous Tissue and Fascia, Left Hand	**Includes:** Palmar fascia (aponeurosis)
Subcutaneous Tissue and Fascia, Left Lower Arm	**Includes:** Antebrachial fascia Bicipital aponeurosis
Subcutaneous Tissue and Fascia, Left Neck	**Includes:** Deep cervical fascia Pretracheal fascia Prevertebral fascia
Subcutaneous Tissue and Fascia, Left Upper Arm	**Includes:** Axillary fascia Deltoid fascia Infraspinatus fascia Subscapular aponeurosis Supraspinatus fascia
Subcutaneous Tissue and Fascia, Left Upper Leg	**Includes:** Crural fascia Fascia lata Iliac fascia Iliotibial tract (band)

ICD-10-PCS Value	Definition
Subcutaneous Tissue and Fascia, Right Foot	**Includes:** Plantar fascia (aponeurosis)
Subcutaneous Tissue and Fascia, Right Hand	**Includes:** Palmar fascia (aponeurosis)
Subcutaneous Tissue and Fascia, Right Lower Arm	**Includes:** Antebrachial fascia Bicipital aponeurosis
Subcutaneous Tissue and Fascia, Right Neck	**Includes:** Deep cervical fascia Pretracheal fascia Prevertebral fascia
Subcutaneous Tissue and Fascia, Right Upper Arm	**Includes:** Axillary fascia Deltoid fascia Infraspinatus fascia Subscapular aponeurosis Supraspinatus fascia
Subcutaneous Tissue and Fascia, Right Upper Leg	**Includes:** Crural fascia Fascia lata Iliac fascia Iliotibial tract (band)
Subcutaneous Tissue and Fascia, Scalp	**Includes:** Galea aponeurotica
Subcutaneous Tissue and Fascia, Trunk	**Includes:** External oblique aponeurosis Transversalis fascia
Submaxillary Gland, Left **Submaxillary Gland, Right**	**Includes:** Submandibular gland
Superior Mesenteric Artery	**Includes:** Ileal artery Ileocolic artery Inferior pancreaticoduodenal artery Jejunal artery
Superior Mesenteric Vein	**Includes:** Right gastroepiploic vein
Superior Vena Cava	**Includes:** Precava
Tarsal Joint, Left **Tarsal Joint, Right**	**Includes:** Calcaneocuboid joint Cuboideonavicular joint Cuneonavicular joint Intercuneiform joint Subtalar (talocalcaneal) joint Talocalcaneal (subtalar) joint Talocalcaneonavicular joint
Tarsal, Left **Tarsal, Right**	**Includes:** Calcaneus Cuboid bone Intermediate cuneiform bone Lateral cuneiform bone Medial cuneiform bone Navicular bone Talus bone
Temporal Artery, Left **Temporal Artery, Right**	**Includes:** Middle temporal artery Superficial temporal artery Transverse facial artery
Temporal Bone, Left **Temporal Bone, Right**	**Includes:** Mastoid process Petrous part of temporal bone Tympanic part of temporal bone Zygomatic process of temporal bone

ICD-10-PCS Value	Definition
Thalamus	**Includes:** Epithalamus Geniculate nucleus Metathalamus Pulvinar
Thoracic Aorta, Ascending/Arch	**Includes:** Aortic arch Ascending aorta
Thoracic Duct	**Includes:** Left jugular trunk Left subclavian trunk
Thoracic Nerve	**Includes:** Intercostal nerve Intercostobrachial nerve Spinal nerve, thoracic Subcostal nerve
Thoracic Sympathetic Nerve	**Includes:** Cardiac plexus Esophageal plexus Greater splanchnic nerve Inferior cardiac nerve Least splanchnic nerve Lesser splanchnic nerve Middle cardiac nerve Pulmonary plexus Superior cardiac nerve Thoracic aortic plexus Thoracic ganglion
Thoracic Vertebra	**Includes:** Spinous process Transverse process Vertebral arch Vertebral body Vertebral foramen Vertebral lamina Vertebral pedicle
Thoracic Vertebral Joint	**Includes:** Costotransverse joint Costovertebral joint Thoracic facet joint
Thoracolumbar Vertebral Joint	**Includes:** Thoracolumbar facet joint
Thorax Muscle, Left **Thorax Muscle, Right**	**Includes:** Intercostal muscle Levatores costarum muscle Pectoralis major muscle Pectoralis minor muscle Serratus anterior muscle Subclavius muscle Subcostal muscle Transverse thoracis muscle
Thymus	**Includes:** Thymus gland
Thyroid Artery, Left **Thyroid Artery, Right**	**Includes:** Cricothyroid artery Hyoid artery Sternocleidomastoid artery Superior laryngeal artery Superior thyroid artery Thyrocervical trunk
Tibia, Left **Tibia, Right**	**Includes:** Lateral condyle of tibia Medial condyle of tibia Medial malleolus
Tibial Nerve	**Includes:** Lateral plantar nerve Medial plantar nerve Medial popliteal nerve Medial sural cutaneous nerve
Toe Nail	**Includes:** Nail bed Nail plate
Toe Phalangeal Joint, Left **Toe Phalangeal Joint, Right**	**Includes:** Interphalangeal (IP) joint
Tongue	**Includes:** Frenulum linguae
Tongue, Palate, Pharynx Muscle	**Includes:** Chondroglossus muscle Genioglossus muscle Hyoglossus muscle Inferior longitudinal muscle Levator veli palatini muscle Palatoglossal muscle Palatopharyngeal muscle Pharyngeal constrictor muscle Salpingopharyngeus muscle Styloglossus muscle Stylopharyngeus muscle Superior longitudinal muscle Tensor veli palatini muscle
Tonsils	**Includes:** Palatine tonsil
Trachea	**Includes:** Cricoid cartilage
Transverse Colon	**Includes:** Hepatic flexure Splenic flexure
Tricuspid Valve	**Includes:** Right atrioventricular valve Tricuspid annulus
Trigeminal Nerve	**Includes:** Fifth cranial nerve Gasserian ganglion Mandibular nerve Maxillary nerve Ophthalmic nerve Trifacial nerve
Trochlear Nerve	**Includes:** Fourth cranial nerve
Trunk Muscle, Left **Trunk Muscle, Right**	**Includes:** Coccygeus muscle Erector spinae muscle Interspinalis muscle Intertransversarius muscle Latissimus dorsi muscle Quadratus lumborum muscle Rhomboid major muscle Rhomboid minor muscle Serratus posterior muscle Transversospinalis muscle Trapezius muscle
Tympanic Membrane, Left **Tympanic Membrane, Right**	**Includes:** Pars flaccida
Ulna, Left **Ulna, Right**	**Includes:** Olecranon process Radial notch

ICD-10-PCS Value	Definition
Ulnar Artery, Left **Ulnar Artery, Right**	**Includes:** Anterior ulnar recurrent artery Common interosseous artery Posterior ulnar recurrent artery
Ulnar Nerve	**Includes:** Cubital nerve
Upper Arm Muscle, Left **Upper Arm Muscle, Right**	**Includes:** Biceps brachii muscle Brachialis muscle Coracobrachialis muscle Triceps brachii muscle
Upper Artery	**Includes:** Aortic intercostal artery Bronchial artery Esophageal artery Subcostal artery
Upper Eyelid, Left **Upper Eyelid, Right**	**Includes:** Lateral canthus Levator palpebrae superioris muscle Orbicularis oculi muscle Superior tarsal plate
Upper Femur, Left **Upper Femur, Right**	**Includes:** Femoral head Greater trochanter Lesser trochanter Neck of femur
Upper Leg Muscle, Left **Upper Leg Muscle, Right**	**Includes:** Adductor brevis muscle Adductor longus muscle Adductor magnus muscle Biceps femoris muscle Gracilis muscle Pectineus muscle Quadriceps (femoris) Rectus femoris muscle Sartorius muscle Semimembranosus muscle Semitendinosus muscle Vastus intermedius muscle Vastus lateralis muscle Vastus medialis muscle
Upper Lip	**Includes:** Frenulum labii superioris Labial gland Vermilion border
Upper Spine Bursa and Ligament	**Includes:** Interspinous ligament, thoracic Intertransverse ligament, thoracic Ligamentum flavum, thoracic Supraspinous ligament
Ureter **Ureter, Left** **Ureter, Right** **Ureters, Bilateral**	**Includes:** Ureteral orifice Ureterovesical orifice
Urethra	**Includes:** Bulbourethral (Cowper's) gland Cowper's (bulbourethral) gland External urethral sphincter Internal urethral sphincter Membranous urethra Penile urethra Prostatic urethra
Uterine Supporting Structure	**Includes:** Broad ligament Infundibulopelvic ligament Ovarian ligament Round ligament of uterus

ICD-10-PCS Value	Definition
Uterus	**Includes:** Fundus uteri Myometrium Perimetrium Uterine cornu
Uvula	**Includes:** Palatine uvula
Vagus Nerve	**Includes:** Anterior vagal trunk Pharyngeal plexus Pneumogastric nerve Posterior vagal trunk Pulmonary plexus Recurrent laryngeal nerve Superior laryngeal nerve Tenth cranial nerve
Vas Deferens **Vas Deferens, Bilateral** **Vas Deferens, Left** **Vas Deferens, Right**	**Includes:** Ductus deferens Ejaculatory duct
Ventricle, Right	**Includes:** Conus arteriosus
Ventricular Septum	**Includes:** Interventricular septum
Vertebral Artery, Left **Vertebral Artery, Right**	**Includes:** Anterior spinal artery Posterior spinal artery
Vertebral Vein, Left **Vertebral Vein, Right**	**Includes:** Deep cervical vein Suboccipital venous plexus
Vestibular Gland	**Includes:** Bartholin's (greater vestibular) gland Greater vestibular (Bartholin's) gland Paraurethral (Skene's) gland Skene's (paraurethral) gland
Vitreous, Left **Vitreous, Right**	**Includes:** Vitreous body
Vocal Cord, Left **Vocal Cord, Right**	**Includes:** Vocal fold
Vulva	**Includes:** Labia majora Labia minora
Wrist Bursa and Ligament, Left **Wrist Bursa and Ligament, Right**	**Includes:** Palmar ulnocarpal ligament Radial collateral carpal ligament Radiocarpal ligament Radioulnar ligament Scapholunate ligament Ulnar collateral carpal ligament
Wrist Joint, Left **Wrist Joint, Right**	**Includes:** Distal radioulnar joint Radiocarpal joint

Appendix F: Device Classification

In most PCS codes, the sixth character of the code classifies the device. The sixth character device value "defines the material or appliance used to accomplish the objective of the procedure that remains in or on the procedure site at the end of the procedure." If the device is the means by which the procedural objective is accomplished, then a specific device value is coded in the sixth character. If no device is used to accomplish the objective of the procedure, the device value No Device is coded in the sixth character. In limited root operations, the classification provides the qualifier values Temporary and Intraoperative, for specific procedures involving clinically significant devices whose purpose is brief use during the procedure or current inpatient stay.

Material that is classified as a PCS device is distinguished from material classified as a PCS substance by its having a specific location. A device is intended to maintain a fixed location at the procedure site where it was put, whereas a substance is intended to disperse or be absorbed in the body. There are circumstances in which a device does not stay where it was put and may need to be "revised" in a subsequent procedure to move the device back to its intended location.

Material classified as a PCS device is also distinguishable by the fact that it is removable. Although it may not be practical to remove some types of devices once they become established at the site, it is physically possible to remove a device for some time after the procedure. A skin graft, for example, once it "takes," may be nearly indistinguishable from the surrounding skin and so is no longer clearly identifiable as a device. Nevertheless, procedures that involve material coded as a device can for the most part be "reversed" by removing the device from the procedure site.

General Device Types

Device Type	Definition	Examples
Grafts	Biological or synthetic material that **takes the place of all or a portion of a body part.**	Full- or partial-thickness skin grafts: • Autologous • Nonautologous • Synthetic • Zooplastic Other tissue grafts: • Bone • Tendon • Vascular
Prosthesis	Biological or synthetic material that **takes the place of all or a portion of a body part.**	Joint prosthesis: • Autologous • Nonautologous • Synthetic
Implants	**Therapeutic** material that is not absorbed by, eliminated by, or incorporated into a body part.	External fixation device Internal fixation device: • Orthopaedic pins • Intramedullary rods Radioactive element implant Mesh
Simple or mechanical appliances	Biological or synthetic material that **assists or prevents a physiological function.**	Drainage device Extraluminal device Endobrachial device Fusion device Intraluminal device (can be temporary) Tracheostomy device IUD
Electronic appliances	Electronic appliances used to **assist, monitor, take the pace of, or prevent a physiological function.**	Cardiac leads Diaphragmatic pacemaker External heart assist system Short-term external heart assist system (Intraoperative) Fetal monitoring Hearing device Monitoring device Neurostimulator
External appliances	Performed without making an incision or a puncture, external appliances are used for the purpose of **protection, immobilization, stretching, compression, or packing.**	Bandage Cast Packing material Pressure dressing Traction apparatus

Transplant/Grafting Tissue Type Terminology

Tissue Type	Terminology
Tissue or organ transferred into a new position in **the body of the same individual**	Autograft Autologous Autoplastic
Having to do with individuals or tissues that have **identical genes**, such as identical twins	Isograft Isologous Syngeneic Syngraft
Tissue or organ taken from **different individuals** of the same species	Allogeneic Allograft Homologous Homograft
Tissue or organ from a **cadaver**	Nonautologous
Tissue or organ from individuals of **different species**	Heterogeneic Heterologous Xenogeneic Xenograft Zooplastic

Appendix G: Device Key and Aggregation Table

Device Key

Term	ICD-10-PCS Value
3f (Aortic) Bioprosthesis valve	Zooplastic Tissue in Heart and Great Vessels
AbioCor® Total Replacement Heart	Synthetic Substitute
Absolute Pro Vascular (OTW) Self-Expanding Stent System	Intraluminal Device
Acculink (RX) Carotid Stent System	Intraluminal Device
Acellular Hydrated Dermis	Nonautologous Tissue Substitute
Acetabular cup	Liner in Lower Joints
Activa PC neurostimulator	Stimulator Generator, Multiple Array for Insertion in Subcutaneous Tissue and Fascia
Activa RC neurostimulator	Stimulator Generator, Multiple Array Rechargeable for Insertion in Subcutaneous Tissue and Fascia
Activa SC neurostimulator	Stimulator Generator, Single Array for Insertion in Subcutaneous Tissue and Fascia
ACUITY™ Steerable Lead	Cardiac Lead, Pacemaker for Insertion in Heart and Great Vessels Cardiac Lead, Defibrillator for Insertion in Heart and Great Vessels
Advisa (MRI)	Pacemaker, Dual Chamber for Insertion in Subcutaneous Tissue and Fascia
AFX® Endovascular AAA System	Intraluminal Device
AMPLATZER® Muscular VSD Occluder	Synthetic Substitute
AMS 800® Urinary Control System	Artificial Sphincter in Urinary System
AneuRx® AAA Advantage®	Intraluminal Device
Annuloplasty ring	Synthetic Substitute
Articulating Spacer (Antibiotic)	Articulating Spacer in Lower Joints
Artificial anal sphincter (AAS)	Artificial Sphincter in Gastrointestinal System
Artificial bowel sphincter (neosphincter)	Artificial Sphincter in Gastrointestinal System
Artificial urinary sphincter (AUS)	Artificial Sphincter in Urinary System
Ascenda Intrathecal Catheter	Infusion Device
Assurant (Cobalt) stent	Intraluminal Device
AtriClip LAA Exclusion System	Extraluminal Device
Attain Ability® Lead	Cardiac Lead, Pacemaker for Insertion in Heart and Great Vessels Cardiac Lead, Defibrillator for Insertion in Heart and Great Vessels
Attain StarFix® (OTW) Lead	Cardiac Lead, Pacemaker for Insertion in Heart and Great Vessels Cardiac Lead, Defibrillator for Insertion in Heart and Great Vessels
Autograft	Autologous Tissue Substitute
Autologous artery graft	Autologous Arterial Tissue in Heart and Great Vessels Autologous Arterial Tissue in Upper Arteries Autologous Arterial Tissue in Lower Arteries Autologous Arterial Tissue in Upper Veins Autologous Arterial Tissue in Lower Veins
Autologous vein graft	Autologous Venous Tissue in Heart and Great Vessels Autologous Venous Tissue in Upper Arteries Autologous Venous Tissue in Lower Arteries Autologous Venous Tissue in Upper Veins Autologous Venous Tissue in Lower Veins
Axial Lumbar Interbody Fusion System	Interbody Fusion Device in Lower Joints
AxiaLIF® System	Interbody Fusion Device in Lower Joints
BAK/C® Interbody Cervical Fusion System	Interbody Fusion Device in Upper Joints
Bard® Composix® (E/X)(LP) mesh	Synthetic Substitute
Bard® Composix® Kugel® patch	Synthetic Substitute
Bard® Dulex™ mesh	Synthetic Substitute
Bard® Ventralex™ hernia patch	Synthetic Substitute
Baroreflex Activation Therapy® (BAT®)	Stimulator Lead in Upper Arteries Stimulator Generator in Subcutaneous Tissue and Fascia
Barricaid® Annular Closure Device (ACD)	Synthetic Substitute
Berlin Heart Ventricular Assist Device	Implantable Heart Assist System in Heart and Great Vessels
Bioactive embolization coil(s)	Intraluminal Device, Bioactive in Upper Arteries
Biventricular external heart assist system	Short-term External Heart Assist System in Heart and Great Vessels
Blood glucose monitoring system	Monitoring Device
Bone anchored hearing device	Hearing Device, Bone Conduction for Insertion in Ear, Nose, Sinus Hearing Device, in Head and Facial Bones
Bone bank bone graft	Nonautologous Tissue Substitute
Bone screw (interlocking)(lag)(pedicle)(recessed)	Internal Fixation Device in Head and Facial Bones Internal Fixation Device in Upper Bones Internal Fixation Device in Lower Bones
Bovine pericardial valve	Zooplastic Tissue in Heart and Great Vessels
Bovine pericardium graft	Zooplastic Tissue in Heart and Great Vessels
Brachytherapy seeds	Radioactive Element
BRYAN® Cervical Disc System	Synthetic Substitute
BVS 5000 Ventricular Assist Device	Short-term External Heart Assist System in Heart and Great Vessels

Term	ICD-10-PCS Value
Cardiac contractility modulation lead	Cardiac Lead in Heart and Great Vessels
Cardiac event recorder	Monitoring Device
Cardiac resynchronization therapy (CRT) lead	Cardiac Lead, Pacemaker for Insertion in Heart and Great Vessels Cardiac Lead, Defibrillator for Insertion in Heart and Great Vessels
CardioMEMS® pressure sensor	Monitoring Device, Pressure Sensor for Insertion in Heart and Great Vessels
Carotid (artery) sinus (baroreceptor) lead	Stimulator Lead in Upper Arteries
Carotid WALLSTENT® Monorail® Endoprosthesis	Intraluminal Device
Centrimag® Blood Pump	Short-term External Heart Assist System in Heart and Great Vessels
Ceramic on ceramic bearing surface	Synthetic Substitute, Ceramic for Replacement in Lower Joints
Cesium-131 Collagen Implant	Radioactive Element, Cesium-131 Collagen Implant for Insertion in Central Nervous System and Cranial Nerves
CivaSheet®	Radioactive Element
Clamp and rod internal fixation system (CRIF)	Internal Fixation Device in Upper Bones Internal Fixation Device in Lower Bones
COALESCE® radiolucent interbody fusion device	Interbody Fusion Device, Radiolucent Porous in New Technology
CoAxia NeuroFlo catheter	Intraluminal Device
Cobalt/chromium head and polyethylene socket	Synthetic Substitute, Metal on Polyethylene for Replacement in Lower Joints
Cobalt/chromium head and socket	Synthetic Substitute, Metal for Replacement in Lower Joints
Cochlear implant (CI), multiple channel (electrode)	Hearing Device, Multiple Channel Cochlear Prosthesis for Insertion in Ear, Nose, Sinus
Cochlear implant (CI), single channel (electrode)	Hearing Device, Single Channel Cochlear Prosthesis for Insertion in Ear, Nose, Sinus
COGNIS® CRT-D	Cardiac Resynchronization Defibrillator Pulse Generator for Insertion in Subcutaneous Tissue and Fascia
COHERE® radiolucent interbody fusion device	Interbody Fusion Device, Radiolucent Porous in New Technology
Colonic Z-Stent®	Intraluminal Device
Complete (SE) stent	Intraluminal Device
Concerto II CRT-D	Cardiac Resynchronization Defibrillator Pulse Generator for Insertion in Subcutaneous Tissue and Fascia
CONSERVE® PLUS Total Resurfacing Hip System	Resurfacing Device in Lower Joints
Consulta CRT-D	Cardiac Resynchronization Defibrillator Pulse Generator for Insertion in Subcutaneous Tissue and Fascia
Consulta CRT-P	Cardiac Resynchronization Pacemaker Pulse Generator for Insertion in Subcutaneous Tissue and Fascia
CONTAK RENEWAL® 3 RF (HE) CRT-D	Cardiac Resynchronization Defibrillator Pulse Generator for Insertion in Subcutaneous Tissue and Fascia
Contegra Pulmonary Valved Conduit	Zooplastic Tissue in Heart and Great Vessels
Continuous Glucose Monitoring (CGM) device	Monitoring Device
Cook Biodesign® Fistula Plug(s)	Nonautologous Tissue Substitute
Cook Biodesign® Hernia Graft(s)	Nonautologous Tissue Substitute
Cook Biodesign® Layered Graft(s)	Nonautologous Tissue Substitute
Cook Zenapro™ Layered Graft(s)	Nonautologous Tissue Substitute
Cook Zenith AAA Endovascular Graft	Intraluminal Device
Cook Zenith® Fenestrated AAA Endovascular Graft	Intraluminal Device, Branched or Fenestrated, One or Two Arteries for Restriction in Lower Arteries Intraluminal Device, Branched or Fenestrated, Three or More Arteries for Restriction in Lower Arteries
CoreValve transcatheter aortic valve	Zooplastic Tissue in Heart and Great Vessels
Cormet Hip Resurfacing System	Resurfacing Device in Lower Joints
CoRoent® XL	Interbody Fusion Device in Lower Joints
Corox (OTW) Bipolar Lead	Cardiac Lead, Pacemaker for Insertion in Heart and Great Vessels Cardiac Lead, Defibrillator for Insertion in Heart and Great Vessels
Cortical strip neurostimulator lead	Neurostimulator Lead in Central Nervous System and Cranial Nerves
Corvia IASD®	Synthetic Substitute
Cultured epidermal cell autograft	Autologous Tissue Substitute
CYPHER® Stent	Intraluminal Device, Drug-eluting in Heart and Great Vessels
Cystostomy tube	Drainage Device
DBS lead	Neurostimulator Lead in Central Nervous System and Cranial Nerves
DeBakey Left Ventricular Assist Device	Implantable Heart Assist System in Heart and Great Vessels
Deep brain neurostimulator lead	Neurostimulator Lead in Central Nervous System and Cranial Nerves
Delta frame external fixator	External Fixation Device, Hybrid for Insertion in Upper Bones External Fixation Device, Hybrid for Reposition in Upper Bones External Fixation Device, Hybrid for Insertion in Lower Bones External Fixation Device, Hybrid for Reposition in Lower Bones
Delta III Reverse shoulder prosthesis	Synthetic Substitute, Reverse Ball and Socket for Replacement in Upper Joints
Diaphragmatic pacemaker generator	Stimulator Generator in Subcutaneous Tissue and Fascia
Direct Lateral Interbody Fusion (DLIF) device	Interbody Fusion Device in Lower Joints
Driver stent (RX) (OTW)	Intraluminal Device
DuraHeart Left Ventricular Assist System	Implantable Heart Assist System in Heart and Great Vessels
Durata® Defibrillation Lead	Cardiac Lead, Defibrillator for Insertion in Heart and Great Vessels
DynaNail®	Internal Fixation Device, Sustained Compression for Fusion in Lower Joints Internal Fixation Device, Sustained Compression for Fusion in Upper Joints

Term	ICD-10-PCS Value
DynaNail Mini®	Internal Fixation Device, Sustained Compression for Fusion in Lower Joints Internal Fixation Device, Sustained Compression for Fusion in Upper Joints
Dynesys® Dynamic Stabilization System	Spinal Stabilization Device, Pedicle-Based for Insertion in Upper Joints Spinal Stabilization Device, Pedicle-Based for Insertion in Lower Joints
E-Luminexx™ (Biliary)(Vascular) Stent	Intraluminal Device
EDWARDS INTUITY Elite valve system	Zooplastic Tissue, Rapid Deployment Technique in New Technology
Electrical bone growth stimulator (EBGS)	Bone Growth Stimulator in Head and Facial Bones Bone Growth Stimulator in Upper Bones Bone Growth Stimulator in Lower Bones
Electrical muscle stimulation (EMS) lead	Stimulator Lead in Muscles
Electronic muscle stimulator lead	Stimulator Lead in Muscles
Eluvia™ Drug-eluting Vascular Stent System	Intraluminal Device, Sustained Release Drug-eluting in New Technology Intraluminal Device, Sustained Release Drug-eluting, Two in New Technology Intraluminal Device, Sustained Release Drug-eluting, Three in New Technology Intraluminal Device, Sustained Release Drug-eluting, Four or More in New Technology
Embolization coil(s)	Intraluminal Device
Endeavor® (III)(IV) (Sprint) Zotarolimus-eluting Coronary Stent System	Intraluminal Device, Drug-eluting in Heart and Great Vessels
Endologix AFX® Endovascular AAA System	Intraluminal Device
EndoSure® sensor	Monitoring Device, Pressure Sensor for Insertion in Heart and Great Vessels
ENDOTAK RELIANCE® (G) Defibrillation Lead	Cardiac Lead, Defibrillator for Insertion in Heart and Great Vessels
Endotracheal tube (cuffed)(double-lumen)	Intraluminal Device, Endotracheal Airway in Respiratory System
Endurant® Endovascular Stent Graft	Intraluminal Device
Endurant® II AAA stent graft system	Intraluminal Device
EnRhythm	Pacemaker, Dual Chamber for Insertion in Subcutaneous Tissue and Fascia
Enterra gastric neurostimulator	Stimulator Generator, Multiple Array for Insertion in Subcutaneous Tissue and Fascia
Epic™ Stented Tissue Valve (aortic)	Zooplastic Tissue in Heart and Great Vessels
Epicel® cultured epidermal autograft	Autologous Tissue Substitute
Esophageal obturator airway (EOA)	Intraluminal Device, Airway in Gastrointestinal System
Esteem® implantable hearing system	Hearing Device in Ear, Nose, Sinus
Evera (XT)(S)(DR/VR)	Defibrillator Generator for Insertion in Subcutaneous Tissue and Fascia
Everolimus-eluting coronary stent	Intraluminal Device, Drug-eluting in Heart and Great Vessels
Ex-PRESS™ mini glaucoma shunt	Synthetic Substitute
EXCLUDER® AAA Endoprosthesis	Intraluminal Device Intraluminal Device, Branched or Fenestrated, One or Two Arteries for Restriction in Lower Arteries Intraluminal Device, Branched or Fenestrated, Three or More Arteries for Restriction in Lower Arteries
EXCLUDER® IBE Endoprosthesis	Intraluminal Device, Branched or Fenestrated, One or Two Arteries for Restriction in Lower Arteries
Express® (LD) Premounted Stent System	Intraluminal Device
Express® Biliary SD Monorail® Premounted Stent System	Intraluminal Device
Express® SD Renal Monorail® Premounted Stent System	Intraluminal Device
External fixator	External Fixation Device in Head and Facial Bones External Fixation Device in Upper Bones External Fixation Device in Lower Bones External Fixation Device in Upper Joints External Fixation Device in Lower Joints
EXtreme Lateral Interbody Fusion (XLIF) device	Interbody Fusion Device in Lower Joints
Facet replacement spinal stabilization device	Spinal Stabilization Device, Facet Replacement for Insertion in Upper Joints Spinal Stabilization Device, Facet Replacement for Insertion in Lower Joints
FLAIR® Endovascular Stent Graft	Intraluminal Device
Flexible Composite Mesh	Synthetic Substitute
Flow Diverter embolization device	Intraluminal Device, Flow Diverter for Restriction in Upper Arteries
Foley catheter	Drainage Device
Formula™ Balloon-Expandable Renal Stent System	Intraluminal Device
Freestyle (Stentless) Aortic Root Bioprosthesis	Zooplastic Tissue in Heart and Great Vessels
Fusion screw (compression)(lag)(locking)	Internal Fixation Device in Upper Joints Internal Fixation Device in Lower Joints
GammaTile™	Radioactive Element, Cesium-131 Collagen Implant for Insertion in Central Nervous System and Cranial Nerves
Gastric electrical stimulation (GES) lead	Stimulator Lead in Gastrointestinal System
Gastric pacemaker lead	Stimulator Lead in Gastrointestinal System
GORE EXCLUDER® AAA Endoprosthesis	Intraluminal Device Intraluminal Device, Branched or Fenestrated, One or Two Arteries for Restriction In Lower Arteries Intraluminal Device, Branched or Fenestrated, Three or More Arteries for Restriction in Lower Arteries
GORE EXCLUDER® IBE Endoprosthesis	Intraluminal Device, Branched or Fenestrated, One or Two Arteries for Restriction in Lower Arteries

Term	ICD-10-PCS Value
GORE TAG® Thoracic Endoprosthesis	Intraluminal Device
GORE® DUALMESH®	Synthetic Substitute
Guedel airway	Intraluminal Device, Airway in Mouth and Throat
Hancock Bioprosthesis (aortic)(mitral) valve	Zooplastic Tissue in Heart and Great Vessels
Hancock Bioprosthetic Valved Conduit	Zooplastic Tissue in Heart and Great Vessels
HeartMate 3™ LVAS	Implantable Heart Assist System in Heart and Great Vessels
HeartMate II® Left Ventricular Assist Device (LVAD)	Implantable Heart Assist System in Heart and Great Vessels
HeartMate XVE® Left Ventricular Assist Device (LVAD)	Implantable Heart Assist System in Heart and Great Vessels
Herculink (RX) Elite Renal Stent System	Intraluminal Device
Hip (joint) liner	Liner in Lower Joints
Holter valve ventricular shunt	Synthetic Substitute
IASD® (InterAtrial Shunt Device), Corvia	Synthetic Substitute
Ilizarov external fixator	External Fixation Device, Ring for Insertion in Upper Bones External Fixation Device, Ring for Reposition in Upper Bones External Fixation Device, Ring for Insertion in Lower Bones External Fixation Device, Ring for Reposition in Lower Bones
Ilizarov-Vecklich device	External Fixation Device, Limb Lengthening for Insertion in Upper Bones External Fixation Device, Limb Lengthening for Insertion in Lower Bones
Impella® heart pump	Short-term External Heart Assist System in Heart and Great Vessels
Implantable cardioverter-defibrillator (ICD)	Defibrillator Generator for Insertion in Subcutaneous Tissue and Fascia
Implantable drug infusion pump (anti-spasmodic) (chemotherapy)(pain)	Infusion Device, Pump in Subcutaneous Tissue and Fascia
Implantable glucose monitoring device	Monitoring Device
Implantable hemodynamic monitor (IHM)	Monitoring Device, Hemodynamic for Insertion in Subcutaneous Tissue and Fascia
Implantable hemodynamic monitoring system (IHMS)	Monitoring Device, Hemodynamic for Insertion in Subcutaneous Tissue and Fascia
Implantable Miniature Telescope™ (IMT)	Synthetic Substitute, Intraocular Telescope for Replacement in Eye
Implanted (venous)(access) port	Vascular Access Device, Totally Implantable in Subcutaneous Tissue and Fascia
InDura, intrathecal catheter (1P) (spinal)	Infusion Device
Injection reservoir, port	Vascular Access Device, Totally Implantable in Subcutaneous Tissue and Fascia
Injection reservoir, pump	Infusion Device, Pump in Subcutaneous Tissue and Fascia

Term	ICD-10-PCS Value
InterAtrial Shunt Device IASD®, Corvia	Synthetic Substitute
Interbody fusion (spine) cage	Interbody Fusion Device in Upper Joints Interbody Fusion Device in Lower Joints
Interspinous process spinal stabilization device	Spinal Stabilization Device, Interspinous Process for Insertion in Upper Joints Spinal Stabilization Device, Interspinous Process for Insertion in Lower Joints
InterStim® Therapy lead	Neurostimulator Lead in Peripheral Nervous System
InterStim® Therapy neurostimulator	Stimulator Generator, Single Array for Insertlon In Subcutaneous Tissue and Fascia
Intramedullary (IM) rod (nail)	Internal Fixation Device, Intramedullary in Upper Bones Internal Fixation Device, Intramedullary in Lower Bones
Intramedullary skeletal kinetic distractor (ISKD)	Internal Fixation Device, Intramedullary in Upper Bones Internal Fixation Device, Intramedullary in Lower Bones
Intrauterine Device (IUD)	Contraceptive Device in Female Reproductive System
INTUITY Elite valve system, EDWARDS	Zooplastic Tissue, Rapid Deployment Technique in New Technology
Itrel (3)(4) neurostimulator	Stimulator Generator, Single Array for Insertion in Subcutaneous Tissue and Fascia
Joint fixation plate	Internal Fixation Device in Upper Joints Internal Fixation Device in Lower Joints
Joint liner (insert)	Liner in Lower Joints
Joint spacer (antibiotic)	Spacer in Upper Joints Spacer in Lower Joints
Kappa	Pacemaker, Dual Chamber for Insertion in Subcutaneous Tissue and Fascia
Kirschner wire (K-wire)	Internal Fixation Device in Head and Facial Bones Internal Fixation Device in Upper Bones Internal Fixation Device in Lower Bones Internal Fixation Device in Upper Joints Internal Fixation Device in Lower Joints
Knee (implant) insert	Liner in Lower Joints
Kuntscher nail	Internal Fixation Device, Intramedullary in Upper Bones Internal Fixation Device, Intramedullary in Lower Bones
LAP-BAND® adjustable gastric banding system	Extraluminal Device
LifeStent® (Flexstar)(XL) Vascular Stent System	Intraluminal Device
LIVIAN™ CRT-D	Cardiac Resynchronization Defibrillator Pulse Generator for Insertion in Subcutaneous Tissue and Fascia
Loop recorder, implantable	Monitoring Device
MAGEC® Spinal Bracing and Distraction System	Magnetically Controlled Growth Rod(s) in New Technology
Mark IV Breathing Pacemaker System	Stimulator Generator in Subcutaneous Tissue and Fascia
Maximo II DR (VR)	Defibrillator Generator for Insertion in Subcutaneous Tissue and Fascia

Term	ICD-10-PCS Value
Maximo II DR CRT-D	Cardiac Resynchronization Defibrillator Pulse Generator for Insertion in Subcutaneous Tissue and Fascia
Medtronic Endurant® II AAA stent graft system	Intraluminal Device
Melody® transcatheter pulmonary valve	Zooplastic Tissue in Heart and Great Vessels
Metal on metal bearing surface	Synthetic Substitute, Metal for Replacement in Lower Joints
Micro-Driver stent (RX) (OTW)	Intraluminal Device
MicroMed HeartAssist	Implantable Heart Assist System in Heart and Great Vessels
Micrus CERECYTE microcoil	Intraluminal Device, Bioactive in Upper Arteries
MIRODERM™ Biologic Wound Matrix	Skin Substitute, Porcine Liver Derived in New Technology
MitraClip valve repair system	Synthetic Substitute
Mitroflow® Aortic Pericardial Heart Valve	Zooplastic Tissue in Heart and Great Vessels
Mosaic Bioprosthesis (aortic) (mitral) valve	Zooplastic Tissue in Heart and Great Vessels
MULTI-LINK (VISION)(MINI-VISION)(ULTRA) Coronary Stent System	Intraluminal Device
nanoLOCK™ interbody fusion device	Interbody Fusion Device, Nanotextured Surface in New Technology
Nasopharyngeal airway (NPA)	Intraluminal Device, Airway in Ear, Nose, Sinus
Neuromuscular electrical stimulation (NEMS) lead	Stimulator Lead in Muscles
Neurostimulator generator, multiple channel	Stimulator Generator, Multiple Array for Insertion in Subcutaneous Tissue and Fascia
Neurostimulator generator, multiple channel rechargeable	Stimulator Generator, Multiple Array Rechargeable for Insertion in Subcutaneous Tissue and Fascia
Neurostimulator generator, single channel	Stimulator Generator, Single Array for Insertion in Subcutaneous Tissue and Fascia
Neurostimulator generator, single channel rechargeable	Stimulator Generator, Single Array Rechargeable for Insertion in Subcutaneous Tissue and Fascia
Neutralization plate	Internal Fixation Device in Head and Facial Bones Internal Fixation Device in Upper Bones Internal Fixation Device in Lower Bones
Nitinol framed polymer mesh	Synthetic Substitute
Non-tunneled central venous catheter	Infusion Device
Novacor Left Ventricular Assist Device	Implantable Heart Assist System in Heart and Great Vessels
Novation® Ceramic AHS® (Articulation Hip System)	Synthetic Substitute, Ceramic for Replacement in Lower Joints
Omnilink Elite Vascular Balloon Expandable Stent System	Intraluminal Device
Open Pivot Aortic Valve Graft (AVG)	Synthetic Substitute
Open Pivot (mechanical) Valve	Synthetic Substitute
Optimizer™ III implantable pulse generator	Contractility Modulation Device for Insertion in Subcutaneous Tissue and Fascia
Oropharyngeal airway (OPA)	Intraluminal Device, Airway in Mouth and Throat
Ovatio™ CRT-D	Cardiac Resynchronization Defibrillator Pulse Generator for Insertion in Subcutaneous Tissue and Fascia
OXINIUM	Synthetic Substitute, Oxidized Zirconium on Polyethylene for Replacement in Lower Joints
Paclitaxel-eluting coronary stent	Intraluminal Device, Drug-eluting in Heart and Great Vessels
Paclitaxel-eluting peripheral stent	Intraluminal Device, Drug-eluting in Upper Arteries Intraluminal Device, Drug-eluting in Lower Arteries
Partially absorbable mesh	Synthetic Substitute
Pedicle-based dynamic stabilization device	Spinal Stabilization Device, Pedicle-Based for Insertion in Upper Joints Spinal Stabilization Device, Pedicle-Based for Insertion in Lower Joints
Perceval sutureless valve	Zooplastic Tissue, Rapid Deployment Technique in New Technology
Percutaneous endoscopic gastrojejunostomy (PEG/J) tube	Feeding Device in Gastrointestinal System
Percutaneous endoscopic gastrostomy (PEG) tube	Feeding Device in Gastrointestinal System
Percutaneous nephrostomy catheter	Drainage Device
Peripherally inserted central catheter (PICC)	Infusion Device
Pessary ring	Intraluminal Device, Pessary in Female Reproductive System
Phrenic nerve stimulator generator	Stimulator Generator in Subcutaneous Tissue and Fascia
Phrenic nerve stimulator lead	Diaphragmatic Pacemaker Lead in Respiratory System
PHYSIOMESH™ Flexible Composite Mesh	Synthetic Substitute
Pipeline™ (Flex) embolization device	Intraluminal Device, Flow Diverter for Restriction in Upper Arteries
Polyethylene socket	Synthetic Substitute, Polyethylene for Replacement in Lower Joints
Polymethylmethacrylate (PMMA)	Synthetic Substitute
Polypropylene mesh	Synthetic Substitute
Porcine (bioprosthetic) valve	Zooplastic Tissue in Heart and Great Vessels
PRECICE intramedullary limb lengthening system	Internal Fixation Device, Intramedullary Limb Lengthening for Insertion in Upper Bones Internal Fixation Device, Intramedullary Limb Lengthening for Insertion in Lower Bones
PRESTIGE® Cervical Disc	Synthetic Substitute
PrimeAdvanced neurostimulator (SureScan)(MRI Safe)	Stimulator Generator, Multiple Array for Insertion in Subcutaneous Tissue and Fascia
PROCEED™ Ventral Patch	Synthetic Substitute
Prodisc-C	Synthetic Substitute
Prodisc-L	Synthetic Substitute

Term	ICD-10-PCS Value
PROLENE Polypropylene Hernia System (PHS)	Synthetic Substitute
Protecta XT CRT-D	Cardiac Resynchronization Defibrillator Pulse Generator for Insertion in Subcutaneous Tissue and Fascia
Protecta XT DR (XT VR)	Defibrillator Generator for Insertion in Subcutaneous Tissue and Fascia
Protégé® RX Carotid Stent System	Intraluminal Device
Pump reservoir	Infusion Device, Pump in Subcutaneous Tissue and Fascia
REALIZE® Adjustable Gastric Band	Extraluminal Device
Rebound HRD® (Hernia Repair Device)	Synthetic Substitute
RestoreAdvanced neurostimulator (SureScan)(MRI Safe)	Stimulator Generator, Multiple Array Rechargeable for Insertion in Subcutaneous Tissue and Fascia
RestoreSensor neurostimulator (SureScan)(MRI Safe)	Stimulator Generator, Multiple Array Rechargeable for Insertion in Subcutaneous Tissue and Fascia
RestoreUltra neurostimulator (SureScan)(MRI Safe)	Stimulator Generator, Multiple Array Rechargeable for Insertion in Subcutaneous Tissue and Fascia
Reveal (LINQ)(DX)(XT)	Monitoring Device
Reverse® Shoulder Prosthesis	Synthetic Substitute, Reverse Ball and Socket for Replacement in Upper Joints
Revo MRI™ SureScan® pacemaker	Pacemaker, Dual Chamber for Insertion in Subcutaneous Tissue and Fascia
Rheos® System device	Stimulator Generator in Subcutaneous Tissue and Fascia
Rheos® System lead	Stimulator Lead in Upper Arteries
RNS System lead	Neurostimulator Lead in Central Nervous System and Cranial Nerves
RNS system neurostimulator generator	Neurostimulator Generator in Head and Facial Bones
S-ICD™ lead	Subcutaneous Defibrillator Lead in Subcutaneous Tissue and Fascia
Sacral nerve modulation (SNM) lead	Stimulator Lead in Urinary System
Sacral neuromodulation lead	Stimulator Lead in Urinary System
SAPIEN transcatheter aortic valve	Zooplastic Tissue in Heart and Great Vessels
SAVAL below-the-knee (BTK) drug-eluting stent system	Intraluminal Device, Sustained Release Drug-eluting in New Technology Intraluminal Device, Sustained Release Drug-eluting, Two in New Technology Intraluminal Device, Sustained Release Drug-eluting, Three in New Technology Intraluminal Device, Sustained Release Drug-eluting, Four or More in New Technology
Secura (DR) (VR)	Defibrillator Generator for Insertion in Subcutaneous Tissue and Fascia
Sheffield hybrid external fixator	External Fixation Device, Hybrid for Insertion in Upper Bones External Fixation Device, Hybrid for Reposition in Upper Bones External Fixation Device, Hybrid for Insertion in Lower Bones External Fixation Device, Hybrid for Reposition in Lower Bones
Sheffield ring external fixator	External Fixation Device, Ring for Insertion in Upper Bones External Fixation Device, Ring for Reposition in Upper Bones External Fixation Device, Ring for Insertion in Lower Bones External Fixation Device, Ring for Reposition in Lower Bones
Single lead pacemaker (atrium)(ventricle)	Pacemaker, Single Chamber for Insertion in Subcutaneous Tissue and Fascia
Single lead rate responsive pacemaker (atrium)(ventricle)	Pacemaker, Single Chamber Rate Responsive for Insertion in Subcutaneous Tissue and Fascia
Sirolimus-eluting coronary stent	Intraluminal Device, Drug-eluting in Heart and Great Vessels
SJM Biocor® Stented Valve System	Zooplastic Tissue in Heart and Great Vessels
Spacer, Articulating (Antibiotic)	Articulating Spacer in Lower Joints
Spacer, Static (Antibiotic)	Spacer in Lower Joints
Spinal cord neurostimulator lead	Neurostimulator Lead in Central Nervous System and Cranial Nerves
Spinal growth rods, magnetically controlled	Magnetically Controlled Growth Rod(s) in New Technology
SpineJack® system	Synthetic Substitute, Mechanically Expandable (Paired) in New Technology
Spiration IBV™ Valve System	Intraluminal Device, Endobronchial Valve in Respiratory System
Static Spacer (Antibiotic)	Spacer in Lower Joints
Stent, intraluminal (cardiovascular) (gastrointestinal) (hepatobiliary)(urinary)	Intraluminal Device
Stented tissue valve	Zooplastic Tissue in Heart and Great Vessels
Stratos LV	Cardiac Resynchronization Pacemaker Pulse Generator for Insertion in Subcutaneous Tissue and Fascia
Subcutaneous injection reservoir, port	Vascular Access Device, Totally Implantable in Subcutaneous Tissue and Fascia
Subcutaneous injection reservoir, pump	Infusion Device, Pump in Subcutaneous Tissue and Fascia
Subdermal progesterone implant	Contraceptive Device in Subcutaneous Tissue and Fascia
Surpass Streamline™ Flow Diverter	Intraluminal Device, Flow Diverter for Restriction in Upper Arteries
Sutureless valve, Perceval	Zooplastic Tissue, Rapid Deployment Technique in New Technology
SynCardia Total Artificial Heart	Synthetic Substitute
Synchra CRT-P	Cardiac Resynchronization Pacemaker Pulse Generator for Insertion in Subcutaneous Tissue and Fascia
SyncroMed Pump	Infusion Device, Pump in Subcutaneous Tissue and Fascia
Talent® Converter	Intraluminal Device
Talent® Occluder	Intraluminal Device
Talent® Stent Graft (abdominal)(thoracic)	Intraluminal Device
TandemHeart® System	Short-term External Heart Assist System in Heart and Great Vessels

Term	ICD-10-PCS Value
TAXUS® Liberté® Paclitaxel-eluting Coronary Stent System	Intraluminal Device, Drug-eluting in Heart and Great Vessels
Therapeutic occlusion coil(s)	Intraluminal Device
Thoracostomy tube	Drainage Device
Thoratec IVAD (Implantable Ventricular Assist Device)	Implantable Heart Assist System in Heart and Great Vessels
Thoratec Paracorporeal Ventricular Assist Device	Short-term External Heart Assist System in Heart and Great Vessels
Tibial insert	Liner in Lower Joints
Tissue bank graft	Nonautologous Tissue Substitute
Tissue expander (inflatable)(injectable)	Tissue Expander in Skin and Breast Tissue Expander in Subcutaneous Tissue and Fascia
Titanium Sternal Fixation System (TSFS)	Internal Fixation Device, Rigid Plate for Insertion in Upper Bones Internal Fixation Device, Rigid Plate for Reposition in Upper Bones
Total artificial (replacement) heart	Synthetic Substitute
Tracheostomy tube	Tracheostomy Device in Respiratory System
Trifecta™ Valve (aortic)	Zooplastic Tissue in Heart and Great Vessels
Tunneled central venous catheter	Vascular Access Device, Tunneled in Subcutaneous Tissue and Fascia
Tunneled spinal (intrathecal) catheter	Infusion Device
Two lead pacemaker	Pacemaker, Dual Chamber for Insertion in Subcutaneous Tissue and Fascia
Ultraflex™ Precision Colonic Stent System	Intraluminal Device
ULTRAPRO Hernia System (UHS)	Synthetic Substitute
ULTRAPRO Partially Absorbable Lightweight Mesh	Synthetic Substitute
ULTRAPRO Plug	Synthetic Substitute
Ultrasonic osteogenic stimulator	Bone Growth Stimulator in Head and Facial Bones Bone Growth Stimulator in Upper Bones Bone Growth Stimulator in Lower Bones
Ultrasound bone healing system	Bone Growth Stimulator in Head and Facial Bones Bone Growth Stimulator in Upper Bones Bone Growth Stimulator in Lower Bones
Uniplanar external fixator	External Fixation Device, Monoplanar for Insertion in Upper Bones External Fixation Device, Monoplanar for Reposition in Upper Bones External Fixation Device, Monoplanar for Insertion in Lower Bones External Fixation Device, Monoplanar for Reposition in Lower Bones
Urinary incontinence stimulator lead	Stimulator Lead in Urinary System
V-Wave Interatrial Shunt System	Synthetic Substitute
Vaginal pessary	Intraluminal Device, Pessary in Female Reproductive System
Valiant Thoracic Stent Graft	Intraluminal Device
Vectra® Vascular Access Graft	Vascular Access Device, Tunneled in Subcutaneous Tissue and Fascia
Ventrio™ Hernia Patch	Synthetic Substitute
Versa	Pacemaker, Dual Chamber for Insertion in Subcutaneous Tissue and Fascia
Virtuoso (II) (DR) (VR)	Defibrillator Generator for Insertion in Subcutaneous Tissue and Fascia
Viva(XT)(S)	Cardiac Resynchronization Defibrillator Pulse Generator for Insertion in Subcutaneous Tissue and Fascia
WALLSTENT® Endoprosthesis	Intraluminal Device
X-STOP® Spacer	Spinal Stabilization Device, Interspinous Process for Insertion in Upper Joints Spinal Stabilization Device, Interspinous Process for Insertion in Lower Joints
Xact Carotid Stent System	Intraluminal Device
Xenograft	Zooplastic Tissue in Heart and Great Vessels
XIENCE Everolimus Eluting Coronary Stent System	Intraluminal Device, Drug-eluting in Heart and Great Vessels
XLIF® System	Interbody Fusion Device in Lower Joints
Zenith® Fenestrated AAA Endovascular Graft	Intraluminal Device, Branched or Fenestrated, One or Two Arteries for Restriction in Lower Arteries Intraluminal Device, Branched or Fenestrated, Three or More Arteries for Restriction in Lower Arteries Intraluminal Device
Zenith Flex® AAA Endovascular Graft	Intraluminal Device
Zenith TX2® TAA Endovascular Graft	Intraluminal Device
Zenith® Renu™ AAA Ancillary Graft	Intraluminal Device
Zilver® PTX® (paclitaxel) Drug-Eluting Peripheral Stent	Intraluminal Device, Drug-eluting in Upper Arteries Intraluminal Device, Drug-eluting in Lower Arteries
Zimmer® NexGen® LPS Mobile Bearing Knee	Synthetic Substitute
Zimmer® NexGen® LPS-Flex Mobile Knee	Synthetic Substitute
Zotarolimus-eluting coronary stent	Intraluminal Device, Drug-eluting in Heart and Great Vessels

Device Aggregation Table

This table crosswalks specific device character value definitions for specific root operations in a specific body system to the more general device character value to be used when the root operation covers a wide range of body parts and the device character represents an entire family of devices.

Specific Device	for Operation	in Body System	General Device
Autologous Arterial Tissue (A)	All applicable	Heart and Great Vessels Lower Arteries Lower Veins Upper Arteries Upper Veins	**7** Autologous Tissue Substitute
Autologous Venous Tissue (9)	All applicable	Heart and Great Vessels Lower Arteries Lower Veins Upper Arteries Upper Veins	**7** Autologous Tissue Substitute
Cardiac Lead, Defibrillator (K)	Insertion	Heart and Great Vessels	**M** Cardiac Lead
Cardiac Lead, Pacemaker (J)	Insertion	Heart and Great Vessels	**M** Cardiac Lead
Cardiac Resynchronization Defibrillator Pulse Generator (9)	Insertion	Subcutaneous Tissue and Fascia	**P** Cardiac Rhythm Related Device
Cardiac Resynchronization Pacemaker Pulse Generator (7)	Insertion	Subcutaneous Tissue and Fascia	**P** Cardiac Rhythm Related Device
Contractility Modulation Device (A)	Insertion	Subcutaneous Tissue and Fascia	**P** Cardiac Rhythm Related Device
Defibrillator Generator (8)	Insertion	Subcutaneous Tissue and Fascia	**P** Cardiac Rhythm Related Device
Epiretinal Visual Prosthesis (5)	All applicable	Eye	**J** Synthetic Substitute
External Fixation Device, Hybrid (D)	Insertion	Lower Bones Upper Bones	**5** External Fixation Device
External Fixation Device, Hybrid (D)	Reposition	Lower Bones Upper Bones	**5** External Fixation Device
External Fixation Device, Limb Lengthening (8)	Insertion	Lower Bones Upper Bones	**5** External Fixation Device
External Fixation Device, Monoplanar (B)	Insertion	Lower Bones Upper Bones	**5** External Fixation Device
External Fixation Device, Monoplanar (B)	Reposition	Lower Bones Upper Bones	**5** External Fixation Device
External Fixation Device, Ring (C)	Insertion	Lower Bones Upper Bones	**5** External Fixation Device
External Fixation Device, Ring (C)	Reposition	Lower Bones Upper Bones	**5** External Fixation Device
Hearing Device, Bone Conduction (4)	Insertion	Ear, Nose, Sinus	**S** Hearing Device
Hearing Device, Multiple Channel Cochlear Prosthesis (6)	Insertion	Ear, Nose, Sinus	**S** Hearing Device
Hearing Device, Single Channel Cochlear Prosthesis (5)	Insertion	Ear, Nose, Sinus	**S** Hearing Device
Internal Fixation Device, Intramedullary (6)	All applicable	Lower Bones Upper Bones	**4** Internal Fixation Device
Internal Fixation Device, Intramedullary Limb Lengthening (7)	Insertion	Lower Bones Upper Bones	**6** Internal Fixation Device, Intramedullary
Internal Fixation Device, Rigid Plate (Ø)	Insertion	Upper Bones	**4** Internal Fixation Device
Internal Fixation Device, Rigid Plate (Ø)	Reposition	Upper Bones	**4** Internal Fixation Device
Intraluminal Device, Airway (B)	All applicable	Ear, Nose, Sinus Gastrointestinal System Mouth and Throat	**D** Intraluminal Device
Intraluminal Device, Bioactive (B)	All applicable	Upper Arteries	**D** Intraluminal Device
Intraluminal Device, Branched or Fenestrated, One or Two Arteries (E)	Restriction	Heart and Great Vessels Lower Arteries	**D** Intraluminal Device
Intraluminal Device, Branched or Fenestrated, Three or More Arteries (F)	Restriction	Heart and Great Vessels Lower Arteries	**D** Intraluminal Device
Intraluminal Device, Drug-eluting (4)	All applicable	Heart and Great Vessels Lower Arteries Upper Arteries	**D** Intraluminal Device
Intraluminal Device, Drug-eluting, Four or More (7)	All applicable	Heart and Great Vessels Lower Arteries Upper Arteries	**D** Intraluminal Device

Specific Device	for Operation	in Body System	General Device
Intraluminal Device, Drug-eluting, Three (6)	All applicable	Heart and Great Vessels Lower Arteries Upper Arteries	**D** Intraluminal Device
Intraluminal Device, Drug-eluting, Two (5)	All applicable	Heart and Great Vessels Lower Arteries Upper Arteries	**D** Intraluminal Device
Intraluminal Device, Endobronchial Valve (G)	All applicable	Respiratory System	**D** Intraluminal Device
Intraluminal Device, Endotracheal Airway (E)	All applicable	Respiratory System	**D** Intraluminal Device
Intraluminal Device, Flow Diverter (H)	Restriction	Upper Arteries	**D** Intraluminal Device
Intraluminal Device, Four or More (G)	All applicable	Heart and Great Vessels Lower Arteries Upper Arteries	**D** Intraluminal Device
Intraluminal Device, Pessary (G)	All applicable	Female Reproductive System	**D** Intraluminal Device
Intraluminal Device, Radioactive (T)	All applicable	Heart and Great Vessels	**D** Intraluminal Device
Intraluminal Device, Three (F)	All applicable	Heart and Great Vessels Lower Arteries Upper Arteries	**D** Intraluminal Device
Intraluminal Device, Two (E)	All applicable	Heart and Great Vessels Lower Arteries Upper Arteries	**D** Intraluminal Device
Monitoring Device, Hemodynamic (Ø)	Insertion	Subcutaneous Tissue and Fascia	**2** Monitoring Device
Monitoring Device, Pressure Sensor (Ø)	Insertion	Heart and Great Vessels	**2** Monitoring Device
Pacemaker, Dual Chamber (6)	Insertion	Subcutaneous Tissue and Fascia	**P** Cardiac Rhythm Related Device
Pacemaker, Single Chamber (4)	Insertion	Subcutaneous Tissue and Fascia	**P** Cardiac Rhythm Related Device
Pacemaker, Single Chamber Rate Responsive (5)	Insertion	Subcutaneous Tissue and Fascia	**P** Cardiac Rhythm Related Device
Spinal Stabilization Device, Facet Replacement (D)	Insertion	Lower Joints Upper Joints	**4** Internal Fixation Device
Spinal Stabilization Device, Interspinous Process (B)	Insertion	Lower Joints Upper Joints	**4** Internal Fixation Device
Spinal Stabilization Device, Pedicle-Based (C)	Insertion	Lower Joints Upper Joints	**4** Internal Fixation Device
Stimulator Generator, Multiple Array (D)	Insertion	Subcutaneous Tissue and Fascia	**M** Stimulator Generator
Stimulator Generator, Multiple Array Rechargeable (E)	Insertion	Subcutaneous Tissue and Fascia	**M** Stimulator Generator
Stimulator Generator, Single Array (B)	Insertion	Subcutaneous Tissue and Fascia	**M** Stimulator Generator
Stimulator Generator, Single Array Rechargeable (C)	Insertion	Subcutaneous Tissue and Fascia	**M** Stimulator Generator
Synthetic Substitute, Ceramic (3)	Replacement	Lower Joints	**J** Synthetic Substitute
Synthetic Substitute, Ceramic on Polyethylene (4)	Replacement	Lower Joints	**J** Synthetic Substitute
Synthetic Substitute, Intraocular Telescope (Ø)	Replacement	Eye	**J** Synthetic Substitute
Synthetic Substitute, Metal (1)	Replacement	Lower Joints	**J** Synthetic Substitute
Synthetic Substitute, Metal on Polyethylene (2)	Replacement	Lower Joints	**J** Synthetic Substitute
Synthetic Substitute, Oxidized Zirconium on Polyethylene (6)	Replacement	Lower Joints	**J** Synthetic Substitute
Synthetic Substitute, Polyethylene (Ø)	Replacement	Lower Joints	**J** Synthetic Substitute
Synthetic Substitute, Reverse Ball and Socket (Ø)	Replacement	Upper Joints	**J** Synthetic Substitute

Appendix H: Device Definitions

ICD-10-PCS Value	Definition
Articulating Spacer in Lower Joints	**Includes:** Articulating Spacer (Antibiotic) Spacer, Articulating (Antibiotic)
Artificial Sphincter in Gastrointestinal System	**Includes:** Artificial anal sphincter (AAS) Artificial bowel sphincter (neosphincter)
Artificial Sphincter in Urinary System	**Includes:** AMS 800® Urinary Control System Artificial urinary sphincter (AUS)
Autologous Arterial Tissue in Heart and Great Vessels	**Includes:** Autologous artery graft
Autologous Arterial Tissue in Lower Arteries	**Includes:** Autologous artery graft
Autologous Arterial Tissue in Lower Veins	**Includes:** Autologous artery graft
Autologous Arterial Tissue in Upper Arteries	**Includes:** Autologous artery graft
Autologous Arterial Tissue in Upper Veins	**Includes:** Autologous artery graft
Autologous Tissue Substitute	**Includes:** Autograft Cultured epidermal cell autograft Epicel® cultured epidermal autograft
Autologous Venous Tissue in Heart and Great Vessels	**Includes:** Autologous vein graft
Autologous Venous Tissue in Lower Arteries	**Includes:** Autologous vein graft
Autologous Venous Tissue in Lower Veins	**Includes:** Autologous vein graft
Autologous Venous Tissue in Upper Arteries	**Includes:** Autologous vein graft
Autologous Venous Tissue in Upper Veins	**Includes:** Autologous vein graft
Bone Growth Stimulator in Head and Facial Bones	**Includes:** Electrical bone growth stimulator (EBGS) Ultrasonic osteogenic stimulator Ultrasound bone healing system
Bone Growth Stimulator in Lower Bones	**Includes:** Electrical bone growth stimulator (EBGS) Ultrasonic osteogenic stimulator Ultrasound bone healing system
Bone Growth Stimulator in Upper Bones	**Includes:** Electrical bone growth stimulator (EBGS) Ultrasonic osteogenic stimulator Ultrasound bone healing system
Cardiac Lead in Heart and Great Vessels	**Includes:** Cardiac contractility modulation lead

ICD-10-PCS Value	Definition
Cardiac Lead, Defibrillator for Insertion in Heart and Great Vessels	**Includes:** ACUITY™ Steerable Lead Attain Ability® lead Attain StarFix® (OTW) lead Cardiac resynchronization therapy (CRT) lead Corox (OTW) Bipolar Lead Durata® Defibrillation Lead ENDOTAK RELIANCE® (G) Defibrillation Lead
Cardiac Lead, Pacemaker for Insertion in Heart and Great Vessels	**Includes:** ACUITY™ Steerable Lead Attain Ability® lead Attain StarFix® (OTW) lead Cardiac resynchronization therapy (CRT) lead Corox (OTW) Bipolar Lead
Cardiac Resynchronization Defibrillator Pulse Generator for Insertion in Subcutaneous Tissue and Fascia	**Includes:** COGNIS® CRT-D Concerto II CRT-D Consulta CRT-D CONTAK RENEWA® 3 RF (HE) CRT-D LIVIAN™ CRT-D Maximo II DR CRT-D Ovatio™ CRT-D Protecta XT CRT-D Viva (XT)(S)
Cardiac Resynchronization Pacemaker Pulse Generator for Insertion in Subcutaneous Tissue and Fascia	**Includes:** Consulta CRT-P Stratos LV Synchra CRT-P
Contraceptive Device in Female Reproductive System	**Includes:** Intrauterine device (IUD)
Contraceptive Device in Subcutaneous Tissue and Fascia	**Includes:** Subdermal progesterone implant
Contractility Modulation Device for Insertion in Subcutaneous Tissue and Fascia	**Includes:** Optimizer™ III implantable pulse generator
Defibrillator Generator for Insertion in Subcutaneous Tissue and Fascia	**Includes:** Evera (XT)(S)(DR/VR) Implantable cardioverter-defibrillator (ICD) Maximo II DR (VR) Protecta XT DR (XT VR) Secura (DR) (VR) Virtuoso (II) (DR) (VR)
Diaphragmatic Pacemaker Lead in Respiratory System	**Includes:** Phrenic nerve stimulator lead
Drainage Device	**Includes:** Cystostomy tube Foley catheter Percutaneous nephrostomy catheter Thoracostomy tube
External Fixation Device in Head and Facial Bones	**Includes:** External fixator
External Fixation Device in Lower Bones	**Includes:** External fixator
External Fixation Device in Lower Joints	**Includes:** External fixator

ICD-10-PCS Value	Definition
External Fixation Device in Upper Bones	**Includes:** External fixator
External Fixation Device in Upper Joints	**Includes:** External fixator
External Fixation Device, Hybrid for Insertion in Lower Bones	**Includes:** Delta frame external fixator Sheffield hybrid external fixator
External Fixation Device, Hybrid for Insertion in Upper Bones	**Includes:** Delta frame external fixator Sheffield hybrid external fixator
External Fixation Device, Hybrid for Reposition in Lower Bones	**Includes:** Delta frame external fixator Sheffield hybrid external fixator
External Fixation Device, Hybrid for Reposition in Upper Bones	**Includes:** Delta frame external fixator Sheffield hybrid external fixator
External Fixation Device, Limb Lengthening for Insertion in Lower Bones	**Includes:** Ilizarov-Vecklich device
External Fixation Device, Limb Lengthening for Insertion in Upper Bones	**Includes:** Ilizarov-Vecklich device
External Fixation Device, Monoplanar for Insertion in Lower Bones	**Includes:** Uniplanar external fixator
External Fixation Device, Monoplanar for Insertion in Upper Bones	**Includes:** Uniplanar external fixator
External Fixation Device, Monoplanar for Reposition in Lower Bones	**Includes:** Uniplanar external fixator
External Fixation Device, Monoplanar for Reposition in Upper Bones	**Includes:** Uniplanar external fixator
External Fixation Device, Ring for Insertion in Lower Bones	**Includes:** Ilizarov external fixator Sheffield ring external fixator
External Fixation Device, Ring for Insertion in Upper Bones	**Includes:** Ilizarov external fixator Sheffield ring external fixator
External Fixation Device, Ring for Reposition in Lower Bones	**Includes:** Ilizarov external fixator Sheffield ring external fixator
External Fixation Device, Ring for Reposition in Upper Bones	**Includes:** Ilizarov external fixator Sheffield ring external fixator
Extraluminal Device	**Includes:** AtriClip LAA Exclusion System LAP-BAND® adjustable gastric banding system REALIZE® Adjustable Gastric Band
Feeding Device in Gastrointestinal System	**Includes:** Percutaneous endoscopic gastrojejunostomy (PEG/J) tube Percutaneous endoscopic gastrostomy (PEG) tube
Hearing Device in Ear, Nose, Sinus	**Includes:** Esteem® implantable hearing system
Hearing Device in Head and Facial Bones	**Includes:** Bone anchored hearing device

ICD-10-PCS Value	Definition
Hearing Device, Bone Conduction for Insertion in Ear, Nose, Sinus	**Includes:** Bone anchored hearing device
Hearing Device, Multiple Channel Cochlear Prosthesis for Insertion in Ear, Nose, Sinus	**Includes:** Cochlear implant (CI), multiple channel (electrode)
Hearing Device, Single Channel Cochlear Prosthesis for Insertion in Ear, Nose, Sinus	**Includes:** Cochlear implant (CI), single channel (electrode)
Implantable Heart Assist System in Heart and Great Vessels	**Includes:** Berlin Heart Ventricular Assist Device DeBakey Left Ventricular Assist Device DuraHeart Left Ventricular Assist System HeartMate 3™ LVAS HeartMate II® Left Ventricular Assist Device (LVAD) HeartMate XVE® Left Ventricular Assist Device (LVAD) MicroMed HeartAssist Novacor Left Ventricular Assist Device Thoratec IVAD (Implantable Ventricular Assist Device)
Infusion Device	**Includes:** Ascenda Intrathecal Catheter InDura, intrathecal catheter (1P) (spinal) Non-tunneled central venous catheter Peripherally inserted central catheter (PICC) Tunneled spinal (intrathecal) catheter
Infusion Device, Pump in Subcutaneous Tissue and Fascia	**Includes:** Implantable drug infusion pump (anti-spasmodic)(chemotherapy)(pain) Injection reservoir, pump Pump reservoir Subcutaneous injection reservoir, pump SynchroMed pump
Interbody Fusion Device in Lower Joints	**Includes:** Axial Lumbar Interbody Fusion System AxiaLIF® System CoRoent® XL Direct Lateral Interbody Fusion (DLIF) device EXtreme Lateral Interbody Fusion (XLIF) device Interbody fusion (spine) cage XLIF® System
Interbody Fusion Device in Upper Joints	**Includes:** BAK/C® Interbody Cervical Fusion System Interbody fusion (spine) cage
Interbody Fusion Device, Nanotextured Surface in New Technology	Includes: nanoLOCK™ interbody fusion device

ICD-10-PCS Value	Definition
Interbody Fusion Device, Radiolucent Porous in New Technology	Includes: COALESCE® radiolucent interbody fusion device COHERE® radiolucent interbody fusion device
Internal Fixation Device in Head and Facial Bones	**Includes:** Bone screw (interlocking)(lag)(pedicle)(recessed) Kirschner wire (K-wire) Neutralization plate
Internal Fixation Device in Lower Bones	**Includes:** Bone screw (interlocking)(lag)(pedicle)(recessed) Clamp and rod internal fixation system (CRIF) Kirschner wire (K-wire) Neutralization plate
Internal Fixation Device in Lower Joints	**Includes:** Fusion screw (compression)(lag)(locking) Joint fixation plate Kirschner wire (K-wire)
Internal Fixation Device in Upper Bones	**Includes:** Bone screw (interlocking)(lag)(pedicle)(recessed) Clamp and rod internal fixation system (CRIF) Kirschner wire (K-wire) Neutralization plate
Internal Fixation Device in Upper Joints	**Includes:** Fusion screw (compression)(lag)(locking) Joint fixation plate Kirschner wire (K-wire)
Internal Fixation Device, Intramedullary in Lower Bones	**Includes:** Intramedullary (IM) rod (nail) Intramedullary skeletal kinetic distractor (ISKD) Kuntscher nail
Internal Fixation Device, Intramedullary in Upper Bones	**Includes:** Intramedullary (IM) rod (nail) Intramedullary skeletal kinetic distractor (ISKD) Kuntscher nail
Internal Fixation Device Intramedullary Limb Lengthening for Insertion in Lower Bones	**Includes:** PRECICE intramedullary limb lengthening system
Internal Fixation Device Intramedullary Limb Lengthening for Insertion in Upper Bones	**Includes:** PRECICE intramedullary limb lengthening system
Internal Fixation Device, Rigid Plate for Insertion in Upper Bones	**Includes:** Titanium Sternal Fixation System (TSFS)
Internal Fixation Device, Rigid Plate for Reposition in Upper Bones	**Includes:** Titanium Sternal Fixation System (TSFS)
Internal Fixation Device, Sustained Compression for Fusion in Lower Joints	**Includes:** DynaNail® DynaNail Mini®
Internal Fixation Device, Sustained Compression for Fusion in Upper Joints	**Includes:** DynaNail® DynaNail Mini®
Intraluminal Device	**Includes:** Absolute Pro Vascular (OTW) Self-Expanding Stent System Acculink (RX) Carotid Stent System AFX® Endovascular AAA System AneuRx® AAA Advantage® Assurant (Cobalt) stent Carotid WALLSTENT® Monorail® Endoprosthesis CoAxia NeuroFlo catheter Colonic Z-Stent® Complete (SE) stent Cook Zenith AAA Endovascular Graft Driver stent (RX) (OTW) E-Luminexx™ (Biliary)(Vascular) Stent Embolization coil(s) Endologix AFX® Endovascular AAA System Endurant® Endovascular Stent Graft Endurant® II AAA stent graft system EXCLUDER® AAA Endoprosthesis Express® (LD) Premounted Stent System Express® Biliary SD Monorail® Premounted Stent System Express® SD Renal Monorail® Premounted Stent System FLAIR® Endovascular Stent Graft Formula™ Balloon-Expandable Renal Stent System GORE EXCLUDER® AAA Endoprosthesis GORE TAG® Thoracic Endoprosthesis Herculink (RX) Elite Renal Stent System LifeStent® (Flexstar)(XL) Vascular Stent System Medtronic Endurant® II AAA stent graft system Micro-Driver stent (RX) (OTW) MULTI-LINK (VISION)(MINI-VISION)(ULTRA) Coronary Stent System Omnilink Elite Vascular Balloon Expandable Stent System Protege® RX Carotid Stent System Stent, intraluminal (cardiovascular)(gastrointestinal)(hepatobiliary)(urinary) Talent® Converter Talent® Occluder Talent® Stent Graft (abdominal)(thoracic) Therapeutic occlusion coil(s) Ultraflex™ Precision Colonic Stent System Valiant Thoracic Stent Graft WALLSTENT® Endoprosthesis Xact Carotid Stent System Zenith AAA Endovascular Graft Zenith Flex® AAA Endovascular Graft Zenith TX2® TAA Endovascular Graft Zenith® Renu™ AAA Ancillary Graft
Intraluminal Device, Airway in Ear, Nose, Sinus	**Includes:** Nasopharyngeal airway (NPA)

ICD-10-PCS Value	Definition
Intraluminal Device, Airway in Gastrointestinal System	**Includes:** Esophageal obturator airway (EOA)
Intraluminal Device, Airway in Mouth and Throat	**Includes:** Guedel airway Oropharyngeal airway (OPA)
Intraluminal Device, Bioactive in Upper Arteries	**Includes:** Bioactive embolization coil(s) Micrus CERECYTE microcoil
Intraluminal Device, Branched or Fenestrated, One or Two Arteries for Restriction in Lower Arteries	**Includes:** Cook Zenith® Fenestrated AAA Endovascular Graft EXCLUDER® AAA Endoprosthesis EXCLUDER® IBE Endoprosthesis GORE EXCLUDER® AAA Endoprosthesis GORE EXCLUDER®IBE Endoprosthesis Zenith® Fenestrated AAA Endovascular Graft
Intraluminal Device, Branched or Fenestrated, Three or More Arteries for Restriction in Lower Arteries	**Includes:** Cook Zenith® Fenestrated AAA Endovascular Graft EXCLUDER® AAA Endoprosthesis GORE EXCLUDER® AAA Endoprosthesis Zenith® Fenestrated AAA Endovascular Graft
Intraluminal Device, Drug-eluting in Heart and Great Vessels	**Includes:** CYPHER® Stent Endeavor® (III)(IV) (Sprint) Zotarolimus-eluting Coronary Stent System Everolimus-eluting coronary stent Paclitaxel-eluting coronary stent Sirolimus-eluting coronary stent TAXUS® Liberte® Paclitaxel-eluting Coronary Stent System XIENCE Everolimus Eluting Coronary Stent System Zotarolimus-eluting coronary stent
Intraluminal Device, Drug-eluting in Lower Arteries	**Includes:** Paclitaxel-eluting peripheral stent Zilver® PTX® (paclitaxel) Drug-Eluting Peripheral Stent
Intraluminal Device, Drug-eluting in Upper Arteries	**Includes:** Paclitaxel-eluting peripheral stent Zilver® PTX® (paclitaxel) Drug-Eluting Peripheral Stent
Intraluminal Device, Endobronchial Valve in Respiratory System	**Includes:** Spiration IBV™ Valve System
Intraluminal Device, Endotracheal Airway in Respiratory System	**Includes:** Endotracheal tube (cuffed)(double-lumen)
Intraluminal Device, Flow Diverter for Restriction in Upper Arteries	**Includes:** Flow Diverter embolization device Pipeline™ (Flex) embolization device Surpass Streamline™ Flow Diverter
Intraluminal Device, Pessary in Female Reproductive System	**Includes:** Pessary ring Vaginal pessary
Intraluminal Device, Sustained Release Drug-eluting in New Technology	**Includes:** Eluvia™ Drug-eluting Vascular Stent System SAVAL below-the-knee (BTK) drug-eluting stent system
Intraluminal Device, Sustained Release Drug-eluting, Four or More in New Technology	**Includes:** Eluvia™ Drug-eluting Vascular Stent System SAVAL below-the-knee (BTK) drug-eluting stent system
Intraluminal Device, Sustained Release Drug-eluting, Three in New Technology	**Includes:** Eluvia™ Drug-eluting Vascular Stent System SAVAL below-the-knee (BTK) drug-eluting stent system
Intraluminal Device, Sustained Release Drug-eluting, Two in New Technology	**Includes:** Eluvia™ Drug-eluting Vascular Stent System SAVAL below-the-knee (BTK) drug-eluting stent system
Liner in Lower Joints	**Includes:** Acetabular cup Hip (joint) liner Joint liner (insert) Knee (implant) insert Tibial insert
Magnetically Controlled Growth Rod(s) in New Technology	**Includes:** MAGEC® Spinal Bracing and Distraction System Spinal growth rods, magnetically controlled
Monitoring Device	**Includes:** Blood glucose monitoring system Cardiac event recorder Continuous Glucose Monitoring (CGM) device Implantable glucose monitoring device Loop recorder, implantable Reveal (LINQ)(DX)(XT)
Monitoring Device, Hemodynamic for Insertion in Subcutaneous Tissue and Fascia	**Includes:** Implantable hemodynamic monitor (IHM) Implantable hemodynamic monitoring system (IHMS)
Monitoring Device, Pressure Sensor for Insertion in Heart and Great Vessels	**Includes:** CardioMEMS® pressure sensor EndoSure® sensor
Neurostimulator Generator in Head and Facial Bones	**Includes:** RNS system neurostimulator generator
Neurostimulator Lead in Central Nervous System and Cranial Nerves	**Includes:** Cortical strip neurostimulator lead DBS lead Deep brain neurostimulator lead RNS System lead Spinal cord neurostimulator lead
Neurostimulator Lead in Peripheral Nervous System	**Includes:** InterStim® Therapy lead

ICD-10-PCS Value	Definition
Nonautologous Tissue Substitute	**Includes:** Acellular Hydrated Dermis Bone bank bone graft Cook Biodesign® Fistula Plug(s) Cook Biodesign® Hernia Graft(s) Cook Biodesign® Layered Graft(s) Cook Zenapro™ Layered Graft(s) Tissue bank graft
Pacemaker, Dual Chamber for Insertion in Subcutaneous Tissue and Fascia	**Includes:** Advisa (MRI) EnRhythm Kappa Revo MRI™ SureScan® pacemaker Two lead pacemaker Versa
Pacemaker, Single Chamber for Insertion in Subcutaneous Tissue and Fascia	**Includes:** Single lead pacemaker (atrium)(ventricle)
Pacemaker, Single Chamber Rate Responsive for Insertion in Subcutaneous Tissue and Fascia	**Includes:** Single lead rate responsive pacemaker (atrium)(ventricle)
Radioactive Element	**Includes:** Brachytherapy seeds CivaSheet®
Radioactive Element, Cesium-131 Collagen Implant for Insertion in Central Nervous System and Cranial Nerves	**Includes:** Cesium-131 Collagen Implant GammaTile™
Resurfacing Device in Lower Joints	**Includes:** CONSERVE® PLUS Total Resurfacing Hip System Cormet Hip Resurfacing System
Short-term External Heart Assist System in Heart and Great Vessels	**Includes:** Biventricular external heart assist system BVS 5000 Ventricular Assist Device Centrimag® Blood Pump Impella® heart pump TandemHeart® System Thoratec Paracorporeal Ventricular Assist Device
Skin Substitute, Porcine Liver Derived in New Technology	**Includes:** MIRODERM™ Biologic Wound Matrix
Spacer in Lower Joints	**Includes:** Joint spacer (antibiotic) Spacer, Static (Antibiotic) Static Spacer (Antibiotic)
Spacer in Upper Joints	**Includes:** Joint spacer (antibiotic)
Spinal Stabilization Device, Facet Replacement for Insertion in Lower Joints	**Includes:** Facet replacement spinal stabilization device
Spinal Stabilization Device, Facet Replacement for Insertion in Upper Joints	**Includes:** Facet replacement spinal stabilization device
Spinal Stabilization Device, Interspinous Process for Insertion in Lower Joints	**Includes:** Interspinous process spinal stabilization device X-STOP® Spacer
Spinal Stabilization Device, Interspinous Process for Insertion in Upper Joints	**Includes:** Interspinous process spinal stabilization device X-STOP® Spacer
Spinal Stabilization Device, Pedicle- Based for Insertion in Lower Joints	**Includes:** Dynesys® Dynamic Stabilization System Pedicle-based dynamic stabilization device
Spinal Stabilization Device, Pedicle-Based for Insertion in Upper Joints	**Includes:** Dynesys® Dynamic Stabilization System Pedicle-based dynamic stabilization device
Stimulator Generator in Subcutaneous Tissue and Fascia	**Includes:** Baroreflex Activation Therapy® (BAT®) Diaphragmatic pacemaker generator Mark IV Breathing Pacemaker System Phrenic nerve stimulator generator Rheos® System device
Stimulator Generator, Multiple Array for Insertion in Subcutaneous Tissue and Fascia	**Includes:** Activa PC neurostimulator Enterra gastric neurostimulator Neurostimulator generator, multiple channel PrimeAdvanced neurostimulator (SureScan)(MRI Safe)
Stimulator Generator, Multiple Array Rechargeable for Insertion in Subcutaneous Tissue and Fascia	**Includes:** Activa RC neurostimulator Neurostimulator generator, multiple channel rechargeable RestoreAdvanced neurostimulator (SureScan)(MRI Safe) RestoreSensor neurostimulator (SureScan)(MRI Safe) RestoreUltra neurostimulator (SureScan)(MRI Safe)
Stimulator Generator, Single Array for Insertion in Subcutaneous Tissue and Fascia	**Includes:** Activa SC neurostimulator InterStim® Therapy neurostimulator Itrel (3)(4) neurostimulator Neurostimulator generator, single channel
Stimulator Generator, Single Array Rechargeable for Insertion in Subcutaneous Tissue and Fascia	**Includes:** Neurostimulator generator, single channel rechargeable
Stimulator Lead in Gastrointestinal System	**Includes:** Gastric electrical stimulation (GES) lead Gastric pacemaker lead
Stimulator Lead in Muscles	**Includes:** Electrical muscle stimulation (EMS) lead Electronic muscle stimulator lead Neuromuscular electrical stimulation (NEMS) lead
Stimulator Lead in Upper Arteries	**Includes:** Baroreflex Activation Therapy® (BAT®) Carotid (artery) sinus (baroreceptor) lead Rheos® System lead

ICD-10-PCS Value	Definition
Stimulator Lead in Urinary System	**Includes:** Sacral nerve modulation (SNM) lead Sacral neuromodulation lead Urinary incontinence stimulator lead
Subcutaneous Defibrillator Lead in Subcutaneous Tissue and Fascia	**Includes:** S-ICD™ lead
Synthetic Substitute	**Includes:** AbioCor® Total Replacement Heart AMPLATZER® Muscular VSD Occluder Annuloplasty ring Bard® Composix® (E/X) (LP) mesh Bard® Composix® Kugel® patch Bard® Dulex™ mesh Bard® Ventralex™ hernia patch Barricaid® Annular Closure Device (ACD) BRYAN® Cervical Disc System Corvia IASD® Ex-PRESS™ mini glaucoma shunt Flexible Composite Mesh GORE® DUALMESH® Holter valve ventricular shunt IASD® (InterAtrial Shunt Device), Corvia InterAtrial Shunt Device IASD®, Corvia MitraClip valve repair system Nitinol framed polymer mesh Open Pivot (mechanical) valve Open Pivot Aortic Valve Graft (AVG) Partially absorbable mesh PHYSIOMESH™ Flexible Composite Mesh Polymethylmethacrylate (PMMA) Polypropylene mesh PRESTIGE® Cervical Disc PROCEED™ Ventral Patch Prodisc-C Prodisc-L PROLENE Polypropylene Hernia System (PHS) Rebound HRD® (Hernia Repair Device) SynCardia Total Artificial Heart Total artificial (replacement) heart ULTRAPRO Hernia System (UHS) ULTRAPRO Partially Absorbable Lightweight Mesh ULTRAPRO Plug V-Wave Interatrial Shunt System Ventrio™ Hernia Patch Zimmer® NexGen® LPS Mobile Bearing Knee Zimmer® NexGen® LPS-Flex Mobile Knee
Synthetic Substitute, Ceramic for Replacement in Lower Joints	**Includes:** Ceramic on ceramic bearing surface Novation® Ceramic AHS® (Articulation Hip System)
Synthetic Substitute, Intraocular Telescope for Replacement in Eye	**Includes:** Implantable Miniature Telescope™ (IMT)
Synthetic Substitute, Mechanically Expandable (Paired) in New Technology	**Includes:** SpineJack® system

ICD-10-PCS Value	Definition
Synthetic Substitute, Metal for Replacement in Lower Joints	**Includes:** Cobalt/chromium head and socket Metal on metal bearing surface
Synthetic Substitute, Metal on Polyethylene for Replacement in Lower Joints	**Includes:** Cobalt/chromium head and polyethylene socket
Synthetic Substitute, Oxidized Zirconium on Polyethylene for Replacement in Lower Joints	**Includes:** OXINIUM
Synthetic Substitute, Polyethylene for Replacement in Lower Joints	**Includes:** Polyethylene socket
Synthetic Substitute, Reverse Ball and Socket for Replacement in Upper Joints	**Includes:** Delta III Reverse shoulder prosthesis Reverse® Shoulder Prosthesis
Tissue Expander in Skin and Breast	**Includes:** Tissue expander (inflatable) (injectable)
Tissue Expander in Subcutaneous Tissue and Fascia	**Includes:** Tissue expander (inflatable) (injectable)
Tracheostomy Device in Respiratory System	**Includes:** Tracheostomy tube
Vascular Access Device, Totally Implantable in Subcutaneous Tissue and Fascia	**Includes:** Implanted (venous)(access) port Injection reservoir, port Subcutaneous injection reservoir, port
Vascular Access Device, Tunneled in Subcutaneous Tissue and Fascia	**Includes:** Tunneled central venous catheter Vectra® Vascular Access Graft
Zooplastic Tissue in Heart and Great Vessels	**Includes:** 3f (Aortic) Bioprosthesis valve Bovine pericardial valve Bovine pericardium graft Contegra Pulmonary Valved Conduit CoreValve transcatheter aortic valve Epic™ Stented Tissue Valve (aortic) Freestyle (Stentless) Aortic Root Bioprosthesis Hancock Bioprosthesis (aortic) (mitral) valve Hancock Bioprosthetic Valved Conduit Melody® transcatheter pulmonary valve Mitroflow® Aortic Pericardial Heart Valve Mosaic Bioprosthesis (aortic) (mitral) valve Porcine (bioprosthetic) valve SAPIEN transcatheter aortic valve SJM Biocor® Stented Valve System Stented tissue valve Trifecta™ Valve (aortic) Xenograft
Zooplastic Tissue, Rapid Deployment Technique in New Technology	**Includes:** EDWARDS INTUITY Elite valve system INTUITY Elite valve system, EDWARDS Perceval sutureless valve Sutureless valve, Perceval

Appendix I: Substance Key/Substance Definitions

Substance Key

This table crosswalks a specific substance, listed by trade name or synonym, to the PCS value that would be used to represent that substance in either the Administration or New Technology section. The ICD-10-PCS value may be located in either the 6th-character Substance column or the 7th-character Qualifier column depending on the section/table to which it is classified. The most specific character is listed in the table.

Trade Name or Synonym	ICD-10-PCS Value	PCS Section
AIGISRx Antibacterial Envelope	Anti-Infective Envelope (A)	Administration (3)
Andexanet Alfa, Factor Xa Inhibitor Reversal Agent	Coagulation Factor Xa, Inactivated (7)	New Technology (X)
Andexxa	Coagulation Factor Xa, Inactivated (7)	New Technology (X)
Angiotensin II	Synthetic Human Angiotensin II (H)	New Technology (X)
Antibacterial Envelope (TYRX) (AIGISRx)	Anti-Infective Envelope (A)	Administration (3)
Antimicrobial envelope	Anti-Infective Envelope (A)	Administration (3)
Axicabtagene Ciloeucel	Engineered Autologous Chimeric Antigen Receptor T-cell Immunotherapy (C)	New Technology (X)
AZEDRA®	Iobenguane I-131 Antineoplastic (S)	New Technology (X)
Bone morphogenetic protein 2 (BMP 2)	Recombinant Bone Morphogenetic Protein (B)	Administration (3)
Brexucabtagene Autoleucel	Brexucabtagene Autoleucel Immunotherapy (4)	New Technology (X)
CBMA (Concentrated Bone Marrow Aspirate)	Concentrated Bone Marrow Aspirate (Ø)	New Technology (X)
Clolar	Clofarabine (P)	Administration (3)
Coagulation Factor Xa, (Recombinant) Inactivated	Coagulation Factor Xa, Inactivated (7)	New Technology (X)
CONTEPO™	Fosfomycin Anti-infective (K)	New Technology (X)
Defitelio	Defibrotide Sodium Anticoagulant (9)	New Technology (X)
DuraGraft® Endothelial Damage Inhibitor	Endothelial Damage Inhibitor (8)	New Technology (X)
ELZONRIS™	Tagraxofusp-erzs Antineoplastic (Q)	New Technology (X)
ERLEADA™	Apalutamide Antineoplastic (J)	New Technology (X)
Factor Xa Inhibitor Reversal Agent, Andexanet Alfa	Coagulation Factor Xa, Inactivated (7)	New Technology (X)
FETROJA®	Cefiderocol Anti-infective (A)	New Technology (X)
Fosfomycin injection	Fosfomycin Anti-infective (K)	New Technology (X)
GIAPREZA™	Synthetic Human AngiotensIn II (H)	New Technology (X)
Hemospray® Endoscopic Hemostat	Mineral-based Topical Hemostatic Agent (8)	New Technology (X)
Human angiotensin II, synthetic	Synthetic Human Angiotensin II (H)	New Technology (X)
IMFINZI®	Durvalumab Antineoplastic (3)	New Technology (X)
IMI/REL	Imipenem-cilastatin-relebactam Anti-infective (U)	New Technology (X)
Iobenguane I-131, High Specific Activity (HSA)	Iobenguane I-131 Antineoplastic (S)	New Technology (X)
Jakafi®	Ruxolitinib (T)	New Technology (X)
Kcentra	4-Factor Prothrombin Complex Concentrate (B)	Administration (3)
KYMRIAH	Engineered Autologous Chimeric Antigen Receptor T-cell Immunotherapy (C)	New Technology (X)
Lisocabtagene Maraleucel	Lisocabtagene Maraleucel Immunotherapy (7)	New Technology (X)
NA-1 (Nerinitide)	Nerinitide (2)	New Technology (X)
Nesiritide	Human B-type Natriuretic Peptide (H)	Administration (3)
NUZYRA™	Omadacycline Anti-infective (B)	New Technology (X)
OTL-101	Hematopoietic Stem/Progenitor Cells, Genetically Modified (C)	Administration (3)
rhBMP-2	Recombinant Bone Morphogenetic Protein (B)	Administration (3)
Seprafilm	Adhesion Barrier (5)	Administration (3)
Soliris®	Eculizumab (C)	New Technology (X)
SPRAVATO™	Esketamine Hydrochloride (M)	New Technology (X)
STELARA®	Other New Technology Therapeutic Substance (F)	New Technology (X)
TECENTRIQ®	Atezolizumab Antineoplastic (D)	New Technology (X)
Tisagenlecleucel	Engineered Autologous Chimeric Antigen Receptor T-cell Immunotherapy (C)	New Technology (X)
Tissue Plasminogen Activator (tPA)(r- tPA)	Other Thrombolytic (7)	Administration (3)
TYRX Antibacterial Envelope	Anti-Infective Envelope (A)	Administration (3)

Trade Name or Synonym	ICD-10-PCS Value	PCS Section
Ustekinumab	Other New Technology Therapeutic Substance (F)	New Technology (X)
Vabomere™	Meropenem-vaborbactam Anti-infective (N)	New Technology (X)
Venclexta®	Ventoclax Antineoplastic (R)	New Technology (X)
Vistogard®	Uridine Triacetate (8)	New Technology (X)
Voraxaze	Glucarpidase (Q)	Administration (3)
VYXEOS™	Cytarabine and Daunorubicin Liposome Antineoplastic (B)	New Technology (X)
XENLETA™	Lefamulin Anti-infective (6)	New Technology (X)
XOSPATA®	Gilteritinib Antineoplastic (V)	New Technology (X)
ZERBAXA®	Ceftolozane/Tazobactam Anti-infective (9)	New Technology (X)
ZINPLAVA™	Bezlotoxumab Monoclonal Antibody (A)	New Technology (X)
ZULRESSO™	Brexanolone (Ø)	New Technology (X)
Zyvox	Oxazolidinones (8)	Administration (3)

Substance Definitions

This table crosswalks a PCS value, used in the Administration or New Technology section, to a specific substance. The specific substances are listed by trade name or synonym. The ICD-10-PCS value may be located in either the 6th-character Substance column or the 7th-character Qualifier column depending on the section/table to which it is classified.

ICD-10-PCS Value	Trade Name or Synonym	PCS Section
4-Factor Prothrombin Complex Concentrate (B)	**Includes:** Kcentra	Administration (3)
Adhesion Barrier (5)	**Includes:** Seprafilm	Administration (3)
Anti-Infective Envelope (A)	**Includes:** AIGISRx Antibacterial Envelope Antimicrobial envelope Antibacterial Envelope (TYRX) (AIGISRx) TYRX Antibacterial Envelope	Administration (3)
Apalutamide Antineoplastic (J)	**Includes:** ERLEADA™	New Technology (X)
Atezolizumab Antineoplastic (D)	**Includes:** TECENTRIQ®	New Technology (X)
Bezlotoxumab Monoclonal Antibody (A)	**Includes:** ZINPLAVA™	New Technology (X)
Brexanolone (Ø)	**Includes:** ZULRESSO™	New Technology (X)
Brexucabtagene Autoleucel Immunotherapy (4)	**Includes:** Brexucabtagene Autoleucel	New Technology (X)
Cefiderocol Anti-infective (A)	**Includes:** FETROJA®	New Technology (X)
Ceftolozane/Tazobactam Anti- infective (9)	**Includes:** ZERBAXA®	New Technology (X)
Clofarabine (P)	**Includes:** Clolar	Administration (3)
Coagulation Factor Xa, Inactivated (7)	**Includes:** Andexanet Alfa, Factor Xa Inhibitor Reversal Agent Andexxa Coagulation Factor Xa, (Recombinant) Inactivated Factor Xa Inhibitor Reversal Agent, Andexanet Alfa	New Technology (X)
Concentrated Bone Marrow Aspirate (Ø)	**Includes:** CBMA (Concentrated Bone Marrow Aspirate)	New Technology (X)
Cytarabine and Daunorubicin Liposome Antineoplastic (B)	**Includes:** VYXEOS™	New Technology (X)
Defibrotide Sodium Anticoagulant (9)	**Includes:** Defitelio	New Technology (X)
Durvalumab Antineoplastic (3)	**Includes:** IMFINZI®	New Technology (X)
Eculizumab (C)	**Includes:** Soliris®	New Technology (X)
Endothelial Damage Inhibitor (8)	**Includes:** DuraGraft® Endothelial Damage Inhibitor	New Technology (X)
Engineered Autologous Chimeric Antigen Receptor T-cell Immunotherapy (C)	**Includes:** Axicabtagene Ciloeucel KYMRIAH Tisagenlecleucel	New Technology (X)
Esketamine Hydrochloride (M)	**Includes:** SPRAVATO™	New Technology (X)
Fosfomycin Anti-infective (K)	**Includes:** CONTEPO™ Fosfomycin injection	New Technology (X)
Gilteritinib Antineoplastic (V)	**Includes:** XOSPATA®	New Technology (X)
Glucarpidase (Q)	**Includes:** Voraxaze	Administration (3)
Hematopoietic Stem/Progenitor Cells, Genetically Modified (C)	**Includes:** OTL-1Ø1	Administration (3)
Human B-type Natriuretic Peptide (H)	**Includes:** Nesiritide	Administration (3)

ICD-10-PCS Value	Trade Name or Synonym	PCS Section
Imipenem-cilastatin-relebactam Anti-infective (U)	**Includes:** IMI/REL	New Technology (X)
Iobenguane I-131 Antineoplastic (S)	**Includes:** AZEDRA® Iobenguane I-131, High Specific Activity (HSA)	New Technology (X)
Lefamulin Anti-infective (6)	**Includes:** XENLETA™	New Technology (X)
Lisocabtagene Maraleucel Immunotherapy (7)	**Includes:** Lisocabtagene Maraleucel	New Technology (X)
Meropenem-vaborbactam Anti-infective (N)	**Includes:** Vabomere™	New Technology (X)
Mineral-based Topical Hemostatic Agent (8)	**Includes:** Hemospray® Endoscopic Hemostat	New Technology (X
Nerinitide (2)	**Includes:** NA-1 (Nerinitide)	New Technology (X
Omadacycline Anti-infective (B)	**Includes:** NUZYRA™	New Technology (X
Other New Technology Therapeutic Substance (F)	**Includes:** STELARA® Ustekinumab	New Technology (X)
Other Thrombolytic (7)	**Includes:** Tissue Plasminogen Activator (tPA)(r-tPA)	Administration (3)
Oxazolidinones (8)	**Includes:** Zyvox	Administration (3)
Recombinant Bone Morphogenetic Protein (B)	**Includes:** Bone morphogenetic protein 2 (BMP 2) rhBMP-2	Administration (3)
Ruxolitinib (T)	**Includes:** Jakafi®	New Technology (X)
Synthetic Human Angiotensin II (H)	**Includes:** Angiotensin II GIAPREZA™ Human angiotensin II, synthetic	New Technology (X)
Tagraxofusp-erzs Antineoplastic (Q)	**Includes:** ELZONRIS™	New Technology (X)
Uridine Triacetate (8)	**Includes:** Vistogard®	New Technology (X)
Venetoclax Antineoplastic (R)	**Includes:** Venclexta®	New Technology (X)

Appendix J: Sections B–H Character Definitions

Sections B-H (Imaging through Substance Abuse Treatment) do not include root operations. Instead, the character 3 value represents the type of procedure performed with additional details about that procedure provided by the character 4 or 5 value, when appropriate. This resource provides the specific ICD-10-PCS value and its associated definition for the character 3, character 4, and character 5 values in the ancillary sections of B-H.

Section B–Imaging

ICD-10-PCS Value (Character 3)	Definition
Computerized Tomography (CT Scan) (2)	Computer reformatted digital display of multiplanar images developed from the capture of multiple exposures of external ionizing radiation
Fluoroscopy (1)	Single plane or bi-plane real time display of an image developed from the capture of external ionizing radiation on a fluorescent screen. The image may also be stored by either digital or analog means.
Magnetic Resonance Imaging (MRI) (3)	Computer reformatted digital display of multiplanar images developed from the capture of radiofrequency signals emitted by nuclei in a body site excited within a magnetic field
Other Imaging (5)	Other specified modality for visualizing a body part
Plain Radiography (Ø)	Planar display of an image developed from the capture of external ionizing radiation on photographic or photoconductive plate
Ultrasonography (4)	Real time display of images of anatomy or flow information developed from the capture of reflected and attenuated high frequency sound waves

Section C–Nuclear Medicine

ICD-10-PCS Value (Character 3)	Definition
Nonimaging Nuclear Medicine Assay (6)	Introduction of radioactive materials into the body for the study of body fluids and blood elements, by the detection of radioactive emissions
Nonimaging Nuclear Medicine Probe (5)	Introduction of radioactive materials into the body for the study of distribution and fate of certain substances by the detection of radioactive emissions; or, alternatively, measurement of absorption of radioactive emissions from an external source
Nonimaging Nuclear Medicine Uptake (4)	Introduction of radioactive materials into the body for measurements of organ function, from the detection of radioactive emissions
Planar Nuclear Medicine Imaging (1)	Introduction of radioactive materials into the body for single plane display of images developed from the capture of radioactive emissions
Positron Emission Tomographic (PET) Imaging (3)	Introduction of radioactive materials into the body for three dimensional display of images developed from the simultaneous capture, 18Ø degrees apart, of radioactive emissions
Systemic Nuclear Medicine Therapy (7)	Introduction of unsealed radioactive materials into the body for treatment
Tomographic (Tomo) Nuclear Medicine Imaging (2)	Introduction of radioactive materials into the body for three dimensional display of images developed from the capture of radioactive emissions

Section F–Physical Rehabilitation and Diagnostic Audiology

ICD-10-PCS Value (Character 3)	Definition
Activities of Daily Living Assessment (2)	Measurement of functional level for activities of daily living
Activities of Daily Living Treatment (8)	Exercise or activities to facilitate functional competence for activities of daily living
Caregiver Training (F)	Training in activities to support patient's optimal level of function
Cochlear Implant Treatment (B)	Application of techniques to improve the communication abilities of individuals with cochlear implant
Device Fitting (D)	Fitting of a device designed to facilitate or support achievement of a higher level of function
Hearing Aid Assessment (4)	Measurement of the appropriateness and/or effectiveness of a hearing device
Hearing Assessment (3)	Measurement of hearing and related functions
Hearing Treatment (9)	Application of techniques to improve, augment, or compensate for hearing and related functional impairment
Motor and/or Nerve Function Assessment (1)	Measurement of motor, nerve, and related functions

Continued on next page

Section F–Physical Rehabilitation and Diagnostic Audiology

Continued from previous page

ICD-10-PCS Value (Character 3)	Definition
Motor Treatment (7)	Exercise or activities to increase or facilitate motor function
Speech Assessment (Ø)	Measurement of speech and related functions
Speech Treatment (6)	Application of techniques to improve, augment, or compensate for speech and related functional impairment
Vestibular Assessment (5)	Measurement of the vestibular system and related functions
Vestibular Treatment (C)	Application of techniques to improve, augment, or compensate for vestibular and related functional impairment

Section F–Physical Rehabilitation and Diagnostic Audiology

ICD-10-PCS Value Qualifier (Character 5)	Definition
Acoustic Reflex Decay (J)	Measures reduction in size/strength of acoustic reflex over time Includes/Examples: Includes site of lesion test
Acoustic Reflex Patterns (G)	Defines site of lesion based upon presence/absence of acoustic reflexes with ipsilateral vs. contralateral stimulation
Acoustic Reflex Threshold (H)	Determines minimal intensity that acoustic reflex occurs with ipsilateral and/or contralateral stimulation
Aerobic Capacity and Endurance (7)	Measures autonomic responses to positional changes; perceived exertion, dyspnea or angina during activity; performance during exercise protocols; standard vital signs; and blood gas analysis or oxygen consumption
Alternate Binaural or Monaural Loudness Balance (7)	Determines auditory stimulus parameter that yields the same objective sensation Includes/Examples: Sound intensities that yield same loudness perception
Anthropometric Characteristics (B)	Measures edema, body,fat composition, height, weight, length and girth
Aphasia (Assessment) (C)	Measures expressive and receptive speech and language function including reading and writing
Aphasia (Treatment) (3)	Applying techniques to improve, augment, or compensate for receptive/ expressive language impairments
Articulation/Phonology (Assessment) (9)	Measures speech production
Articulation/Phonology (Treatment) (4)	Applying techniques to correct, improve, or compensate for speech productive impairment
Assistive Listening Device (5)	Assists in use of effective and appropriate assistive listening device/system
Assistive Listening System/Device Selection (4)	Measures the effectiveness and appropriateness of assistive listening systems/devices
Assistive, Adaptive, Supportive or Protective Devices (9)	Explanation: Devices to facilitate or support achievement of a higher level of function in wheelchair mobility; bed mobility; transfer or ambulation ability; bath and showering ability; dressing; grooming; personal hygiene; play or leisure
Auditory Evoked Potentials (L)	Measures electric responses produced by the VIIIth cranial nerve and brainstem following auditory stimulation
Auditory Processing (Assessment) (Q)	Evaluates ability to receive and process auditory information and comprehension of spoken language
Auditory Processing (Treatment) (2)	Applying techniques to improve the receiving and processing of auditory information and comprehension of spoken language
Augmentative/Alternative Communication System (Assessment) (L)	Determines the appropriateness of aids, techniques, symbols, and/or strategies to augment or replace speech and enhance communication Includes/Examples: Includes the use of telephones, writing equipment, emergency equipment, and TDD
Augmentative/Alternative Communication System (Treatment) (3)	Includes/Examples: Includes augmentative communication devices and aids
Aural Rehabilitation (5)	Applying techniques to improve the communication abilities associated with hearing loss
Aural Rehabilitation Status (P)	Measures impact of a hearing loss including evaluation of receptive and expressive communication skills

Continued on next page

Section F–Physical Rehabilitation and Diagnostic Audiology

Continued from previous page

ICD-10-PCS Value Qualifier (Character 5)	Definition
Bathing/Showering (Ø)	Includes/Examples: Includes obtaining and using supplies; soaping, rinsing, and drying body parts; maintaining bathing position; and transferring to and from bathing positions
Bathing/Showering Techniques (Ø)	Activities to facilitate obtaining and using supplies, soaping, rinsing and drying body parts, maintaining bathing position, and transferring to and from bathing positions
Bed Mobility (Assessment) (B)	Transitional movement within bed
Bed Mobility (Treatment) (5)	Exercise or activities to facilitate transitional movements within bed
Bedside Swallowing and Oral Function (H)	Includes/Examples: Bedside swallowing includes assessment of sucking, masticating, coughing, and swallowing. Oral function includes assessment of musculature for controlled movements, structures, and functions to determine coordination and phonation.
Bekesy Audiometry (3)	Uses an instrument that provides a choice of discrete or continuously varying pure tones; choice of pulsed or continuous signal
Binaural Electroacoustic Hearing Aid Check (6)	Determines mechanical and electroacoustic function of bilateral hearing aids using hearing aid test box
Binaural Hearing Aid (Assessment) (3)	Measures the candidacy, effectiveness, and appropriateness of a hearing aid Explanation: Measures bilateral fit
Binaural Hearing Aid (Treatment) (2)	Explanation: Assists in achieving maximum understanding and performance
Bithermal, Binaural Caloric Irrigation (Ø)	Measures the rhythmic eye movements stimulated by changing the temperature of the vestibular system
Bithermal, Monaural Caloric Irrigation (1)	Measures the rhythmic eye movements stimulated by changing the temperature of the vestibular system in one ear
Brief Tone Stimuli (R)	Measures specific central auditory process
Cerumen Management (3)	Includes examination of external auditory canal and tympanic membrane and removal of cerumen from external ear canal
Cochlear Implant (Ø)	Measures candidacy for cochlear implant
Cochlear Implant Rehabilitation (Ø)	Applying techniques to improve the communication abilities of individuals with cochlear implant; includes programming the device, providing patients/families with information
Communicative/Cognitive Integration Skills (Assessment) (G)	Measures ability to use higher cortical functions Includes/Examples: Includes orientation, recognition, attention span, initiation and termination of activity, memory, sequencing, categorizing, concept formation, spatial operations, judgment, problem solving, generalization and pragmatic communication
Communicative/Cognitive Integration Skills (Treatment) (6)	Activities to facilitate the use of higher cortical functions Includes/Examples: Includes level of arousal, orientation, recognition, attention span, initiation and termination of activity, memory sequencing, judgment and problem solving, learning and generalization, and pragmatic communication
Computerized Dynamic Posturography (6)	Measures the status of the peripheral and central vestibular system and the sensory/motor component of balance; evaluates the efficacy of vestibular rehabilitation
Conditioned Play Audiometry (4)	Behavioral measures using nonspeech and speech stimuli to obtain frequency-specific and ear-specific information on auditory status from the patient Explanation: Obtains speech reception threshold by having patient point to pictures of spondaic words
Coordination/Dexterity (Assessment) (3)	Measures large and small muscle groups for controlled goal-directed movements Explanation: Dexterity includes object manipulation
Coordination/Dexterity (Treatment) (2)	Exercise or activities to facilitate gross coordination and fine coordination
Cranial Nerve Integrity (9)	Measures cranial nerve sensory and motor functions, including tastes, smell and facial expression
Dichotic Stimuli (T)	Measures specific central auditory process
Distorted Speech (S)	Measures specific central auditory process
Dix-Hallpike Dynamic (5)	Measures nystagmus following Dix-Hallpike maneuver

Continued on next page

Section F–Physical Rehabilitation and Diagnostic Audiology

Continued from previous page

ICD-10-PCS Value Qualifier (Character 5)	Definition
Dressing (1)	Includes/Examples: Includes selecting clothing and accessories, obtaining clothing from storage, dressing, fastening and adjusting clothing and shoes, and applying and removing personal devices, prosthesis or orthosis
Dressing Techniques (1)	Activities to facilitate selecting clothing and accessories, dressing and undressing, adjusting clothing and shoes, applying and removing devices, prostheses or orthoses
Dynamic Orthosis (6)	Includes/Examples: Includes customized and prefabricated splints, inhibitory casts, spinal and other braces, and protective devices; allows motion through transfer of movement from other body parts or by use of outside forces
Ear Canal Probe Microphone (1)	Real ear measures
Ear Protector Attentuation (7)	Measures ear protector fit and effectiveness
Electrocochleography (K)	Measures the VIIIth cranial nerve action potential
Environmental, Home, Work Barriers (B)	Measures current and potential barriers to optimal function, including safety hazards, access problems and home or office design
Ergonomics and Body Mechanics (C)	Ergonomic measurement of job tasks, work hardening or work conditioning needs; functional capacity; and body mechanics
Eustachian Tube Function (F)	Measures eustachian tube function and patency of eustachian tube
Evoked Otoacoustic Emissions, Diagnostic (N)	Measures auditory evoked potentials in a diagnostic format
Evoked Otoacoustic Emissions, Screening (M)	Measures auditory evoked potentials in a screening format
Facial Nerve Function (7)	Measures electrical activity of the VIIth cranial nerve (facial nerve)
Feeding/Eating (Assessment) (2)	Includes/Examples: Includes setting up food, selecting and using utensils and tableware, bringing food or drink to mouth, cleaning face, hands, and clothing, and management of alternative methods of nourishment
Feeding/Eating (Treatment) (3)	Exercise or activities to facilitate setting up food, selecting and using utensils and tableware, bringing food or drink to mouth, cleaning face, hands, and clothing, and management of alternative methods of nourishment
Filtered Speech (Ø)	Uses high or low pass filtered speech stimuli to assess central auditory processing disorders, site of lesion testing
Fluency (Assessment) (D)	Measures speech fluency or stuttering
Fluency (Treatment) (7)	Applying techniques to improve and augment fluent speech
Gait and/or Balance (D)	Measures biomechanical, arthrokinematic and other spatial and temporal characteristics of gait and balance
Gait Training/Functional Ambulation (9)	Exercise or activities to facilitate ambulation on a variety of surfaces and in a variety of environments
Grooming/Personal Hygiene (Assessment) (3)	Includes/Examples: Includes ability to obtain and use supplies in a sequential fashion, general grooming, oral hygiene, toilet hygiene, personal care devices, including care for artificial airways
Grooming/Personal Hygiene (Treatment) (2)	Activities to facilitate obtaining and using supplies in a sequential fashion: general grooming, oral hygiene, toilet hygiene, cleaning body, and personal care devices, including artificial airways
Hearing and Related Disorders Counseling (Ø)	Provides patients/families/caregivers with information, support, referrals to facilitate recovery from a communication disorder Includes/Examples: Includes strategies for psychosocial adjustment to hearing loss for clients and families/caregivers
Hearing and Related Disorders Prevention (1)	Provides patients/families/caregivers with information and support to prevent communication disorders
Hearing Screening (Ø)	Pass/refer measures designed to identify need for further audiologic assessment
Home Management (Assessment) (4)	Obtaining and maintaining personal and household possessions and environment Includes/Examples: Includes clothing care, cleaning, meal preparation and cleanup, shopping, money management, household maintenance, safety procedures, and childcare/parenting

Continued on next page

Section F–Physical Rehabilitation and Diagnostic Audiology

Continued from previous page

ICD-10-PCS Value Qualifier (Character 5)	Definition
Home Management (Treatment) (4)	Activities to facilitate obtaining and maintaining personal household possessions and environment Includes/Examples: Includes clothing care, cleaning, meal preparation and clean-up, shopping, money management, household maintenance, safety procedures, childcare/parenting
Instrumental Swallowing and Oral Function (J)	Measures swallowing function using instrumental diagnostic procedures Explanation: Methods include videofluoroscopy, ultrasound, manometry, endoscopy
Integumentary Integrity (1)	Includes/Examples: Includes burns, skin conditions, ecchymosis, bleeding, blisters, scar tissue, wounds and other traumas, tissue mobility, turgor and texture
Manual Therapy Techniques (7)	Techniques in which the therapist uses his/her hands to administer skilled movements Includes/Examples: Includes connective tissue massage, joint mobilization and manipulation, manual lymph drainage, manual traction, soft tissue mobilization and manipulation
Masking Patterns (W)	Measures central auditory processing status
Monaural Electroacoustic Hearing Aid Check (8)	Determines mechanical and electroacoustic function of one hearing aid using hearing aid test box
Monaural Hearing Aid (Assessment) (2)	Measures the candidacy, effectiveness, and appropriateness of a hearing aid Explanation: Measures unilateral fit
Monaural Hearing Aid (Treatment) (1)	Explanation: Assists in achieving maximum understanding and performance
Motor Function (Assessment) (4)	Measures the body's functional and versatile movement patterns Includes/Examples: Includes motor assessment scales, analysis of head, trunk and limb movement, and assessment of motor learning
Motor Function (Treatment) (3)	Exercise or activities to facilitate crossing midline, laterality, bilateral integration, praxis, neuromuscular relaxation, inhibition, facilitation, motor function and motor learning
Motor Speech (Assessment) (B)	Measures neurological motor aspects of speech production
Motor Speech (Treatment) (8)	Applying techniques to improve and augment the impaired neurological motor aspects of speech production
Muscle Performance (Assessment) (Ø)	Measures muscle strength, power and endurance using manual testing, dynamometry or computer-assisted electromechanical muscle test; functional muscle strength, power and endurance; muscle pain, tone, or soreness; or pelvic-floor musculature Explanation: Muscle endurance refers to the ability to contract a muscle repeatedly over time
Muscle Performance (Treatment) (1)	Exercise or activities to increase the capacity of a muscle to do work in terms of strength, power, and/or endurance Explanation: Muscle strength is the force exerted to overcome resistance in one maximal effort. Muscle power is work produced per unit of time, or the product of strength and speed. Muscle endurance is the ability to contract a muscle repeatedly over time.
Neuromotor Development (D)	Measures motor development, righting and equilibrium reactions, and reflex and equilibrium reactions
Non-invasive Instrumental Status (N)	Instrumental measures of oral, nasal, vocal, and velopharyngeal functions as they pertain to speech production
Nonspoken Language (Assessment) (7)	Measures nonspoken language (print, sign, symbols) for communication
Nonspoken Language (Treatment) (Ø)	Applying techniques that improve, augment, or compensate spoken communication
Oral Peripheral Mechanism (P)	Structural measures of face, jaw, lips, tongue, teeth, hard and soft palate, pharynx as related to speech production
Orofacial Myofunctional (Assessment) (K)	Measures orofacial myofunctional patterns for speech and related functions
Orofacial Myofunctional (Treatment) (9)	Applying techniques to improve, alter, or augment impaired orofacial myofunctional patterns and related speech production errors
Oscillating Tracking (3)	Measures ability to visually track
Pain (F)	Measures muscle soreness, pain and soreness with joint movement, and pain perception Includes/Examples: Includes questionnaires, graphs, symptom magnification scales or visual analog scales
Perceptual Processing (Assessment) (5)	Measures stereognosis, kinesthesia, body schema, right-left discrimination, form constancy, position in space, visual closure, figure-ground, depth perception, spatial relations and topographical orientation

Continued on next page

Section F–Physical Rehabilitation and Diagnostic Audiology

Continued from previous page

ICD-10-PCS Value Qualifier (Character 5)	Definition
Perceptual Processing (Treatment) (1)	Exercise and activities to facilitate perceptual processing Explanation: Includes stereognosis, kinesthesia, body schema, right-left discrimination, form constancy, position in space, visual closure, figure-ground, depth perception, spatial relations, and topographical orientation Includes/Examples: Includes stereognosis, kinesthesia, body schema, right-left discrimination, form constancy, position in space, visual closure, figure-ground, depth perception, spatial relations, and topographical orientation
Performance Intensity Phonetically Balanced Speech Discrimination (Q)	Measures word recognition over varying intensity levels
Postural Control (3)	Exercise or activities to increase postural alignment and control
Prosthesis (8)	Explanation: Artificial substitutes for missing body parts that augment performance or function Includes/Examples: Limb prosthesis, ocular prosthesis
Psychosocial Skills (Assessment) (6)	The ability to interact in society and to process emotions Includes/Examples: Includes psychological (values, interests, self-concept); social (role performance, social conduct, interpersonal skills, self expression); self-management (coping skills, time management, self-control)
Psychosocial Skills (Treatment) (6)	The ability to interact in society and to process emotions Includes/Examples: Includes psychological (values, interests, self-concept); social (role performance, social conduct, interpersonal skills, self expression); self-management (coping skills, time management, self-control)
Pure Tone Audiometry, Air (1)	Air-conduction pure tone threshold measures with appropriate masking
Pure Tone Audiometry, Air and Bone (2)	Air-conduction and bone-conduction pure tone threshold measures with appropriate masking
Pure Tone Stenger (C)	Measures unilateral nonorganic hearing loss based on simultaneous presentation of pure tones of differing volume
Range of Motion and Joint Integrity (5)	Measures quantity, quality, grade, and classification of joint movement and/or mobility Explanation: Range of Motion is the space, distance or angle through which movement occurs at a joint or series of joints. Joint integrity is the conformance of joints to expected anatomic, biomechanical and kinematic norms.
Range of Motion and Joint Mobility (Ø)	Exercise or activities to increase muscle length and joint mobility
Receptive/Expressive Language (Assessment) (8)	Measures receptive and expressive language
Receptive/Expressive Language (Treatment) (B)	Applying techniques to improve and augment receptive/expressive language
Reflex Integrity (G)	Measures the presence, absence, or exaggeration of developmentally appropriate, pathologic or normal reflexes
Select Picture Audiometry (5)	Establishes hearing threshold levels for speech using pictures
Sensorineural Acuity Level (4)	Measures sensorineural acuity masking presented via bone conduction
Sensory Aids (5)	Determines the appropriateness of a sensory prosthetic device, other than a hearing aid or assistive listening system/device
Sensory Awareness/ Processing/ Integrity (6)	Includes/Examples: Includes light touch, pressure, temperature, pain, sharp/dull, proprioception, vestibular, visual, auditory, gustatory, and olfactory
Short Increment Sensitivity Index (9)	Measures the ear's ability to detect small intensity changes; site of lesion test requiring a behavioral response
Sinusoidal Vertical Axis Rotational (4)	Measures nystagmus following rotation
Somatosensory Evoked Potentials (9)	Measures neural activity from sites throughout the body
Speech/Language Screening (6)	Identifies need for further speech and/or language evaluation
Speech Threshold (1)	Measures minimal intensity needed to repeat spondaic words

Continued on next page

Section F–Physical Rehabilitation and Diagnostic Audiology

Continued from previous page

ICD-10-PCS Value Qualifier (Character 5)	Definition
Speech-Language Pathology and Related Disorders Counseling (1)	Provides patients/families with information, support, referrals to facilitate recovery from a communication disorder
Speech-Language Pathology and Related Disorders Prevention (2)	Applying techniques to avoid or minimize onset and/or development of a communication disorder
Speech/Word Recognition (2)	Measures ability to repeat/identify single syllable words; scores given as a percentage; includes word recognition/speech discrimination
Staggered Spondaic Word (3)	Measures central auditory processing site of lesion based upon dichotic presentation of spondaic words
Static Orthosis (7)	Includes/Examples: Includes customized and prefabricated splints, inhibitory casts, spinal and other braces, and protective devices; has no moving parts, maintains joint(s) in desired position
Stenger (B)	Measures unilateral nonorganic hearing loss based on simultaneous presentation of signals of differing volume
Swallowing Dysfunction (D)	Activities to improve swallowing function in coordination with respiratory function Includes/Examples: Includes function and coordination of sucking, mastication, coughing, swallowing
Synthetic Sentence Identification (5)	Measures central auditory dysfunction using identification of third order approximations of sentences and competing messages
Temporal Ordering of Stimuli (V)	Measures specific central auditory process
Therapeutic Exercise (6)	Exercise or activities to facilitate sensory awareness, sensory processing, sensory integration, balance training, conditioning, reconditioning Includes/Examples: Includes developmental activities, breathing exercises, aerobic endurance activities, aquatic exercises, stretching and ventilatory muscle training
Tinnitus Masker (Assessment) (7)	Determines candidacy for tinnitus masker
Tinnitus Masker (Treatment) (Ø)	Explanation: Used to verify physical fit, acoustic appropriateness, and benefit; assists in achieving maximum benefit
Tone Decay (8)	Measures decrease in hearing sensitivity to a tone; site of lesion test requiring a behavioral response
Transfer (C)	Transitional movement from one surface to another
Transfer Training (8)	Exercise or activities to facilitate movement from one surface to another
Tympanometry (D)	Measures the integrity of the middle ear; measures ease at which sound flows through the tympanic membrane while air pressure against the membrane is varied
Unithermal Binaural Screen (2)	Measures the rhythmic eye movements stimulated by changing the temperature of the vestibular system in both ears using warm water, screening format
Ventilation/Respiration/Circulation (G)	Measures ventilatory muscle strength, power and endurance, pulmonary function and ventilatory mechanics Includes/Examples: Includes ability to clear airway, activities that aggravate or relieve edema, pain, dyspnea or other symptoms, chest wall mobility, cardiopulmonary response to performance of ADL and IAD, cough and sputum, standard vital signs
Vestibular (Ø)	Applying techniques to compensate for balance disorders; includes habituation, exercise therapy, and balance retraining
Visual Motor Integration (Assessment) (2)	Coordinating the interaction of information from the eyes with body movement during activity
Visual Motor Integration (Treatment) (2)	Exercise or activities to facilitate coordinating the interaction of information from eyes with body movement during activity
Visual Reinforcement Audiometry (6)	Behavioral measures using nonspeech and speech stimuli to obtain frequency/ear-specific information on auditory status Includes/Examples: Includes a conditioned response of looking toward a visual reinforcer (e.g., lights, animated toy) every time auditory stimuli are heard
Vocational Activities and Functional Community or Work Reintegration Skills (Assessment) (H)	Measures environmental, home, work (job/school/play) barriers that keep patients from functioning optimally in their environment Includes/Examples: Includes assessment of vocational skills and interests, environment of work (job/school/play), injury potential and injury prevention or reduction, ergonomic stressors, transportation skills, and ability to access and use community resources

Continued on next page

Section F–Physical Rehabilitation and Diagnostic Audiology

Continued from previous page

ICD-10-PCS Value Qualifier (Character 5)	Definition
Vocational Activities and Functional Community or Work Reintegration Skills (Treatment) (7)	Activities to facilitate vocational exploration, body mechanics training, job acquisition, and environmental or work (job/school/play) task adaptation Includes/Examples: Includes injury prevention and reduction, ergonomic stressor reduction, job coaching and simulation, work hardening and conditioning, driving training, transportation skills, and use of community resources
Voice (Assessment) (F)	Measures vocal structure, function and production
Voice (Treatment) (C)	Applying techniques to improve voice and vocal function
Voice Prosthetic (Assessment) (M)	Determines the appropriateness of voice prosthetic/adaptive device to enhance or facilitate communication
Voice Prosthetic (Treatment) (4)	Includes/Examples: Includes electrolarynx, and other assistive, adaptive, supportive devices
Wheelchair Mobility (Assessment) (F)	Measures fit and functional abilities within wheelchair in a variety of environments
Wheelchair Mobility (Treatment) (4)	Management, maintenance and controlled operation of a wheelchair, scooter or other device, in and on a variety of surfaces and environments
Wound Management (5)	Includes/Examples: Includes non-selective and selective debridement (enzymes, autolysis, sharp debridement), dressings (wound coverings, hydrogel, vacuum-assisted closure), topical agents, etc.

Section G–Mental Health

ICD-10-PCS Value (Character 3)	Definition
Biofeedback (C)	Provision of information from the monitoring and regulating of physiological processes in conjunction with cognitive-behavioral techniques to improve patient functioning or well-being Includes/Examples: Includes EEG, blood pressure, skin temperature or peripheral blood flow, ECG, electrooculogram, EMG, respirometry or capnometry, GSR/EDR, perineometry to monitor/regulate bowel/bladder activity, electrogastrogram to monitor/regulate gastric motility
Counseling (6)	The application of psychological methods to treat an individual with normal developmental issues and psychological problems in order to increase function, improve well-being, alleviate distress, maladjustment or resolve crises
Crisis Intervention (2)	Treatment of a traumatized, acutely disturbed or distressed individual for the purpose of short-term stabilization Includes/Examples: Includes defusing, debriefing, counseling, psychotherapy and/or coordination of care with other providers or agencies
Electroconvulsive Therapy (B)	The application of controlled electrical voltages to treat a mental health disorder Includes/Examples: Includes appropriate sedation and other preparation of the individual
Family Psychotherapy (7)	Treatment that includes one or more family members of an individual with a mental health disorder by behavioral, cognitive, psychoanalytic, psychodynamic or psychophysiological means to improve functioning or well-being Explanation: Remediation of emotional or behavioral problems presented by one or more family members in cases where psychotherapy with more than one family member is indicated
Group Psychotherapy (H)	Treatment of two or more individuals with a mental health disorder by behavioral, cognitive, psychoanalytic, psychodynamic or psychophysiological means to improve functioning or well-being
Hypnosis (F)	Induction of a state of heightened suggestibility by auditory, visual and tactile techniques to elicit an emotional or behavioral response
Individual Psychotherapy (5)	Treatment of an individual with a mental health disorder by behavioral, cognitive, psychoanalytic, psychodynamic or psychophysiological means to improve functioning or well-being
Light Therapy (J)	Application of specialized light treatments to improve functioning or well-being
Medication Management (3)	Monitoring and adjusting the use of medications for the treatment of a mental health disorder
Narcosynthesis (G)	Administration of intravenous barbiturates in order to release suppressed or repressed thoughts
Psychological Tests (1)	The administration and interpretation of standardized psychological tests and measurement instruments for the assessment of psychological function

Continued on next page

Section G–Mental Health

ICD-10-PCS Value Qualifier (Character 4)	Definition
Behavioral (1)	Primarily to modify behavior Includes/Examples: Includes modeling and role playing, positive reinforcement of target behaviors, response cost, and training of self-management skills
Cognitive (2)	Primarily to correct cognitive distortions and errors
Cognitive-Behavioral (8)	Combining cognitive and behavioral treatment strategies to improve functioning Explanation: Maladaptive responses are examined to determine how cognitions relate to behavior patterns in response to an event. Uses learning principles and information-processing models.
Developmental (Ø)	Age-normed developmental status of cognitive, social and adaptive behavior skills
Intellectual and Psychoeducational (2)	Intellectual abilities, academic achievement and learning capabilities (including behaviors and emotional factors affecting learning)
Interactive (Ø)	Uses primarily physical aids and other forms of non-oral interaction with a patient who is physically, psychologically or developmentally unable to use ordinary language for communication Includes/Examples: Includes the use of toys in symbolic play
Interpersonal (3)	Helps an individual make changes in interpersonal behaviors to reduce psychological dysfunction Includes/Examples: Includes exploratory techniques, encouragement of affective expression, clarification of patient statements, analysis of communication patterns, use of therapy relationship and behavior change techniques
Neurobehavioral and Cognitive Status (4)	Includes neurobehavioral status exam, interview(s), and observation for the clinical assessment of thinking, reasoning and judgment, acquired knowledge, attention, memory, visual spatial abilities, language functions, and planning
Neuropsychological (3)	Thinking, reasoning and judgment, acquired knowledge, attention, memory, visual spatial abilities, language functions, planning
Personality and Behavioral (1)	Mood, emotion, behavior, social functioning, psychopathological conditions, personality traits and characteristics
Psychoanalysis (4)	Methods of obtaining a detailed account of past and present mental and emotional experiences to determine the source and eliminate or diminish the undesirable effects of unconscious conflicts Explanation: Accomplished by making the individual aware of their existence, origin, and inappropriate expression in emotions and behavior
Psychodynamic (5)	Exploration of past and present emotional experiences to understand motives and drives using insight-oriented techniques to reduce the undesirable effects of internal conflicts on emotions and behavior Explanation: Techniques include empathetic listening, clarifying self-defeating behavior patterns, and exploring adaptive alternatives
Psychophysiological (9)	Monitoring and alteration of physiological processes to help the individual associate physiological reactions combined with cognitive and behavioral strategies to gain improved control of these processes to help the individual cope more effectively
Supportive (6)	Formation of therapeutic relationship primarily for providing emotional support to prevent further deterioration in functioning during periods of particular stress Explanation: Often used in conjunction with other therapeutic approaches
Vocational (1)	Exploration of vocational interests, aptitudes and required adaptive behavior skills to develop and carry out a plan for achieving a successful vocational placement Includes/Examples: Includes enhancing work related adjustment and/or pursuing viable options in training education or preparation

Section H–Substance Abuse Treatment

ICD-10-PCS Value (Character 3)	Definition
Detoxification Services (2)	Detoxification from alcohol and/or drugs Explanation: Not a treatment modality, but helps the patient stabilize physically and psychologically until the body becomes free of drugs and the effects of alcohol
Family Counseling (6)	The application of psychological methods that includes one or more family members to treat an individual with addictive behavior Explanation: Provides support and education for family members of addicted individuals. Family member participation is seen as a critical area of substance abuse treatment.
Group Counseling (4)	The application of psychological methods to treat two or more individuals with addictive behavior Explanation: Provides structured group counseling sessions and healing power through the connection with others
Individual Counseling (3)	The application of psychological methods to treat an individual wlth addictive behavior Explanation: Comprised of several different techniques, which apply various strategies to address drug addiction
Individual Psychotherapy (5)	Treatment of an individual with addictive behavior by behavioral, cognitive, psychoanalytic, psychodynamic or psychophysiological means
Medication Management (8)	Monitoring and adjusting the use of replacement medications for the treatment of addiction
Pharmacotherapy (9)	The use of replacement medications for the treatment of addiction

Appendix K: Hospital Acquired Conditions

Hospital acquired conditions (HACs) are conditions considered reasonably preventable through the application of evidence-based guidelines. Although it is the ICD-10-CM diagnosis code that drives a HAC designation, in some cases a specific ICD-10-PCS procedure code must also be present before that diagnosis code can be considered a HAC. This resource provides only those HAC categories that require both an ICD-10-PCS code and an ICD-10-CM diagnosis code. The official descriptions for each code are also provided. To see all 14 HAC categories and their corresponding codes, refer to Optum360's *ICD-10-CM Expert for Hospitals*.

Note: The resource used to compile this list is the proposed, version 38, MS-DRG Grouper software and Definitions Manual files published with the fiscal 2021 IPPS proposed rule. For the final, version 38, MS-DRG Grouper software and Definitions Manual files, refer to the following: https://www.cms.gov/Medicare/Medicare-Fee-for-Service-Payment/AcuteInpatientPPS/MS-DRG-Classifications-and-Software.

HAC 08: Surgical Site Infection of Mediastinitis After Coronary Bypass Graft (CABG) Procedures

Secondary diagnosis not POA:

J98.51 Mediastinitis
J98.59 Other diseases of mediastinum, not elsewhere classified

AND

Any of the following procedures:

0210083 Bypass Coronary Artery, One Artery from Coronary Artery with Zooplastic Tissue, Open Approach
0210088 Bypass Coronary Artery, One Artery from Right Internal Mammary with Zooplastic Tissue, Open Approach
0210089 Bypass Coronary Artery, One Artery from Left Internal Mammary with Zooplastic Tissue, Open Approach
021008C Bypass Coronary Artery, One Artery from Thoracic Artery with Zooplastic Tissue, Open Approach
021008F Bypass Coronary Artery, One Artery from Abdominal Artery with Zooplastic Tissue, Open Approach
021008W Bypass Coronary Artery, One Artery from Aorta with Zooplastic Tissue, Open Approach
0210093 Bypass Coronary Artery, One Artery from Coronary Artery with Autologous Venous Tissue, Open Approach
0210098 Bypass Coronary Artery, One Artery from Right Internal Mammary with Autologous Venous Tissue, Open Approach
0210099 Bypass Coronary Artery, One Artery from Left Internal Mammary with Autologous Venous Tissue, Open Approach
021009C Bypass Coronary Artery, One Artery from Thoracic Artery with Autologous Venous Tissue, Open Approach
021009F Bypass Coronary Artery, One Artery from Abdominal Artery with Autologous Venous Tissue, Open Approach
021009W Bypass Coronary Artery, One Artery from Aorta with Autologous Venous Tissue, Open Approach
02100A3 Bypass Coronary Artery, One Artery from Coronary Artery with Autologous Arterial Tissue, Open Approach
02100A8 Bypass Coronary Artery, One Artery from Right Internal Mammary with Autologous Arterial Tissue, Open Approach
02100A9 Bypass Coronary Artery, One Artery from Left Internal Mammary with Autologous Arterial Tissue, Open Approach
02100AC Bypass Coronary Artery, One Artery from Thoracic Artery with Autologous Arterial Tissue, Open Approach
02100AF Bypass Coronary Artery, One Artery from Abdominal Artery with Autologous Arterial Tissue, Open Approach
02100AW Bypass Coronary Artery, One Artery from Aorta with Autologous Arterial Tissue, Open Approach
02100J3 Bypass Coronary Artery, One Artery from Coronary Artery with Synthetic Substitute, Open Approach
02100J8 Bypass Coronary Artery, One Artery from Right Internal Mammary with Synthetic Substitute, Open Approach
02100J9 Bypass Coronary Artery, One Artery from Left Internal Mammary with Synthetic Substitute, Open Approach
02100JC Bypass Coronary Artery, One Artery from Thoracic Artery with Synthetic Substitute, Open Approach
02100JF Bypass Coronary Artery, One Artery from Abdominal Artery with Synthetic Substitute, Open Approach
02100JW Bypass Coronary Artery, One Artery from Aorta with Synthetic Substitute, Open Approach
02100K3 Bypass Coronary Artery, One Artery from Coronary Artery with Nonautologous Tissue Substitute, Open Approach
02100K8 Bypass Coronary Artery, One Artery from Right Internal Mammary with Nonautologous Tissue Substitute, Open Approach
02100K9 Bypass Coronary Artery, One Artery from Left Internal Mammary with Nonautologous Tissue Substitute, Open Approach
02100KC Bypass Coronary Artery, One Artery from Thoracic Artery with Nonautologous Tissue Substitute, Open Approach
02100KF Bypass Coronary Artery, One Artery from Abdominal Artery with Nonautologous Tissue Substitute, Open Approach
02100KW Bypass Coronary Artery, One Artery from Aorta with Nonautologous Tissue Substitute, Open Approach
02100Z3 Bypass Coronary Artery, One Artery from Coronary Artery, Open Approach
02100Z8 Bypass Coronary Artery, One Artery from Right Internal Mammary, Open Approach
02100Z9 Bypass Coronary Artery, One Artery from Left Internal Mammary, Open Approach
02100ZC Bypass Coronary Artery, One Artery from Thoracic Artery, Open Approach
02100ZF Bypass Coronary Artery, One Artery from Abdominal Artery, Open Approach
0210483 Bypass Coronary Artery, One Artery from Coronary Artery with Zooplastic Tissue, Percutaneous Endoscopic Approach
0210488 Bypass Coronary Artery, One Artery from Right Internal Mammary with Zooplastic Tissue, Percutaneous Endoscopic Approach
0210489 Bypass Coronary Artery, One Artery from Left Internal Mammary with Zooplastic Tissue, Percutaneous Endoscopic Approach
021048C Bypass Coronary Artery, One Artery from Thoracic Artery with Zooplastic Tissue, Percutaneous Endoscopic Approach
021048F Bypass Coronary Artery, One Artery from Abdominal Artery with Zooplastic Tissue, Percutaneous Endoscopic Approach
021048W Bypass Coronary Artery, One Artery from Aorta with Zooplastic Tissue, Percutaneous Endoscopic Approach
0210493 Bypass Coronary Artery, One Artery from Coronary Artery with Autologous Venous Tissue, Percutaneous Endoscopic Approach
0210498 Bypass Coronary Artery, One Artery from Right Internal Mammary with Autologous Venous Tissue, Percutaneous Endoscopic Approach
0210499 Bypass Coronary Artery, One Artery from Left Internal Mammary with Autologous Venous Tissue, Percutaneous Endoscopic Approach
021049C Bypass Coronary Artery, One Artery from Thoracic Artery with Autologous Venous Tissue, Percutaneous Endoscopic Approach
021049F Bypass Coronary Artery, One Artery from Abdominal Artery with Autologous Venous Tissue, Percutaneous Endoscopic Approach
021049W Bypass Coronary Artery, One Artery from Aorta with Autologous Venous Tissue, Percutaneous Endoscopic Approach
02104A3 Bypass Coronary Artery, One Artery from Coronary Artery with Autologous Arterial Tissue, Percutaneous Endoscopic Approach
02104A8 Bypass Coronary Artery, One Artery from Right Internal Mammary with Autologous Arterial Tissue, Percutaneous Endoscopic Approach
02104A9 Bypass Coronary Artery, One Artery from Left Internal Mammary with Autologous Arterial Tissue, Percutaneous Endoscopic Approach
02104AC Bypass Coronary Artery, One Artery from Thoracic Artery with Autologous Arterial Tissue, Percutaneous Endoscopic Approach

HAC 08: Surgical Site Infection of Mediastinitis After Coronary Bypass Graft (CABG) Procedures (continued)

Ø2104AF Bypass Coronary Artery, One Artery from Abdominal Artery with Autologous Arterial Tissue, Percutaneous Endoscopic Approach
Ø2104AW Bypass Coronary Artery, One Artery from Aorta with Autologous Arterial Tissue, Percutaneous Endoscopic Approach
Ø2104J3 Bypass Coronary Artery, One Artery from Coronary Artery with Synthetic Substitute, Percutaneous Endoscopic Approach
Ø2104J8 Bypass Coronary Artery, One Artery from Right Internal Mammary with Synthetic Substitute, Percutaneous Endoscopic Approach
Ø2104J9 Bypass Coronary Artery, One Artery from Left Internal Mammary with Synthetic Substitute, Percutaneous Endoscopic Approach
Ø2104JC Bypass Coronary Artery, One Artery from Thoracic Artery with Synthetic Substitute, Percutaneous Endoscopic Approach
Ø2104JF Bypass Coronary Artery, One Artery from Abdominal Artery with Synthetic Substitute, Percutaneous Endoscopic Approach
Ø2104JW Bypass Coronary Artery, One Artery from Aorta with Synthetic Substitute, Percutaneous Endoscopic Approach
Ø2104K3 Bypass Coronary Artery, One Artery from Coronary Artery with Nonautologous Tissue Substitute, Percutaneous Endoscopic Approach
Ø2104K8 Bypass Coronary Artery, One Artery from Right Internal Mammary with Nonautologous Tissue Substitute, Percutaneous Endoscopic Approach
Ø2104K9 Bypass Coronary Artery, One Artery from Left Internal Mammary with Nonautologous Tissue Substitute, Percutaneous Endoscopic Approach
Ø2104KC Bypass Coronary Artery, One Artery from Thoracic Artery with Nonautologous Tissue Substitute, Percutaneous Endoscopic Approach
Ø2104KF Bypass Coronary Artery, One Artery from Abdominal Artery with Nonautologous Tissue Substitute, Percutaneous Endoscopic Approach
Ø2104KW Bypass Coronary Artery, One Artery from Aorta with Nonautologous Tissue Substitute, Percutaneous Endoscopic Approach
Ø2104Z3 Bypass Coronary Artery, One Artery from Coronary Artery, Percutaneous Endoscopic Approach
Ø2104Z8 Bypass Coronary Artery, One Artery from Right Internal Mammary, Percutaneous Endoscopic Approach
Ø2104Z9 Bypass Coronary Artery, One Artery from Left Internal Mammary, Percutaneous Endoscopic Approach
Ø2104ZC Bypass Coronary Artery, One Artery from Thoracic Artery, Percutaneous Endoscopic Approach
Ø2104ZF Bypass Coronary Artery, One Artery from Abdominal Artery, Percutaneous Endoscopic Approach
Ø211083 Bypass Coronary Artery, Two Arteries from Coronary Artery with Zooplastic Tissue, Open Approach
Ø211088 Bypass Coronary Artery, Two Arteries from Right Internal Mammary with Zooplastic Tissue, Open Approach
Ø211089 Bypass Coronary Artery, Two Arteries from Left Internal Mammary with Zooplastic Tissue, Open Approach
Ø21108C Bypass Coronary Artery, Two Arteries from Thoracic Artery with Zooplastic Tissue, Open Approach
Ø21108F Bypass Coronary Artery, Two Arteries from Abdominal Artery with Zooplastic Tissue, Open Approach
Ø21108W Bypass Coronary Artery, Two Arteries from Aorta with Zooplastic Tissue, Open Approach
Ø211093 Bypass Coronary Artery, Two Arteries from Coronary Artery with Autologous Venous Tissue, Open Approach
Ø211098 Bypass Coronary Artery, Two Arteries from Right Internal Mammary with Autologous Venous Tissue, Open Approach
Ø211099 Bypass Coronary Artery, Two Arteries from Left Internal Mammary with Autologous Venous Tissue, Open Approach
Ø21109C Bypass Coronary Artery, Two Arteries from Thoracic Artery with Autologous Venous Tissue, Open Approach
Ø21109F Bypass Coronary Artery, Two Arteries from Abdominal Artery with Autologous Venous Tissue, Open Approach
Ø21109W Bypass Coronary Artery, Two Arteries from Aorta with Autologous Venous Tissue, Open Approach
Ø2110A3 Bypass Coronary Artery, Two Arteries from Coronary Artery with Autologous Arterial Tissue, Open Approach
Ø2110A8 Bypass Coronary Artery, Two Arteries from Right Internal Mammary with Autologous Arterial Tissue, Open Approach
Ø2110A9 Bypass Coronary Artery, Two Arteries from Left Internal Mammary with Autologous Arterial Tissue, Open Approach
Ø2110AC Bypass Coronary Artery, Two Arteries from Thoracic Artery with Autologous Arterial Tissue, Open Approach
Ø2110AF Bypass Coronary Artery, Two Arteries from Abdominal Artery with Autologous Arterial Tissue, Open Approach
Ø2110AW Bypass Coronary Artery, Two Arteries from Aorta with Autologous Arterial Tissue, Open Approach
Ø2110J3 Bypass Coronary Artery, Two Arteries from Coronary Artery with Synthetic Substitute, Open Approach
Ø2110J8 Bypass Coronary Artery, Two Arteries from Right Internal Mammary with Synthetic Substitute, Open Approach
Ø2110J9 Bypass Coronary Artery, Two Arteries from Left Internal Mammary with Synthetic Substitute, Open Approach
Ø2110JC Bypass Coronary Artery, Two Arteries from Thoracic Artery with Synthetic Substitute, Open Approach
Ø2110JF Bypass Coronary Artery, Two Arteries from Abdominal Artery with Synthetic Substitute, Open Approach
Ø2110JW Bypass Coronary Artery, Two Arteries from Aorta with Synthetic Substitute, Open Approach
Ø2110K3 Bypass Coronary Artery, Two Arteries from Coronary Artery with Nonautologous Tissue Substitute, Open Approach
Ø2110K8 Bypass Coronary Artery, Two Arteries from Right Internal Mammary with Nonautologous Tissue Substitute, Open Approach
Ø2110K9 Bypass Coronary Artery, Two Arteries from Left Internal Mammary with Nonautologous Tissue Substitute, Open Approach
Ø2110KC Bypass Coronary Artery, Two Arteries from Thoracic Artery with Nonautologous Tissue Substitute, Open Approach
Ø2110KF Bypass Coronary Artery, Two Arteries from Abdominal Artery with Nonautologous Tissue Substitute, Open Approach
Ø2110KW Bypass Coronary Artery, Two Arteries from Aorta with Nonautologous Tissue Substitute, Open Approach
Ø2110Z3 Bypass Coronary Artery, Two Arteries from Coronary Artery, Open Approach
Ø2110Z8 Bypass Coronary Artery, Two Arteries from Right Internal Mammary, Open Approach
Ø2110Z9 Bypass Coronary Artery, Two Arteries from Left Internal Mammary, Open Approach
Ø2110ZC Bypass Coronary Artery, Two Arteries from Thoracic Artery, Open Approach
Ø2110ZF Bypass Coronary Artery, Two Arteries from Abdominal Artery, Open Approach
Ø211483 Bypass Coronary Artery, Two Arteries from Coronary Artery with Zooplastic Tissue, Percutaneous Endoscopic Approach
Ø211488 Bypass Coronary Artery, Two Arteries from Right Internal Mammary with Zooplastic Tissue, Percutaneous Endoscopic Approach
Ø211489 Bypass Coronary Artery, Two Arteries from Left Internal Mammary with Zooplastic Tissue, Percutaneous Endoscopic Approach
Ø21148C Bypass Coronary Artery, Two Arteries from Thoracic Artery with Zooplastic Tissue, Percutaneous Endoscopic Approach
Ø21148F Bypass Coronary Artery, Two Arteries from Abdominal Artery with Zooplastic Tissue, Percutaneous Endoscopic Approach
Ø21148W Bypass Coronary Artery, Two Arteries from Aorta with Zooplastic Tissue, Percutaneous Endoscopic Approach
Ø211493 Bypass Coronary Artery, Two Arteries from Coronary Artery with Autologous Venous Tissue, Percutaneous Endoscopic Approach
Ø211498 Bypass Coronary Artery, Two Arteries from Right Internal Mammary with Autologous Venous Tissue, Percutaneous Endoscopic Approach
Ø211499 Bypass Coronary Artery, Two Arteries from Left Internal Mammary with Autologous Venous Tissue, Percutaneous Endoscopic Approach
Ø21149C Bypass Coronary Artery, Two Arteries from Thoracic Artery with Autologous Venous Tissue, Percutaneous Endoscopic Approach

HAC 08: Surgical Site Infection of Mediastinitis After Coronary Bypass Graft (CABG) Procedures (continued)

Ø21149F Bypass Coronary Artery, Two Arteries from Abdominal Artery with Autologous Venous Tissue, Percutaneous Endoscopic Approach
Ø21149W Bypass Coronary Artery, Two Arteries from Aorta with Autologous Venous Tissue, Percutaneous Endoscopic Approach
Ø2114A3 Bypass Coronary Artery, Two Arteries from Coronary Artery with Autologous Arterial Tissue, Percutaneous Endoscopic Approach
Ø2114A8 Bypass Coronary Artery, Two Arteries from Right Internal Mammary with Autologous Arterial Tissue, Percutaneous Endoscopic Approach
Ø2114A9 Bypass Coronary Artery, Two Arteries from Left Internal Mammary with Autologous Arterial Tissue, Percutaneous Endoscopic Approach
Ø2114AC Bypass Coronary Artery, Two Arteries from Thoracic Artery with Autologous Arterial Tissue, Percutaneous Endoscopic Approach
Ø2114AF Bypass Coronary Artery, Two Arteries from Abdominal Artery with Autologous Arterial Tissue, Percutaneous Endoscopic Approach
Ø2114AW Bypass Coronary Artery, Two Arteries from Aorta with Autologous Arterial Tissue, Percutaneous Endoscopic Approach
Ø2114J3 Bypass Coronary Artery, Two Arteries from Coronary Artery with Synthetic Substitute, Percutaneous Endoscopic Approach
Ø2114J8 Bypass Coronary Artery, Two Arteries from Right Internal Mammary with Synthetic Substitute, Percutaneous Endoscopic Approach
Ø2114J9 Bypass Coronary Artery, Two Arteries from Left Internal Mammary with Synthetic Substitute, Percutaneous Endoscopic Approach
Ø2114JC Bypass Coronary Artery, Two Arteries from Thoracic Artery with Synthetic Substitute, Percutaneous Endoscopic Approach
Ø2114JF Bypass Coronary Artery, Two Arteries from Abdominal Artery with Synthetic Substitute, Percutaneous Endoscopic Approach
Ø2114JW Bypass Coronary Artery, Two Arteries from Aorta with Synthetic Substitute, Percutaneous Endoscopic Approach
Ø2114K3 Bypass Coronary Artery, Two Arteries from Coronary Artery with Nonautologous Tissue Substitute, Percutaneous Endoscopic Approach
Ø2114K8 Bypass Coronary Artery, Two Arteries from Right Internal Mammary with Nonautologous Tissue Substitute, Percutaneous Endoscopic Approach
Ø2114K9 Bypass Coronary Artery, Two Arteries from Left Internal Mammary with Nonautologous Tissue Substitute, Percutaneous Endoscopic Approach
Ø2114KC Bypass Coronary Artery, Two Arteries from Thoracic Artery with Nonautologous Tissue Substitute, Percutaneous Endoscopic Approach
Ø2114KF Bypass Coronary Artery, Two Arteries from Abdominal Artery with Nonautologous Tissue Substitute, Percutaneous Endoscopic Approach
Ø2114KW Bypass Coronary Artery, Two Arteries from Aorta with Nonautologous Tissue Substitute, Percutaneous Endoscopic Approach
Ø2114Z3 Bypass Coronary Artery, Two Arteries from Coronary Artery, Percutaneous Endoscopic Approach
Ø2114Z8 Bypass Coronary Artery, Two Arteries from Right Internal Mammary, Percutaneous Endoscopic Approach
Ø2114Z9 Bypass Coronary Artery, Two Arteries from Left Internal Mammary, Percutaneous Endoscopic Approach
Ø2114ZC Bypass Coronary Artery, Two Arteries from Thoracic Artery, Percutaneous Endoscopic Approach
Ø2114ZF Bypass Coronary Artery, Two Arteries from Abdominal Artery, Percutaneous Endoscopic Approach
Ø212Ø83 Bypass Coronary Artery, Three Arteries from Coronary Artery with Zooplastic Tissue, Open Approach
Ø212Ø88 Bypass Coronary Artery, Three Arteries from Right Internal Mammary with Zooplastic Tissue, Open Approach
Ø212Ø89 Bypass Coronary Artery, Three Arteries from Left Internal Mammary with Zooplastic Tissue, Open Approach
Ø212Ø8C Bypass Coronary Artery, Three Arteries from Thoracic Artery with Zooplastic Tissue, Open Approach
Ø212Ø8F Bypass Coronary Artery, Three Arteries from Abdominal Artery with Zooplastic Tissue, Open Approach
Ø212Ø8W Bypass Coronary Artery, Three Arteries from Aorta with Zooplastic Tissue, Open Approach
Ø212Ø93 Bypass Coronary Artery, Three Arteries from Coronary Artery with Autologous Venous Tissue, Open Approach
Ø212Ø98 Bypass Coronary Artery, Three Arteries from Right Internal Mammary with Autologous Venous Tissue, Open Approach
Ø212Ø99 Bypass Coronary Artery, Three Arteries from Left Internal Mammary with Autologous Venous Tissue, Open Approach
Ø212Ø9C Bypass Coronary Artery, Three Arteries from Thoracic Artery with Autologous Venous Tissue, Open Approach
Ø212Ø9F Bypass Coronary Artery, Three Arteries from Abdominal Artery with Autologous Venous Tissue, Open Approach
Ø212Ø9W Bypass Coronary Artery, Three Arteries from Aorta with Autologous Venous Tissue, Open Approach
Ø212ØA3 Bypass Coronary Artery, Three Arteries from Coronary Artery with Autologous Arterial Tissue, Open Approach
Ø212ØA8 Bypass Coronary Artery, Three Arteries from Right Internal Mammary with Autologous Arterial Tissue, Open Approach
Ø212ØA9 Bypass Coronary Artery, Three Arteries from Left Internal Mammary with Autologous Arterial Tissue, Open Approach
Ø212ØAC Bypass Coronary Artery, Three Arteries from Thoracic Artery with Autologous Arterial Tissue, Open Approach
Ø212ØAF Bypass Coronary Artery, Three Arteries from Abdominal Artery with Autologous Arterial Tissue, Open Approach
Ø212ØAW Bypass Coronary Artery, Three Arteries from Aorta with Autologous Arterial Tissue, Open Approach
Ø212ØJ3 Bypass Coronary Artery, Three Arteries from Coronary Artery with Synthetic Substitute, Open Approach
Ø212ØJ8 Bypass Coronary Artery, Three Arteries from Right Internal Mammary with Synthetic Substitute, Open Approach
Ø212ØJ9 Bypass Coronary Artery, Three Arteries from Left Internal Mammary with Synthetic Substitute, Open Approach
Ø212ØJC Bypass Coronary Artery, Three Arteries from Thoracic Artery with Synthetic Substitute, Open Approach
Ø212ØJF Bypass Coronary Artery, Three Arteries from Abdominal Artery with Synthetic Substitute, Open Approach
Ø212ØJW Bypass Coronary Artery, Three Arteries from Aorta with Synthetic Substitute, Open Approach
Ø212ØK3 Bypass Coronary Artery, Three Arteries from Coronary Artery with Nonautologous Tissue Substitute, Open Approach
Ø212ØK8 Bypass Coronary Artery, Three Arteries from Right Internal Mammary with Nonautologous Tissue Substitute, Open Approach
Ø212ØK9 Bypass Coronary Artery, Three Arteries from Left Internal Mammary with Nonautologous Tissue Substitute, Open Approach
Ø212ØKC Bypass Coronary Artery, Three Arteries from Thoracic Artery with Nonautologous Tissue Substitute, Open Approach
Ø212ØKF Bypass Coronary Artery, Three Arteries from Abdominal Artery with Nonautologous Tissue Substitute, Open Approach
Ø212ØKW Bypass Coronary Artery, Three Arteries from Aorta with Nonautologous Tissue Substitute, Open Approach
Ø212ØZ3 Bypass Coronary Artery, Three Arteries from Coronary Artery, Open Approach
Ø212ØZ8 Bypass Coronary Artery, Three Arteries from Right Internal Mammary, Open Approach
Ø212ØZ9 Bypass Coronary Artery, Three Arteries from Left Internal Mammary, Open Approach
Ø212ØZC Bypass Coronary Artery, Three Arteries from Thoracic Artery, Open Approach
Ø212ØZF Bypass Coronary Artery, Three Arteries from Abdominal Artery, Open Approach
Ø212483 Bypass Coronary Artery, Three Arteries from Coronary Artery with Zooplastic Tissue, Percutaneous Endoscopic Approach
Ø212488 Bypass Coronary Artery, Three Arteries from Right Internal Mammary with Zooplastic Tissue, Percutaneous Endoscopic Approach
Ø212489 Bypass Coronary Artery, Three Arteries from Left Internal Mammary with Zooplastic Tissue, Percutaneous Endoscopic Approach
Ø21248C Bypass Coronary Artery, Three Arteries from Thoracic Artery with Zooplastic Tissue, Percutaneous Endoscopic Approach

HAC 08: Surgical Site Infection of Mediastinitis After Coronary Bypass Graft (CABG) Procedures (continued)

Ø21248F Bypass Coronary Artery, Three Arteries from Abdominal Artery with Zooplastic Tissue, Percutaneous Endoscopic Approach
Ø21248W Bypass Coronary Artery, Three Arteries from Aorta with Zooplastic Tissue, Percutaneous Endoscopic Approach
Ø212493 Bypass Coronary Artery, Three Arteries from Coronary Artery with Autologous Venous Tissue, Percutaneous Endoscopic Approach
Ø212498 Bypass Coronary Artery, Three Arteries from Right Internal Mammary with Autologous Venous Tissue, Percutaneous Endoscopic Approach
Ø212499 Bypass Coronary Artery, Three Arteries from Left Internal Mammary with Autologous Venous Tissue, Percutaneous Endoscopic Approach
Ø21249C Bypass Coronary Artery, Three Arteries from Thoracic Artery with Autologous Venous Tissue, Percutaneous Endoscopic Approach
Ø21249F Bypass Coronary Artery, Three Arteries from Abdominal Artery with Autologous Venous Tissue, Percutaneous Endoscopic Approach
Ø21249W Bypass Coronary Artery, Three Arteries from Aorta with Autologous Venous Tissue, Percutaneous Endoscopic Approach
Ø2124A3 Bypass Coronary Artery, Three Arteries from Coronary Artery with Autologous Arterial Tissue, Percutaneous Endoscopic Approach
Ø2124A8 Bypass Coronary Artery, Three Arteries from Right Internal Mammary with Autologous Arterial Tissue, Percutaneous Endoscopic Approach
Ø2124A9 Bypass Coronary Artery, Three Arteries from Left Internal Mammary with Autologous Arterial Tissue, Percutaneous Endoscopic Approach
Ø2124AC Bypass Coronary Artery, Three Arteries from Thoracic Artery with Autologous Arterial Tissue, Percutaneous Endoscopic Approach
Ø2124AF Bypass Coronary Artery, Three Arteries from Abdominal Artery with Autologous Arterial Tissue, Percutaneous Endoscopic Approach
Ø2124AW Bypass Coronary Artery, Three Arteries from Aorta with Autologous Arterial Tissue, Percutaneous Endoscopic Approach
Ø2124J3 Bypass Coronary Artery, Three Arteries from Coronary Artery with Synthetic Substitute, Percutaneous Endoscopic Approach
Ø2124J8 Bypass Coronary Artery, Three Arteries from Right Internal Mammary with Synthetic Substitute, Percutaneous Endoscopic Approach
Ø2124J9 Bypass Coronary Artery, Three Arteries from Left Internal Mammary with Synthetic Substitute, Percutaneous Endoscopic Approach
Ø2124JC Bypass Coronary Artery, Three Arteries from Thoracic Artery with Synthetic Substitute, Percutaneous Endoscopic Approach
Ø2124JF Bypass Coronary Artery, Three Arteries from Abdominal Artery with Synthetic Substitute, Percutaneous Endoscopic Approach
Ø2124JW Bypass Coronary Artery, Three Arteries from Aorta with Synthetic Substitute, Percutaneous Endoscopic Approach
Ø2124K3 Bypass Coronary Artery, Three Arteries from Coronary Artery with Nonautologous Tissue Substitute, Percutaneous Endoscopic Approach
Ø2124K8 Bypass Coronary Artery, Three Arteries from Right Internal Mammary with Nonautologous Tissue Substitute, Percutaneous Endoscopic Approach
Ø2124K9 Bypass Coronary Artery, Three Arteries from Left Internal Mammary with Nonautologous Tissue Substitute, Percutaneous Endoscopic Approach
Ø2124KC Bypass Coronary Artery, Three Arteries from Thoracic Artery with Nonautologous Tissue Substitute, Percutaneous Endoscopic Approach
Ø2124KF Bypass Coronary Artery, Three Arteries from Abdominal Artery with Nonautologous Tissue Substitute, Percutaneous Endoscopic Approach
Ø2124KW Bypass Coronary Artery, Three Arteries from Aorta with Nonautologous Tissue Substitute, Percutaneous Endoscopic Approach
Ø2124Z3 Bypass Coronary Artery, Three Arteries from Coronary Artery, Percutaneous Endoscopic Approach
Ø2124Z8 Bypass Coronary Artery, Three Arteries from Right Internal Mammary, Percutaneous Endoscopic Approach
Ø2124Z9 Bypass Coronary Artery, Three Arteries from Left Internal Mammary, Percutaneous Endoscopic Approach
Ø2124ZC Bypass Coronary Artery, Three Arteries from Thoracic Artery, Percutaneous Endoscopic Approach
Ø2124ZF Bypass Coronary Artery, Three Arteries from Abdominal Artery, Percutaneous Endoscopic Approach
Ø213Ø83 Bypass Coronary Artery, Four or More Arteries from Coronary Artery with Zooplastic Tissue, Open Approach
Ø213Ø88 Bypass Coronary Artery, Four or More Arteries from Right Internal Mammary with Zooplastic Tissue, Open Approach
Ø213Ø89 Bypass Coronary Artery, Four or More Arteries from Left Internal Mammary with Zooplastic Tissue, Open Approach
Ø213Ø8C Bypass Coronary Artery, Four or More Arteries from Thoracic Artery with Zooplastic Tissue, Open Approach
Ø213Ø8F Bypass Coronary Artery, Four or More Arteries from Abdominal Artery with Zooplastic Tissue, Open Approach
Ø213Ø8W Bypass Coronary Artery, Four or More Arteries from Aorta with Zooplastic Tissue, Open Approach
Ø213Ø93 Bypass Coronary Artery, Four or More Arteries from Coronary Artery with Autologous Venous Tissue, Open Approach
Ø213Ø98 Bypass Coronary Artery, Four or More Arteries from Right Internal Mammary with Autologous Venous Tissue, Open Approach
Ø213Ø99 Bypass Coronary Artery, Four or More Arteries from Left Internal Mammary with Autologous Venous Tissue, Open Approach
Ø213Ø9C Bypass Coronary Artery, Four or More Arteries from Thoracic Artery with Autologous Venous Tissue, Open Approach
Ø213Ø9F Bypass Coronary Artery, Four or More Arteries from Abdominal Artery with Autologous Venous Tissue, Open Approach
Ø213Ø9W Bypass Coronary Artery, Four or More Arteries from Aorta with Autologous Venous Tissue, Open Approach
Ø213ØA3 Bypass Coronary Artery, Four or More Arteries from Coronary Artery with Autologous Arterial Tissue, Open Approach
Ø213ØA8 Bypass Coronary Artery, Four or More Arteries from Right Internal Mammary with Autologous Arterial Tissue, Open Approach
Ø213ØA9 Bypass Coronary Artery, Four or More Arteries from Left Internal Mammary with Autologous Arterial Tissue, Open Approach
Ø213ØAC Bypass Coronary Artery, Four or More Arteries from Thoracic Artery with Autologous Arterial Tissue, Open Approach
Ø213ØAF Bypass Coronary Artery, Four or More Arteries from Abdominal Artery with Autologous Arterial Tissue, Open Approach
Ø213ØAW Bypass Coronary Artery, Four or More Arteries from Aorta with Autologous Arterial Tissue, Open Approach
Ø213ØJ3 Bypass Coronary Artery, Four or More Arteries from Coronary Artery with Synthetic Substitute, Open Approach
Ø213ØJ8 Bypass Coronary Artery, Four or More Arteries from Right Internal Mammary with Synthetic Substitute, Open Approach
Ø213ØJ9 Bypass Coronary Artery, Four or More Arteries from Left Internal Mammary with Synthetic Substitute, Open Approach
Ø213ØJC Bypass Coronary Artery, Four or More Arteries from Thoracic Artery with Synthetic Substitute, Open Approach
Ø213ØJF Bypass Coronary Artery, Four or More Arteries from Abdominal Artery with Synthetic Substitute, Open Approach
Ø213ØJW Bypass Coronary Artery, Four or More Arteries from Aorta with Synthetic Substitute, Open Approach
Ø213ØK3 Bypass Coronary Artery, Four or More Arteries from Coronary Artery with Nonautologous Tissue Substitute, Open Approach
Ø213ØK8 Bypass Coronary Artery, Four or More Arteries from Right Internal Mammary with Nonautologous Tissue Substitute, Open Approach
Ø213ØK9 Bypass Coronary Artery, Four or More Arteries from Left Internal Mammary with Nonautologous Tissue Substitute, Open Approach
Ø213ØKC Bypass Coronary Artery, Four or More Arteries from Thoracic Artery with Nonautologous Tissue Substitute, Open Approach
Ø213ØKF Bypass Coronary Artery, Four or More Arteries from Abdominal Artery with Nonautologous Tissue Substitute, Open Approach

HAC 08: Surgical Site Infection of Mediastinitis After Coronary Bypass Graft (CABG) Procedures (continued)

Ø2130KW Bypass Coronary Artery, Four or More Arteries from Aorta with Nonautologous Tissue Substitute, Open Approach
Ø2130Z3 Bypass Coronary Artery, Four or More Arteries from Coronary Artery, Open Approach
Ø2130Z8 Bypass Coronary Artery, Four or More Arteries from Right Internal Mammary, Open Approach
Ø2130Z9 Bypass Coronary Artery, Four or More Arteries from Left Internal Mammary, Open Approach
Ø2130ZC Bypass Coronary Artery, Four or More Arteries from Thoracic Artery, Open Approach
Ø2130ZF Bypass Coronary Artery, Four or More Arteries from Abdominal Artery, Open Approach
Ø213483 Bypass Coronary Artery, Four or More Arteries from Coronary Artery with Zooplastic Tissue, Percutaneous Endoscopic Approach
Ø213488 Bypass Coronary Artery, Four or More Arteries from Right Internal Mammary with Zooplastic Tissue, Percutaneous Endoscopic Approach
Ø213489 Bypass Coronary Artery, Four or More Arteries from Left Internal Mammary with Zooplastic Tissue, Percutaneous Endoscopic Approach
Ø21348C Bypass Coronary Artery, Four or More Arteries from Thoracic Artery with Zooplastic Tissue, Percutaneous Endoscopic Approach
Ø21348F Bypass Coronary Artery, Four or More Arteries from Abdominal Artery with Zooplastic Tissue, Percutaneous Endoscopic Approach
Ø21348W Bypass Coronary Artery, Four or More Arteries from Aorta with Zooplastic Tissue, Percutaneous Endoscopic Approach
Ø213493 Bypass Coronary Artery, Four or More Arteries from Coronary Artery with Autologous Venous Tissue, Percutaneous Endoscopic Approach
Ø213498 Bypass Coronary Artery, Four or More Arteries from Right Internal Mammary with Autologous Venous Tissue, Percutaneous Endoscopic Approach
Ø213499 Bypass Coronary Artery, Four or More Arteries from Left Internal Mammary with Autologous Venous Tissue, Percutaneous Endoscopic Approach
Ø21349C Bypass Coronary Artery, Four or More Arteries from Thoracic Artery with Autologous Venous Tissue, Percutaneous Endoscopic Approach
Ø21349F Bypass Coronary Artery, Four or More Arteries from Abdominal Artery with Autologous Venous Tissue, Percutaneous Endoscopic Approach
Ø21349W Bypass Coronary Artery, Four or More Arteries from Aorta with Autologous Venous Tissue, Percutaneous Endoscopic Approach
Ø2134A3 Bypass Coronary Artery, Four or More Arteries from Coronary Artery with Autologous Arterial Tissue, Percutaneous Endoscopic Approach
Ø2134A8 Bypass Coronary Artery, Four or More Arteries from Right Internal Mammary with Autologous Arterial Tissue, Percutaneous Endoscopic Approach
Ø2134A9 Bypass Coronary Artery, Four or More Arteries from Left Internal Mammary with Autologous Arterial Tissue, Percutaneous Endoscopic Approach
Ø2134AC Bypass Coronary Artery, Four or More Arteries from Thoracic Artery with Autologous Arterial Tissue, Percutaneous Endoscopic Approach
Ø2134AF Bypass Coronary Artery, Four or More Arteries from Abdominal Artery with Autologous Arterial Tissue, Percutaneous Endoscopic Approach
Ø2134AW Bypass Coronary Artery, Four or More Arteries from Aorta with Autologous Arterial Tissue, Percutaneous Endoscopic Approach
Ø2134J3 Bypass Coronary Artery, Four or More Arteries from Coronary Artery with Synthetic Substitute, Percutaneous Endoscopic Approach
Ø2134J8 Bypass Coronary Artery, Four or More Arteries from Right Internal Mammary with Synthetic Substitute, Percutaneous Endoscopic Approach
Ø2134J9 Bypass Coronary Artery, Four or More Arteries from Left Internal Mammary with Synthetic Substitute, Percutaneous Endoscopic Approach
Ø2134JC Bypass Coronary Artery, Four or More Arteries from Thoracic Artery with Synthetic Substitute, Percutaneous Endoscopic Approach
Ø2134JF Bypass Coronary Artery, Four or More Arteries from Abdominal Artery with Synthetic Substitute, Percutaneous Endoscopic Approach
Ø2134JW Bypass Coronary Artery, Four or More Arteries from Aorta with Synthetic Substitute, Percutaneous Endoscopic Approach
Ø2134K3 Bypass Coronary Artery, Four or More Arteries from Coronary Artery with Nonautologous Tissue Substitute, Percutaneous Endoscopic Approach
Ø2134K8 Bypass Coronary Artery, Four or More Arteries from Right Internal Mammary with Nonautologous Tissue Substitute, Percutaneous Endoscopic Approach
Ø2134K9 Bypass Coronary Artery, Four or More Arteries from Left Internal Mammary with Nonautologous Tissue Substitute, Percutaneous Endoscopic Approach
Ø2134KC Bypass Coronary Artery, Four or More Arteries from Thoracic Artery with Nonautologous Tissue Substitute, Percutaneous Endoscopic Approach
Ø2134KF Bypass Coronary Artery, Four or More Arteries from Abdominal Artery with Nonautologous Tissue Substitute, Percutaneous Endoscopic Approach
Ø2134KW Bypass Coronary Artery, Four or More Arteries from Aorta with Nonautologous Tissue Substitute, Percutaneous Endoscopic Approach
Ø2134Z3 Bypass Coronary Artery, Four or More Arteries from Coronary Artery, Percutaneous Endoscopic Approach
Ø2134Z8 Bypass Coronary Artery, Four or More Arteries from Right Internal Mammary, Percutaneous Endoscopic Approach
Ø2134Z9 Bypass Coronary Artery, Four or More Arteries from Left Internal Mammary, Percutaneous Endoscopic Approach
Ø2134ZC Bypass Coronary Artery, Four or More Arteries from Thoracic Artery, Percutaneous Endoscopic Approach
Ø2134ZF Bypass Coronary Artery, Four or More Arteries from Abdominal Artery, Percutaneous Endoscopic Approach

HAC 10: Deep Vein Thrombosis (DVT) or Pulmonary Embolism (PE) with Total Knee or Hip Replacement

Secondary diagnosis not POA:

I26.Ø2 Saddle embolus of pulmonary artery with acute cor pulmonale
I26.Ø9 Other pulmonary embolism with acute cor pulmonale
I26.92 Saddle embolus of pulmonary artery without acute cor pulmonale
I26.93 Single subsegmental pulmonary embolism without acute cor pulmonale
I26.94 Multiple subsegmental pulmonary emboli without acute cor pulmonale
I26.99 Other pulmonary embolism without acute cor pulmonale
I82.4Ø1 Acute embolism and thrombosis of unspecified deep veins of right lower extremity
I82.4Ø2 Acute embolism and thrombosis of unspecified deep veins of left lower extremity
I82.4Ø3 Acute embolism and thrombosis of unspecified deep veins of lower extremity, bilateral
I82.4Ø9 Acute embolism and thrombosis of unspecified deep veins of unspecified lower extremity
I82.411 Acute embolism and thrombosis of right femoral vein
I82.412 Acute embolism and thrombosis of left femoral vein
I82.413 Acute embolism and thrombosis of femoral vein, bilateral
I82.419 Acute embolism and thrombosis of unspecified femoral vein
I82.421 Acute embolism and thrombosis of right iliac vein
I82.422 Acute embolism and thrombosis of left iliac vein
I82.423 Acute embolism and thrombosis of iliac vein, bilateral
I82.429 Acute embolism and thrombosis of unspecified iliac vein
I82.431 Acute embolism and thrombosis of right popliteal vein
I82.432 Acute embolism and thrombosis of left popliteal vein
I82.433 Acute embolism and thrombosis of popliteal vein, bilateral
I82.439 Acute embolism and thrombosis of unspecified popliteal vein
I82.441 Acute embolism and thrombosis of right tibial vein
I82.442 Acute embolism and thrombosis of left tibial vein
I82.443 Acute embolism and thrombosis of tibial vein, bilateral
I82.449 Acute embolism and thrombosis of unspecified tibial vein
I82.451 Acute embolism and thrombosis of right peroneal vein
I82.452 Acute embolism and thrombosis of left peroneal vein
I82.453 Acute embolism and thrombosis of peroneal vein, bilateral

HAC 10: Deep Vein Thrombosis (DVT) or Pulmonary Embolism (PE) with Total Knee or Hip Replacement (continued)

I82.459 Acute embolism and thrombosis of unspecified peroneal vein
I82.491 Acute embolism and thrombosis of other specified deep vein of right lower extremity
I82.492 Acute embolism and thrombosis of other specified deep vein of left lower extremity
I82.493 Acute embolism and thrombosis of other specified deep vein of lower extremity, bilateral
I82.499 Acute embolism and thrombosis of other specified deep vein of unspecified lower extremity
I82.4Y1 Acute embolism and thrombosis of unspecified deep veins of right proximal lower extremity
I82.4Y2 Acute embolism and thrombosis of unspecified deep veins of left proximal lower extremity
I82.4Y3 Acute embolism and thrombosis of unspecified deep veins of proximal lower extremity, bilateral
I82.4Y9 Acute embolism and thrombosis of unspecified deep veins of unspecified proximal lower extremity
I82.4Z1 Acute embolism and thrombosis of unspecified deep veins of right distal lower extremity
I82.4Z2 Acute embolism and thrombosis of unspecified deep veins of left distal lower extremity
I82.4Z3 Acute embolism and thrombosis of unspecified deep veins of distal lower extremity, bilateral
I82.4Z9 Acute embolism and thrombosis of unspecified deep veins of unspecified distal lower extremity

AND

Any of the following procedures:

ØSR9Ø19 Replacement of Right Hip Joint with Metal Synthetic Substitute, Cemented, Open Approach
ØSR9Ø1A Replacement of Right Hip Joint with Metal Synthetic Substitute, Uncemented, Open Approach
ØSR9Ø1Z Replacement of Right Hip Joint with Metal Synthetic Substitute, Open Approach
ØSR9Ø29 Replacement of Right Hip Joint with Metal on Polyethylene Synthetic Substitute, Cemented, Open Approach
ØSR9Ø2A Replacement of Right Hip Joint with Metal on Polyethylene Synthetic Substitute, Uncemented, Open Approach
ØSR9Ø2Z Replacement of Right Hip Joint with Metal on Polyethylene Synthetic Substitute, Open Approach
ØSR9Ø39 Replacement of Right Hip Joint with Ceramic Synthetic Substitute, Cemented, Open Approach
ØSR9Ø3A Replacement of Right Hip Joint with Ceramic Synthetic Substitute, Uncemented, Open Approach
ØSR9Ø3Z Replacement of Right Hip Joint with Ceramic Synthetic Substitute, Open Approach
ØSR9Ø49 Replacement of Right Hip Joint with Ceramic on Polyethylene Synthetic Substitute, Cemented, Open Approach
ØSR9Ø4A Replacement of Right Hip Joint with Ceramic on Polyethylene Synthetic Substitute, Uncemented, Open Approach
ØSR9Ø4Z Replacement of Right Hip Joint with Ceramic on Polyethylene Synthetic Substitute, Open Approach
ØSR9Ø69 Replacement of Right Hip Joint with Oxidized Zirconium on Polyethylene Synthetic Substitute, Cemented, Open Approach
ØSR9Ø6A Replacement of Right Hip Joint with Oxidized Zirconium on Polyethylene Synthetic Substitute, Uncemented, Open Approach
ØSR9Ø6Z Replacement of Right Hip Joint with Oxidized Zirconium on Polyethylene Synthetic Substitute, Open Approach
ØSR9Ø7Z Replacement of Right Hip Joint with Autologous Tissue Substitute, Open Approach
ØSR9ØEZ Replacement of Right Hip Joint with Articulating Spacer, Open Approach
ØSR9ØJ9 Replacement of Right Hip Joint with Synthetic Substitute, Cemented, Open Approach
ØSR9ØJA Replacement of Right Hip Joint with Synthetic Substitute, Uncemented, Open Approach
ØSR9ØJZ Replacement of Right Hip Joint with Synthetic Substitute, Open Approach
ØSR9ØKZ Replacement of Right Hip Joint with Nonautologous Tissue Substitute, Open Approach
ØSRAØØ9 Replacement of Right Hip Joint, Acetabular Surface with Polyethylene Synthetic Substitute, Cemented, Open Approach
ØSRAØØA Replacement of Right Hip Joint, Acetabular Surface with Polyethylene Synthetic Substitute, Uncemented, Open Approach
ØSRAØØZ Replacement of Right Hip Joint, Acetabular Surface with Polyethylene Synthetic Substitute, Open Approach
ØSRAØ19 Replacement of Right Hip Joint, Acetabular Surface with Metal Synthetic Substitute, Cemented, Open Approach
ØSRAØ1A Replacement of Right Hip Joint, Acetabular Surface with Metal Synthetic Substitute, Uncemented, Open Approach
ØSRAØ1Z Replacement of Right Hip Joint, Acetabular Surface with Metal Synthetic Substitute, Open Approach
ØSRAØ39 Replacement of Right Hip Joint, Acetabular Surface with Ceramic Synthetic Substitute, Cemented, Open Approach
ØSRAØ3A Replacement of Right Hip Joint, Acetabular Surface with Ceramic Synthetic Substitute, Uncemented, Open Approach
ØSRAØ3Z Replacement of Right Hip Joint, Acetabular Surface with Ceramic Synthetic Substitute, Open Approach
ØSRAØ7Z Replacement of Right Hip Joint, Acetabular Surface with Autologous Tissue Substitute, Open Approach
ØSRAØJ9 Replacement of Right Hip Joint, Acetabular Surface with Synthetic Substitute, Cemented, Open Approach
ØSRAØJA Replacement of Right Hip Joint, Acetabular Surface with Synthetic Substitute, Uncemented, Open Approach
ØSRAØJZ Replacement of Right Hip Joint, Acetabular Surface with Synthetic Substitute, Open Approach
ØSRAØKZ Replacement of Right Hip Joint, Acetabular Surface with Nonautologous Tissue Substitute, Open Approach
ØSRBØ19 Replacement of Left Hip Joint with Metal Synthetic Substitute, Cemented, Open Approach
ØSRBØ1A Replacement of Left Hip Joint with Metal Synthetic Substitute, Uncemented, Open Approach
ØSRBØ1Z Replacement of Left Hip Joint with Metal Synthetic Substitute, Open Approach
ØSRBØ29 Replacement of Left Hip Joint with Metal on Polyethylene Synthetic Substitute, Cemented, Open Approach
ØSRBØ2A Replacement of Left Hip Joint with Metal on Polyethylene Synthetic Substitute, Uncemented, Open Approach
ØSRBØ2Z Replacement of Left Hip Joint with Metal on Polyethylene Synthetic Substitute, Open Approach
ØSRBØ39 Replacement of Left Hip Joint with Ceramic Synthetic Substitute, Cemented, Open Approach
ØSRBØ3A Replacement of Left Hip Joint with Ceramic Synthetic Substitute, Uncemented, Open Approach
ØSRBØ3Z Replacement of Left Hip Joint with Ceramic Synthetic Substitute, Open Approach
ØSRBØ49 Replacement of Left Hip Joint with Ceramic on Polyethylene Synthetic Substitute, Cemented, Open Approach
ØSRBØ4A Replacement of Left Hip Joint with Ceramic on Polyethylene Synthetic Substitute, Uncemented, Open Approach
ØSRBØ4Z Replacement of Left Hip Joint with Ceramic on Polyethylene Synthetic Substitute, Open Approach
ØSRBØ69 Replacement of Left Hip Joint with Oxidized Zirconium on Polyethylene Synthetic Substitute, Cemented, Open Approach
ØSRBØ6A Replacement of Left Hip Joint with Oxidized Zirconium on Polyethylene Synthetic Substitute, Uncemented, Open Approach
ØSRBØ6Z Replacement of Left Hip Joint with Oxidized Zirconium on Polyethylene Synthetic Substitute, Open Approach
ØSRBØ7Z Replacement of Left Hip Joint with Autologous Tissue Substitute, Open Approach
ØSRBØEZ Replacement of Left Hip Joint with Articulating Spacer, Open Approach
ØSRBØJ9 Replacement of Left Hip Joint with Synthetic Substitute, Cemented, Open Approach
ØSRBØJA Replacement of Left Hip Joint with Synthetic Substitute, Uncemented, Open Approach
ØSRBØJZ Replacement of Left Hip Joint with Synthetic Substitute, Open Approach
ØSRBØKZ Replacement of Left Hip Joint with Nonautologous Tissue Substitute, Open Approach
ØSRCØ69 Replacement of Right Knee Joint with Oxidized Zirconium on Polyethylene Synthetic Substitute, Cemented, Open Approach

HAC 10: Deep Vein Thrombosis (DVT) or Pulmonary Embolism (PE) with Total Knee or Hip Replacement (continued)

ØSRCØ6A Replacement of Right Knee Joint with Oxidized Zirconium on Polyethylene Synthetic Substitute, Uncemented, Open Approach
ØSRCØ6Z Replacement of Right Knee Joint with Oxidized Zirconium on Polyethylene Synthetic Substitute, Open Approach
ØSRCØ7Z Replacement of Right Knee Joint with Autologous Tissue Substitute, Open Approach
ØSRCØEZ Replacement of Right Knee Joint with Articulating Spacer, Open Approach
ØSRCØJ9 Replacement of Right Knee Joint with Synthetic Substitute, Cemented, Open Approach
ØSRCØJA Replacement of Right Knee Joint with Synthetic Substitute, Uncemented, Open Approach
ØSRCØJZ Replacement of Right Knee Joint with Synthetic Substitute, Open Approach
ØSRCØKZ Replacement of Right Knee Joint with Nonautologous Tissue Substitute, Open Approach
ØSRCØL9 Replacement of Right Knee Joint with Medial Unicondylar Synthetic Substitute, Cemented, Open Approach
ØSRCØLA Replacement of Right Knee Joint with Medial Unicondylar Synthetic Substitute, Uncemented, Open Approach
ØSRCØLZ Replacement of Right Knee Joint with Medial Unicondylar Synthetic Substitute, Open Approach
ØSRCØM9 Replacement of Right Knee Joint with Lateral Unicondylar Synthetic Substitute, Cemented, Open Approach
ØSRCØMA Replacement of Right Knee Joint with Lateral Unicondylar Synthetic Substitute, Uncemented, Open Approach
ØSRCØMZ Replacement of Right Knee Joint with Lateral Unicondylar Synthetic Substitute, Open Approach
ØSRCØN9 Replacement of Right Knee Joint with Patellofemoral Synthetic Substitute, Cemented, Open Approach
ØSRCØNA Replacement of Right Knee Joint with Patellofemoral Synthetic Substitute, Uncemented, Open Approach
ØSRCØNZ Replacement of Right Knee Joint with Patellofemoral Synthetic Substitute, Open Approach
ØSRDØ69 Replacement of Left Knee Joint with Oxidized Zirconium on Polyethylene Synthetic Substitute, Cemented, Open Approach
ØSRDØ6A Replacement of Left Knee Joint with Oxidized Zirconium on Polyethylene Synthetic Substitute, Uncemented, Open Approach
ØSRDØ6Z Replacement of Left Knee Joint with Oxidized Zirconium on Polyethylene Synthetic Substitute, Open Approach
ØSRDØ7Z Replacement of Left Knee Joint with Autologous Tissue Substitute, Open Approach
ØSRDØEZ Replacement of Left Knee Joint with Articulating Spacer, Open Approach
ØSRDØJ9 Replacement of Left Knee Joint with Synthetic Substitute, Cemented, Open Approach
ØSRDØJA Replacement of Left Knee Joint with Synthetic Substitute, Uncemented, Open Approach
ØSRDØJZ Replacement of Left Knee Joint with Synthetic Substitute, Open Approach
ØSRDØKZ Replacement of Left Knee Joint with Nonautologous Tissue Substitute, Open Approach
ØSRDØL9 Replacement of Left Knee Joint with Medial Unicondylar Synthetic Substitute, Cemented, Open Approach
ØSRDØLA Replacement of Left Knee Joint with Medial Unicondylar Synthetic Substitute, Uncemented, Open Approach
ØSRDØLZ Replacement of Left Knee Joint with Medial Unicondylar Synthetic Substitute, Open Approach
ØSRDØM9 Replacement of Left Knee Joint with Lateral Unicondylar Synthetic Substitute, Cemented, Open Approach
ØSRDØMA Replacement of Left Knee Joint with Lateral Unicondylar Synthetic Substitute, Uncemented, Open Approach
ØSRDØMZ Replacement of Left Knee Joint with Lateral Unicondylar Synthetic Substitute, Open Approach
ØSRDØN9 Replacement of Left Knee Joint with Patellofemoral Synthetic Substitute, Cemented, Open Approach
ØSRDØNA Replacement of Left Knee Joint with Patellofemoral Synthetic Substitute, Uncemented, Open Approach
ØSRDØNZ Replacement of Left Knee Joint with Patellofemoral Synthetic Substitute, Open Approach
ØSREØØ9 Replacement of Left Hip Joint, Acetabular Surface with Polyethylene Synthetic Substitute, Cemented, Open Approach
ØSREØØA Replacement of Left Hip Joint, Acetabular Surface with Polyethylene Synthetic Substitute, Uncemented, Open Approach
ØSREØØZ Replacement of Left Hip Joint, Acetabular Surface with Polyethylene Synthetic Substitute, Open Approach
ØSREØ19 Replacement of Left Hip Joint, Acetabular Surface with Metal Synthetic Substitute, Cemented, Open Approach
ØSREØ1A Replacement of Left Hip Joint, Acetabular Surface with Metal Synthetic Substitute, Uncemented, Open Approach
ØSREØ1Z Replacement of Left Hip Joint, Acetabular Surface with Metal Synthetic Substitute, Open Approach
ØSREØ39 Replacement of Left Hip Joint, Acetabular Surface with Ceramic Synthetic Substitute, Cemented, Open Approach
ØSREØ3A Replacement of Left Hip Joint, Acetabular Surface with Ceramic Synthetic Substitute, Uncemented, Open Approach
ØSREØ3Z Replacement of Left Hip Joint, Acetabular Surface with Ceramic Synthetic Substitute, Open Approach
ØSREØ7Z Replacement of Left Hip Joint, Acetabular Surface with Autologous Tissue Substitute, Open Approach
ØSREØJ9 Replacement of Left Hip Joint, Acetabular Surface with Synthetic Substitute, Cemented, Open Approach
ØSREØJA Replacement of Left Hip Joint, Acetabular Surface with Synthetic Substitute, Uncemented, Open Approach
ØSREØJZ Replacement of Left Hip Joint, Acetabular Surface with Synthetic Substitute, Open Approach
ØSREØKZ Replacement of Left Hip Joint, Acetabular Surface with Nonautologous Tissue Substitute, Open Approach
ØSRRØ19 Replacement of Right Hip Joint, Femoral Surface with Metal Synthetic Substitute, Cemented, Open Approach
ØSRRØ1A Replacement of Right Hip Joint, Femoral Surface with Metal Synthetic Substitute, Uncemented, Open Approach
ØSRRØ1Z Replacement of Right Hip Joint, Femoral Surface with Metal Synthetic Substitute, Open Approach
ØSRRØ39 Replacement of Right Hip Joint, Femoral Surface with Ceramic Synthetic Substitute, Cemented, Open Approach
ØSRRØ3A Replacement of Right Hip Joint, Femoral Surface with Ceramic Synthetic Substitute, Uncemented, Open Approach
ØSRRØ3Z Replacement of Right Hip Joint, Femoral Surface with Ceramic Synthetic Substitute, Open Approach
ØSRRØ7Z Replacement of Right Hip Joint, Femoral Surface with Autologous Tissue Substitute, Open Approach
ØSRRØJ9 Replacement of Right Hip Joint, Femoral Surface with Synthetic Substitute, Cemented, Open Approach
ØSRRØJA Replacement of Right Hip Joint, Femoral Surface with Synthetic Substitute, Uncemented, Open Approach
ØSRRØJZ Replacement of Right Hip Joint, Femoral Surface with Synthetic Substitute, Open Approach
ØSRRØKZ Replacement of Right Hip Joint, Femoral Surface with Nonautologous Tissue Substitute, Open Approach
ØSRSØ19 Replacement of Left Hip Joint, Femoral Surface with Metal Synthetic Substitute, Cemented, Open Approach
ØSRSØ1A Replacement of Left Hip Joint, Femoral Surface with Metal Synthetic Substitute, Uncemented, Open Approach
ØSRSØ1Z Replacement of Left Hip Joint, Femoral Surface with Metal Synthetic Substitute, Open Approach
ØSRSØ39 Replacement of Left Hip Joint, Femoral Surface with Ceramic Synthetic Substitute, Cemented, Open Approach
ØSRSØ3A Replacement of Left Hip Joint, Femoral Surface with Ceramic Synthetic Substitute, Uncemented, Open Approach
ØSRSØ3Z Replacement of Left Hip Joint, Femoral Surface with Ceramic Synthetic Substitute, Open Approach
ØSRSØ7Z Replacement of Left Hip Joint, Femoral Surface with Autologous Tissue Substitute, Open Approach
ØSRSØJ9 Replacement of Left Hip Joint, Femoral Surface with Synthetic Substitute, Cemented, Open Approach
ØSRSØJA Replacement of Left Hip Joint, Femoral Surface with Synthetic Substitute, Uncemented, Open Approach
ØSRSØJZ Replacement of Left Hip Joint, Femoral Surface with Synthetic Substitute, Open Approach

HAC 10: Deep Vein Thrombosis (DVT) or Pulmonary Embolism (PE) with Total Knee or Hip Replacement (continued)

ØSRSØKZ Replacement of Left Hip Joint, Femoral Surface with Nonautologous Tissue Substitute, Open Approach
ØSRTØ7Z Replacement of Right Knee Joint, Femoral Surface with Autologous Tissue Substitute, Open Approach
ØSRTØJ9 Replacement of Right Knee Joint, Femoral Surface with Synthetic Substitute, Cemented, Open Approach
ØSRTØJA Replacement of Right Knee Joint, Femoral Surface with Synthetic Substitute, Uncemented, Open Approach
ØSRTØJZ Replacement of Right Knee Joint, Femoral Surface with Synthetic Substitute, Open Approach
ØSRTØKZ Replacement of Right Knee Joint, Femoral Surface with Nonautologous Tissue Substitute, Open Approach
ØSRUØ7Z Replacement of Left Knee Joint, Femoral Surface with Autologous Tissue Substitute, Open Approach
ØSRUØJ9 Replacement of Left Knee Joint, Femoral Surface with Synthetic Substitute, Cemented, Open Approach
ØSRUØJA Replacement of Left Knee Joint, Femoral Surface with Synthetic Substitute, Uncemented, Open Approach
ØSRUØJZ Replacement of Left Knee Joint, Femoral Surface with Synthetic Substitute, Open Approach
ØSRUØKZ Replacement of Left Knee Joint, Femoral Surface with Nonautologous Tissue Substitute, Open Approach
ØSRVØ7Z Replacement of Right Knee Joint, Tibial Surface with Autologous Tissue Substitute, Open Approach
ØSRVØJ9 Replacement of Right Knee Joint, Tibial Surface with Synthetic Substitute, Cemented, Open Approach
ØSRVØJA Replacement of Right Knee Joint, Tibial Surface with Synthetic Substitute, Uncemented, Open Approach
ØSRVØJZ Replacement of Right Knee Joint, Tibial Surface with Synthetic Substitute, Open Approach
ØSRVØKZ Replacement of Right Knee Joint, Tibial Surface with Nonautologous Tissue Substitute, Open Approach
ØSRWØ7Z Replacement of Left Knee Joint, Tibial Surface with Autologous Tissue Substitute, Open Approach
ØSRWØJ9 Replacement of Left Knee Joint, Tibial Surface with Synthetic Substitute, Cemented, Open Approach
ØSRWØJA Replacement of Left Knee Joint, Tibial Surface with Synthetic Substitute, Uncemented, Open Approach
ØSRWØJZ Replacement of Left Knee Joint, Tibial Surface with Synthetic Substitute, Open Approach
ØSRWØKZ Replacement of Left Knee Joint, Tibial Surface with Nonautologous Tissue Substitute, Open Approach
ØSU9ØBZ Supplement Right Hip Joint with Resurfacing Device, Open Approach
ØSUAØBZ Supplement Right Hip Joint, Acetabular Surface with Resurfacing Device, Open Approach
ØSUBØBZ Supplement Left Hip Joint with Resurfacing Device, Open Approach
ØSUEØBZ Supplement Left Hip Joint, Acetabular Surface with Resurfacing Device, Open Approach
ØSURØBZ Supplement Right Hip Joint, Femoral Surface with Resurfacing Device, Open Approach
ØSUSØBZ Supplement Left Hip Joint, Femoral Surface with Resurfacing Device, Open Approach

HAC 11: Surgical Site Infection-Bariatric Surgery

Principal diagnosis of:

E66.Ø1 Morbid (severe) obesity due to excess calories

AND

Secondary diagnosis not POA:

K68.11 Postprocedural retroperitoneal abscess
K95.Ø1 Infection due to gastric band procedure
K95.81 Infection due to other bariatric procedure
T81.40XA Infection following a procedure, unspecified, initial encounter
T81.41XA Infection following a procedure, superficial incisional surgical site, initial encounter
T81.42XA Infection following a procedure, deep incisional surgical site, initial encounter
T81.43XA Infection following a procedure, organ and space surgical site, initial encounter
T81.44XA Sepsis following a procedure, initial encounter
T81.49XA Infection following a procedure, other surgical site, initial encounter

AND

Any of the following procedures:

ØD16Ø79 Bypass Stomach to Duodenum with Autologous Tissue Substitute, Open Approach
ØD16Ø7A Bypass Stomach to Jejunum with Autologous Tissue Substitute, Open Approach
ØD16Ø7B Bypass Stomach to Ileum with Autologous Tissue Substitute, Open Approach
ØD16Ø7L Bypass Stomach to Transverse Colon with Autologous Tissue Substitute, Open Approach
ØD16ØJ9 Bypass Stomach to Duodenum with Synthetic Substitute, Open Approach
ØD16ØJA Bypass Stomach to Jejunum with Synthetic Substitute, Open Approach
ØD16ØJB Bypass Stomach to Ileum with Synthetic Substitute, Open Approach
ØD16ØJL Bypass Stomach to Transverse Colon with Synthetic Substitute, Open Approach
ØD16ØK9 Bypass Stomach to Duodenum with Nonautologous Tissue Substitute, Open Approach
ØD16ØKA Bypass Stomach to Jejunum with Nonautologous Tissue Substitute, Open Approach
ØD16ØKB Bypass Stomach to Ileum with Nonautologous Tissue Substitute, Open Approach
ØD16ØKL Bypass Stomach to Transverse Colon with Nonautologous Tissue Substitute, Open Approach
ØD16ØZ9 Bypass Stomach to Duodenum, Open Approach
ØD16ØZA Bypass Stomach to Jejunum, Open Approach
ØD16ØZB Bypass Stomach to Ileum, Open Approach
ØD16ØZL Bypass Stomach to Transverse Colon, Open Approach
ØD16479 Bypass Stomach to Duodenum with Autologous Tissue Substitute, Percutaneous Endoscopic Approach
ØD1647A Bypass Stomach to Jejunum with Autologous Tissue Substitute, Percutaneous Endoscopic Approach
ØD1647B Bypass Stomach to Ileum with Autologous Tissue Substitute, Percutaneous Endoscopic Approach
ØD1647L Bypass Stomach to Transverse Colon with Autologous Tissue Substitute, Percutaneous Endoscopic Approach
ØD164J9 Bypass Stomach to Duodenum with Synthetic Substitute, Percutaneous Endoscopic Approach
ØD164JA Bypass Stomach to Jejunum with Synthetic Substitute, Percutaneous Endoscopic Approach
ØD164JB Bypass Stomach to Ileum with Synthetic Substitute, Percutaneous Endoscopic Approach
ØD164JL Bypass Stomach to Transverse Colon with Synthetic Substitute, Percutaneous Endoscopic Approach
ØD164K9 Bypass Stomach to Duodenum with Nonautologous Tissue Substitute, Percutaneous Endoscopic Approach
ØD164KA Bypass Stomach to Jejunum with Nonautologous Tissue Substitute, Percutaneous Endoscopic Approach
ØD164KB Bypass Stomach to Ileum with Nonautologous Tissue Substitute, Percutaneous Endoscopic Approach
ØD164KL Bypass Stomach to Transverse Colon with Nonautologous Tissue Substitute, Percutaneous Endoscopic Approach
ØD164Z9 Bypass Stomach to Duodenum, Percutaneous Endoscopic Approach
ØD164ZA Bypass Stomach to Jejunum, Percutaneous Endoscopic Approach
ØD164ZB Bypass Stomach to Ileum, Percutaneous Endoscopic Approach
ØD164ZL Bypass Stomach to Transverse Colon, Percutaneous Endoscopic Approach
ØD16879 Bypass Stomach to Duodenum with Autologous Tissue Substitute, Via Natural or Artificial Opening Endoscopic
ØD1687A Bypass Stomach to Jejunum with Autologous Tissue Substitute, Via Natural or Artificial Opening Endoscopic
ØD1687B Bypass Stomach to Ileum with Autologous Tissue Substitute, Via Natural or Artificial Opening Endoscopic
ØD1687L Bypass Stomach to Transverse Colon with Autologous Tissue Substitute, Via Natural or Artificial Opening Endoscopic
ØD168J9 Bypass Stomach to Duodenum with Synthetic Substitute, Via Natural or Artificial Opening Endoscopic
ØD168JA Bypass Stomach to Jejunum with Synthetic Substitute, Via Natural or Artificial Opening Endoscopic
ØD168JB Bypass Stomach to Ileum with Synthetic Substitute, Via Natural or Artificial Opening Endoscopic
ØD168JL Bypass Stomach to Transverse Colon with Synthetic Substitute, Via Natural or Artificial Opening Endoscopic
ØD168K9 Bypass Stomach to Duodenum with Nonautologous Tissue Substitute, Via Natural or Artificial Opening Endoscopic
ØD168KA Bypass Stomach to Jejunum with Nonautologous Tissue Substitute, Via Natural or Artificial Opening Endoscopic

HAC 11: Surgical Site Infection-Bariatric Surgery (continued)

ØD168KB Bypass Stomach to Ileum with Nonautologous Tissue Substitute, Via Natural or Artificial Opening Endoscopic
ØD168KL Bypass Stomach to Transverse Colon with Nonautologous Tissue Substitute, Via Natural or Artificial Opening Endoscopic
ØD168Z9 Bypass Stomach to Duodenum, Via Natural or Artificial Opening Endoscopic
ØD168ZA Bypass Stomach to Jejunum, Via Natural or Artificial Opening Endoscopic
ØD168ZB Bypass Stomach to Ileum, Via Natural or Artificial Opening Endoscopic
ØD168ZL Bypass Stomach to Transverse Colon, Via Natural or Artificial Opening Endoscopic
ØDV64CZ Restriction of Stomach with Extraluminal Device, Percutaneous Endoscopic Approach

HAC 12: Surgical Site Infection-Certain Orthopedic Procedures of the Spine, Shoulder, and Elbow

Secondary diagnosis not POA:

K68.11 Postprocedural retroperitoneal abscess
T81.4ØXA Infection following a procedure, unspecified, initial encounter
T81.41XA Infection following a procedure, superficial incisional surgical site, initial encounter
T81.42XA Infection following a procedure, deep incisional surgical site, initial encounter
T81.43XA Infection following a procedure, organ and space surgical site, initial encounter
T81.44XA Sepsis following a procedure, initial encounter
T81.49XA Infection following a procedure, other surgical site, initial encounter
T84.6ØXA Infection and inflammatory reaction due to internal fixation device of unspecified site, initial encounter
T84.61ØA Infection and inflammatory reaction due to internal fixation device of right humerus, initial encounter
T84.611A Infection and inflammatory reaction due to internal fixation device of left humerus, initial encounter
T84.612A Infection and inflammatory reaction due to internal fixation device of right radius, initial encounter
T84.613A Infection and inflammatory reaction due to internal fixation device of left radius, initial encounter
T84.614A Infection and inflammatory reaction due to internal fixation device of right ulna, initial encounter
T84.615A Infection and inflammatory reaction due to internal fixation device of left ulna, initial encounter
T84.619A Infection and inflammatory reaction due to internal fixation device of unspecified bone of arm, initial encounter
T84.63XA Infection and inflammatory reaction due to internal fixation device of spine, initial encounter
T84.69XA Infection and inflammatory reaction due to internal fixation device of other site, initial encounter
T84.7XXA Infection and inflammatory reaction due to other internal orthopedic prosthetic devices, implants and grafts, initial encounter

AND

Any of the following procedures:

ØRGØØ7Ø Fusion of Occipital-cervical Joint with Autologous Tissue Substitute, Anterior Approach, Anterior Column, Open Approach
ØRGØØ71 Fusion of Occipital-cervical Joint with Autologous Tissue Substitute, Posterior Approach, Posterior Column, Open Approach
ØRGØØ7J Fusion of Occipital-cervical Joint with Autologous Tissue Substitute, Posterior Approach, Anterior Column, Open Approach
ØRGØØAØ Fusion of Occipital-cervical Joint with Interbody Fusion Device, Anterior Approach, Anterior Column, Open Approach
ØRGØØAJ Fusion of Occipital-cervical Joint with Interbody Fusion Device, Posterior Approach, Anterior Column, Open Approach
ØRGØØJØ Fusion of Occipital-cervical Joint with Synthetic Substitute, Anterior Approach, Anterior Column, Open Approach
ØRGØØJ1 Fusion of Occipital-cervical Joint with Synthetic Substitute, Posterior Approach, Posterior Column, Open Approach
ØRGØØJJ Fusion of Occipital-cervical Joint with Synthetic Substitute, Posterior Approach, Anterior Column, Open Approach
ØRGØØKØ Fusion of Occipital-cervical Joint with Nonautologous Tissue Substitute, Anterior Approach, Anterior Column, Open Approach
ØRGØØK1 Fusion of Occipital-cervical Joint with Nonautologous Tissue Substitute, Posterior Approach, Posterior Column, Open Approach
ØRGØØKJ Fusion of Occipital-cervical Joint with Nonautologous Tissue Substitute, Posterior Approach, Anterior Column, Open Approach
ØRGØ37Ø Fusion of Occipital-cervical Joint with Autologous Tissue Substitute, Anterior Approach, Anterior Column, Percutaneous Approach
ØRGØ371 Fusion of Occipital-cervical Joint with Autologous Tissue Substitute, Posterior Approach, Posterior Column, Percutaneous Approach
ØRGØ37J Fusion of Occipital-cervical Joint with Autologous Tissue Substitute, Posterior Approach, Anterior Column, Percutaneous Approach
ØRGØ3AØ Fusion of Occipital-cervical Joint with Interbody Fusion Device, Anterior Approach, Anterior Column, Percutaneous Approach
ØRGØ3AJ Fusion of Occipital-cervical Joint with Interbody Fusion Device, Posterior Approach, Anterior Column, Percutaneous Approach
ØRGØ3JØ Fusion of Occipital-cervical Joint with Synthetic Substitute, Anterior Approach, Anterior Column, Percutaneous Approach
ØRGØ3J1 Fusion of Occipital-cervical Joint with Synthetic Substitute, Posterior Approach, Posterior Column, Percutaneous Approach
ØRGØ3JJ Fusion of Occipital-cervical Joint with Synthetic Substitute, Posterior Approach, Anterior Column, Percutaneous Approach
ØRGØ3KØ Fusion of Occipital-cervical Joint with Nonautologous Tissue Substitute, Anterior Approach, Anterior Column, Percutaneous Approach
ØRGØ3K1 Fusion of Occipital-cervical Joint with Nonautologous Tissue Substitute, Posterior Approach, Posterior Column, Percutaneous Approach
ØRGØ3KJ Fusion of Occipital-cervical Joint with Nonautologous Tissue Substitute, Posterior Approach, Anterior Column, Percutaneous Approach
ØRGØ47Ø Fusion of Occipital-cervical Joint with Autologous Tissue Substitute, Anterior Approach, Anterior Column, Percutaneous Endoscopic Approach
ØRGØ471 Fusion of Occipital-cervical Joint with Autologous Tissue Substitute, Posterior Approach, Posterior Column, Percutaneous Endoscopic Approach
ØRGØ47J Fusion of Occipital-cervical Joint with Autologous Tissue Substitute, Posterior Approach, Anterior Column, Percutaneous Endoscopic Approach
ØRGØ4AØ Fusion of Occipital-cervical Joint with Interbody Fusion Device, Anterior Approach, Anterior Column, Percutaneous Endoscopic Approach
ØRGØ4AJ Fusion of Occipital-cervical Joint with Interbody Fusion Device, Posterior Approach, Anterior Column, Percutaneous Endoscopic Approach
ØRGØ4JØ Fusion of Occipital-cervical Joint with Synthetic Substitute, Anterior Approach, Anterior Column, Percutaneous Endoscopic Approach
ØRGØ4J1 Fusion of Occipital-cervical Joint with Synthetic Substitute, Posterior Approach, Posterior Column, Percutaneous Endoscopic Approach
ØRGØ4JJ Fusion of Occipital-cervical Joint with Synthetic Substitute, Posterior Approach, Anterior Column, Percutaneous Endoscopic Approach
ØRGØ4KØ Fusion of Occipital-cervical Joint with Nonautologous Tissue Substitute, Anterior Approach, Anterior Column, Percutaneous Endoscopic Approach
ØRGØ4K1 Fusion of Occipital-cervical Joint with Nonautologous Tissue Substitute, Posterior Approach, Posterior Column, Percutaneous Endoscopic Approach
ØRGØ4KJ Fusion of Occipital-cervical Joint with Nonautologous Tissue Substitute, Posterior Approach, Anterior Column, Percutaneous Endoscopic Approach
ØRG1Ø7Ø Fusion of Cervical Vertebral Joint with Autologous Tissue Substitute, Anterior Approach, Anterior Column, Open Approach
ØRG1Ø71 Fusion of Cervical Vertebral Joint with Autologous Tissue Substitute, Posterior Approach, Posterior Column, Open Approach
ØRG1Ø7J Fusion of Cervical Vertebral Joint with Autologous Tissue Substitute, Posterior Approach, Anterior Column, Open Approach
ØRG1ØAØ Fusion of Cervical Vertebral Joint with Interbody Fusion Device, Anterior Approach, Anterior Column, Open Approach
ØRG1ØAJ Fusion of Cervical Vertebral Joint with Interbody Fusion Device, Posterior Approach, Anterior Column, Open Approach

HAC 12: Surgical Site Infection-Certain Orthopedic Procedures of the Spine, Shoulder, and Elbow (continued)

ØRG10JØ Fusion of Cervical Vertebral Joint with Synthetic Substitute, Anterior Approach, Anterior Column, Open Approach

ØRG10J1 Fusion of Cervical Vertebral Joint with Synthetic Substitute, Posterior Approach, Posterior Column, Open Approach

ØRG10JJ Fusion of Cervical Vertebral Joint with Synthetic Substitute, Posterior Approach, Anterior Column, Open Approach

ØRG10KØ Fusion of Cervical Vertebral Joint with Nonautologous Tissue Substitute, Anterior Approach, Anterior Column, Open Approach

ØRG10K1 Fusion of Cervical Vertebral Joint with Nonautologous Tissue Substitute, Posterior Approach, Posterior Column, Open Approach

ØRG10KJ Fusion of Cervical Vertebral Joint with Nonautologous Tissue Substitute, Posterior Approach, Anterior Column, Open Approach

ØRG137Ø Fusion of Cervical Vertebral Joint with Autologous Tissue Substitute, Anterior Approach, Anterior Column, Percutaneous Approach

ØRG1371 Fusion of Cervical Vertebral Joint with Autologous Tissue Substitute, Posterior Approach, Posterior Column, Percutaneous Approach

ØRG137J Fusion of Cervical Vertebral Joint with Autologous Tissue Substitute, Posterior Approach, Anterior Column, Percutaneous Approach

ØRG13AØ Fusion of Cervical Vertebral Joint with Interbody Fusion Device, Anterior Approach, Anterior Column, Percutaneous Approach

ØRG13AJ Fusion of Cervical Vertebral Joint with Interbody Fusion Device, Posterior Approach, Anterior Column, Percutaneous Approach

ØRG13JØ Fusion of Cervical Vertebral Joint with Synthetic Substitute, Anterior Approach, Anterior Column, Percutaneous Approach

ØRG13J1 Fusion of Cervical Vertebral Joint with Synthetic Substitute, Posterior Approach, Posterior Column, Percutaneous Approach

ØRG13JJ Fusion of Cervical Vertebral Joint with Synthetic Substitute, Posterior Approach, Anterior Column, Percutaneous Approach

ØRG13KØ Fusion of Cervical Vertebral Joint with Nonautologous Tissue Substitute, Anterior Approach, Anterior Column, Percutaneous Approach

ØRG13K1 Fusion of Cervical Vertebral Joint with Nonautologous Tissue Substitute, Posterior Approach, Posterior Column, Percutaneous Approach

ØRG13KJ Fusion of Cervical Vertebral Joint with Nonautologous Tissue Substitute, Posterior Approach, Anterior Column, Percutaneous Approach

ØRG147Ø Fusion of Cervical Vertebral Joint with Autologous Tissue Substitute, Anterior Approach, Anterior Column, Percutaneous Endoscopic Approach

ØRG1471 Fusion of Cervical Vertebral Joint with Autologous Tissue Substitute, Posterior Approach, Posterior Column, Percutaneous Endoscopic Approach

ØRG147J Fusion of Cervical Vertebral Joint with Autologous Tissue Substitute, Posterior Approach, Anterior Column, Percutaneous Endoscopic Approach

ØRG14AØ Fusion of Cervical Vertebral Joint with Interbody Fusion Device, Anterior Approach, Anterior Column, Percutaneous Endoscopic Approach

ØRG14AJ Fusion of Cervical Vertebral Joint with Interbody Fusion Device, Posterior Approach, Anterior Column, Percutaneous Endoscopic Approach

ØRG14JØ Fusion of Cervical Vertebral Joint with Synthetic Substitute, Anterior Approach, Anterior Column, Percutaneous Endoscopic Approach

ØRG14J1 Fusion of Cervical Vertebral Joint with Synthetic Substitute, Posterior Approach, Posterior Column, Percutaneous Endoscopic Approach

ØRG14JJ Fusion of Cervical Vertebral Joint with Synthetic Substitute, Posterior Approach, Anterior Column, Percutaneous Endoscopic Approach

ØRG14KØ Fusion of Cervical Vertebral Joint with Nonautologous Tissue Substitute, Anterior Approach, Anterior Column, Percutaneous Endoscopic Approach

ØRG14K1 Fusion of Cervical Vertebral Joint with Nonautologous Tissue Substitute, Posterior Approach, Posterior Column, Percutaneous Endoscopic Approach

ØRG14KJ Fusion of Cervical Vertebral Joint with Nonautologous Tissue Substitute, Posterior Approach, Anterior Column, Percutaneous Endoscopic Approach

ØRG207Ø Fusion of 2 or more Cervical Vertebral Joints with Autologous Tissue Substitute, Anterior Approach, Anterior Column, Open Approach

ØRG2071 Fusion of 2 or more Cervical Vertebral Joints with Autologous Tissue Substitute, Posterior Approach, Posterior Column, Open Approach

ØRG207J Fusion of 2 or more Cervical Vertebral Joints with Autologous Tissue Substitute, Posterior Approach, Anterior Column, Open Approach

ØRG20AØ Fusion of 2 or more Cervical Vertebral Joints with Interbody Fusion Device, Anterior Approach, Anterior Column, Open Approach

ØRG20AJ Fusion of 2 or more Cervical Vertebral Joints with Interbody Fusion Device, Posterior Approach, Anterior Column, Open Approach

ØRG20JØ Fusion of 2 or more Cervical Vertebral Joints with Synthetic Substitute, Anterior Approach, Anterior Column, Open Approach

ØRG20J1 Fusion of 2 or more Cervical Vertebral Joints with Synthetic Substitute, Posterior Approach, Posterior Column, Open Approach

ØRG20JJ Fusion of 2 or more Cervical Vertebral Joints with Synthetic Substitute, Posterior Approach, Anterior Column, Open Approach

ØRG20KØ Fusion of 2 or more Cervical Vertebral Joints with Nonautologous Tissue Substitute, Anterior Approach, Anterior Column, Open Approach

ØRG20K1 Fusion of 2 or more Cervical Vertebral Joints with Nonautologous Tissue Substitute, Posterior Approach, Posterior Column, Open Approach

ØRG20KJ Fusion of 2 or more Cervical Vertebral Joints with Nonautologous Tissue Substitute, Posterior Approach, Anterior Column, Open Approach

ØRG237Ø Fusion of 2 or more Cervical Vertebral Joints with Autologous Tissue Substitute, Anterior Approach, Anterior Column, Percutaneous Approach

ØRG2371 Fusion of 2 or more Cervical Vertebral Joints with Autologous Tissue Substitute, Posterior Approach, Posterior Column, Percutaneous Approach

ØRG237J Fusion of 2 or more Cervical Vertebral Joints with Autologous Tissue Substitute, Posterior Approach, Anterior Column, Percutaneous Approach

ØRG23AØ Fusion of 2 or more Cervical Vertebral Joints with Interbody Fusion Device, Anterior Approach, Anterior Column, Percutaneous Approach

ØRG23AJ Fusion of 2 or more Cervical Vertebral Joints with Interbody Fusion Device, Posterior Approach, Anterior Column, Percutaneous Approach

ØRG23JØ Fusion of 2 or more Cervical Vertebral Joints with Synthetic Substitute, Anterior Approach, Anterior Column, Percutaneous Approach

ØRG23J1 Fusion of 2 or more Cervical Vertebral Joints with Synthetic Substitute, Posterior Approach, Posterior Column, Percutaneous Approach

ØRG23JJ Fusion of 2 or more Cervical Vertebral Joints with Synthetic Substitute, Posterior Approach, Anterior Column, Percutaneous Approach

ØRG23KØ Fusion of 2 or more Cervical Vertebral Joints with Nonautologous Tissue Substitute, Anterior Approach, Anterior Column, Percutaneous Approach

ØRG23K1 Fusion of 2 or more Cervical Vertebral Joints with Nonautologous Tissue Substitute, Posterior Approach, Posterior Column, Percutaneous Approach

ØRG23KJ Fusion of 2 or more Cervical Vertebral Joints with Nonautologous Tissue Substitute, Posterior Approach, Anterior Column, Percutaneous Approach

ØRG247Ø Fusion of 2 or more Cervical Vertebral Joints with Autologous Tissue Substitute, Anterior Approach, Anterior Column, Percutaneous Endoscopic Approach

ØRG2471 Fusion of 2 or more Cervical Vertebral Joints with Autologous Tissue Substitute, Posterior Approach, Posterior Column, Percutaneous Endoscopic Approach

ØRG247J Fusion of 2 or more Cervical Vertebral Joints with Autologous Tissue Substitute, Posterior Approach, Anterior Column, Percutaneous Endoscopic Approach

ØRG24AØ Fusion of 2 or more Cervical Vertebral Joints with Interbody Fusion Device, Anterior Approach, Anterior Column, Percutaneous Endoscopic Approach

HAC 12: Surgical Site Infection-Certain Orthopedic Procedures of the Spine, Shoulder, and Elbow (continued)

ØRG24AJ Fusion of 2 or more Cervical Vertebral Joints with Interbody Fusion Device, Posterior Approach, Anterior Column, Percutaneous Endoscopic Approach
ØRG24JØ Fusion of 2 or more Cervical Vertebral Joints with Synthetic Substitute, Anterior Approach, Anterior Column, Percutaneous Endoscopic Approach
ØRG24J1 Fusion of 2 or more Cervical Vertebral Joints with Synthetic Substitute, Posterior Approach, Posterior Column, Percutaneous Endoscopic Approach
ØRG24JJ Fusion of 2 or more Cervical Vertebral Joints with Synthetic Substitute, Posterior Approach, Anterior Column, Percutaneous Endoscopic Approach
ØRG24KØ Fusion of 2 or more Cervical Vertebral Joints with Nonautologous Tissue Substitute, Anterior Approach, Anterior Column, Percutaneous Endoscopic Approach
ØRG24K1 Fusion of 2 or more Cervical Vertebral Joints with Nonautologous Tissue Substitute, Posterior Approach, Posterior Column, Percutaneous Endoscopic Approach
ØRG24KJ Fusion of 2 or more Cervical Vertebral Joints with Nonautologous Tissue Substitute, Posterior Approach, Anterior Column, Percutaneous Endoscopic Approach
ØRG4Ø7Ø Fusion of Cervicothoracic Vertebral Joint with Autologous Tissue Substitute, Anterior Approach, Anterior Column, Open Approach
ØRG4Ø71 Fusion of Cervicothoracic Vertebral Joint with Autologous Tissue Substitute, Posterior Approach, Posterior Column, Open Approach
ØRG4Ø7J Fusion of Cervicothoracic Vertebral Joint with Autologous Tissue Substitute, Posterior Approach, Anterior Column, Open Approach
ØRG4ØAØ Fusion of Cervicothoracic Vertebral Joint with Interbody Fusion Device, Anterior Approach, Anterior Column, Open Approach
ØRG4ØAJ Fusion of Cervicothoracic Vertebral Joint with Interbody Fusion Device, Posterior Approach, Anterior Column, Open Approach
ØRG4ØJØ Fusion of Cervicothoracic Vertebral Joint with Synthetic Substitute, Anterior Approach, Anterior Column, Open Approach
ØRG4ØJ1 Fusion of Cervicothoracic Vertebral Joint with Synthetic Substitute, Posterior Approach, Posterior Column, Open Approach
ØRG4ØJJ Fusion of Cervicothoracic Vertebral Joint with Synthetic Substitute, Posterior Approach, Anterior Column, Open Approach
ØRG4ØKØ Fusion of Cervicothoracic Vertebral Joint with Nonautologous Tissue Substitute, Anterior Approach, Anterior Column, Open Approach
ØRG4ØK1 Fusion of Cervicothoracic Vertebral Joint with Nonautologous Tissue Substitute, Posterior Approach, Posterior Column, Open Approach
ØRG4ØKJ Fusion of Cervicothoracic Vertebral Joint with Nonautologous Tissue Substitute, Posterior Approach, Anterior Column, Open Approach
ØRG437Ø Fusion of Cervicothoracic Vertebral Joint with Autologous Tissue Substitute, Anterior Approach, Anterior Column, Percutaneous Approach
ØRG4371 Fusion of Cervicothoracic Vertebral Joint with Autologous Tissue Substitute, Posterior Approach, Posterior Column, Percutaneous Approach
ØRG437J Fusion of Cervicothoracic Vertebral Joint with Autologous Tissue Substitute, Posterior Approach, Anterior Column, Percutaneous Approach
ØRG43AØ Fusion of Cervicothoracic Vertebral Joint with Interbody Fusion Device, Anterior Approach, Anterior Column, Percutaneous Approach
ØRG43AJ Fusion of Cervicothoracic Vertebral Joint with Interbody Fusion Device, Posterior Approach, Anterior Column, Percutaneous Approach
ØRG43JØ Fusion of Cervicothoracic Vertebral Joint with Synthetic Substitute, Anterior Approach, Anterior Column, Percutaneous Approach
ØRG43J1 Fusion of Cervicothoracic Vertebral Joint with Synthetic Substitute, Posterior Approach, Posterior Column, Percutaneous Approach
ØRG43JJ Fusion of Cervicothoracic Vertebral Joint with Synthetic Substitute, Posterior Approach, Anterior Column, Percutaneous Approach
ØRG43KØ Fusion of Cervicothoracic Vertebral Joint with Nonautologous Tissue Substitute, Anterior Approach, Anterior Column, Percutaneous Approach
ØRG43K1 Fusion of Cervicothoracic Vertebral Joint with Nonautologous Tissue Substitute, Posterior Approach, Posterior Column, Percutaneous Approach
ØRG43KJ Fusion of Cervicothoracic Vertebral Joint with Nonautologous Tissue Substitute, Posterior Approach, Anterior Column, Percutaneous Approach
ØRG447Ø Fusion of Cervicothoracic Vertebral Joint with Autologous Tissue Substitute, Anterior Approach, Anterior Column, Percutaneous Endoscopic Approach
ØRG4471 Fusion of Cervicothoracic Vertebral Joint with Autologous Tissue Substitute, Posterior Approach, Posterior Column, Percutaneous Endoscopic Approach
ØRG447J Fusion of Cervicothoracic Vertebral Joint with Autologous Tissue Substitute, Posterior Approach, Anterior Column, Percutaneous Endoscopic Approach
ØRG44AØ Fusion of Cervicothoracic Vertebral Joint with Interbody Fusion Device, Anterior Approach, Anterior Column, Percutaneous Endoscopic Approach
ØRG44AJ Fusion of Cervicothoracic Vertebral Joint with Interbody Fusion Device, Posterior Approach, Anterior Column, Percutaneous Endoscopic Approach
ØRG44JØ Fusion of Cervicothoracic Vertebral Joint with Synthetic Substitute, Anterior Approach, Anterior Column, Percutaneous Endoscopic Approach
ØRG44J1 Fusion of Cervicothoracic Vertebral Joint with Synthetic Substitute, Posterior Approach, Posterior Column, Percutaneous Endoscopic Approach
ØRG44JJ Fusion of Cervicothoracic Vertebral Joint with Synthetic Substitute, Posterior Approach, Anterior Column, Percutaneous Endoscopic Approach
ØRG44KØ Fusion of Cervicothoracic Vertebral Joint with Nonautologous Tissue Substitute, Anterior Approach, Anterior Column, Percutaneous Endoscopic Approach
ØRG44K1 Fusion of Cervicothoracic Vertebral Joint with Nonautologous Tissue Substitute, Posterior Approach, Posterior Column, Percutaneous Endoscopic Approach
ØRG44KJ Fusion of Cervicothoracic Vertebral Joint with Nonautologous Tissue Substitute, Posterior Approach, Anterior Column, Percutaneous Endoscopic Approach
ØRG6Ø7Ø Fusion of Thoracic Vertebral Joint with Autologous Tissue Substitute, Anterior Approach, Anterior Column, Open Approach
ØRG6Ø71 Fusion of Thoracic Vertebral Joint with Autologous Tissue Substitute, Posterior Approach, Posterior Column, Open Approach
ØRG6Ø7J Fusion of Thoracic Vertebral Joint with Autologous Tissue Substitute, Posterior Approach, Anterior Column, Open Approach
ØRG6ØAØ Fusion of Thoracic Vertebral Joint with Interbody Fusion Device, Anterior Approach, Anterior Column, Open Approach
ØRG6ØAJ Fusion of Thoracic Vertebral Joint with Interbody Fusion Device, Posterior Approach, Anterior Column, Open Approach
ØRG6ØJØ Fusion of Thoracic Vertebral Joint with Synthetic Substitute, Anterior Approach, Anterior Column, Open Approach
ØRG6ØJ1 Fusion of Thoracic Vertebral Joint with Synthetic Substitute, Posterior Approach, Posterior Column, Open Approach
ØRG6ØJJ Fusion of Thoracic Vertebral Joint with Synthetic Substitute, Posterior Approach, Anterior Column, Open Approach
ØRG6ØKØ Fusion of Thoracic Vertebral Joint with Nonautologous Tissue Substitute, Anterior Approach, Anterior Column, Open Approach
ØRG6ØK1 Fusion of Thoracic Vertebral Joint with Nonautologous Tissue Substitute, Posterior Approach, Posterior Column, Open Approach
ØRG6ØKJ Fusion of Thoracic Vertebral Joint with Nonautologous Tissue Substitute, Posterior Approach, Anterior Column, Open Approach
ØRG637Ø Fusion of Thoracic Vertebral Joint with Autologous Tissue Substitute, Anterior Approach, Anterior Column, Percutaneous Approach
ØRG6371 Fusion of Thoracic Vertebral Joint with Autologous Tissue Substitute, Posterior Approach, Posterior Column, Percutaneous Approach
ØRG637J Fusion of Thoracic Vertebral Joint with Autologous Tissue Substitute, Posterior Approach, Anterior Column, Percutaneous Approach
ØRG63AØ Fusion of Thoracic Vertebral Joint with Interbody Fusion Device, Anterior Approach, Anterior Column, Percutaneous Approach

HAC 12: Surgical Site Infection-Certain Orthopedic Procedures of the Spine, Shoulder, and Elbow (continued)

ØRG63AJ Fusion of Thoracic Vertebral Joint with Interbody Fusion Device, Posterior Approach, Anterior Column, Percutaneous Approach
ØRG63JØ Fusion of Thoracic Vertebral Joint with Synthetic Substitute, Anterior Approach, Anterior Column, Percutaneous Approach
ØRG63J1 Fusion of Thoracic Vertebral Joint with Synthetic Substitute, Posterior Approach, Posterior Column, Percutaneous Approach
ØRG63JJ Fusion of Thoracic Vertebral Joint with Synthetic Substitute, Posterior Approach, Anterior Column, Percutaneous Approach
ØRG63KØ Fusion of Thoracic Vertebral Joint with Nonautologous Tissue Substitute, Anterior Approach, Anterior Column, Percutaneous Approach
ØRG63K1 Fusion of Thoracic Vertebral Joint with Nonautologous Tissue Substitute, Posterior Approach, Posterior Column, Percutaneous Approach
ØRG63KJ Fusion of Thoracic Vertebral Joint with Nonautologous Tissue Substitute, Posterior Approach, Anterior Column, Percutaneous Approach
ØRG647Ø Fusion of Thoracic Vertebral Joint with Autologous Tissue Substitute, Anterior Approach, Anterior Column, Percutaneous Endoscopic Approach
ØRG6471 Fusion of Thoracic Vertebral Joint with Autologous Tissue Substitute, Posterior Approach, Posterior Column, Percutaneous Endoscopic Approach
ØRG647J Fusion of Thoracic Vertebral Joint with Autologous Tissue Substitute, Posterior Approach, Anterior Column, Percutaneous Endoscopic Approach
ØRG64AØ Fusion of Thoracic Vertebral Joint with Interbody Fusion Device, Anterior Approach, Anterior Column, Percutaneous Endoscopic Approach
ØRG64AJ Fusion of Thoracic Vertebral Joint with Interbody Fusion Device, Posterior Approach, Anterior Column, Percutaneous Endoscopic Approach
ØRG64JØ Fusion of Thoracic Vertebral Joint with Synthetic Substitute, Anterior Approach, Anterior Column, Percutaneous Endoscopic Approach
ØRG64J1 Fusion of Thoracic Vertebral Joint with Synthetic Substitute, Posterior Approach, Posterior Column, Percutaneous Endoscopic Approach
ØRG64JJ Fusion of Thoracic Vertebral Joint with Synthetic Substitute, Posterior Approach, Anterior Column, Percutaneous Endoscopic Approach
ØRG64KØ Fusion of Thoracic Vertebral Joint with Nonautologous Tissue Substitute, Anterior Approach, Anterior Column, Percutaneous Endoscopic Approach
ØRG64K1 Fusion of Thoracic Vertebral Joint with Nonautologous Tissue Substitute, Posterior Approach, Posterior Column, Percutaneous Endoscopic Approach
ØRG64KJ Fusion of Thoracic Vertebral Joint with Nonautologous Tissue Substitute, Posterior Approach, Anterior Column, Percutaneous Endoscopic Approach
ØRG7070 Fusion of 2 to 7 Thoracic Vertebral Joints with Autologous Tissue Substitute, Anterior Approach, Anterior Column, Open Approach
ØRG7071 Fusion of 2 to 7 Thoracic Vertebral Joints with Autologous Tissue Substitute, Posterior Approach, Posterior Column, Open Approach
ØRG707J Fusion of 2 to 7 Thoracic Vertebral Joints with Autologous Tissue Substitute, Posterior Approach, Anterior Column, Open Approach
ØRG70AØ Fusion of 2 to 7 Thoracic Vertebral Joints with Interbody Fusion Device, Anterior Approach, Anterior Column, Open Approach
ØRG70AJ Fusion of 2 to 7 Thoracic Vertebral Joints with Interbody Fusion Device, Posterior Approach, Anterior Column, Open Approach
ØRG70JØ Fusion of 2 to 7 Thoracic Vertebral Joints with Synthetic Substitute, Anterior Approach, Anterior Column, Open Approach
ØRG70J1 Fusion of 2 to 7 Thoracic Vertebral Joints with Synthetic Substitute, Posterior Approach, Posterior Column, Open Approach
ØRG70JJ Fusion of 2 to 7 Thoracic Vertebral Joints with Synthetic Substitute, Posterior Approach, Anterior Column, Open Approach
ØRG70KØ Fusion of 2 to 7 Thoracic Vertebral Joints with Nonautologous Tissue Substitute, Anterior Approach, Anterior Column, Open Approach
ØRG70K1 Fusion of 2 to 7 Thoracic Vertebral Joints with Nonautologous Tissue Substitute, Posterior Approach, Posterior Column, Open Approach
ØRG70KJ Fusion of 2 to 7 Thoracic Vertebral Joints with Nonautologous Tissue Substitute, Posterior Approach, Anterior Column, Open Approach
ØRG737Ø Fusion of 2 to 7 Thoracic Vertebral Joints with Autologous Tissue Substitute, Anterior Approach, Anterior Column, Percutaneous Approach
ØRG7371 Fusion of 2 to 7 Thoracic Vertebral Joints with Autologous Tissue Substitute, Posterior Approach, Posterior Column, Percutaneous Approach
ØRG737J Fusion of 2 to 7 Thoracic Vertebral Joints with Autologous Tissue Substitute, Posterior Approach, Anterior Column, Percutaneous Approach
ØRG73AØ Fusion of 2 to 7 Thoracic Vertebral Joints with Interbody Fusion Device, Anterior Approach, Anterior Column, Percutaneous Approach
ØRG73AJ Fusion of 2 to 7 Thoracic Vertebral Joints with Interbody Fusion Device, Posterior Approach, Anterior Column, Percutaneous Approach
ØRG73JØ Fusion of 2 to 7 Thoracic Vertebral Joints with Synthetic Substitute, Anterior Approach, Anterior Column, Percutaneous Approach
ØRG73J1 Fusion of 2 to 7 Thoracic Vertebral Joints with Synthetic Substitute, Posterior Approach, Posterior Column, Percutaneous Approach
ØRG73JJ Fusion of 2 to 7 Thoracic Vertebral Joints with Synthetic Substitute, Posterior Approach, Anterior Column, Percutaneous Approach
ØRG73KØ Fusion of 2 to 7 Thoracic Vertebral Joints with Nonautologous Tissue Substitute, Anterior Approach, Anterior Column, Percutaneous Approach
ØRG73K1 Fusion of 2 to 7 Thoracic Vertebral Joints with Nonautologous Tissue Substitute, Posterior Approach, Posterior Column, Percutaneous Approach
ØRG73KJ Fusion of 2 to 7 Thoracic Vertebral Joints with Nonautologous Tissue Substitute, Posterior Approach, Anterior Column, Percutaneous Approach
ØRG747Ø Fusion of 2 to 7 Thoracic Vertebral Joints with Autologous Tissue Substitute, Anterior Approach, Anterior Column, Percutaneous Endoscopic Approach
ØRG7471 Fusion of 2 to 7 Thoracic Vertebral Joints with Autologous Tissue Substitute, Posterior Approach, Posterior Column, Percutaneous Endoscopic Approach
ØRG747J Fusion of 2 to 7 Thoracic Vertebral Joints with Autologous Tissue Substitute, Posterior Approach, Anterior Column, Percutaneous Endoscopic Approach
ØRG74AØ Fusion of 2 to 7 Thoracic Vertebral Joints with Interbody Fusion Device, Anterior Approach, Anterior Column, Percutaneous Endoscopic Approach
ØRG74AJ Fusion of 2 to 7 Thoracic Vertebral Joints with Interbody Fusion Device, Posterior Approach, Anterior Column, Percutaneous Endoscopic Approach
ØRG74JØ Fusion of 2 to 7 Thoracic Vertebral Joints with Synthetic Substitute, Anterior Approach, Anterior Column, Percutaneous Endoscopic Approach
ØRG74J1 Fusion of 2 to 7 Thoracic Vertebral Joints with Synthetic Substitute, Posterior Approach, Posterior Column, Percutaneous Endoscopic Approach
ØRG74JJ Fusion of 2 to 7 Thoracic Vertebral Joints with Synthetic Substitute, Posterior Approach, Anterior Column, Percutaneous Endoscopic Approach
ØRG74KØ Fusion of 2 to 7 Thoracic Vertebral Joints with Nonautologous Tissue Substitute, Anterior Approach, Anterior Column, Percutaneous Endoscopic Approach
ØRG74K1 Fusion of 2 to 7 Thoracic Vertebral Joints with Nonautologous Tissue Substitute, Posterior Approach, Posterior Column, Percutaneous Endoscopic Approach
ØRG74KJ Fusion of 2 to 7 Thoracic Vertebral Joints with Nonautologous Tissue Substitute, Posterior Approach, Anterior Column, Percutaneous Endoscopic Approach
ØRG807Ø Fusion of 8 or More Thoracic Vertebral Joints with Autologous Tissue Substitute, Anterior Approach, Anterior Column, Open Approach
ØRG8071 Fusion of 8 or More Thoracic Vertebral Joints with Autologous Tissue Substitute, Posterior Approach, Posterior Column, Open Approach
ØRG807J Fusion of 8 or More Thoracic Vertebral Joints with Autologous Tissue Substitute, Posterior Approach, Anterior Column, Open Approach
ØRG80AØ Fusion of 8 or More Thoracic Vertebral Joints with Interbody Fusion Device, Anterior Approach, Anterior Column, Open Approach
ØRG80AJ Fusion of 8 or More Thoracic Vertebral Joints with Interbody Fusion Device, Posterior Approach, Anterior Column, Open Approach

HAC 12: Surgical Site Infection-Certain Orthopedic Procedures of the Spine, Shoulder, and Elbow (continued)

ØRG80JØ Fusion of 8 or More Thoracic Vertebral Joints with Synthetic Substitute, Anterior Approach, Anterior Column, Open Approach
ØRG80J1 Fusion of 8 or More Thoracic Vertebral Joints with Synthetic Substitute, Posterior Approach, Posterior Column, Open Approach
ØRG80JJ Fusion of 8 or More Thoracic Vertebral Joints with Synthetic Substitute, Posterior Approach, Anterior Column, Open Approach
ØRG80KØ Fusion of 8 or More Thoracic Vertebral Joints with Nonautologous Tissue Substitute, Anterior Approach, Anterior Column, Open Approach
ØRG80K1 Fusion of 8 or More Thoracic Vertebral Joints with Nonautologous Tissue Substitute, Posterior Approach, Posterior Column, Open Approach
ØRG80KJ Fusion of 8 or More Thoracic Vertebral Joints with Nonautologous Tissue Substitute, Posterior Approach, Anterior Column, Open Approach
ØRG837Ø Fusion of 8 or More Thoracic Vertebral Joints with Autologous Tissue Substitute, Anterior Approach, Anterior Column, Percutaneous Approach
ØRG8371 Fusion of 8 or More Thoracic Vertebral Joints with Autologous Tissue Substitute, Posterior Approach, Posterior Column, Percutaneous Approach
ØRG837J Fusion of 8 or More Thoracic Vertebral Joints with Autologous Tissue Substitute, Posterior Approach, Anterior Column, Percutaneous Approach
ØRG83AØ Fusion of 8 or More Thoracic Vertebral Joints with Interbody Fusion Device, Anterior Approach, Anterior Column, Percutaneous Approach
ØRG83AJ Fusion of 8 or More Thoracic Vertebral Joints with Interbody Fusion Device, Posterior Approach, Anterior Column, Percutaneous Approach
ØRG83JØ Fusion of 8 or More Thoracic Vertebral Joints with Synthetic Substitute, Anterior Approach, Anterior Column, Percutaneous Approach
ØRG83J1 Fusion of 8 or More Thoracic Vertebral Joints with Synthetic Substitute, Posterior Approach, Posterior Column, Percutaneous Approach
ØRG83JJ Fusion of 8 or More Thoracic Vertebral Joints with Synthetic Substitute, Posterior Approach, Anterior Column, Percutaneous Approach
ØRG83KØ Fusion of 8 or More Thoracic Vertebral Joints with Nonautologous Tissue Substitute, Anterior Approach, Anterior Column, Percutaneous Approach
ØRG83K1 Fusion of 8 or More Thoracic Vertebral Joints with Nonautologous Tissue Substitute, Posterior Approach, Posterior Column, Percutaneous Approach
ØRG83KJ Fusion of 8 or More Thoracic Vertebral Joints with Nonautologous Tissue Substitute, Posterior Approach, Anterior Column, Percutaneous Approach
ØRG847Ø Fusion of 8 or More Thoracic Vertebral Joints with Autologous Tissue Substitute, Anterior Approach, Anterior Column, Percutaneous Endoscopic Approach
ØRG8471 Fusion of 8 or More Thoracic Vertebral Joints with Autologous Tissue Substitute, Posterior Approach, Posterior Column, Percutaneous Endoscopic Approach
ØRG847J Fusion of 8 or More Thoracic Vertebral Joints with Autologous Tissue Substitute, Posterior Approach, Anterior Column, Percutaneous Endoscopic Approach
ØRG84AØ Fusion of 8 or More Thoracic Vertebral Joints with Interbody Fusion Device, Anterior Approach, Anterior Column, Percutaneous Endoscopic Approach
ØRG84AJ Fusion of 8 or More Thoracic Vertebral Joints with Interbody Fusion Device, Posterior Approach, Anterior Column, Percutaneous Endoscopic Approach
ØRG84JØ Fusion of 8 or More Thoracic Vertebral Joints with Synthetic Substitute, Anterior Approach, Anterior Column, Percutaneous Endoscopic Approach
ØRG84J1 Fusion of 8 or More Thoracic Vertebral Joints with Synthetic Substitute, Posterior Approach, Posterior Column, Percutaneous Endoscopic Approach
ØRG84JJ Fusion of 8 or More Thoracic Vertebral Joints with Synthetic Substitute, Posterior Approach, Anterior Column, Percutaneous Endoscopic Approach
ØRG84KØ Fusion of 8 or More Thoracic Vertebral Joints with Nonautologous Tissue Substitute, Anterior Approach, Anterior Column, Percutaneous Endoscopic Approach
ØRG84K1 Fusion of 8 or More Thoracic Vertebral Joints with Nonautologous Tissue Substitute, Posterior Approach, Posterior Column, Percutaneous Endoscopic Approach
ØRG84KJ Fusion of 8 or More Thoracic Vertebral Joints with Nonautologous Tissue Substitute, Posterior Approach, Anterior Column, Percutaneous Endoscopic Approach
ØRGAØ7Ø Fusion of Thoracolumbar Vertebral Joint with Autologous Tissue Substitute, Anterior Approach, Anterior Column, Open Approach
ØRGAØ71 Fusion of Thoracolumbar Vertebral Joint with Autologous Tissue Substitute, Posterior Approach, Posterior Column, Open Approach
ØRGAØ7J Fusion of Thoracolumbar Vertebral Joint with Autologous Tissue Substitute, Posterior Approach, Anterior Column, Open Approach
ØRGAØAØ Fusion of Thoracolumbar Vertebral Joint with Interbody Fusion Device, Anterior Approach, Anterior Column, Open Approach
ØRGAØAJ Fusion of Thoracolumbar Vertebral Joint with Interbody Fusion Device, Posterior Approach, Anterior Column, Open Approach
ØRGAØJØ Fusion of Thoracolumbar Vertebral Joint with Synthetic Substitute, Anterior Approach, Anterior Column, Open Approach
ØRGAØJ1 Fusion of Thoracolumbar Vertebral Joint with Synthetic Substitute, Posterior Approach, Posterior Column, Open Approach
ØRGAØJJ Fusion of Thoracolumbar Vertebral Joint with Synthetic Substitute, Posterior Approach, Anterior Column, Open Approach
ØRGAØKØ Fusion of Thoracolumbar Vertebral Joint with Nonautologous Tissue Substitute, Anterior Approach, Anterior Column, Open Approach
ØRGAØK1 Fusion of Thoracolumbar Vertebral Joint with Nonautologous Tissue Substitute, Posterior Approach, Posterior Column, Open Approach
ØRGAØKJ Fusion of Thoracolumbar Vertebral Joint with Nonautologous Tissue Substitute, Posterior Approach, Anterior Column, Open Approach
ØRGA37Ø Fusion of Thoracolumbar Vertebral Joint with Autologous Tissue Substitute, Anterior Approach, Anterior Column, Percutaneous Approach
ØRGA371 Fusion of Thoracolumbar Vertebral Joint with Autologous Tissue Substitute, Posterior Approach, Posterior Column, Percutaneous Approach
ØRGA37J Fusion of Thoracolumbar Vertebral Joint with Autologous Tissue Substitute, Posterior Approach, Anterior Column, Percutaneous Approach
ØRGA3AØ Fusion of Thoracolumbar Vertebral Joint with Interbody Fusion Device, Anterior Approach, Anterior Column, Percutaneous Approach
ØRGA3AJ Fusion of Thoracolumbar Vertebral Joint with Interbody Fusion Device, Posterior Approach, Anterior Column, Percutaneous Approach
ØRGA3JØ Fusion of Thoracolumbar Vertebral Joint with Synthetic Substitute, Anterior Approach, Anterior Column, Percutaneous Approach
ØRGA3J1 Fusion of Thoracolumbar Vertebral Joint with Synthetic Substitute, Posterior Approach, Posterior Column, Percutaneous Approach
ØRGA3JJ Fusion of Thoracolumbar Vertebral Joint with Synthetic Substitute, Posterior Approach, Anterior Column, Percutaneous Approach
ØRGA3KØ Fusion of Thoracolumbar Vertebral Joint with Nonautologous Tissue Substitute, Anterior Approach, Anterior Column, Percutaneous Approach
ØRGA3K1 Fusion of Thoracolumbar Vertebral Joint with Nonautologous Tissue Substitute, Posterior Approach, Posterior Column, Percutaneous Approach
ØRGA3KJ Fusion of Thoracolumbar Vertebral Joint with Nonautologous Tissue Substitute, Posterior Approach, Anterior Column, Percutaneous Approach
ØRGA47Ø Fusion of Thoracolumbar Vertebral Joint with Autologous Tissue Substitute, Anterior Approach, Anterior Column, Percutaneous Endoscopic Approach
ØRGA471 Fusion of Thoracolumbar Vertebral Joint with Autologous Tissue Substitute, Posterior Approach, Posterior Column, Percutaneous Endoscopic Approach
ØRGA47J Fusion of Thoracolumbar Vertebral Joint with Autologous Tissue Substitute, Posterior Approach, Anterior Column, Percutaneous Endoscopic Approach

HAC 12: Surgical Site Infection-Certain Orthopedic Procedures of the Spine, Shoulder, and Elbow (continued)

ØRGA4AØ Fusion of Thoracolumbar Vertebral Joint with Interbody Fusion Device, Anterior Approach, Anterior Column, Percutaneous Endoscopic Approach
ØRGA4AJ Fusion of Thoracolumbar Vertebral Joint with Interbody Fusion Device, Posterior Approach, Anterior Column, Percutaneous Endoscopic Approach
ØRGA4JØ Fusion of Thoracolumbar Vertebral Joint with Synthetic Substitute, Anterior Approach, Anterior Column, Percutaneous Endoscopic Approach
ØRGA4J1 Fusion of Thoracolumbar Vertebral Joint with Synthetic Substitute, Posterior Approach, Posterior Column, Percutaneous Endoscopic Approach
ØRGA4JJ Fusion of Thoracolumbar Vertebral Joint with Synthetic Substitute, Posterior Approach, Anterior Column, Percutaneous Endoscopic Approach
ØRGA4KØ Fusion of Thoracolumbar Vertebral Joint with Nonautologous Tissue Substitute, Anterior Approach, Anterior Column, Percutaneous Endoscopic Approach
ØRGA4K1 Fusion of Thoracolumbar Vertebral Joint with Nonautologous Tissue Substitute, Posterior Approach, Posterior Column, Percutaneous Endoscopic Approach
ØRGA4KJ Fusion of Thoracolumbar Vertebral Joint with Nonautologous Tissue Substitute, Posterior Approach, Anterior Column, Percutaneous Endoscopic Approach
ØRGEØ4Z Fusion of Right Sternoclavicular Joint with Internal Fixation Device, Open Approach
ØRGEØ7Z Fusion of Right Sternoclavicular Joint with Autologous Tissue Substitute, Open Approach
ØRGEØJZ Fusion of Right Sternoclavicular Joint with Synthetic Substitute, Open Approach
ØRGEØKZ Fusion of Right Sternoclavicular Joint with Nonautologous Tissue Substitute, Open Approach
ØRGE34Z Fusion of Right Sternoclavicular Joint with Internal Fixation Device, Percutaneous Approach
ØRGE37Z Fusion of Right Sternoclavicular Joint with Autologous Tissue Substitute, Percutaneous Approach
ØRGE3JZ Fusion of Right Sternoclavicular Joint with Synthetic Substitute, Percutaneous Approach
ØRGE3KZ Fusion of Right Sternoclavicular Joint with Nonautologous Tissue Substitute, Percutaneous Approach
ØRGE44Z Fusion of Right Sternoclavicular Joint with Internal Fixation Device, Percutaneous Endoscopic Approach
ØRGE47Z Fusion of Right Sternoclavicular Joint with Autologous Tissue Substitute, Percutaneous Endoscopic Approach
ØRGE4JZ Fusion of Right Sternoclavicular Joint with Synthetic Substitute, Percutaneous Endoscopic Approach
ØRGE4KZ Fusion of Right Sternoclavicular Joint with Nonautologous Tissue Substitute, Percutaneous Endoscopic Approach
ØRGFØ4Z Fusion of Left Sternoclavicular Joint with Internal Fixation Device, Open Approach
ØRGFØ7Z Fusion of Left Sternoclavicular Joint with Autologous Tissue Substitute, Open Approach
ØRGFØJZ Fusion of Left Sternoclavicular Joint with Synthetic Substitute, Open Approach
ØRGFØKZ Fusion of Left Sternoclavicular Joint with Nonautologous Tissue Substitute, Open Approach
ØRGF34Z Fusion of Left Sternoclavicular Joint with Internal Fixation Device, Percutaneous Approach
ØRGF37Z Fusion of Left Sternoclavicular Joint with Autologous Tissue Substitute, Percutaneous Approach
ØRGF3JZ Fusion of Left Sternoclavicular Joint with Synthetic Substitute, Percutaneous Approach
ØRGF3KZ Fusion of Left Sternoclavicular Joint with Nonautologous Tissue Substitute, Percutaneous Approach
ØRGF44Z Fusion of Left Sternoclavicular Joint with Internal Fixation Device, Percutaneous Endoscopic Approach
ØRGF47Z Fusion of Left Sternoclavicular Joint with Autologous Tissue Substitute, Percutaneous Endoscopic Approach
ØRGF4JZ Fusion of Left Sternoclavicular Joint with Synthetic Substitute, Percutaneous Endoscopic Approach
ØRGF4KZ Fusion of Left Sternoclavicular Joint with Nonautologous Tissue Substitute, Percutaneous Endoscopic Approach
ØRGGØ4Z Fusion of Right Acromioclavicular Joint with Internal Fixation Device, Open Approach
ØRGGØ7Z Fusion of Right Acromioclavicular Joint with Autologous Tissue Substitute, Open Approach
ØRGGØJZ Fusion of Right Acromioclavicular Joint with Synthetic Substitute, Open Approach
ØRGGØKZ Fusion of Right Acromioclavicular Joint with Nonautologous Tissue Substitute, Open Approach
ØRGG34Z Fusion of Right Acromioclavicular Joint with Internal Fixation Device, Percutaneous Approach
ØRGG37Z Fusion of Right Acromioclavicular Joint with Autologous Tissue Substitute, Percutaneous Approach
ØRGG3JZ Fusion of Right Acromioclavicular Joint with Synthetic Substitute, Percutaneous Approach
ØRGG3KZ Fusion of Right Acromioclavicular Joint with Nonautologous Tissue Substitute, Percutaneous Approach
ØRGG44Z Fusion of Right Acromioclavicular Joint with Internal Fixation Device, Percutaneous Endoscopic Approach
ØRGG47Z Fusion of Right Acromioclavicular Joint with Autologous Tissue Substitute, Percutaneous Endoscopic Approach
ØRGG4JZ Fusion of Right Acromioclavicular Joint with Synthetic Substitute, Percutaneous Endoscopic Approach
ØRGG4KZ Fusion of Right Acromioclavicular Joint with Nonautologous Tissue Substitute, Percutaneous Endoscopic Approach
ØRGHØ4Z Fusion of Left Acromioclavicular Joint with Internal Fixation Device, Open Approach
ØRGHØ7Z Fusion of Left Acromioclavicular Joint with Autologous Tissue Substitute, Open Approach
ØRGHØJZ Fusion of Left Acromioclavicular Joint with Synthetic Substitute, Open Approach
ØRGHØKZ Fusion of Left Acromioclavicular Joint with Nonautologous Tissue Substitute, Open Approach
ØRGH34Z Fusion of Left Acromioclavicular Joint with Internal Fixation Device, Percutaneous Approach
ØRGH37Z Fusion of Left Acromioclavicular Joint with Autologous Tissue Substitute, Percutaneous Approach
ØRGH3JZ Fusion of Left Acromioclavicular Joint with Synthetic Substitute, Percutaneous Approach
ØRGH3KZ Fusion of Left Acromioclavicular Joint with Nonautologous Tissue Substitute, Percutaneous Approach
ØRGH44Z Fusion of Left Acromioclavicular Joint with Internal Fixation Device, Percutaneous Endoscopic Approach
ØRGH47Z Fusion of Left Acromioclavicular Joint with Autologous Tissue Substitute, Percutaneous Endoscopic Approach
ØRGH4JZ Fusion of Left Acromioclavicular Joint with Synthetic Substitute, Percutaneous Endoscopic Approach
ØRGH4KZ Fusion of Left Acromioclavicular Joint with Nonautologous Tissue Substitute, Percutaneous Endoscopic Approach
ØRGJØ4Z Fusion of Right Shoulder Joint with Internal Fixation Device, Open Approach
ØRGJØ7Z Fusion of Right Shoulder Joint with Autologous Tissue Substitute, Open Approach
ØRGJØJZ Fusion of Right Shoulder Joint with Synthetic Substitute, Open Approach
ØRGJØKZ Fusion of Right Shoulder Joint with Nonautologous Tissue Substitute, Open Approach
ØRGJ34Z Fusion of Right Shoulder Joint with Internal Fixation Device, Percutaneous Approach
ØRGJ37Z Fusion of Right Shoulder Joint with Autologous Tissue Substitute, Percutaneous Approach
ØRGJ3JZ Fusion of Right Shoulder Joint with Synthetic Substitute, Percutaneous Approach
ØRGJ3KZ Fusion of Right Shoulder Joint with Nonautologous Tissue Substitute, Percutaneous Approach
ØRGJ44Z Fusion of Right Shoulder Joint with Internal Fixation Device, Percutaneous Endoscopic Approach
ØRGJ47Z Fusion of Right Shoulder Joint with Autologous Tissue Substitute, Percutaneous Endoscopic Approach
ØRGJ4JZ Fusion of Right Shoulder Joint with Synthetic Substitute, Percutaneous Endoscopic Approach
ØRGJ4KZ Fusion of Right Shoulder Joint with Nonautologous Tissue Substitute, Percutaneous Endoscopic Approach
ØRGKØ4Z Fusion of Left Shoulder Joint with Internal Fixation Device, Open Approach
ØRGKØ7Z Fusion of Left Shoulder Joint with Autologous Tissue Substitute, Open Approach
ØRGKØJZ Fusion of Left Shoulder Joint with Synthetic Substitute, Open Approach
ØRGKØKZ Fusion of Left Shoulder Joint with Nonautologous Tissue Substitute, Open Approach
ØRGK34Z Fusion of Left Shoulder Joint with Internal Fixation Device, Percutaneous Approach

HAC 12: Surgical Site Infection-Certain Orthopedic Procedures of the Spine, Shoulder, and Elbow (continued)

ØRGK37Z Fusion of Left Shoulder Joint with Autologous Tissue Substitute, Percutaneous Approach
ØRGK3JZ Fusion of Left Shoulder Joint with Synthetic Substitute, Percutaneous Approach
ØRGK3KZ Fusion of Left Shoulder Joint with Nonautologous Tissue Substitute, Percutaneous Approach
ØRGK44Z Fusion of Left Shoulder Joint with Internal Fixation Device, Percutaneous Endoscopic Approach
ØRGK47Z Fusion of Left Shoulder Joint with Autologous Tissue Substitute, Percutaneous Endoscopic Approach
ØRGK4JZ Fusion of Left Shoulder Joint with Synthetic Substitute, Percutaneous Endoscopic Approach
ØRGK4KZ Fusion of Left Shoulder Joint with Nonautologous Tissue Substitute, Percutaneous Endoscopic Approach
ØRGLØ4Z Fusion of Right Elbow Joint with Internal Fixation Device, Open Approach
ØRGLØ5Z Fusion of Right Elbow Joint with External Fixation Device, Open Approach
ØRGLØ7Z Fusion of Right Elbow Joint with Autologous Tissue Substitute, Open Approach
ØRGLØJZ Fusion of Right Elbow Joint with Synthetic Substitute, Open Approach
ØRGLØKZ Fusion of Right Elbow Joint with Nonautologous Tissue Substitute, Open Approach
ØRGL34Z Fusion of Right Elbow Joint with Internal Fixation Device, Percutaneous Approach
ØRGL35Z Fusion of Right Elbow Joint with External Fixation Device, Percutaneous Approach
ØRGL37Z Fusion of Right Elbow Joint with Autologous Tissue Substitute, Percutaneous Approach
ØRGL3JZ Fusion of Right Elbow Joint with Synthetic Substitute, Percutaneous Approach
ØRGL3KZ Fusion of Right Elbow Joint with Nonautologous Tissue Substitute, Percutaneous Approach
ØRGL44Z Fusion of Right Elbow Joint with Internal Fixation Device, Percutaneous Endoscopic Approach
ØRGL45Z Fusion of Right Elbow Joint with External Fixation Device, Percutaneous Endoscopic Approach
ØRGL47Z Fusion of Right Elbow Joint with Autologous Tissue Substitute, Percutaneous Endoscopic Approach
ØRGL4JZ Fusion of Right Elbow Joint with Synthetic Substitute, Percutaneous Endoscopic Approach
ØRGL4KZ Fusion of Right Elbow Joint with Nonautologous Tissue Substitute, Percutaneous Endoscopic Approach
ØRGMØ4Z Fusion of Left Elbow Joint with Internal Fixation Device, Open Approach
ØRGMØ5Z Fusion of Left Elbow Joint with External Fixation Device, Open Approach
ØRGMØ7Z Fusion of Left Elbow Joint with Autologous Tissue Substitute, Open Approach
ØRGMØJZ Fusion of Left Elbow Joint with Synthetic Substitute, Open Approach
ØRGMØKZ Fusion of Left Elbow Joint with Nonautologous Tissue Substitute, Open Approach
ØRGM34Z Fusion of Left Elbow Joint with Internal Fixation Device, Percutaneous Approach
ØRGM35Z Fusion of Left Elbow Joint with External Fixation Device, Percutaneous Approach
ØRGM37Z Fusion of Left Elbow Joint with Autologous Tissue Substitute, Percutaneous Approach
ØRGM3JZ Fusion of Left Elbow Joint with Synthetic Substitute, Percutaneous Approach
ØRGM3KZ Fusion of Left Elbow Joint with Nonautologous Tissue Substitute, Percutaneous Approach
ØRGM44Z Fusion of Left Elbow Joint with Internal Fixation Device, Percutaneous Endoscopic Approach
ØRGM45Z Fusion of Left Elbow Joint with External Fixation Device, Percutaneous Endoscopic Approach
ØRGM47Z Fusion of Left Elbow Joint with Autologous Tissue Substitute, Percutaneous Endoscopic Approach
ØRGM4JZ Fusion of Left Elbow Joint with Synthetic Substitute, Percutaneous Endoscopic Approach
ØRGM4KZ Fusion of Left Elbow Joint with Nonautologous Tissue Substitute, Percutaneous Endoscopic Approach
ØRQEØZZ Repair Right Sternoclavicular Joint, Open Approach
ØRQE3ZZ Repair Right Sternoclavicular Joint, Percutaneous Approach
ØRQE4ZZ Repair Right Sternoclavicular Joint, Percutaneous Endoscopic Approach
ØRQEXZZ Repair Right Sternoclavicular Joint, External Approach
ØRQFØZZ Repair Left Sternoclavicular Joint, Open Approach
ØRQF3ZZ Repair Left Sternoclavicular Joint, Percutaneous Approach
ØRQF4ZZ Repair Left Sternoclavicular Joint, Percutaneous Endoscopic Approach
ØRQFXZZ Repair Left Sternoclavicular Joint, External Approach
ØRQGØZZ Repair Right Acromioclavicular Joint, Open Approach
ØRQG3ZZ Repair Right Acromioclavicular Joint, Percutaneous Approach
ØRQG4ZZ Repair Right Acromioclavicular Joint, Percutaneous Endoscopic Approach
ØRQGXZZ Repair Right Acromioclavicular Joint, External Approach
ØRQHØZZ Repair Left Acromioclavicular Joint, Open Approach
ØRQH3ZZ Repair Left Acromioclavicular Joint, Percutaneous Approach
ØRQH4ZZ Repair Left Acromioclavicular Joint, Percutaneous Endoscopic Approach
ØRQHXZZ Repair Left Acromioclavicular Joint, External Approach
ØRQJØZZ Repair Right Shoulder Joint, Open Approach
ØRQJ3ZZ Repair Right Shoulder Joint, Percutaneous Approach
ØRQJ4ZZ Repair Right Shoulder Joint, Percutaneous Endoscopic Approach
ØRQJXZZ Repair Right Shoulder Joint, External Approach
ØRQKØZZ Repair Left Shoulder Joint, Open Approach
ØRQK3ZZ Repair Left Shoulder Joint, Percutaneous Approach
ØRQK4ZZ Repair Left Shoulder Joint, Percutaneous Endoscopic Approach
ØRQKXZZ Repair Left Shoulder Joint, External Approach
ØRQLØZZ Repair Right Elbow Joint, Open Approach
ØRQL3ZZ Repair Right Elbow Joint, Percutaneous Approach
ØRQL4ZZ Repair Right Elbow Joint, Percutaneous Endoscopic Approach
ØRQLXZZ Repair Right Elbow Joint, External Approach
ØRQMØZZ Repair Left Elbow Joint, Open Approach
ØRQM3ZZ Repair Left Elbow Joint, Percutaneous Approach
ØRQM4ZZ Repair Left Elbow Joint, Percutaneous Endoscopic Approach
ØRQMXZZ Repair Left Elbow Joint, External Approach
ØRUEØ7Z Supplement Right Sternoclavicular Joint with Autologous Tissue Substitute, Open Approach
ØRUEØJZ Supplement Right Sternoclavicular Joint with Synthetic Substitute, Open Approach
ØRUEØKZ Supplement Right Sternoclavicular Joint with Nonautologous Tissue Substitute, Open Approach
ØRUE37Z Supplement Right Sternoclavicular Joint with Autologous Tissue Substitute, Percutaneous Approach
ØRUE3JZ Supplement Right Sternoclavicular Joint with Synthetic Substitute, Percutaneous Approach
ØRUE3KZ Supplement Right Sternoclavicular Joint with Nonautologous Tissue Substitute, Percutaneous Approach
ØRUE47Z Supplement Right Sternoclavicular Joint with Autologous Tissue Substitute, Percutaneous Endoscopic Approach
ØRUE4JZ Supplement Right Sternoclavicular Joint with Synthetic Substitute, Percutaneous Endoscopic Approach
ØRUE4KZ Supplement Right Sternoclavicular Joint with Nonautologous Tissue Substitute, Percutaneous Endoscopic Approach
ØRUFØ7Z Supplement Left Sternoclavicular Joint with Autologous Tissue Substitute, Open Approach
ØRUFØJZ Supplement Left Sternoclavicular Joint with Synthetic Substitute, Open Approach
ØRUFØKZ Supplement Left Sternoclavicular Joint with Nonautologous Tissue Substitute, Open Approach
ØRUF37Z Supplement Left Sternoclavicular Joint with Autologous Tissue Substitute, Percutaneous Approach
ØRUF3JZ Supplement Left Sternoclavicular Joint with Synthetic Substitute, Percutaneous Approach
ØRUF3KZ Supplement Left Sternoclavicular Joint with Nonautologous Tissue Substitute, Percutaneous Approach
ØRUF47Z Supplement Left Sternoclavicular Joint with Autologous Tissue Substitute, Percutaneous Endoscopic Approach
ØRUF4JZ Supplement Left Sternoclavicular Joint with Synthetic Substitute, Percutaneous Endoscopic Approach
ØRUF4KZ Supplement Left Sternoclavicular Joint with Nonautologous Tissue Substitute, Percutaneous Endoscopic Approach
ØRUGØ7Z Supplement Right Acromioclavicular Joint with Autologous Tissue Substitute, Open Approach

HAC 12: Surgical Site Infection-Certain Orthopedic Procedures of the Spine, Shoulder, and Elbow (continued)

ØRUGØJZ Supplement Right Acromioclavicular Joint with Synthetic Substitute, Open Approach
ØRUGØKZ Supplement Right Acromioclavicular Joint with Nonautologous Tissue Substitute, Open Approach
ØRUG37Z Supplement Right Acromioclavicular Joint with Autologous Tissue Substitute, Percutaneous Approach
ØRUG3JZ Supplement Right Acromioclavicular Joint with Synthetic Substitute, Percutaneous Approach
ØRUG3KZ Supplement Right Acromioclavicular Joint with Nonautologous Tissue Substitute, Percutaneous Approach
ØRUG47Z Supplement Right Acromioclavicular Joint with Autologous Tissue Substitute, Percutaneous Endoscopic Approach
ØRUG4JZ Supplement Right Acromioclavicular Joint with Synthetic Substitute, Percutaneous Endoscopic Approach
ØRUG4KZ Supplement Right Acromioclavicular Joint with Nonautologous Tissue Substitute, Percutaneous Endoscopic Approach
ØRUHØ7Z Supplement Left Acromioclavicular Joint with Autologous Tissue Substitute, Open Approach
ØRUHØJZ Supplement Left Acromioclavicular Joint with Synthetic Substitute, Open Approach
ØRUHØKZ Supplement Left Acromioclavicular Joint with Nonautologous Tissue Substitute, Open Approach
ØRUH37Z Supplement Left Acromioclavicular Joint with Autologous Tissue Substitute, Percutaneous Approach
ØRUH3JZ Supplement Left Acromioclavicular Joint with Synthetic Substitute, Percutaneous Approach
ØRUH3KZ Supplement Left Acromioclavicular Joint with Nonautologous Tissue Substitute, Percutaneous Approach
ØRUH47Z Supplement Left Acromioclavicular Joint with Autologous Tissue Substitute, Percutaneous Endoscopic Approach
ØRUH4JZ Supplement Left Acromioclavicular Joint with Synthetic Substitute, Percutaneous Endoscopic Approach
ØRUH4KZ Supplement Left Acromioclavicular Joint with Nonautologous Tissue Substitute, Percutaneous Endoscopic Approach
ØRUJØ7Z Supplement Right Shoulder Joint with Autologous Tissue Substitute, Open Approach
ØRUJØJZ Supplement Right Shoulder Joint with Synthetic Substitute, Open Approach
ØRUJØKZ Supplement Right Shoulder Joint with Nonautologous Tissue Substitute, Open Approach
ØRUJ37Z Supplement Right Shoulder Joint with Autologous Tissue Substitute, Percutaneous Approach
ØRUJ3JZ Supplement Right Shoulder Joint with Synthetic Substitute, Percutaneous Approach
ØRUJ3KZ Supplement Right Shoulder Joint with Nonautologous Tissue Substitute, Percutaneous Approach
ØRUJ47Z Supplement Right Shoulder Joint with Autologous Tissue Substitute, Percutaneous Endoscopic Approach
ØRUJ4JZ Supplement Right Shoulder Joint with Synthetic Substitute, Percutaneous Endoscopic Approach
ØRUJ4KZ Supplement Right Shoulder Joint with Nonautologous Tissue Substitute, Percutaneous Endoscopic Approach
ØRUKØ7Z Supplement Left Shoulder Joint with Autologous Tissue Substitute, Open Approach
ØRUKØJZ Supplement Left Shoulder Joint with Synthetic Substitute, Open Approach
ØRUKØKZ Supplement Left Shoulder Joint with Nonautologous Tissue Substitute, Open Approach
ØRUK37Z Supplement Left Shoulder Joint with Autologous Tissue Substitute, Percutaneous Approach
ØRUK3JZ Supplement Left Shoulder Joint with Synthetic Substitute, Percutaneous Approach
ØRUK3KZ Supplement Left Shoulder Joint with Nonautologous Tissue Substitute, Percutaneous Approach
ØRUK47Z Supplement Left Shoulder Joint with Autologous Tissue Substitute, Percutaneous Endoscopic Approach
ØRUK4JZ Supplement Left Shoulder Joint with Synthetic Substitute, Percutaneous Endoscopic Approach
ØRUK4KZ Supplement Left Shoulder Joint with Nonautologous Tissue Substitute, Percutaneous Endoscopic Approach
ØRULØ7Z Supplement Right Elbow Joint with Autologous Tissue Substitute, Open Approach
ØRULØJZ Supplement Right Elbow Joint with Synthetic Substitute, Open Approach
ØRULØKZ Supplement Right Elbow Joint with Nonautologous Tissue Substitute, Open Approach
ØRUL37Z Supplement Right Elbow Joint with Autologous Tissue Substitute, Percutaneous Approach
ØRUL3JZ Supplement Right Elbow Joint with Synthetic Substitute, Percutaneous Approach
ØRUL3KZ Supplement Right Elbow Joint with Nonautologous Tissue Substitute, Percutaneous Approach
ØRUL47Z Supplement Right Elbow Joint with Autologous Tissue Substitute, Percutaneous Endoscopic Approach
ØRUL4JZ Supplement Right Elbow Joint with Synthetic Substitute, Percutaneous Endoscopic Approach
ØRUL4KZ Supplement Right Elbow Joint with Nonautologous Tissue Substitute, Percutaneous Endoscopic Approach
ØRUMØ7Z Supplement Left Elbow Joint with Autologous Tissue Substitute, Open Approach
ØRUMØJZ Supplement Left Elbow Joint with Synthetic Substitute, Open Approach
ØRUMØKZ Supplement Left Elbow Joint with Nonautologous Tissue Substitute, Open Approach
ØRUM37Z Supplement Left Elbow Joint with Autologous Tissue Substitute, Percutaneous Approach
ØRUM3JZ Supplement Left Elbow Joint with Synthetic Substitute, Percutaneous Approach
ØRUM3KZ Supplement Left Elbow Joint with Nonautologous Tissue Substitute, Percutaneous Approach
ØRUM47Z Supplement Left Elbow Joint with Autologous Tissue Substitute, Percutaneous Endoscopic Approach
ØRUM4JZ Supplement Left Elbow Joint with Synthetic Substitute, Percutaneous Endoscopic Approach
ØRUM4KZ Supplement Left Elbow Joint with Nonautologous Tissue Substitute, Percutaneous Endoscopic Approach
ØSGØØ7Ø Fusion of Lumbar Vertebral Joint with Autologous Tissue Substitute, Anterior Approach, Anterior Column, Open Approach
ØSGØØ71 Fusion of Lumbar Vertebral Joint with Autologous Tissue Substitute, Posterior Approach, Posterior Column, Open Approach
ØSGØØ7J Fusion of Lumbar Vertebral Joint with Autologous Tissue Substitute, Posterior Approach, Anterior Column, Open Approach
ØSGØØAØ Fusion of Lumbar Vertebral Joint with Interbody Fusion Device, Anterior Approach, Anterior Column, Open Approach
ØSGØØAJ Fusion of Lumbar Vertebral Joint with Interbody Fusion Device, Posterior Approach, Anterior Column, Open Approach
ØSGØØJØ Fusion of Lumbar Vertebral Joint with Synthetic Substitute, Anterior Approach, Anterior Column, Open Approach
ØSGØØJ1 Fusion of Lumbar Vertebral Joint with Synthetic Substitute, Posterior Approach, Posterior Column, Open Approach
ØSGØØJJ Fusion of Lumbar Vertebral Joint with Synthetic Substitute, Posterior Approach, Anterior Column, Open Approach
ØSGØØKØ Fusion of Lumbar Vertebral Joint with Nonautologous Tissue Substitute, Anterior Approach, Anterior Column, Open Approach
ØSGØØK1 Fusion of Lumbar Vertebral Joint with Nonautologous Tissue Substitute, Posterior Approach, Posterior Column, Open Approach
ØSGØØKJ Fusion of Lumbar Vertebral Joint with Nonautologous Tissue Substitute, Posterior Approach, Anterior Column, Open Approach
ØSGØ37Ø Fusion of Lumbar Vertebral Joint with Autologous Tissue Substitute, Anterior Approach, Anterior Column, Percutaneous Approach
ØSGØ371 Fusion of Lumbar Vertebral Joint with Autologous Tissue Substitute, Posterior Approach, Posterior Column, Percutaneous Approach
ØSGØ37J Fusion of Lumbar Vertebral Joint with Autologous Tissue Substitute, Posterior Approach, Anterior Column, Percutaneous Approach
ØSGØ3AØ Fusion of Lumbar Vertebral Joint with Interbody Fusion Device, Anterior Approach, Anterior Column, Percutaneous Approach
ØSGØ3AJ Fusion of Lumbar Vertebral Joint with Interbody Fusion Device, Posterior Approach, Anterior Column, Percutaneous Approach
ØSGØ3JØ Fusion of Lumbar Vertebral Joint with Synthetic Substitute, Anterior Approach, Anterior Column, Percutaneous Approach

HAC 12: Surgical Site Infection-Certain Orthopedic Procedures of the Spine, Shoulder, and Elbow (continued)

ØSGØ3J1 Fusion of Lumbar Vertebral Joint with Synthetic Substitute, Posterior Approach, Posterior Column, Percutaneous Approach
ØSGØ3JJ Fusion of Lumbar Vertebral Joint with Synthetic Substitute, Posterior Approach, Anterior Column, Percutaneous Approach
ØSGØ3KØ Fusion of Lumbar Vertebral Joint with Nonautologous Tissue Substitute, Anterior Approach, Anterior Column, Percutaneous Approach
ØSGØ3K1 Fusion of Lumbar Vertebral Joint with Nonautologous Tissue Substitute, Posterior Approach, Posterior Column, Percutaneous Approach
ØSGØ3KJ Fusion of Lumbar Vertebral Joint with Nonautologous Tissue Substitute, Posterior Approach, Anterior Column, Percutaneous Approach
ØSGØ47Ø Fusion of Lumbar Vertebral Joint with Autologous Tissue Substitute, Anterior Approach, Anterior Column, Percutaneous Endoscopic Approach
ØSGØ471 Fusion of Lumbar Vertebral Joint with Autologous Tissue Substitute, Posterior Approach, Posterior Column, Percutaneous Endoscopic Approach
ØSGØ47J Fusion of Lumbar Vertebral Joint with Autologous Tissue Substitute, Posterior Approach, Anterior Column, Percutaneous Endoscopic Approach
ØSGØ4AØ Fusion of Lumbar Vertebral Joint with Interbody Fusion Device, Anterior Approach, Anterior Column, Percutaneous Endoscopic Approach
ØSGØ4AJ Fusion of Lumbar Vertebral Joint with Interbody Fusion Device, Posterior Approach, Anterior Column, Percutaneous Endoscopic Approach
ØSGØ4JØ Fusion of Lumbar Vertebral Joint with Synthetic Substitute, Anterior Approach, Anterior Column, Percutaneous Endoscopic Approach
ØSGØ4J1 Fusion of Lumbar Vertebral Joint with Synthetic Substitute, Posterior Approach, Posterior Column, Percutaneous Endoscopic Approach
ØSGØ4JJ Fusion of Lumbar Vertebral Joint with Synthetic Substitute, Posterior Approach, Anterior Column, Percutaneous Endoscopic Approach
ØSGØ4KØ Fusion of Lumbar Vertebral Joint with Nonautologous Tissue Substitute, Anterior Approach, Anterior Column, Percutaneous Endoscopic Approach
ØSGØ4K1 Fusion of Lumbar Vertebral Joint with Nonautologous Tissue Substitute, Posterior Approach, Posterior Column, Percutaneous Endoscopic Approach
ØSGØ4KJ Fusion of Lumbar Vertebral Joint with Nonautologous Tissue Substitute, Posterior Approach, Anterior Column, Percutaneous Endoscopic Approach
ØSG1Ø7Ø Fusion of 2 or More Lumbar Vertebral Joints with Autologous Tissue Substitute, Anterior Approach, Anterior Column, Open Approach
ØSG1Ø71 Fusion of 2 or More Lumbar Vertebral Joints with Autologous Tissue Substitute, Posterior Approach, Posterior Column, Open Approach
ØSG1Ø7J Fusion of 2 or More Lumbar Vertebral Joints with Autologous Tissue Substitute, Posterior Approach, Anterior Column, Open Approach
ØSG1ØAØ Fusion of 2 or More Lumbar Vertebral Joints with Interbody Fusion Device, Anterior Approach, Anterior Column, Open Approach
ØSG1ØAJ Fusion of 2 or More Lumbar Vertebral Joints with Interbody Fusion Device, Posterior Approach, Anterior Column, Open Approach
ØSG1ØJØ Fusion of 2 or More Lumbar Vertebral Joints with Synthetic Substitute, Anterior Approach, Anterior Column, Open Approach
ØSG1ØJ1 Fusion of 2 or More Lumbar Vertebral Joints with Synthetic Substitute, Posterior Approach, Posterior Column, Open Approach
ØSG1ØJJ Fusion of 2 or More Lumbar Vertebral Joints with Synthetic Substitute, Posterior Approach, Anterior Column, Open Approach
ØSG1ØKØ Fusion of 2 or More Lumbar Vertebral Joints with Nonautologous Tissue Substitute, Anterior Approach, Anterior Column, Open Approach
ØSG1ØK1 Fusion of 2 or More Lumbar Vertebral Joints with Nonautologous Tissue Substitute, Posterior Approach, Posterior Column, Open Approach
ØSG1ØKJ Fusion of 2 or More Lumbar Vertebral Joints with Nonautologous Tissue Substitute, Posterior Approach, Anterior Column, Open Approach
ØSG137Ø Fusion of 2 or More Lumbar Vertebral Joints with Autologous Tissue Substitute, Anterior Approach, Anterior Column, Percutaneous Approach
ØSG1371 Fusion of 2 or More Lumbar Vertebral Joints with Autologous Tissue Substitute, Posterior Approach, Posterior Column, Percutaneous Approach
ØSG137J Fusion of 2 or More Lumbar Vertebral Joints with Autologous Tissue Substitute, Posterior Approach, Anterior Column, Percutaneous Approach
ØSG13AØ Fusion of 2 or More Lumbar Vertebral Joints with Interbody Fusion Device, Anterior Approach, Anterior Column, Percutaneous Approach
ØSG13AJ Fusion of 2 or More Lumbar Vertebral Joints with Interbody Fusion Device, Posterior Approach, Anterior Column, Percutaneous Approach
ØSG13JØ Fusion of 2 or More Lumbar Vertebral Joints with Synthetic Substitute, Anterior Approach, Anterior Column, Percutaneous Approach
ØSG13J1 Fusion of 2 or More Lumbar Vertebral Joints with Synthetic Substitute, Posterior Approach, Posterior Column, Percutaneous Approach
ØSG13JJ Fusion of 2 or More Lumbar Vertebral Joints with Synthetic Substitute, Posterior Approach, Anterior Column, Percutaneous Approach
ØSG13KØ Fusion of 2 or More Lumbar Vertebral Joints with Nonautologous Tissue Substitute, Anterior Approach, Anterior Column, Percutaneous Approach
ØSG13K1 Fusion of 2 or More Lumbar Vertebral Joints with Nonautologous Tissue Substitute, Posterior Approach, Posterior Column, Percutaneous Approach
ØSG13KJ Fusion of 2 or More Lumbar Vertebral Joints with Nonautologous Tissue Substitute, Posterior Approach, Anterior Column, Percutaneous Approach
ØSG147Ø Fusion of 2 or More Lumbar Vertebral Joints with Autologous Tissue Substitute, Anterior Approach, Anterior Column, Percutaneous Endoscopic Approach
ØSG1471 Fusion of 2 or More Lumbar Vertebral Joints with Autologous Tissue Substitute, Posterior Approach, Posterior Column, Percutaneous Endoscopic Approach
ØSG147J Fusion of 2 or More Lumbar Vertebral Joints with Autologous Tissue Substitute, Posterior Approach, Anterior Column, Percutaneous Endoscopic Approach
ØSG14AØ Fusion of 2 or More Lumbar Vertebral Joints with Interbody Fusion Device, Anterior Approach, Anterior Column, Percutaneous Endoscopic Approach
ØSG14AJ Fusion of 2 or More Lumbar Vertebral Joints with Interbody Fusion Device, Posterior Approach, Anterior Column, Percutaneous Endoscopic Approach
ØSG14JØ Fusion of 2 or More Lumbar Vertebral Joints with Synthetic Substitute, Anterior Approach, Anterior Column, Percutaneous Endoscopic Approach
ØSG14J1 Fusion of 2 or More Lumbar Vertebral Joints with Synthetic Substitute, Posterior Approach, Posterior Column, Percutaneous Endoscopic Approach
ØSG14JJ Fusion of 2 or More Lumbar Vertebral Joints with Synthetic Substitute, Posterior Approach, Anterior Column, Percutaneous Endoscopic Approach
ØSG14KØ Fusion of 2 or More Lumbar Vertebral Joints with Nonautologous Tissue Substitute, Anterior Approach, Anterior Column, Percutaneous Endoscopic Approach
ØSG14K1 Fusion of 2 or More Lumbar Vertebral Joints with Nonautologous Tissue Substitute, Posterior Approach, Posterior Column, Percutaneous Endoscopic Approach
ØSG14KJ Fusion of 2 or More Lumbar Vertebral Joints with Nonautologous Tissue Substitute, Posterior Approach, Anterior Column, Percutaneous Endoscopic Approach
ØSG3Ø7Ø Fusion of Lumbosacral Joint with Autologous Tissue Substitute, Anterior Approach, Anterior Column, Open Approach
ØSG3Ø71 Fusion of Lumbosacral Joint with Autologous Tissue Substitute, Posterior Approach, Posterior Column, Open Approach
ØSG3Ø7J Fusion of Lumbosacral Joint with Autologous Tissue Substitute, Posterior Approach, Anterior Column, Open Approach
ØSG3ØAØ Fusion of Lumbosacral Joint with Interbody Fusion Device, Anterior Approach, Anterior Column, Open Approach

HAC 12: Surgical Site Infection-Certain Orthopedic Procedures of the Spine, Shoulder, and Elbow (continued)

ØSG3ØAJ Fusion of Lumbosacral Joint with Interbody Fusion Device, Posterior Approach, Anterior Column, Open Approach

ØSG3ØJØ Fusion of Lumbosacral Joint with Synthetic Substitute, Anterior Approach, Anterior Column, Open Approach

ØSG3ØJ1 Fusion of Lumbosacral Joint with Synthetic Substitute, Posterior Approach, Posterior Column, Open Approach

ØSG3ØJJ Fusion of Lumbosacral Joint with Synthetic Substitute, Posterior Approach, Anterior Column, Open Approach

ØSG3ØKØ Fusion of Lumbosacral Joint with Nonautologous Tissue Substitute, Anterior Approach, Anterior Column, Open Approach

ØSG3ØK1 Fusion of Lumbosacral Joint with Nonautologous Tissue Substitute, Posterior Approach, Posterior Column, Open Approach

ØSG3ØKJ Fusion of Lumbosacral Joint with Nonautologous Tissue Substitute, Posterior Approach, Anterior Column, Open Approach

ØSG337Ø Fusion of Lumbosacral Joint with Autologous Tissue Substitute, Anterior Approach, Anterior Column, Percutaneous Approach

ØSG3371 Fusion of Lumbosacral Joint with Autologous Tissue Substitute, Posterior Approach, Posterior Column, Percutaneous Approach

ØSG337J Fusion of Lumbosacral Joint with Autologous Tissue Substitute, Posterior Approach, Anterior Column, Percutaneous Approach

ØSG33AØ Fusion of Lumbosacral Joint with Interbody Fusion Device, Anterior Approach, Anterior Column, Percutaneous Approach

ØSG33AJ Fusion of Lumbosacral Joint with Interbody Fusion Device, Posterior Approach, Anterior Column, Percutaneous Approach

ØSG33JØ Fusion of Lumbosacral Joint with Synthetic Substitute, Anterior Approach, Anterior Column, Percutaneous Approach

ØSG33J1 Fusion of Lumbosacral Joint with Synthetic Substitute, Posterior Approach, Posterior Column, Percutaneous Approach

ØSG33JJ Fusion of Lumbosacral Joint with Synthetic Substitute, Posterior Approach, Anterior Column, Percutaneous Approach

ØSG33KØ Fusion of Lumbosacral Joint with Nonautologous Tissue Substitute, Anterior Approach, Anterior Column, Percutaneous Approach

ØSG33K1 Fusion of Lumbosacral Joint with Nonautologous Tissue Substitute, Posterior Approach, Posterior Column, Percutaneous Approach

ØSG33KJ Fusion of Lumbosacral Joint with Nonautologous Tissue Substitute, Posterior Approach, Anterior Column, Percutaneous Approach

ØSG347Ø Fusion of Lumbosacral Joint with Autologous Tissue Substitute, Anterior Approach, Anterior Column, Percutaneous Endoscopic Approach

ØSG3471 Fusion of Lumbosacral Joint with Autologous Tissue Substitute, Posterior Approach, Posterior Column, Percutaneous Endoscopic Approach

ØSG347J Fusion of Lumbosacral Joint with Autologous Tissue Substitute, Posterior Approach, Anterior Column, Percutaneous Endoscopic Approach

ØSG34AØ Fusion of Lumbosacral Joint with Interbody Fusion Device, Anterior Approach, Anterior Column, Percutaneous Endoscopic Approach

ØSG34AJ Fusion of Lumbosacral Joint with Interbody Fusion Device, Posterior Approach, Anterior Column, Percutaneous Endoscopic Approach

ØSG34JØ Fusion of Lumbosacral Joint with Synthetic Substitute, Anterior Approach, Anterior Column, Percutaneous Endoscopic Approach

ØSG34J1 Fusion of Lumbosacral Joint with Synthetic Substitute, Posterior Approach, Posterior Column, Percutaneous Endoscopic Approach

ØSG34JJ Fusion of Lumbosacral Joint with Synthetic Substitute, Posterior Approach, Anterior Column, Percutaneous Endoscopic Approach

ØSG34KØ Fusion of Lumbosacral Joint with Nonautologous Tissue Substitute, Anterior Approach, Anterior Column, Percutaneous Endoscopic Approach

ØSG34K1 Fusion of Lumbosacral Joint with Nonautologous Tissue Substitute, Posterior Approach, Posterior Column, Percutaneous Endoscopic Approach

ØSG34KJ Fusion of Lumbosacral Joint with Nonautologous Tissue Substitute, Posterior Approach, Anterior Column, Percutaneous Endoscopic Approach

ØSG7Ø4Z Fusion of Right Sacroiliac Joint with Internal Fixation Device, Open Approach

ØSG7Ø7Z Fusion of Right Sacroiliac Joint with Autologous Tissue Substitute, Open Approach

ØSG7ØJZ Fusion of Right Sacroiliac Joint with Synthetic Substitute, Open Approach

ØSG7ØKZ Fusion of Right Sacroiliac Joint with Nonautologous Tissue Substitute, Open Approach

ØSG734Z Fusion of Right Sacroiliac Joint with Internal Fixation Device, Percutaneous Approach

ØSG737Z Fusion of Right Sacroiliac Joint with Autologous Tissue Substitute, Percutaneous Approach

ØSG73JZ Fusion of Right Sacroiliac Joint with Synthetic Substitute, Percutaneous Approach

ØSG73KZ Fusion of Right Sacroiliac Joint with Nonautologous Tissue Substitute, Percutaneous Approach

ØSG744Z Fusion of Right Sacroiliac Joint with Internal Fixation Device, Percutaneous Endoscopic Approach

ØSG747Z Fusion of Right Sacroiliac Joint with Autologous Tissue Substitute, Percutaneous Endoscopic Approach

ØSG74JZ Fusion of Right Sacroiliac Joint with Synthetic Substitute, Percutaneous Endoscopic Approach

ØSG74KZ Fusion of Right Sacroiliac Joint with Nonautologous Tissue Substitute, Percutaneous Endoscopic Approach

ØSG8Ø4Z Fusion of Left Sacroiliac Joint with Internal Fixation Device, Open Approach

ØSG8Ø7Z Fusion of Left Sacroiliac Joint with Autologous Tissue Substitute, Open Approach

ØSG8ØJZ Fusion of Left Sacroiliac Joint with Synthetic Substitute, Open Approach

ØSG8ØKZ Fusion of Left Sacroiliac Joint with Nonautologous Tissue Substitute, Open Approach

ØSG834Z Fusion of Left Sacroiliac Joint with Internal Fixation Device, Percutaneous Approach

ØSG837Z Fusion of Left Sacroiliac Joint with Autologous Tissue Substitute, Percutaneous Approach

ØSG83JZ Fusion of Left Sacroiliac Joint with Synthetic Substitute, Percutaneous Approach

ØSG83KZ Fusion of Left Sacroiliac Joint with Nonautologous Tissue Substitute, Percutaneous Approach

ØSG844Z Fusion of Left Sacroiliac Joint with Internal Fixation Device, Percutaneous Endoscopic Approach

ØSG847Z Fusion of Left Sacroiliac Joint with Autologous Tissue Substitute, Percutaneous Endoscopic Approach

ØSG84JZ Fusion of Left Sacroiliac Joint with Synthetic Substitute, Percutaneous Endoscopic Approach

ØSG84KZ Fusion of Left Sacroiliac Joint with Nonautologous Tissue Substitute, Percutaneous Endoscopic Approach

XRGØØ92 Fusion of Occipital-cervical Joint using Nanotextured Surface Interbody Fusion Device, Open Approach, New Technology Group 2

XRGØØF3 Fusion of Occipital-cervical Joint using Radiolucent Porous Interbody Fusion Device, Open Approach, New Technology Group 3

XRG1Ø92 Fusion of Cervical Vertebral Joint using Nanotextured Surface Interbody Fusion Device, Open Approach, New Technology Group 2

XRG1ØF3 Fusion of Cervical Vertebral Joint using Radiolucent Porous Interbody Fusion Device, Open Approach, New Technology Group 3

XRG2Ø92 Fusion of 2 or more Cervical Vertebral Joints using Nanotextured Surface Interbody Fusion Device, Open Approach, New Technology Group 2

XRG2ØF3 Fusion of 2 or more Cervical Vertebral Joints using Radiolucent Porous Interbody Fusion Device, Open Approach, New Technology Group 3

XRG4Ø92 Fusion of Cervicothoracic Vertebral Joint using Nanotextured Surface Interbody Fusion Device, Open Approach, New Technology Group 2

XRG4ØF3 Fusion of Cervicothoracic Vertebral Joint using Radiolucent Porous Interbody Fusion Device, Open Approach, New Technology Group 3

XRG6Ø92 Fusion of Thoracic Vertebral Joint using Nanotextured Surface Interbody Fusion Device, Open Approach, New Technology Group 2

HAC 12: Surgical Site Infection-Certain Orthopedic Procedures of the Spine, Shoulder, and Elbow (continued)

XRG60F3 Fusion of Thoracic Vertebral Joint using Radiolucent Porous Interbody Fusion Device, Open Approach, New Technology Group 3
XRG7092 Fusion of 2 to 7 Thoracic Vertebral Joints using Nanotextured Surface Interbody Fusion Device, Open Approach, New Technology Group 2
XRG70F3 Fusion of 2 to 7 Thoracic Vertebral Joints using Radiolucent Porous Interbody Fusion Device, Open Approach, New Technology Group 3
XRG8092 Fusion of 8 or more Thoracic Vertebral Joints using Nanotextured Surface Interbody Fusion Device, Open Approach, New Technology Group 2
XRG80F3 Fusion of 8 or more Thoracic Vertebral Joints using Radiolucent Porous Interbody Fusion Device, Open Approach, New Technology Group 3
XRGA092 Fusion of Thoracolumbar Vertebral Joint using Nanotextured Surface Interbody Fusion Device, Open Approach, New Technology Group 2
XRGA0F3 Fusion of Thoracolumbar Vertebral Joint using Radiolucent Porous Interbody Fusion Device, Open Approach, New Technology Group 3
XRGB092 Fusion of Lumbar Vertebral Joint using Nanotextured Surface Interbody Fusion Device, Open Approach, New Technology Group 2
XRGB0F3 Fusion of Lumbar Vertebral Joint using Radiolucent Porous Interbody Fusion Device, Open Approach, New Technology Group 3
XRGC092 Fusion of 2 or more Lumbar Vertebral Joints using Nanotextured Surface Interbody Fusion Device, Open Approach, New Technology Group 2
XRGC0F3 Fusion of 2 or more Lumbar Vertebral Joints using Radiolucent Porous Interbody Fusion Device, Open Approach, New Technology Group 3
XRGD092 Fusion of Lumbosacral Joint using Nanotextured Surface Interbody Fusion Device, Open Approach, New Technology Group 2
XRGD0F3 Fusion of Lumbosacral Joint using Radiolucent Porous Interbody Fusion Device, Open Approach, New Technology Group 3

HAC 13: Surgical Site Infection (SSI) Following Cardiac Implantable Electronic Device (CIED) Procedures

Secondary diagnosis not POA:

K68.11 Postprocedural retroperitoneal abscess
T81.40XA Infection following a procedure, unspecified, initial encounter
T81.41XA Infection following a procedure, superficial incisional surgical site, initial encounter
T81.42XA Infection following a procedure, deep incisional surgical site, initial encounter
T81.43XA Infection following a procedure, organ and space surgical site, initial encounter
T81.44XA Sepsis following a procedure, initial encounter
T81.49XA Infection following a procedure, other surgical site, initial encounter
T82.6XXA Infection and inflammatory reaction due to cardiac valve prosthesis, initial encounter
T82.7XXA Infection and inflammatory reaction due to other internal orthopedic prosthetic devices, implants and grafts, initial encounter

AND

Any of the following procedures:

02H43JZ Insertion of Pacemaker Lead into Coronary Vein, Percutaneous Approach
02H43KZ Insertion of Defibrillator Lead into Coronary Vein, Percutaneous Approach
02H43MZ Insertion of Cardiac Lead into Coronary Vein, Percutaneous Approach
02H63JZ Insertion of Pacemaker Lead into Right Atrium, Percutaneous Approach
02H63MZ Insertion of Cardiac Lead into Right Atrium, Percutaneous Approach
02H73JZ Insertion of Pacemaker Lead into Left Atrium, Percutaneous Approach
02H73MZ Insertion of Cardiac Lead into Left Atrium, Percutaneous Approach
02HK3JZ Insertion of Pacemaker Lead into Right Ventricle, Percutaneous Approach
02HL3JZ Insertion of Pacemaker Lead into Left Ventricle, Percutaneous Approach
02HN0JZ Insertion of Pacemaker Lead into Pericardium, Open Approach
02HN0MZ Insertion of Cardiac Lead into Pericardium, Open Approach
02HN3JZ Insertion of Pacemaker Lead into Pericardium, Percutaneous Approach
02HN3MZ Insertion of Cardiac Lead into Pericardium, Percutaneous Approach
02HN4JZ Insertion of Pacemaker Lead into Pericardium, Percutaneous Endoscopic Approach
02HN4MZ Insertion of Cardiac Lead into Pericardium, Percutaneous Endoscopic Approach
02PA0MZ Removal of Cardiac Lead from Heart, Open Approach
02PA3MZ Removal of Cardiac Lead from Heart, Percutaneous Approach
02PA4MZ Removal of Cardiac Lead from Heart, Percutaneous Endoscopic Approach
02PAXMZ Removal of Cardiac Lead from Heart, External Approach
02WA0MZ Revision of Cardiac Lead in Heart, Open Approach
02WA3MZ Revision of Cardiac Lead in Heart, Percutaneous Approach
02WA4MZ Revision of Cardiac Lead in Heart, Percutaneous Endoscopic Approach
0JH604Z Insertion of Pacemaker, Single Chamber into Chest Subcutaneous Tissue and Fascia, Open Approach
0JH605Z Insertion of Pacemaker, Single Chamber Rate Responsive into Chest Subcutaneous Tissue and Fascia, Open Approach
0JH606Z Insertion of Pacemaker, Dual Chamber into Chest Subcutaneous Tissue and Fascia, Open Approach
0JH607Z Insertion of Cardiac Resynchronization Pacemaker Pulse Generator into Chest Subcutaneous Tissue and Fascia, Open Approach
0JH608Z Insertion of Defibrillator Generator into Chest Subcutaneous Tissue and Fascia, Open Approach
0JH609Z Insertion of Cardiac Resynchronization Defibrillator Pulse Generator into Chest Subcutaneous Tissue and Fascia, Open Approach
0JH60PZ Insertion of Cardiac Rhythm Related Device into Chest Subcutaneous Tissue and Fascia, Open Approach
0JH634Z Insertion of Pacemaker, Single Chamber into Chest Subcutaneous Tissue and Fascia, Percutaneous Approach
0JH635Z Insertion of Pacemaker, Single Chamber Rate Responsive into Chest Subcutaneous Tissue and Fascia, Percutaneous Approach
0JH636Z Insertion of Pacemaker, Dual Chamber into Chest Subcutaneous Tissue and Fascia, Percutaneous Approach
0JH637Z Insertion of Cardiac Resynchronization Pacemaker Pulse Generator into Chest Subcutaneous Tissue and Fascia, Percutaneous Approach
0JH638Z Insertion of Defibrillator Generator into Chest Subcutaneous Tissue and Fascia, Percutaneous Approach
0JH639Z Insertion of Cardiac Resynchronization Defibrillator Pulse Generator into Chest Subcutaneous Tissue and Fascia, Percutaneous Approach
0JH63PZ Insertion of Cardiac Rhythm Related Device into Chest Subcutaneous Tissue and Fascia, Percutaneous Approach
0JH804Z Insertion of Pacemaker, Single Chamber into Abdomen Subcutaneous Tissue and Fascia, Open Approach
0JH805Z Insertion of Pacemaker, Single Chamber Rate Responsive into Abdomen Subcutaneous Tissue and Fascia, Open Approach
0JH806Z Insertion of Pacemaker, Dual Chamber into Abdomen Subcutaneous Tissue and Fascia, Open Approach
0JH807Z Insertion of Cardiac Resynchronization Pacemaker Pulse Generator into Abdomen Subcutaneous Tissue and Fascia, Open Approach
0JH808Z Insertion of Defibrillator Generator into Abdomen Subcutaneous Tissue and Fascia, Open Approach
0JH809Z Insertion of Cardiac Resynchronization Defibrillator Pulse Generator into Abdomen Subcutaneous Tissue and Fascia, Open Approach
0JH80PZ Insertion of Cardiac Rhythm Related Device into Abdomen Subcutaneous Tissue and Fascia, Open Approach
0JH834Z Insertion of Pacemaker, Single Chamber into Abdomen Subcutaneous Tissue and Fascia, Percutaneous Approach
0JH835Z Insertion of Pacemaker, Single Chamber Rate Responsive into Abdomen Subcutaneous Tissue and Fascia, Percutaneous Approach
0JH836Z Insertion of Pacemaker, Dual Chamber into Abdomen Subcutaneous Tissue and Fascia, Percutaneous Approach
0JH837Z Insertion of Cardiac Resynchronization Pacemaker Pulse Generator into Abdomen Subcutaneous Tissue and Fascia, Percutaneous Approach
0JH838Z Insertion of Defibrillator Generator into Abdomen Subcutaneous Tissue and Fascia, Percutaneous Approach
0JH839Z Insertion of Cardiac Resynchronization Defibrillator Pulse Generator into Abdomen Subcutaneous Tissue and Fascia, Percutaneous Approach

HAC 13: Surgical Site Infection (SSI) Following Cardiac Implantable Electronic Device (CIED) Procedures (continued)

ØJH83PZ Insertion of Cardiac Rhythm Related Device into Abdomen Subcutaneous Tissue and Fascia, Percutaneous Approach
ØJPTØFZ Removal of Subcutaneous Defibrillator Lead from Trunk Subcutaneous Tissue and Fascia, Open Approach
ØJPTØPZ Removal of Cardiac Rhythm Related Device from Trunk Subcutaneous Tissue and Fascia, Open Approach
ØJPT3FZ Removal of Subcutaneous Defibrillator Lead from Trunk Subcutaneous Tissue and Fascia, Percutaneous Approach
ØJPT3PZ Removal of Cardiac Rhythm Related Device from Trunk Subcutaneous Tissue and Fascia, Percutaneous Approach
ØJWTØFZ Revision of Subcutaneous Defibrillator Lead in Trunk Subcutaneous Tissue and Fascia, Open Approach
ØJWTØPZ Revision of Cardiac Rhythm Related Device in Trunk Subcutaneous Tissue and Fascia, Open Approach
ØJWT3FZ Revision of Subcutaneous Defibrillator Lead in Trunk Subcutaneous Tissue and Fascia, Percutaneous Approach
ØJWT3PZ Revision of Cardiac Rhythm Related Device in Trunk Subcutaneous Tissue and Fascia, Percutaneous Approach

HAC 14: Iatrogenic Pneumothorax with Venous Catheterization

Secondary diagnosis not POA:

J95.811 Postprocedural pneumothorax

AND

Any of the following procedures:

Ø2H633Z Insertion of Infusion Device into Right Atrium, Percutaneous Approach
Ø2HK33Z Insertion of Infusion Device into Right Ventricle, Percutaneous Approach
Ø2HS33Z Insertion of Infusion Device into Right Pulmonary Vein, Percutaneous Approach
Ø2HS43Z Insertion of Infusion Device into Right Pulmonary Vein, Percutaneous Endoscopic Approach
Ø2HT33Z Insertion of Infusion Device into Left Pulmonary Vein, Percutaneous Approach
Ø2HT43Z Insertion of Infusion Device into Left Pulmonary Vein, Percutaneous Endoscopic Approach
Ø2HV33Z Insertion of Infusion Device into Superior Vena Cava, Percutaneous Approach
Ø2HV43Z Insertion of Infusion Device into Superior Vena Cava, Percutaneous Endoscopic Approach
Ø5HØ33Z Insertion of Infusion Device into Azygos Vein, Percutaneous Approach
Ø5HØ43Z Insertion of Infusion Device into Azygos Vein, Percutaneous Endoscopic Approach
Ø5H133Z Insertion of Infusion Device into Hemiazygos Vein, Percutaneous Approach
Ø5H143Z Insertion of Infusion Device into Hemiazygos Vein, Percutaneous Endoscopic Approach
Ø5H333Z Insertion of Infusion Device into Right Innominate Vein, Percutaneous Approach
Ø5H343Z Insertion of Infusion Device into Right Innominate Vein, Percutaneous Endoscopic Approach
Ø5H433Z Insertion of Infusion Device into Left Innominate Vein, Percutaneous Approach
Ø5H443Z Insertion of Infusion Device into Left Innominate Vein, Percutaneous Endoscopic Approach
Ø5H533Z Insertion of Infusion Device into Right Subclavian Vein, Percutaneous Approach
Ø5H543Z Insertion of Infusion Device into Right Subclavian Vein, Percutaneous Endoscopic Approach
Ø5H633Z Insertion of Infusion Device into Left Subclavian Vein, Percutaneous Approach
Ø5H643Z Insertion of Infusion Device into Left Subclavian Vein, Percutaneous Endoscopic Approach
Ø5HM33Z Insertion of Infusion Device into Right Internal Jugular Vein, Percutaneous Approach
Ø5HN33Z Insertion of Infusion Device into Left Internal Jugular Vein, Percutaneous Approach
Ø5HP33Z Insertion of Infusion Device into Right External Jugular Vein, Percutaneous Approach
Ø5HQ33Z Insertion of Infusion Device into Left External Jugular Vein, Percutaneous Approach
ØJH63XZ Insertion of Vascular Access Device into Chest Subcutaneous Tissue and Fascia, Percutaneous Approach

Appendix L: Procedure Combination Tables

The tables below were developed to help simplify the relationship between ICD-10-PCS coding and MS-DRG assignment. The Centers for Medicare & Medicaid Services (CMS) has identified in the MS-DRG Definitions Manual certain procedure combinations that must occur in order to assign a specific MS-DRG. There are many factors influencing MS-DRG assignment, including principal and secondary diagnoses, MCC or CC use, sex of the patient, and discharge status. These tables should be used only as a guide. These tables were created based on the proposed, version 38, MS-DRG Grouper software and Definitions Manual files published with the fiscal 2021 IPPS proposed rule. To view the final, version 38, MS-DRG Grouper software and Definitions Manual files, refer to the following: https://www.cms.gov/Medicare/Medicare-Fee-for-Service-Payment/AcuteInpatientPPS/MS-DRG-Classifications-and-Software.

DRG ØØ1-ØØ2 Heart Transplant or Implant of Heart Assist System

Heart Transplant

Replacement of Right and Left Ventricle Ø2RKØJZ and Ø2RLØJZ

Insertion With Removal of Heart Assist System

Type of Heart Assist System	Code as appropriate Insertion by approach	Code also as appropriate Removal of Heart Assist System by approach
Biventricular External	Ø2HA[Ø,3,4]RS	Ø2PA[Ø,3,4]RZ
External	Ø2HA[Ø,4]RZ	Ø2PA[Ø,3,4]RZ

Revision With Removal of Heart Assist System

Type of Heart Assist System	Code as appropriate Revision by approach	Code also as appropriate Removal of Heart Assist System by approach
Implantable	Ø2WA[Ø,3,4]QZ	Ø2PA[Ø,3,4]RZ
External	Ø2WA[Ø,3,4]RZ	Ø2PA[Ø,3,4]RZ

DRG ØØ8 Simultaneous Pancreas/Kidney Transplant

Transplanted Body Part	Code Transplant as appropriate by tissue type			Code also Pancreas Transplant as appropriate by tissue type		
	Allogeneic	Syngeneic	Zooplastic	Allogeneic	Syngeneic	Zooplastic
Kidney, Right	ØTYØØZØ	ØTYØØZ1	ØTYØØZ2	ØFYGØZØ	ØFYGØZ1	ØFYGØZ2
Kidney, Left	ØTY1ØZØ	ØTY1ØZ1	ØTY1ØZ2			

DRG Ø19 Simultaneous Pancreas/Kidney Transplant with Hemodialysis

Transplanted Body Part	Code Transplant as appropriate by tissue type			Code also Pancreas Transplant as appropriate by tissue type			Code also Hemodialysis		
	Allogeneic	Syngeneic	Zooplastic	Allogeneic	Syngeneic	Zooplastic	< 6 Hours	6-18 Hours	> 18 Hours
Kidney, Right	ØTYØØZØ	ØTYØØZ1	ØTYØØZ2	ØFYGØZØ	ØFYGØZ1	ØFYGØZ2	5A1DØ7Z	5A1D8ØZ	5A1D9ØZ
Kidney, Left	ØTY1ØZØ	ØTY1ØZ1	ØTY1ØZ2						

DRG Ø23-Ø27 Craniotomy

Site of Neurostimulator Lead	Code as appropriate Insertion of Lead by approach	Code also as appropriate Insertion of Device by type and subcutaneous site						
		Neuro-stimulator Generator	Stimulator Multiple Array Code as appropriate by approach			Stimulator Multiple Array, Rechargeable Code as appropriate by approach		
		Skull	Chest	Back	Abdomen	Chest	Back	Abdomen
Brain	ØØHØ[Ø,3,4]MZ	ØNHØØNZ	ØJH6[Ø,3]DZ	ØJH7[Ø,3]DZ	ØJH8[Ø,3]DZ	ØJH6[Ø,3]EZ	ØJH7[Ø,3]EZ	ØJH8[Ø,3]EZ
Cerebral Ventricle	ØØH6[Ø,3,4]MZ	ØNHØØNZ	ØJH6[Ø,3]DZ	ØJH7[Ø,3]DZ	ØJH8[Ø,3]DZ	ØJH6[Ø,3]EZ	ØJH7[Ø,3]EZ	ØJH8[Ø,3]EZ

DRG Ø28-Ø3Ø Spinal Procedures

Generator Type	Insertion of Generator by Site			Code also as appropriate Insertion of Neurostimulator Lead by approach	
	Chest	Abdomen	Back	Spinal Canal	Spinal Cord
Single Array	ØJH6[Ø,3]BZ	ØJH8[Ø,3]BZ	ØJH7[Ø,3]BZ	ØØHU[Ø,3,4]MZ	ØØHV[Ø,3,4]MZ
Single Array, Rechargeable	ØJH6[Ø,3]CZ	ØJH8[Ø,3]CZ	ØJH7[Ø,3]CZ	ØØHU[Ø,3,4]MZ	ØØHV[Ø,3,4]MZ
Multiple Array	ØJH6[Ø,3]DZ	ØJH8[Ø,3]DZ	ØJH7[Ø,3]DZ	ØØHU[Ø,3,4]MZ	ØØHV[Ø,3,4]MZ
Multiple Array, Rechargable	ØJH6[Ø,3]EZ	—	ØJH7[Ø,3]EZ	ØØHU[Ø,3,4]MZ	ØØHV[Ø,3,4]MZ
Multiple Array, Rechargable	—	ØJH8[Ø,3]EZ	—	ØØHU[Ø,3,4]MZ	ØØHV[Ø,3,4]MZ

DRG Ø4Ø-Ø42 Peripheral and Cranial Nerve and Other Nervous System Procedures

Insertion of Neurostimulator Lead With Device

Site of Neurostimulator Lead	Code as appropriate Insertion by approach	Code also as appropriate Insertion of Device by type and subcutaneous site					
		Stimulator Single Array Code as appropriate by approach			Stimulator Single Array, Rechargeable Code as appropriate by approach		
		Chest	Back	Abdomen	Chest	Back	Abdomen
Cranial Nerve	ØØHE[Ø,3,4]MZ	ØJH6[Ø,3]BZ	ØJH7[Ø,3]BZ	ØJH8[Ø,3]BZ	ØJH6[Ø,3]CZ	ØJH7[Ø,3]CZ	ØJH8[Ø,3]CZ
Peripheral Nerve	Ø1HY[Ø,3,4]MZ	ØJH6[Ø,3]BZ	ØJH7[Ø,3]BZ	ØJH8[Ø,3]BZ	ØJH6[Ø,3]CZ	ØJH7[Ø,3]CZ	ØJH8[Ø,3]CZ
Stomach	ØDH6[Ø,3,4]MZ	ØJH6[Ø,3]BZ	ØJH7[Ø,3]BZ	ØJH8[Ø,3]BZ	ØJH6[Ø,3]CZ	ØJH7[Ø,3]CZ	ØJH8[Ø,3]CZ
Azygos vein	Ø5HØ[Ø,3,4]MZ	ØJH6[Ø,3]BZ	ØJH7[Ø,S]BZ	ØJH8[Ø,3]BZ	ØJH6[Ø,3]CZ	ØJH7[Ø,S]CZ	ØJH8[Ø,3]CZ
Innominate Vein, Right	Ø5H3[Ø,3,4]MZ	ØJH6[Ø,3]BZ	ØJH7[Ø,S]BZ	ØJH8[Ø,3]BZ	ØJH6[Ø,3]CZ	ØJH7[Ø,S]CZ	ØJH8[Ø,3]CZ
Innominate Vein, Left	Ø5H4[Ø,3,4]MZ	ØJH6[Ø,3]BZ	ØJH7[Ø,S]BZ	ØJH8[Ø,3]BZ	ØJH6[Ø,3]CZ	ØJH7[Ø,S]CZ	ØJH8[Ø,3]CZ
		Stimulator Multiple Array Code as appropriate by approach			Stimulator Multiple Array, Rechargeable Code as appropriate by approach		
		Chest	Back	Abdomen	Chest	Back	Abdomen
Cranial Nerve	ØØHE[Ø,3,4]MZ	ØJH6[Ø,3]DZ	ØJH7[Ø,3]DZ	ØJH8[Ø,3]DZ	ØJH6[Ø,3]EZ	ØJH7[Ø,3]EZ	ØJH8[Ø,3]EZ
Peripheral Nerve	Ø1HY[Ø,3,4]MZ	ØJH6[Ø,3]DZ	ØJH7[Ø,3]DZ	ØJH8[Ø,3]DZ	ØJH6[Ø,3]EZ	ØJH7[Ø,3]EZ	ØJH8[Ø,3]EZ
Stomach	ØDH6[Ø,3,4]MZ	ØJH6[Ø,3]DZ	ØJH7[Ø,3]DZ	ØJH8[Ø,3]DZ	ØJH6[Ø,3]EZ	ØJH7[Ø,3]EZ	ØJH8[Ø,3]EZ
Azygos vein	Ø5HØ[Ø,3,4]MZ	ØJH6[Ø,3]DZ	ØJH7[Ø,S]DZ	ØJH8[Ø,3]DZ	ØJH6[Ø,3]EZ	ØJH7[Ø,S]EZ	ØJH8[Ø,3]EZ
Innominate Vein, Right	Ø5H3[Ø,3,4]MZ	ØJH6[Ø,3]DZ	ØJH7[Ø,S]DZ	ØJH8[Ø,3]DZ	ØJH6[Ø,3]EZ	ØJH7[Ø,S]EZ	ØJH8[Ø,3]EZ
Innominate Vein, Left	Ø5H4[Ø,3,4]MZ	ØJH6[Ø,3]DZ	ØJH7[Ø,S]DZ	ØJH8[Ø,3]DZ	ØJH6[Ø,3]EZ	ØJH7[Ø,S]EZ	ØJH8[Ø,3]EZ

DRG 222-227 Cardiac Defibrillator Implant

Insertion of Generator With Insertion of Lead(s) into Coronary Vein, Atrium or Ventricle

Generator Type	Insertion of Generator by Site		Code also as appropriate Insertion of Leads by site				
	Chest	Abdomen	Coronary Vein	Atrium		Ventricle	
				Right	Left	Right	Left
Defibrillator	ØJH6[Ø,3]8Z	ØJH8[Ø,3]8Z	Ø2H4[Ø,4]KZ	Ø2H6[Ø,3,4]KZ	Ø2H7[Ø,3,4]KZ	Ø2HK[Ø,3,4]KZ	Ø2HL[Ø,3,4]KZ
Cardiac Resynch Defibrillator Pulse Generator	ØJH6[Ø,3]9Z	ØJH8[Ø,3]9Z	Ø2H4[Ø,3,4]KZ or Ø2H43[J,M]Z	Ø2H6[Ø,3,4]KZ	Ø2H7[Ø,3,4]KZ	Ø2HK[Ø,3,4]KZ	Ø2HL[Ø,3,4]KZ
Contractility Modulation Device	ØJH6[Ø,3]AZ	ØJH8[Ø,3]AZ	—	Ø2H6[Ø,3,4]MZ	—	Ø2HK[Ø,3,4]MZ	—

Insertion of Generator with Insertion of Lead(s) into Pericardium or Chest

Generator Type	Insertion of Generator by Site		Code also as appropriate Insertion of Leads by Site and Type			
			Pericardium			Chest
	Chest	Abdomen	Pacemaker	Defibrillator	Cardiac	Subcutaneous
Defibrillator	ØJH6[Ø,3]8Z	ØJH8[Ø,3]8Z	Ø2HN[Ø,3,4]JZ	Ø2HN[Ø,3,4]KZ	Ø2HN[Ø,3,4]MZ	ØJH6[Ø,3]FZ
Cardiac Resynch Defibrillator Pulse Generator	ØJH6[Ø,3]9Z	ØJH8[Ø,3]9Z	Ø2HN[Ø,3,4]JZ	Ø2HN[Ø,3,4]KZ	Ø2HN[Ø,3,4]MZ	ØJH6[Ø,3]FZ

DRG 242-244 Permanent Cardiac Pacemaker Implant

Insertion of Generator and Lead(s) Only

Generator Type	Insertion of Generator by Site		Code also as appropriate Insertion of Leads by site					
			Coronary Vein	Atrium		Ventricle		Pericardium
	Chest	Abdomen		Right	Left	Right	Left	
Single Chamber	ØJH6[Ø,3]4Z	ØJH8[Ø,3]4Z	Ø2H4[Ø,3,4][J,M]Z	Ø2H6[Ø,3,4][J,M]Z	Ø2H7[Ø,3,4][J,M]Z	Ø2HK[Ø,3,4][J,M]Z	Ø2HL[Ø,3,4][J,M]Z	Ø2HN[Ø,3,4][J,M]Z
Single Chamber RR	ØJH6[Ø,3]5Z	ØJH8[Ø,3]5Z	Ø2H4[Ø,3,4][J,M]Z	Ø2H6[Ø,3,4][J,M]Z	Ø2H7[Ø,3,4][J,M]Z	Ø2HK[Ø,3,4][J,M]Z	Ø2HL[Ø,3,4][J,M]Z	Ø2HN[Ø,3,4][J,M]Z
Dual Chamber	ØJH6[Ø,3]6Z	ØJH8[Ø,3]6Z	Ø2H4[Ø,3,4][J,M]Z	Ø2H6[Ø,3,4][J,M]Z	Ø2H7[Ø,3,4][J,M]Z	Ø2HK[Ø,3,4][J,M]Z	Ø2HL[Ø,3,4][J,M]Z	Ø2HN[Ø,3,4][J,M]Z
Cardiac Resynch Pulse Generator	ØJH6[Ø,3]7Z	ØJH8[Ø,3]7Z	Ø2H4[Ø,3,4][J,M]Z	Ø2H6[Ø,3,4][J,M]Z	Ø2H7[Ø,3,4][J,M]Z	Ø2HK[Ø,3,4][J,M]Z	Ø2HL[Ø,3,4][J,M]Z	Ø2HN[Ø,3,4][J,M]Z
Cardiac Rhythm Related	ØJH6[Ø,3]PZ	ØJH8[Ø,3]PZ	Ø2H4[Ø,3,4][J,M]Z	Ø2H6[Ø,3,4][J,M]Z	Ø2H7[Ø,3,4][J,M]Z	Ø2HK[Ø,3,4][J,M]Z	Ø2HL[Ø,3,4][J,M]Z	Ø2HN[Ø,3,4][J,M]Z

DRG 326-328 Stomach, Esophageal and Duodenal Procedures

Site	Resection by Open Approach	Code also as appropriate Resection of Pancreas by Open Approach
Duodenum	ØDT9ØZZ	ØFTGØZZ

DRG 344-346 Minor Small and Large Bowel Procedures

Site	Repair by Open Approach	Code also as appropriate Repair by external approach of Abdominal Wall Stoma
Small Intestine	ØDQ8ØZZ	ØWQFXZ2
Duodenum	ØDQ9ØZZ	ØWQFXZ2
Jejunum	ØDQAØZZ	ØWQFXZ2
Ileum	ØDQBØZZ	ØWQFXZ2
Large Intestine	ØDQEØZZ	ØWQFXZ2
Large Intestine, Right	ØDQFØZZ	ØWQFXZ2
Large Intestine, Left	ØDQGØZZ	ØWQFXZ2
Cecum	ØDQHØZZ	ØWQFXZ2
Ascending Colon	ØDQKØZZ	ØWQFXZ2
Transverse Colon	ØDQLØZZ	ØWQFXZ2
Descending Colon	ØDQMØZZ	ØWQFXZ2
Sigmoid Colon	ØDQNØZZ	ØWQFXZ2

DRG 456-458 Spinal Fusion Except Cervical with Spinal Curvature/Malignancy/ Infection or Extensive Fusions

Fusion of Thoracic and Lumbar Vertebra, Anterior Column

2 to 7 Thoracic Vertebra		Code also 2 or more Lumbar Vertebra	
ØRG[Ø,3,4][7,A,J,K]Ø	XRG7ØF3	ØSG1[Ø,3,4][7,A,J,K]Ø	XRGCØF3

Fusion of Thoracic and Lumbar Vertebra, Posterior Column

2 to 7 Thoracic Vertebra			Code also 2 or more Lumbar Vertebra		
Posterior Approach	**Anterior Approach**	**New Technology**	**Posterior Approach**	**Anterior Approach**	**New Technology**
ØRG7[Ø,3,4][7,J,K]1	ØRG7[Ø,3,4][7,A,J,K]J	XRG7Ø92 XRG7ØF3	ØSG1[Ø,3,4][7,J,K]1	ØSG1[Ø,3,4][7,A,J,K]J	XRGCØ92 XRGCØF3

DRG 461-462 Bilateral or Multiple Major Joint Procedures of Lower Extremity

For procedures to qualify as bilateral or multiple joint procedures, at least one replacement code or combination removal and replacement code from two different lower extremity sites from the following table(s) must be reported.

Examples: Left hip and right hip codes (bilateral); left hip and left knee codes (multiple); left hip and right ankle codes (multiple); left knee and right knee codes (bilateral); right hip removal and replacement, with right knee replacement

Hip, RT	Hip, LT	Knee, RT	Knee, LT	Ankle, RT	Ankle, LT
ØSR9Ø19	ØSRBØ19	ØSRCØ69	ØSRDØ69	ØSRFØ7Z	ØSRGØ7Z
ØSR9Ø1A	ØSRBØ1A	ØSRCØ6A	ØSRDØ6A	ØSRFØJ9	ØSRGØJ9
ØSR9Ø1Z	ØSRBØ1Z	ØSRCØ6Z	ØSRDØ6Z	ØSRFØJA	ØSRGØJA
ØSR9Ø29	ØSRBØ29	ØSRCØ7Z	ØSRDØ7Z	ØSRFØJZ	ØSRGØJZ
ØSR9Ø2A	ØSRBØ2A	ØSRCØJ9	ØSRDØJ9	ØSRFØKZ	ØSRGØKZ
ØSR9Ø2Z	ØSRBØ2Z	ØSRCØJA	ØSRDØJA		
ØSR9Ø39	ØSRBØ39	ØSRCØJZ	ØSRDØJZ		
ØSR9Ø3A	ØSRBØ3A	ØSRCØKZ	ØSRDØKZ		
ØSR9Ø3Z	ØSRBØ3Z	ØSRCØL9	ØSRDØL9		
ØSR9Ø49	ØSRBØ49	ØSRCØLA	ØSRDØLA		
ØSR9Ø4A	ØSRBØ4A	ØSRCØLZ	ØSRDØLZ		
ØSR9Ø4Z	ØSRBØ4Z	ØSRCØM9	ØSRDØM9		
ØSR9Ø69	ØSRBØ69	ØSRCØMA	ØSRDØMA		
ØSR9Ø6A	ØSRBØ6A	ØSRCØMZ	ØSRDØMZ		
ØSR9Ø6Z	ØSRBØ6Z	ØSRCØN9	ØSRDØN9		
ØSR9Ø7Z	ØSRBØ7Z	ØSRCØNA	ØSRDØNA		
ØSR9ØJ9	ØSRBØJ9	ØSRCØNZ	ØSRDØNZ		
ØSR9ØJA	ØSRBØJA	ØSRTØ7Z	ØSRUØ7Z		
ØSR9ØJZ	ØSRBØJZ	ØSRTØJ9	ØSRUØJ9		
ØSR9ØKZ	ØSRBØKZ	ØSRTØJA	ØSRUØJA		
ØSRAØØ9	ØSREØØ9	ØSRTØJZ	ØSRUØJZ		
ØSRAØØA	ØSREØØA	ØSRTØKZ	ØSRUØKZ		
ØSRAØØZ	ØSREØØZ	ØSRVØ7Z	ØSRWØ7Z		
ØSRAØ19	ØSREØ19	ØSRVØJ9	ØSRWØJ9		
ØSRAØ1A	ØSREØ1A	ØSRVØJA	ØSRWØJA		
ØSRAØ1Z	ØSREØ1Z	ØSRVØJZ	ØSRWØJZ		
ØSRAØ39	ØSREØ39	ØSRVØKZ	ØSRWØKZ		
ØSRAØ3A	ØSREØ3A	ØSPCØJZ	ØSPDØJZ		
ØSRAØ3Z	ØSREØ3Z				
ØSRAØ7Z	ØSREØ7Z				
ØSRAØJ9	ØSREØJ9				
ØSRAØJA	ØSREØJA				
ØSRAØJZ	ØSREØJZ				
ØSRAØKZ	ØSREØKZ				
ØSRRØ19	ØSRSØ19				

Hip, RT	Hip, LT	Knee, RT	Knee, LT	Ankle, RT	Ankle, LT
ØSRRØ1A	ØSRSØ1A				
ØSRRØ1Z	ØSRSØ1Z				
ØSRRØ39	ØSRSØ39				
ØSRRØ3A	ØSRSØ3A				
ØSRRØ3Z	ØSRSØ3Z				
ØSRRØ7Z	ØSRSØ7Z				
ØSRRØJ9	ØSRSØJ9				
ØSRRØJA	ØSRSØJA				
ØSRRØJZ	ØSRSØJZ				
ØSRRØKZ	ØSRSØKZ				
ØSU9ØBZ	ØSUBØBZ				
ØSUAØBZ	ØSUEØBZ				
ØSURØBZ	ØSUSØBZ				
ØSP9ØJZ	ØSPBØJZ				

Hip Procedure Combinations

Open Removal of Hip Spacer with Replacement

Removal of Spacer		Code also as appropriate Replacement by Device Type					
		Metal	Metal on Poly	Ceramic	Ceramic on Poly	Oxidized Zirc on Poly	Synth Subst
Hip, RT	ØSP9Ø8Z	ØSR9Ø1[9,A,Z]	ØSR9Ø2[9,A,Z]	ØSR9Ø3[9,A,Z]	ØSR9Ø4[9,A,Z]	ØSR9Ø6[9,A,Z]	ØSR9ØJ[9,A,Z]
Hip, LT	ØSPBØ8Z	ØSRBØ1[9,A,Z]	ØSRBØ2[9,A,Z]	ØSRBØ3[9,A,Z]	ØSRBØ4[9,A,Z]	ØSRBØ6[9,A,Z]	ØSRBØJ[9,A,Z]

Open Removal of Hip Spacer with Replacement

Removal of Spacer		Code also as appropriate Replacement by Device Type						
		Acetabular Surface				Femoral Surface		
		Poly	Metal	Ceramic	Synthetic	Metal	Ceramic	Synth
Hip, RT	ØSP9Ø8Z	ØSRAØØ[9,A,Z]	ØSRAØ1[9,A,Z]	ØSRAØ3[9,A,Z]	ØSRAØJ[9,A,Z]	ØSRRØ1[9,A,Z]	ØSRRØ3[9,A,Z]	ØSRRØJ[9,A,Z]
Hip, LT	ØSPBØ8Z	ØSREØØ[9,A,Z]	ØSREØ1[9,A,Z]	ØSREØ3[9,A,Z]	ØSREØJ[9,A,Z]	ØSRSØ1[9,A,Z]	ØSRSØ3[9,A,Z]	ØSRSØJ[9,A,Z]

Open Removal of Hip Liner with Replacement

Removal of Liner		Code also as appropriate Replacement by Device Type					
		Metal	Metal on Poly	Ceramic	Ceramic on Poly	Oxidized Zirc on Poly	Synth Subst
Hip, RT	ØSP9Ø9Z	ØSR9Ø1[9,A,Z]	ØSR9Ø2[9,A,Z]	ØSR9Ø3[9,A,Z]	ØSR9Ø4[9,A,Z]	ØSR9Ø6[9,A,Z]	ØSR9ØJ[9,A,Z]
Hip, LT	ØSPBØ9Z	ØSRBØ1[9,A,Z]	ØSRBØ2[9,A,Z]	ØSRBØ3[9,A,Z]	ØSRBØ4[9,A,Z]	ØSRBØ6[9,A,Z]	ØSRBØJ[9,A,Z]

Open Removal of Hip Liner with Replacement

Removal of Liner		Code also as appropriate Replacement by Device Type						
		Acetabular Surface				Femoral Surface		
		Poly	Metal	Ceramic	Synthetic	Metal	Ceramic	Synth
Hip, RT	ØSP9Ø9Z	ØSRAØØ[9,A,Z]	ØSRAØ1[9,A,Z]	ØSRAØ3[9,A,Z]	ØSRAØJ[9,A,Z]	ØSRRØ1[9,A,Z]	ØSRRØ3[9,A,Z]	ØSRRØJ[9,A,Z]
Hip, LT	ØSPBØ9Z	ØSREØØ[9,A,Z]	ØSREØ1[9,A,Z]	ØSREØ3[9,A,Z]	ØSREØJ[9,A,Z]	ØSRSØ1[9,A,Z]	ØSRSØ3[9,A,Z]	ØSRSØJ[9,A,Z]

Open Removal of Hip Resurfacing Device with Replacement

Removal of Resurfacing Device		Code also as appropriate Replacement by Device Type					
		Metal	Metal on Poly	Ceramic	Ceramic on Poly	Oxidized Zirc on Poly	Synth Subst
Hip, RT	ØSP9ØBZ	ØSR9Ø1[9,A,Z]	ØSR9Ø2[9,A,Z]	ØSR9Ø3[9,A,Z]	ØSR9Ø4[9,A,Z]	ØSR9Ø6[9,A,Z]	ØSR9ØJ[9,A,Z]
Hip, LT	ØSPBØBZ	ØSRBØ1[9,A,Z]	ØSRBØ2[9,A,Z]	ØSRBØ3[9,A,Z]	ØSRBØ4[9,A,Z]	ØSRBØ6[9,A,Z]	ØSRBØJ[9,A,Z]

Open Removal of Hip Resurfacing Device with Replacement

Removal of Resurfacing Device		Code also as appropriate Replacement by Device Type						
		Acetabular Surface				Femoral Surface		
		Poly	Metal	Ceramic	Synthetic	Metal	Ceramic	Synth
Hip, RT	ØSP9ØBZ	ØSRAØØ[9,A,Z]	ØSRAØ1[9,A,Z]	ØSRAØ3[9,A,Z]	ØSRAØJ[9,A,Z]	ØSRRØ1[9,A,Z]	ØSRRØ3[9,A,Z]	ØSRRØJ[9,A,Z]
Hip, LT	ØSPBØBZ	ØSREØØ[9,A,Z]	ØSREØ1[9,A,Z]	ØSREØ3[9,A,Z]	ØSREØJ[9,A,Z]	ØSRSØ1[9,A,Z]	ØSRSØ3[9,A,Z]	ØSRSØJ[9,A,Z]

Open Removal of Hip Articulating Spacer with Replacement

Removal of Articulating Spacer		Code also as appropriate Replacement by Device Type					
		Metal	Metal on Poly	Ceramic	Ceramic on Poly	Oxidized Zirc on Poly	Synth Subst
Hip, RT	ØSP9ØEZ	ØSR9Ø1[9,A,Z]	ØSR9Ø2[9,A,Z]	ØSR9Ø3[9,A,Z]	ØSR9Ø4[9,A,Z]	ØSR9Ø6[9,A,Z]	ØSR9ØJ[9,A,Z]
Hip, LT	ØSPBØEZ	ØSRBØ1[9,A,Z]	ØSRBØ2[9,A,Z]	ØSRBØ3[9,A,Z]	ØSRBØ4[9,A,Z]	ØSRBØ6[9,A,Z]	ØSRBØJ[9,A,Z]

Open Removal of Hip Articulating Spacer with Replacement

Removal of Articulating Spacer		Code also as appropriate Replacement by Device Type						
		Acetabular Surface				Femoral Surface		
		Poly	Metal	Ceramic	Synthetic	Metal	Ceramic	Synth
Hip, RT	ØSP9ØEZ	ØSRAØØ[9,A,Z]	ØSRAØ1[9,A,Z]	ØSRAØ3[9,A,Z]	ØSRAØJ[9,A,Z]	ØSRRØ1[9,A,Z]	ØSRRØ3[9,A,Z]	ØSRRØJ[9,A,Z]
Hip, LT	ØSPBØEZ	ØSREØØ[9,A,Z]	ØSREØ1[9,A,Z]	ØSREØ3[9,A,Z]	ØSREØJ[9,A,Z]	ØSRSØ1[9,A,Z]	ØSRSØ3[9,A,Z]	ØSRSØJ[9,A,Z]

Open Removal of Hip Synthetic Substitute with Replacement

Removal of Synthetic Substitute		Code also as appropriate Replacement by Device Type					
		Metal	Metal on Poly	Ceramic	Ceramic on Poly	Oxidized Zirc on Poly	Synth Subst
Hip, RT	ØSP[9,A,R]ØJZ	ØSR9Ø1[9,A,Z]	ØSR9Ø2[9,A,Z]	ØSR9Ø3[9,A,Z]	ØSR9Ø4[9,A,Z]	ØSR9Ø6[9,A,Z]	ØSR9ØJ[9,A,Z]
Hip, LT	ØSP[B,E,S]ØJZ	ØSRBØ1[9,A,Z]	ØSRBØ2[9,A,Z]	ØSRBØ3[9,A,Z]	ØSRBØ4[9,A,Z]	ØSRBØ6[9,A,Z]	ØSRBØJ[9,A,Z]

Open Removal of Hip Synthetic Substitute with Replacement

Removal of Synthetic Substitute		Code also as appropriate Replacement by Device Type						
		Acetabular Surface				Femoral Surface		
		Poly	Metal	Ceramic	Synthetic	Metal	Ceramic	Synth
Hip, RT	ØSP[9,A,R]ØJZ	ØSRAØØ[9,A,Z]	ØSRAØ1[9,A,Z]	ØSRAØ3[9,A,Z]	ØSRAØJ[9,A,Z]	ØSRRØ1[9,A,Z]	ØSRRØ3[9,A,Z]	ØSRRØJ[9,A,Z]
Hip, LT	ØSP[B,E,S]ØJZ	ØSREØØ[9,A,Z]	ØSREØ1[9,A,Z]	ØSREØ3[9,A,Z]	ØSREØJ[9,A,Z]	ØSRSØ1[9,A,Z]	ØSRSØ3[9,A,Z]	ØSRSØJ[9,A,Z]

Percutaneous Endoscopic Removal of Hip Spacer with Open Replacement

Removal of Spacer		Code also as appropriate Replacement by Device Type					
		Metal	Metal on Poly	Ceramic	Ceramic on Poly	Oxidized Zirc on Poly	Synth Subst
Hip, RT	ØSP948Z	ØSR9Ø1[9,A,Z]	ØSR9Ø2[9,A,Z]	ØSR9Ø3[9,A,Z]	ØSR9Ø4[9,A,Z]	ØSR9Ø6[9,A,Z]	ØSR9ØJ[9,A,Z]
Hip, LT	ØSPB48Z	ØSRBØ1[9,A,Z]	ØSRBØ2[9,A,Z]	ØSRBØ3[9,A,Z]	ØSRBØ4[9,A,Z]	ØSRBØ6[9,A,Z]	ØSRBØJ[9,A,Z]

Percutaneous Endoscopic Removal of Hip Spacer with Open Replacement

Removal of Spacer		Code also as appropriate Replacement by Device Type						
		Acetabular Surface				Femoral Surface		
		Poly	Metal	Ceramic	Synthetic	Metal	Ceramic	Synth
Hip, RT	ØSP948Z	ØSRAØØ[9,A,Z]	ØSRAØ1[9,A,Z]	ØSRAØ3[9,A,Z]	ØSRAØJ[9,A,Z]	ØSRRØ1[9,A,Z]	ØSRRØ3[9,A,Z]	ØSRRØJ[9,A,Z]
Hip, LT	ØSPB48Z	ØSREØØ[9,A,Z]	ØSREØ1[9,A,Z]	ØSREØ3[9,A,Z]	ØSREØJ[9,A,Z]	ØSRSØ1[9,A,Z]	ØSRSØ3[9,A,Z]	ØSRSØJ[9,A,Z]

Percutaneous Endoscopic Removal of Hip Synthetic Substitute with Open Replacement

Removal of Synthetic Substitute		Code also as appropriate Replacement by Device Type					
		Metal	Metal on Poly	Ceramic	Ceramic on Poly	Oxidized Zirc on Poly	Synth Subst
Hip, RT	ØSP[9,A,R]4JZ	ØSR9Ø1[9,A,Z]	ØSR9Ø2[9,A,Z]	ØSR9Ø3[9,A,Z]	ØSR9Ø4[9,A,Z]	ØSR9Ø6[9,A,Z]	ØSR9ØJ[9,A,Z]
Hip, LT	ØSP[B,E,S]4JZ	ØSRBØ1[9,A,Z]	ØSRBØ2[9,A,Z]	ØSRBØ3[9,A,Z]	ØSRBØ4[9,A,Z]	ØSRBØ6[9,A,Z]	ØSRBØJ[9,A,Z]

Percutaneous Endoscopic Removal of Hip Synthetic Substitute with Open Replacement

Removal of Synthetic Substitute		Code also as appropriate Replacement by Device Type						
		Acetabular Surface				Femoral Surface		
		Poly	Metal	Ceramic	Synthetic	Metal	Ceramic	Synth
Hip, RT	ØSP[9,A,R]4JZ	ØSRAØØ[9,A,Z]	ØSRAØ1[9,A,Z]	ØSRAØ3[9,A,Z]	ØSRAØJ[9,A,Z]	ØSRRØ1[9,A,Z]	ØSRRØ3[9,A,Z]	ØSRRØJ[9,A,Z]
Hip, LT	ØSP[B,E,S]4JZ	ØSREØØ[9,A,Z]	ØSREØ1[9,A,Z]	ØSREØ3[9,A,Z]	ØSREØJ[9,A,Z]	ØSRSØ1[9,A,Z]	ØSRSØ3[9,A,Z]	ØSRSØJ[9,A,Z]

Knee Procedure Combinations

Open Removal of Knee Spacer with Synthetic Substitute Replacement

Removal of Spacer		Code also as appropriate Replacement by Type of Synthetic Substitute				
		Oxidized Zircon on Poly	Synth Subst	Patello-femoral	Femoral Surface	Tibial Surface
Knee, RT	ØSPCØ8Z	ØSRCØ6[9,A,Z]	ØSRCØJ[9,A,Z]	ØSRCØN[9,A,Z]	ØSRTØJ[9,A,Z]	ØSRVØJ[9,A,Z]
Knee, LT	ØSPDØ8Z	ØSRDØ6[9,A,Z]	ØSRDØJ[9,A,Z]	ØSRDØN[9,A,Z]	ØSRUØJ[9,A,Z]	ØSRWØJ[9,A,Z]

Open Removal of Knee Liner with Synthetic Substitute Replacement

Removal of Liner		Code also as appropriate Replacement by Type of Synthetic Substitute						
		Oxidized Zircon on Poly	Synth Subst	Medial Unicondylar	Lateral Unicondylar	Patello-femoral	Femoral Surface	Tibial Surface
Knee, RT	ØSPCØ9Z	ØSRCØ6[9,A,Z]	ØSRCØJ[9,A,Z]	ØSRCØL[9,A,Z]	ØSRCØM[9,A,Z]	ØSRCØN[9,A,Z]	ØSRTØJ[9,A,Z]	ØSRVØJ[9,A,Z]
Knee, LT	ØSPDØ9Z	ØSRDØ6[9,A,Z]	ØSRDØJ[9,A,Z]	ØSRDØL[9,A,Z]	ØSRDØM[9,A,Z]	ØSRDØN[9,A,Z]	ØSRUØJ[9,A,Z]	ØSRWØJ[9,A,Z]

Open Removal of Knee Articulating Spacer with Synthetic Substitute Replacement

Removal of Articulating Spacer		Code also as appropriate Replacement by Type of Synthetic Substitute			
		Oxidized Zircon on Poly	Synth Subst	Femoral Surface	Tibial Surface
Knee, RT	ØSPCØEZ	ØSRCØ6[9,A,Z]	ØSRCØJ[9,A,Z]	ØSRTØJ[9,A,Z]	ØSRVØJ[9,A,Z]
Knee, LT	ØSPDØEZ	ØSRDØ6[9,A,Z]	ØSRDØJ[9,A,Z]	ØSRUØJ[9,A,Z]	ØSRWØJ[9,A,Z]

Open Removal of Patellar Surface of Knee with Synthetic Substitute Replacement

Removal of Patellar Surface		Code also as appropriate Replacement by Type of Synthetic Substitute				
		Oxidized Zircon on Poly	Synth Subst	Patello-femoral	Femoral Surface	Tibial Surface
Knee, RT	ØSPCØJC	ØSRCØ6[9,A,Z]	ØSRCØJ[9,A,Z]	ØSRCØN[9,A,Z]	ØSRTØJ[9,A,Z]	ØSRVØJ[9,A,Z]
Knee, LT	ØSPDØJC	ØSRDØ6[9,A,Z]	ØSRDØJ[9,A,Z]	ØSRDØN[9,A,Z]	ØSRUØJ[9,A,Z]	ØSRWØJ[9,A,Z]

Open Removal of Knee Synthetic Substitute with Synthetic Substitute Replacement

Removal of Synthetic Substitute		Code also as appropriate Replacement by Type of Synthetic Substitute						
		Oxidized Zircon on Poly	Synth Subst	Medial Unicondylar	Lateral Unicondylar	Patello-femoral	Femoral Surface	Tibial Surface
Knee, RT	ØSPCØJZ	ØSRCØ6[9,A,Z]	ØSRCØJ[9,A,Z]	ØSRCØL[9,A,Z]	ØSRCØM[9,A,Z]	ØSRCØN[9,A,Z]	ØSRTØJ[9,A,Z]	ØSRVØJ[9,A,Z]
Knee, LT	ØSPDØJZ	ØSRDØ6[9,A,Z]	ØSRDØJ[9,A,Z]	ØSRDØL[9,A,Z]	ØSRDØM[9,A,Z]	ØSRDØN[9,A,Z]	ØSRUØJ[9,A,Z]	ØSRWØJ[9,A,Z]

Open Removal of Medial or Lateral Unicondylar Knee with Synthetic Substitute Replacement

Removal of Medial/Lateral Unicondylar Knee		Code also as appropriate Replacement by Type of Synthetic Substitute				
		Oxidized Zircon on Poly	Synth Subst	Medial Unicondylar	Femoral Surface	Tibial Surface
Knee, RT	ØSPCØ[L,M]Z	ØSRCØ6[9,A,Z]	ØSRCØJ[9,A,Z]	ØSRCØL[9,A,Z]	ØSRTØJ[9,A,Z]	ØSRVØJ[9,A,Z]
Knee, LT	ØSPDØ[L,M]Z	ØSRDØ6[9,A,Z]	ØSRDØJ[9,A,Z]	ØSRDØL[9,A,Z]	ØSRUØJ[9,A,Z]	ØSRWØJ[9,A,Z]

Open Removal of Patellofemoral Knee with Synthetic Substitute Replacement

Removal of Patellofemoral Knee		Code also as appropriate Replacement by Type of Synthetic Substitute				
		Oxidized Zircon on Poly	Synth Subst	Medial Unicondylar	Femoral Surface	Tibial Surface
Knee, RT	ØSPCØNZ	ØSRCØ6[9,A,Z]	ØSRCØJ[9,A,Z]	ØSRCØL[9,A,Z]	ØSRTØJ[9,A,Z]	ØSRVØJ[9,A,Z]
Knee, LT	ØSPDØNZ	ØSRDØ6[9,A,Z]	ØSRDØJ[9,A,Z]	ØSRDØL[9,A,Z]	ØSRUØJ[9,A,Z]	ØSRWØJ[9,A,Z]

Open Removal of Femoral/Tibial Surface of Knee with Synthetic Substitute Replacement

Removal of Femoral/Tibial Surface of Knee		Code also as appropriate Replacement by Type of Synthetic Substitute					
		Oxidized Zircon on Poly	Synth Subst	Articulating Spacer	Patello-femoral	Femoral Surface	Tibial Surface
Knee, RT	ØSP[T,V]ØJZ	ØSRCØ6[9,A,Z]	ØSRCØJ[9,A,Z]	ØSRCØEZ	ØSRCØN[9,A,Z]	ØSRTØJ[9,A,Z]	ØSRVØJ[9,A,Z]
Knee, LT	ØSP[U,W]ØJZ	ØSRDØ6[9,A,Z]	ØSRDØJ[9,A,Z]	ØSRDØEZ	ØSRDØN[9,A,Z]	ØSRUØJ[9,A,Z]	ØSRWØJ[9,A,Z]

Percutaneous/Percutaneous Endoscopic Removal of Knee Spacer with Open Synthetic Substitute Replacement

Removal of Spacer		Code also as appropriate Replacement by Type of Synthetic Substitute				
		Oxidized Zircon on Poly	Synth Subst	Patello-femoral	Femoral Surface	Tibial Surface
Knee, RT	ØSPC[3,4]8Z	ØSRCØ6[9,A,Z]	ØSRCØJ[9,A,Z]	ØSRCØN[9,A,Z]	ØSRTØJ[9,A,Z]	ØSRVØJ[9,A,Z]
Knee, LT	ØSPD[3,4]8Z	ØSRDØ6[9,A,Z]	ØSRDØJ[9,A,Z]	ØSRDØN[9,A,Z]	ØSRUØJ[9,A,Z]	ØSRWØJ[9,A,Z]

Percutaneous Endoscopic Removal of Patellar Surface of Knee with Synthetic Substitute Replacement

Removal of Patellar Surface		Code also as appropriate Replacement by Type of Synthetic Substitute				
		Oxidized Zircon on Poly	Synth Subst	Patello-femoral	Femoral Surface	Tibial Surface
Knee, RT	ØSPC4JC	ØSRCØ6[9,A,Z]	ØSRCØJ[9,A,Z]	ØSRCØN[9,A,Z]	ØSRTØJ[9,A,Z]	ØSRVØJ[9,A]
Knee, LT	ØSPD4JC	ØSRDØ6[9,A,Z]	ØSRDØJ[9,A,Z]	ØSRDØN[9,A,Z]	ØSRUØJ[9,A]	ØSRWØJ[9,A,Z]

Percutaneous Endoscopic Removal of Knee Synthetic Substitute with Synthetic Substitute Replacement

Removal of Synthetic Substitute		Code also as appropriate Replacement by Type of Synthetic Substitute						
		Oxidized Zircon on Poly	Synth Subst	Medial Unicondylar	Lateral Unicondylar	Patello-femoral	Femoral Surface	Tibial Surface
Knee, RT	ØSPC4JZ	ØSRCØ6[9,A,Z]	ØSRCØJ[9,A,Z]	ØSRCØL[9,A,Z]	ØSRCØM[9,A,Z]	ØSRCØN[9,A,Z]	ØSRTØJ[9,A,Z]	ØSRVØJ[9,A,Z]
Knee, LT	ØSPD4JZ	ØSRDØ6[9,A,Z]	ØSRDØJ[9,A,Z]	ØSRDØL[9,A,Z]	ØSRDØM[9,A,Z]	ØSRDØN[9,A,Z]	ØSRUØJ[9,A,Z]	ØSRWØJ[9,A,Z]

Percutaneous Endoscopic Removal of Medial or Lateral Unicondylar Knee with Synthetic Substitute Replacement

Removal of Medial/Lateral Unicondylar Knee		Code also as appropriate Replacement by Type of Synthetic Substitute				
		Oxidized Zircon on Poly	Synth Subst	Medial Unicondylar	Femoral Surface	Tibial Surface
Knee, RT	ØSPC4[L,M]Z	ØSRCØ6[9,A,Z]	ØSRCØJ[9,A,Z]	ØSRCØL[9,A,Z]	ØSRTØJ[9,A,Z]	ØSRVØJ[9,A,Z]
Knee, LT	ØSPD4[L,M]Z	ØSRDØ6[9,A,Z]	ØSRDØJ[9,A,Z]	ØSRDØL[9,A,Z]	ØSRUØJ[9,A,Z]	ØSRWØJ[9,A,Z]

Percutaneous Endoscopic Removal of Patellofemoral Knee with Synthetic Substitute Replacement

Removal of Patellofemoral Knee		Code also as appropriate Replacement by Type of Synthetic Substitute				
		Oxidized Zircon on Poly	Synth Subst	Medial Unicondylar	Femoral Surface	Tibial Surface
Knee, RT	ØSPC4NZ	ØSRCØ6[9,A,Z]	ØSRCØJ[9,A,Z]	ØSRCØL[9,A,Z]	ØSRTØJ[9,A,Z]	ØSRVØJ[9,A,Z]
Knee, LT	ØSPD4NZ	ØSRDØ6[9,A,Z]	ØSRDØJ[9,A,Z]	ØSRDØL[9,A,Z]	ØSRUØJ[9,A,Z]	ØSRWØJ[9,A,Z]

Percutaneous Endoscopic Removal of Femoral/Tibial Surface of Knee with Synthetic Substitute Replacement

Removal of Femoral/Tibial Surface of Knee		Code also as appropriate Replacement by Type of Synthetic Substitute					
		Oxidized Zircon on Poly	Synth Subst	Articulating Spacer	Patello-femoral	Femoral Surface	Tibial Surface
Knee, RT	ØSP[T,V]4JZ	ØSRCØ6[9,A,Z]	ØSRCØJ[9,A,Z]	ØSRCØEZ	ØSRCØN[9,A,Z]	ØSRTØJ[9,A,Z]	ØSRVØJ[9,A]
Knee, LT	ØSP[U,W]4JZ	ØSRDØ6[9,A,Z]	ØSRDØJ[9,A,Z]	ØSRDØEZ	ØSRDØN[9,A,Z]	ØSRUØJ[9,A,Z]	ØSRWØJ[9,A,Z]

466-468 Revision of Hip or Knee Replacement

Hip Procedures

Open Removal of Hip Spacer with Replacement

Removal of Spacer		Code also as appropriate Replacement by Device Type						
		Metal	Metal on Poly	Ceramic	Ceramic on Poly	Oxidized Zirc on Poly	Articulating Spacer	Synth Subst
Hip, RT	ØSP9Ø8Z	ØSR9Ø1[9,A,Z]	ØSR9Ø2[9,A,Z]	ØSR9Ø3[9,A,Z]	ØSR9Ø4[9,A,Z]	ØSR9Ø6[9,A,Z]	ØSR9ØEZ	ØSR9ØJ[9,A,Z]
Hip, LT	ØSPBØ8Z	ØSRBØ1[9,A,Z]	ØSRBØ2[9,A,Z]	ØSRBØ3[9,A,Z]	ØSRBØ4[9,A,Z]	ØSRBØ6[9,A,Z]	ØSRBØEZ	ØSRBØJ[9,A,Z]

Open Removal of Hip Spacer with Replacement

Removal of Spacer		Code also as appropriate Replacement by Device Type						
		Acetabular Surface				Femoral Surface		
		Poly	Metal	Ceramic	Synthetic	Metal	Ceramic	Synth
Hip, RT	ØSP9Ø8Z	ØSRAØØ[9,A,Z]	ØSRAØ1[9,A,Z]	ØSRAØ3[9,A,Z]	ØSRAØJ[9,A,Z]	ØSRRØ1[9,A,Z]	ØSRRØ3[9,A,Z]	ØSRRØJ[9,A,Z]
Hip, LT	ØSPBØ8Z	ØSREØØ[9,A,Z]	ØSREØ1[9,A,Z]	ØSREØ3[9,A,Z]	ØSREØJ[9,A,Z]	ØSRSØ1[9,A,Z]	ØSRSØ3[9,A,Z]	ØSRSØJ[9,A,Z]

Open Removal of Hip Spacer with Liner Insertion (supplement)

Removal of Spacer		Code also as appropriate Supplement of Body Part by Site		
		Joint	Acetabular Surface	Femoral Surface
Hip, RT	ØSP9Ø8Z	ØSU9Ø9Z	ØSUAØ9Z	ØSURØ9Z
Hip, LT	ØSPBØ8Z	ØSUBØ9Z	ØSUEØ9Z	ØSUSØ9Z

Open Removal of Hip Liner with Replacement

Removal of Liner		Code also as appropriate Replacement by Device Type						
		Metal	Metal on Poly	Ceramic	Ceramic on Poly	Oxidized Zirc on Poly	Articulating Spacer	Synth Subst
Hip, RT	ØSP9Ø9Z	ØSR9Ø1[9,A,Z]	ØSR9Ø2[9,A,Z]	ØSR9Ø3[9,A,Z]	ØSR9Ø4[9,A,Z]	ØSR9Ø6[9,A,Z]	ØSR9ØEZ	ØSR9ØJ[9,A,Z]
Hip, LT	ØSPBØ9Z	ØSRBØ1[9,A,Z]	ØSRBØ2[9,A,Z]	ØSRBØ3[9,A,Z]	ØSRBØ4[9,A,Z]	ØSRBØ6[9,A,Z]	ØSRBØEZ	ØSRBØJ[9,A,Z]

Open Removal of Hip Liner with Replacement

Removal of Liner		Code also as appropriate Replacement by Device Type						
		Acetabular Surface				Femoral Surface		
		Poly	Metal	Ceramic	Synthetic	Metal	Ceramic	Synth
Hip, RT	ØSP9Ø9Z	ØSRAØØ[9,A,Z]	ØSRAØ1[9,A,Z]	ØSRAØ3[9,A,Z]	ØSRAØJ[9,A,Z]	ØSRRØ1[9,A,Z]	ØSRRØ3[9,A,Z]	ØSRRØJ[9,A,Z]
Hip, LT	ØSPBØ9Z	ØSREØØ[9,A,Z]	ØSREØ1[9,A,Z]	ØSREØ3[9,A,Z]	ØSREØJ[9,A,Z]	ØSRSØ1[9,A,Z]	ØSRSØ3[9,A,Z]	ØSRSØJ[9,A,Z]

Open Removal of Hip Liner with Liner Insertion (supplement)

Removal of Liner		Code also as appropriate Supplement of Body Part by Site		
		Joint	Acetabular Surface	Femoral Surface
Hip, RT	ØSP9Ø9Z	ØSU9Ø9Z	ØSUAØ9Z	ØSURØ9Z
Hip, LT	ØSPBØ9Z	ØSUBØ9Z	ØSUEØ9Z	ØSUSØ9Z

Open Removal of Hip Resurfacing Device with Replacement

Removal of Resurfacing Device		Code also as appropriate Replacement by Device Type						
		Metal	Metal on Poly	Ceramic	Ceramic on Poly	Oxidized Zirc on Poly	Articulating Spacer	Synth Subst
Hip, RT	ØSP9ØBZ	ØSR9Ø1[9,A,Z]	ØSR9Ø2[9,A,Z]	ØSR9Ø3[9,A,Z]	ØSR9Ø4[9,A,Z]	ØSR9Ø6[9,A,Z]	ØSR9ØEZ	ØSR9ØJ[9,A,Z]
Hip, LT	ØSPBØBZ	ØSRBØ1[9,A,Z]	ØSRBØ2[9,A,Z]	ØSRBØ3[9,A,Z]	ØSRBØ4[9,A,Z]	ØSRBØ6[9,A,Z]	ØSRBØEZ	ØSRBØJ[9,A,Z]

Open Removal of Hip Resurfacing Device with Replacement

Removal of Resurfacing Device		Code also as appropriate Replacement by Device Type						
		Acetabular Surface				Femoral Surface		
		Poly	Metal	Ceramic	Synthetic	Metal	Ceramic	Synth
Hip, RT	ØSP9ØBZ	ØSRAØØ[9,A,Z]	ØSRAØ1[9,A,Z]	ØSRAØ3[9,A,Z]	ØSRAØJ[9,A,Z]	ØSRRØ1[9,A,Z]	ØSRRØ3[9,A,Z]	ØSRRØJ[9,A,Z]
Hip, LT	ØSPBØBZ	ØSREØØ[9,A,Z]	ØSREØ1[9,A,Z]	ØSREØ3[9,A,Z]	ØSREØJ[9,A,Z]	ØSRSØ1[9,A,Z]	ØSRSØ3[9,A,Z]	ØSRSØJ[9,A,Z]

Open Removal of Hip Resurfacing Device with Liner Insertion (supplement)

Removal of Resurfacing Device		Code also as appropriate Supplement of Body Part by Site		
		Joint	Acetabular Surface	Femoral Surface
Hip, RT	ØSP9ØBZ	ØSU9Ø9Z	ØSUAØ9Z	ØSURØ9Z
Hip, LT	ØSPBØBZ	ØSUBØ9Z	ØSUEØ9Z	ØSUSØ9Z

Open Removal of Hip Articulating Spacer with Replacement

Removal of Articulating Spacer		Code also as appropriate Replacement by Device Type					
		Metal	Metal on Poly	Ceramic	Ceramic on Poly	Oxidized Zirc on Poly	Synth Subst
Hip, RT	ØSP9ØEZ	ØSR9Ø1[9,A,Z]	ØSR9Ø2[9,A,Z]	ØSR9Ø3[9,A,Z]	ØSR9Ø4[9,A,Z]	ØSR9Ø6[9,A,Z]	ØSR9ØJ[9,A,Z]
Hip, LT	ØSPBØEZ	ØSRBØ1[9,A,Z]	ØSRBØ2[9,A,Z]	ØSRBØ3[9,A,Z]	ØSRBØ4[9,A,Z]	ØSRBØ6[9,A,Z]	ØSRBØJ[9,A,Z]

Open Removal of Hip Articulating Spacer with Replacement

Removal of Articulating Spacer		Code also as appropriate Replacement by Device Type						
		Acetabular Surface				Femoral Surface		
		Poly	Metal	Ceramic	Synthetic	Metal	Ceramic	Synth
Hip, RT	ØSP9ØEZ	ØSRAØØ[9,A,Z]	ØSRAØ1[9,A,Z]	ØSRAØ3[9,A,Z]	ØSRAØJ[9,A,Z]	ØSRRØ1[9,A,Z]	ØSRRØ3[9,A,Z]	ØSRRØJ[9,A,Z]
Hip, LT	ØSPBØEZ	ØSREØØ[9,A,Z]	ØSREØ1[9,A,Z]	ØSREØ3[9,A,Z]	ØSREØJ[9,A,Z]	ØSRSØ1[9,A,Z]	ØSRSØ3[9,A,Z]	ØSRSØJ[9,A,Z]

Open Removal of Hip Articulating Spacer with Liner Insertion (supplement)

Removal of Articulating Spacer		Code also as appropriate Supplement of Body Part by Site		
		Joint	Acetabular Surface	Femoral Surface
Hip, RT	ØSP9ØEZ	ØSU9Ø9Z	ØSUAØ9Z	ØSURØ9Z
Hip, LT	ØSPBØEZ	ØSUBØ9Z	ØSUEØ9Z	ØSUSØ9Z

Open Removal of Hip Synthetic Substitute with Replacement

Removal of Synthetic Substitute		Code also as appropriate Replacement by Device Type						
		Metal	Metal on Poly	Ceramic	Ceramic on Poly	Oxidized Zirc on Poly	Articulating Spacer	Synth Subst
Hip, RT	ØSP[9,A,R]ØJZ	ØSR9Ø1[9,A,Z]	ØSR9Ø2[9,A,Z]	ØSR9Ø3[9,A,Z]	ØSR9Ø4[9,A,Z]	ØSR9Ø6[9,A,Z]	ØSR9ØEZ	ØSR9ØJ[9,A,Z]
Hip, LT	ØSP[B,E,S]ØJZ	ØSRBØ1[9,A,Z]	ØSRBØ2[9,A,Z]	ØSRBØ3[9,A,Z]	ØSRBØ4[9,A,Z]	ØSRBØ6[9,A,Z]	ØSRBØEZ	ØSRBØJ[9,A,Z]

Open Removal of Hip Synthetic Substitute with Replacement

Removal of Synthetic Substitute		Code also as appropriate Replacement by Device Type						
		Acetabular Surface				Femoral Surface		
		Poly	Metal	Ceramic	Synthetic	Metal	Ceramic	Synth
Hip, RT	ØSP[9,A,R]ØJZ	ØSRAØØ[9,A,Z]	ØSRAØ1[9,A,Z]	ØSRAØ3[9,A,Z]	ØSRAØJ[9,A,Z]	ØSRRØ1[9,A,Z]	ØSRRØ3[9,A,Z]	ØSRRØJ[9,A,Z]
Hip, LT	ØSP[B,E,S]ØJZ	ØSREØØ[9,A,Z]	ØSREØ1[9,A,Z]	ØSREØ3[9,A,Z]	ØSREØJ[9,A,Z]	ØSRSØ1[9,A,Z]	ØSRSØ3[9,A,Z]	ØSRSØJ[9,A,Z]

Percutaneous Endoscopic Removal of Hip Spacer with Open Replacement

Removal of Spacer		Code also as appropriate Replacement by Device Type						
		Metal	Metal on Poly	Ceramic	Ceramic on Poly	Oxidized Zirc on Poly	Articulating Spacer	Synth Subst
Hip, RT	ØSP948Z	ØSR9Ø1[9,A,Z]	ØSR9Ø2[9,A,Z]	ØSR9Ø3[9,A,Z]	ØSR9Ø4[9,A,Z]	ØSR9Ø6[9,A,Z]	ØSR9ØEZ	ØSR9ØJ[9,A,Z]
Hip, LT	ØSPB48Z	ØSRBØ1[9,A,Z]	ØSRBØ2[9,A,Z]	ØSRBØ3[9,A,Z]	ØSRBØ4[9,A,Z]	ØSRBØ6[9,A,Z]	ØSRBØEZ	ØSRBØJ[9,A,Z]

Percutaneous Endoscopic Removal of Hip Spacer with Open Replacement

Removal of Spacer		Code also as appropriate Replacement by Device Type						
		Acetabular Surface				Femoral Surface		
		Poly	Metal	Ceramic	Synthetic	Metal	Ceramic	Synth
Hip, RT	ØSP948Z	ØSRAØØ[9,A,Z]	ØSRAØ1[9,A,Z]	ØSRAØ3[9,A,Z]	ØSRAØJ[9,A,Z]	ØSRRØ1[9,A,Z]	ØSRRØ3[9,A,Z]	ØSRRØJ[9,A,Z]
Hip, LT	ØSPB48Z	ØSREØØ[9,A,Z]	ØSREØ1[9,A,Z]	ØSREØ3[9,A,Z]	ØSREØJ[9,A,Z]	ØSRSØ1[9,A,Z]	ØSRSØ3[9,A,Z]	ØSRSØJ[9,A,Z]

Percutaneous Endoscopic Removal of Hip Spacer with Open Liner Insertion (supplement)

Removal of Spacer		Code also as appropriate Supplement of Body Part by Site		
		Joint	Acetabular Surface	Femoral Surface
Hip, RT	ØSP948Z	ØSU9Ø9Z	ØSUAØ9Z	ØSURØ9Z
Hip, LT	ØSPB48Z	ØSUBØ9Z	ØSUEØ9Z	ØSUSØ9Z

Percutaneous Endoscopic Removal of Hip Synthetic Substitute with Open Replacement

Removal of Synthetic Substitute		Code also as appropriate Replacement by Device Type						
		Metal	Metal on Poly	Ceramic	Ceramic on Poly	Oxidized Zirc on Poly	Articulating Spacer	Synth Subst
Hip, RT	ØSP[9,A,R]4JZ	ØSR9Ø1[9,A,Z]	ØSR9Ø2[9,A,Z]	ØSR9Ø3[9,A,Z]	ØSR9Ø4[9,A,Z]	ØSR9Ø6[9,A,Z]	ØSR9ØEZ	ØSR9ØJ[9,A,Z]
Hip, LT	ØSP[B,E,S]4JZ	ØSRBØ1[9,A,Z]	ØSRBØ2[9,A,Z]	ØSRBØ3[9,A,Z]	ØSRBØ4[9,A,Z]	ØSRBØ6[9,A,Z]	ØSRBØEZ	ØSRBØJ[9,A,Z]

Percutaneous Endoscopic Removal of Hip Synthetic Substitute with Open Replacement

Removal of Synthetic Substitute		Code also as appropriate Replacement by Device Type						
		Acetabular Surface				Femoral Surface		
		Poly	Metal	Ceramic	Synthetic	Metal	Ceramic	Synth
Hip, RT	ØSP[9,A,R]4JZ	ØSRAØØ[9,A,Z]	ØSRAØ1[9,A,Z]	ØSRAØ3[9,A,Z]	ØSRAØJ[9,A,Z]	ØSRRØ1[9,A,Z]	ØSRRØ3[9,A,Z]	ØSRRØJ[9,A,Z]
Hip, LT	ØSP[B,E,S]4JZ	ØSREØØ[9,A,Z]	ØSREØ1[9,A,Z]	ØSREØ3[9,A,Z]	ØSREØJ[9,A,Z]	ØSRSØ1[9,A,Z]	ØSRSØ3[9,A,Z]	ØSRSØJ[9,A,Z]

Percutaneous Endoscopic Removal of Hip Synthetic Substitute with Open Liner Insertion (supplement)

Removal of Synthetic Substitute		Code also as appropriate Supplement of Body Part by Site		
		Joint	Acetabular Surface	Femoral Surface
Hip, RT	ØSP[9,A,R]4JZ	ØSU9Ø9Z	ØSUAØ9Z	ØSURØ9Z
Hip, LT	ØSP[B,E,S]4JZ	ØSUBØ9Z	ØSUEØ9Z	ØSUSØ9Z

Knee Procedures

Open Removal of Knee Spacer with Articulating Spacer Replacement

Removal of Spacer		Code also as appropriate Replacement with Articulating Spacer
Knee, RT	ØSPCØ8Z	ØSRCØEZ
Knee, LT	ØSPDØ8Z	ØSRDØEZ

Open Removal of Knee Spacer with Synthetic Substitute Replacement

Removal of Spacer		Code also as appropriate Replacement by Type of Synthetic Substitute				
		Oxidized Zircon on Poly	Synth Subst	Patello-femoral	Femoral Surface	Tibial Surface
Knee, RT	ØSPCØ8Z	ØSRCØ6[9,A,Z]	ØSRCØJ[9,A,Z]	ØSRCØN[9,A,Z]	ØSRTØJ[9,A,Z]	ØSRVØJ[9,A,Z]
Knee, LT	ØSPDØ8Z	ØSRDØ6[9,A,Z]	ØSRDØJ[9,A,Z]	ØSRDØN[9,A,Z]	ØSRUØJ[9,A,Z]	ØSRWØJ[9,A,Z]

Open Removal of Knee Liner with Articulating Spacer Replacement

Removal of Liner		Code also as appropriate Replacement with Articulating Spacer
Knee, RT	ØSPCØ9Z	ØSRCØEZ
Knee, LT	ØSPDØ9Z	ØSRDØEZ

Open Removal of Knee Liner with Synthetic Substitute Replacement

Removal of Liner		Code also as appropriate Replacement by Type of Synthetic Substitute						
		Oxidized Zircon on Poly	Synth Subst	Medial Unicondylar	Lateral Unicondylar	Patello-femoral	Femoral Surface	Tibial Surface
Knee, RT	ØSPCØ9Z	ØSRCØ6[9,A,Z]	ØSRCØJ[9,A,Z]	ØSRCØL[9,A,Z]	ØSRCØM[9,A,Z]	ØSRCØN[9,A,Z]	ØSRTØJ[9,A,Z]	ØSRVØJ[9,A,Z]
Knee, LT	ØSPDØ9Z	ØSRDØ6[9,A,Z]	ØSRDØJ[9,A,Z]	ØSRDØL[9,A,Z]	ØSRDØM[9,A,Z]	ØSRDØN[9,A,Z]	ØSRUØJ[9,A,Z]	ØSRWØJ[9,A,Z]

Open Removal of Knee Articulating Spacer with Synthetic Substitute Replacement

Removal of Articulating Spacer		Code also as appropriate Replacement by Type of Synthetic Substitute			
		Oxidized Zircon on Poly	Synth Subst	Femoral Surface	Tibial Surface
Knee, RT	ØSPCØEZ	ØSRCØ6[9,A,Z]	ØSRCØJ[9,A,Z]	ØSRTØJ[9,A,Z]	ØSRVØJ[9,A,Z]
Knee, LT	ØSPDØEZ	ØSRDØ6[9,A,Z]	ØSRDØJ[9,A,Z]	ØSRUØJ[9,A,Z]	ØSRWØJ[9,A,Z]

Open Removal of Patellar Surface of Knee with Synthetic Substitute Replacement

Removal of Patellar Surface		Code also as appropriate Replacement by Type of Synthetic Substitute				
		Oxidized Zircon on Poly	Synth Subst	Patello-femoral	Femoral Surface	Tibial Surface
Knee, RT	ØSPCØJC	ØSRCØ6[9,A,Z]	ØSRCØJ[9,A,Z]	ØSRCØN[9,A,Z]	ØSRTØJ[9,A,Z]	ØSRVØJ[9,A,Z]
Knee, LT	ØSPDØJC	ØSRDØ6[9,A,Z]	ØSRDØJ[9,A,Z]	ØSRDØN[9,A,Z]	ØSRUØJ[9,A,Z]	ØSRWØJ[9,A,Z]

Open Removal of Patellar Surface of Knee with Articulating Spacer Replacement

Removal of Patellar Surface		Code also as appropriate Replacement with Articulating Spacer
Knee, RT	ØSPCØJC	ØSRCØEZ
Knee, LT	ØSPDØJC	ØSRDØEZ

Open Removal of Knee Synthetic Substitute with Synthetic Substitute Replacement

Removal of Synthetic Substitute		Code also as appropriate Replacement by Type of Synthetic Substitute						
		Oxidized Zircon on Poly	Synth Subst	Medial Unicondylar	Lateral Unicondylar	Patello-femoral	Femoral Surface	Tibial Surface
Knee, RT	ØSPCØJZ	ØSRCØ6[9,A,Z]	ØSRCØJ[9,A,Z]	ØSRCØL[9,A,Z]	ØSRCØM[9,A,Z]	ØSRCØN[9,A,Z]	ØSRTØJ[9,A,Z]	ØSRVØJ[9,A,Z]
Knee, LT	ØSPDØJZ	ØSRDØ6[9,A,Z]	ØSRDØJ[9,A,Z]	ØSRDØL[9,A,Z]	ØSRDØM[9,A,Z]	ØSRDØN[9,A,Z]	ØSRUØJ[9,A,Z]	ØSRWØJ[9,A,Z]

Open Removal of Knee Synthetic Substitute with Articulating Spacer Replacement

Removal of Synthetic Substitute		Code also as appropriate Replacement with Articulating Spacer
Knee, RT	ØSPCØJZ	ØSRCØEZ
Knee, LT	ØSPDØJZ	ØSRDØEZ

Open Removal of Medial or Lateral Unicondylar Knee with Synthetic Substitute Replacement

Removal of Medial/Lateral Unicondylar Knee		Code also as appropriate Replacement by Type of Synthetic Substitute				
		Oxidized Zircon on Poly	Synth Subst	Medial Unicondylar	Femoral Surface	Tibial Surface
Knee, RT	ØSPCØ[L,M]Z	ØSRCØ6[9,A,Z]	ØSRCØJ[9,A,Z]	ØSRCØL[9,A,Z]	ØSRTØJ[9,A,Z]	ØSRVØJ[9,A,Z]
Knee, LT	ØSPDØ[L,M]Z	ØSRDØ6[9,A,Z]	ØSRDØJ[9,A,Z]	ØSRDØL[9,A,Z]	ØSRUØJ[9,A,Z]	ØSRWØJ[9,A,Z]

Open Removal of Patellofemoral Knee with Synthetic Substitute Replacement

Removal of Patellofemoral Knee		Code also as appropriate Replacement by Type of Synthetic Substitute				
		Oxidized Zircon on Poly	Synth Subst	Medial Unicondylar	Femoral Surface	Tibial Surface
Knee, RT	ØSPCØNZ	ØSRCØ6[9,A,Z]	ØSRCØJ[9,A,Z]	ØSRCØL[9,A,Z]	ØSRTØJ[9,A,Z]	ØSRVØJ[9,A,Z]
Knee, LT	ØSPDØNZ	ØSRDØ6[9,A,Z]	ØSRDØJ[9,A,Z]	ØSRDØL[9,A,Z]	ØSRUØJ[9,A,Z]	ØSRWØJ[9,A,Z]

Open Removal of Femoral/Tibial Surface of Knee with Synthetic Substitute Replacement

Removal of Femoral/Tibial Surface of Knee		Code also as appropriate Replacement by Type of Synthetic Substitute					
		Oxidized Zircon on Poly	Synth Subst	Articulating Spacer	Patello-femoral	Femoral Surface	Tibial Surface
Knee, RT	ØSP[T,V]ØJZ	ØSRCØ6[9,A,Z]	ØSRCØJ[9,A,Z]	ØSRCØEZ	ØSRCØN[9,A,Z]	ØSRTØJ[9,A,Z]	ØSRVØJ[9,A,Z]
Knee, LT	ØSP[U,W]ØJZ	ØSRDØ6[9,A,Z]	ØSRDØJ[9,A,Z]	ØSRDØEZ	ØSRDØN[9,A,Z]	ØSRUØJ[9,A,Z]	ØSRWØJ[9,A,Z]

Percutaneous/Percutaneous Endoscopic Removal of Knee Spacer with Open Synthetic Substitute Replacement

Removal of Spacer		Code also as appropriate Replacement by Type of Synthetic Substitute				
		Oxidized Zircon on Poly	Synth Subst	Patello-femoral	Femoral Surface	Tibial Surface
Knee, RT	ØSPC[3,4]8Z	ØSRCØ6[9,A,Z]	ØSRCØJ[9,A,Z]	ØSRCØN[9,A,Z]	ØSRTØJ[9,A,Z]	ØSRVØJ[9,A,Z]
Knee, LT	ØSPD[3,4]8Z	ØSRDØ6[9,A,Z]	ØSRDØJ[9,A,Z]	ØSRDØN[9,A,Z]	ØSRUØJ[9,A,Z]	ØSRWØJ[9,A,Z]

Percutaneous/Percutaneous Endoscopic Removal of Knee Spacer with Open Articulating Spacer Replacement

Removal of Spacer		Code also as appropriate Replacement with Articulating Spacer
Knee, RT	ØSPC[3,4]8Z	ØSRCØEZ
Knee, LT	ØSPD[3,4]8Z	ØSRDØEZ

Percutaneous Endoscopic Removal of Patellar Surface of Knee with Synthetic Substitute Replacement

Removal of Patellar Surface		Code also as appropriate Replacement by Type of Synthetic Substitute				
		Oxidized Zircon on Poly	Synth Subst	Patello-femoral	Femoral Surface	Tibial Surface
Knee, RT	ØSPC4JC	ØSRCØ6[9,A,Z]	ØSRCØJ[9,A,Z]	ØSRCØN[9,A,Z]	ØSRTØJ[9,A,Z]	ØSRVØJ[9,A]
Knee, LT	ØSPD4JC	ØSRDØ6[9,A,Z]	ØSRDØJ[9,A,Z]	ØSRDØN[9,A,Z]	ØSRUØJ[9,A,Z]	ØSRWØJ[9,A,Z]

Percutaneous Endoscopic Removal of Patellar Surface of Knee with Articulating Spacer Replacement

Removal of Patellar Surface		Code also as appropriate Replacement with Articulating Spacer
Knee, RT	ØSPC4JC	ØSRCØEZ
Knee, LT	ØSPD4JC	ØSRDØEZ

Percutaneous Endoscopic Removal of Knee Synthetic Substitute with Synthetic Substitute Replacement

Removal of Synthetic Substitute		Code also as appropriate Replacement by Type of Synthetic Substitute						
		Oxidized Zircon on Poly	Synth Subst	Medial Unicondylar	Lateral Unicondylar	Patello-femoral	Femoral Surface	Tibial Surface
Knee, RT	ØSPC4JZ	ØSRCØ6[9,A,Z]	ØSRCØJ[9,A,Z]	ØSRCØL[9,A,Z]	ØSRCØM[9,A,Z]	ØSRCØN[9,A,Z]	ØSRTØJ[9,A,Z]	ØSRVØJ[9,A,Z]
Knee, LT	ØSPD4JZ	ØSRDØ6[9,A,Z]	ØSRDØJ[9,A,Z]	ØSRDØL[9,A,Z]	ØSRDØM[9,A,Z]	ØSRDØN[9,A,Z]	ØSRUØJ[9,A,Z]	ØSRWØJ[9,A,Z]

Percutaneous Endoscopic Removal of Knee Synthetic Substitute with Articulating Spacer Replacement

Removal of Synthetic Substitute		Code also as appropriate Replacement with Articulating Spacer
Knee, RT	ØSPC4JZ	ØSRCØEZ
Knee, LT	ØSPD4JZ	ØSRDØEZ

Percutaneous Endoscopic Removal of Medial or Lateral Unicondylar Knee with Synthetic Substitute Replacement

Removal of Medial/Lateral Unicondylar Knee		Code also as appropriate Replacement by Type of Synthetic Substitute				
		Oxidized Zircon on Poly	Synth Subst	Medial Unicondylar	Femoral Surface	Tibial Surface
Knee, RT	ØSPC4[L,M]Z	ØSRCØ6[9,A,Z]	ØSRCØJ[9,A,Z]	ØSRCØL[9,A,Z]	ØSRTØJ[9,A,Z]	ØSRVØJ[9,A,Z]
Knee, LT	ØSPD4[L,M]Z	ØSRDØ6[9,A,Z]	ØSRDØJ[9,A,Z]	ØSRDØL[9,A,Z]	ØSRUØJ[9,A,Z]	ØSRWØJ[9,A,Z]

Percutaneous Endoscopic Removal of Patellofemoral Knee with Synthetic Substitute Replacement

Removal of Patellofemoral Knee		Code also as appropriate Replacement by Type of Synthetic Substitute				
		Oxidized Zircon on Poly	Synth Subst	Medial Unicondylar	Femoral Surface	Tibial Surface
Knee, RT	ØSPC4NZ	ØSRCØ6[9,A,Z]	ØSRCØJ[9,A,Z]	ØSRCØL[9,A,Z]	ØSRTØJ[9,A,Z]	ØSRVØJ[9,A,Z]
Knee, LT	ØSPD4NZ	ØSRDØ6[9,A,Z]	ØSRDØJ[9,A,Z]	ØSRDØL[9,A,Z]	ØSRUØJ[9,A,Z]	ØSRWØJ[9,A,Z]

Percutaneous Endoscopic Removal of Femoral/Tibial Surface of Knee with Synthetic Substitute Replacement

Removal of Femoral/Tibial Surface of Knee		Code also as appropriate Replacement by Type of Synthetic Substitute					
		Oxidized Zircon on Poly	Synth Subst	Articulating Spacer	Patello-femoral	Femoral Surface	Tibial Surface
Knee, RT	ØSP[T,V]4JZ	ØSRCØ6[9,A,Z]	ØSRCØJ[9,A,Z]	ØSRCØEZ	ØSRCØN[9,A,Z]	ØSRTØJ[9,A,Z]	ØSRVØJ[9,A]
Knee, LT	ØSP[U,W]4JZ	ØSRDØ6[9,A,Z]	ØSRDØJ[9,A,Z]	ØSRDØEZ	ØSRDØN[9,A,Z]	ØSRUØJ[9,A,Z]	ØSRWØJ[9,A,Z]

DRG 485-489 Knee Procedures

Joint	Removal of Liner by open approach	Code also as appropriate Supplement of Tibial Surface by Site
Knee, RT	ØSPCØ9Z	ØSUVØ9Z
Knee, LT	ØSPDØ9Z	ØSUWØ9Z

DRG 515-517 Other Musculoskeletal System and Connective Tissue Procedures

Site	Reposition of Vertebra by percutaneous approach	Code also as appropriate Supplement With Synthetic Substitute by Percutaneous Approach at site of Repositioned Vertebra
Cervical	ØPS33ZZ	ØPU33JZ
Coccyx	ØQSS3ZZ	ØQUS3JZ
Lumbar	ØQSØ3ZZ	ØQUØ3JZ
Sacrum	ØQS13ZZ	ØQU13JZ
Thoracic	ØPS43ZZ	ØPU43JZ

DRG 518-52Ø Back and Neck Procedures, Except Spinal Fusion, or Disc Devices/Neurostimulators

Generator Type	Insertion of Generator by Site			Code also as appropriate Insertion Neurostimulator Lead by approach and Site	
	Chest	Abdomen	Back	Spinal Canal	Spinal Cord
Single Array	ØJH6[Ø,3]BZ	ØJH8[Ø,3]BZ	ØJH7[Ø,3]BZ	ØØHU[Ø,3,4]MZ	ØØHV[Ø,3,4]MZ
Single Array, Rechargeable	ØJH6[Ø,3]CZ	ØJH8[Ø,3]CZ	ØJH7[Ø,3]CZ	ØØHU[Ø,3,4]MZ	ØØHV[Ø,3,4]MZ
Multiple Array	ØJH6[Ø,3]DZ	ØJH8[Ø,3]DZ	ØJH7[Ø,3]DZ	ØØHU[Ø,3,4]MZ	ØØHV[Ø,3,4]MZ
Multiple Array, Rechargable	ØJH6[Ø,3]EZ	—	ØJH7[Ø,3]EZ	ØØHU[Ø,3,4]MZ	ØØHV[Ø,3,4]MZ
Multiple Array, Rechargable	—	ØJH8[Ø,3]EZ	—	ØØHU[Ø,3,4]MZ	ØØHV[Ø,3,4]MZ

DRG 582-583 Mastectomy for Malignancy

Site	Resection by Open approach	Code also as appropriate Resection of Lymph Nodes by Open approach by site			Code also as appropriate Resection of Thorax Muscle by Open approach	
		Axillary	Internal Mammary	Thorax	Right	Left
Breast, Right	ØHTTØZZ	Ø7T5ØZZ	Ø7T8ØZZ	Ø7T7ØZZ	ØKTHØZZ	—
Breast, Left	ØHTUØZZ	Ø7T6ØZZ	Ø7T9ØZZ	Ø7T7ØZZ	—	ØKTJØZZ
Breast, Bilateral	ØHTVØZZ	Ø7T5ØZZ and Ø7T6ØZZ	Ø7T8ØZZ and Ø7T9ØZZ	Ø7T7ØZZ	ØKTHØZZ	ØKTJØZZ

DRG 584-585 Breast Biopsy, Local Excision and Other Breast procedures

Resection of Breast With Resection of Lymph Nodes and Thorax Muscle

Site	Resection by Open approach	Code also as appropriate Resection of Lymph Nodes by Open approach by site			Code also as appropriate Resection of Thorax Muscle by Open approach	
		Axillary	Internal Mammary	Thorax	Right	Left
Breast, Right	ØHTTØZZ	Ø7T5ØZZ	Ø7T8ØZZ	Ø7T7ØZZ	ØKTHØZZ	—
Breast, Left	ØHTUØZZ	Ø7T6ØZZ	Ø7T9ØZZ	Ø7T7ØZZ	—	ØKTJØZZ
Breast, Bilateral	ØHTVØZZ	Ø7T5ØZZ and Ø7T6ØZZ	Ø7T8ØZZ and Ø7T9ØZZ	Ø7T7ØZZ	ØKTHØZZ	ØKTJØZZ

Replacement of Breast Tissue

Site	Replacement by Percutaneous approach with Autologous Tissue	Code also as appropriate Extraction of Subcutaneous Tissue by Percutaneous approach					
		Abdomen	Back	Buttock	Chest	Leg, Upper, Right	Leg, Upper, Left
Breast, Right	ØHRT37Z	ØJD83ZZ	ØJD73ZZ	ØJD93ZZ	ØJD63ZZ	ØJDL3ZZ	ØJDM3ZZ
Breast, Left	ØHRU37Z	ØJD83ZZ	ØJD73ZZ	ØJD93ZZ	ØJD63ZZ	ØJDL3ZZ	ØJDM3ZZ
Breast, Bilateral	ØHRV37Z	ØJD83ZZ	ØJD73ZZ	ØJD93ZZ	ØJD63ZZ	ØJDL3ZZ	ØJDM3ZZ

DRG 628-63Ø Other Endocrine, Nutritional and Metabolic Procedures

Hip Procedures

Open Removal of Hip Spacer with Replacement

Removal of Spacer		Code also as appropriate Replacement by Device Type					
		Metal	Metal on Poly	Ceramic	Ceramic on Poly	Oxidized Zirc on Poly	Synthetic Substitute
Hip, RT	ØSP9Ø8Z	ØSR9Ø1[9,A,Z]	ØSR9Ø2[9,A,Z]	ØSR9Ø3[9,A,Z]	ØSR9Ø4[9,A,Z]	ØSR9Ø6[9,A,Z]	ØSR9ØJ[9,A,Z]
Hip, LT	ØSPBØ8Z	ØSRBØ1[9,A,Z]	ØSRBØ2[9,A,Z]	ØSRBØ3[9,A,Z]	ØSRBØ4[9,A,Z]	ØSRBØ6[9,A,Z]	ØSRBØJ[9,A,Z]

Open Removal of Hip Spacer with Replacement

Removal of Spacer		Code also as appropriate Replacement by Device Type						
		Acetabular Surface				Femoral Surface		
		Poly	Metal	Ceramic	Synthetic	Metal	Ceramic	Synthetic
Hip, RT	ØSP9Ø8Z	ØSRAØØ[9,A,Z]	ØSRAØ1[9,A,Z]	ØSRAØ3[9,A,Z]	ØSRAØJ[9,A,Z]	ØSRRØ1[9,A,Z]	ØSRRØ3[9,A,Z]	ØSRRØJ[9,A,Z]
Hip, LT	ØSPBØ8Z	ØSREØØ[9,A,Z]	ØSREØ1[9,A,Z]	ØSREØ3[9,A,Z]	ØSREØJ[9,A,Z]	ØSRSØ1[9,A,Z]	ØSRSØ3[9,A,Z]	ØSRSØJ[9,A,Z]

Open Removal of Hip Spacer with Liner Insertion (supplement)

Removal of Spacer		Code also as appropriate Supplement of Body Part by Site		
		Joint	Acetabular Surface	Femoral Surface
Hip, RT	ØSP9Ø8Z	ØSU9Ø9Z	ØSUAØ9Z	ØSURØ9Z
Hip, LT	ØSPBØ8Z	ØSUBØ9Z	ØSUEØ9Z	ØSUSØ9Z

Open Removal of Hip Liner with Replacement

Removal of Liner		Code also as appropriate Replacement by Device Type					
		Metal	Metal on Poly	Ceramic	Ceramic on Poly	Oxidized Zirc on Poly	Synthetic Substitute
Hip, RT	ØSP9Ø9Z	ØSR9Ø1[9,A,Z]	ØSR9Ø2[9,A,Z]	ØSR9Ø3[9,A,Z]	ØSR9Ø4[9,A,Z]	ØSR9Ø6[9,A,Z]	ØSR9ØJ[9,A,Z]
Hip, LT	ØSPBØ9Z	ØSRBØ1[9,A,Z]	ØSRBØ2[9,A,Z]	ØSRBØ3[9,A,Z]	ØSRBØ4[9,A,Z]	ØSRBØ6[9,A,Z]	ØSRBØJ[9,A,Z]

Open Removal of Hip Liner with Replacement

Removal of Liner		Code also as appropriate Replacement by Device Type						
		Acetabular Surface				Femoral Surface		
		Poly	Metal	Ceramic	Synthetic	Metal	Ceramic	Synthetic
Hip, RT	ØSP9Ø9Z	ØSRAØØ[9,A,Z]	ØSRAØ1[9,A,Z]	ØSRAØ3[9,A,Z]	ØSRAØJ[9,A,Z]	ØSRRØ1[9,A,Z]	ØSRRØ3[9,A,Z]	ØSRRØJ[9,A,Z]
Hip, LT	ØSPBØ9Z	ØSREØØ[9,A,Z]	ØSREØ1[9,A,Z]	ØSREØ3[9,A,Z]	ØSREØJ[9,A,Z]	ØSRSØ1[9,A,Z]	ØSRSØ3[9,A,Z]	ØSRSØJ[9,A,Z]

Open Removal of Hip Liner with Liner Insertion (supplement)

Removal of Liner		Code also as appropriate Supplement of Body Part by Site		
		Joint	Acetabular Surface	Femoral Surface
Hip, RT	ØSP9Ø9Z	ØSU9Ø9Z	ØSUAØ9Z	ØSURØ9Z
Hip, LT	ØSPBØ9Z	ØSUBØ9Z	ØSUEØ9Z	ØSUSØ9Z

Open Removal of Hip Resurfacing Device with Replacement

Removal of Resurfacing Device		Code also as appropriate Replacement by Device Type					
		Metal	Metal on Poly	Ceramic	Ceramic on Poly	Oxidized Zirc on Poly	Synthetic Substitute
Hip, RT	ØSP9ØBZ	ØSR9Ø1[9,A,Z]	ØSR9Ø2[9,A,Z]	ØSR9Ø3[9,A,Z]	ØSR9Ø4[9,A,Z]	ØSR9Ø6[9,A,Z]	ØSR9ØJ[9,A,Z]
Hip, LT	ØSPBØBZ	ØSRBØ1[9,A,Z]	ØSRBØ2[9,A,Z]	ØSRBØ3[9,A,Z]	ØSRBØ4[9,A,Z]	ØSRBØ6[9,A,Z]	ØSRBØJ[9,A,Z]

Open Removal of Hip Resurfacing Device with Replacement

Removal of Resurfacing Device		Code also as appropriate Replacement by Device Type						
		Acetabular Surface				Femoral Surface		
		Poly	Metal	Ceramic	Synthetic	Metal	Ceramic	Synthetic
Hip, RT	ØSP9ØBZ	ØSRAØØ[9,A,Z]	ØSRAØ1[9,A,Z]	ØSRAØ3[9,A,Z]	ØSRAØJ[9,A,Z]	ØSRRØ1[9,A,Z]	ØSRRØ3[9,A,Z]	ØSRRØJ[9,A,Z]
Hip, LT	ØSPBØBZ	ØSREØØ[9,A,Z]	ØSREØ1[9,A,Z]	ØSREØ3[9,A,Z]	ØSREØJ[9,A,Z]	ØSRSØ1[9,A,Z]	ØSRSØ3[9,A,Z]	ØSRSØJ[9,A,Z]

Open Removal of Hip Resurfacing Device with Liner Insertion (supplement)

Removal of Resurfacing Device		Code also as appropriate Supplement of Body Part by Site		
		Joint	Acetabular Surface	Femoral Surface
Hip, RT	ØSP9ØBZ	ØSU9Ø9Z	ØSUAØ9Z	ØSURØ9Z
Hip, LT	ØSPBØBZ	ØSUBØ9Z	ØSUEØ9Z	ØSUSØ9Z

Open Removal of Hip Synthetic Substitute with Replacement

Removal of Synthetic Substitute		Code also as appropriate Replacement by Device Type					
		Metal	Metal on Poly	Ceramic	Ceramic on Poly	Oxidized Zirc on Poly	Synthetic Substitute
Hip, RT	ØSP9ØJZ	ØSR9Ø1[9,A,Z]	ØSR9Ø2[9,A,Z]	ØSR9Ø3[9,A,Z]	ØSR9Ø4[9,A,Z]	ØSR9Ø6[9,A,Z]	ØSR9ØJ[9,A,Z]
Hip, LT	ØSPBØJZ	ØSRBØ1[9,A,Z]	ØSRBØ2[9,A,Z]	ØSRBØ3[9,A,Z]	ØSRBØ4[9,A,Z]	ØSRBØ6[9,A,Z]	ØSRBØJ[9,A,Z]

Open Removal of Hip Synthetic Substitute with Replacement

Removal of Synthetic Substitute		Code also as appropriate Replacement by Device Type						
		Acetabular Surface				Femoral Surface		
		Poly	Metal	Ceramic	Synthetic	Metal	Ceramic	Synthetic
Hip, RT	ØSP9ØJZ	ØSRAØØ[9,A,Z]	ØSRAØ1[9,A,Z]	ØSRAØ3[9,A,Z]	ØSRAØJ[9,A,Z]	ØSRRØ1[9,A,Z]	ØSRRØ3[9,A,Z]	ØSRRØJ[9,A,Z]
Hip, LT	ØSPBØJZ	ØSREØØ[9,A,Z]	ØSREØ1[9,A,Z]	ØSREØ3[9,A,Z]	ØSREØJ[9,A,Z]	ØSRSØ1[9,A,Z]	ØSRSØ3[9,A,Z]	ØSRSØJ[9,A,Z]

Open Removal of Hip Acetabular/Femoral Surface with Replacement

Removal of Acetabular/Femoral Surface		Code also as appropriate Replacement by Device Type					
		Metal	Metal on Poly	Ceramic	Ceramic on Poly	Oxidized Zirc on Poly	Synthetic Substitute
Hip, RT	ØSP[A,R]ØJZ	ØSR9Ø1[9,A,Z]	ØSR9Ø2[9,A,Z]	ØSR9Ø3[9,A,Z]	ØSR9Ø4[9,A,Z]	ØSR9Ø6[9,A,Z]	ØSR9ØJ[9,A,Z]
Hip, LT	ØSP[E,S]ØJZ	ØSRBØ1[9,A,Z]	ØSRBØ2[9,A,Z]	ØSRBØ3[9,A,Z]	ØSRBØ4[9,A,Z]	ØSRBØ6[9,A,Z]	ØSRBØJ[9,A,Z]

Open Removal of Hip Acetabular/Femoral Surface with Replacement

Removal of Acetabular/Femoral Surface		Code also as appropriate Replacement by Device Type						
		Acetabular Surface				Femoral Surface		
		Poly	Metal	Ceramic	Synthetic	Metal	Ceramic	Synthetic
Hip, RT	ØSP[A,R]ØJZ	ØSRAØØ[9,A,Z]	ØSRAØ1[9,A,Z]	ØSRAØ3[9,A,Z]	ØSRAØJ[9,A,Z]	ØSRRØ1[9,A,Z]	ØSRRØ3[9,A,Z]	ØSRRØJ[9,A,Z]
Hip, LT	ØSP[E,S]ØJZ	ØSREØØ[9,A,Z]	ØSREØ1[9,A,Z]	ØSREØ3[9,A,Z]	ØSREØJ[9,A,Z]	ØSRSØ1[9,A,Z]	ØSRSØ3[9,A,Z]	ØSRSØJ[9,A,Z]

Percutaneous Endoscopic Removal of Hip Spacer with Replacement

Removal of Spacer		Code also as appropriate Replacement by Device Type					
		Metal	Metal on Poly	Ceramic	Ceramic on Poly	Oxidized Zirc on Poly	Synthetic Substitute
Hip, RT	ØSP948Z	ØSR9Ø1[9,A,Z]	ØSR9Ø2[9,A,Z]	ØSR9Ø3[9,A,Z]	ØSR9Ø4[9,A,Z]	ØSR9Ø6[9,A,Z]	ØSR9ØJ[9,A,Z]
Hip, LT	ØSPB48Z	ØSRBØ1[9,A,Z]	ØSRBØ2[9,A,Z]	ØSRBØ3[9,A,Z]	ØSRBØ4[9,A,Z]	ØSRBØ6[9,A,Z]	ØSRBØJ[9,A,Z]

Percutaneous Endoscopic Removal of Hip Spacer with Replacement

Removal of Spacer		Code also as appropriate Replacement by Device Type						
		Acetabular Surface				Femoral Surface		
		Poly	Metal	Ceramic	Synthetic	Metal	Ceramic	Synthetic
Hip, RT	ØSP948Z	ØSRAØØ[9,A,Z]	ØSRAØ1[9,A,Z]	ØSRAØ3[9,A,Z]	ØSRAØJ[9,A,Z]	ØSRRØ1[9,A,Z]	ØSRRØ3[9,A,Z]	ØSRRØJ[9,A,Z]
Hip, LT	ØSPB48Z	ØSREØØ[9,A,Z]	ØSREØ1[9,A,Z]	ØSREØ3[9,A,Z]	ØSREØJ[9,A,Z]	ØSRSØ1[9,A,Z]	ØSRSØ3[9,A,Z]	ØSRSØJ[9,A,Z]

Percutaneous Endoscopic Removal of Hip Spacer with Liner Insertion (supplement)

Removal of Spacer		Code also as appropriate Supplement of Body Part by Site		
		Joint	Acetabular Surface	Femoral Surface
Hip, RT	ØSP948Z	ØSU9Ø9Z	ØSUAØ9Z	ØSURØ9Z
Hip, LT	ØSPB48Z	ØSUBØ9Z	ØSUEØ9Z	ØSUSØ9Z

Percutaneous Endoscopic Removal of Hip Synthetic Substitute with Replacement

Removal of Synthetic Substitute		Code also as appropriate Replacement by Device Type					
		Metal	Metal on Poly	Ceramic	Ceramic on Poly	Oxidized Zirc on Poly	Synthetic Substitute
Hip, RT	ØSP94JZ	ØSR9Ø1[9,A,Z]	ØSR9Ø2[9,A,Z]	ØSR9Ø3[9,A,Z]	ØSR9Ø4[9,A,Z]	ØSR9Ø6[9,A,Z]	ØSR9ØJ[9,A,Z]
Hip, LT	ØSPB4JZ	ØSRBØ1[9,A,Z]	ØSRBØ2[9,A,Z]	ØSRBØ3[9,A,Z]	ØSRBØ4[9,A,Z]	ØSRBØ6[9,A,Z]	ØSRBØJ[9,A,Z]

Percutaneous Endoscopic of Hip Synthetic Substitute with Replacement

Removal of Synthetic Substitute		Code also as appropriate Replacement by Device Type						
		Acetabular Surface				Femoral Surface		
		Poly	Metal	Ceramic	Synthetic	Metal	Ceramic	Synthetic
Hip, RT	ØSP94JZ	ØSRAØØ[9,A,Z]	ØSRAØ1[9,A,Z]	ØSRAØ3[9,A,Z]	ØSRAØJ[9,A,Z]	ØSRRØ1[9,A,Z]	ØSRRØ3[9,A,Z]	ØSRRØJ[9,A,Z]
Hip, LT	ØSPB4JZ	ØSREØØ[9,A,Z]	ØSREØ1[9,A,Z]	ØSREØ3[9,A,Z]	ØSREØJ[9,A,Z]	ØSRSØ1[9,A,Z]	ØSRSØ3[9,A,Z]	ØSRSØJ[9,A,Z]

Percutaneous Endoscopic Removal of Hip Synthetic Substitute with Liner Insertion (supplement)

Removal of Synthetic Substitute		Code also as appropriate Supplement of Body Part by Site		
		Joint	Acetabular Surface	Femoral Surface
Hip, RT	ØSP94JZ	ØSU9Ø9Z	ØSUAØ9Z	ØSURØ9Z
Hip, LT	ØSPB4JZ	ØSUBØ9Z	ØSUEØ9Z	ØSUSØ9Z

Percutaneous Endoscopic Removal of Hip Acetabular/Femoral Surface with Replacement

Removal of Acetabular/Femoral Surface		Code also as appropriate Replacement by Device Type					
		Metal	Metal on Poly	Ceramic	Ceramic on Poly	Oxidized Zirc on Poly	Synthetic Substitute
Hip, RT	ØSP[A,R]4JZ	ØSR9Ø1[9,A,Z]	ØSR9Ø2[9,A,Z]	ØSR9Ø3[9,A,Z]	ØSR9Ø4[9,A,Z]	ØSR9Ø6[9,A,Z]	ØSR9ØJ[9,A,Z]
Hip, LT	ØSP[E,S]4JZ	ØSRBØ1[9,A,Z]	ØSRBØ2[9,A,Z]	ØSRBØ3[9,A,Z]	ØSRBØ4[9,A,Z]	ØSRBØ6[9,A,Z]	ØSRBØJ[9,A,Z]

Percutaneous Endoscopic of Hip Acetabular/Femoral Surface with Replacement

Removal of Acetabular/Femoral Surface		Code also as appropriate Replacement by Device Type						
		Acetabular Surface				Femoral Surface		
		Poly	Metal	Ceramic	Synthetic	Metal	Ceramic	Synthetic
Hip, RT	ØSP[A,R]4JZ	ØSRAØØ[9,A,Z]	ØSRAØ1[9,A,Z]	ØSRAØ3[9,A,Z]	ØSRAØJ[9,A,Z]	ØSRRØ1[9,A,Z]	ØSRRØ3[9,A,Z]	ØSRRØJ[9,A,Z]
Hip, LT	ØSP[E,S]4JZ	ØSREØØ[9,A,Z]	ØSREØ1[9,A,Z]	ØSREØ3[9,A,Z]	ØSREØJ[9,A,Z]	ØSRSØ1[9,A,Z]	ØSRSØ3[9,A,Z]	ØSRSØJ[9,A,Z]

Percutaneous Endoscopic Removal of Hip Acetabular/Femoral Surface with Liner Insertion (supplement)

Removal of Acetabular/Femoral Surface		Code also as appropriate Supplement of Body Part by Site		
		Joint	Acetabular Surface	Femoral Surface
Hip, RT	ØSP[A,R]4JZ	ØSU9Ø9Z	ØSUAØ9Z	ØSURØ9Z
Hip, LT	ØSP[E,S]4JZ	ØSUBØ9Z	ØSUEØ9Z	ØSUSØ9Z

Knee Procedures

Open Removal of Knee Liner with Synthetic Substitute Replacement

Removal of Liner		Code also as appropriate Replacement by Type of Synthetic Substitute						
		Oxidized Zircon on Poly	Synthetic Substitute	Medial Unicondylar	Lateral Unicondylar	Patello-femoral	Femoral Surface	Tibial Surface
Knee, RT	ØSPCØ9Z	ØSRCØ6[9,A,Z]	ØSRCØJ[9,A,Z]	ØSRCØL[9,A,Z]	ØSRCØM[9,A,Z]	ØSRCØN[9,A,Z]	ØSRTØJ[9,A,Z]	ØSRVØJ[9,A,Z]
Knee, LT	ØSPDØ9Z	ØSRDØ6[9,A,Z]	ØSRDØJ[9,A,Z]	ØSRDØL[9,A,Z]	ØSRDØM[9,A,Z]	ØSRDØN[9,A,Z]	ØSRUØJ[9,A,Z]	ØSRWØJ[9,A,Z]

Open Removal of Patellar Surface of Knee with Synthetic Substitute Replacement

Removal of Patellar Surface		Code also as appropriate Replacement by Type of Synthetic Substitute	
		Femoral Surface	Tibial Surface
Knee, RT	ØSPCØJC	ØSRTØJ[9,A]	ØSRVØJ[9,A]
Knee, LT	ØSPDØJC	ØSRUØJ[9,A]	ØSRWØJ[9,A,Z]

Open Removal of Knee Synthetic Substitute with Synthetic Substitute Replacement

Removal of Synthetic Substitute		Code also as appropriate Replacement by Type of Synthetic Substitute	
		Femoral Surface	Tibial Surface
Knee, RT	ØSPCØJZ	ØSRTØJ[9,A]	ØSRVØJ[9,A]
Knee, LT	ØSPDØJZ	ØSRUØJ[9,A]	ØSRWØJ[9,A,Z]

Open Removal of Knee Medial/Lateral Unicondylar Device with Synthetic Substitute Replacement

Removal of Medial/Lateral Unicondylar Device		Code also as appropriate Replacement by Type of Synthetic Substitute	
		Femoral Surface	Tibial Surface
Knee, Medial Unicondylar, RT	ØSPCØLZ	ØSRTØJ[9,A]	ØSRVØJ[9,A]
Knee, Medial Unicondylar, LT	ØSPDØLZ	ØSRUØJ[9,A]	ØSRWØJ[9,A,Z]
Knee, Lateral Unicondylar, RT	ØSPCØMZ	ØSRTØJ[9,A]	ØSRVØJ[9,A]
Knee, Lateral Unicondylar, LT	ØSPDØMZ	ØSRUØJ[9,A]	ØSRWØJ[9,A,Z]

Open Removal of Knee Patellofemoral Device with Synthetic Substitute Replacement

Removal of Patellofemoral Device		Code also as appropriate Replacement by Type of Synthetic Substitute	
		Femoral Surface	Tibial Surface
Knee, RT	ØSPCØNZ	ØSRTØJ[9,A]	ØSRVØJ[9,A]
Knee, LT	ØSPDØNZ	ØSRUØJ[9,A]	ØSRWØJ[9,A,Z]

Open Removal of Femoral/Tibial Surface of Knee with Synthetic Substitute Replacement

Removal of Femoral/Tibial Surface		Code also as appropriate Replacement by Type of Synthetic Substitute	
		Femoral Surface	Tibial Surface
Knee, RT	ØSP[T,V]ØJZ	ØSRTØJ[9,A]	ØSRVØJ[9,A]
Knee, LT	ØSP[U,W]ØJZ	ØSRUØJ[9,A]	ØSRWØJ[9,A,Z]

Percutaneous Endoscopic Removal of Patellar Surface of Knee with Synthetic Substitute Replacement

Removal of Patellar Surface		Code also as appropriate Replacement by Type of Synthetic Substitute	
		Femoral Surface	Tibial Surface
Knee, RT	ØSPC4JC	ØSRTØJ[9,A]	ØSRVØJ[9,A]
Knee, LT	ØSPD4JC	ØSRUØJ[9,A]	ØSRWØJ[9,A,Z]

Percutaneous Endoscopic Removal of Knee Synthetic Substitute with Synthetic Substitute Replacement

Removal of Synthetic Substitute		Code also as appropriate Replacement by Type of Synthetic Substitute	
		Femoral Surface	Tibial Surface
Knee, RT	ØSPC4JZ	ØSRTØJ[9,A]	ØSRVØJ[9,A]
Knee, LT	ØSPD4JZ	ØSRUØJ[9,A]	ØSRWØJ[9,A,Z]

Percutaneous Endoscopic Removal of Knee Medial/Lateral Unicondylar Device with Synthetic Substitute Replacement

Removal of Medial/Lateral Unicondylar Device		Code also as appropriate Replacement by Type of Synthetic Substitute	
		Femoral Surface	Tibial Surface
Knee, Medial Unicondylar, RT	ØSPC4LZ	ØSRTØJ[9,A]	ØSRVØJ[9,A]
Knee, Medial Unicondylar, LT	ØSPD4LZ	ØSRUØJ[9,A]	ØSRWØJ[9,A,Z]
Knee, Lateral Unicondylar, RT	ØSPC4MZ	ØSRTØJ[9,A]	ØSRVØJ[9,A]
Knee, Lateral Unicondylar, LT	ØSPD4MZ	ØSRUØJ[9,A]	ØSRWØJ[9,A,Z]

Percutaneous Endoscopic Removal of Knee Patellofemoral Device with Synthetic Substitute Replacement

Removal of Patellofemoral Device		Code also as appropriate Replacement by Type of Synthetic Substitute	
		Femoral Surface	Tibial Surface
Knee, RT	ØSPC4NZ	ØSRTØJ[9,A]	ØSRVØJ[9,A]
Knee, LT	ØSPD4NZ	ØSRUØJ[9,A]	ØSRWØJ[9,A,Z]

Percutaneous Endoscopic Removal of Femoral/Tibial Surface of Knee with Synthetic Substitute Replacement

Removal of Femoral/Tibial Surface		Code also as appropriate Replacement by Type of Synthetic Substitute	
		Femoral Surface	Tibial Surface
Knee, RT	ØSP[T,V]4JZ	ØSRTØJ[9,A]	ØSRVØJ[9,A]
Knee, LT	ØSP[U,W]4JZ	ØSRUØJ[9,A]	ØSRWØJ[9,A,Z]

DRG 662-664 Minor Bladder Procedure

Repair of Bladder	Code also as appropriate Repair of Abdominal Wall	
	with Stoma	without Stoma
ØTQB[Ø,3,4]ZZ	ØWQFXZ2	ØWQFXZZ

DRG 665-667 Prostatectomy

Site	Resection by approach				Code also as appropriate Resection of Seminal Vesicles, Bilateral by approach	
	Open	Percutaneous Endoscopic	Via Natural or Artificial Opening	Via Natural or Artificial Opening Endoscopic	Open	Percutaneous Endoscopic
Prostate	ØVTØØZZ	ØVTØ4ZZ	ØVTØ7ZZ	ØVTØ8ZZ	ØVT3ØZZ	ØVT34ZZ

DRG 7Ø7-7Ø8 Major Male Pelvic Procedures

Site	Resection by approach				Code also as appropriate Resection of Seminal Vesicles, Bilateral by approach	
	Open	Percutaneous Endoscopic	Via Natural or Artificial Opening	Via Natural or Artificial Opening Endoscopic	Open	Percutaneous Endoscopic
Prostate	ØVTØØZZ	ØVTØ4ZZ	ØVTØ7ZZ	ØVTØ8ZZ	ØVT3ØZZ	ØVT34ZZ

DRG 734-735 Pelvic Evisceration, Radical Hysterectomy and Radical Vulvectomy

Pelvic Evisceration

Resection by Site						
Bladder	Cervix	Fallopian Tubes, Bilateral	Ovaries, Bilateral	Urethra	Uterus	Vagina
ØTTBØZZ	ØUTCØZZ	ØUT7ØZZ	ØUT2ØZZ	ØTTDØZZ	ØUT9ØZZ	ØUTGØZZ

Radical Hysterectomy

Approach	Resection by Site		
	Cervix	Uterus	Uterine Support Structure
Vaginal	ØUTC[7,8]ZZ	ØUT9[7,8]ZZ	ØUT4[7,8]ZZ
Abdominal, Endoscopic	ØUTC4ZZ	ØUT9[4,F]ZZ	ØUT44ZZ
Abdominal, Open	ØUTCØZZ	ØUT9ØZZ	ØUT4ØZZ

Radical Vulvectomy

Resection by Site	Code also as appropriate Excision of Inguinal Lymph Nodes by Approach	
Vulva	Right	Left
ØUTM[Ø,X]ZZ	Ø7BH[Ø,4]ZZ	Ø7BJ[Ø,4]ZZ

Non-OR procedure combinations

Note: The following table identifies procedure combinations that are considered Non-OR even though one or more procedures of the combination are considered valid DRG OR procedures

Insertion With Removal of Intraluminal Device

Code as appropriate Insertion of Intraluminal Device into Hepatobiliary Duct	Code also as appropriate Removal of Intraluminal Device by Approach and Site			
	Via Natural or Artificial Opening		External	
	Hepatobiliary Duct	Pancreatic Duct	Hepatobiliary Duct	Pancreatic Duct
ØFHB7DZ	ØFPB[7,8]DZ	ØFPD[7,8]DZ	ØFPBXDZ	ØFPDXDZ

Appendix M: Coding Exercises and Answers

Using the ICD-10-PCS tables construct the code that accurately represents the procedure performed.

Medical Surgical Section

Procedure	Code
1. Excision of malignant melanoma from skin of right ear	
2. Laparoscopy with excision of endometrial implant from left ovary	
3. Percutaneous needle core biopsy of right kidney	
4. EGD with gastric biopsy	
5. Open endarterectomy of left common carotid artery	
6. Excision of basal cell carcinoma of lower lip	
7. Open excision of tail of pancreas	
8. Percutaneous biopsy of right gastrocnemius muscle	
9. Sigmoidoscopy with sigmoid polypectomy	
10. Open excision of lesion from right Achilles tendon	
11. Open resection of cecum	
12. Total excision of pituitary gland, open	
13. Explantation of left failed kidney, open	
14. Open left axillary total lymphadenectomy	
15. Laparoscopic-assisted vaginal hysterectomy	
16. Right total mastectomy, open	
17. Open resection of papillary muscle	
18. Total retropubic prostatectomy, open	
19. Laparoscopic cholecystectomy	
20. Endoscopic bilateral total maxillary sinusectomy	
21. Amputation at right elbow level	
22. Right below-knee amputation, proximal tibia/fibula	
23. Fifth ray carpometacarpal joint amputation, left hand	
24. Right leg and hip amputation through ischium	
25. DIP joint amputation of right thumb	
26. Right wrist joint amputation	
27. Trans-metatarsal amputation of foot at left big toe	
28. Mid-shaft amputation, right humerus	
29. Left fourth toe amputation, mid-proximal phalanx	
30. Right above-knee amputation, distal femur	
31. Cryotherapy of wart on left hand	
32. Percutaneous radiofrequency ablation of right vocal cord lesion	
33. Left heart catheterization with laser destruction of arrhythmogenic focus, A-V node	
34. Cautery of nosebleed	
35. Transurethral endoscopic laser ablation of prostate	
36. Percutaneous cautery of oozing varicose vein, left calf	

Procedure	Code
37. Laparoscopy with destruction of endometriosis, bilateral ovaries	
38. Laser coagulation of right retinal vessel hemorrhage, percutaneous	
39. Thoracoscopic pleurodesis, left side	
40. Percutaneous insertion of Greenfield IVC filter	
41. Forceps total mouth extraction, upper and lower teeth	
42. Removal of left thumbnail	
43. Extraction of right intraocular lens without replacement, percutaneous	
44. Laparoscopy with needle aspiration of ova for in vitro fertilization	
45. Nonexcisional debridement of skin ulcer, right foot	
46. Open stripping of abdominal fascia, right side	
47. Hysteroscopy with D&C, diagnostic	
48. Liposuction for medical purposes, left upper arm	
49. Removal of tattered right ear drum fragments with tweezers	
50. Microincisional phlebectomy of spider veins, right lower leg	
51. Routine Foley catheter placement	
52. Incision and drainage of external anal abscess	
53. Percutaneous drainage of ascites	
54. Laparoscopy with left ovarian cystotomy and drainage	
55. Laparotomy and drain placement for liver abscess, right lobe	
56. Right knee arthrotomy with drain placement	
57. Thoracentesis of left pleural effusion	
58. Phlebotomy of left median cubital vein for polycythemia vera	
59. Percutaneous chest tube placement for right pneumothorax	
60. Endoscopic drainage of left ethmoid sinus	
61. External ventricular CSF drainage catheter placement via burr hole	
62. Removal of foreign body, right cornea	
63. Percutaneous mechanical thrombectomy, left brachial artery	
64. Esophagogastroscopy with removal of bezoar from stomach	
65. Foreign body removal, skin of left thumb	
66. Transurethral cystoscopy with removal of bladder stone	
67. Forceps removal of foreign body in right nostril	
68. Laparoscopy with excision of old suture from mesentery	
69. Incision and removal of right lacrimal duct stone	
70. Nonincisional removal of intraluminal foreign body from vagina	
71. Right common carotid endarterectomy, open	
72. Open excision of retained sliver, subcutaneous tissue of left foot	
73. Extracorporeal shockwave lithotripsy (ESWL), bilateral ureters	

Procedure	Code
74. Endoscopic retrograde cholangiopancreatography (ERCP) with lithotripsy of common bile duct stone	
75. Thoracotomy with crushing of pericardial calcifications	
76. Transurethral cystoscopy with fragmentation of bladder calculus	
77. Hysteroscopy with intraluminal lithotripsy of left fallopian tube calcification	
78. Division of right foot tendon, percutaneous	
79. Left heart catheterization with division of bundle of HIS	
80. Open osteotomy of capitate, left hand	
81. EGD with esophagotomy of esophagogastric junction	
82. Sacral rhizotomy for pain control, percutaneous	
83. Laparotomy with exploration and adhesiolysis of right ureter	
84. Incision of scar contracture, right elbow	
85. Frenulotomy for treatment of tongue-tie syndrome	
86. Right shoulder arthroscopy with coracoacromial ligament release	
87. Mitral valvulotomy for release of fused leaflets, open approach	
88. Percutaneous left Achilles tendon release	
89. Laparoscopy with lysis of peritoneal adhesions	
90. Manual rupture of right shoulder joint adhesions under general anesthesia	
91. Open posterior tarsal tunnel release	
92. Laparoscopy with freeing of left ovary and fallopian tube	
93. Liver transplant with donor matched liver	
94. Orthotopic heart transplant using porcine heart	
95. Right lung transplant, open, using organ donor match	
96. Transplant of large intestine, organ donor match	
97. Left kidney/pancreas organ bank transplant	
98. Replantation of avulsed scalp	
99. Reattachment of severed right ear	
100. Reattachment of traumatic left gastrocnemius avulsion, open	
101. Closed replantation of three avulsed teeth, lower jaw	
102. Reattachment of severed left hand	
103. Right open palmaris longus tendon transfer	
104. Endoscopic radial to median nerve transfer	
105. Fasciocutaneous flap closure of left thigh, open	
106. Transfer left index finger to left thumb position, open	
107. Percutaneous fascia transfer to fill defect, right neck	
108. Trigeminal to facial nerve transfer, percutaneous endoscopic	
109. Endoscopic left leg flexor hallucis longus tendon transfer	
110. Right scalp advancement flap to right temple	

Procedure	Code
111. Bilateral TRAM pedicle flap reconstruction status post mastectomy, muscle only, open	
112. Skin transfer flap closure of complex open wound, left lower back	
113. Open fracture reduction, right tibia	
114. Laparoscopy with gastropexy for malrotation	
115. Left knee arthroscopy with reposition of anterior cruciate ligament	
116. Open transposition of ulnar nerve	
117. Closed reduction with percutaneous internal fixation of right femoral neck fracture	
118. Trans-vaginal intraluminal cervical cerclage	
119. Cervical cerclage using Shirodkar technique	
120. Thoracotomy with banding of left pulmonary artery using extraluminal device	
121. Restriction of thoracic duct with intraluminal stent, percutaneous	
122. Craniotomy with clipping of cerebral aneurysm	
123. Nonincisional, transnasal placement of restrictive stent in right lacrimal duct	
124. Catheter-based temporary restriction of blood flow in abdominal aorta for treatment of cerebral ischemia	
125. Percutaneous ligation of esophageal vein	
126. Percutaneous embolization of left internal carotid-cavernous fistula	
127. Laparoscopy with bilateral occlusion of fallopian tubes using Hulka extraluminal clips	
128. Open suture ligation of failed AV graft, left brachial artery	
129. Percutaneous embolization of vascular supply, intracranial meningioma	
130. Percutaneous embolization of right uterine artery, using coils	
131. Open occlusion of left atrial appendage, using extraluminal pressure clips	
132. Percutaneous suture exclusion of left atrial appendage, via femoral artery access	
133. ERCP with balloon dilation of common bile duct	
134. PTCA of two coronary arteries, LAD with stent placement, RCA with no stent	
135. Cystoscopy with intraluminal dilation of bladder neck stricture	
136. Open dilation of old anastomosis, left femoral artery	
137. Dilation of upper esophageal stricture, direct visualization, with Bougie sound	
138. PTA of right brachial artery stenosis	
139. Transnasal dilation and stent placement in right lacrimal duct	
140. Hysteroscopy with balloon dilation of bilateral fallopian tubes	
141. Tracheoscopy with intraluminal dilation of tracheal stenosis	
142. Cystoscopy with dilation of left ureteral stricture, with stent placement	
143. Open gastric bypass with Roux-en-Y limb to jejunum	
144. Right temporal artery to intracranial artery bypass using Gore-Tex graft, open	

Procedure	Code
145. Tracheostomy formation with tracheostomy tube placement, percutaneous	
146. PICVA (percutaneous in situ coronary venous arterialization) of single coronary artery	
147. Open left femoral-popliteal artery bypass using cadaver vein graft	
148. Shunting of intrathecal cerebrospinal fluid to peritoneal cavity using synthetic shunt	
149. Colostomy formation, open, transverse colon to abdominal wall	
150. Open urinary diversion, left ureter, using ileal conduit to skin	
151. CABG of LAD using pedicled left internal mammary artery, open off-bypass	
152. Open pleuroperitoneal shunt, right pleural cavity, using synthetic device	
153. Percutaneous placement of ventriculoperitoneal shunt for treatment of hydrocephalus	
154. End-of-life replacement of spinal neurostimulator generator, multiple array, in lower abdomen	
155. Percutaneous insertion of spinal neurostimulator lead, lumbar spinal cord	
156. Percutaneous replacement of broken pacemaker lead in left atrium	
157. Open placement of dual chamber pacemaker generator in chest wall	
158. Percutaneous placement of venous central line in right internal jugular, with tip in superior vena cava	
159. Open insertion of multiple channel cochlear implant, left ear	
160. Percutaneous placement of Swan-Ganz catheter in pulmonary trunk	
161. Bronchoscopy with insertion of Low Dose, Pd-103 brachytherapy seeds, right lung	
162. Open insertion of interspinous process device into lumbar vertebral joint	
163. Open placement of bone growth stimulator, left femoral shaft	
164. Cystoscopy with placement of brachytherapy seeds in prostate gland	
165. Percutaneous insertion of Greenfield IVC filter	
166. Full-thickness skin graft to right lower arm, autograft (do not code graft harvest for this exercise)	
167. Excision of necrosed left femoral head with bone bank bone graft to fill the defect, open	
168. Penetrating keratoplasty of right cornea with donor matched cornea, percutaneous approach	
169. Excision of abdominal aorta with Gore-Tex graft replacement, open	
170. Total right knee arthroplasty with insertion of total knee prosthesis	
171. Tenonectomy with graft to right ankle using cadaver graft, open	
172. Mitral valve replacement using porcine valve, open	
173. Percutaneous phacoemulsification of right eye cataract with prosthetic lens insertion	
174. Transcatheter replacement of pulmonary valve using of bovine jugular vein valve	

Procedure	Code
175. Total left hip replacement using ceramic on ceramic prosthesis, without bone cement	
176. Aortic valve annuloplasty using ring, open	
177. Laparoscopic repair of left inguinal hernia with marlex plug	
178. Autograft nerve graft to right median nerve, percutaneous endoscopic (do not code graft harvest for this exercise)	
179. Exchange of liner in femoral component of previous left hip replacement, open approach	
180. Anterior colporrhaphy with polypropylene mesh reinforcement, open approach	
181. Implantation of CorCap cardiac support device, open approach	
182. Abdominal wall herniorrhaphy, open, using synthetic mesh	
183. Tendon graft to strengthen injured left shoulder using autograft, open (do not code graft harvest for this exercise)	
184. Onlay lamellar keratoplasty of left cornea using autograft, external approach	
185. Resurfacing procedure on right femoral head, open approach	
186. Exchange of drainage tube from right hip joint	
187. Tracheostomy tube exchange	
188. Change chest tube for left pneumothorax	
189. Exchange of cerebral ventriculostomy drainage tube	
190. Foley urinary catheter exchange	
191. Open removal of lumbar sympathetic neurostimulator lead	
192. Nonincisional removal of Swan-Ganz catheter from right pulmonary artery	
193. Laparotomy with removal of pancreatic drain	
194. Extubation, endotracheal tube	
195. Nonincisional PEG tube removal	
196. Transvaginal removal of brachytherapy seeds	
197. Transvaginal removal of extraluminal cervical cerclage	
198. Incision with removal of K-wire fixation, right first metatarsal	
199. Cystoscopy with retrieval of left ureteral stent	
200. Removal of nasogastric drainage tube for decompression	
201. Removal of external fixator, left radial fracture	
202. Trimming and reanastomosis of stenosed femorofemoral synthetic bypass graft, open	
203. Open revision of right hip replacement, with readjustment of prosthesis	
204. Adjustment of position, pacemaker lead in left ventricle, percutaneous	
205. External repositioning of Foley catheter to bladder	
206. Taking out loose screw and putting larger screw in fracture repair plate, left tibia	
207. Revision of totally implantable VAD port placement in chest wall, causing patient discomfort, open	
208. Thoracotomy with exploration of right pleural cavity	
209. Diagnostic laryngoscopy	

Procedure	Code
210. Exploratory arthrotomy of left knee	
211. Colposcopy with diagnostic hysteroscopy	
212. Digital rectal exam	
213. Diagnostic arthroscopy of right shoulder	
214. Endoscopy of maxillary sinus	
215. Laparotomy with palpation of liver	
216. Transurethral diagnostic cystoscopy	
217. Colonoscopy, discontinued at sigmoid colon	
218. Percutaneous mapping of basal ganglia	
219. Heart catheterization with cardiac mapping	
220. Intraoperative whole brain mapping via craniotomy	
221. Mapping of left cerebral hemisphere, percutaneous endoscopic	
222. Intraoperative cardiac mapping during open heart surgery	
223. Hysteroscopy with cautery of post-hysterectomy oozing and evacuation of clot	
224. Open exploration and ligation of post-op arterial bleeder, left forearm	
225. Control of post-operative retroperitoneal bleeding via laparotomy	
226. Reopening of thoracotomy site with drainage and control of post-op hemopericardium	
227. Arthroscopy with drainage of hemarthrosis at previous operative site, right knee	
228. Radiocarpal fusion of left hand with internal fixation, open	
229. Posterior approach spinal fusion at L1-L3 level with BAK cage interbody fusion device, open	
230. Intercarpal fusion of right hand with bone bank bone graft, open	
231. Sacrococcygeal fusion with bone graft from same operative site, open	
232. Interphalangeal fusion of left great toe, percutaneous pin fixation	
233. Suture repair of left radial nerve laceration	
234. Laparotomy with suture repair of blunt force duodenal laceration	
235. Perineoplasty with repair of old obstetric laceration, open	
236. Suture repair of right biceps tendon (upper arm) laceration, open	
237. Closure of abdominal wall stab wound	
238. Cosmetic face lift, open, no other information available	
239. Bilateral breast augmentation with silicone implants, open	
240. Cosmetic rhinoplasty with septal reduction and tip elevation using local tissue graft, open	
241. Abdominoplasty (tummy tuck), open	
242. Liposuction of bilateral thighs	
243. Creation of penis in female patient using tissue bank donor graft	
244. Creation of vagina in male patient using synthetic material	
245. Laparoscopic vertical (sleeve) gastrectomy	
246. Left uterine artery embolization with intraluminal biosphere injection	

Obstetrics

Procedure	Code
1. Abortion by dilation and evacuation following laminaria insertion	
2. Manually assisted spontaneous abortion	
3. Abortion by abortifacient insertion	
4. Bimanual pregnancy examination	
5. Extraperitoneal C-section, low transverse incision	
6. Fetal spinal tap, percutaneous	
7. Fetal kidney transplant, laparoscopic	
8. Open in utero repair of congenital diaphragmatic hernia	
9. Laparoscopy with total excision of tubal pregnancy	
10. Transvaginal removal of fetal monitoring electrode	

Placement

Procedure	Code
1. Placement of packing material, right ear	
2. Mechanical traction of entire left leg	
3. Removal of splint, right shoulder	
4. Placement of neck brace	
5. Change of vaginal packing	
6. Packing of wound, chest wall	
7. Sterile dressing placement to left groin region	
8. Removal of packing material from pharynx	
9. Placement of intermittent pneumatic compression device, covering entire right arm	
10. Exchange of pressure dressing to left thigh	

Administration

Procedure	Code
1. Peritoneal dialysis via indwelling catheter	
2. Transvaginal artificial insemination	
3. Infusion of total parenteral nutrition via central venous catheter	
4. Esophagogastroscopy with Botox injection into esophageal sphincter	
5. Percutaneous irrigation of knee joint	
6. Systemic infusion of recombinant tissue plasminogen activator (r-tPA) via peripheral venous catheter	
7. Transabdominal in vitro fertilization, implantation of donor ovum	
8. Autologous bone marrow transplant via central venous line	
9. Implantation of anti-microbial envelope with cardiac defibrillator placement, open	
10. Sclerotherapy of brachial plexus lesion, alcohol injection	
11. Percutaneous peripheral vein injection, glucarpidase	
12. Introduction of anti-infective envelope into subcutaneous tissue, open	

Measurement and Monitoring

Procedure	Code
1. Cardiac stress test, single measurement	
2. EGD with biliary flow measurement	
3. Right and left heart cardiac catheterization with bilateral sampling and pressure measurements	
4. Temperature monitoring, rectal	
5. Peripheral venous pulse, external, single measurement	
6. Holter monitoring	
7. Respiratory rate, external, single measurement	
8. Fetal heart rate monitoring, transvaginal	
9. Visual mobility test, single measurement	
10. Left ventricular cardiac output monitoring from pulmonary artery wedge (Swan-Ganz) catheter	
11. Olfactory acuity test, single measurement	

Extracorporeal or Systemic Assistance and Performance

Procedure	Code
1. Intermittent mechanical ventilation, 16 hours	
2. Liver dialysis, single encounter	
3. Cardiac countershock with successful conversion to sinus rhythm	
4. IPPB (intermittent positive pressure breathing) for mobilization of secretions, 22 hours	
5. Renal dialysis, 12 hours	
6. IABP (intra-aortic balloon pump) continuous	
7. Intra-operative cardiac pacing, continuous	
8. Intraoperative ECMO (extracorporeal membrane oxygenation), central	
9. Controlled mechanical ventilation (CMV), 45 hours	
10. Pulsatile compression boot with intermittent inflation	

Extracorporeal or Systemic Therapies

Procedure	Code
1. Donor thrombocytapheresis, single encounter	
2. Bili-lite phototherapy, series treatment	
3. Whole body hypothermia, single treatment	
4. Circulatory phototherapy, single encounter	
5. Shock wave therapy of plantar fascia, single treatment	
6. Antigen-free air conditioning, series treatment	
7. TMS (transcranial magnetic stimulation), series treatment	
8. Therapeutic ultrasound of peripheral vessels, single treatment	
9. Plasmapheresis, series treatment	
10. Extracorporeal electromagnetic stimulation (EMS) for urinary incontinence, single treatment	

Osteopathic

Procedure	Code
1. Isotonic muscle energy treatment of right leg	
2. Low velocity-high amplitude osteopathic treatment of head	
3. Lymphatic pump osteopathic treatment of left axilla	
4. Indirect osteopathic treatment of sacrum	
5. Articulatory osteopathic treatment of cervical region	

Other Procedures

Procedure	Code
1. Near infrared spectroscopy of leg vessels	
2. CT computer assisted sinus surgery	
3. Suture removal, abdominal wall	
4. Isolation after infectious disease exposure	
5. Robotic assisted open prostatectomy	
6. In vitro fertilization	

Chiropractic

Procedure	Code
1. Chiropractic treatment of lumbar region using long lever specific contact	
2. Chiropractic manipulation of abdominal region, indirect visceral	
3. Chiropractic extra-articular treatment of hip region	
4. Chiropractic treatment of sacrum using long and short lever specific contact	
5. Mechanically-assisted chiropractic manipulation of head	

Imaging

Procedure	Code
1. Noncontrast CT of abdomen and pelvis	
2. Intravascular ultrasound, left subclavian artery	
3. Fluoroscopic guidance for insertion of central venous catheter in SVC, low osmolar contrast	
4. Chest x-ray, AP/PA and lateral views	
5. Endoluminal ultrasound of gallbladder and bile ducts	
6. MRI of thyroid gland, contrast unspecified	
7. Esophageal videofluoroscopy study with oral barium contrast	
8. Portable x-ray study of right radius/ulna shaft, standard series	
9. Routine fetal ultrasound, second trimester twin gestation	
10. CT scan of bilateral lungs, high osmolar contrast with densitometry	
11. Fluoroscopic guidance for percutaneous transluminal angioplasty (PTA) of left common femoral artery, low osmolar contrast	

Nuclear Medicine

Procedure	Code
1. Tomo scan of right and left heart, unspecified radiopharmaceutical, qualitative gated rest	
2. Technetium pentetate assay of kidneys, ureters, and bladder	
3. Uniplanar scan of spine using technetium oxidronate, with first-pass study	
4. Thallous chloride tomographic scan of bilateral breasts	
5. PET scan of myocardium using rubidium	
6. Gallium citrate scan of head and neck, single plane imaging	
7. Xenon gas nonimaging probe of brain	
8. Upper GI scan, radiopharmaceutical unspecified, for gastric emptying	
9. Carbon 11 PET scan of brain with quantification	
10. Iodinated albumin nuclear medicine assay, blood plasma volume study	

Radiation Therapy

Procedure	Code
1. Plaque radiation of left eye, single port	
2. 8 MeV photon beam radiation to brain	
3. IORT of colon, 3 ports	
4. HDR brachytherapy of prostate using low dose palladium-103, unidirectional source	
5. Electron radiation treatment of right breast, with custom device	
6. Hyperthermia oncology treatment of pelvic region	
7. Contact radiation of tongue	
8. Heavy particle radiation treatment of pancreas, four risk sites	
9. LDR brachytherapy to spinal cord using iodine	
10. Whole body Phosphorus 32 administration with risk to hematopoetic system	

Physical Rehabilitation and Diagnostic Audiology

Procedure	Code
1. Bekesy assessment using audiometer	
2. Individual fitting of left eye prosthesis	
3. Physical therapy for range of motion and mobility, patient right hip, no special equipment	
4. Bedside swallow assessment using assessment kit	
5. Caregiver training in airway clearance techniques	
6. Application of short arm cast in rehabilitation setting	
7. Verbal assessment of patient's pain level	
8. Caregiver training in communication skills using manual communication board	
9. Group musculoskeletal balance training exercises, whole body, no special equipment	
10. Individual therapy for auditory processing using tape recorder	

Mental Health

Procedure	Code
1. Cognitive-behavioral psychotherapy, individual	
2. Narcosynthesis	
3. Light therapy	
4. ECT (electroconvulsive therapy), unilateral, multiple seizure	
5. Crisis intervention	
6. Neuropsychological testing	
7. Hypnosis	
8. Developmental testing	
9. Vocational counseling	
10. Family psychotherapy	

Substance Abuse Treatment

Procedure	Code
1. Naltrexone treatment for drug dependency	
2. Substance abuse treatment family counseling	
3. Medication monitoring of patient on methadone maintenance	
4. Individual interpersonal psychotherapy for drug abuse	
5. Patient in for alcohol detoxification treatment	
6. Group motivational counseling	
7. Individual 12-step psychotherapy for substance abuse	
8. Post-test infectious disease counseling for IV drug abuser	
9. Psychodynamic psychotherapy for drug dependent patient	
10. Group cognitive-behavioral counseling for substance abuse	

New Technology

Procedure	Code
1. Infusion of ceftazidime via peripheral venous catheter	
2. Transcatheter dilation of left peroneal artery with 2 SAVAL stents	

Answers to Coding Exercises

Medical Surgical Section

Procedure	Code
1. Excision of malignant melanoma from skin of right ear	ØHB2XZZ
2. Laparoscopy with excision of endometrial implant from left ovary	ØUB14ZZ
3. Percutaneous needle core biopsy of right kidney	ØTBØ3ZX
4. EGD with gastric biopsy	ØDB68ZX
5. Open endarterectomy of left common carotid artery	Ø3CJØZZ
6. Excision of basal cell carcinoma of lower lip	ØCB1XZZ
7. Open excision of tail of pancreas	ØFBGØZZ
8. Percutaneous biopsy of right gastrocnemius muscle	ØKBS3ZX
9. Sigmoidoscopy with sigmoid polypectomy	ØDBN8ZZ
10. Open excision of lesion from right Achilles tendon	ØLBNØZZ
11. Open resection of cecum	ØDTHØZZ
12. Total excision of pituitary gland, open	ØGTØØZZ
13. Explantation of left failed kidney, open	ØTT1ØZZ
14. Open left axillary total lymphadenectomy	Ø7T6ØZZ (RESECTION is coded for cutting out a chain of lymph nodes.)
15. Laparoscopic-assisted vaginal hysterectomy	ØUT9FZZ
16. Right total mastectomy, open	ØHTTØZZ
17. Open resection of papillary muscle	Ø2TDØZZ (The papillary muscle refers to the heart and is found in the *Heart and Great Vessels* body system.)
18. Total retropubic prostatectomy, open	ØVTØØZZ
19. Laparoscopic cholecystectomy	ØFT44ZZ
20. Endoscopic bilateral total maxillary sinusectomy	Ø9TQ8ZZ, Ø9TR8ZZ
21. Amputation at right elbow level	ØX6BØZZ
22. Right below-knee amputation, proximal tibia/fibula	ØY6HØZ1 (The qualifier *High* here means the portion of the tib/fib closest to the knee.)
23. Fifth ray carpometacarpal joint amputation, left hand	ØX6KØZ8 (A *complete* ray amputation is through the carpometacarpal joint.)
24. Right leg and hip amputation through ischium	ØY62ØZZ (The *Hindquarter* body part includes amputation along any part of the hip bone.)
25. DIP joint amputation of right thumb	ØX6LØZ3 (The qualifier *low* here means through the distal interphalangeal joint.)
26. Right wrist joint amputation	ØX6JØZØ (Amputation at the wrist joint is actually complete amputation of the hand.)
27. Trans-metatarsal amputation of foot at left big toe	ØY6NØZ9 (A *partial* amputation is through the shaft of the metatarsal bone.)
28. Mid-shaft amputation, right humerus	ØX68ØZ2

Procedure	Code
29. Left fourth toe amputation, mid-proximal phalanx	ØY6WØZ1 (The qualifier *High* here means anywhere along the proximal phalanx.)
30. Right above-knee amputation, distal femur	ØY6CØZ3
31. Cryotherapy of wart on left hand	ØH5GXZZ
32. Percutaneous radiofrequency ablation of right vocal cord lesion	ØC5T3ZZ
33. Left heart catheterization with laser destruction of arrhythmogenic focus, A-V node	Ø2583ZZ
34. Cautery of nosebleed	Ø95KXZZ
35. Transurethral endoscopic laser ablation of prostate	ØV5Ø8ZZ
36. Percutaneous cautery of oozing varicose vein, left calf	Ø65Y3ZZ
37. Laparoscopy with destruction of endometriosis, bilateral ovaries	ØU524ZZ
38. Laser coagulation of right retinal vessel hemorrhage, percutaneous	Ø85G3ZZ (The *Retinal Vessel* body-part values are in the *Eye* body system.)
39. Thoracoscopic pleurodesis, left side	ØB5P4ZZ
40. Percutaneous insertion of Greenfield IVC filter	Ø6HØ3DZ
41. Forceps total mouth extraction, upper and lower teeth	ØCDWXZ2, ØCDXXZ2
42. Removal of left thumbnail	ØHDQXZZ (No separate body-part value is given for thumbnail, so this is coded to *Fingernail*.)
43. Extraction of right intraocular lens without replacement, percutaneous	Ø8DJ3ZZ
44. Laparoscopy with needle aspiration of ova for in vitro fertilization	ØUDN4ZZ
45. Nonexcisional debridement of skin ulcer, right foot	ØHDMXZZ
46. Open stripping of abdominal fascia, right side	ØJD8ØZZ
47. Hysteroscopy with D&C, diagnostic	ØUDB8ZX
48. Liposuction for medical purposes, left upper arm	ØJDF3ZZ (The *Percutaneous* approach is inherent in the liposuction technique.)
49. Removal of tattered right ear drum fragments with tweezers	Ø9D77ZZ
50. Microincisional phlebectomy of spider veins, right lower leg	Ø6DY3ZZ
51. Routine Foley catheter placement	ØT9B7ØZ
52. Incision and drainage of external anal abscess	ØD9QXZZ
53. Percutaneous drainage of ascites	ØW9G3ZZ (This is drainage of the cavity and not the peritoneal membrane itself.)
54. Laparoscopy with left ovarian cystotomy and drainage	ØU914ZZ
55. Laparotomy and drain placement for liver abscess, right lobe	ØF91ØØZ
56. Right knee arthrotomy with drain placement	ØS9CØØZ
57. Thoracentesis of left pleural effusion	ØW9B3ZZ (This is drainage of the pleural cavity)
58. Phlebotomy of left median cubital vein for polycythemia vera	Ø59C3ZZ (The median cubital vein is a branch of the basilic vein)

Procedure	Code
59. Percutaneous chest tube placement for right pneumothorax	ØW993ØZ
60. Endoscopic drainage of left ethmoid sinus	Ø99V4ZZ
61. External ventricular CSF drainage catheter placement via burr hole	ØØ963ØZ
62. Removal of foreign body, right cornea	Ø8C8XZZ
63. Percutaneous mechanical thrombectomy, left brachial artery	Ø3C83ZZ
64. Esophagogastroscopy with removal of bezoar from stomach	ØDC68ZZ
65. Foreign body removal, skin of left thumb	ØHCGXZZ (There is no specific value for thumb skin, so the procedure is coded to *Hand*.)
66. Transurethral cystoscopy with removal of bladder stone	ØTCB8ZZ
67. Forceps removal of foreign body in right nostril	Ø9CKXZZ (Nostril is coded to the *Nasal muscosa and soft tissue* body-part value.)
68. Laparoscopy with excision of old suture from mesentery	ØDCV4ZZ
69. Incision and removal of right lacrimal duct stone	Ø8CXØZZ
70. Nonincisional removal of intraluminal foreign body from vagina	ØUCG7ZZ (The approach *External* is also a possibility. It is assumed here that since the patient went to the doctor to have the object removed, that it was not in the vaginal orifice.)
71. Right common carotid endarterectomy, open	Ø3CHØZZ
72. Open excision of retained sliver, subcutaneous tissue of left foot	ØJCRØZZ
73. Extracorporeal shockwave lithotripsy (ESWL), bilateral ureters	ØTF6XZZ, ØTF7XZZ (The *Bilateral Ureter* body-part value is not available for the root operation FRAGMENTATION, so the procedures are coded separately.)
74. Endoscopic retrograde cholangiopancreatography (ERCP) with lithotripsy of common bile duct stone	ØFF98ZZ (ERCP is performed through the mouth to the biliary system via the duodenum, so the approach value is *Via Natural or Artificial Opening Endoscopic*.)
75. Thoracotomy with crushing of pericardial calcifications	Ø2FNØZZ
76. Transurethral cystoscopy with fragmentation of bladder calculus	ØTFB8ZZ
77. Hysteroscopy with intraluminal lithotripsy of left fallopian tube calcification	ØUF68ZZ
78. Division of right foot tendon, percutaneous	ØL8V3ZZ
79. Left heart catheterization with division of bundle of HIS	Ø2883ZZ
80. Open osteotomy of capitate, left hand	ØP8NØZZ (The capitate is one of the carpal bones of the hand.)
81. EGD with esophagotomy of esophagogastric junction	ØD948ZZ
82. Sacral rhizotomy for pain control, percutaneous	Ø18R3ZZ
83. Laparotomy with exploration and adhesiolysis of right ureter	ØTN6ØZZ

Procedure	Code
84. Incision of scar contracture, right elbow	ØHNDXZZ (The skin of the elbow region is coded to *Lower Arm*.)
85. Frenulotomy for treatment of tongue-tie syndrome	ØCN7XZZ (The frenulum is coded to the body-part value *Tongue*.)
86. Right shoulder arthroscopy with coracoacromial ligament release	ØMN14ZZ
87. Mitral valvulotomy for release of fused leaflets, open approach	Ø2NGØZZ
88. Percutaneous left Achilles tendon release	ØLNP3ZZ
89. Laparoscopy with lysis of peritoneal adhesions	ØDNW4ZZ
90. Manual rupture of right shoulder joint adhesions under general anesthesia	ØRNJXZZ
91. Open posterior tarsal tunnel release	Ø1NGØZZ (The nerve released in the posterior tarsal tunnel is the tibial nerve.)
92. Laparoscopy with freeing of left ovary and fallopian tube	ØUN14ZZ, ØUN64ZZ
93. Liver transplant with donor matched liver	ØFYØØZØ
94. Orthotopic heart transplant using porcine heart	Ø2YAØZ2 (The donor heart comes from an animal [pig], so the qualifier value is *Zooplastic*.)
95. Right lung transplant, open, using organ donor match	ØBYKØZØ
96. Transplant of large intestine, organ donor match	ØDYEØZØ
97. Left kidney/pancreas organ bank transplant	ØFYGØZØ, ØTY1ØZØ
98. Replantation of avulsed scalp	ØHMØXZZ
99. Reattachment of severed right ear	Ø9MØXZZ
100. Reattachment of traumatic left gastrocnemius avulsion, open	ØKMTØZZ
101. Closed replantation of three avulsed teeth, lower jaw	ØCMXXZ1
102. Reattachment of severed left hand	ØXMKØZZ
103. Right open palmaris longus tendon transfer	ØLX5ØZZ
104. Endoscopic radial to median nerve transfer	Ø1X64Z5
105. Fasciocutaneous flap closure of left thigh, open	ØJXMØZC (The qualifier identifies the body layers in addition to fascia included in the procedure.)
106. Transfer left index finger to left thumb position, open	ØXXPØZM
107. Percutaneous fascia transfer to fill defect, right neck	ØJX43ZZ
108. Trigeminal to facial nerve transfer, percutaneous endoscopic	ØØXK4ZM
109. Endoscopic left leg flexor hallucis longus tendon transfer	ØLXP4ZZ
110. Right scalp advancement flap to right temple	ØHXØXZZ
111. Bilateral TRAM pedicle flap reconstruction status post mastectomy, muscle only, open	ØKXKØZ6, ØKXLØZ6 (The transverse rectus abdominus muscle (TRAM) flap is coded for each flap developed.)
112. Skin transfer flap closure of complex open wound, left lower back	ØHX6XZZ
113. Open fracture reduction, right tibia	ØQSGØZZ
114. Laparoscopy with gastropexy for malrotation	ØDS64ZZ
115. Left knee arthroscopy with reposition of anterior cruciate ligament	ØMSP4ZZ

Procedure	Code
116. Open transposition of ulnar nerve	Ø1S4ØZZ
117. Closed reduction with percutaneous internal fixation of right femoral neck fracture	ØQS634Z
118. Trans-vaginal intraluminal cervical cerclage	ØUVC7DZ
119. Cervical cerclage using Shirodkar technique	ØUVC7ZZ
120. Thoracotomy with banding of left pulmonary artery using extraluminal device	Ø2VRØCZ
121. Restriction of thoracic duct with intraluminal stent, percutaneous	Ø7VK3DZ
122. Craniotomy with clipping of cerebral aneurysm	Ø3VGØCZ (The clip is placed lengthwise on the outside wall of the widened portion of the vessel.)
123. Nonincisional, transnasal placement of restrictive stent in right lacrimal duct	Ø8VX7DZ
124. Catheter-based temporary restriction of blood flow in abdominal aorta for treatment of cerebral ischemia	Ø4VØ3DJ
125. Percutaneous ligation of esophageal vein	Ø6L33ZZ
126. Percutaneous embolization of left internal carotid-cavernous fistula	Ø3LL3DZ
127. Laparoscopy with bilateral occlusion of fallopian tubes using Hulka extraluminal clips	ØUL74CZ
128. Open suture ligation of failed AV graft, left brachial artery	Ø3L8ØZZ
129. Percutaneous embolization of vascular supply, intracranial meningioma	Ø3LG3DZ
130. Percutaneous embolization of right uterine artery, using coils	Ø4LE3DT
131. Open occlusion of left atrial appendage, using extraluminal pressure clips	Ø2L7ØCK
132. Percutaneous suture exclusion of left atrial appendage, via femoral artery access	Ø2L73ZK
133. ERCP with balloon dilation of common bile duct	ØF798ZZ
134. PTCA of two coronary arteries, LAD with stent placement, RCA with no stent	Ø27Ø3DZ, Ø27Ø3ZZ (A separate procedure is coded for each artery dilated, since the device value differs for each artery.)
135. Cystoscopy with intraluminal dilation of bladder neck stricture	ØT7C8ZZ
136. Open dilation of old anastomosis, left femoral artery	Ø47LØZZ
137. Dilation of upper esophageal stricture, direct visualization, with Bougie sound	ØD717ZZ
138. PTA of right brachial artery stenosis	Ø3773ZZ
139. Transnasal dilation and stent placement in right lacrimal duct	Ø87X7DZ
140. Hysteroscopy with balloon dilation of bilateral fallopian tubes	ØU778ZZ
141. Tracheoscopy with intraluminal dilation of tracheal stenosis	ØB718ZZ
142. Cystoscopy with dilation of left ureteral stricture, with stent placement	ØT778DZ
143. Open gastric bypass with Roux-en-Y limb to jejunum	ØD16ØZA
144. Right temporal artery to intracranial artery bypass using Gore-Tex graft, open	Ø31SØJG
145. Tracheostomy formation with tracheostomy tube placement, percutaneous	ØB113F4
146. PICVA (percutaneous in situ coronary venous arterialization) of single coronary artery	Ø21Ø3D4
147. Open left femoral-popliteal artery bypass using cadaver vein graft	Ø41LØKL
148. Shunting of intrathecal cerebrospinal fluid to peritoneal cavity using synthetic shunt	ØØ16ØJ6
149. Colostomy formation, open, transverse colon to abdominal wall	ØD1LØZ4
150. Open urinary diversion, left ureter, using ileal conduit to skin	ØT17ØZC
151. CABG of LAD using pedicled left internal mammary artery, open off-bypass	Ø21ØØZ9
152. Open pleuroperitoneal shunt, right pleural cavity, using synthetic device	ØW19ØJG
153. Percutaneous placement of ventriculoperitoneal shunt for treatment of hydrocephalus	ØØ163J6
154. End-of-life replacement of spinal neurostimulator generator, multiple array, in lower abdomen	ØJH8ØDZ (Taking out of the old generator is coded separately to the root operation *Removal*)
155. Percutaneous insertion of spinal neurostimulator lead, lumbar spinal cord	ØØHV3MZ
156. Percutaneous replacement of broken pacemaker lead in left atrium	Ø2H73JZ (Taking out the broken pacemaker lead is coded separately to the root operation *Removal*.)
157. Open placement of dual chamber pacemaker generator in chest wall	ØJH6Ø6Z
158. Percutaneous placement of venous central line in right internal jugular, with tip in superior vena cava	Ø2HV33Z
159. Open insertion of multiple channel cochlear implant, left ear	Ø9HEØ6Z
160. Percutaneous placement of Swan-Ganz catheter in pulmonary trunk	Ø2HP32Z (The Swan-Ganz catheter is coded to the device value *Monitoring Device* because it monitors pulmonary artery output.)
161. Bronchoscopy with insertion of Low Dose Pd-103 brachytherapy seeds, right lung	ØBHK81Z, DB11BBZ
162. Open insertion of interspinous process device into lumbar vertebral joint	ØSHØØBZ
163. Open placement of bone growth stimulator, left femoral shaft	ØQHYØMZ
164. Cystoscopy with placement of brachytherapy seeds in prostate gland	ØVHØ81Z
165. Percutaneous insertion of Greenfield IVC filter	Ø6HØ3DZ
166. Full-thickness skin graft to right lower arm, autograft (do not code graft harvest for this exercise)	ØHRDX73
167. Excision of necrosed left femoral head with bone bank bone graft to fill the defect, open	ØQR7ØKZ
168. Penetrating keratoplasty of right cornea with donor matched cornea, percutaneous approach	Ø8R83KZ
169. Excision of abdominal aorta with Gore-Tex graft replacement, open	Ø4RØØJZ
170. Total right knee arthroplasty with insertion of total knee prosthesis	ØSRCØJZ
171. Tenonectomy with graft to right ankle using cadaver graft, open	ØLRSØKZ
172. Mitral valve replacement using porcine valve, open	Ø2RGØ8Z
173. Percutaneous phacoemulsification of right eye cataract with prosthetic lens insertion	Ø8RJ3JZ
174. Transcatheter replacement of pulmonary valve using of bovine jugular vein valve	Ø2RH38Z

Procedure	Code
175. Total left hip replacement using ceramic on ceramic prosthesis, without bone cement	ØSRBØ3A
176. Aortic valve annuloplasty using ring, open	Ø2UFØJZ
177. Laparoscopic repair of left inguinal hernia with marlex plug	ØYU64JZ
178. Autograft nerve graft to right median nerve, percutaneous endoscopic (do not code graft harvest for this exercise)	Ø1U547Z
179. Exchange of liner in femoral component of previous left hip replacement, open approach	ØSUSØ9Z (Taking out of the old liner is coded separately to the root operation *Removal*)
180. Anterior colporrhaphy with polypropylene mesh reinforcement, open approach	ØJUCØJZ
181. Implantation of CorCap cardiac support device, open approach	Ø2UAØJZ
182. Abdominal wall herniorrhaphy, open, using synthetic mesh	ØWUFØJZ
183. Tendon graft to strengthen injured left shoulder using autograft, open (do not code graft harvest for this exercise)	ØLU2Ø7Z
184. Onlay lamellar keratoplasty of left cornea using autograft, external approach	Ø8U9X7Z
185. Resurfacing procedure on right femoral head, open approach	ØSURØBZ
186. Exchange of drainage tube from right hip joint	ØS2YXØZ
187. Tracheostomy tube exchange	ØB21XFZ
188. Change chest tube for left pneumothorax	ØW2BXØZ
189. Exchange of cerebral ventriculostomy drainage tube	ØØ2ØXØZ
190. Foley urinary catheter exchange	ØT2BXØZ (This is coded to *Drainage Device* because urine is being drained.)
191. Open removal of lumbar sympathetic neurostimulator lead	Ø1PYØMZ
192. Nonincisional removal of Swan-Ganz catheter from right pulmonary artery	Ø2PYX2Z
193. Laparotomy with removal of pancreatic drain	ØFPGØØZ
194. Extubation, endotracheal tube	ØBP1XDZ
195. Nonincisional PEG tube removal	ØDP6XUZ
196. Transvaginal removal of brachytherapy seeds	ØUPH71Z
197. Transvaginal removal of extraluminal cervical cerclage	ØUPD7CZ
198. Incision with removal of K-wire fixation, right first metatarsal	ØQPNØ4Z
199. Cystoscopy with retrieval of left ureteral stent	ØTP98DZ
200. Removal of nasogastric drainage tube for decompression	ØDP6XØZ
201. Removal of external fixator, left radial fracture	ØPPJX5Z
202. Trimming and reanastomosis of stenosed femorofemoral synthetic bypass graft, open	Ø4WYØJZ
203. Open revision of right hip replacement, with readjustment of prosthesis	ØSW9ØJZ
204. Adjustment of position, pacemaker lead in left ventricle, percutaneous	Ø2WA3MZ
205. External repositioning of Foley catheter to bladder	ØTWBXØZ
206. Taking out loose screw and putting larger screw in fracture repair plate, left tibia	ØQWHØ4Z
207. Revision of totally implantable VAD port placement in chest wall, causing patient discomfort, open	ØJWTØWZ
208. Thoracotomy with exploration of right pleural cavity	ØWJ9ØZZ

Procedure	Code
209. Diagnostic laryngoscopy	ØCJS8ZZ
210. Exploratory arthrotomy of left knee	ØSJDØZZ
211. Colposcopy with diagnostic hysteroscopy	ØUJD8ZZ
212. Digital rectal exam	ØDJD7ZZ
213. Diagnostic arthroscopy of right shoulder	ØRJJ4ZZ
214. Endoscopy of maxillary sinus	Ø9JY4ZZ
215. Laparotomy with palpation of liver	ØFJØØZZ
216. Transurethral diagnostic cystoscopy	ØTJB8ZZ
217. Colonoscopy, discontinued at sigmoid colon	ØDJD8ZZ
218. Percutaneous mapping of basal ganglia	ØØK83ZZ
219. Heart catheterization with cardiac mapping	Ø2K83ZZ
220. Intraoperative whole brain mapping via craniotomy	ØØKØØZZ
221. Mapping of left cerebral hemisphere, percutaneous endoscopic	ØØK74ZZ
222. Intraoperative cardiac mapping during open heart surgery	Ø2K8ØZZ
223. Hysteroscopy with cautery of post-hysterectomy oozing and evacuation of clot	ØW3R8ZZ
224. Open exploration and ligation of post-op arterial bleeder, left forearm	ØX3FØZZ
225. Control of post-operative retroperitoneal bleeding via laparotomy	ØW3HØZZ
226. Reopening of thoracotomy site with drainage and control of post-op hemopericardium	ØW3DØZZ
227. Arthroscopy with drainage of hemarthrosis at previous operative site, right knee	ØY3F4ZZ
228. Radiocarpal fusion of left hand with internal fixation, open	ØRGPØ4Z
229. Posterior approach spinal fusion at L1-L3 level with BAK cage interbody fusion device, open	ØSG1ØAJ
230. Intercarpal fusion of right hand with bone bank bone graft, open	ØRGQØKZ
231. Sacrococcygeal fusion with bone graft from same operative site, open	ØSG5Ø7Z
232. Interphalangeal fusion of left great toe, percutaneous pin fixation	ØSGQ34Z
233. Suture repair of left radial nerve laceration	Ø1Q6ØZZ (The approach value is *Open*, though the surgical exposure may have been created by the wound itself.)
234. Laparotomy with suture repair of blunt force duodenal laceration	ØDQ9ØZZ
235. Perineoplasty with repair of old obstetric laceration, open	ØWQNØZZ
236. Suture repair of right biceps tendon (upper arm) laceration, open	ØLQ3ØZZ
237. Closure of abdominal wall stab wound	ØWQFØZZ
238. Cosmetic face lift, open, no other information available	ØWØ2ØZZ
239. Bilateral breast augmentation with silicone implants, open	ØHØVØJZ
240. Cosmetic rhinoplasty with septal reduction and tip elevation using local tissue graft, open	Ø9ØKØ7Z
241. Abdominoplasty (tummy tuck), open	ØWØFØZZ
242. Liposuction of bilateral thighs	ØJØL3ZZ, ØJØM3ZZ
243. Creation of penis in female patient using tissue bank donor graft	ØW4NØK1
244. Creation of vagina in male patient using synthetic material	ØW4MØJØ

Procedure	Code
245. Laparoscopic vertical (sleeve) gastrectomy	ØDB64Z3
246. Left uterine artery embolization with intraluminal biosphere injection	Ø4LF3DU

Obstetrics

Procedure	Code
1. Abortion by dilation and evacuation following laminaria insertion	1ØAØ7ZW
2. Manually assisted spontaneous abortion	1ØEØXZZ (Since the pregnancy was not artificially terminated, this is coded to *Delivery* because it captures the procedure objective. The fact that it was an abortion will be identified in the diagnosis code.)
3. Abortion by abortifacient insertion	1ØAØ7ZX
4. Bimanual pregnancy examination	1ØJØ7ZZ
5. Extraperitoneal C-section, low transverse incision	1ØDØØZ1
6. Fetal spinal tap, percutaneous	1Ø9Ø3ZA
7. Fetal kidney transplant, laparoscopic	1ØYØ4ZS
8. Open in utero repair of congenital diaphragmatic hernia	1ØQØØZK (Diaphragm is classified to the *Respiratory* body system in the *Medical and Surgical* section.)
9. Laparoscopy with total excision of tubal pregnancy	1ØT24ZZ
10. Transvaginal removal of fetal monitoring electrode	1ØPØ73Z

Placement

Procedure	Code
1. Placement of packing material, right ear	2Y42X5Z
2. Mechanical traction of entire left leg	2W6MXØZ
3. Removal of splint, right shoulder	2W5AX1Z
4. Placement of neck brace	2W32X3Z
5. Change of vaginal packing	2YØ4X5Z
6. Packing of wound, chest wall	2W44X5Z
7. Sterile dressing placement to left groin region	2W27X4Z
8. Removal of packing material from pharynx	2Y5ØX5Z
9. Placement of intermittent pneumatic compression device, covering entire right arm	2W18X7Z
10. Exchange of pressure dressing to left thigh	2WØPX6Z

Administration

Procedure	Code
1. Peritoneal dialysis via indwelling catheter	3E1M39Z
2. Transvaginal artificial insemination	3EØP7LZ
3. Infusion of total parenteral nutrition via central venous catheter	3EØ436Z
4. Esophagogastroscopy with Botox injection into esophageal sphincter	3EØG8GC (Botulinum toxin is a paralyzing agent with temporary effects; it does not sclerose or destroy the nerve.)
5. Percutaneous irrigation of knee joint	3E1U38Z
6. Systemic infusion of recombinant tissue plasminogen activator (r-tPA) via peripheral venous catheter	3EØ3317
7. Transabdominal in vitro fertilization, implantation of donor ovum	3EØP3Q1
8. Autologous bone marrow transplant via central venous line	3Ø243GØ
9. Implantation of anti-microbial envelope with cardiac defibrillator placement, open	3EØ1Ø2A
10. Sclerotherapy of brachial plexus lesion, alcohol injection	3EØT3TZ
11. Percutaneous peripheral vein injection, glucarpidase	3EØ33GQ
12. Introduction of anti-infective envelope into subcutaneous tissue, open	3EØ1Ø2A

Measurement and Monitoring

Procedure	Code
1. Cardiac stress test, single measurement	4AØ2XM4
2. EGD with biliary flow measurement	4AØC85Z
3. Right and left heart cardiac catheterization with bilateral sampling and pressure measurements	4AØ23N8
4. Temperature monitoring, rectal	4A1Z7KZ
5. Peripheral venous pulse, external, single measurement	4AØ4XJ1
6. Holter monitoring	4A12X45
7. Respiratory rate, external, single measurement	4AØ9XCZ
8. Fetal heart rate monitoring, transvaginal	4A1H7CZ
9. Visual mobility test, single measurement	4AØ7X7Z
10. Left ventricular cardiac output monitoring from pulmonary artery wedge (Swan-Ganz) catheter	4A1239Z
11. Olfactory acuity test, single measurement	4AØ8XØZ

Extracorporeal or Systemic Assistance and Performance

Procedure	Code
1. Intermittent mechanical ventilation, 16 hours	5A1935Z
2. Liver dialysis, single encounter	5A1C00Z
3. Cardiac countershock with successful conversion to sinus rhythm	5A2204Z
4. IPPB (intermittent positive pressure breathing) for mobilization of secretions, 22 hours	5A09358
5. Renal dialysis, 12 hours	5A1D80Z
6. IABP (intra-aortic balloon pump) continuous	5A02210
7. Intra-operative cardiac pacing, continuous	5A1223Z
8. Intraoperative ECMO (extracorporeal membrane oxygenation), central	5A15A2F
9. Controlled mechanical ventilation (CMV), 45 hours	5A1945Z
10. Pulsatile compression boot with intermittent inflation	5A02115 (This is coded to the function value *Cardiac Output*, because the purpose of such compression devices is to return blood to the heart faster.)

Extracorporeal or Systemic Therapies

Procedure	Code
1. Donor thrombocytapheresis, single encounter	6A550Z2
2. Bili-lite phototherapy, series treatment	6A601ZZ
3. Whole body hypothermia, single treatment	6A4Z0ZZ
4. Circulatory phototherapy, single encounter	6A650ZZ
5. Shock wave therapy of plantar fascia, single treatment	6A930ZZ
6. Antigen-free air conditioning, series treatment	6A0Z1ZZ
7. TMS (transcranial magnetic stimulation), series treatment	6A221ZZ
8. Therapeutic ultrasound of peripheral vessels, single treatment	6A750Z6
9. Plasmapheresis, series treatment	6A551Z3
10. Extracorporeal electromagnetic stimulation (EMS) for urinary incontinence, single treatment	6A210ZZ

Osteopathic

Procedure	Code
1. Isotonic muscle energy treatment of right leg	7W06X8Z
2. Low velocity-high amplitude osteopathic treatment of head	7W00X5Z
3. Lymphatic pump osteopathic treatment of left axilla	7W07X6Z
4. Indirect osteopathic treatment of sacrum	7W04X4Z
5. Articulatory osteopathic treatment of cervical region	7W01X0Z

Other Procedures

Procedure	Code
1. Near infrared spectroscopy of leg vessels	8E023DZ
2. CT computer assisted sinus surgery	8E09XBG (The primary procedure is coded separately.)
3. Suture removal, abdominal wall	8E0WXY8
4. Isolation after infectious disease exposure	8E0ZXY6
5. Robotic assisted open prostatectomy	8E0W0CZ (The primary procedure is coded separately.)
6. In vitro fertilization	8E0ZXY1

Chiropractic

Procedure	Code
1. Chiropractic treatment of lumbar region using long lever specific contact	9WB3XGZ
2. Chiropractic manipulation of abdominal region, indirect visceral	9WB9XCZ
3. Chiropractic extra-articular treatment of hip region	9WB6XDZ
4. Chiropractic treatment of sacrum using long and short lever specific contact	9WB4XJZ
5. Mechanically-assisted chiropractic manipulation of head	9WB0XKZ

Imaging

Procedure	Code
1. Noncontrast CT of abdomen and pelvis	BW21ZZZ
2. Intravascular ultrasound, left subclavian artery	B342ZZ3
3. Fluoroscopic guidance for insertion of central venous catheter in SVC, low osmolar contrast	B5181ZA
4. Chest x-ray, AP/PA and lateral views	BW03ZZZ
5. Endoluminal ultrasound of gallbladder and bile ducts	BF43ZZZ
6. MRI of thyroid gland, contrast unspecified	BG34YZZ
7. Esophageal videofluoroscopy study with oral barium contrast	BD11YZZ
8. Portable x-ray study of right radius/ulna shaft, standard series	BP0JZZZ
9. Routine fetal ultrasound, second trimester twin gestation	BY4DZZZ
10. CT scan of bilateral lungs, high osmolar contrast with densitometry	BB240ZZ
11. Fluoroscopic guidance for percutaneous transluminal angioplasty (PTA) of left common femoral artery, low osmolar contrast	B41G1ZZ

Nuclear Medicine

Procedure	Code
1. Tomo scan of right and left heart, unspecified radiopharmaceutical, qualitative gated rest	C226YZZ
2. Technetium pentetate assay of kidneys, ureters, and bladder	CT631ZZ
3. Uniplanar scan of spine using technetium oxidronate, with first-pass study	CP151ZZ
4. Thallous chloride tomographic scan of bilateral breasts	CH22SZZ
5. PET scan of myocardium using rubidium	C23GQZZ
6. Gallium citrate scan of head and neck, single plane imaging	CW1BLZZ
7. Xenon gas nonimaging probe of brain	CØ5ØVZZ
8. Upper GI scan, radiopharmaceutical unspecified, for gastric emptying	CD15YZZ
9. Carbon 11 PET scan of brain with quantification	CØ3ØBZZ
10. Iodinated albumin nuclear medicine assay, blood plasma volume study	C763HZZ

Radiation Therapy

Procedure	Code
1. Plaque radiation of left eye, single port	D8YØFZZ
2. 8 MeV photon beam radiation to brain	DØØ11ZZ
3. IORT of colon, 3 ports	DDY5CZZ
4. HDR brachytherapy of prostate using low dose palladium-103, unidirectional source	DV1ØBB1
5. Electron radiation treatment of right breast, with custom device	DMØ13ZZ
6. Hyperthermia oncology treatment of pelvic region	DWY68ZZ
7. Contact radiation of tongue	D9Y57ZZ
8. Heavy particle radiation treatment of pancreas, four risk sites	DFØ34ZZ
9. LDR brachytherapy to spinal cord using iodine	DØ16B9Z
10. Whole body Phosphorus 32 administration with risk to hematopoetic system	DWY5GFZ

Physical Rehabilitation and Diagnostic Audiology

Procedure	Code
1. Bekesy assessment using audiometer	F13Z31Z
2. Individual fitting of left eye prosthesis	FØDZ8UZ
3. Physical therapy for range of motion and mobility, patient right hip, no special equipment	FØ7LØZZ
4. Bedside swallow assessment using assessment kit	FØØZHYZ
5. Caregiver training in airway clearance techniques	FØFZ8ZZ
6. Application of short arm cast in rehabilitation setting	FØDZ7EZ (Inhibitory cast is listed in the equipment reference table under E, *Orthosis*.)
7. Verbal assessment of patient's pain level	FØ2ZFZZ
8. Caregiver training in communication skills using manual communication board	FØFZJMZ (Manual communication board is listed in the equipment reference table under M, *Augmentative/Alternative Communication*.)
9. Group musculoskeletal balance training exercises, whole body, no special equipment	FØ7M6ZZ (Balance training is included in the motor treatment reference table under *Therapeutic Exercise*.)
10. Individual therapy for auditory processing using tape recorder	FØ9Z2KZ (Tape recorder is listed in the equipment reference table under *Audiovisual Equipment*.)

Mental Health

Procedure	Code
1. Cognitive-behavioral psychotherapy, individual	GZ58ZZZ
2. Narcosynthesis	GZGZZZZ
3. Light therapy	GZJZZZZ
4. ECT (electroconvulsive therapy), unilateral, multiple seizure	GZB1ZZZ
5. Crisis intervention	GZ2ZZZZ
6. Neuropsychological testing	GZ13ZZZ
7. Hypnosis	GZFZZZZ
8. Developmental testing	GZ1ØZZZ
9. Vocational counseling	GZ61ZZZ
10. Family psychotherapy	GZ72ZZZ

Substance Abuse Treatment

Procedure	Code
1. Naltrexone treatment for drug dependency	HZ94ZZZ
2. Substance abuse treatment family counseling	HZ63ZZZ
3. Medication monitoring of patient on methadone maintenance	HZ81ZZZ
4. Individual interpersonal psychotherapy for drug abuse	HZ54ZZZ
5. Patient in for alcohol detoxification treatment	HZ2ZZZZ
6. Group motivational counseling	HZ47ZZZ
7. Individual 12-step psychotherapy for substance abuse	HZ53ZZZ
8. Post-test infectious disease counseling for IV drug abuser	HZ3CZZZ
9. Psychodynamic psychotherapy for drug dependent patient	HZ5CZZZ
10. Group cognitive-behavioral counseling for substance abuse	HZ42ZZZ

New Technology

Procedure	Code
1. Infusion of ceftazidime via peripheral venous catheter	XWØ3321
2. Transcatheter dilation of left peroneal artery with 2 SAVAL stents	X27U395